Tobacco: The Growing Epidemic

Springer

London
Berlin
Heidelberg
New York
Barcelona
Hong Kong
Milan
Paris
Singapore
Tokyo

Rushan Lu, Judith Mackay, Shiru Niu,
and Richard Peto (Eds)

Tobacco: The Growing Epidemic

Proceedings of the Tenth World Conference on Tobacco or
Health, 24-28 August 1997, Beijing, China

With 65 Figures

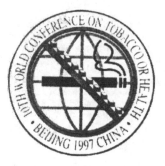

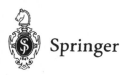 Springer

Rushan Lu, MD
Institute of Medical Information, Chinese Academy of Medical Sciences, Beijing, China

Judith Mackay, MD
Asian Consultancy on Tobacco Control, Kowloon, Hong Kong

Shiru Niu, MD, PhD
Institute of Environmental Health and Engineering, Nan Wei Road, Xuan Wu District, Beijing, China

Richard Peto, MD
Clinical Trial Service Unit, Radcliffe Infirmary, Oxford, UK

ISBN-13: 978-1-85233-296-9   e-ISBN-13: 978-1-4471-0769-9
DOI: 10.1007/978-1-4471-0769-9

British Library Cataloguing in Publication Data
Tobacco : the growing epidemic : proceedings of the tenth
    World Conference on Tobacco or Health, 24-28 August 1997,
    Beijing, China
    1.Tobacco habit - Health aspects - Congresses 2.Tobacco
    habit - Social aspects - Congresses 3.Tobacco habit -
    Treatment - Congresses
    I.Lu, Rushan II.World Conference on Tobacco or Health (10th
    :1997 : Beijing, China)
    362.2'96
ISBN-13: 978-1-85233-296-9

Library of Congress Cataloging-in-Publication Data
World Conference on Tobacco and Health (10th : 1997 : Beijing, China)
    Tobacco, the growing epidemic : proceedings of the Tenth World Conference on
    Tobacco or Health, 24-28 August 1997, Beijing, China / Rushan Lu... [et al.](eds.).
        p.;cm.
    Includes bibliographical references and index.
    ISBN-13: 978-1-85233-296-9
        1. Tobacco habit--Health aspects--Congresses. I. Lu, Rushan. II. Title.
    [DNLM: 1. Tobacco Use Disorder--epidemiology--Congresses. 2. Smoking--adverse
    effects--Congresses. 3. Tobacco Use Disorder--prevention & control--Congresses. WM
    290 W927 2000]
    RA645.T62 T63 2000
    616.86'5--dc21   00-030054

Typesetting: Camera ready by contributors
Printed and bound by Athenæum Press Ltd., Gateshead, Tyne & Wear
34/3830-543210 Printed on acid-free paper SPIN 10753029

Foreword and resolutions

The triennial world conference held in Beijing in 1997 marked 30 years of the tobacco control movement and was the first to be held in a developing Asian country. The choice of 'Tobacco: The Growing Epidemic' as the title of the conference and of Beijing as its venue acknowledged both the spread of the epidemic to developing countries in general and the huge size of the tobacco problem in China in particular.

The conference was opened by China's President, Jiang Zemin, in the Great Hall of the People. Some 2000 delegates from 110 countries attended the Conference, including 800 from China.

Although 'Tobacco: The Growing Epidemic' was the major theme of the Conference, 'Women and tobacco' and 'Developing countries' were the twin sub-themes. In deference to these themes, the conference made an unprecedented effort to involve women at all levels, with about 50% representation on the many planning committees and as chairs, speakers, discussants and funded delegates at the conference itself. Equally, a considerable effort was made to fund delegates from developing countries. All of the invited speakers were asked to include these perspectives in their presentations.

In a few countries, there have been substantial decreases in smoking prevalence over the past few decades that are now resulting in substantial decreases in premature death due to tobacco use. Worldwide, however, the general pattern is of an increase. If current high uptake rates and low cessation rates persist, then, partly because of population growth, the current 1.1 thousand million smokers will increase to 1.6 thousand million, and the 3 to 4 million deaths from tobacco use per year during the 1990s will rise to 10 million by 2030.

Large epidemiological studies were released at the conference that show the current patterns of smoking in China, current mortality rates from tobacco and the way in which the epidemic is evolving. Already, one in three of the world's cigarettes is smoked in China, and one in three young men in China will be killed by tobacco use, unless many of the 300 million current smokers stop. For, in China, as in the west, about half of all cigarette smokers will eventually be killed by their habit—but western experience shows that stopping smoking works remarkably well, even after smoking for many years.

Emphasis was placed on different methods of cessation, for if efforts are concentrated only on preventing children from smoking there will be no reduction in the 200 million smoking-related deaths expected to occur before 2030 in people who smoke already.

There were nearly 100 presentations in the plenary and symposium sessions alone, covering tobacco issues in every continent and from diverse viewpoints. The topics included: litigation, legislation, tobacco promotion, world trade and smuggling, addiction and cessation, youth, school, families, passive smoking, occupational health, religion and the effect of tobacco on economies and on the environment. The role of health professionals, the United Nations and, particularly, governments, in tobacco control also came under scrutiny. There is a clear need for governmental regulation of many aspects of tobacco production and use and for inter-governmental action on issues such as transnational tobacco marketing and promotion and on cigarette smuggling and the corruption that accompanies it.

Sports organizations were urged to boycott tobacco sponsorship, as has already been agreed by the Olympics Committee. The economic analyses showed that when all the direct and indirect economic consequences are considered, a reduction in tobacco consumption is good not only for health but also for a country's economy.

One novelty at the conference was the 'how-to' workshops—how to lobby, raise funds, prepare and present papers, introduce tobacco issues into the medical curriculum, free sports from tobacco and network electronically. In relation to the last, the conference had two Internet sites, and the UICC Globalink computers were used by delegates throughout the conference. Even before the conference, three workshops on preparing abstracts and presenting papers, specifically for delegates to the conference, were held around Asia. Delegates were also offered expert help in the presentation of their papers before their sessions, and an on-the-spot slide-making machine was available.

One controversial decision was that to invite a tobacco-industry scientist, who stated in his abstract that he believes 'the data do not demonstrate that ETS exposure increases the risk of lung cancer or heart disease'.

A session had been held 'empty' until three weeks before the conference for any last-minute issue of importance, and there was no doubt that this had to be the United States settlement agreement with the tobacco companies. Indeed, the Resolutions Committee received more submissions on this than on any other topic.

The conference was organized by the Chinese Association on Smoking and Health and the Chinese Medical Association under the auspices of several international organizations, including the World Health Organization (WHO), the United Nations Conference on Trade and Development (UNCTAD), the United Nations Children's Fund (UNICEF), the International Union Against Cancer (UICC) and the American Cancer Society .

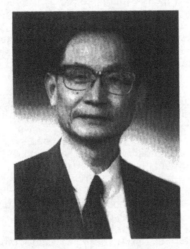

Chen Ming Zhang (1931–1999)

During his decade as Minister of Public Health, the late Dr Chen Ming Zhang contributed greatly to official recognition of the hazards of tobacco in China, to legislation on tobacco advertising and promotion, to establishment of the nationwide Chinese Association on Smoking and Health and to support for the preparatory work and conduct of the 10th World Congress on Tobacco or Health. His initiatives on tobacco in this century will prevent many premature deaths next century.

The editors would like to note the outstanding contribution of the late Minister of Health, Dr Chen Min-zhang, to the improvement of health in China. His early recognition of the tobacco problem led to important action, especially legislation and the establishment of the Chinese Association on Smoking and Health. We would also like to thank him for his support for the 10th World Conference on Tobacco or Health.

Lu Rushan, Niu Shiru, Judith Mackay and Richard Peto, Editors

The manuscripts were edited and prepared for publication by Professor E. Heseltine.

The views presented at the conference and in these proceedings represent the views of the authors and not necessarily those of the editors or the conference. The following resolutions were, however, adopted at the closing ceremony:

Resolutions of the Tenth World Conference on Tobacco or Health

The Conference notes that the current 3.5 million deaths from tobacco annually will increase to 10 million deaths by about 2030 and that the epidemic is expanding, especially in developing countries and among women. Given the overwhelming scientific evidence that tobacco use is responsible for this growing global epidemic of death and disease and that passive smoking is harmful, the Tenth World Conference on Tobacco or Health makes the following resolutions:

1. Stopping tobacco use
The Conference recommends that, since the only way to save millions of lives is by reducing the projected global tobacco-related death toll over the next 20 years, which is over 100 million deaths:
– the public health community should make strenuous efforts to help people stop using tobacco products.

2. WHO International Framework Convention on Tobacco Control
The Conference recommends that:
i. WHO and governments formulate an international framework convention to include protocols for comprehensive tobacco control programmes and the recommendations from previous world conferences, which could be made broader and more restrictive over time;
ii. governments make the necessary financial and technical resources available to WHO to enable it to develop a framework convention on tobacco control, as requested by the Forty-ninth World Health Assembly in 1996;
iii. WHO undertake urgent work to develop a comprehensive framework convention in time for agreement at the Fifty-third World Health Assembly in 2000;
iv. all governments agree on the text of a framework convention at the Fifty-third World Health Assembly in 2000 and ratify and bring the convention into force promptly.

3. United Nations
The Conference recommends that:
i. the United Nations Secretary-General ensure that the issue of tobacco control is a priority at the highest level in the United Nations and its agencies;
ii. governments take up the issue of international tobacco control at the highest level in the United Nations and secure adequate funding and political commitment for this task throughout the world.

4. International implications of domestic tobacco control measures
The Conference recommends that governments consider the international implications of tobacco control policies or settlements with the tobacco industry, and to ensure that:
i. such measures do not contribute to an increase in the worldwide epidemic of tobacco-related death and disease;
ii. the legal rights of those not party to any agreement or policy are fully protected;
iii. such measures do not inhibit full public scrutiny of the past, present and future activities of the tobacco industry;
iv. the tobacco industry pays the costs of damage caused by tobacco.

5. Participation of women and representatives of developing countries and countries in transition

The Conference recommends that:

i. all bodies concerned with strategic planning and tobacco control policy development, implementation and evaluation, such as the WHO Expert Advisory Panel, increase the involvement and representation of women and of people from developing countries and countries in transition;

ii. future world conferences on tobacco or health follow the successful example of the Tenth World Conference and ensure:

    a. equal representation of women and strong representation of people from developing countries and countries in transition as committee members, plenary speakers, chairpersons and discussants;

    b. that support be provided to allow all key constituencies, including women, minorities and people from developing countries and countries in transition, to participate at all levels.

6. Reflecting the full human, social and environmental costs of tobacco

The Conference recommends:

i. the establishment and maintenance of a worldwide system to monitor the tobacco epidemic and the provision of appropriate resources to this end;

ii. that appropriate multilateral agencies and development banks finance and undertake cooperative research programmes to establish a full economic analysis of tobacco growing, production and use, taking into account the costs of damage to the environment, harm to workers, damage to smokers and passive smokers and all other tobacco-induced costs that fall on society;

iii. that those responsible for economic policy and advice, including finance ministries and agencies such as development banks and the International Monetary Fund, ensure that the full health, environmental, social and economic costs of tobacco are represented in the price of tobacco products through taxation.

7. Denormalization and regulation of tobacco as a harmful substance

The Conference recommends that:

i. all governments recognize that tobacco is uniquely dangerous and cannot be treated like a normal consumer product because it is the only substance that is both extremely harmful and powerfully addictive when used as intended by its manufacturers, while remaining legal and in widespread use;

ii. all governments subject the contents of tobacco products and smoke and all aspects of the tobacco business to strict and legally binding regulatory control.

8. Expanding partnerships for a tobacco-free world

The Conference recommends:

i. that all non-governmental organizations involved in tobacco control support the International Non-governmental Coalition Against Tobacco;

ii. that international networking be established in all sectors involved in tobacco control, such as nursing professionals and religious sectors.

TABLE OF CONTENTS

PART I. THE GLOBAL EPIDEMIC

1. The growing epidemic

Smoking in China 5
    G. Yang, K. Becker, L. Fan, Y. Zhang, G. Qi, C.E. Taylor & J. Samet
Emerging tobacco hazards in China: Results on early mortality from a
prospective study of 224 500 men 10
    S.-R. Niu, G.-H. Yang, Z.-M. Chen, J.-L. Wang, G.-H. Wang, X.-Z. He,
    H. Schoepff, J. Boreham, H.-C. Pan & R. Peto
Health effects of tobacco use in women 14
    A.J. Sasco
Women: The second wave of the tobacco epidemic 18
    M. Haglund
Oral cancer and tobacco use in India: A new epidemic 20
    P.C. Gupta

2. Studies on tobacco use

The prevalence of tobacco use

Tobacco use in Japan 27
    N. Yamaguchi, Y. Mochizuki-Kobayashi & S. Watanabe
The tobacco epidemic in Viet Nam 33
    C.N.H. Jenkins, P.X. Dai, D.H. Ngoc, T.T. Hoang, H.V. Kinh, S. Bales,
    S. Stewart & S.J. McPhee
Population survey of smoking in Macao, 1997 37
    C. Lam & A. Joao Maia
Tobacco smoking in Malaysia 39
    H. Habil
Pilot studies on tobacco use in Chennai (Madras), India 40
    C.K. Gajalakshmi, V. Shanta & R. Peto
Tobacco use in India 41
    R. Thanhawla & R. Thanseia
High prevalence of obesity, hypertension and smoking in an Egyptian 43
    population
    F. Hassan, H. Gelband & R. Peto
Tobacco consumption and prevalence of smoking in Cuba 45
    M. Bonet Gorbea, G. Roche, N. Suarez Lugo & P. Varona Perez
Characteristics of tobacco prevalence in Venezuela: Use of a new parameter 47
    M. Adrianza, T. Villamizar, B. López & N. Herrera
Expected trends in the prevalence of cigarette smoking in the United States 48
    D. Méndez, K.E. Warner & P.N. Courant
Epidemiology of smoking and some determinants of smoking behaviour 51
    V. Levshin, V. Drojachih, T. Fedichkina & N. Slepchenko
Epidemiology of smoking in Slovakia 55
    S. Urban & J. Luha
Smoking behaviour and attitudes of key at-risk groups in Turkey 57
    N. Bilir, A. Naci Yildiz, B. Güçiz Dogan & F. Kalyoncu
The growing tobacco epidemic in Palau 59
    C. Otto
Epidemiological transition: Infectious to chronic diseases 59
    R. Tapia-Conyer
Changing perceptions that influence tobacco smoking in central Sri Lanka:
Preliminary findings from a qualitative investigation 60
    G.L. Mehl, T. Seimon, E.K. Rodrigo, K.T. Silva & R. Uyanwatte
Population attitudes to smoking in Chelyabinsk region, Russian Federation 62
    E.G. Volkova, T.B. Karasikova, S.U. Levashov, G.B. Tkachenko,
    T.V. Kamantina, S.U. Pnomareva, D.A. Dmitriev & A.M. Levin

Mortality and morbidity due to tobacco use

A pilot study on mortality and smoking in Hong Kong 67
S.Y. Ho, T.H. Lam, A.J. Hedley & K.H. Mak

Deaths attributable to smoking in Taiwan, 1995 69
S.P. Tsai, C.-P. Wen & D.D. Yen

Life loss related to cigarette smoking in Taiwan: A 12-year follow-up study 72
K. Liaw

Mortality due to cigarette smoking by district in New Zealand, estimated from
national and district deaths 72
H. Glasgow & M. Laugesen

Cigarette smoking-attributable mortality in Norway 75
T. Sanner

Effects of smoking on the epidemiology of obstructive lung disease in an older
population in the United States 78
E.A. Frazier, W.M. Voller, A.D. Haywant, S.R. Wilson & A.S. Buist

Tobacco and cancer

Tobacco-attributable cancer burden: A global review 81
D.M. Parkin, P. Pisani & E. Masuyer

Smoking and mortality in China: A prospective study of 9351 middle-aged
adults with a 16-year follow-up in Shanghai 84
Z. Chen, Z. Xu, R. Collins, W.-X. Li & R. Peto

Smoking-related cancers and other diseases: Results of a 10-year prospective
study in Shanghai, China 90
*Y.-T. Gao, J. Deng, Y.-B. Xiang, Z.-X. Ruan, Z.-X. Wang, B.-Y. Hu, M.-R.,
Guo, W.-K. Teng, J.-J. Han & Y.-S. Zhang*

A review of case–control studies on smoking and lung cancer in China 94
T.H. Lam & Y. He

Analysis of the lung cancer epidemic in Taiwan: A crisis? 98
C.P. Wen, S.P. Tsai & D.D. Yen

Additive interaction between tobacco smoking and domestic radon on the
occurrence of lung cancer: A Spanish case–control study 100
B. Takkouche, A. Montes-Martinez, A. Barreiro-Carracedo & J. Barros-Dios

Tobacco smoking and lung cancer in Viet Nam 102
N.V. Co, H.L. Phat, D.K. Hung, T.K. Dung & N.V. Nhung

Tobacco smoking and hepatocellular carcinoma 103
C. Chen

Laryngeal cancer and tobacco smoking 103
A.N. Zubritsky

Naswar (snuff) dipping and oral cancer in north-west Pakistan 104
S.M. Khan, S. Nasreen & S. Zai

Epidemiology of smoking-related cancers in South Africa 104
*F. Sitas, H.R.O. Carrara, M. Patel, M. Hale, W. Bozwoda, P. Ruff, R. Laikier,
R. Newton & V. Beral*

Cardiovascular disease

Cigarette smoking, tar yields and non-fatal myocardial infarct: 14 000 cases and
32 000 controls in the United Kingdom 111
*S. Parish, R. Collins, R. Peto, L. Youngman, J. Barton, K. Jayne, R. Clarke,
P. Appleby, V. Lyon, S. Cederhom-Williams, J. Marshall & P. Sleight
for the International Studies of Infarct Survival Collaborators*

Prospective study on the relationship between smoking and and death from
cardiovascular disease among retired men in Xi'an, China 111
Q. Shi, L. Li, C. Sun, Y. He & J. Huang

Cigarette smoking and coronary heart disease 113
J. Huang, L. Li, D. Xu, G. Jia, L. Li, H. Yao & Q. Shi

Smoking and coronary changes in patients with documented coronary artery
disease 115
J. Majewski & K. Moczurad

3. Experimental studies on effects of tobacco
Experimental animals
Uterotrophic effect of oestrogens in rats is modified by exposure to cigarette
smoke 123
    L.M. Berstein, E.V. Tsyrlina, O.S. Kolesnik, O.G. Krjukova,
    S.V. Dzhumasultanova & V.B. Gamajunova
Generation of mammalian cell lines that stably express rat neuronal nicotinic
acetylcholine receptor subtypes 125
    Y. Xiao, E.L. Meyer, R.A. Houghtling, J.M. Thompson & K.J. Kellar
Survival index of offspring of smoking mothers: An animal model 128
    E. Florek & A. Marszalek
Influence of tobacco smoke on gas stabilization in newborn rat lung 129
    A Marszalek, W. Biczysko, M. Wasowicz & E. Florek
Effects of environmental tobacco smoke on eustachian tube surfactant in
guinea-pigs 130
    B. Jiang, Y. He & L.N. Feng

Humans
Inhibition of natural killer cell activity by alveolar macrophages in smokers 135
    M. Takeuchi, S. Nagai & T. Izumi
Free radical production in Indian smokers of cigarettes, bidis and hookah 137
    D. Behera, D. Deva, R. Sharma & K.L. Khanduja
Effect of cigarette smoking on lipid profile: Analysis of mass screening of
29 519 middle-aged Japanese men 137
    W. Chun, A. Sano, H. Nishida, S. Urano & K. Sakagami
Effects of smoking on serum lipids and the blood pressure response to a
rehabilitation exercise programme in cardiac patients 138
    N. Sarrafzadegan, K. Sadegi, M. Boshtam & N. Mohammadifar
Effect of smoking on mean systolic and diastolic blood pressure 138
    N. Sarrafzadegan & S. Mostafavi
Effects of smoking on the response of blood pressure to exercise and physical
activity 139
    N. Sarrafzadegan, S. Mostafavi & M. Boshtam
Mean value of blood lipids, body mass index and fasting blood glucose in
smokers and non-smokers in Isfahan, Iran 140
    M. Boshtam, M. Rafie & N. Sarrafzadegan

4. Passive smoking
Passive smoking and the risk for lung cancer 143
    D. Zaridze
Environmental tobacco smoke, lung cancer and heart disease 145
    P.N. Lee
Environmental tobacco smoke, air pollution and respiratory symptoms in
non-smoking housewives in Hong Kong 150
    C.M. Wong, Z.G. Hu, T.H. Lam, A.J. Hedley & J. Peters
Passive smoking from husbands as a risk factor for coronary heart disease in
women in Xi'an, China, who have never smoked 153
    Y. He, T.H. Lam, L.S. Li, L.S. Li, R.Y. Du, G.L. Jia, J.Y. Huang, Q.L. Shi
    & J.S. Zheng
Lesser known and minor effects of active smoking on non-smokers 156
    M. Whidden
Effects of passive smoking on fibrinogen and lipids 158
    N. Sarrafzadegan, N. Mohammadifar & M. Bagheri
Measurement of nicotine in indoor air as an indicator of passive smoking 159
    M. Rothberg, A. Heloma, J. Svinhufvud, E. Kähkönen & K. Reijula
Project for public awareness of indoor exposure to tobacco smoke in Hungary 159
    T. Demjén, B. Buda & L. Galley

Effects on children and young people
Exposure of non-smoking pregnant women to environmental tobacco smoke
in Guangzhou, China 163
    A. Yuen Loke, T.H. Lam, C.L. Betson, S.C. Pan, S.Y. Li, X.J. Gao, Q.S. Xuan
    & Y.Y. Song

Prenatal exposure to tobacco smoke and maldevelopment of the brain 167
    H. Tanaka
Living with smoking grandparents and upper respiratory symptoms of children
    aged 3–6 years in Hong Kong 167
    S.F. Chung & T.H. Lam
Smoking behaviour of parents of children born in 1990–94 in Agaete, Canary
    Islands, Spain 170
    J.M. Segura, A. López, M. López, M. Torres, J.R. Calvo, M.C. Navarro,
    J. Calvo, J.C. Orengo, M. Marrero, S. Flórez, A. Ramos, O. Rojas, S. Solano
    & C. Jiménez
Prevalence of passive smoking among adolescents and its relation to the
    education and socioeconomic status of parents in Isfahan, Iran 171
    N. Sarrafzadegan, S. Mostafavi & F. Tafazzoly
Smoking in the home: Changing attitudes and current practices 172
    M.J. Ashley, J. Cohen, R. Ferrence, S.B. Bull, S. Bondy, B. Poland &
    L.L. Pederson
Passive smoking: Public opinion and behaviour in Victoria, Australia 172
    J. Martin, R. Mullins & M. Morand
Children's residential exposure to environmental tobacco smoke in the
    Nordic countries 175
    K. Lund & A.R. Helgason
Passive smoking and children: A three Nordic country intervention and
    evaluation project 175
    K. Lund, A.R. Helgason, B. Hessult, A.P. Hudtloff & T. Kolset
Knowledge, attitudes and education are independent factors that protect
    children against environmental tobacco smoke: A population-based survey 176
    A.R. Helgason, A. Skrondal & K.E. Lund

5. Tobacco and the environment
Damage to the environment: Environmentalism and health 181
    C. Loh
Tobacco and the environment 184
    S. Parkin
Attitudes of smoking and non-smoking Estonian schoolchildren towards the
    environment 190
    D. Eensoo, A. Saava & K. Pärna
Carbon dioxide in the expired air of smokers and nonsmokers in urban and
    suburban Mexico City 192
    J. Perez-Neria, L. Martinez-Rossier, R. Quezada-Zambrano,
    E. Hernandez-Garduno, M. Catalan-Vazquez & J. Villalba-Caloca

6. Tobacco addiction
Consumption of cigarettes, nicotine dependence and health status 197
    H. Sovinová & L. Csémy
The future of nicotine delivery: Technology, policy and public health 199
    K.E. Warner, J. Slade & D.T. Sweanor
Reflection on alternative nicotine delivery systems 202
    M.C. Taylor
Context stimuli can modify the craving generated by smoking-related cues 205
    B. Willems, M. Dols, R. Bittoun, M. van den Hout & H. Adriaanse
Tobacco manufacturers manipulate nicotine content of cigarettes to cause and 209
    sustain addiction
    C.E. Douglas
Super tobacco cultivated in southern Brazil 211
    J.E. Murad
The family as a cornerstone of tobacco addiction 212
    J. van Reek, H. Adriaanse & F. Vergeer
Are the smoking habits and nicotine dependence of psychiatric patients
    related to medication or diagnosis? 213
    A. Batra, I. Hehl, I. Garfami, G. Farger & G. Buchkremer

Smoking: A predictor or even a promoter of opiate dependence? 214
   P.M. Liebmann, M. Lehofer, M. Moser, T. Legl, G. Pernhaupt &
   K. Schauenstein
Potentiating effect of heroin on smoking rates 216
   M. Lehofer, P.M. Liebmann, M. Moser, T. Legl, G. Pernhaupt &
   H.G. Zapotoczky
Smoking is associated with other types of risk behaviour 217
   D. Hrubá, E. Nová & P. Kachlík
The epidemiology of nicotine dependence 218
   K.O. Fagerstrom
Tobacco dependence and other drug dependences: Similarities and differences 218
   S. Shiffman & J.E. Henningfield

7. Women and tobacco
Prevalence and attitudes
Changes in smoking behaviour among pregnant women in England, 1992–97 227
   L. Owen & A. McNeill
Smoking among pregnant women: Epidemiology and cessation 229
   A. Batra, V. Heuer-Jung, P.E. Schupp, B. Eckert & G. Buchkremer
Tobacco and the Indian woman 231
   M.B. Aghi
Tobacco dependence: Issues and concerns of women, children and families
   in South Asia 233
   M.B. Aghi
Influence of sex on smoking behaviour in Turkey 234
   N. Bilir, B. Güçiz Dodan & A. Naci Yyldyz
Attitudes towards cigarette smoking among women of child-bearing age in
   Poland 235
   J. Szymborski, B. Chazan, W. Zatoński, M. Komar-Szymborski,
   J. Niezurawski & T. Kowalczyk
Tobacco habits among Bajau and Kadazan women in Sabah, Malaysia 236
   C.-Y. Gan
Hubble-bubble (narguilch): A female pattern of smoking 236
   Y. Mohammad

Health effects
Risk for multiple prior miscarriages among middle-aged women who smoke 241
   M. Schofield, G. Mishra & A. Dobson
Risk for early menopause among Australian women who smoke 243
   M. Schofield, G. Mishra & A. Dobson
Tobacco and the health of women 246
   M.A. Pope, M.J. Ashley & R. Ferrence
Smoking in pregnancy 246
   I. Nerin, L. Sanchez Agudo, D. Guillén, M.J. Ruiz, R. Vicente & C. Toyas

8. Youth and tobacco
Prevalence
Tobacco use among French children 252
   A.J. Sasco, M. Poncet, I. Gendre, R. Ah-Song & V. Benhaïm-Luzon
Smoking habits among eighth- and ninth-grade schoolchildren in Halland
   County, Sweden 255
   A. Baigi & T. Melin
Smoking trends among young adults in the United Kingdom 258
   L. Owen & K. Bolling
Smoking in transition: A longitudinal study of Scottish adolescents 260
   S. Pavis, R. Bell, A. Amos & S. Cunningham-Burley
Tobacco use among adolescents aged 10–16 in Gran Canaria, Canary Islands, Spain 263
   J.M. Segura, J.R. Calvo, M.C. Navarro, M. Torres, M. López, A. López,
   J.C. Orengo, J. Calvo, M. Marrero, S. Flórez, A. Ramos, O. Rojas, S. Solano
   & C. Jiménez

Incidence of tobacco smoking among students in Slovenian secondary schools 264
  E. Stergar & M. Tomori
Smoking prevalence among Moscow schoolchildren and approaches to prevention 266
  A.A. Alexandrov, V.Yu. Alexandrova & E.I. Ivanova
Patterns of tobacco use among Russian students 268
  M.R. Torabi & J.W. Crowe
Prevalence and trends of cigarette smoking among children and adolescents 270
  in Siberia
  D. Denisova
Smoking among secondary-school students in Bangladesh 271
  N. Islam
Smoking: A rising ill among Malaysian youth 272
  M.A. Kolandai
Smoking behaviour of Taiwanese adolescents: A case study of a senior technical
  high-school 274
  N.-Y. Chiu, L.-Y. Hsieh & S. Mo
Tobacco use among adolescents in Mongolia 275
  T.S. Sodnompil, Sh. Ouynbileg & D. Lhkaijav
Comparative survey among smoking and non-smoking students in Mongolia 277
  G. Dashzeveg, G. Sukhbat & N. Khurelbaatar
Frequency of tobacco and alcohol use among first-year university students in
  the United States, 1996 278
  J. Lee, S. Parrott, W. Feigelman, R. Wu & M. Forouzeah
Prevalence of current smoking among Iranian adolescents estimated from
  plasma cotinine 278
  N. Sarrafzadegan, M. Boshtam, G.R. Naderi, S. Asgari & F. Tafazoli

Attitudes
Why they smoke: A qualitative study among Taiwanese university students 281
  S.-J. Huang
Smoking behaviour and mental health status among senior high-school and
  vocational high-school students in Taiwan metropolitan areas 282
  D.D. Yen, S.-Y. Huang, A.-P. Ma, H.-H. Chou, M.-H Yang & T.-P. Lo
Smoking behaviour of schoolteachers in Mie Prefecture, Japan 284
  Y. Osaki, T. Ohida & M. Minowa
Factors that contribute to adolescent smoking 285
  K. Pärna, A. Saava & D. Eensoo
An adolescent's perspective on adolescent smoking 288
  K. Koplan
Why young people in Switzerland smoke 289
  H. Krebs, D. Hänggi &V. El Fehri
School education, smoking habits of parents and children and children's
  attitudes towards smoking: Results of the Heidelberg Children Study 291
  M. Pötschke-Langer, L.R. Pilz & L. Edler
Speculations on cigarette smoking among youngsters in Greece 295
  K. Athanasiou
Influence of youth culture on smoking: Two surveys in Ostrobothnia, Finland 297
  P. Rautama
Smoking behaviour of ninth-form pupils in Pitkäranta (Russian Federation)
  and in North Karelia (Finland) 299
  K. Tossavainen, U. Kemppainen, E. Vartiainen, V. Pantelejev & P. Puška
Psychosocial aspects of acquisition and cessation of tobacco habits in India 301
  M.B. Aghi
Exploring children's perceptions of smoking with the 'draw and write'
  investigative technique 303
  L. Porcellato, L. Dugdill, J. Springett & F. Sanderson
Do parents and children know each other's smoking experience and attitudes
  towards children's smoking? 306
  S.F. Chung, Z.M. Wat, S.H. Tong, S.L. Tsang, Y.H. Tsang, C.H. Wong,
  C.Y. Wong, H.S. Wong, H. Wong, K.C. Wong, M.K. Wong, S.T. Wong,
  S.H. Wong & W.Y. Wong

Five-year-old urban children's perceptions, attitudes and expressed intentions
regarding cigarette use (The Birth-to-ten Study) 308
    T. De Wet, K. Steyn, I. Richter & D. Yach
Tobacco smoking and music preferences of students 308
    J. Posluszna & R. Palusiński
Youth culture and smoking: How to find out who does what and why 309
    P. Schofield, D. Hill & P. Pattison
The social symbolism of smoking 309
    T. Bechmann Jensen

Health effects
Smoking and lung function in Hong Kong Chinese schoolchildren 313
    J. Peters, A. Hedley, T.H. Lam & C.-M. Wong

9. Tobacco and occupational health
Smoking and occupational exposure of workers in Guangzhou, China 319
    C.Q. Jiang, T.H. Lam, S.Y. Ho, W.W. Liu, W.S. Zhang, J.M. He & C.Q. Zhu
Smoking cessation at the worksite: Taking the viewpoint of employers into account 321
    M.C. Willemsen
Structure and effectiveness of an in-company non-smoking programme 323
    G. Zeeman
Tobacco use among police personnel in Indore, India 325
    B.M. Shrivastava
Five-year study of the smoking habits of taxi drivers 325
    H.C.O. Ogbulu, R.C. Azinge, P. Owen, D.E. Sawyer, A.E. Van-Santos &
    V.I. Omeruwa
Toxicological data sheet for tobacco smoke: A proposal for smoke-free workplaces 326
    J. Tostain

10. Tobacco promotion
Impact of cigarette marketing on female smoking 331
    Y. Mochizuki-Kobayashi
Policies of the editors of magazines for young women with regard to tobacco 335
    N. Nakano
Women's magazines and tobacco in Europe: Preliminary findings 336
    A. Amos, Y. Bostock & C. Bostock
    Tobacco advertisements were associated with positive attitudes to smoking
    among children who had never smoked 338
    T.H. Lam, S.F. Chung, C.L. Betson, C.M. Wong & A.J. Hedley
Effects of targeted advertising by the tobacco industry 341
    J.P. Pierce
Children's perceptions of cigarette advertisements in Malaysia 343
    J. Rogayah, A. Zulkifli, M. Razlan & N.N. Naing
Strategies used by the tobacco industry to target young consumers: The Canary
Islands experience 347
    J.R. Calvo, J. Calvo-Rosales, A. Lopez-Cabañas, M. Lopez, M. Torres,
    M.C. Navarro, J.M. Segura, M. Marrero & J.C. Orengo
Tobacco promotion in Ghana 348
    S. Koranteng
Tobacco promotion in Nepal 348
    M.R. Pandey
Effect of tobacco loyalty programmes on low-income smokers 351
    D.R. Eadie, A.M. MacKintosh & G.B. Hastings
Influence of cigarette promotion on mediators of smoking 353
    H. Lee, D. Buller, L. Chassin, J. Kronenfeld & D. MacKinnon
Health sponsorship of sport: What are the rules of the game? 357
    S.K. Frizzell & A.M. Carroll
Influence of sports sponsorship by cigarette companies on the adolescent mind:
A national survey in India 360
    S.G. Vaidya, U.D. Naik & J.S. Vaidya

11. Tobacco economics

Economics of tobacco consumption 365
  K.E. Warner
Estimation of direct smoking-related costs in China 369
  S. Jin & Y. Jiang
Economy and diseconomy of tobacco use 369
  S. Watanabe, K. Goto & N. Yamaguchi
Estimated social costs of active and passive smoking in Japan 371
  T. Nakahara & Y.M. Kobayashi
Impact of the tobacco farm policy on cigarette consumption in the United States 373
  P. Zhang, C. Husten, G. Giovino & T. Pechacek
United States farm policy on tobacco and tobacco control: Consistent or conflicting? ... 374
  P. Zhang, C. Husten & T. Pechacek
Tobacco or health: The grower's perspective 376
  T.J. Stamps

12. World trade and smuggling

Success in the West—Disaster in the East 379
  G.N. Connolly
Cigarette trade and smuggling in Europe 381
  L. Joossens
Do trade pressures lead to market expansion? 387
  F.J. Chaloupka & A. Laixuthai
Investigation and prosecution of smuggling 390
  A.A. Godfrey
A comprehensive strategy to reduce and prevent tobacco smuggling 392
  R. Cunningham

PART II. STEMMING THE EPIDEMIC

13.   International and government options

Global tobacco policy 401
  N. Gray
International action for tobacco control 407
  R. Roemer
An international framework convention for tobacco control 410
  N.E. Collishaw
The World Health Organization and a framework convention–protocol
  approach to global tobacco control 422
  A.L. Taylor
Understanding the role of governments in global tobacco control 425
  P. Jha, T.E. Novotny & R.G.A. Feachem
Stages of change: Moving countries towards comprehensive tobacco policies
  and programmes 429
  B. Zolty

14. Tobacco control programmes
Regional and national

China: Tobacco control 435
  M. Chen
China: Tobacco control campaign 436
  X. Weng
Africa: Challenges for tobacco control 439
  W.F.T. Muna
Asia: Research network for tobacco control policy 439
  S. Hamman
Australia: The Western Australia smoking and health programme:
  Persistence pays dividends 440
  M.G. Swanson

Australia: A firm foundation for tobacco control: The Victorian Health
Promotion Foundation model 441
R. Galbally
Australia: Sports and arts: Tobacco-free, tobacco control and health promotion 443
R. Galbally, C. Borthwick & M. Blackburn
Australia: Banquo's ghost: A case study of the corruption of public policy
on exposure to environmental tobacco smoke 447
K. Jamrozik, S. Chapman & A. Woodward
Bangladesh: Anti-smoking education programme 450
S.M. Abdus Sattar
Bolivia: Tobacco control 450
J. Rios-Dalenz
Cambodia: Tobacco or health: An overview 451
C. Radford, K. Baldwin Radford, S. Pun & M. Spedding
Canada: Public attitudes towards tobacco control policies: Current attitudes
and changes in support over time 453
J.E. Cohen, M.J. Ashley, L.L. Pederson, P.D. Poland, S.B. Bull
& R.G. Ferrence
Canada: Public attitudes towards tobacco control policies: How different
are smokers and non-smokers? 453
M.J. Ashley
Cuba: Programme for tobacco prevention and control 454
N. Suarez Lugo
Europe: Smoking, risk behaviour and attitudes to coronary heart disease
in five European countries: The HELP study 456
P. Schioldborg on behalf of the HELP Study Group
Europe: Creating the European Network for Smoking Prevention 456
S. Fleitmann
Europe: Smoke-free Europe: A forum for networks 458
P. Puška, L. Elovainio, H. Vertio & S. Lipponen
India: Tobacco control: A perspective 459
K. Chaudhry & K.P. Unnikrishnan
Macao: Tobacco or health 462
A. Ho
New Zealand: Tobacco control, 1990–97 464
M. Allen
New Zealand: Smoking is not a disease of poverty 468
M. Glover
Norway: Tobacco-free Norway: A five-year action plan 470
S. Stenmarck, E. Juul Andersen & T. Sanner
Norway: 'Tobacco-free': A coalition for reducing use of tobacco 473
E. Juul Andersen, S. Stenmarck, S. Jacobsen & T. Sanner
Russian Federation:Tobacco smoking control 476
A.N. Zubritsky
Russian Federation: Use of computers in tobacco control 478
L. Dartau
Singapore. National smoking control programme, 1986–96 480
C.Y. Chng
Slovakia: Evaluation of tobacco control initiatives 483
Z. Honzátková
Slovenia: United in non-smoking: New thinking, model and philosophy 485
V. Rehar
South Africa: Development of a comprehensive tobacco control policy 488
D. Swart, P. Reddy, Y. Saloojee & K. Steyn
Taiwan area: Anti-smoking activities 488
L. Ho & C.-L. Lin
United Kingdom: Impact of No Smoking Day 491
L. Owen
United Kingdom: No Smoking Day 493
J. Buckler

United Kingdom: The post of smoking prevention coordinator:
A strategic coordinated approach to reducing smoking prevalence 494
C. Owens
United States: Achieving an effective national tobacco control policy 495
J.R. Seffrin
United States: Money against tobacco *versus* money for tobacco 497
J. Cook, D.G. Bal, R. Todd, M. Morra, N. Lins & J. Seffrin
Venezuela: 'World No Tobacco Day': Ten years of experience 501
M. Adrianza, T. Villamizar & N. Herrera
Viet Nam: Action plan on tobacco control, 1995–97 503
T.T. Thuy
Yugoslavia: Smoking prevention and control with special reference to the
Novi Sad MONICA project 505
B. Legetic, M. Planojevic & D. Jakovljevic
Tobacco control networks in Latin America, sub-Saharan Africa and
communities of colour in the United States 508
R.G. Robinson

Local
The Khush Dil Stop Smoking Initiative: A project to raise awareness and reduce
smoking in a predominantly Asian community in Birmingham, England 515
C. Farren
Development of an anti-smoking policy in Novosibirsk, Russian Federation 518
N.V. Alexeeva, A.L. Molokov, S.K. Malyutina, O.L. Alexeev & T.A. Kovalenko
Lessons from nine years of a quit campaign 520
L. Roberts & M. Wakefield
Prevention of smoking in the Veneto Region, Italy 521
E. Tamang, G. Pilati, M. Boschiero, M. Fridegotto & F. Michieletto
Anti-smoking campaign in Shanghai Medical University, China 523
T. Yao, F.-J. Xiong, H.-F. Xia, J.-H. Huang & L. Zhou
Community approach to tobacco control in Thailand 525
B.-O. Ritthiphakdee
Smoking intervention programme in the Mamre community, South Africa 528
K. Steyn, N.S. Levitt, J.M. Fourie, G. Reagan, K. Rossouw & M.N. Hoffman
The journal *Tobacco Front*, a cooperative project in building tobacco control
networks 529
C. Holm
The Badvertising workshop 530
B. Vierthaler
Smoke-free sport—More than a banner! Local activities in Birmingham,
United Kingdom 531
P. Hooper

Women
The role of public policy in reducing tobacco use among women 535
H. Selin
The International Network of Women Against Tobacco 539
M. Haglund
Beauties beating the beast: Working with women against tobacco in Sweden 540
M. Haglund & A. Duckmark
Women, low income and smoking: Developing community-based initiatives 542
P. Gaunt-Richardson, A. Amos, E. Crossan & M. Moore
Involving women's organizations in tobacco control: What are the challenges? 544
A. Amos

Youth
Health-promoting schools and the prevention of tobacco use 553
R. Erben
The European Network on Young People and Tobacco: Activities,
experiences and interactions among networks in Europe 555
S. Ratte

Youth-centred tobacco control 558
  W.D. Novelli
How pupils themselves can work towards a tobacco-free society 560
  I. Talu
Young people and tobacco: The Belgian experience of the 'Smokebusters'
  movement 561
  F. Bourgeois
Health education and changes in students' smoking habits at vocational
  institutions and senior secondary schools in Finland 563
  A.-E. Liimatainen-Lamberg
Intervention against smoking among boys in urban junior middle schools
  in China 564
  H. Ma, Y. Hu & B.-Y Zhang
A programme to prevent Indonesian youth from smoking 565
  L.A. Hanafiah
Life education: Prevention starts in primary school 566
  M.M.H. Yu-Chan
No-smoking competitions for young people in Finland 568
  M. Paavola, E. Vartianinen & P. Puska
Towards smoke-free schools 569
  T. Fraser
Youth are the leaders of today 570
  D. Grande
Educating third-graders against smoking 573
  A. Winder, M. Barnes & A. Geller
'Staying safe': Smoking education for adolescents 574
  L. Wiseman
Swedish Teachers against Tobacco 576
  C. Sätterberg
Sixteen years' experience of tobacco prevention among children in Sweden 577
  G. Steinwall
Engaging schools and families in tobacco prevention and control 579
  T. Chen
Restricting smoking among young students in global smoking control 580
  W.K. Liao
The family: The key to tobacco control 581
  G.Y. Tsang
Youth and prevention: A comprehensive approach 582
  C.A. Moyer & C. Sutherland-Brown
Smoke-free soccer: Healthy kids, healthy communities 585
  E.R. Forbes
Tobacco art and children 587
  K. Yavuz
An educational anti-tobacco programme for preschool children: 'Clean
  air around us' 589
  J. Szymborski, W. Zatoński, Z. Juczyński, T. Kowalczyk, M. Lewandowska,
  A. Dobrowolska & N. Ogińska-Bulik
Anti-tobacco education programme for children and adolescents in Cuba 590
  N. Suarez Lugo
Effect of a school-based smoking prevention programme on recruitment
  of smokers: A multi-level analysis 592
  O. Jøsendal
The tobacco industry is not a popular sponsor among youth in Switzerland 592
  V. El Fehri & H. Krebs
Tackling smoking among 16–24-year olds through a large-scale art, design
  and fashion project 593
  P. Hooper
Books on tobacco and smoking in the Danish education system 594
  K. Trangbek
Smoking by adolescents: Three years later, there's an even larger revenue
  but little for prevention 594
  C.M. Doran, A. Girgis & R.W. Sanson-Fisher

15. Tobacco legislation and regulation

Legislation: A key component of a comprehensive tobacco control plan 599
   G. Mahood
Trends over time and international variation in tobacco-control legislation:
   Experience of the European Union 604
   A.J. Sasco, R. Ah-Song, I. Gendre & V. Bourdès
Strategies for successful legislation 606
   C.H. Leong
Measures to kick out and keep out transnational tobacco companies from a
   national market 608
   R. Cunningham
The Canadian set-back: Tobacco use in Canada 1986–97 610
   C. Callard
Tobacco control and Cuban legislation 616
   N. Suarez Lugo
Legislation against tobacco smoking in France, 1996 617
   G. Dubois
Movement for a people-friendly tobacco law in the Republic of Slovenia 619
   E. Stergar, M. Bevc Stankovic & S. Dizdarevic
Results of a legislative approach to tobacco control: Thailand's experience 621
   P. Vateesatokit
Tobacco legislation in the Ukraine: Advertising and other issues 623
   K. Krasovsky
Analysis of tobacco policy in Viet Nam 624
   D. Efroymson & D.T. Phuong
Smoking bans in domestic environments in South Australia 625
   L. Roberts, C. Miller, M. Wakefield & C. Reynolds
Public opinion in Australia about the adequacy of tobacco health warnings
   and information on tobacco-related harm, in the context of the introduction
   of stronger warnings on packs 627
   R. Borland & D. Hill
Headmasters' views of the effectiveness of tobacco laws in vocational and
   commercial institutions 631
   A.-E. Liimatainen-Lamberg
Negotiating legislation to discourage use of tobacco in a Pacific Island country 633
   A. Vakacegu, Mrs Hong Tiy, Dr Brough & Dr Phillips
Canadian legislators' support for tobacco control policies 633
   J.E. Cohen, M.J. Ashley, R.G. Ferrence, D.A. Northrup, J.S. Pollard
   & D.L. Alexander
Canadian legislators' knowledge of and attitudes towards tobacco and
   tobacco control 634
   M.J. Ashley, J.E. Cohen, R.G. Ferrence, D.A. Northrup, J.S. Pollard
   & D.L. Alexander
Legislation to prevent circumvention of bans on direct tobacco advertising 635
   Z.M. Zain & M. Assunta
Tobacco advertising ban in Lithuania 636
   T. Stanikas

Regulatory measures

Regulation of tobacco and nicotine 641
   D.T. Sweanor
Dedicated regulation of nicotine use: It is time! 645
   R. Borland

Smoke-free areas

Tobacco-free, healthy cities: Multi-city action plan 653
   G. Pilati & E. Tamang
Attitudes and experiences of restaurant owners regarding smoking bans in
   Adelaide, South Australia 655
   D. Turnbull, K. Jones, M. Wakefield & D. Teusner
Are the bars in Glasgow, Scotland, ready to ban smoking? 658
   D. McIntyre

Will Birmingham become the United Kingdon's first smoke-free city? 663
   P. Hooper
Effectiveness of Thailand's non-smokers' protection law in restaurants 664
   C. Supawongse
Creating smoke-free facilities 666
   L.L. Fairbanks, R.D. Hurt & B. Watanabe
Tobacco-free venues 667
   S.B. Cohen
A completely smoke-free university? 669
   P. Schioldborg

Youth access

A comprehensive approach to reducing the supply of tobacco to children in
   Western Australia 673
   D. Sullivan & T. Jackiewicz
Reducing young people's access to tobacco: An evaluation of policies and
   laws in New South Wales, Australia 676
   K. Purcell. L. Burns, B. O'Hara & C. O'Neil
Measurement of retailers' compliance with legislation on tobacco sales to
   minors in Canada 678
   J. King & M.J. Kaiserman
New Zealand cigarette manufacturers compete on nicotine and price for
   young smokers 681
   M. Laugesen
Community context of minors' access to tobacco in 20 communities in the
   United States 682
   D. Sharp, P. Mowery, J. Myllyluoma, G. Giovino. T. Pechacek & M. Erilsen

16. Economic measures to control tobacco use

Annual submission by the Tobacco Control Alliance in the United Kingdom
   to the Finance Ministry 685
   P. White, K. Aston & L. Joossens
Smoking in disadvantaged communities: Assessing motivation and ability
   to quit 686
   G.B. Hastings, M. Stead, D.R. Eadie, A.M. MacKintosh & P. Graham
The case for profit control of the tobacco industry 689
   R. Cunningham
Socio-epidemiological data underlying the programme for control of
   tobacco use in Romania, 1997–2000 691
   C. Didilescu & C. Marica
Economic aspects of tobacco smoking in Romania 692
   C. Marica & C. Didilescu
Effect of cigarette advertising bans and warning labels on cigarette smoking:
   Evidence from aggregate and individual data 692
   H. Saffer

Taxation and pricing

Price, tobacco control policies and smoking among young people in the
   United States 697
   M. Grossman & F.J. Chaloupka
Cigarette taxation in China: Lessons from international experience 698
   T. Hu
Empirical analysis of the output effects of cigarette taxes in South Africa
   and the regional impact 699
   R. van der Merwe & I. Abedian
Empirical analysis of cigarette taxes and advertising in South Africa, 1970–95 699
   I. Abedian & N. Annett
Global approaches to active tobacco taxing and pricing: Initiative for
   standardization 699
   N. Krstic

17. Approaches to cessation
Pharmacological methods

Pharmacological approaches to smoking cessation 705
  M.J. Jarvis
Improving the effectiveness of the transdermal nicotine patch: A multicentre study 708
  J. González Quintana, D. Marín Tuyà, M.J. Consuegra Manzanares
  & A. Garcia Baena
Review of nicotine replacement therapy in helping people stop smoking 710
  J.-L. Tang & J.L.Y. Liu
Smoking cessation programme with nicotine patches for employees of a
  teaching hospital 711
  T.E. Jones
Pharmaceutical approach to smoking cessation: Public health benefit of
  over-the-counter nicotine medications—Experience in the United States 713
  G.M. Quesnelle, S.L. Burton, K.E. Kemper & J. Gitchell
Continuously up-dated, systematic reviews of nicotine replacement therapy:
  The latest evidence of effectiveness 714
  C.A. Silagy & T. Lancaster
Overview of nicotine replacement therapy 715
  M. A.H. Russell, J.A. Stapleton & G. Sutherland
Real-world efficacy of computer-tailored smoking cessation material as a
  supplement to nicotine replacement 715
  S. Shiffman, J. Gitchell & V. Strecher
Determining who will benefit from nicotine replacement therapy and choosing
  a product 716
  A. Hjalmarson
Determination of concentration of cotinine associated with smoking cessation 716
  M. Abe, E. Midorikawa, T. Takubo, K. Yoshino, A. Nagai & K. Konno
Urinary cotinine: An indicator for smoking quitting therapy 718
  L. Martinez-Rossier, J. Villalba-Caloca, R. Montes-Vizuet,
  S. Flores-Sanchez & L. Teran-Ortiz

Behavioural methods

Behavioural approaches to smoking cessation 723
  K. Slama
Self-efficacy theory, locus of control and smoking cessation among Asians 728
  W.C. Andress
Quitline® 731
  P. McCabe
Quitline in Thailand 732
  B.O. Ritthiphadkee & S. Suwanrasami
Tabac Info Línea: Implementation and first results 733
  T. Marin, A. Garcia & J. González
Smoking cessation programme in Catalonia, Spain: A 10-year retrospective study 734
  D. Marín Tuyà, J. Gonzàlez-Quintana & M.J. Consuegra Manzanares
Evaluation of a multi-component behavioural programme for smoking
  cessation in Spain after 36 months' follow-up, with survival analysis 735
  E. Becoña, F.L. Vázquez & A. Montes
Smoking cessation intervention with a multiple-component programme for the
  general population of Gran Canaria, Spain: Evaluation after six months'
  follow-up 739
  A. López, M. López, J.R. Calvo, M. Torres, J.M. Segura, M.C. Navarro,
  J. Calvo, M.P. García, C. Jiménez, A. Ramos, O. Rojas & S. Solano
Effectiveness of a five-day plan to eliminate the smoking habit in France 740
  R. Romand
Seven years of smoking cessation campaigns in the Netherlands 741
  G. Zeeman
Quit and Win contest for daily smoking mothers of children 0–6 years of age
  in Stockholm County, Sweden 743
  P. Tillgren, L. Eriksson, K. Guldbrandsson, A. Reimers, M. Spiik,
  T. Ainetdin & M.-L. Stjerna

Effectiveness in Poland of the second international 'Quit and Win' anti-smoking campaign 745
W. Drygas, A. Kowalska & E. Dziankowska-Stachowiak
A study of smoking cessation in Egypt: Perspective for success 746
H.M. El Shahat, A.A.M.T. Mobasher, L.A. Zaki, M.H. Fawzy & E.I.D. Nour
Implementation of a smoking cessation programme for adolescents in Israel:
Lessons learnt 750
S. Gan-Noy, M. Blitner, A. Aizik-Kelem & M. Michaeli
A randomized controlled trial of smoking cessation in Government outpatient
clinics in Hong Kong 751
C.L. Betson, T.H. Lam, T.W.H. Chung & S.F. Chung
Stop smoking contest in Japan 756
T. Kinoshita & M. Nakamura
Smoking cessation for patients with heart disease 757
H. Nurkkala, U.-R. Pentillä & M. Romo
Short-term effectiveness of a multi-media smoking cessation programme
for pregnant women 758
M.J. Bakker & H. de Vries
Smoking and smoking cessation among men whose partners are pregnant 759
M. Wakefield, Y. Reid, L. Roberts, R. Mullins & P. Gillies
Intervention for cessation of use of smokeless tobacco in a dental office 761
H.H. Severson, J.A. Andrews, E. Lichtenstein & J.S. Gordon
Multi-faceted treatment of tobacco addiction in a group of health professionals 762
L. Sanchez-Agudo, J.M. Carreras-Castellet, M.P. Jiménez-Santolaya
& F.J. Iñigo-Barrera
Multi-component smoking treatment in a pneumological unit: Methods, results
and predictors of success 764
L. Sánchez-Agudo, J.M. Carreras-Castellet & B. Maldonado-Arostegui
Community-based smoking cessation 767
P. Tvaermose
Effectiveness of teaching advice on smoking cessation 767
L.C.Y. Tsang
Workshop in smoking cessation 768
A. Carr & R. Hayley
Using diffusion research for participatory tobacco cessation 769
A.B. Lund
A stepped-care plus matching model for community smoking cessation 770
R.S. Niaura & D.B. Abrams
A new, effective smoking cessation programme based on the Internet 770
Y. Takahashi
Tobacco control measures and smoking cessation therapy: Different
strategies for different types of smokers 771
R. Schoberberger & M. Kunze
Experiences with alternative means and indirect cessation 772
A. Lund
Future of smoking cessation 773
M. Kunze
Public policy as a cessation tool: A framework for discussion 774
H. Selin

Methods for young people

Call for a new approach to tobacco 'cessation' programming among youth 781
J.J. Librett & H.R. Borski
Adolescent smoking cessation: A multi-level approach 783
S. Thomas & E. Choi
'Quit because you can': The Western Australian 'Young women and smoking'
campaign 783
D. Sullivan & C. Thompson
Tobacco use cessation among children and young people 789
T. Glynn

18. Health education

Health promotion in tobacco control: Widening our horizons 793
  D. Tan
The African experience: Present difficulties and future possibilities 794
  Y. Saloojee
The shifting tobacco paradigm and the role of the American Cancer Society 796
  D.G. Bal, J. Cook, R. Todd, M. Morra, N. Lins & H. Eyre
Cost–benefits of health promotion 797
  J.R. Terborg
Soul City: A health promotion initiative against tobacco 799
  S. Goldstein, G. Japhet, S. Usdin, P. Esterhuysen & T. Shongwe
Evaluation of Soul City: A multi-media health promotion initiative against
  tobacco 803
  S. Goldstein, G. Japhet, S. Usdin, P. Esterhuysen & T. Shongwe
Giving smokers what they want: Certainties not probabilities 805
  T. Cotter, D. Hill, J. Watt & J. Boulter
Health education and smoking cessation 807
  R. Sadek, S. Mostafa, M. Dydamony & L. Zarief
A systematic approach to setting up a health promotion organization in Thailand 808
  B. Supakorn
Rural community health promotion for tobacco control in Thailand 811
  N. Charoenca & S. Hamann
Changes in adult smoking prevalence after a three-year community health
  education: The Nose Town Project in Japan 812
  M. Nakamura & S. Masui
Awareness initiatives on the negative effects of smokeless tobacco 812
  C. Grant
A survey of sportsmens' attitudes to tobacco 813
  J. Talmud

19. Litigation

Litigation by individuals against the tobacco industry 817
  J. Banzhaf
Legal protection for child victims of adult smoking: A call for action 819
  M. Whidden
Litigation by states against the tobacco industry 821
  R.A. Daynard
International implications of the United States 'global settlement' of tobacco
  litigation 826
  B. Fox, J. Lightwood & S.A. Glantz

20. Lobbying, advocacy and use of mass media for tobacco control

Lighting up locally and not burning out: Tobacco control activism in a tobacco
  industry town 833
  C. Farren
Role of a national cancer society in lobbying for tobacco control legislation:
  A case study from Canada in the campaign for the 1997 Tobacco Act 838
  K. Kyle
Smokeline: Australia's Internet library 840
  P. Markham & C. Hilder
Countering Philip Morris in The Netherlands 842
  B. de Blij
The 'reality check': A way to make tobacco shareholders aware 844
  G. Boëthius, Y. Bergmark-Bröske, B.-M. Lindblad, G. Steinwall & I. Talu
A framework for using the media for tobacco control 845
  R.J. Donovan
Family smoking campaign: Evaluation of a mass media campaign in England 847
  L. Owen, D. McVey, A. McNeill, J. Stapleton & K. Bolling
Which media to use to promote your message about smoking 849
  K. Aston

A most potent weapon: Three case studies of media advocacy by the medical
  profession in the fight for tobacco control 851
  K. Woollard
Using television and other mass media to counter the threat of tobacco to
  women and children 854
  M. Palmer, S. Palmer, W. Zatonski & D. Zaridze
GLOBALink 856
  R.J. Israel
Consumer pressure as a counter-measure to tobacco promotion 857
  K. Mulvey, L. Wykle-Rosenberg & W. Fassett
Advocating for a total tobacco advertising ban in Hong Kong 858
  S.H. Lee
Evidence-based lobbying for stronger legislation: Inputs versus outcomes 860
  H. Glasgow, B. Swinburn & M. Laugesen
Reducing passive smoking in public places 863
  R. Burton & S. Woodward
The Swedish war against the tobacco industry: A Non Smoking Generation 864
  G. Steinwall
Lobbying for tobacco control: Attitudes and experiences of Canadian legislators 865
  J.E. Cohen, M.J. Ashley, R.G. Ferrence, D.A. Northrup, J.S. Pollard &
  D.L. Alexander

21. The role of health professionals
Practising health professionals
The role of doctors in tobacco prevention 871
  G. Boëthius
The role of health professionals: Caring for the victims 872
  L. Sarna & P. McCarthy
Teaching about tobacco in medical schools 877
  R. Richmond
Putting an end to tobacco use in hospitals: A tribute to Dr Takeshi Hirayama 879
  L.L. Fairbanks
Changes in tobacco habits and attitudes to tobacco prevention among
  Swedish dental personnel, 1991–96 881
  E. Uhrbom
World Dentistry against Tobacco 883
  O. Akerberg
Habits and opinions about smoking among health professionals in Denmark 884
  T. Clement
New approach to improving the effectiveness of anti-smoking interventions
  in primary health care.. 884
  W.K. Drygas & W. Sapiński
Doctors' opinions about education for smoking control in Nairobi, 1996 887
  B. Fiévez, W. Lore, H. de Vries & H. Adriaanse
Developing the contribution of health professionals to smoking cessation 887
  M. Raw, A. McNeill, L. Owen & K. Aston
Role of paediatricians and obstetricians in preventing and combating tobacco
  smoking 889
  J. Szymborski, W. Zatoński & B. Chazan
An approach by community physicians to quitting smoking 890
  D.-Y. Yan & L.Q. Cheng
Integrating tobacco education and provider advice into clinical practice
  in community-orientated primary care settings... 891
  D.I. Bahrs
Cigarette smoking and anti-smoking counselling among Chinese physicians 893
  H.Z. Li, D. Fish & X. Zhou
Categorical, clear and helpful approach to smoking cessation by health
  professionals in the Czech Republic 893
  E. Králíková & J.T. Kozák

Quantitative research among doctors in Nairobi, Kenya, about their smoking
  behaviour and their opinions on smoking control education 895
  H. de Vries, W. Lore, B. Fiévez & H. Adriaanse
Smoking cessation in general practice 897
  R. Borge, D. Skylstad & E. Aaserud
Behaviour and attitude of Turkish physicians to smoking 897
  N. Bilir, A. Naci Yyldyz, B. Güçiz Dogan & S. Emri
Helping health professionals to help smokers 898
  F. Bass
Creating awareness about the effects of smoking through community-based
  health-care providers in Nigeria 900
  O.A. Abosede, E. Bandele, G. Essien & N. Olupona
General practitioners' role in preventive medicine: Scenario analysis with
  smoking as a case study 902
  C. Doran, B. Pekarsky, M. Gordon & R. Sanson-Fisher
Prevalence of smoking among pneumologists in Romania 903
  F. Mihaltan
Smoking among professors at medical schools in Spain 903
  I. Nerin
General practitioners and smoking prevention 904
  C. Doran
Health education on tobacco or health: The role of professional nurses
  in Hong Kong 904
  S. Chan, C. Betson & T.H. Lam
Smoking habits of Finnish public health nurses 907
  A.-E. Liimatainen-Lamberg
Swedish Nurses against Tobacco: How to build an organization 907
  Y. Höijer & I. Nordström Torpenberg
Smoking behaviour among midwives in some hospitals in Japan 909
  F. Fukushima, K. Miyasato, Y. Osaki & M. Minowa
Nurses and tobacco control: Need for a strategic plan 911
  L. Sarna
Prevalence of smoking among staff of chemists' shops in Romania 912
  F. Mihaltan

Health-care students
Evaluation of a smoking prevention and cessation support programme for
  student nurses and their patients in Japan 915
  K. Okada, C. Kawata, M. Nakamura & A. Oshima
Cigarette smoking among Polish medical students 916
  R. Palusiński, A. Bilan, J. Mosiewicz, W. Myśliński & J. Hanzlik
Social environment and tobacco smoking among Polish medical students 918
  A. Bilan, R. Palusiński, A. Witczak, S. Ostrowski, E. Rymarz, J. Zdanowska
  & J. Hanzlik
Smoking habits and knowledge of its harmful effects among medical students
  in the Slovak Republic 920
  E. Kavcová, E. Rozborilová, R. Vysehradský, J. Kollár, J. Zucha & M. Bronis
Tobacco habits among medical students in Spain: An 11-year study 921
  A. Montes-Martinez & J.J. Gestal-Otero
Smoking among medical students in Spain 922
  I. Nerin, L. Sánchez Agudo, D. Guillén, C. Toyas, R. Vicente & A. Más
Prevalence and attitudes of medical students in Spain towards smokers 923
  I. Nerin, L. Sánchez Agudo, A. Mas, D. Guillén, C. Toyas & R. Vicente
Smoking among medical students and student nurses in the Russian Federation:
  Educational problems 923
  K.P. Hanson, A.S. Barchuk & M.A. Zabezhinski
Prevalence of smoking among medical students at Makerere University,
  Kampala, Uganda 924
  E.K. Kanyesigye, R. Basiraha, A. Ampaire, G. Wabwire, J.B. Waniaye,
  S. Muchuro & E. Nkangi
Smoking behaviour of first-year student nurses in Canada 927
  A. Draffin Jones

22. Religion and tobacco

Islamic beliefs and practices in tobacco control 931
    E. Dagli
Buddhist belief in tobacco control 932
    P.C. Khongchinda
Survey of the knowledge, attitudes and practices of Cambodian Buddhist
    monks with regard to tobacco 936
    M. Smith, T. Umenai & C. Radford
Religious influences on tobacco investments: The Judaeo–Christian
    perspective 938
    M.H. Crosby
Smoking control and religion 939
    H. Gimbel
The tobacco plantation system in the extreme south of Brazil 941
    L. Prado

23. Discussants' remarks

The tobacco holocausts 947
    T.H. Lam
Tobacco use in the developing world 948
    J.P. Koplan
Passive smoking: The industry sows doubt behind epidemiology's plough 949
    A.J. Hedley
The strategic role of smoking cessation 955
    L.M. Ramström
Practical approaches to smoking cessation 957
    A. Hillhouse
Tobacco control programmes 959
    K. Bjartveit
Health promotion in tobacco control 961
    E. Protacio-Marcelino
Effective use of the mass media for tobacco control 962
    J. Watt
Tobacco economics 964
    D.J. Collins
Litigation for tobacco control 966
    P. Boucher
Settlements with the tobacco industry 967
    R. Weissman

Closing remarks

Lessons from the Conference: The next 25 years 973
    J. Mackay

Author index 977

Subject index 989

THE GLOBAL EPIDEMIC

The growing epidemic

Smoking in China

G. Yang[1], K. Becker[2], L. Fan[1], Y. Zhang[3], G. Qi[1], C.E. Taylor[2] & J. Samet[2]

[1]*Chinese Academy of Preventive Medicine, Beijing, China;* [2]*The Johns Hopkins University School of Hygiene and Public Health, Department of Epidemiology, Baltimore, Maryland, United States;* [3]*Chinese Association on Smoking and Health, Beijing, China*

Abstract

This paper contains the results of the 1996 National Smoking Prevalence Survey. Of a representative sample of 120 000 adults aged 15 or over, 67% of the men and 4.2% of the women smoked. The rates for people aged 15–24 were lower, since it is in this age range that most smokers start the habit. Thus, 300 million people in China are current smokers. Among people aged 25–49, the prevalence of smoking was 69% among males (66% urban, 71% rural) and 2% among females (1% urban, 3% rural). In addition, 53% of non-smokers are exposed to passive smoking. Data from the prevalence survey were cross-tabulated by level of education, occupation, region, ethnic group and numerous variables related to knowledge and attitudes about smoking.

Background

Almost 1 million people in China die every year from diseases caused by tobacco. If current smoking patterns persist, however, tobacco will cause about 2 million deaths annually by the year 2025, and about 50 million of people now living will eventually die from smoking in middle age (Liu *et al.*, 1998; Niu *et al.*, 1998). The 1996 Smoking Prevalence Survey provides the first nationwide information since 1984 (Weng *et al.*, 1997) on patterns of tobacco use, and the methods used ensure data of high quality that are representative of the adult population of China (Yang, 1997; Yang *et al.*, 1999).

Methods

The survey was conducted in a population covered by the 'disease surveillance points' system, which covers a representative sample of rural and urban areas in China. One thousand households were selected from each of 145 disease surveillance points in 30 provinces by a randomized, three-stage sampling method. A total of 123 030 people over the age of 15 were interviewed; 122 700 (99.7%) were included in the final analysis, of whom 53% were men and 47% women, and 34% lived in urban and 66% in rural areas. When compared with the 1990 census, persons aged 15–24 were under-represented, but the survey sample was otherwise similar with regard to the distribution of characteristics such as age, sex, rural:urban ratio, level of education, occupation and geographical distribution. The survey questionnaire elicited information on demographics, the prevalence of smoking, passive smoking, smoking cessation, health status and knowledge and attitudes towards smoking. After trained interviewers had surveyed each household, a random sample of 5% of the respondents was selected for independent re-interview, to ensure reliability. Statistical analysis was done with the SAS software package.

Results

In China, smoking is chiefly a male activity, with 67% of men and only 4.2% of women ever having smoked, giving an overall rate of 38%. The prevalence of current smokers is 63% of men, 4% of women and 35% overall. Table 1 shows the current smoking rates by age for men and women living in urban and rural areas. As smoking is usually initiated between the ages of 15 and 24, the prevalence among people in this age range was misleadingly low, but that among people aged 25–49 was 69% for men

Table 1. Current smoking rates by age among women and men in urban and rural areas of China

Age group (years)	Male		Female	
	Urban (%)	Rural (%)	Urban (%)	Rural (%)
15–19	14	18	0.49	0.20
20–24	55	52	0.59	0.69
25–29	64	66	1.0	1.4
30–34	68	70	1.2	2.2
35–39	68	73	1.4	3.0
40–44	66	73	1.4	4.1
45–49	62	73	3.2	5.0
50–54	59	73	4.6	6.8
55–59	55	71	10.0	7.4
60–64	51	69	11.3	8.7
65–69	47	67	14.2	11.3
≥ 70	45	59	9.0	4.9

(66% urban, 71% rural) and 2% for women (1% urban, 3% rural). Although the mean consumption per smoker was 15 cigarettes per day (a figure that is also suggested by national cigarette sales), there was strong 'digit preference' in the responses, with many smokers reporting 20 cigarettes a day and few reporting more than this number. Smokers who reported smoking more than 20 cigarettes per day represented 7.5% of the men, 0.2% of the women and 4% of the total population. Among men, particularly in rural areas, the prevalence is high throughout adult life, but among women it is substantially lower among those aged under 50 (i.e. those born after 1945) than among women who were born earlier. Smoking rates decline with level of education, from about 70% among men with little or no schooling to 54% among those with university education and more. Among women, the rates by educational level are between 7.6 and 1.1%, the latter rate representing the most highly educated women.

Smoking rates by occupation show that, among men, the following groups have rates of 70% or more: farmers, factory workers, service personnel, employees of private companies, the self-employed and the 'floating population' (with no fixed residence). The rates among male teachers, health workers, researchers and officials are about 60%, which is still substantial; this high prevalence is of special concern because these groups are primary role models for other people, especially the young. Among women, the distribution is distinctly different, with the highest rate of about 10% among retired people and those doing housework. The lowest rates are for female teachers, researchers and students, with health workers in the mid-range.

Among older men, the smoking rates are higher in rural than in urban areas. Among women up to 50 years of age, the rural rates are also higher, but older urban women have slightly higher rates than rural women, reaching a peak of 14% for urban women over the age of 65. Differences in smoking by region show that male rates are high everywhere but are slightly higher than average in the southwest, which is where much of the tobacco in China is grown. The regional differences among women are much greater, with much higher rates in the north-east. Different patterns were found among the minority groups, which together make up about 7% of China's population. The highest rates in the country are among the Yao in the southwest, with 90% of men and 13% of women smoking, although in this area there is extensive use of traditional bamboo pipes, which filter the smoke through water. Other groups with smoking rates higher than 60% are the Mongols and Koreans in the north and the Zhuang and Dai in the south. The lowest rates are found among Muslim minorities in the north-west, such as the Uighur and Hui. The rates are much lower among minority women, but rates above 10% are found among the Yi, Mongol and Yao peoples.

Starting to smoke

Table 2 shows the proportions of men and women who began smoking before the age of 25, by birth year. Of those who smoked, the men reported that they had started to smoke at a median age of about 20 years and the women that they had started at about 25 years of age. Hence, the results for people born since 1971 under-represent the proportion of those birth cohorts who will eventually start before age 25. Among males, the proportion who started to smoke before the age of 25 was 66% for those born 1947–71 and somewhat less for those born earlier, but for women it was 2% for those born in 1947–71 and substantially more for those born earlier.

Fifty-eight percent of men and 46% of women said they had started just to experiment but had then developed the habit. Among men who smoked, 18% said that they had started because of social pressure, but only 5% of women who smoked agreed that this was an important reason. By contrast, more women (34%) than men (14%) said that they had started smoking to overcome fatigue, and 4% of both men and women said they had started because it was fashionable. In comparison with smokers aged 20 or older, more of the 15–19-year-old smokers (13%) said they had started because it was fashionable.

Educational levels greatly influence the reasons given for starting to smoke. Overcoming fatigue was twice as important for people of lower educational levels. Social pressure was reported as four times more important for smokers who were university graduates than for smokers with less schooling. University graduates also had lower rates of just experimenting. Similar differences are seen in selected occupational groups. About 60% of farmers and factory workers, 50% of health workers and 45% of teachers said they had been just experimenting when they started to smoke. Among health workers and teachers, 30 and 35% said that social pressure got them started, while only 13 and 14% of farmers and factory workers mentioned this reason for adopting the habit.

Amounts and types of tobacco smoked

Tobacco is smoked in several different ways in China: filtered, unfiltered and hand-rolled cigarettes; cigars and cigarillos; and two types of pipe—the traditional Chinese pipe with a small bowl and a long stem and the bamboo pipe in which smoke is filtered through water. Filtered cigarettes account for 73% of total tobacco use and now dominate the market, especially among young people. Hand-rolled cigarettes are used mainly in the northeast and the water-filter bamboo pipe mainly in the south-west.

Table 2. Populations of Chinese males and females who began smoking at less than 25 years of age

Birth year	Started smoking when < 25 /total population (%)	
	Males	Females
1977–81[a]	722/4011 (18)	10/3571 (0.3)
1972–76[a]	2839/5201 (55)	32/4667 (0.7)
1967–71	5527/8281 (67)	98/7647 (1.3)
1962–66	6707/9896 (68)	153/9427 (1.6)
1957–61	5683/8379 (68)	139/7185 (1.9)
1952–56	5396/8204 (66)	153/6261 (2.5)
1947–51	3156/5037 (63)	116/4029 (2.9)
1942–46	2246/3877 (58)	105/3253 (3.2)
1937–41	2179/3899 (56)	163/3365 (4.8)
1932–36	2122/3883 (55)	237/3724 (5.8)
1927–31	1658/3125 (53)	207/2887 (7.2)
< 1926	684/1348 (51)	35/997 (3.5)

[a]Since people in these birth cohorts were all under 25 years at the time of the 1996 survey, the smoking rates do not show how many people in this group will actually have started to smoke by their 25th birthday.

The numbers of cigarettes smoked daily per smoker varied by age and sex. Both men and women smokers aged from 15 to 20 years smoked about two per day, while older men and women typically smoked about 10–15 cigarettes per day, so that students had the lowest daily consumption per smoker. Adults smoked a fairly uniform number of cigarettes per day across all levels of education. Unfiltered cigarettes and traditional pipes were used mainly by less well educated and rural populations. There was considerable variation in cigarette use by occupation, the highest rates beingamong self-employed men and among women teachers and officials. Both men and women who had never married had a slightly higher consumption per smoker than those who had married.

Knowledge and attitudes about smoking

Awareness of the harm caused by tobacco use is one of the first stages in changing social norms. Twenty-three percent of smokers and 36% of non-smokers knew that tobacco causes serious harm to health, while 8% of smokers and 2% of non-smokers responded that it caused no harm. There was a steadily increasing awareness of the harm caused by smoking at higher educational levels, with 22% of people with no schooling and 56% at university level acknowledging harmful risks; 22% of farmers, 41% of factory workers, 53% of teachers and 59% of health workers said that smoking causes serious harm.

Sharp differences were found in knowledge about whether three representative diseases were caused by smoking. About 70% of both smokers and non-smokers recognized the relationship with bronchitis, presumably because there is a close relationship in time between smoking and symptoms, but only 42% of non-smokers and 36% of smokers knew of the causal relationship with lung cancer. Only 4% of both smokers and non-smokers knew that smoking can cause heart disease, suggesting the need for health education. A steep relationship between educational level and knowledge that smoking causes lung cancer was found, ranging from about 15% in people with no schooling to about 70% in those with university education and above. The causal relationship with lung cancer was recognized by 80% of health workers, 68% of teachers, 56% of factory workers and only 28% of farmers. Knowledge about smoking risks also differed by geographical area, with 58% of urban populations and only 30% of rural people aware of the association between smoking and lung cancer.

People were aware of the impact that doctors and teachers have as role models on smoking behaviour. The influence that role models can have on smoking behaviour was widely accepted, about 80% of female and male non-smokers agreeing with the statement that 'Doctors and teachers and parents should not smoke in front of children'. About 75% of both male and female smokers agreed with the statement concerning doctors and teachers, but only 68% agreed with the statement in relation to parents. Ninety-two percent of people with university education and above agreed with the statement concerning smoking by doctors and teachers, but the percentage dropped to 68% of people with no schooling. Similarly, 87% of those with a university education and 64% of those with no schooling responded that parents should not smoke in front of their children. Over 80% of people in all occupations agreed with the statement about doctors and teachers smoking, although smaller percentages were found among farmers, self-employed, 'floating' people and houseworkers. More urban than rural people responded that doctors and teachers should not smoke.

In setting public policy, it is important to know how people would react to changes in laws, such as control measures to limit the public health effects of passive smoking. The support for legal action was strongly associated with educational level. Support for banning smoking in public places went from 59% of people with no schooling to 94% of people with university education and above. Banning sales to young people had the approval of 75% of people with no schooling and 95% of people with university education and above. About 53% of smokers and 62% of non-smokers were in favour of banning cigarette advertising. Raising the price of cigarettes had the least support, with 23% of people with no schooling and 43% of those with university and above being in favour. For each of these policies, the strongest support was from health workers, teachers and factory workers, suggesting that these may be groups of people who could lead advocacy efforts to implement anti-smoking policies.

Smoking among women

Although smoking is chiefly practised by older women, often among minorities using traditional methods, a particular concern about smoking among women is awareness of danger to the foetus when mothers smoke during pregnancy. In the survey question about knowledge of harm during pregnancy, 22% of smokers and 30% of non-smokers said that such harm could be serious, and 3 and 5% of smokers and non-smokers, respectively, said there it caused no harm. About 32% of smokers and 27% of non-smokers said that they did not know whether smoking during pregnancy is harmful, indicating a need for public education. The need for education is also demonstrated by the finding that 35% of the 15–19-year-old group said they did not know that smoking during pregnancy was harmful, as compared with 29% of the total population. About 46% of people with no schooling said they did not know about possible harm to the foetus, while only 8% of the respondents with a university education were unaware of foetal risk. Fewer farmers and factory workers than health workers or teachers knew about the risk of smoking to the foetus. Differences in knowledge were also evident by geographic area, with more urban than rural people recognizing the risk of smoking to the foetus.

A sharp difference between men and women was observed in responses to a question about the public image of people who smoked. Only 3–5% said that it was fashionable for a young woman to smoke; 8% of female smokers and 12% of male smokers agreed with the statement, 'A man who does not smoke is not a real man', while only 4% of both male and female non-smokers agreed. Among smokers, 47% of men and 43% of women agreed with the statement, 'Smoking can help relaxation and increase efficiency in exhausted people', while only 19% of non-smokers agreed.

Smoking among youth

Sampling for the national prevalence survey started with people 15 years of age. The smoking rates at ages 15–19 were already 18% among males, and climbed steeply to over 50% by the ages of 20–24 years. Although young people showed essentially the same awareness of the harmful effects of smoking and passive smoking as non-smoking adults, fewer knew that smoking during pregnancy is harmful to the foetus. Young people had about the same knowledge as adults about the disease-specific risks of smoking and reflected essentially the same attitudes as older people in responses to statements about the public image of smokers.

The attitudes of young people towards new laws that would change policies to control smoking are relevant to future trends. For four of the five proposed tobacco control laws, young people were somewhat more positive than older people, particularly with regard to banning smoking in public places, banning cigarette advertising, requiring warnings on cigarette packs and raising the price of cigarettes. There was even almost 80% agreement on a new law banning sales of cigarettes to young people.

Discussion

The 1996 National Smoking Prevalence Survey indicates China's need and potential for national action. Indeed, in many respects the effort to create awareness of and commitment to smoking control through public education and the mass media has hardly begun. Nevertheless, there is strong public support for effective implementation of control programmes, in spite of wide recognition of the economic implications of the proposed policy changes. National and community-based action to promote smoking cessation will have to proceed in parallel with continuing field research to find out how such programmes can best be applied. Smoking prevention campaigns should perhaps be targeted to particular groups, such as doctors and teachers, in ways that are adapted to Chinese conditions.

Although the smoking rates in China are currently much higher in males than in females, experience elsewhere shows that the potential exists for large increases among women, emphasizing the importance of prevention among both females and males who do not yet smoke. The emphasis in tobacco control among males should include not only prevention but also effective cessation programmes. The 1996 National Smoking Prevalence Survey confirms the importance of giving smoking control high priority among public health services in China, bringing together health-care professionals, researchers, policy-makers and administrators in many disciplines and services.

References

Liu, B.-Q., Peto, R., Chen, Z.-M., et al. (1998) Emerging tobacco hazards in China: 1. Retrospective proportional mortality study of one million deaths. Br. Med. J., 317, 1411–1422

Niu, S.-R., Yang, G.-H., Chen, Z.-M., et al. (1998) Emerging tobacco hazards in China: 2. Early mortality results from a prospective study. Br. Med. J., 317, 1423–1424

Weng, X., Hong, Z. & Chen, D. (1987) Smoking prevalence in Chinese aged 15 and above. Chin. Med. J., 100, 886–892

Yang, G.-H., Fan, L., Jian, T., et al. (1999) Smoking in China: Findings of the 1996 National Prevalence Survey. JAMA (in press)

Yang, G.-H., chief editor (1997) Smoking and Health in China: 1996 National Prevalence Survey of Smoking Patterns, Beijing: Chinese Science Technology Press

Emerging tobacco hazards in China:
Results on early mortality from a prospective study of 224 500 men

S.-R. Niu[1], G.-H. Yang[1], Z.-M. Chen[2], J.-L. Wang[1], G.-H. Wang[1], X.-Z. He[1],
H. Schoepff[2], J. Boreham[2], H.-C. Pan[2] & R. Peto[2]

[1] Chinese Academy of Preventive Medicine, Beijing, China, and [2] Clinical Trials
Service Unit and Epidemiological Studies Unit, Nuffield Department of Clinical
Medicine, Radcliffe Infirmary, Oxford, United Kingdom

Abstract

Objective: To monitor the evolving epidemic of mortality due to tobacco use in China that has followed the large increase in cigarette use among males in recent decades.

Design: A prospective study of cigarette smoking and mortality, starting with interviews with 224 500 men who will be followed-up for some decades.

Setting: 45 nationally representative, small, urban or rural areas distributed across China.

Subjects: Male population aged 40 or over in 1991, of whom about 80% were interviewed about smoking, drinking and medical history.

Main outcome measure: Cause-specific mortality, initially up to 1995 but to be continued, measured as risk ratios for smokers versus non-smokers and standardized for area, age and use of alcohol.

Results: 74% were smokers (73% current, only 1% former), but few men of this generation would have smoked substantial numbers of cigarettes since early adult life. The overall mortality rate has increased among smokers (risk ratio, 1.2; 95% confidence interval, 1.1–1.2; $p < 0.0001$). Almost all the increased mortality was due to neoplastic, respiratory or vascular disease. The overall risk ratios associated with smoking are less extreme in rural areas (1.3 for smokers who started before the age of 20, 1.1 for those who began at 20–24 and 1.0 for those who began at older ages) than in urban areas (1.7, 1.4 and 1.2, respectively).

Conclusion: This prospective study and the accompanying retrospective study show that by 1990 smoking was already causing about 12% of deaths among Chinese men in middle age. This proportion is predicted to rise to about 33% by 2030. Long-term continuation of the prospective study (with periodic re-surveys) will allow the evolution of this epidemic to be monitored.

Introduction

The recent substantial increase in cigarette consumption by Chinese men will eventually cause a substantial increase in mortality (Peto, 1987). To monitor the long-term evolution of this epidemic, a large, nationally representative, prospective study has begun which will continue for some decades. We describe here the early (1992–95) results with respect to mortality.

Methods

In 1987, the Chinese Academy of Preventive Medicine established 145 nationally representative 'disease surveillance points', each involving about 100 000 registered residents in five to eight units (urban street committees or rural villages) (Yang *et al.*, 1991). All men aged ≥ 40 in two or three units in 45 representative disease surveillance points were enlisted in 1990–91 for this prospective study, and about 80% (224 500) were interviewed about their smoking, drinking, and medical history. In all, 30% of the men lived in urban areas, which is the same proportion as in China as a whole. Mortality was monitored prospectively from local residential records. Causes of death from official death certificates were supplemented by medical notes and were coded (according to *The International Classification of Diseases*, Ninth Revision) by trained staff who were unaware of the baseline information. By January 1996, 3608 (2%) of the men had not been traced and 13 412 (6%) had died from neoplastic, respiratory, vascular and other causes in roughly equally proportions.

Results

In 1990, 73% of the men (68% urban, 75% rural) smoked; just 1% were former smokers, many having stopped because they were ill. Of the smokers, 55% used only cigarettes in 1990 (87% urban, 43% rural; 67% at ages 40–49, 37% at ≥ 65), and 30% had begun before the age of 20 (26% urban, 32% rural). The overall mortality rate among the smokers was significantly higher than that among men who had never smoked (relative risk 1.2; 95% confidence interval, 1.1–1.2; $p < 0.00001$) and was highest among men who had begun smoking before the age of 20, particularly in urban areas (Table 1). The excess mortality among smokers was due mainly to neoplastic (1.3; $p < 0.0001$), respiratory (1.4; $p < 0.00001$) and vascular (1.1; $p = 0.01$) disease. If these associations with smoking are largely causal, then tobacco is the cause of about 12% of all deaths among men in China (Table 2).

Table 1. Mortality rates from all causes of mortality by age at starting to smoke among middle-aged men in China

Age began smoking (years)	Proportion (%)		Age-standardized mortality risk ratio[a] (smoker/non-smoker)		
	Urban	Rural	Urban	Rural	Total
< 20	6	32	1.73 ± 0.06	1.26 ± 0.03	1.34
20–24	39	42	1.40 ± 0.05	1.12 ± 0.02	1.18
≥ 25	35	26	1.16 ± 0.05	1.02 ± 0.03	1.05
Never			1.00 ± 0.05	1.00 ± 0.03	

[a]Risk ratios and floated standard errors

Table 2. Numbers of deaths among Chinese men aged 40–79 during 1992–95[a]: mortality, mortality risk ratios (95% confidence intervals) and percentages of deaths attributed to smoking

Cause of death	No. of deaths	Annual mortality/1000[b]		Mortality ratio for ever smokers vs non-smokers[c]	% of deaths attributed to smoking
		Smoker	Non-smoker		
Neoplastic	2018	3.1	2.5	1.3 (1.1–1.6)**	16
Respiratory	2530	3.8	2.7	1.4 (1.2–1.6)**	22
Vascular	2543	3.8	3.4	1.1 (1.1–1.2)*	9
Other	2142	2.9	2.9	1.0 (0.92–1.1)	0
All causes[d]	9233	14	12	1.2 (1.1–1.2)**	12

[a] Deaths before 1992 or after age 80 are omitted; 6997 deaths among smokers and 2236 among people who never smoked are included.
[b] Standardized to the age distribution of non-smokers, so that the rate in smokers is the relative risk times that in non-smokers.
[c] Relative risk and 95% confidence interval. Estimated by maximum likelihood, stratified for area, age and alcohol. Such stratified analyses of this nationally representative study allow for the heterogeneity between urban and rural populations and between particular areas.
[d] Including tuberculosis and respiratory heart disease

Discussion

This nationally representative, prospective study shows that smoking is already an important cause of neoplastic, respiratory and vascular death among Chinese men. This finding is consistent with the results of smaller prospective studies in particular parts of China (Chen et al., 1997) and with those of a retrospective study of 1 million deaths (Liu et al., 1998). For many conditions that can be caused by tobacco, the smoker:non-smoker mortality ratio is less extreme in China than in countries where cigarettes have been used widely for several decades. However, since the background mortality (except from ischaemic heart disease) among non-smokers is particularly high in China, the mortality from tobacco-related diseases is already substantial. By about 1990, smoking was already responsible for about 12% of deaths among Chinese men, which corresponds to 0.7 million male deaths in the year 2000 from tobacco (or somewhat more as the percentage increases) (Liu et al., 1998).

The current health effects, however, chiefly reflect the consequences of past smoking patterns, and the future health effects of current smoking patterns will be much greater. In countries such as the United Kingdom and the United States, where most smokers start before the age of 20, about half of all persistent cigarette smokers are eventually killed by tobacco (Doll et al., 1994). Yet, it is only recently that the full extent of the hazard in the United States became evident. Although the main increase in cigarette use in the United States took place before 1950 (the mean consumption among adults aged over 15 was 1 cigarette a day in 1910, 4 cigarettes a day in 1930 and 10 cigarettes a day in 1950), the main increase in mortality from tobacco-related disease took place after 1950, when those who had started smoking substantial numbers of cigarettes in early adult life reached middle and old age. Of all deaths in the United States among men aged 35–69, the proportion attributable to tobacco in 1950 was only 12%, but this percentage rose to 33% in 1990, when the increase in tobacco-related deaths had been completed (Peto et al., 1994). Recent prospective studies of male smokers in the United Kingdom and the United States correctly indicate that about half are killed by tobacco, but similar studies in those countries in the 1960s, before the main increase in mortality was completed, misleadingly indicated that 'only' one-quarter of the deaths would be due to tobacco (Peto, 1994). In China as a whole, the ratio for deaths from all causes for smokers who began before the age of 20 is already 1.3, indicating that even at the current death rates about one smoker in 4 (0.34/1.3) would be killed by tobacco. This low risk ratio reflects the fact that older men may not have smoked persistently in the past (Chen et al., 1997) or may have smoked forms of tobacco that are associated with a lower risk than cigarettes. In urban areas, however, where a greater proportion of tobacco use is from cigarettes, the risk ratio for those who began before the age of 20 is already approaching 2, suggesting that about half will be killed by tobacco.

The main increase in cigarette consumption in China took place only recently (the mean consumption among Chinese men was 1 cigarette a day in 1952, 4 cigarettes a day in 1972 and 10 cigarettes a day in 1992); on the basis of present-day smoking patterns, mortality from tobacco-related disease in China will increase substantially. Of all deaths among men aged 35–69, the proportion attributable to tobacco will rise between 1990 and 2030 from 12% to about 33% (as happened previously in the United States; Peto *et al.*, 1994), because both in urban and in rural China two-thirds of young men (but currently few young women) become cigarette smokers, and cessation is rare. Long-term continuation of this prospective study, with periodic re-surveys of all middle-aged adults living in the study areas will allow monitoring of the evolution of the epidemic.

The epidemiological studies give four key messages:

- In recent years, most young men in China have become persistent cigarette smokers and started at about the age of 20; this will cause high mortality rates in middle age and old age.
- Currently, however, most middle-aged and older smokers (particularly in rural areas) have not persistently used substantial numbers of cigarettes daily ever since they were young adults, so their current tobacco-attributed mortality rate is lower.
- Nationally representative retrospective and prospective studies now show that in about 1990 'only' about 12% of deaths among middle-aged men were caused by smoking.
- Continuation of the present prospective study will consist of monitoring the growth of the epidemic of tobacco-related deaths in China over the next few decades.

Acknowledgements

After the conference, this article was published in *The British Medical Journal*, from which it is reproduced with permission, and in which fuller acknowledgements may be found. The papers by Liu *et al.* (1998) and Niu *et al.* (1998) are also available in Chinese in the February 1999 Chinese edition of *The British Medical Journal*.

References

Chen, Z.M., Xu, Z., Collins, R., Li, W.X. & Peto, R. (1997) The early health effects of the emerging tobacco epidemic in China: 16-year prospective study. *JAMA*, **278**, 1500–1504

Doll, R., Peto, R., Wheatley, K., Gray, R. & Sutherland, I. (1994) Mortality in relation to smoking: 40 years' observations on male British doctors. *Br. Med. J.*, **309**, 901–911

Liu, B.Q., Peto, R., Chen, Z.M., Boreham, J., Wu, Y.P., Li, J.Y., *et al.* (1998) Emerging tobacco hazards in China: 1. Retrospective proportional mortality study of one million deaths. *BMJ*, **317**, 1411–1422

Peto, R. (1987) Tobacco-related death in China. *Lancet*, ii, 211

Peto, R. (1994) Smoking and death: The past 40 years and the next 40. *Br. Med. J.*, 309, 937–939

Peto, R., Lopez, A.D., Boreham, J., Health, C. & Thun, M. (1994) *Mortality from Tobacco in Developed Countries, 1950–2000*, Oxford: Oxford University Press

Yang, G.H., Murray, C.J.L. & Zhang, Z. (1991) *Exploring Adult Mortality in China: Levels, Patterns and Causes*, Beijing: Hua Xia Press

Health effects of tobacco use in women

A.J. Sasco

Unit of Epidemiology for Cancer Prevention,
International Agency for Research on Cancer, Lyon, France[1]

[1]At the time of the conference, Dr Sasco was also Acting Chief, Programme for Cancer Control, World Health Organization, and is currently director of research at the Institut National de la Santé et de la Recherche Médicale, France.

Introduction

A large amount of data is currently available on the myriad diseases linked to tobacco use (Doll *et al.*, 1994). The deleterious effects of smoking were suspected in the last century or even before, but it is only recently that the magnitude of the negative impact of tobacco on health has become clear, and the evidence is becoming stronger every day. During the second half of this century, hundreds of studies became available that allowed us to estimate correctly the full burden of tobacco-related morbidity and mortality. Yet, as a woman, even more than as a cancer specialist or public health expert, I am greatly concerned by the relative scarcity of valid studies dealing specifically with women. I wish to describe the current state of knowledge on the health effects of tobacco use in women and, from this assessment, to derive recommendations on action to be taken to promote health in the population of the world at large.

Tobacco and women's health

For a long time, diseases linked to tobacco use were seen as a male attribute, and the tobacco industry, always prompt at taking advantage of figures that at first appear favourable to them, let women believe that they were immune to the effects of tobacco. Whereas this type of argument was prevalent in the West in the 1950s and 1960s, exactly the same strategy is now seen in the developing countries.

If the annual number of tobacco-related deaths is evaluated at 3 million, 'only' 500 000 occurred in women, most of them in the western world. Such a statistic does not give any cause for reassurance, as this low proportion of deaths among all deaths in women is merely a reflection of the tobacco use patterns prevailing in the world 20–30 years ago. If more and more women smoke and use other forms of tobacco, they will be equally and even predominantly affected by tobacco-related morbidity and mortality during the next century. This dark prediction is firmly grounded on a simple fact: if women are exposed to tobacco as men were, they will be equally affected and even more. Any comparison of rates of disease between the two sexes must therefore be made in the light of careful consideration of exposure. Keeping this crucial distinction in mind, we can now review the effects of tobacco on the health of women.

Effects on cancer

Cancer of the lung has been the traditional marker of disease linked to tobacco, for both historical and scientific reasons. Currently, about 1.2 million deaths from lung cancer occur annually in the world, making it the most frequent cause of death from cancer worldwide. Of these, about 282 000 cases occur in women (World Health Organization, 1998). The variation in age-adjusted (to the world population standard) incidence rates of lung cancer among women goes from a low of 0.33 in Barshi, Paranda and Bhum in India to a high of 72.9 per 100 000 woman–years in the Maori population of New Zealand (Parkin *et al.*, 1997). Countries with current high incidence rates of lung cancer among women include those of North America, northern Europe and Australia, whereas intermediate rates are seen in other parts of Europe and low rates in Asia and Africa.

Unfortunately, this currently rather mild global picture will not remain mild. Time trends clearly indicate that the rates of lung cancer are increasing dramatically in most countries of the world. In Europe, for example, the total number of deaths from lung cancer increased only slightly between 1973 and 1992 among men, from 107 056 to 140 782 deaths, whereas the number has approximately doubled among women, from 18 822 to 36 772 (World Health Organization, 1998). All European countries have seen an increase in the figures for women, whereas some decrease is seen for men in Austria, Finland and the United Kingdom. Yet, large disparities still persist in Europe, where the highest rates are seen in the English-speaking and Nordic countries and much lower rates in French-speaking and southern countries. In the United States, mortality from lung cancer has already overtaken the traditionally important cause of death from cancer in women, namely cancer of the breast. In other countries, such as France, a similar change in cancer mortality rates is expected to occur around the year 2020; even in countries with low rates, increases are being observed. In those with a long history of smoking, such as the United States, it is interesting and at the same time very worrying to note that the death rates from lung cancer among smokers are greater in more recent than in older studies, even after adjustment for current amount and duration of smoking. For example, in the prospective cohort 'Cancer Prevention Studies' (CPS I and II), the death rates from lung cancer increased between 1959–65 and 1982–88, with a greater proportionate increase in women than in men (Thun & Heath, 1997). The reasons for this trend are not clear. They may relate to an effect of earlier age at initiation of smoking and clearly counteract the argument that 'light' cigarettes are 'safer' than regular ones.

Also from the United States comes evidence that if the amount and duration of smoking are equal women may be more sensitive than men to lung cancer. Although the cohort or time period effect previously described cannot be easily disentangled from other potential explanations such as earlier age at initiation of smoking or a different tobacco composition, this aspect must be thoroughly studied in the years to come, also in relation to the increase in the incidence of specific histological forms of lung cancer such as adenocarcinoma (Thun et al., 1997), which may be partly hormone-dependent. This is of special relevance to populations such as that of China, where Dr Liu Qing from Sun Yat Sen University has demonstrated, in collaboration with IARC, the role of passive smoking and home indoor air pollution in the occurrence of lung cancers that are frequently of the adenocarcinoma type (Liu et al., 1993). Similarly, consideration of susceptibility should be evaluated in populations which currently have low rates of lung cancer but where tobacco use is now exploding, such as in Africa. In my view, the question of the association between lung cancer and tobacco use is still a valid and potentially promising scientific endeavour and may also be a public health tool of crucial importance.

The incidences of other cancers linked to tobacco use (Sasco, 1991) have also been found to have increased among women smokers. This applies to cancers of the urinary bladder, renal pelvis and kidney and pancreatic cancer. Clearly, all urinary sites come into close contact with tobacco metabolites which exert a carcinogenic action. Cancers at other sites that are causally linked to tobacco use are those of the upper aero-digestive tract, comprising cancers of the oral cavity, lip, larynx, pharynx and oesophagus. According to the most prevalent form of tobacco use in a given population, lung cancer may be an inadequate universal marker of exposure to tobacco. For example, the highest reported rates of cancer of the mouth in the world are those for women in India, a country where tobacco is mostly chewed and only rarely and recently smoked (Parkin et al., 1997; Gupta, this volume). Furthermore, there is an interaction between tobacco and alcohol, with a potentiation of risk when the two exposures are combined. As women generally drink less alcohol than men, they are less frequently affected by these cancers, and the male to female ratio is generally higher than that for lung cancer. Again, the more women smoke in the future, the higher their risk will be of developing all tobacco-related cancers. If their alcohol consumption also increases, the multiplicative effect often described in men will also be seen in women.

The classical cancers of women deserve special attention. An increased risk for cancer of the cervix uteri is seen among smokers; the relative risk is small and has been the object of continued controversy. It has long been argued that any increased risk for cervical cancer among women smokers is the result of confounding by sexual activity: women smokers were deemed to have more sexual partners than non-smokers and therefore a greater likelihood of contracting sexually transmitted diseases. As cervical cancer is linked to infection by the human papillomavirus (IARC, 1995), smoking is considered by some to be only a confounder and not a causal factor. Others advance arguments that smoking has at least a facilitating role in the development of cervical cancer, since cotinine, a marker of exposure to tobacco, has been found in the cervical fluid of smokers and even of women passively exposed to tobacco smoke. Furthermore, tobacco has a negative effect on immunity and may therefore play a role in the response of the individual to sexually transmitted viruses. Although the causal role of smoking in the occurrence of cervical cancer cannot be fully demonstrated, it cannot be completely discarded.

Similarly controversial is the effect of smoking on the occurrence of breast cancer. For a long time, smoking was considered to be slightly protective against breast cancer, the rationale being that tobacco behaves like an anti-oestrogen in women. This effect is linked to an earlier age at menopause of smokers than non-smokers and an increased risk for osteoporosis. More recent studies found no such protective effect, and some even found an increased risk for breast cancer among smokers in relation to a specific N-acetylation phenotype. Studies have been initiated, especially in China, on the role of passive smoking in the etiology of breast cancer. The data on cancer of the ovary are as yet too limited to provide a conclusive answer. Again because of the anti-oestrogenic effect of tobacco, smokers have a slightly reduced risk for cancer of the corpus uteri.

Effects on the circulatory system

In women, as in men, tobacco use is linked to coronary heart disease, in particular myocardial infarct, chronic heart disease, peripheral vascular disease and cerebrovascular diseases. As the etiology of cardio-cerebrovascular diseases is multifactorial, it is much more difficult to isolate the role of tobacco from other risk factors. Most of the studies have been done in countries where there is a high risk for the disease. In contrast to the situation for lung cancer in the United States, the death rate from coronary heart disease has decreased among both smokers and non-smokers, with a less marked effect in women than in men (Thun & Heath, 1997). These contrasting temporal trends between lung cancer and coronary disease reflect the change in risk factors other than smoking for the latter.

A specific interaction for women that should be thoroughly studied is smoking and use of exogenous hormones, such as oral contraceptives. Among older women who smoke, the excess risk for cancer associated with oral contraceptive use is substantial.

Effects on the pulmonary system

Chronic obstructive pulmonary disease, such as emphysema and chronic bronchitis, is linked to tobacco use. These diseases may not be immediately fatal, but they are extremely debilitating. The trends are similar to those observed for lung cancer. In the United States, an increase in the incidence of these diseases is seen over time in smokers, which is more marked in women than in men (Thun & Heath, 1997).

Other health effects

Smoking has been reliably linked to facial wrinkling and the general aspect of the skin. Through a negative effect on the microcirculation of the skin, more tissue damage accumulates more rapidly in smokers than in non-smokers. Effects such as these, yellow fingers and teeth and a malodorant smell may not appeal to young girls and might therefore be used as additional arguments for not initiating smoking.

In older women, the effects on age at menopause and on osteoporosis with its associated fractures should be emphasized.

Effects on reproductive health

Smoking affects the fertility of both women and men, with a longer delay to conception in smokers than non-smokers. In more extreme cases, in-vitro fertilization is less successful in smokers than non-smokers. Smoking is also associated with an increased risk for pelvic inflammatory disease, even after adjustment for other risk factors and potential confounders, leading in turn to higher risks for total infertility and ectopic pregnancy. Once a woman who smokes becomes pregnant, she has increased risks for low birthweight infants and for spontaneous abortions.

Tobacco use has been reliably associated with an increase in perinatal mortality, as well as with sudden infant death syndrome. Anaemia, which is known to be more frequent in developing countries, further compounds the risk and therefore can be expected to have even more severe health consequences among undernourished women of child-bearing age. The negative impact on children's health extends beyond the neonatal period, with more frequent and more severe infections among passively exposed children, in diseases of the ear, nose and throat and of the pulmonary system. Asthma is also more severe among these children, who may suffer from a slower general development.

Conclusion

In the face of so many diseases, the best route is clearly prevention. Primary prevention may be effected in three ways: action on genes (maybe in the future), chemoprevention (still experimental) and avoidance of recognized carcinogens (Sasco, 1995). The public health message is very clear and simple: in order to have a healthy population, the world must become tobacco-free. Women, as the givers of life and providers of care, have the major role to play; the future of humankind lies in their hands. Given their pivotal role in the family, they will be the actors in a holistic approach to health promotion, encouraging a healthy lifestyle and avoidance of recognized carcinogens, such as tobacco. If women could also assume more leadership in society, the achievement of this goal would be greatly facilitated.

Even more important for our future is the fight for the health of tomorrow's world: our children. The idea of a 'Child Health Day', originally proclaimed in 1928 by Calvin Coolidge in the United States and recently given special attention in that country by Dr Ernst Wynder, President of the American Health Foundation, could be extended worldwide. On the first Monday of October, the 'Healthy Practices Pledge' should be publicized in as many countries as possible. Children and their families should take time to have a healthy breakfast together, engage in physical activity, live and play safely, take care of their health and, last but not least, not smoke.

References

Doll, R., Peto, R., Wheatley, K., Gray, R. &Sutherland, I. (1994) Mortality in relation to smoking: 40 years' observation on male British doctors. Br. Med. J., 309, 901–911

International Agency for Research on Cancer (1995) IARC Monographs on the Evaluation of Carcinogenic Risk to Humans, Vol. 64, Human Papillomaviruses, Lyon

Liu, Q., Sasco, A.J., Riboli, E. & Hu, M.X. (1993) Indoor air pollution and lung cancer in Guangzhou, People's Republic of China. Am. J. Epidemiol., 137, 145–154

Parkin, D.M., Whelan, S.L., Ferlay, J., Raymond, L. & Young, J., eds (1997) Cancer Incidence in Five Continents, Vol. VII (IARC Scientific Publications No. 143), Lyon: International Agency for Research on Cancer

Sasco, A.J. (1991) World burden of tobacco related cancer. Lancet, 338, 123–124

Sasco, A.J. (1995) [Epidemiology and prevention of cancer: Reflections on the ethics of public health approaches.] Bull. Acad. Natl Méd., 179, 987–1007 (in French)

Thun, M.J. & Heath, C.W., Jr (1997) Changes in mortality from smoking in two American Cancer Society prospective studies since 1950. Prev. Med., 26, 422–426

Thun, M.J., Lally, C.A., Flannery, J.T., Calle, E.E., Flanders, W.D. & Heath, C.W., Jr (1997) Cigarette smoking and changes in the histopathology of lung cancer. J. Natl Cancer Inst., 89, 1580–1586

World Health Organization (1998) The World Health Report 1998. Life in the Twenty-first Century: A Vision for All, Geneva

Women: The second wave of the tobacco epidemic

M. Haglund

National Institute of Public Health, Stockholm, Sweden

When the American singer Rudy Vallee composed a song about his favourite woman, 'My cigarette lady', in 1931, smoking among women was still not well accepted in American or any other western society. Few could foresee the tragic development that we are now facing, with women as the next wave of the tobacco epidemic. Many projections have been made of the dire trends in smoking among women in developed nations, but we can only begin to make estimates for developing nations. Currently, 2–10% of women in developing countries smoke in comparison with 25–30% in developed countries. WHO's estimate of those more than 1 million women who will be killed by tobacco by 2020 is not just a faceless statistic but represents the girls and women of today. What is even more tragic is that we have seen only the tip of the iceberg.

In developed countries such as Sweden, there has been a trend towards more smoking among girls than among boys. Sweden is one of the few countries in the world where smoking is now more common among women than men. Several years ago in Beijing, Sweden was recognized as the most emancipated country in the world, but isn´t our smoking trend the ultimate backlash of equality? Our experience in developed countries gives us strong reason to believe that the smoking habits of women in developing countries will soon become similar to those of men and then follow the same trend. It seems to be only a question of time and of a country's phase of development before the tragic tobacco history of women and smoking that started in the United States in the 1920s repeats itself in country after country. The number of women who smoke will also increase for demographic reasons, as the female population in developing countries will rise by more than 1 billion by the year 2025.

In many developing countries, including the new democracies in central and eastern Europe, the situation is now explosive. For example, in one of Sweden´s neighbours, Lithuania, only 10% of women used to smoke before the beginning of the 1990s, but in the last five years the proportion of women smokers has doubled. The increase in Lithuania was much faster than in Sweden, where it took almost 20 years for the prevalence among women to double. The value of persuading women in Sweden and the United States to quit smoking is neutralized if women in China, Brazil and South Africa take up smoking at the same time.

While we are hesitating to take action, the transnational tobacco companies are finding new markets, and their prime target is women. Since the 1920s, women have been heavily targeted by the tobacco industry with advertising that exploits our ideas of liberation, power and other values important for women. Dr Mochizuki-Kobayashi gave examples of the ruthless marketing activities of the tobacco companies, who are trying to hook women with their misleading messages. Tobacco advertising is nothing less than seduction! If the dire smoking trends are not enough to inspire us to further action, we also have the strong medical arguments, so well described by Dr Sasco. Smoking may be even worse for women than for men, as the female body may be even more sensitive to tobacco than that of males, as in the case of alcohol. There are also risks related to our reproductive function. The effects of tobacco consumption on men have been extensively documented, but further research is needed on women.

The challenge is tremendous, but luckily the solution is very simple! We just have to do more, and the sooner we act the sooner we will get results. There is still a chance to maintain the relatively low rates of women´s smoking in, for example, Asia, where the tobacco companies are perfectly aware of their potential market of approximately 1 thousand million women. Unfortunately, until recently, there was a perception in many countries that smoking was mainly a male problem and that women were more resistant to tobacco than men. This is not suprising, as smoking-related diseases have become common among women in only a few countries, like the Denmark, the United Kingdom and the United States, where women have smoked for decades. At present, as many as 50% of the women killed by tobacco every year die in the United States, which has only 5% of the world's female population. This fact clearly demonstrates the magnitude of the smoking epidemic among women.

Of course there is no alternative; Beauty must beat the Beast! First of all, however, we must realize that our task cannot be done either quickly or easily, but that we must change the negatives into positives and the problems into possibilities! So why let it get worse before it gets better? Each of us has an important role to play in educating people. Like many mediaeval women, it is our responsibility to educate ourselves and to teach others that women who smoke like men will also die like men.

My first recommendation for action is to identify women's tobacco use as a major health problem and to build an international consensus round this issue. As the President of the International Network of Women Against Tobacco, I am very pleased to see women and smoking as one of the main themes at this conference.

My second recommendation is to combine tobacco control policies and measures, such as the ban on promotion and tobacco price policies, with a comprehensive tobacco control strategy which includes 'gender sensitivity' in every aspect of tobacco research, cessation and prevention. Worldwide patterns, trends and prevalence of tobacco use and the exposure of women should be determined. We also need to know how tobacco control policies, laws and regulations differentially affect women and about women-specific risk factors that affect prevention, initiation, maintenance, cessation and relapse. As not even the most powerful legislation will eliminate the need for public education, we will also need woman-specific campaigns and programmes, which are so far rare or non-existent except those concentrating on smoking during pregnancy. Of course quitting during pregnancy is very important, but we also need programmes that encourage women to quit smoking for their own sakes or, even better, never to start.

In developing health education programmes for women, I strongly believe that we must not rely on our traditional working methods. We must also involve new partners. In Sweden, our prime target is teenage girls, mainly those with parents who are blue-collar workers. The involvement of Miss Sweden in our tobacco control activities in Sweden appears to be one of our most effective health education campaigns for girls. It is important to define and use the most effective role models for each target group. We should be much more inventive in our efforts and not forget that even health educators can fail.

In order to implement strategies and action on women and tobacco issues, we will need the help of many organizations at different levels, such as the International Network of Women Against Tobacco, the American Medical Women's Association's Strategic Coalition of Girls and Women against Tobacco and the Swedish Nurses Against Tobacco, which are responsible for advocacy and coordinaton. We will also need the further involvement of women organizations, which, according to Dr Amos, will require time, understanding and resources.

My third and last recommendation is to increase the number and power of women leaders in the tobacco control movement. Like Joan of Arc, who led the French army in many battles during the Hundred Years' War, many more women should lead in the tobacco control movement all over the world. This is not a competition between men and women, but tobacco is an important women's health issue in which women can play a key role in raising awareness within women's movements and among other women.

Since the World Conference in Perth, Australia, in 1990, where only about 5% of the speakers were women, there has been a significant increase in female presenters at plenary sessions of world conferences. In this conference, we have almost reached our final goal of at least 50% of invited speakers, chairs and discussant.

Finally, I shall quote something I read when I was a student at the university more than 20 years ago, which clearly demonstrates the dilemma of being a leader and a woman: 'If a woman invests in her intelligence you will find her unwomanly, but if she invests in her womanhood she will be seen as ignorant'. Dear colleagues, you are welcome to join our forces; women's lives are at stake, and we will need all of you to fight the tobacco epidemic among women!

Oral cancer and tobacco use in India: A new epidemic

P.C. Gupta

Tata Institute of Fundamental Research
Mumbai, India

Oral submucous fibrosis is a chronic, progressive, debilitating disease in which the oral mucosa loses its elasticity, fibrous bands develop, and there is a marked intolerance to spicy food. The size of the opening of the mouth is progressively reduced. The disease is also precancerous and is associated with a high relative risk (397 after control for tobacco use) for malignant transformation (Gupta *et al.*, 1989). Spontaneous regression has not been reported, and there is no effective or widely accepted treatment.

Chewing of areca nut has now clearly been shown to be the most important etiological factor for oral sub-mucous fibrosis (Murti *et al.*, 1995). In case–control studies from Bhavnagar, Gujarat, and from Karachi, Pakistan, very high relative risks for areca-nut chewing were reported (110 and 94). Population-based studies in India do not indicate that this is a very common disease. Health professionals, especially dentists and ear-nose-and-throat surgeons, in northern India have noted, however, a manifold increase in the prevalence of oral submucous fibrosis.

The present study was undertaken in Bhavnagar district, Gujarat, to investigate whether the prevalence of this disease has increased and, if so, whether it could be attributed to use of areca nuts.

Subjects and methods

Bhavnagar district lies between 71° 15' and 72° 18' E and 22° 18' and 21° 18' N, on the western coast of India in the State of Gujarat. It has an area of 9259 km². Twenty geographically contiguous villages were selected in *Palitana taluka* of this district, and all individuals aged 15 and older were questioned about their use of areca nut and chewing and smoking of tobacco by trained investigators during house-to-house visits. Men who reported some kind of chewing or smoking habit were examined for the presence of oral submucous fibrosis. The criterion for a diagnosis of this condition was the presence of palpable fibrous bands in the oral mucosa, as in all of our studies since 1966. The visits and examinations were discontinued after 5018 examinations, for logistical reasons.

The most popular method of chewing areca nut in the region was as *mawa*, a combination of areca nut, tobacco and slaked lime (calcium hydroxide). Areca nut is also chewed in betel quid. Some of the men chewed tobacco and lime without areca nut. More information on these and other chewing and smoking habits can be found elsewhere (Bhonsle *et al.*, 1992).

Results

Among 11 262 men who were screened, 68% reported using tobacco. A variety of habits was prevalent, the commonest being *bidi* smoking (31%), followed by *mawa* chewing (19%); smoking was slightly more popular than use of smokeless tobacco (35% vs. 28%), with 4.8% of the men reporting both types of use. Cigarette smoking was uncommon (0.2%). Use of smokeless tobacco was concentrated in the lower age groups: 76% of all smokeless tobacco users were under 35.

Oral submucous fibrosis was diagnosed in 164 men, 71% of whom were solely *mawa* chewers; an additional 22% used tobacco in other forms as well. Only four men (2%) reported no current use of areca nut but had used it in the past. The disease seemed to be concentrated in young men, 84% of the cases occurring in men under the age of 35.

The highest prevalence of oral submucous fibrosis was found among *mawa* users (11%) and the lowest among those who did not use areca nut (0.12%). The relative risk associated with any kind of areca nut use was 75.

Discussion

In a population-based house-to-house survey carried out in early 1967 of 10 071 individuals aged 15 or older, the prevalence of oral submucous fibrosis in Bhavnagar district was 0.16%. In the current survey, carried out in 1993–94 with the same criteria, 164 cases of this disease were diagnosed in 5018 tobacco and/or areca nut users (3.2%) who were examined. If the prevalence among men who were not examined is assumed to be zero, the prevalence among the 21 852 men interviewed would be 0.75%.

The real difference in prevalence is higher than it appears to be at first glance. In the older sample, not a single case of oral submucous fibrosis was found, although 5227 men were examined, 71% of whom were tobacco users (Mehta *et al.*, 1971). Thus, the prevalence of this disease among men has increased from zero in 1967 to at least 1.5% in 1993–94 (164 cases among 11 262 men).

The trend in prevalence closely followed the trend in areca-nut chewing. Oral submucous fibrosis was diagnosed only in areca-nut chewers, as the four patients who were not currently users had chewed areca nut in the past. The age distribution followed the pattern of smokeless tobacco use. This study also confirms that areca-nut chewing in India almost always involves tobacco chewing as well.

Our findings clearly indicate an evolving epidemic of oral submucous fibrosis in the rural population of Bhavnagar district. Although there is no cure for this disease, 84% of the patients were under 35 and 44% were under 25. The prevalence of *mawa* chewing followed a similar pattern. The age-specific prevalence of oral submucous fibrosis among smokeless tobacco users thus indicates a close, direct link.

The reasons for the increased use of areca nut, and thus the increased prevalence of oral submucous fibrosis, are hard to identify. Areca nut is the main constituent of all *pan masala* (betel-quid mixture). Government taxes on these products, unlike cigarettes, are low, and there is no restriction on advertising for *pan masala*. As a consequence, the earnings of the *pan masala* industry have increased to several thousand million rupees within less than three decades of its initiation. Use of areca nut and all types of smokeless tobacco has therefore increased enormously, especially in northern India where most of the industry is concentrated.

The perceived substantial increase in the incidence of oral submucous fibrosis in northern India thus appears to be real. Given the tobacco use of areca-nut chewers and the high relative risk for malignant transformation of oral submucous fibrosis, there is a clear probability of an increase in the incidence of oral cancer. The epidemic must be stemmed by specific measures to discourage use of products containing tobacco and/or areca nut.

References

Bhonsle, R.B., Murti, P.R. & Gupta, P.C. (1992) Tobacco habits in India. In: Gupta, P.C/, Hamner, J.E. & Murti, P.E., eds, *Control of Tobacco-related Cancers and Other Diseases*, Bombay: Oxford University Press, pp. 25–46

Gupta, P.C., Bhonsle, R.B., Murti, P.R., Daftary, D.K., Mehta, F.S. & Pindborg, J.J. (1989) An epidemiologic assessment of cancer risk in oral precancerous lesions in India with special reference to nodular leukoplakia. *Cancer*, 63, 2247–2251

Mehta, F.S., Pindborg, J.J., Hamner, J.E., Gupta, P.C., Daftary, D.K., Sahiar, B.E. et al. (1971) *Report on Investigations of Oral Cancer and Precancerous Conditions in Indian Rural Populations 1966–69*, Copenhagen: Munksgaard

Murti, P.R., Bhonsle, R.B., Gupta, P.C., Daftary, D.K., Pindborg, J.J. & Mehta, F.S. (1995) Etiology of oral submucous fibrosis: Role of areca-nut chewing. *J. Oral Pathol. Med.*, 24, 145–152

STUDIES ON TOBACCO USE

The prevalence of tobacco use

Tobacco use in Japan

N. Yamaguchi[1], Y. Mochizuki-Kobayashi[2] & S. Watanabe[3]

[1]*WHO Collaborating Centre for Reference on Smoking and Health, National Cancer Center;* [2]*Ministry of Health and Welfare; and* [3]*Tokyo University of Agriculture, Tokyo, Japan*

Summary

The prevalence of smoking among Japanese men decreased from over 80% in 1965 to less than 60% in 1996, but the prevalence among women remained fairly constant during that time, at about 15%. In contrast to the decreasing prevalence of smoking, the annual consumption of cigarettes and the average consumption per smoker has been increasing for decades. The burden of tobacco use on the health status of the Japanese should therefore be evaluated by taking into account not only smoking prevalence but also daily cigarette consumption per smoker. We propose the use of a measure, the 'cumulative cigarette consumption', for estimating life-long cumulative exposure to tobacco smoke. The cumulative cigarette consumption can be calculated by adding up the annual, age-specific consumption of cigarettes of a specific birth cohort. The death rate from lung cancer was found to correlate linearly with cumulative cigarette consumption. Tobacco control in Japan is also discussed, with emphasis on the prevention of smoking among minors.

Introduction

Although cigarette consumption is high in Japan, the rates of mortality and morbidity for tobacco-related diseases are lower than would be expected. Three aspects of tobacco and health in Japan are important. First, cigarette smoking became popular in Japan after the Second World War, so that there is a time lag of 20–30 years in comparison with many western European countries and the United States, where smoking became popular after the First World War. Secondly, a number of people in Japan became concerned about the health effects of tobacco use in the 1960s; for instance, the health effects of environmental tobacco smoke were first addressed in a large-scale prospective study launched by the late Dr T. Hirayama after publication of the Surgeon-General's report in 1964, supported by the Ministry of Health and Welfare (Hirayama, 1984). Thirdly, tobacco sales were monopolized by the Government up to 1985. This did not necessarily mean that the Government promoted tobacco sales, but the long-standing monopoly formed a solid, stable structure of economic support for tobacco-producing farmers, which has been a major obstacle to change in the Government policy on smoking. Nonetheless, the efforts of many people involved in tobacco control have resulted in a decrease in the prevalence of smoking among men over the last few decades (Figure 1). The smoking prevalence thus decreased from over 80% in 1965 to less than 60% in 1996, although the prevalence among women remained stable over those 30 years, at 15%.

Trends in smoking prevalence

The trends in smoking prevalence in 10-year age groups are shown in Figure 2. The data on age-specific prevalence were provided by Japan Tobacco, Inc., the former Japan Tobacco Monopoly Bureau. We depended on these unpublished data because no other figures are available for the period 1965–96. For males, decreasing trends of similar magnitude are seen in all age groups; for females, on the other hand, the prevalence among women aged 40 to ≥ 60 appears to be decreasing, whereas that for 20–30-year-olds is increasing.

Figure 1. Trends in smoking prevalence in Japan

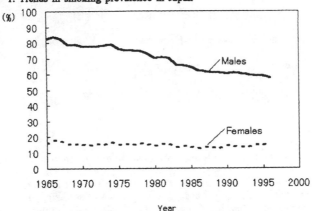

Figure 2. Trends in smoking prevalence in Japan in 10-year age groups

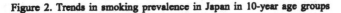
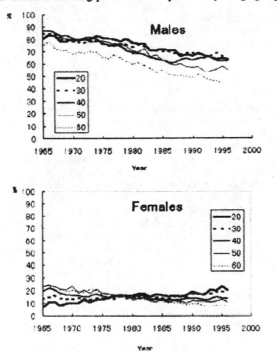

The changes in smoking prevalence by year of birth are shown for 10-year age groups in Figure 3. For this figure, the prevalence for each 10-year age group was assumed to represent that of the mid-point: 25 for the age group 20–29, 35 for 30–39, 45 for 40–49, 55 for 50–59 and 65 for ≥ 60. In all age groups of men, the prevalence shows a clear decline in later birth cohorts (born more recently). For women, the figure shows a clear U shape. Thus, the prevalence among women aged 40 to ≥ 60 shows a decrease between those born in 1900 and those born in 1930–40, whereas the prevalence among women in their 20s and 30s shows an increase for those born in 1940–71. This indicates that cigarette smoking became popular in the post-war generation.

Figure 3. Changes in smoking prevalence in Japan in 10-year age groups by year of birth

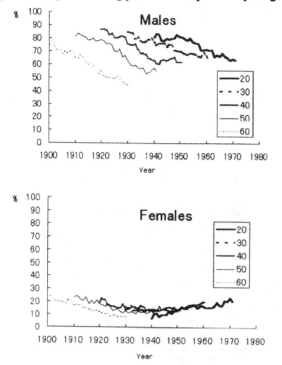

The future trend can be predicted by extrapolating the smoking prevalence in each age group to future generations. The prevalence among men can be predicted to continue to decrease, but that among women can be predicted to begin increasing when the post-war generation forms the majority of the female population.

Trends in cigarette consumption

The annual sales of tobacco in Japan are shown in Figure 4. Although the smoking prevalence has shown a decrease, especially among men, total tobacco sales have increased since 1920, except for a temporary deficit after the Second World War. On the basis of the total sales and the smoking prevalence among men and women, the number of cigarettes consumed daily by one smoker can be estimated (Figure 5), assuming that daily consumption is equal for men and women. It can be seen that the daily consumption has also increased, from fewer than 10 cigarettes in the 1950s to nearly 25 cigarettes in the 1990s.

It is widely argued that the increase in mortality from lung cancer in Japan cannot be explained adequaltely by smoking. Nevertheless, although the smoking prevalence among men has been decreasing and that among women has been relatively stable, rapid, sizable increases in mortality from lung cancer have been observed in both sexes. Figure 5 shows clearly that not only the smoking prevalence but also the number of cigarettes smoked daily should be taken into account in relating cigarette smoking to its health outcomes.

Cumulative cigarette consumption

In an attempt to integrate smoking prevalence and daily cigarette consumption for assessing the risk of cigarette use, we propose a quantity called the 'cumulative cigarette

Figure 4. Annual sales of cigarettes in Japan, 1920–96

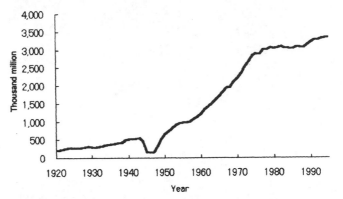

Figure 5. Average daily consumption of cigarettes among Japanese smokers

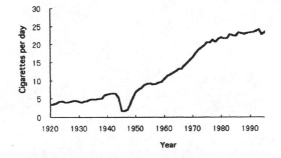

Consumption by men and women is considered to be equal.

consumption'. This quantity is estimated by summing the age-specific cigarette consumption of each birth cohort, which is obtained by multiplying the average cigarette consumption of a smoker by the smoking prevalence at each age. The cumulative cigarette consumption is an indicator of the lifetime cigarette consumption of a birth cohort weighted by the smoking prevalence. The advantage of this indicator is that it can be estimated from data on smoking prevalence and cigarette sales.

For this report, the cumulative cigarette consumption up to age 70 was estimated separately for men and women in cohorts born in 1900–51 (Figure 6). Data on smoking prevalence were available for persons in their 20s, 30s, 40s, 50s and ≥ 60 for 1940–71, 1930–61, 1920–51, 1910–41 and 1900–31, respectively. The smoking prevalence in earlier years for which no data were available for younger age groups were assumed to be the same as the earliest available value. For example, the smoking prevalence for people in their 20s in 1900–39 was assumed to be same as that in 1940. The smoking prevalence in recent years for which no data were available for older age groups was obtained by extrapolation for each birth cohort. For example, the smoking prevalence among people born in 1951 is available only for those in their 20s, 30s and 40s, because they had reached age 45 as of 1996. The smoking prevalence for the future, when they would be in their 50s and ≥ 60s, was projected by assuming that the trend observed over the previous 10 years would continue.

The daily cigarette consumption was available up to 1995 (Figure 5); in order to estimate future cumulative cigarette consumption, the daily cigarette consumption after

Figure 6. Estimated ciumulative cigarette consumption for people born 1900–51

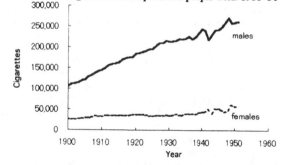

1995 was assumed to remain stable. The cumulative cigarette consumption of men between the ages of 20 and 70 doubled, from 106 100 for those born in 1900 to 213 200 for those born in 1930. That of women showed a smaller increase, from 25 600 for those born in 1900 to 36 700 for those born in 1930—a 1.43-fold increase. The cumulative cigarette consumption of both men and women is predicted to continue to increase if the current trends in smoking prevalence and daily cigarette consumption continue. The predicted values of cumulative cigarette consumption for men and women born in 1951 are 262 300 and 60 800, respectively. When compared with the values for those born in 1930, a 1.23-fold increase is predicted for men and a 1.66-fold increase for women.

Correlation between cumulative cigarette consumption and lung cancer mortality

To examine the validity of cumulative cigarette consumption for assessing the risk of adverse health effects of cigarette smoking, we studied the relationship between cumulative cigarette consumption from age 20 to 70 and the death rate from lung cancer among people aged 70–74. The death rate showed a trend similar to that of cumulative cigarette consumption for both men and women (Figure 7). The rates per 100 000 for men and women born in 1922 are 304.9 and 69.1, respectively. As compared with the rates for those born in 1900, 175.9 for men and 48.9 for women, the increases are 1.73-fold for men and 1.41-fold for women. The corresponding increases in the cumulative cigarette consumption between birth years 1900 and 1922 are 1.77-fold for men and 1.46-fold for women. Furthermore, when the correlation between cumulative cigarette

Figure 7. Trends in death rates from lung cancer in Japan among people aged 70–74 who were born in 1900–23

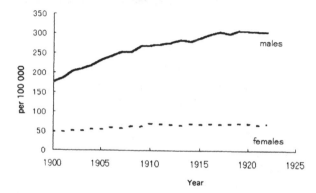

consumption and death rates from lung cancer was examined by linear regression analysis, the rate was found to increase in proportion to the cumulative cigarette consumption (Figure 8). The squared correlation coefficient is 0.9935, indicating that more than 99% of the change in the death rate from lung cancer can be explained by the cumulative cigarette consumption. The slope of the regression equation, 0.0017, indicates that one cigarette consumed will increase the death rate from lung cancer by 0.0017 per 100 000 among people aged 70–74, which represents approximately two persons in the whole country. This also indicates that one lung cancer death per 100 000 in the age group 70–74 can be attributed to the consumption of 588 cigarettes over 50 years.

This linear equation can also be used to predict future mortality from lung cancer in Japan. For example, the death rate at age 70–74 among men and women born in 1951 can be predicted to be 454 and 111 per 100 000, respectively, by incorporating the values for cumulative cigarette consumption (262 300 and 60 800) into the regression equation. It can therefore be predicted that the death rate from lung cancer will continue to increase during the coming 20–30 years, unless effective countermeasures to reduce the prevalence of smoking are introduced.

Tobacco control in Japan

As shown by the projection for future mortality from lung cancer, the health effects of cigarette smoking have not yet reached their peak in Japan, and it is therefore of paramount importance to strengthen anti-smoking activities as soon as possible. Minors are the primary target in the prevention of initiation of smoking (Yamaguchi *et al.*, 1991, 1992). In Japan, the sale of any type of tobacco to minors is prohibited by law, and strict penalties, such as suspension from school, are imposed on pupils found smoking; nevertheless, since there are no regulations against tobacco-vending machines, minors can buy cigarettes easily. The number of tobacco-vending machines increased from 227 244 in 1975 to 498 800 in 1995. The average price of a pack of 20 cigarettes is US$ 1.9, which does not appear to be expensive enough to prevent young people from smoking. Although the Ministry of Finance has issued guidelines on the basic principles of tobacco advertising and the Japan Tobacco Association has imposed voluntary rules on itself on that basis, the situation of advertisement control is still far from ideal.

The Ministry of Health and Welfare of Japan recently decided to place more emphasis on primary prevention of chronic diseases such as cancer and cardiovascular diseases by improvements in lifestyle. Needless to say, cigarette smoking is the most important lifestyle target for primary prevention (Doll & Peto, 1978). As the first step of the Government's commitment, national goals for tobacco control should be set, and achievement of tobacco control should be monitored nationally.

Figure 8. Linear correlation between cumulative cigarette consumption at ages 20–70 and death rate from lung cancer at age 70–74

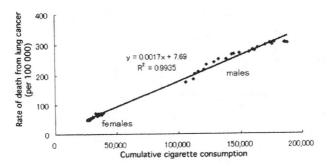

Discussion

Among the so-called developed countries, Japan is one of the few in which the prevalence of smoking among men exceeds one half of the adult population. The lower prevalence among women is typical of east Asian countries, but it can be predicted to increase in the future. A continuing increase in the burden of tobacco use on the health of the Japanese can be predicted from the cumulative cigarette consumption, which we propose as a new measure of tobacco use on a national level. Other reports presented at this meeting indicate that the situation in other Asian countries is strikingly similar, with high smoking prevalences among males and lower but increasing prevalences among females. In many Asian countires, effective national countermeasures against tobacco use are yet to be introduced. International collaboration, especially among Asian–Pacific countries, would seem to be a promising approach, and the role of international organizations such as the World Health Organization should be important.

References

Doll, R. & Peto, R. (1978) Cigarette smoking and bronchial carcinoma: Dose and time relationships among regular smokers and lifelong non-smokers. *J. Epidemiol. Community Health*, **32**, 303–313

Hirayama, T. (1984) Cancer mortality in nonsmoking women with smoking husbands based on a large-scale cohort study in Japan. *Prev. Med.*, **13**, 680–690

Yamaguchi, N., Tamura, Y., Sobue, T., Akiba, S., Ohtaki, M., Baba, Y., Mizuno, S. & Watanabe, S. (1991) Evaluation of cancer prevention strategies by computerized simulation model: An approach to lung cancer. *Cancer Causes Control*, **2**, 147–155

Yamaguchi, N., Mizuno, S., Akiba, S., Sobue, T. & Watanabe, S. (1992) A 50-year projection of lung cancer deaths among Japanese males and potential impact evaluation of anti-smoking measures and screening using a computerized simulation model. *Jpn J. Cancer Res.*, **83**, 251–257

The tobacco epidemic in Viet Nam

C.N.H. Jenkins, P.X. Da, D.H. Ngoc, T.T. Hoang, H.V. Kinh, S. Bales, S. Stewart & S.J. McPhee

University of California at San Francisco, San Francisco, California, United States

No reliable data are available on the prevalence of cigarette smoking in Viet Nam. In this study, we present the results of a survey of tobacco use in Viet Nam and the impact of transnational tobacco corporations.

Methods

We conducted face-to-face interviews with 2004 men and women aged 18 or over in the two largest cities of the country, Hanoi and Ho Chi Minh City, and in two neighbouring rural communes, Phu Linh in the north and Phuoc Vinh An in the south, during the autumn of 1995.

Results

More than one-third of the respondents (36%) reported that they were current smokers, but the prevalence of smoking was much higher among men (73%) than among women (4.3%). Smoking was related to age for both men ($p < 0.001$) and women ($p = 0.002$), although the patterns of this relationship differed by sex (Figure 1).

Except where indicated, the results presented below are for males, who accounted for 95% of the current smokers. Most of them smoked manufactured cigarettes (65%); another 8.9% smoked loose tobacco rolled into cigarettes, 15% smoked loose tobacco in a water pipe, and 11% reported smoking both manufactured cigarettes and water pipes. Those who smoked cigarettes (manufactured or rolled, $n = 526$) smoked a mean of 9.6 cigarettes per day (SE, 0.4). Current smokers of all forms of tobacco reported

Figure 1. Proportions of males (n = 970) and females (n = 1031) in Viet Nam who smoke any kind of tobacco, by age group

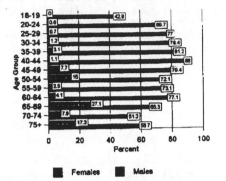

having smoked for a mean of 15.5 years (SE, 0.7). The median age of beginning to smoke was 19.5 years.

Over one third of the respondents (38%) could recall seeing or reading any cigarette advertising. Among these, men (41%) were more likely to recall advertising than women (23%); current smokers (40%) recalled more than non-smokers (26%); and those living in cities (65%) recalled more than those living in rural areas (22%). The rates of recall of cigarette advertising declined with age (p = 0.005) but rose with income (p < 0.001) and years of education (p < 0.001).

The cigarette brands most commonly smoked were domestic . Foreign brands (Jet, 555, Dunhill, Marlboro and others) accounted for only 16% of brands currently smoked. More than twice as many people (38%), however, said that they preferred smoking a foreign brand when they could afford it. Among those who recalled cigarette advertising, foreign brands were recalled by a wide majority (71%) as the most commonly advertised.

On average, cigarette smokers spent about 1.5 times as much on cigarettes as on education and five times as much as on health care; cigarette expenditure represented about one third that for food (Figure 2). As might be expected, the amount spent on cigarettes rose significantly with income (p < 0.001) and with the number of cigarettes smoked per day (p < 0.001). The mean expenditure on cigarettes could have bought 136 kg of rice at 1995 prices (US$ 0.36/kg), nearly enough to feed one person for one year.

In multiple logistic regression analyses (Table 1), we found that the males who were more likely to smoke were in the three 10-year age cohorts from 25 to 54 and had

Figure 2. Mean annual expenditure of current cigarette smokers in Viet Nam

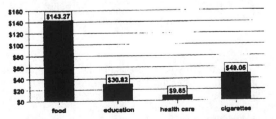

The numbers of cigarette smokers on which the estimate of annual food expenditure was based was 398 (SE, 7.03); for education, n = 222 (SE, 2.21); for health care, n = 227 (SE, 1.08); for cigarettes, n = 486 (SE, 2.75). Expenditure for food, education and health care was adjusted for respondents' household size to represent annual per capita expenditures. Vietnamese dong have been converted to US dollars at the rate of 11 000 dong per US dollar.

Table 1. Multiple logistic regression analysis of predictors of current smoking (all forms of tobacco), smoking foreign-brand cigarettes and preferring foreign-brand cigarettes, Viet Nam, males only

Predictor	Current smoker (n = 970)		Smokes foreign brand (n = 533)		Prefers foreign brand (n = 533)	
	OR	95% CI	OR	95% CI	OR	95% CI
Age (years)						
18–24	1.6	0.6, 4.5	7.0	1.0, 50.4	14.9	4.1, 53.9
25–34	3.8	1.5, 9.3	5.0	0.8, 30.0	14.2	4.0, 50.1
35–44	4.9	2.0, 12.0	1.7	0.3, 10.5	7.5	2.1, 26.2
45–54	3.1	1.3, 7.6	4.2	0.5, 32.6	6.3	1.8, 21.7
55–64	2.4	1.0, 5.7	0.8	0.1, 5.4	2.1	0.5, 9.9
≥ 65	Referent		Referent		Referent	
Occupation						
Not in labour force	0.7	0.3, 1.5	3.9	0.6, 25.8	2.3	0.8, 6.5
Blue collar	0.8	0.4, 1.6	10.0	2.5, 40.5	1.8	0.8, 4.0
Business/service	0.9	0.3, 2.3	23.2	3.3, 164.1	2.2	0.7, 7.5
White collar	0.4	0.2, 0.9	3.9	0.5, 29.7	1.2	0.4, 3.1
Peasant	Referent	Referent	Referent			
Urban/rural,						
Urban	1.1	0.6, 1.8	8.8	3.6, 21.9	3.1	1.5, 6.6
Rural	Referent		Referent		Referent	
Region						
South	0.7	0.4, 1.3	256.8	40.4, 1633.1	6.3	2.9, 13.5
North	Referent		Referent		Referent	
Education (years)						
0–5	3.4	1.2, 9.4	0.1	0.0, 1.2	0.1	0.0, 0.3
6–8	2.3	1.0, 5.3	0.3	0.0, 2.3	0.2	0.1, 0.7
9–11	2.5	1.1, 5.9	0.3	0.1, 2.3	0.3	0.1, 1.1
12–15	2.5	1.1, 5.4	0.4	0.1, 2.1	0.3	0.1, 1.1
≥ 16	Referent		Referent		Referent	
Per capita monthly income (dong)						
Refused to answer	1.2	0.6, 2.5	0.3	0.1, 1.2	1.7	0.7, 4.2
8000–11,000	1.0	0.5, 2.1	0.1	0.0, 0.8	1.1	0.4, 3.0
113 000–179 000	0.6	0.4, 1.2	0.1	0.0, 0.5	0.9	0.4, 2.2
≥ 180 000	Referent		Referent		Referent	
Marital status						
Married	1.2	0.6, 2.2	0.5	0.2, 1.2	0.6	0.3, 1.2
Not married	Referent		Referent		Referent	

OR, odds ratio; CI, confidence interva

The analysis of "current smoker" is based on all males; analyses of 'smokes foreign brand' and 'prefers foreign brand' are based on all male cigarette smokers, manufactured and rolled.

less than a university education. White-collar workers, however, were less likely to smoke. In a second regression analysis, living in the southern survey sites was overwhelmingly associated with smoking foreign-brand cigarettes. Other predictors of smoking foreign brands were working in business or service or blue-collar occupations and living in the urban survey sites. Men with lower incomes, however, were less likely to smoke foreign brands. In the final regression analysis, the strongest predictor of preferring to smoke foreign brands was belonging to the youngest age cohorts. Other predictors included being aged 35–44 or 45–54 and coming from an urban or southern survey site. The less educated men were less likely to prefer foreign brands.

Comment

In comparison with the smoking prevalence rates reported by the World Health Organization for 87 countries for which national data are available (Murray & Lopez, 1996), males in Viet Nam have the highest prevalence rate in the world, whereas the rates for Vietnamese females are among the world's lowest. On the basis of the smoking prevalence rates reported here and Vietnamese population data for 1994, there are approximately 15 500 000 smokers in Viet Nam. Reports from developed countries indicate that about one half of all lifetime smokers will die from tobacco-related diseases; half of these deaths will occur in people between the ages of 35 and 69 (Peto *et al.*, 1994). From this evidence, we can project that approximately 7 325 000 Vietnamese (about 10% of the population) will die from tobacco use, about 3 660 000 of these between the ages of 35 and 69. Furthermore, if children start to smoke at the rates their parents smoke, more than 5 000 000 of those aged under 15 in 1995 will die prematurely from smoking-related diseases.

In the data we report, the rate of smoking foreign-brand cigarettes in Viet Nam was relatively low, although future trends may be discerned in the higher rate of smokers who expressed a desire to smoke these brands if they could afford them and the overwhelming recognition commanded by foreign brands on the advertising market. Foreign-brand cigarettes have established their largest market niche in the urban south, perhaps a legacy of taste preferences established during the United States presence there before 1975. It is also noteworthy that it was the younger urban males who were more likely to notice tobacco advertising and want to smoke foreign brands if they could afford them. It is these segments of the population which have been most successfully targeted by the transnational tobacco corporations to date. Although the female smoking rate is now low, especially among younger women, it may rise as these women enter the industrial workforce, and their incomes rise, especially if transnational tobacco corporation advertising targets women more successfully.

Although cigarette advertising has been banned in the print, electronic and outdoor media in Viet Nam, the transnational tobacco corporations promote their products aggressively through point-of-purchase advertising, sponsorship of sports and cultural events and the provision of logo-bearing baseball caps, T-shirts, umbrellas and other merchandise in exchange for empty cigarette packs. Young women distribute free samples in restaurants, hotels, karaoke bars and sports arenas. The manufacturers of Dunhill cigarettes provide US$ 470 000 in aid annually to the development of professional football in Viet Nam (Reuters, 1994). In addition, Dunhill sponsors television broadcasts of Saturday-night football, slipping through an advertising ban by showing only its logo with the slogan 'the best taste in the world', without showing the actual cigarette.

Unless forceful steps are taken to reduce smoking among men and prevent the uptake of smoking by youth and women, Viet Nam will face a tremendous health and economic burden in the near future. Health education and information campaigns should be tailored for rural communities, where most of the population—and most smokers—live. Smoking bans already in place must be more strictly enforced. Advertising bans should be modified to include point-of-purchase advertising, the donation of free samples and sponsorship of sporting and cultural events. To discourage the uptake of smoking, especially by youth, taxes on cigarettes should be raised and sales of cigarettes to minors should be banned. Prominent health warnings should be required on all cigarette packs. Multinational efforts to control the illegal import of foreign cigarettes are needed. Finally, special attention must be focused on the transnational tobacco corporations in order to monitor and control their activities there. Exporting countries, which have made admirable progress in recent years in controlling tobacco at home, should take steps to ensure that they do not permit the export of the tobacco epidemic to countries such as Viet Nam and the rest of the developing world.

References

Murray, C.L.J. & Lopez, A.D., eds (1996) *The Global Burden of Disease: A Comprehensive Assessment of Mortality and Disability from Diseases, Injuries and Risk Factors in 1990 and Projected to 2020,* Cambridge, Massachusetts: Harvard School of Public Health, World Health Organization, World Bank

Peto, R., Lopez, A.D., Boreham, J., Thun, M. & Health, C., Jr (1994) *Mortality from Smoking in Developed Countries 1950–2000: Indirect Estimates from National Vitality Statistics,* Oxford: Oxford University Press

Reuters (1994) Cigarette firm financing soccer in Vietnam. 19 December

Population survey of smoking in Macao, 1997

C. Lam & A. Joao Maia

Macao Medical and Health Department, Macao

Introduction

Macao is a Chinese territory currently administered by the Portuguese Government, with a population of about 420 000, more than 95% of whom are Chinese. Cardiovascular disease is the predominant cause of death, and lung cancer is the predominant cause of death from cancer. Until this survey was conducted, there was no reliable information on tobacco use in Macao. The objectives of the survey were to identify the prevalence of tobacco use, the characteristics of tobacco consumers, relevant opinions on and attitudes to tobacco use and knowledge about the health effects of tobacco use in Macao among the population aged ≥ 15 years.

Method

The target population was that of Macao residents aged ≥ 15; boat dwellers and residents who were not in Macao during the interviewing period but were living in institutions such as prisons, military camps and universities were not included. A stratified proportional random sample of 1500 dwellings was provided by the local census department. One household in each sample was selected by a simple random-number table, and then one person aged ≥ 15 in each sample household was selected as a participant by the Kish and Leslie grid method (1965). The participants were interviewed personally and given a questionnaire based on that recommended by the World Health Organization Regional Office for Europe and the Commission of the European Communities (1989). Efforts were made to reduce non-response, for example by announcements in the mass media, mailing notices to the sample dwellings and at least three visits to non-responders. Randomly selected questionnaires were verified by telephone or household interviews by the senior interviewer. The data were entered in Microsoft Excel 7.0 for Windows 95 and then imported to SPSS 7.0 for Windows 95 for further analysis; 95% confidence intervals (CIs) of proportion were computed by the exact binominal method with Epi Info 6.0 (Centers for Disease Control, World Health Organization, 1996).

Main results

The prevalence of current smokers was 32% (95% CI, 28–36) among males and 4.2% (2.7–6.2) among females aged ≥ 15. Among young people aged 15–24, the prevalences of current smokers were 14% (7.9–22) in men and 3.2% (0.66–9.0) in women. In people aged ≥ 25, there were 36% (31–40) current smokers among men and 4.4% (2.7–6.2) among women. The cumulative prevalence (including smokers and ex-smokers) at age 19 and 24 was lower in young men than in adult men (19 vs 29% and 25 vs 49%, respectively; both $p < 0.05$), while the cumulative prevalence at age 19 and 24 was higher in young women than in adult women (7 vs 3% and 10 vs 6%, respectively, both $p < 0.05$).

Of the current smokers, 96% consumed manufactured cigarettes with filters; no one used smokeless tobacco. The daily cigarette consumption was 15–24 cigarettes for 54% of smokers; the average consumption was 14.5 cigarettes per day.

In men, the smoking rate was conversely related to educational level; among women, those with the highest and lowest educational levels had higher smoking rates than women with secondary education.

The percentage of smokers was higher among the family or friends of the smokers than the non-smokers (45 vs. 25%; $p = 0.004$). Smoking by young people was significantly associated with the smoking status of their best friends but not with that of their family members.

On average, 64% of the participants gave correct answers to the seven questions related to the health effects of tobacco use. Non-smokers gave slightly more correct answers than smokers (66 vs. 54%; $p = 0.000$). There was little difference in knowledge between men and women. Opinions were sought on eight items referring to smoking control legislation. On average, the participants completely agreed with 69% of the items and agreed to some extent with 21%, and 53% of the smokers and 73% of the non-smokers completely agreed (Mann-Whitney rank test, $p = 0.000$).

Discussion

Only one person was selected from each household because members of a household often share attitudes, opinions and behaviour and also because one person's answer will often affect that of another in the same household. The probability of a person in a larger household being selected will be lower than the probability of a person in a smaller household; according to Kish and Leslie (1965), however, this bias can be ignored when the grid is used.

The results of this survey indicate that the prevalence of smoking is lower in Macao than in developing countries—42% in men and 7% in women (World Health Organization, 1996)—and in mainland China—63% in men and 4.2% in women in 1996 (Chinese Academy of Preventive Medicine, 1997). The result is similar to that in Singapore (32% in men and 2.7% in women in 1995 (World Health Organization, 1996).

The fact that the cumulative prevalence at the same age was higher among young women than that adult women and the smoking prevalence among young women and adult women was similar may indicate that there is an increasing prevalence among women. The finding that the prevalence among women with the highest educational level was higher than that of women with an intermediate educational level may also imply that the smoking prevalence may increase in this area, accompanying socioeconomic development.

Conclusion

Although the smoking prevalence is lower in Macao than in nearby areas, everyeffort to reduce the smoking prevalence must be continued and even increased, because of the trend towards increasing prevalence among young women. Effective surveillance must be established to monitor the trend in smoking patterns and to evaluate the effectiveness of the control methods.

Acknowledgements
We wish to thank the Macao Medical and Health Department for financial support and the Macao Consumer Council for personnel support. We also wish to thank Professor Tak-sun Ignatius Yu for comments on this paper. Any comment and questions on this paper are welcome: e-mail to: lamc@macau.ctm.net

References
Centers for Disease Control, World Health Organization (1996) Epi Infor 6, version 6.04
Chinese Academy of Preventive Medicine (1996) *Smoking and Health in China—1996 National Prevalence Survey of Smoking Pattern*, Beijing: China Science and Technology Press
Kish & Leslie (1965) *Survey Sampling*, New York: John Wiley & Sons
World Health Organization (1996) The Tobacco Epidemic: A Global Public Health Emergency, Geneva
World Health Organization Regional Office for Europe and Commission of the European Communities (1989) *Evaluation and Monitoring of Public Action on Tobacco*, Geneva

Tobacco smoking in Malaysia

H. Habil

*Department of Psychological Medicine, Faculty of Medicine,
University of Malaya Lembai and Pantai, Kuala Lumpur, Malaysia*

Like other developing countries, Malaysia is currently experiencing disorders related to cigarette smoking. The prevalence of smoking in the adult population has been about 60% since the 1980s, and a national morbidity study in 1987 showed that such cigarette smoking-related diseases as myocardial infarct, lung cancer and other respiratory diseases are the tenth most common cause of death in the country.

In response to the impact of cigarette smoking on health, the Ministry of Health has implemented a number of plans to reduce the number of smokers. These include public education to raise awareness about the hazards of smoking, the banning of cigarette advertisements on radio and television and the 1990 *Tobacco Act* which prohibits smoking in designated areas such as hospitals and airports. The main result of these programmes has been to increase public understanding of the effects on health, but not to reduce cigarette smoking: Knowledge about the harmful effects of smoking have not been enough to stop people from reaching for their cigarettes. We therefore looked at the possible reasons why there is still resistance to the smoking cessation programme in Malaysia.

It is now clear that nicotine is a drug that can induce addiction, which is why some smokers find it hard to give up their habit. Nevertheless, according to the interaction model of addiction, the drug should be complemented by individual factors, such as sex, age and health, and environmental factors, such as culture, time of day and place of smoking, in order to explain its continued use. Evidence has shown that culture might be the ultimate determining factor that determines the choice of drug in a community.

Malays in lower income groups are those most at risk from smoking. A major reason for their increased risk is that, unlike alcohol, cigarette smoking has a special cultural connotation. Thus, tobacco is used to give thanks for the birth of a child, is offered during any feast or celebration and is offered to the bride during wedding ceremonies.

Another reason why tobacco has managed to penetrate Malay culture is that it is considered not to be intoxicating; it is popular wisdom that only substances that induce intoxication need to be avoided. This belief has even influenced some policy-makers, who define drugs only on the basis of their intoxicating potential. The medical profession therefore finds itself giving a confrontational view when it tries to convince the public about the similarity between the effects and addictive properties of nicotine and those of other drugs of abuse. The time has therefore come to review the definition of 'drug of abuse', so as to be able to take more effective measures. World bodies such as WHO should take a lead in this redefinition, so that universal regulations can be enacted to minimize the use of nicotine throughout the world and especially in the vulnerable developing countries.

Although direct advertising of cigarettes on radio and television has been banned, the Government cannot stop cigarette companies from promoting their products through indirect advertising. Some of the techniques used are to associate cultural events and traditional games such as *sepak takraw* with cigarettes, perhaps in order to reinforce cigarette use as 'culturally OK'. Once they have fulfilled this objective, they will count on the public to defend them against organizations that wish to stop cigarette use in communities.

Our understanding of the cultural issues that place Malays at risk from cigarette smoking has led us to seek an antidote. Since religion can counteract certain cultural beliefs and even modify cultural behaviour, and since virtually all Malays are Muslims, we sought a solution in the religion of Islam. Although initially we experienced some difficulty in persuading religious leaders to help redefine smoking as prohibited behaviour, like alcohol drinking, they have finally enacted a *fatwa* that prohibits Muslims from smoking cigarettes.

There has also been an attempt to associate cigarette use with use of hard drugs, such as heroin. This initiative was based on the results of a study which showed that many heroin addicts initially smoke cigarettes. Although more research is needed, this argument may help convince the public to recognize the danger of cigarettes, especially to their children. There has recently been much emphasis in Malaysia on family-related issues. As passive smoking harms children's health, an effort has been made to motivate married smokers who bring their children to the clinic for respiratory conditions to stop smoking. Similarly, encouraging non-smokers to advise family members to stop smoking may help them to give up.

Pilot studies on tobacco use in Chennai (Madras), India

C.K. Gajalakshmi[1], V. Shanta[1] and R. Peto[2]

[1]*Cancer Institute, Chennai, India*
[2]*Clinical Trial Service and Epidemiological Studies Unit, Oxford, United Kingdom*

We have carried out two pilot studies to determine the feasibility of a study on tobacco use in Chennai (Madras), India.

A retrospective study was perfomed in late 1995 in Chennai, in which data on dead people were collected from their surviving spouses. A total of 36 844 deaths occurred in Chennai in 1994, with 2226 in the randomly selected study area. People who were under 25 years of age at the time of their death, had never married, did not have a surviving spouse at the time of the interview or had died from unnatural causes were not included in the study; 1154 fulfilled the study criteria. As about 25% of the deceased could not be traced because of change of address of the surviving spouse, the final analysis comprised 569 deceased spouses (456 men and 113 women) and 569 surviving spouses. All of the women were non-smokers. If we assume that the surviving spouses were representative of the general population of Chennai, 42% of the male population smoke, 7% chew tobacco and 12% snuff tobacco; and 8% of the female population chew tobacco and 4% snuff. A significantly higher risk (odds ratio adjusted for age, 1.8; 95% confidence interval, 1.2–2.6) of death from all causes was seen for smokers relative to non-smokers, and the risk appeared to be higher for those who smoked *bidis* than for those who smoked cigarettes. The proportion of deaths attributable to tobacco smoking was 45%, and the population attributable risk was 25%, based on both prevalence and relative risk. A similar but larger study is needed to compute the hazards of tobacco use in India.

The second pilot study was a prospective study, with the objectives of establishing a cohort in Chennai, collecting data on their tobacco habits and following them up by record linkage with databases on cancer morbidity and mortality at the population-based cancer registry located at the Cancer Institute. The study was carried out by conducting a house-to-house survey in 1996 in a randomly chosen area of Chennai and interviewing residents who were ≥ 40 years of age. The criteria for residence were listing on the voters' register or possession of a ration card. The data collected were: height, weight, blood pressure, level of education, current and past occupations, vegetarian or non-vegetarian, history of any major disease in the last five years, smoking, chewing, snuffing and drinking alcohol, and data to assess socioeconomic status. A total of 1003 subjects were interviewed (503 men and 500 women); 98% were married. Data were collected on 835 subjects at single visits, and these data were used to analyse sociodemographic characteristics and tobacco use. The mean age at interview was 55 years for men and 53 years for women, and the distribution of age groups was similar to that of the population of Chennai. The men had a higher level of education than the women. Hindus represented 90% of the participants, 6% were Muslims and 3% were Christians. All of the women were non-smokers, but 14% chewed tobacco and/or took snuff. Of the men, 43% were smokers, including 32% current smokers and 11% ex-smokers, and 12% chewed tobacco and/or took snuff; 45% did not use tobacco in any form. The percentages of non-smokers and cigarette smokers increased with the level of education, but a reverse pattern was seen for *bidi* smokers, and the prevalence of tobacco chewing decreased with educational level. A similar picture was seen among women. A higher percentage of non-smokers was found among Hindus, but with a higher percentage of tobacco chewers. Higher percentages of *bidi* and *bidi* plus cigarette smokers were seen among Muslims, and a higher percentage of cigarette smokers among Christians.

Tobacco use in India

R. Thanhawla & R. Thanseia

Indian Society on Tobacco and Health, Mizoram Chapter, Mizoram, India

The Indian scenario

India is the third largest tobacco-producing country in the world: China produces 30%, the United States 9% and India 7.9% of the world's tobacco. Out of a total of 6 million million kg of tobacco produced globally, 450–500 million kg are grown in India. In our country, 30% is used in manufacturing *bidis* or *biris*, 20% for chewing, 15% for cigarettes and 6% for export. We produce 900 million million *bidis* and about 120 million million cigarettes per day.

In the West, cigarettes contain 19–21 mg nicotine and 27 mg tar. *Bidis* have a 3–3.4 mg nicotine and 27–46 mg tar content, but the smoke provides more nicotine and tar because it is inhaled deeply and rapidly (four to nine puffs per minute). *Bidis* are cheap and therefore many more are smoked than cigarettes.

It is well known that smoking causes lung cancer, heart disease, chronic bronchitis, emphysema, vascular disease and cancer of the cervix. Women who smoke have frequent abortions, stillbirths, miscarriages, infants with a low birthweight, painful monthly periods, early menopause, wrinkles, fragile hair, bad teeth and bad breath. The health consequences of *bidi* smoking and tobacco chewing have been studied extensively in India and have been associated with cancers of the mouth, pharynx, larynx, oesophagus and lungs. Cancers of the mouth and throat constitute 33% of all cancers in India as compared with 4% in the West. *Bidi* smokers are twice as likely as non-smokers to have heart disease, three times more likely to have a heart attack and seven times more likely to have a second heart attack.

Some children aged 10–12 smoke, because their parents smoke; they are usually school drop-outs. Children in schools and colleges smoke because their friends and parents smoke. About 2–3 million Indian children are addicted to smoking. Many infants and children are passive smokers and have frequent coughs, colds, pneumonia, asthma, tonsillitis, bad breath, earaches, stomach aches and headaches. When they start smoking, they also have higher rates of absenteeism from school and reduced fitness, reaction time, vigilance and concentration; they have delayed physical and mental growth and increased risks for death from lung cancer, heart disease, bronchitis and mouth cancer later in life.

Women smokers are usually found in rural areas and among daily wage earners in the cities. Women in urban areas who smoke usually work for airlines, international organizations or the media. They demand emancipation and equality with men, and their number has increased in recent years. They have fragile hair, wrinkled skin, low fertility rates, two times more abortions, three times more stillbirths, early menopause, sickly, low-weight babies, easily broken bones, bad breath, bad teeth, hoarseness and cancer of the mouth or uterus.

Eating and chewing tobacco in various forms is prevalent in many states of India, especially in the north-east and in Mizoram in particular. The habit is increasing and has spread to well-to-do, educated families.

Tobacco use in Mizoram State and control activities

In the villages of Mizoram, villagers used to cut down the jungle, burn the trees and use the land to cultivate rice. To drive away the mosquitoes, parents and children alike smoked tobacco (*Nicotina percica*) rolled in maize leaves or waste paper. The practice of smoking then became part of their lifestyle; a young woman's ability to smoke a pipe was considered to be an added attribute of a good bride, or a young girl offered rolled cigarettes to a young man at her house to smoke together as part of the courtship ritual. Furthermore, women in the region retain *tuibur*, the nicotine-infused water from bamboo water pipes, smoked only by women, in their mouths until it loses its savour.

It was against this culural and social background that the Mizoram Chapter of the Indian Society on Tobacco and Health was constituted. Over the five years of its existence, the Society has been promoting the concept of a tobacco-free society and has seen substantial success. In a survey carried out with the largest women's organization in Mizoram, the Society found that 50% of the population was still smoking. The members of Society make frequent visits to Government departments and to religious and social organizations, where discussions and lectures are arranged. During such events, pamphlets on the evils of tobacco are distributed. Members of the Society are also in close contact with church leaders to convince them of the hazards of smoking and to ask them to propogate the knowledge among their members. Joint meetings are held with members of the largest social organization of young people in the State, and appeals were sent to branches of the organization throughout the State asking them to propogate information about the harmful effects of smoking, through individual contacts, on hoardings and in other publicity materials.

Other members of the Society are meeting with doctors in various hospitals, urging them to set a personal example of not smoking and to spread the idea to their patients. Each year, the Society conducts public meetings on 'World No-Tobacco Day', which are attended by ministers, senior officials and common people. To implement the motto 'Catch them young', the Society arranges various activities to inculcate the idea of not smoking among schoolchildren. Visits have been made to 400 educational institutions, and essay-writing competitions, plays and similar activities are organized by the student community in the campaign against use of tobacco.

One sign of the effectiveness of these measures and activities is that many people have begun to seek permission to smoke in the presence of others. Such considerate behaviour was unthinkable until recently.

High prevalences of obesity, hypertension and smoking in an Egyptian population

F. Hassan[1], H. Gelband[2] and R. Peto[3]

[1] *Community Medicine Department, Faculty of Medicine, Suez Canal University, Ismailia, Egypt*
[2] *Health Technology Consulting, Takoma Park, Maryland, United States*
[3] *Clinical Trials Service Unit & Epidemiological Studies Unit, Nuffield Department of Clinical Medicine, Radcliffe Infirmary, Oxford, United Kingdom*

Summary

A high prevalence of risk factors for chronic disease was found in a sample of 1300 urban adult Egyptians; grade II obesity was common—26% of men and 65% of women had a body mass index > 30 kg/m²—as was hypertension—59% of men 63% of women had a systolic blood pressure > 140 mm Hg and 64% of men and 67% of women had a diastolic blood pressure > 90 mm Hg—and 54% of the men and 2% of the women were cigarette smokers.

Introduction

Chronic diseases are of increasing relative importance in Egypt. Of particular concern is the evolving epidemic of smoking-related disease among men and problems such as hypertension, obesity and diabetes in both men and women. We report here on the prevalences of certain risk factors in population-based survey of 1300 adults. Although it was undertaken chiefly for other purposes, this survey provides a useful description of the prevalence of smoking and other risk factors in the population of this area.

Methods

In a cross-sectional survey, body mass index (kg/m²), blood pressure (systolic/diastolic) and the use of tobacco products were recorded in El-Herfieen, a relatively new residential area within the city of Ismailia, situated near the middle of the Suez Canal in Egypt. El-Herfieen was chosen as the study site because it is easily defined geographically and the population includes a range of socioeconomic levels. All adults 30 years and older were eligible for the survey, which consisted of a questionnaire about tobacco use, health problems and treatment for hypertension and diabetes, and measurement of blood pressure, weight and height. The questionnaire was completed by interviewers who met with each participant. Blood pressure was measured twice, once at the beginning of the interview and again at the end, while the participant was seated (Perloff *et al.*, 1993). Weight was measured with a portable balance and height with an inflexible scale. All instruments were checked and calibrated before the interviewers entered the field each day.

The study population consisted of all 500 households in the area, which were visited on up to three occasions, until it was established that either no people aged ≥ 30 lived there or at least one such person was present. All persons aged ≥ 30 who were then present were included. No refusals were encountered and, with help from conversations with neighbours, none of the selected households was missed. Men, however, were more likely to be out at work or absent for other reasons than were women. There were 1300 participants in the survey, comprising 588 men and 712 women. Smoking status was ascertained for all individuals and height, weight and blood pressure were measured in all except 13 individuals.

The average of the two blood pressure measurements is reported in this paper, classified according to both systolic and diastolic hypertension. For systolic blood pressure (in mm Hg), mild, moderate and severe hypertension are defined as 140–159, 160–179 and ≥ 180, respectively. For diastolic blood pressure, the corresponding figures are 90–99, 100–109 and ≥ 110. Body mass index, calculated as weight (kg) divided by the square of height (m), gives a useful measure of adiposity (World Health Organization, 1990). A body mass index < 19 is considered underweight, and grades I, II and III obesity correspond to body mass indexes of 25–30, > 30–39, and ≥ 40, respectively. The Epi-Info 5 program was used for data management.

Results

The age range of the survey population was 30–89 years (Table 1). Age was sometimes not known exactly; the means were 50.6 years (SD, 13.2) for the 582 men and 48.5 years (SD, 11.6) for the 671 women for whom it was known. Most of the women (87%) reported their occupation as housewife, but 7% had clerical jobs, 3% were professionals and fewer than 2% were administrative, industrial or sales employees. Of the men, 32% reported industrial jobs, 23% were on pensions, 15% were professionals, 13% had clerical jobs, 7% had administrative jobs, 5% reported jobs in sales and 4% were in service industries.

Just over half (54%) of the men were regular smokers, and this prevalence did not vary much among the 10-year age groups in the survey (Table 2). Smoking was rare among women, with less than 2% reporting regular smoking and again no substantial differences among age groups. Among men, 13% were former smokers, with higher percentages in the older age groups.

The mean height of men was 168 cm (SD, 7.6) and the mean weight was 77.5 kg (SD, 14.8). The corresponding values for women were 156 cm (SD, 7.2) and 80.7 kg (SD = 16.2). Only 29% of the men and 10% of the women were not overweight (body mass index, < 25); 45% of the men were in the grade I category of obesity, but 25% were in grade II and 1% were in grade III. Of the women, 25% were in grade I, 53% in grade II and 12% in grade III (body mass index, > 40 kg/m^2).

Only 40% of the men and 37% of the women had 'normal' systolic blood pressure, and 36% of the men and 33% of the women had 'normal' diastolic blood pressure. The women tended to have more severe grades of both systolic and diastolic hypertension than the men. For systolic blood pressure, the mean of the first measurement was 145.7 mm Hg, the mean of the second measurement was 145.6 mm Hg. For diastolic blood pressure, the corresponding figures were 91.4 and 91.1 mm Hg. Thus, there was no

Table 1. Distribution of the surveyed sample of 1278 persons in El-Herfieen by age and sex

Sex	Age group (years)												Total
	30–		40–		50–		60–		70–		80–89		
	No.	%	No.	%	No.	%	No.	%	No.	%	No.	%	
Male	149	25.4	136	23.1	130	22.1	126	21.4	39	6.6	8	1.4	588
Female	164	23.8	240	34.8	147	21.3	90	13	41	5.9	8	1.2	690
Total	313	24.5	376	29.4	277	21.76	216	16.9	80	6.3	16	1.2	1278

Table 2. Smoking habits of men in El-Herfieen by age group

Age group (years)	Smoking status						Total
	Regular smoker		Ex-smoker		Never smoked regularly		
	No.	%	No.	%	No.	%	
30–	83	55.7	7	4.7	59	39.6	149
40–	67	49.3	21	15.4	48	35.3	136
50–	76	58.5	17	13.1	37	28.4	130
60–	67	53.2	21	16.6	38	30.2	126
70–	20	51.3	8	20.5	11	28.2	39
80–	4	50			4	50	8
Total	317	53.9	74	12.6	197	33.5	588

substantial difference between the two measurements, even though at the end of the interview the participant was more relaxed than at the beginning.

Discussion

More than half of the adult males in El-Herfieen smoke cigarettes, but few women smoke. This pattern reflects the norms of Egyptian society, in which it is acceptable for men but not for women to smoke. The population has a remarkably high rate of obesity: the weights of fewer than one third of the men and only 10% of the women was within the 'normal' range, and 26 and 65% was of at least grade II obesity. By contrast, in a study in Saudi Arabia, Kordy *et al.* (1993) found only 11 and 13% of men and women who had at least grade II obesity. The high prevalence of obesity may be attributable to the generally sedentary lifestyle and lack of exercise among both men and women. Most of the women were housewives who had had repeated pregnancies, which might also have contributed to their overweight. High blood pressure is also common in El-Herfieen. The mean values in the entire population exceed the values of 140/90 that are commonly used to define mild hypertension, and many individual values exceeded 160/100. These high rates of hypertension are due in part to the high rates of obesity.

The high rates of smoking among men and the high rates of obesity and hypertension in the population as a whole suggest that this is a population at substantial risk of premature death from tobacco use. A large, long-term longitudinal study is planned to assess the relevance of smoking, obesity and reproductive history to adult mortality.

References

Kordy, M.N.S., Ibrahim, M.A., Saleh, A., Bahnsy, A., Zaghloul, N. & Gamal, F.M. (1993) Obesity: The epidemiological aspects and the associated risks in Queza district, Jeddah, Saudi Arabia. *Egypt. J. Commun. Med.*, **2**, 39–48

Perloff, D., Grim, C., Flack, J., Frohlich, E.D., Hill, M., McDonald, M. & Morgensern, B. (1993) Human blood pressure determination by spygmomanometery. *Circulation*, **88**, 2460–2470

World Health Organization (1990) Diet, nutrition and the prevention of chronic disease. *Bull. World Health Organ.*, **797**, 25–26

Tobacco consumption and prevalence of smoking in Cuba

M. Bonet Gorbea, G. Roche, N. Suarez Lugo & P. Varona Perez

National Institute of Hygiene, Epidemiology and Microbiology, Carlos J. Finlay National School in Public Health and Ministry of Public Health, Havana, Cuba

Methods

Data on the prevalence of smoking in Cuba in 1978–95 were obtained from three sources: for 1978, from the Ministry of Internal Commerce; for 1980–90, from the Cuban Institute for Research and Orientation of Internal Demand; and for 1995, from the National Institute of Hygiene, Epidemiology and Microbiology, the Ministry of Health and the National Statistics Office. National surveys were conducted by three institutions, using representative sampling techniques in which current smokers were defined as daily smokers at the time of the survey. For reliable comparisons of prevalence over time, the same sampling frame was used in all of the surveys.

Data on the consumption of tobacco in 1975–95 were obtained from the Cuban Institute for Research and Orientation of Internal Demand, the Ministry of Agriculture and the Ministry of Internal Commerce.

Results

The trends in cigarette consumption by persons aged ≥ 15 are shown in Table 1. A steady decrease in consumption can be seen, with a reduction of 0.1% between 1975

Table 1. Trends in
cigarette smoking by
persons aged ≥ 15, Cuba,
1975–95

Year	No. of cigarettes/person
1975	2669
1980	2237
1985	2164
1990	1934
1995	1395

and 1980, 0.3% between 1980 and 1985, 1% between 1985 and 1990 and 1.5% between 1990 and 1995, for a decrease of 4.7% over the entire period. The trends in tobacco consumption show a different picture (Table 2), but still with an overall decrease of 7.1%. The prevalence of smoking in Cuba decreased annually by 0.5% between 1984 and 1995 (Table 3); the decrease was observed mainly among men, with an increase among women. Analysis of smoking prevalence in 1995 showed that 48% of males and 37% of females aged ≥ 15 were smokers, 40 and 53% had never smoked, and 12 and 10% were ex-smokers. Little difference was seen by level of education, but economic status affected the rate of smoking, with prevalences of 42% for workers, 43% for unemployed, 37% for pensioners, 26% for housewives, 13% among students and 38% for other categories. The proportions by race were 46% among blacks, 39% among people of mixed race and 35% among whites.

The age at which people started smoking was stable between 1984 and 1990, with 77% starting to smoke before the age of 19, but in 1995 75% started to smoke before that age (Table 4). In 1995, 48% of men and 54% of women considered that they should stop smoking (3.3 and 3.2% considering that it would be easy to do so), 10 and 9.8% were undecided, and 38 and 33% did not wish to stop. The population was aware of the hazard associated with smoking (98% in 1990) but was unaware of the magnitude of the risk.

Table 2. Trends in
tobacco consumption
by persons aged ≥ 15,
Cuba, 1975–95

Year	Tobacco (g)/person
1975	43.7
1980	22.2
1985	35.5
1990	29.2
1995	12.4

Table 3. Prevalence of
smoking among persons
aged ≥ 15, Cuba, 1984–95

Year	% smokers
1984	42
1988	40
1989	38
1990	36
1995	37

Table 4. Prevalence of initiation of smoking at < 19 years of age, Cuba, 1990 and 1995

Year	< 10 (%)			10–14 (%)			15–19 (%)			Total (%)		
	Boys	Girls	Total	Boys	Girls	Total	Boys	Girls	Total	Boys	Girls	Total
1990	11.0	10.4	10.8	24.3	23.5	24.0	44.5	37.2	41.9	79.8	71.2	76.7
1995	5.4	5.1	5.1	30.8	29.1	29.1	44.6	41.2	41.2	80.8	75.4	75.4

Characteristics of tobacco prevalence in Venezuela: Use of a new parameter

M. Adrianza, T. Villamizar, B. López & N. Herrera

Fundacion Antitabaquica de Venezuela, Instituto Diagnostico, Caracas, Venezuela

Introduction

Since 1984, we have periodically evaluated the characteristics of smoking in Venezuela using amplified models from the questionnaires for youth and adults presented by Daniel Horn at a special epidemiological workshop organized by the UICC in São Paulo, Brazil, in 1983. These surveys were initiated before the anti-tobacco activities of the public health programme within the Integrated Programme against Risk Factors of the Division of Chronic Non-transmissible Diseases of the Ministry of Health and Social Assistance.

The objectives of these investigations are to elucidate the relationship between socioeconomic and cultural characteristics and smoking, to establish categories of smoking and the types and quantities of tobacco use, to define the smoking population and its attitudes and beliefs, and to observe the epidemiological evolution of the social process and the impact of the activities of the programme.

Methods

We adapted the sampling technique mentioned above to our country. All of the studies were conducted in population centres of 5000 inhabitants or more. A probabilistic sampling design in multiple stages was used so that the total number of interviews would correspond to the size of the population studied, with an estimation error of 2.5% and a reliability of 95%. We studied children aged 12, 13 and 14 and persons aged $\geq$ 15 in each geographical area, the field work being carried out over an average of 12 days in the three months after 31 May in 1984, 1988 and 1996. We also conducted five investigations in metropolitan Caracas, which contains about 25% of the population of the country, in 1989, 1991, 1993, 1994 and 1996, using the same methods.

Results

We present here the analyses of the answers to the first three questions of the questionnaire: 'Have you ever smoked, even once?', 'Do you currently smoke daily?' and 'Do you currently smoke occasionally?'. The last two categories constitute the prevalence and represent people who have been smoking for six months or more. The answer to the first question represents the first contact with a cigarette.

The percentage of children who had any contact with cigarettes doubled between 1984 and 1996 (Table 1), whereas the number of adults responding positively to the first question decreased by almost 8% over that period (Table 2), the reduction being more pronounced among men than among women. In 1984, 9.6% of the first contacts occurred at the age of 12, 13 or 14, whereas in 1996 the percentage was 25%. Thus, in one quarter of the subjects, the first contact occurred before the age of 15.

Table 1. First smoking contact (%) at age 12–14, Venezuela, 1984–96

Sex	Year of survey		
	1984	1988	1996
Boys	6.5	12.8	14.7
Girls	6.8	10.8	13.7
Total	6.7	11.8	14.2

Table 2. First smoking contact at age
≥ 15, Venezuela, 1984–96

Sex	Year of survey		
	1984	1988	1996
Male	67.6	63.5	59.1
Female	48.7	40.9	41.5
Total	58.1	52.1	50.4

The prevalence of smoking among the young rose by 2.5-fold, with a faster rise in boys than in girls (Table 3). The prevalence in adults has decreased by 9.2%, with a 10% decrease in women and 8% in men (Table 4). There is a considerable increase in prevalence after the age of 15, from 7 to 31%, which is probably due to the greater independence of individuals after that age, especially among boys.

Conclusions

Reliable periodic opinion surveys, in which young and older people are separated, is an ideal instrument for monitoring the characteristics of smoking and its prevalence and, therefore, also for evaluating the impact of the advertising strategies of the tobacco industry and the success of national programmes to combat them.

The young population has progressively increased its first contact with cigarettes, the prevalence having doubled in the last 12 years, as has the smoking prevalence. In the adult population, however, first contacts with smoking have decreased, as has the smoking prevalence, especially among women.

The use of periodic prevalence surveys in the same population, based on reliable techniques, is fundamental for elucidating the tendencies towards nicotine addiction and the effect of control measures. Investigating the causes of changes in behaviour helps in evaluating the impact of advertising and the effectiveness of control. More and better specific control programmes are needed for homes and schools in order to reduce opportunities for first contacts with cigarettes, thereby avoiding an increased prevalence among children under 15 years of age. Special programmes should be designed for institutes of higher education, companies and informal work areas to decrease the prevalence of smoking.

Table 3. Smoking prevalence among
children aged 12–14, Venezuela, 1984–96

Sex	Year of survey		
	1984	1988	1996
Boys	1.9	3.2	6.4
Girls	3.4	3.4	7.5
Total	2.7	3.3	7.0

Table 4. Smoking prevalence among
persons aged ≥ 15, Venezuela, 1984–96

Sex	Year of survey		
	1984	1988	1996
Male	45.4	42.9	37.4
Female	34.1	25.2	23.8
Total	39.8	33.9	30.6

The greatest effort should be made to design a legal instrument for the control of production, sales and promotion of tobacco. The last is of particular importance, since it is advertising that is responsible for the increase in the number of first contacts of young people with cigarettes.

Expected trends in the prevalence of cigarette smoking in the United States

D. Méndez, K.E. Warner & P.N. Courant

School of Public Health, University of Michigan
Ann Arbor, Michigan, United States

The prevalence of smoking among adults in the United States fell steadily and substantially for a quarter of a century after publication of the first Surgeon General's report on smoking and health in 1964 (Department of Health and Human Services, 1964). Recent data suggest that the decline may have stalled, however. Government surveys through 1994 show that the prevalence among adults remained at about 25% (Department of Health and Human Services, 1994). Thirty-day data on smoking prevalence among high-school and junior high-school students, the harbinger of future smoking patterns, show annual increases since the beginning of the decade (Kluger, 1996).

Although the decline in smoking prevalence may slow down, the demographics of smoking imply that it will inexorably continue to decline over the next several decades, even in the absence of any intensified efforts at tobacco control. Indeed, assuming that nothing changes in terms of contemporary patterns of smoking initiation and quitting, the prevalence among adults will automatically fall to about 16% by the end of the first quarter of the next century. This will be the inevitable result of the ageing of the population and anticipated birth and mortality patterns, combined with cohort-specific rates of peak smoking prevalence, contemporary prevalence and quitting rates.

Methods

We have developed a dynamic forecasting model to predict the prevalence of smoking among adults. The principal characteristics of the model are as follows: the number of people of age a in year t is computed by multiplying the number of people of age $a-1$ in year $t-1$ by the appropriate survival rate; birth cohort sizes are supplied exogenously to the model; death rates are differentiated by year, age and smoking status; current smokers in any given year are estimated as the number of current smokers in the previous year who survived to the current year and did not quit smoking; the smoking prevalence of 18-year-olds, supplied exogenously to the model for each cohort, is used to calculate the size of each year's cohort of new adult smokers; the prevalence for a specific age group in a specific year is computed by taking the ratio of current smokers to the total number of people within the group in that year.

The model assumes that smoking is not initiated after the age of 18, when the prevalence attains its peak value for the cohort. After that age, smoking cessation drives the dynamics of the model. Smoking cessation rates are estimated from historical data on smoking prevalence by the generalized least-squares method (Judge *et al.*, 1985). The R^2 for the model was 0.98. The observed prevalence rates and those predicted from the model are shown in Figure 1.

Figure 1. Observed versus predicted prevalence of smoking

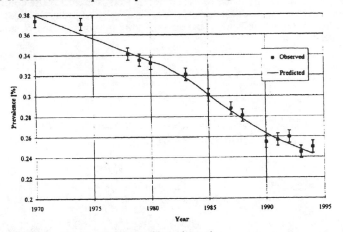

Observed values are shown with 95% confidence intervals.

Model

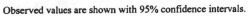

$$P_{a,t} = P_{a-1,t-1} \times (1 - \delta_{a-1,t-1}) \qquad a = 1,...,110 \qquad (1)$$
$$P_{0,t} = \alpha_t \qquad\qquad\qquad\qquad\qquad\qquad\qquad (2)$$
$$C_{a,t} = C_{a-1,t-1} \times (1 - \mu_{a-1,t-1}) \times (1 - \beta_{a-1,t-1}) \qquad a = 19,...,110 \qquad (3)$$
$$C_{18,t} = \gamma_t \times P_{18,t} \qquad\qquad\qquad\qquad\qquad\qquad (4)$$

$$R_{(a_i:a_f),t} = \frac{\sum\limits_{a=a_i}^{a_f} C_{a,t}}{\sum\limits_{a=a_i}^{a_f} P_{a,t}} \qquad (5)$$

$$\mu_{a,t} =$$

		18–30	31–50	> 50
Year (t)	1970–80	v_1	v_2	v_3
	1981–	v_4	v_5	v_6

where:
$P_{a,t}$ = size of cohort aged a in year t
$C_{a,t}$ = current smokers aged a in year t
$R_{(a_i:a_f),t}$ = prevalence of smoking between ages a_i and a_f in year t
$\delta_{a,t}$ = death rate in year t for individuals aged a in the general population
$\beta_{a,t}$ = death rate in year t for smokers aged a
$\mu_{a,t}$ = smoking cessation rate in year t for smokers aged a
γ_t = prevalence of smoking among 18-year olds in year t
α_t = size of the birth cohort in year t

Results

The estimated values and confidence intervals for the six cessation rates specified in the model are shown in Table 1. The smoking cessation rate rises sharply with age and increased between the 1970s and the 1980s. The coefficients for the rates corresponding to the two older age groups are significantly different from zero after 1980; for the period 1970–80, only the coefficient for the older age group was statistically significant. Particularly in the earlier period, the estimates of the cessation rate are confounded by initiation rates. This confounding has the effect of biasing the estimates downwards and might partially account for the lack of significance of some of the coefficients.

Using the estimated cessation rates for the period after 1980, we forecast the smoking prevalence in the United States to the year 2100. The size of all future birth cohorts was held constant at the size of the average birth cohort for the period 1981–90: 3 643 582. In order to forecast future prevalence, we examined the behaviour of the model when it was assumed that the smoking prevalence among 18-year-olds remains constant at 20, 25, 30 or 35% Figure 2). At 27%, the current prevalence among 18-year-olds lies between the two middle figures. The other two prevalences were selected as extreme cases for sensitivity analyses. In particular, 35% represents a worst-case scenario. Use of 20% prevalence among the young indicates the potential impact on the eventual smoking prevalence among adults of modestly successful policies directed towards reducing smoking among young people.

This analysis shows that if cessation rates do not decrease from those during the 1980s, the overall prevalence of smoking among adults in the United States will continue to fall, even with an unlikely extreme value of 35% for the smoking prevalence of 18-year-olds. The results show that if current quitting conditions persist, with a prevalence of 25% at age 18, the adult smoking prevalence will decline from its current level of 25% to a steady-state value of 15–16% after the first quarter of the next century. Prevalence rates of 20, 30 and 35% would produce steady-state adult smoking prevalence rates of 12, 18 and 22%, respectively.

Discussion

The nearly steady prevalence of smoking among adults observed in the United States during the 1990s has led many to believe that, short of dramatic new smoking control policies, the prevalence will no longer decline. We examined the necessary rise in initiation rate (peak prevalence at 18) to keep smoking prevalence constant at the current level of 25% on the basis of cessation rates estimated for the post-1980 period and for the lower limit of their 95% confidence intervals, which corresponds to a very unlikely worst-case scenario. The 18-year-old prevalence rate necessary to maintain the current adult smoking prevalence (25%) is 41% for the first set of cessation rates and 35% for the second. The current rates of smoking initiation are about 27%, which implies that, unless initiation rates rise well above 35%, the overall adult smoking prevalence will continue to decline.

Even though initiation rates may be rising at present and may continue to rise in the near future, we are still likely to observe a decline in overall adult smoking prevalence

Table 1. Estimated annual smoking cessation rates

Period	Age group	Estimate	95% confidence interval	
			Lower bound	Higher bound
1970–80	18–30	−0.00953	−0.02221	0.00315
	31–50	0.00718	−0.00125	0.01560
	≥ 51	0.04528	0.03531	0.05525
1981–	18–30	0.00209	−0.00689	0.01107
	31–50	0.02147	0.01588	0.02706
	≥ 51	0.05958	0.05441	0.06475

Figure 2. Forecast overall smoking prevalence by peak prevalence at the age of 18

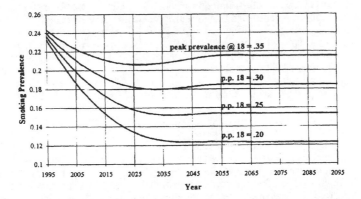

because older smokers who joined the pool at extremely high prevalence rates continue to boost the aggregate rate of smoking. These smokers are rapidly disappearing from the pool, due to death and smoking cessation, and their disappearance will continue to reduce the overall prevalence. Although we anticipate that the adult smoking prevalence will continue to decline even if the initiation rate rises to 35%, the eventual decline will be modest, to a rate of about 22%. If, in contrast, the initiation rate can be brought down to 20%, the adult prevalence will decline to a steady-state rate of just over 12%. The difference is substantial in terms of the burden that smoking will place on the health of Americans. Through aggressive education and policy, the toll of tobacco can be brought well below the course it is on at present. We note, however, that even if our most optimistic assumption about smoking initiation is realized, nearly one-eighth of Americans will be smokers in the middle of the next century. The health toll of smoking will remain extraordinarily high. The health of our children and their children depends on continuation of tobacco control.

References
Department of Health and Human Services (1964) *Smoking and Health: Report of the Advisory Committee to the Surgeon General of the Public Health Service,* Washington DC
Department of Health and Human Services (1994) *National Health Interview Survey,* Washington DC, National Center for Health Statistics
Judge, G.G., Griffiths, W.E., Hill, R.C., Lutkepohl, H. & Lee, T.C. (1985) *The Theory and Practice of Econometrics,* New York: John Wiley & Sons
Kluger, R. (1996) *Ashes to Ashes: America's Hundred-year Cigarette War, the Public Health, and the Unabashed Triumph of Philip Morris,* New York: Alfred A. Knopf

Epidemiology of smoking and some determinants of smoking behaviour

V. Levshin, V. Drojachih, T. Fedichkina & N. Slepchenko

Implementation and Evaluation of Cancer Prevention Measures Cancer Research Centre, Moscow, Russian Federation

We present data from several population- and clinic-based surveys in Moscow conducted during 1995–97, covering more than 5000 residents of the city. All of the subjects were interviewed with questionnaires eliciting information on complex social and biological factors and smoking history. The smoking rates among adults in Moscow are 59% for men and 18% for women. The rate for men is one of the highest in the world, and that for women is relatively low.

Since health professionals are looked upon as role models for healthy behaviour, they have a special opportunity to influence the community. A decrease in the rate of smoking among health professionals generally precedes a similar decrease in the general population (Table 1). The smoking rates among physicians are three times lower than those of the general population in countries such as Finland, Luxembourg and the United States, where significant decreases in smoking prevalence have been observed during the past few decades. In Moscow, the smoking rates among physicians and the general population in the same age groups are the same for males, and that of female physicians exceeds that of the population. Unless smoking can be discouraged among health professionals, there is little hope that tobacco use by other sectors of the population can be effectively discouraged.

Table 2 shows the smoking prevalence by subgroups of family status, level of education and body mass index. The proportions of current smokers are highest among widowed men and women who have never married, twice as high among less well-educated men and three times as high among lean men.

A group of 106 current smokers and the same number of people who had never smoked, matched for age, sex, education and residence, were asked about the smoking habits of their father, mother, spouse or friend. The proportions of smokers with a relative or friend who smoked was markedly higher than among non-smokers (Table 3), confirming the impact of a family history of smoking.

Table 4 gives data on the attitudes of 200 current smokers aged 40–59. Most current smokers (75% of men and 95% of women) knew that 'smoking causes some kinds of cancer'; moreover, half of them considered that smoking harmed their health, and most wanted to change their habit. Most had attempted to quit.one or more times. Most of the current male smokers had a nicotine dependence score of five or more points in Fagerström's test; as many as 57% of males under the age of 20 had nicotine dependence, indicating that dependence develops during the first years of smoking. The majority of smokers therefore need more help and treatment of tobacco dependence than knowledge or motivation to give up.

Conclusion

The tobacco smoking situation in Moscow is alarming: 59% of men and 18% of women are current smokers. There are definite relationships between smoking and social, familial and biological factors which should be taken into account in smoking prevention. The great majority of current smokers have contracted nicotine dependence, which is clearly a barrier to successful cessation. The development of more effective anti-smoking measures requires detailed studies of the epidemiology and nature of smoking.

Table 1. Prevalence of smoking among physicians

| Region | Proportion of smokers (%) | | | |
| | Physicians | | Population | |
	Male	Female	Male	Female
Albania	39	9	50	8
China	45	–	61	–
Finland	7	3	27	18
France	40	32	40	27
Greece	41	45	53	27
Lithuania	38	4	52	10
Luxembourg	12		34	
United States	9		29	
Moscow	41	13	42	8

Table 2. Prevalence of smoking in men and women aged 40–59, Moscow

Subgroup	Smoking prevalence (%)					
	Males ($n = 483$)			Females ($n = 465$)		
	Current smoker	Ex-smoker	Never smoked	Current smoker	Ex-smoker	Never smoked
Married	50	22	28	8	6	86
Widowed	71	23	6	11	5	84
Divorced	40	40	20	6	9	85
Never married	–	50	50	17	9	74
Years of schooling						
≤ 7	70	10	20	–	2	98
8–10	55	23	22	12	6	82
11–14	55	27	18	12	12	76
≥ 15	36	29	35	7	8	85
Weight (kg)/height (m)						
≤ 24	63	19	18	8	6	86
25–29	47	22	31	9	6	85
≥ 30	21	41	38	7	7	86

Table 3. Family history of smoking

Family member	Proportion (%) of subjects with family member who smokes					
	Male			Female		
	Smokers ($n = 62$)	Never smoked ($n = 62$)	p	Smokers ($n = 54$)	Never smoked ($n = 54$)	p
Father	72.6	38.5	< 0.001	61.1	46.3	< 0.01
Mother	9.7	0	–	14.8	5.6	–
Spouse or friend	61.3	15.4	< 0.001	75.9	46.3	< 0.05

Table 4. Smokers' attitudes regarding quitting (200 current smokers aged 40–59)

Question	Answer	Proportion (%) of smokers	
		Male	Female
Does smoking cause cancer?	Yes	75	90
	No	19	10
	Don't know	6	–
Do you feel that smoking is harming your health?	Yes	47	58
	No	15	17
	Don't know	38	25
Would you like to change your habit?	Quit	58	62
	Cut down	26	28
	No	16	10
Have you tried to quit?	Yes	78	75
	No	22	25
Would you need help to quit?	Yes	46	55
	No	54	45

Epidemiology of smoking in Slovakia

S. Urban[1] & J. Luha[2]

[1]Clinic of Pneumology and Phthisiology, Comenius University, Bratislava, and
[2]Research Institute of Public Opinion, Bratislava, Slovak Republic

Objectives

Slovakia is a central European country of 5.3 million people formed after the split of Czechoslovakia in 1993. The aims of the study were to review the prevalence of smoking and trends in the last decade and the numbers of cigarettes smoked per day by people in the main socioeconomic groups according to sex and level of education. The success of smoking cessation was evaluated for different age groups, levels of education and socioeconomic status.

Approach and methods

The sample consisted of 1322 respondents from all regions and socioeconomic groups in Slovakia in 1996. Persons who smoked one cigarette per day or seven per week were considered to be smokers. The rates were derived from the Slovak Research Institute of Public Opinion.

Results

The prevalence of smoking among adults in Slovakia in 1996 was 42%, with 55% among men and 30% among women. These rates correspond to increases of more than 12% for men and 2% for women since 1986. The rates in 1996 broken down by age group and sex are shown in Table 1.

The highest prevalences according to socioeconomic status were among unemployed persons (62%) and unskilled manual workers (56%), and the lowest prevalences were those of pensioners (30%) and civil and public employees (38%); businessmen (47%) and members of agricultural companies (48%) had intermediate rates.

Table 1. Prevalence of smoking, Slovakia, 1996, by age and sex

Age group (years)	Sex	Prevalence (%)
15–17	Both	37
	Male	45
	Female	29
18–24	Both	46
	Male	59
	Female	33
25–29	Both	50
	Male	67
	Female	32
30–39	Both	49
	Male	58
	Female	42
40–49	Both	43
	Male	54
	Female	36
50–59	Both	39
	Male	49
	Female	29
≥ 60	Both	29
	Male	48
	Female	11

Persons who had finished higher education were less likely to smoke than those with lower levels of education, the prevalences being 32% for university graduates, 38% for high-school graduates, 44% for primary or elementary school leavers and 47% for technical-school leavers.

Analysis of the number of cigarettes smoked per day showed that 41% of men smoked 11–20 cigarettes per day and about 25% smoked 1–5 or 6–10 per day, while 50% of women smoked 1–5 per day and about 25% smoked 6–10 per day. Ten percent of men and 4% of women smoked 21–30 cigarettes per day, and 1% of men and 2% of women smoked ≥ 31 per day.

The success rates of quitting were higher (35–40%) among people aged 30 and over than among younger people and higher among graduates of universities (52%) and high schools (40%) than among leavers of technical schools (35%) and primary or elementary schools (25%).

Discussion

The proportion of smokers is higher in Slovakia than in other European countries (Joossens et al., 1994), the rates being 42% for men in the European Union and 28% for women, in comparison with 55 and 30% in Slovakia. There are also large differences in prevalence between similar populations, such as that of Finland, with rates of 27 and 19% for men and women, respectively (Helakorpi et al., 1994). The high rate (37%) of regular or occasional smokers among young people aged 15–17 in Slovakia and the increasing numbers of smokers in the population between 1986 and 1996 are particularly alarming.

Whereas cigarette consumption declined in Canada during the last decade (Collishaw, 1996), the manufacture and sales of cigarettes in Slovakia have increased (Kavcová et al., 1994). Public health authorities are well aware that children and adolescents are the tobacco industry's primary source of potential new customers (Kessler, 1995); however, despite new restrictions in Slovakia, the authorities have been unable to prohibit aggressive advertising campaigns of tobacco products.

Our findings with regard to the relationship between level of education and socioeconomic status and reduced smoking are similar to those of an analagous study in Finland (Puska et al., 1997).

Conclusions

The prevalence of smoking has increased in Slovakia over the last decade. The largest numbers of smokers are the unemployed and unskilled manual workers, whereas the rate of smoking has increased among children and adolescents. Smoking cessation is most successful among well-educated men. The increase in smoking rates may be due in part to the extremely aggressive advertising by multinational tobacco companies.

References

Collishaw, N.E. (1996) Comprehensive tobacco policies in Canada. Stud. Pneumol. Phtisel., 56, 101–105
Helakorpi, S., Berg, M.A., Uutela, A. & Puska, P. (1994) Health Behaviour among Finnish Adult Population (Publication B6/1994), Helsinki, National Public Health Institute
Joossens, L., Naett, C., Howie, C. & Muldoon (1994) Tobacco and Health in the European Union: An Overview, Brussels, European Bureau for Action on Smoking Prevention
Kavcová, E. Rozborilová, E., Babál, M. & Zucha, J. (1994) Smoking problems in Slovak Republic. Abstracts of the 8th Congress of Slovak and Czech Pneumologic and Phthisiologic Societies, 7–10 September 1994
Kessler, D.A. (1995) Nicotine addiction in young people. New Engl. J. Med., 333, 186–189
Puska, P., Korhonen, H.J., Uutela, A., Helakorpi, S. & Piha, T. (1997) Anti-smoking policy in Finland. In: Waller, M. & Lipponen, S., eds, Smokefree Europe. A Forum for Networks, Helsinki, Finnish Centre for Health Promotion, pp. 26–42

Smoking behaviour and attitudes of key at-risk groups in Turkey

N. Bilir, A. Naci Yyldyz, B. Güçiz Doğan & F. Kalyoncu

Hacettepe University, Department of Public Health, Ankara, Turkey

Rationale and objectives

Smoking is the most important cause of death from cancer, and 40–45% of cancers in males and 30% of cancers in the whole population are caused by smoking. There is significant correlation between smoking status and the development of cardiovascular disease, cancer and chronic bronchitis. Smoking is very common in Turkey. Although the smoking rates among children, adolescents and women are relatively low, those are the main risk groups that should be protected against smoking. Cigarette smoking not only affects the smoker but other people in the same environment as well. Thus, measures have been taken during the last decade in developed countries to prevent passive exposure to smoke, and achievements were made in this respect in our country in 1996.

The objectives of this study are to determine the smoking prevalence in various segments of the population, to define the background characteristics of smokers related to smoking behaviour, to obtain the opinions of these individuals about smoking in certain situations or environments and to increase awareness in the population about a draft law against smoking, which was currently on the agenda of the Parliament.

Methods

The Province of Ankara, the capital city of Turkey, was chosen as the region for this descriptive study. Groups that were considered to be particularly important with regard to their smoking status were selected, and 2503 subjects from nine segments of the community were interviewed:
- 1064 secondary and high-school students (512 secondary, 552 high-school students) and 254 teachers in the same schools as the students;
- the mothers of 499 students;
- 237 physicians registered with the Ankara Chamber of the Turkish Medical Association chosen by simple random sampling;
- 130 performers from the State opera and ballet;
- 149 sportsmen, included when they applied for license renewal;
- 109 persons working in the Ankara offices of newspapers and television stations;
- 61 parliamentarians.

All 550 parliamentarians were intended to be included in the study, but the contribution from this sector was very low (11%). Data were collected by a pre-tested questionnaire developed for this study. The artists, sportsmen and mothers were interviewed personally, whereas the physicians, parliamentarians, journalists, students and teachers filled in the questionnaires themselves. Data were collected by 20 interviewers trained and supervised by a field coordinator.

SPSS 5.0 statistical software was used for the analyses.

Results

The mean age was about 35 for the mothers, teachers, physicians and artists, 30.9 for journalists, 23.7 for sportsmen and 47.2 for parliamentarians. The years of education completed were 7.6 for the mothers and 11.2 for the sportsmen. The lowest smoking prevalence was found among secondary-school students (3.5%), while the highest was among journalists (64%), then teachers (51%), artists (46%) and physicians (44%). Approximately one third of high-school students were current smokers (Table 1).

The mean age of starting to smoke was 20–30 for teachers, mothers, physicians, artists and parliamentarians. The starting age decreased with the years, from 12.2 for secondary-school students and 14.2 for high-school students. The average duration of smoking was 20.3 years for parliamentarians and 15.5 for artists; that of teachers and mothers was nearly the same (14.1 and 14.9, respectively). Parliamentarians smoked more than a pack and mothers nearly a pack; physicians and journalists smoked more than half a pack of cigarettes per day. The average number of cigarette smoked was 7.3 per day for high-school students, 3.2 for secondary-school students and 9.6 for sportsmen (Table 2).

With regard to attitudes to smoking, 16–39% of the smokers stated that they did not regret smoking. The percentage of subjects who regretted smoking was highest among parliamentarians (57%), secondary-school students (56%), sportsmen (51%) and high-school students (51%) (Table 3). Hospitals and schools are the places in which smoking is not approved of by all groups, regardless of their smoking status. Most of the smokers approved of smoking in restaurants, some public places, offices and public transport under certain conditions.

Table 1. Characteristics of sociodemographic groups and smoking prevalence, Ankara, 1996

Group	No.	Age (mean ± SD)	Education (years)	Smoking prevalence (%)	
				Current	Ever
Secondary-school students	512	13.7 ± 0.8	7.0	3.5	8.2
High-school students	552	16.5 ± 1.0	10.0	28.3	32.5
Teachers	254	35.4 ± 7.1	15.0	50.8	61.8
Mothers of students	499	39.8 ± 6.1	7.6	30.2	36.9
Physicians	237	36.3 ± 9.1	17.0	43.9	62.0
Sportsmen	149	23.7 ± 5.4	11.2	34.9	43.1
Artists	130	37.7 ± 10.5	14.4	46.2	60.8
Journalists	109	30.9 ± 7.6	13.3	63.9	70.4
Parliamentarians	61	47.2 ± 8.5	14.8	27.1	57.6

Table 2. Characteristics of smokers in various groups, Ankara, 1996

Group	Mean age at starting smoking (years)	Average duration of smoking (years)	Average no. of cigarettes smoked per day
Secondary-school students	12.2 ± 1.8	1.3 ± 1.2	3.2 ± 3.3
High-school students	14.2 ± 2.0	2.4 ± 2.0	7.3 ± 7.3
Teachers	20.5 ± 4.9	14.1 ± 7.5	12.3 ± 9.8
Mothers of students	22.8 ± 6.2	14.9 ± 6.9	19.3 ± 8.4
Physicians	21.0 ± 5.0	13.9 ± 7.9	15.1 ± 10.6
Sportsmen	17.9 ± 3.8	5.3 ± 4.4	9.6 ± 7.8
Artists	20.3 ± 5.8	15.5 ± 9.8	13.6 ± 9.1
Journalists	18.9 ± 4.0	11.9 ± 8.0	16.2 ± 9.0
Parliamentarians	21.3 ± 5.4	20.3 ± 8.9	22.9 ± 12.7

Table 3. Distribution of smokers according to regret about smoking, Ankara, 1996

Group	No.	Regret		
		Never	Sometimes	Frequently
Secondary-school students	16	25.0	18.8	56.2
High-school students	143	16.8	32.2	51.0
Teachers	121	18.2	44.6	37.1
Mothers of students	146	23.3	33.6	43.2
Physicians	87	23.0	31.0	46.0
Sportsmen	37	16.2	32.4	51.4
Artists	49	38.7	32.7	28.6
Journalists	69	20.3	33.3	46.4
Parliamentarians	14	21.4	21.4	57.2

The growing tobacco epidemic in Palau

C. Otto & A. Lyman

Ministry of Health
Koro, Palau

In a small paradise in the Pacific, the lives of young people are gradually being destroyed by the slowly permeating use of tobacco. In the island nation of Palau, in the westernmost part of Micronesia with a total population of about 17 000, tobacco use has crept into the lives of young people by attaching itself to the traditional habit of betel-nut chewing. Betel-nut chewing has long been practised by adults in this island paradise, much as it has been throughout south-west Asia, including Viet Nam and the Indian subcontinent, but chewing with tobacco as an additive is a more recent phenomenon, dating only to the introduction of tobacco by westerners, especially since the Second World War. Insidiously, it has reached such epidemic proportions that it was one of the main topics of the Fourth Annual Conference of Women of Palau, which took place in March 1997.

Three studies that have been conducted document the wide use of tobacco in betel-nut chewing among the young. One study of pupils in grades 4–8 in a Catholic school showed that 72% of them chewed betel nut regularly, and 78% of them added tobacco. A study of a similar population indicated that 19.3% of the pupils regularly chewed with tobacco. A study in 1995 found that 55% of 5–14 year-olds and 77% of 15–24 year-olds chewed betel nut regularly. Of these, 87 and 96%, respectively, added tobacco to their betel nut.

Efforts to address this problem have included the creation of a 'Coalition for Tobacco-free Palau', whose members have been instrumental in the passage of a law prohibiting the sale of tobacco products to people under 19 years of age. So ingrained is the habit, however, that when the Coalition members conducted a compliance survey in December 1996, they found that 73% of the local merchants were still selling cigarettes to minors. The Coalition members have conducted a vendor education programme regarding tobacco, written articles for local newspapers, given radio talks, held community outreach meetings, erected billboards and printed slogans on payroll checks, all in an effort to stem the tide of this epidemic. The Coalition's five-year action plan calls for activities that include bans on tobacco product advertisements and of sports sponsorship by tobacco companies and increasing the excise tax on tobacco and earmarking the revenue for activities to control and prevent the use of tobacco in any form in Palau, especially among the young.

Epidemiological transition: Infectious to chronic diseases

R. Tapia-Conyer

Ministry of Health, Mexico City, Mexico

The objective of this communication is to explain and demonstrate the process of epidemiological transition, using Mexico's experience as an example. The concept of 'epidemiological transition' has been in use for at least 25 years; the phrase, coined by Abdel Omran in 1971, refers to a series of changes that all societies undergo with regard to illness and death in the population; epidemiological methods are applied to the study of populations. Epidemiological transition occurs in parallel with a demographic and technological transition. It consist of four main patterns of change: in causes of death (from infectious to chronic diseases), age at death, relationship between morbidity and mortality (communicable to non-communicable diseases) and the social importance of disease. There are three models of transition: classical, accelerated and contemporary; another model called 'extended' has been observed and includes polarization, mosaic and countertransition. Some indicators that give a clear idea of the transition in Mexico during this century are increases in the population size, a decrease in the number of deaths and an increase in the number of deaths due to chronic diseases, with estimated projections that follow the same trend.

Epidemiological transition is the most conspicuous form of health change in societies today. Populations now acquire and die from more chronic diseases. The integrated study of populations allows a general analysis of health and disease and their variation in time.

Changing perceptions that influence tobacco smoking in central Sri Lanka: Preliminary findings from a qualitative investigation

G.L. Mehl[1,2,3], T. Seimon[1], E.K. Rodrigo[2], K.T. Silva[2] & R. Uyanwatte[3]

[1]*Center for International Community-based Health Research, The Johns Hopkins School of Hygiene and Public Health, Baltimore, Maryland, United States;* [2]*The Centre for Intersectoral Community Health Studies, Peradeniya, and* [3]*LIFE Drug Prevention Movement, Kandy, Sri Lanka*

Abstract

We present the initial findings of an ongoing ethnographic study of tobacco smoking among urban youth in central Sri Lanka. We have explored an apparent disparity in smoking rates among males in high- and low-income communities, focusing on research conducted thus far in the low-income area. Multiple ethnographic interviews and systematic collection of qualitative data were used to investigate the influences on smoking among youth in this poor urban community. The preliminary findings suggest that the combined effect of the health transition and the country's stagnant economy is influencing smoking by the young in this community in a paradoxical manner. On the one hand, the informants seemed to be well aware of the negative health effects of smoking; in addition, smoking is not tolerated by families, neighbours, community members or prospective spouses. On the other hand, smoking is encouraged by peers, reinforced by difficult work situations and promoted at community events. In the current economic and social climate, these young males appear to be more strongly influenced by pro-smoking social influences.

Introduction

The study encompasses one low-income and one high-income urban community; this paper focuses on research conducted thus far in the low-income community of approximately 6000 persons. The majority (~ 80%) of this community's residents are Tamil-speaking Hindus of Indian descent, although Sinhalese Buddhists (~ 10%), Moor Muslims (~ 9%) Burghers and Malays also reside in the community. Historically, community residents have worked for the municipality, living in Government-provided 'line houses', which are retained throughout the period of employment. This is the most densely populated urban community in Sri Lanka's central province.

Sri Lanka is considered a model for health-care delivery in the developing world (Jamison & Mosly, 1991). Despite a low gross national product *per capita* (US$ 500; UNICEF, 1997), the health indicators in the country are comparable to those of industrialized countries: life expectancy is 69.7 years for males and 74.2 years for females, and the infant mortality rate is 18/1000 live births (World Health Organization,

1997). This is attributable in part to a uniformly distributed, effective, accessible health-care system that emphasizes primary health care and a sound educational system, evidenced by a literacy rate close to 90% (Bjorklan, 1985; World Bank, 1993). Sri Lanka is one of the first developing countries to experience changes associated with the 'health transition' (the shift from a 'young' population experiencing acute infectious diseases to an 'ageing' population experiencing chronic diseases). Tobacco smoking threatens these hard-won advances in public health (Orntan, 1971; Olshansky & Ault, 1986; Stanley, 1993; World Bank, 1993; D. Samarasinghe, personal communication).

Until the middle of this century, life expectancy was so low in Sri Lanka that the chronic health effects of tobacco smoking, such as heart disease, respiratory illness and cancer, which usually manifest themselves only after 20–25 years of smoking (Stanley, 1993), were barely noticeable in comparison with the problems of undernutrition and infectious diseases. Now, chronic illness has surpassed infectious disease and malnutrition as a public health problem (Registrar General, 1984; Mendis, 1992; D.B. Nugegoda, personal communication; D. Samarasinghe, personal communication). Currently, the two leading causes of death in Sri Lanka are ischaemic heart disease and cerebrovascular disease, for both of which tobacco smoking is the main risk factor (Jamison *et al.*, 1993). Several community-based organizations are conducting health education activities for smoking prevention.

Tobacco was introduced into Sri Lanka by the Portuguese in the late sixteenth century and is now used in various forms (Uragoda & Senewiratne, 1971): it is smoked as cigarettes and hand-rolled *bidis* and cheroots and chewed in betel quid. Today, the preferred form of smoking tobacco is machine-rolled cigarettes (F.K. Rodrigo, personal communication). The smoking rates are negligible among Sri Lankan women (World Health Organization, 1997). Periodic surveys among men indicate a slight increase in per capita consumption of cigarettes during the 1980s and early 1990s, although the prevalence rate is still high (55%; World Health Organization, 1997). Low-income populations are not part of the downward trend in tobacco smoking, the prevalence rate among low-income males remaining at approximlately 80% (F.K. Rodgrigo, personal communication). The aim of this study was to examine the reasons for the apparent disparity in smoking rates between high- and low-income populations.

Methods

Three male interviewers are using in-depth, semi-structured interviews and methods of systematic data collection (Weller & Romney, 1988; Russell, 1994) to elicit personal, family and community information from 85 smoking and non-smoking males aged 16–30. Two follow-up interviews are conducted with each informant to extend the information. One female interviewer is interviewing the mother, sister or wife of each Sinhalese male informant to elicit further information about individual and community smoking behaviour. All interviews are being conducted in the informant's native language, and data are collected as written notes and tape recordings. The field notes are subsequently expanded, translated into English, entered into the qualitative analysis software package ATLAS/ti (Muhr, 1997) and coded for analysis.

Preliminary findings

During primary and secondary schooling, young men usually associate themselves with a *gantze* or gang of 15–20 boys in their community. There is considerable peer pressure to smoke, especially when participating in special events such as birthday parties, community funerals, religious and cultural events and 'jolly' trips, all of which are important community events.

The epidemiological transition is bringing about a heightened awareness of the effects of tobacco smoking and a concomitant change in perceptions of 'health'. The informants seem to be well aware of the health effects of smoking: they have seen or heard cautionary advice from doctors, Government warnings and the messages of tobacco control organizations and have witnessed chronic illness in others. Many of them reported that their fathers, other close relatives or neighbours had died as a result of smoking; some even tended to overestimate the effect of smoking in the community. Despite this widespread recognition, smoking is expected of men.

Before marriage, young men living with their parents are heavily supervised—by their parents, other family members, neighbours and other adults in the community. Smoking is seen as an excessive expenditure, inappropriate for a youth without a permanent job; it is considered shameful to smoke in the presence of elders. Unmarried men who smoke take pains to avoid being identified as smokers. Smoking is thus encouraged by peers, and important community events facilitate and invite smoking; yet smoking is not tolerated by the family, the community or prospective wives, and the young men are well aware of the hazards of tobacco smoking. They have therefore devised numerous ways of hiding their smoking from a disapproving community. Notably, during this study, many of the informants initially identified themselves as non-smokers; subsequent in-depth interviews and observations revealed that more than 70% of them smoke.

References

Bernard, H.R. (1994) *Research Methods in Anthropology*, Newbury Park, California: Sage Publications
Bjorkman, J.W. (1985) Health policy and politics in Sri Lanka: Developments in the south Asian welfare state. *Asian Surv.*, **25**, 537–552
Jamison, D. & Mosly, W.H. (1991) Disease control priorities in developing countries: Health policy responses to epidemiological change. *Am. J. Public Health*, **81**, 15–22
Jamison, D., Mosly, W.H. *et al.*, eds (1993) *Disease Control Priotrities in Developing Countries*, Oxford: Oxford University Press
Mendis, S. (1992) Prevention of coronary heart disease: Putting theory into practice. *Ceylon Med. J.*, **37**, 9–11
Muhr, T. (1997) *ATLAS/ti: Release 4.0*, Berlin: Scientific Software Development
Olshansky, S.F. & Ault, A.B. (1986) The fourth stage of the epidemiological transition: The age of degenerative diseases. *Milbank Fund Q.*, **64**, 355–391
Orntan, A.R. (1971) The epidemiological transition: A theory of the epidemiology of population change. *Milbank Mem. Fund Q.*, **49**, 509–538
Registrar General (1984) *Morbidity and Mortality Statistics*, Colombo, Ministry of Plan Implementation
Stanley, K. (1993) Appendix A: Control of tobacco production and use. In: *Disease Control Priorities in Developing Countries*, Oxford: Oxford University Press, pp. 703–722
UNICEF (1007) *Country Profile 1997*, World Wide Web, February, p. 6
Uragoda, C.G. & Senewiratne, B. (1971) Tobacco smoking in Ceylon. *J. Trop. Med. Hyg.*, **74**, 145–147
Weller, S.C. & Romney, A.K. (1988) *Systematic data Collection*, Newbury Park, California: Sage Publications
World Health Organization (1997) *Tobacco or Health: A Global Status Report*, Geneva
World Bank (1993) *World Development Report*, Oxford: Oxford University Press

Population attitudes to smoking in Chelyabinsk region, Russian Federation

E.G. Volkova, T.B. Karasikova, S.U. Levashov, G.B. Tkachenko, T.V. Kamardina, S.U. Pnomareva, D.A. Dmitriev & A.M. Levin

Ural Institute of Postgraduate Medical Training, Chelyabinsk, Russian Federation

Earlier investigations showed high prevalences of smoking in the Ural region of the Russian Federation: 66% in men and 8–12% in women; a pilot investigation among students aged 12–17 showed a prevalence of 26%. In collaboration with American scientists, we conducted a randomized investigation of smoking in various age groups of employees, medical workers and students. Of the 447 respondents to a questionnaire, 70% considered smoking to be one of the major risk factors for poor health; 59% said that smoking cessation was essential for health promotion; 68% considered that a healthy lifestyle meant not smoking; and 49% indicated that tobacco advertising prevented them from stopping smoking. The majority of the respondents said that the cost of cigarettes represented a large part of the family budget but agreed that tobacco should be taxed in order to finance preventive programmes. Even if cigarettes became more expensive, however, 45% of the respondents would not change their habit. Current smoking was reported by 40%, and only 34% of these had been advised by their physician to stop smoking during the previous 12 months. Attempts to quit had been made by 29% of the respondents, but only 4.2% had completely stopped smoking. Our participation in the international 'Quit and Win' campaign raised interest in smoking cessation in the population and showed the economic advantages of such smoking control. The investigation demonstrated the magnitude of the smoking problem and allowed us to determine priorities and to develop a programme called 'Chelyabinsk steps into Europe without tobacco'.

Mortality and morbidity due to tobacco use

A pilot study on mortality and smoking in Hong Kong

S.Y. Ho[1], T.H. Lam[1], A.J. Hedley[1] & K.H. Mak[2]

[1] *Department of Community Medicine, The University of Hong Kong, and*
[2] *Department of Health, Hong Kong SAR, China*

Introduction

No epidemiological study on the mortality attributable to smoking has been carried out in Hong Kong. Indirect local estimates have been derived from western data, but these figures may be subject to flaws caused by differences between Hong Kong and the West in the stage of the smoking epidemic, background disease rates and exposure to other risk factors. The weakness of these indirect estimates had been challenged by the Tobacco Institute in Hong Kong (Fletcher, 1995). Epidemiological studies are urgently needed to produce more direct evidence on the burden of local deaths attributable to tobacco. The results would provide the first assessment of the tobacco epidemic and provide strong support for tobacco control measures in Hong Kong.

The case–control method of Liu *et al.*(this volume) of interviewing the relatives of deceased persons ('cases') to obtain smoking histories and to compare these with the smoking histories of the surviving spouses ('controls') is potentially a very useful method for estimating the risks of deaths attributable to smoking. In the study of Liu *et al.*, the interviews were conducted in the early 1990s by visiting the relatives of about 1 million persons who had died in 1986–88. There was a gap of a few years between the death and the interview, and the costs of the home visits were very high. As a modification, we aimed to carry out interviews at death registries for deaths that had occurred within a few days. In 1996, we used this method to conduct a pilot study on mortality due to smoking in Hong Kong, to test the feasibility of carrying out a full-scale study.

Methods

There were four death registries in Hong Kong where the relatives of deceased persons were required by law to go to obtain a death certificate. In 1996, we conducted interviews in three of the registries and distributed self-administered questionnaires to one registry in which few deaths were registered. In all registries, the questionnaires were handed out by the registry staff when the relatives first came to the counter. While the relatives were waiting for the death certificate, an interviewer would approach them. If the deceased persons had been aged 30 or older, the relatives were invited to complete the questionnaire by themselves or with the interviewer's assistance.

The questionnaire was standardized and structured, designed to elicit information on sociodemographic factors, past smoking and other lifestyle factors about 10 years previously. The causes of death as listed on the death certificates were also recorded. Information on the cases was obtained from the relative in the registry who was most familiar with the deceased. Two types of relatives were used as sources of controls: live spouses of decedents and relatives of the opposite sex and of similar age (± 10 years) to the cases. Relatives of the opposite sex were selected so that in the analysis we could compare male cases with male controls and female cases with female controls. Because the sample size was small, we also compared the age-specific smoking prevalence data from the 1986 General Household Survey (Census and Statistics Department, 1986; GHS) with the cases in the estimation of odds ratios. The 1986 GHS data provided the smoking prevalence of the population about 10 years ago.

Results

There were 99 male cases and 57 male controls and 88 female cases and 73 female controls (Table 1). Most of the cases were over 60 years old, but it was difficult to find

Table 1. Age distribution of cases and controls by sex

Age (years)	Males		Females	
	Cases	Controls	Cases	Controls
30–59	19	29	11	45
≥ 60	80	28	77	28
Total	99	57	88	73

sufficient controls who were above this age. Despite the difficulties of interviewing relatives in death registries, a satisfactory response rate of 83% was obtained for the three busy registries in each of which an interviewer was placed.

Table 2 shows the daily smoking rates and odds ratios for all deaths due to smoking in males. Among younger males (aged 30–59), the daily smoking prevalence was 58% for cases, which was higher than that for controls (31%) and in the GHS data (38%). The crude odds ratios were 3.1 and 2.3, respectively. In older males (aged ≥ 60), the daily smoking prevalence was 54% for both cases and the controls but was only 39% in the GHS data. The crude odds ratios were 1.0 and 1.9 relative to the controls and the GHS data, respectively. The age-weighted odds ratio was smaller relative to the controls (1.5) than to the GHS data (1.9).

Table 3 shows the daily smoking rates and crude odds ratios for all deaths due to smoking in females. Among younger females (aged 30–59), there were no smokers among either the cases or the controls. Assuming that one smoker was present in each group, the daily smoking rates were 9% for the cases and 2% for the controls. The crude odds ratio was 4.1, which was much higher than that of 1.9 based on the GHS daily smoking rate of 5%. In older females (aged ≥ 60), daily smoking was more prevalent among cases (18%) than among controls (7%) and in the GHS data (11%). Again, the crude odds ratio was higher relative to the controls (2.9) than to the GHS data (1.9). The age-weighted odds ratio was 3.1 relative to controls but only 1.9 relative to the GHS data.

Table 2. Deaths due to smoking in males

Age (years)	Daily smoking (%)		Crude odds ratios (Control / GHS)
	Cases (n = 99)	Control / GHS (n = 57)	
30–59	58	31 / 38	3.1 / 2.3
≥ 60	54	54 / 39	1.0 / 1.9
Weighted average	55	42 / 38	1.5 / 1.9

GHS, 1986 General Household Survey

Table 3. Deaths due to smoking in females

Age (years)	Daily smoking (%)		Odds ratios (Control / GHS)
	Cases (n = 88)	Control / GHS (n = 73)	
30–59	9[a]	2[a] / 5	4.1 / 1.9
≥ 60	18	7 / 11	2.9 / 1.9
Weighted average	16	3 / 8	3.1 / 1.9

GHS, 1986 General Household Survey
[a] Actually zero, but assuming one smoker

Discussion

As Hong Kong is mostly urbanized and the reporting of deaths is virtually complete, information on deceased persons is more easily obtained at death registries than at homes and at a lower cost. The support of the death registry was crucial in two respects: the distribution of questionnaires by the registry staff increased the likelihood of participation by the relatives, and the death registry provided us with official causes of deaths.

While cases were not difficult to obtain, it was difficult to find enough old controls, particularly for males. This is because Chinese husbands are generally older than their wives, and men usually die earlier than women. Consequently, when a woman dies, it is likely that her husband is already dead, and there are therefore insufficient male spouse controls. In the future main study, more controls will be obtained through other channels, such as from random telephone interviews, resulting in additional costs. As the sample size in this pilot study was small, the estimates of smoking prevalence and odds ratios are not reliable, especially for younger subjects (30–59 years), as there were fewer deaths and the females had low smoking rates. The results for older subjects are reasonable and therefore encouraging.

As part of China, Hong Kong is unique not only in its economic development but also its early westernization of lifestyle, including smoking. As other parts of China develop and become westernized, other Chinese cities may show similar mortality patterns due to tobacco. If this is the case, our study will be not only of local relevance but could also contribute data for predicting mortality due to tobacco in other parts of China.

Conclusion

This modified method of conducting a case–control study in death registries is innovative and operationally feasible. It is an economic and efficient way of gathering information on deaths and relatives quickly and it is acceptable to the subjects and the death registries. The main study will begin in January 1998, and we are testing other methods for recruitment of a more representative control group.

Acknowledgements

We thank the Health and Welfare Branch of the Hong Kong Government for funding this pilot study and the Immigration Department for its kind arrangements in the death registries.

References

Fletcher, R.J. (1995) Mathematical speculation (Letter to the Editor). *South China Morning Post,* 11 September 1995

Census and Statistics Department (1986) Cigarette smoking pattern. In: Special Topics Report No. 11, Hong Kong, pp. 71–96.

Deaths attributable to smoking in Taiwan, 1995

S.P. Tsai, C.P. Wen & D.D. Yen

John Tung Foundation, Taipei, Taiwan, China

The impact of smoking in a society is multifactorial and can be measured in several dimensions. One of the most important is the burden of mortality, i.e. the number of smoking-attributable deaths. The purpose of this study is to estimate the number of deaths due to smoking in Taiwan in 1995 by calculating the smoking-attributable mortality.

Materials and methods

The cause-specific mortality rates in Taiwan were extracted from the official publication of vital statistics for 1995 (Department of Health, 1995). The age- and sex-specific rates of smoking were derived from the statistics of the Taiwan Provincial Tobacco and Liquor Monopoly Bureau (1965, 1994) for 1965–94. The risks for current smokers relative to non-smokers were based on the results of a large-scale census-based cohort study in Japan (Hirayama, 1990). Smoking-attributable mortality was calculated by a standard method published by the United States Department of Health and Human Services (Shultz et al., 1992). Deaths from lung cancer due to exposure to environmental tobacco smoke were estimated by a method presented by the United States Environmental Protection Agency (1992). The numbers of deaths from other cancers and from cardiovascular disease due to exposure to environmental tobacco smoke were based on the estimate of Wells (1988).

Results

The prevalence of smoking in Taiwan has remained at approximately 60% for men and only about 4% for women for the last 30 years, but the rates among men aged 30 or less have increased substantially (Figure 1). An increase of similar magnitude was seen among young women, with a more than twofold increase for the 16–25-year-old group. The rates among men and women over 30 years of age decreased. The per capita cigarette consumption increased by 70%, from 1040 cigarettes per year in 1954 to 1776 per year in 1992.

The numbers of deaths attributable to smoking by disease category in 1995 are shown in Table 1. There were 14 421 smoking-attributable deaths, which was twice as many as those due to motor accidents in the same year. Deaths due to exposure to environmental tobacco smoke constituted 38% of all smoking-attributable mortality, or one of every three smoking-related deaths. This proportion was much higher among women (82%) than men (18%). The total number of deaths attributable to active smoking and environmental tobacco smoke represented 15% of all causes of death for males and 14% for females; in other words, one out of seven deaths in Taiwan was related to smoking. Nearly one third (31%) of deaths of males from cancer could be attributed to smoking, in contrast to 3% of female deaths from cancer. Of the cases of lung cancer, 66% of those in males and 9% of those in females could be attributed to active smoking.

Discussion

Cigarette smoking is the single most readily preventable cause of premature death in Taiwan. The estimated impact on health is alarming: one out of seven people died

Figure 1. Age-specific prevalence rates of smoking per 100 men, Taiwan, 1965 and 1994

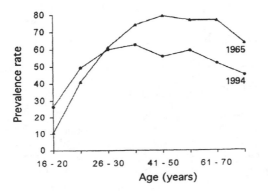

Table 1. Smoking-attributable mortality (SAM), Taiwan, 1995

Cause of death	Men		Women		Total SAM
	RR	SAM	RR	SAM	
Neoplasms					
Lip, oral cavity and pharynx	3.00	808	1.5	1	809
Oesophagus	2.24	273	1.75	5	278
Stomach	1.45	302	1.18	9	311
Liver	1.50	890	1.66	51	941
Pancreas	156	113	1.44	8	121
Larynx	32.5	175	3.29	3	178
Lung	4.45	2322	2.34	127	2449
Urinary bladder	1.61	85	2.29	15	100
Other sites	–	213	–	51	264
Cardiovascular disease					
Cerebrovascular	1.08	350	1.18	82	432
Ischaemic heart	1.73	982	1.90	136	1118
Hypertensive heart	1.66	167	1.25	13	180
Other heart	1.37	587	1.43	101	688
Peripheral vascular	3.83	153	1.75	7	160
Asthma	1.83	250	4.02	89	339
Gastric ulcer	1.86	94	2.48	16	110
Liver cirrhosis	1.21	354	1.49	37	391
Burns	–	70	–	39	109
environmental tobacco smoke	–	1794	–	3649	5443
Total		9982		4439	14 421

RR, relative risk: risks relative to those of non-smokers

from smoking-attributable causes in 1995. The effect of environmental tobacco smoke on health among females has received little attention in this male-dominated society, but there were more deaths due to such exposure among females, and substantially more women died from exposure to environmental tobacco smoke than from active smoking. Men (60%) who smoked caused non-smoking women (96%) to inhale cigarette smoke involuntarily at home, at work and in public places.

While banning tobacco is feasible, every possible step must be taken to prevent young people in Taiwan from starting to use tobacco products. In 1986, an anti-smoking campaign launched by the John Tung Foundation, a private organization known for its anti-smoking activities, made some progress: the rate of quitting smoking that year was about 3%, whereas it was only 1% in other years. Recently, the Department of Health in Taiwan intensified its smoking cessation campaign. It established a new policy on smoking in public places, added warning labels on cigarette packs and limited the promotional activities of cigarette manufacturers. The commitment of the Government will result in more innovative programmes to combat smoking. Finally, the Government announced its goal of a smoke-free nation by the year 2010 could have an important effect in reducing smoking, as this pronouncement will force the public to focus on the urgency of the problem and create social pressure for smokers to quit.

References

Department of Health (1995) *Health Statistics 2. Vital Statistics*, Taipei

Environmental Protection Agency (1992) *Respiratory Health Effects of Passive Smoking: Lung Cancer and Other Disorders* (EPA/600/6-90/006F), Washington DC: Office of Health and Environmental Assessment

Hirayama, T. (1990) *Life-style and Mortality: A Large Census-based Cohort Study in Japan*, Basel: Karger

Shultz, J.M., Novotny, T.E. & Rice, D.P. (1992) *Smoking Attributable Mortality, Morbidity, and Economic Cost*, Atlanta: Centers for Disease Control

Taiwan Provincial Tobacco and Liquor Monopoly Bureau (1965) *Tobacco and Liquor Consumption Survey for Taiwan Area, 1965*, Taipei (in Chinese)

Taiwan Provincial Tobacco and Liquor Monopoly Bureau (1994) *Tobacco and Liquor Consumption Survey for Taiwan Area, 1994*, Taipei (in Chinese)

Wells, A.J. (1988) An estimate of adult mortality in the United States from passive smoking. *Environ. Int.*, 14, 249–265

Loss of life related to cigarette smoking in Taiwan: A 12-year follow up study

K.-M. Liaw

Graduate Institute of Epidemiology, College of Public Health, National Taiwan University, Taipei, Taiwan

Objectives: This study was carried out to examine the relative risks of dying from various diseases associated with cigarette smoking and to estimate annual life loss attributable to cigarette smoking in Taiwan.

Methods: A cohort of 17 538 male and female residents were recruited from 12 townships and precincts in Taiwan during 1982–86. Information on history of cigarette smoking, including duration and quantity, was collected from each study subject at a standardized personal interview based on a structured questionnaire. The participants were followed-up regularly to ascertain their vital status until 1994; the follow-up rate was as high as 96%. Cox's proportional hazards regression was used to derive risks for cause-specific mortality of cigarette smokers relative to non-smokers and to examine the dose–response relationship between cumulative cigarette smoking and mortality from various causes.

Results: A total of 2640 persons died during the study period. After adjustment for age and sex, a significant dose–response relationship was observed between cumulative cigarette smoking and deaths from all causes combined, cancers at all sites combined, oral cancer, gastric cancer, lung cancer, liver cancer and pneumonia and other lung diseases. It was estimated that 8072 deaths of 7552 males and 520 females were attributable to cigarette smoking annually in Taiwan. If all deaths related to cigarette smoking were categorized under a classification code for cause of death, cigarette smoking-related diseases would become the fourth leading cause of death in Taiwan.

Conclusions: Cigarette smoking has a striking impact on mortality from various causes in the Taiwanese population. Tobacco control should be the first priority among public health programmes in Taiwan.

Mortality due to cigarette smoking by district in New Zealand, estimated from national and district deaths

H. Glasgow[1] & M. Laugesen[2]

[1]Cancer Society of New Zealand, Wellington, and
[2]Health New Zealand, Auckland, New Zealand

Abstract

Aim: To estimate mortality due to tobacco use in districts of 10 000 to 1 million population and build local support for tobacco control.

Method: The Big Kill Continues (Cancer Society, 1996) is based on numbers of deaths by cause, nationally, for each district and national population by census. The first was multiplied by the national fractions of cigarette-attributable mortality (Peto et al., 1994) to obtain the numbers of deaths due to cigarette smoking for 70 districts and 20 health districts in 1989–93. Formatting and planned publicity maximized the media impact.

Results: The toll of tobacco is graphically presented and shows the serious effects of smoking, particularly among Maori, the indigenous population. One in three deaths among Maori were due to smoking; 15% more Maori would survive to middle age (35–69 years) if they all quit smoking at the age of 25. The publication is useful for lobbying politicians, district tobacco control staff, school libraries and generating local publicity. 'One in six of all deaths due to smoking' was the top story on the morning news. Media interest quickly moved to policies to reduce the toll.

Conclusions: District mortality can be calculated from district deaths-by-cause. The results for smoking prevalence were in line with previous estimates based on census district. The method can be applied widely, as most developed countries have district mortality data, but few have cigarette smoking prevalence by district.

Introduction

In 1996, the Cancer Society of New Zealand published two books of tobacco statistics, written by Murray Laugesen. One report, *Tobacco Statistics 1996* (Laugesen, 1996a), published jointly with the Ministry of Health, contains a wide range of information about tobacco and smoking. The other, *The Big Kill Continues* (Laugesen, 1996b), contains statistics on deaths due to tobacco and followed an earlier edition in 1988, published by the Department of Health. With this report, we aimed to provide regional staff with estimates of mortality due to tobacco in each district, city and health district. We wanted to make the most of the opportunity these publications offered to gain maximum publicity and to create a good climate for the tobacco control legislation that was in process of being passed in Parliament.

Method

In 1994, Peto *et al.* published estimates of mortality due to tobacco for 46 countries, including New Zealand. These estimates are based on lung cancer rates for each country and year and differences in the rates for respiratory and cardiovascular disease and cancer between smokers and non-smokers in the American Cancer Society follow-up of 1 million Americans in the 1980s. *The Big Kill Continues* uses this method to verify the results for New Zealand, then calculates fractions for each cause of death due to cigarette smoking in 1989–93. These national fractions for each age and sex group are then multiplied by the number of district deaths for each age and sex, to give the number of deaths due to cigarette smoking by age and sex for each district.

The Big Kill Continues has a strong visual impact. It presents a wide range of data and graphs in a well-designed, standard format, with one page per population: one for New Zealand, two for typical parliamentary electorates, 20 for health districts and 73 for districts or cities. Each district page was designed to show the fractions of all deaths from cancer, heart and respiratory disease due to cigarettes, how cigarettes contribute to deaths in middle age, the percentage of deaths due to cigarettes at each age, how many more people would survive middle age if everyone quit smoking at age 25, the number of 15-year olds who smoke and the number of 15-year olds who bought cigarettes from shops (which is illegal) (Ford *et al.*, 1995).

We designed the book with an eye-catching cover and a dramatic title. The Cancer Society employed a journalist to give as much publicity as possible to the release of the report. The news releases prepared by the journalist focused on the most newsworthy items but also called for a variety of Government interventions. The media releases highlighted the need for a tax increase and for quitting and prevention campaigns. The news releases served a variety of purposes: some were sent out electronically to national radio, television and newspapers; a report and news release were sent to the 36 daily newspapers throughout the country; and sample media releases were sent to district staff, who provided them to their local newspapers and other media. The Cancer Society also prepared letters for all Members of Parliament and provided them with a copy of the report.

Results

We found that smoking caused 17% of deaths in New Zealand, or approximately one in six deaths.

- It caused 25% of all cancer deaths and kills one in two life-long smokers.
- Among New Zealand Maori, smoking caused one in three deaths and 42% of all deaths from cancer.

- 15% more Maori would survive to middle age (35–69 years) if they all quit smoking at age 25.
- Among 15-year olds, 11% smoked daily, but 24% of Maori 15-year olds smoked daily.
- Comparisons between districts show that 20% of deaths are due to smoking in the districts with the highest rates and 13% of deaths in those with the lowest rates.

'One in six of all deaths due to smoking' was the top story on the national morning radio news and many of the major newspapers. The media quickly moved on to ask 'Why?' and 'What can be done to reduce this shocking death toll?' In the districts, the news of the local statistics followed. There was more emphasis on districts with highest mortality but overall the main picture was of high mortality due to cigarette smoking in all districts. In some areas, weekly community newspapers published reports days, weeks and sometimes a month or two later. Combining its release with *Tobacco Statistics 1996* increased the impact considerably.

One fifth of all Members of Parliament replied to our letters, responding positively to the information. The Minister of Health and other Members of Parliament have quoted figures from *The Big Kill* in speeches and during a recent debate on tobacco legislation. Other Members of Parliament referred to *The Big Kill* during recent debates in Parliament on tobacco legislation, and the Minister of Health had it with him when giving a speech at a tobacco conference.

The Big Kill Continues can be used to give politicians local reasons to take action on cigarettes, in talks to groups (each page can be used for an overhead transparency), to provide to media (each district A4 page was easy to photocopy), for health planning (for example, senior health managers and non-government organizations can monitor whether local anti-smoking publicity and enforcement is reaching districts with high mortality) and in school libraries for projects.

Conclusions

District mortality can be caluated from district deaths-by-cause for populations > 10 000. The method used produced credible results which were in line with previous estimates based on smoking prevalence in district censuses. The method can be used widely, as most developed countries have district data on mortality but few have the prevalence of cigarette smoking by district.

The Big Kill Continues created a media opportunity for tobacco control. Mortality due to cigarette smoking is still news, but as the public accepts that cigarettes kill, the media are moving on to ask 'What are you (health experts) going to do about it?' It provides sets of statistics on tobacco which have been purchased by the libraries of a large proportion of New Zealand secondary schools. The impact of this edition, *The Big Kill Continues*', is just as great as that of *The Big Kill*, published in 1988.

Enquiries to: Helen Glasgow heleng@cancernz.org.na

References

Ford, D.J., Scragg, R., Weir, J. & Gaiser, J. (1995) A national survey of cigarette smoking in fourth-form school children in New Zealand. *NZ Med. J.*, **108**, 454–457
Laugesen, M. (1996a) *Tobacco Statistics 1996*, Wellington: Cancer Society of NZ Inc. and Ministry of Health
Laugesen, M. (1996b) *The Big Kill Continues*, Wellington: Cancer Society of NZ Inc.
Peto, R., Lopez, A.D., Boreham, J., et al. (1994) *Mortality from Smoking in Developed Countries, 1950–2000*, Oxford: Oxford University Press

Cigarette smoking-attributable mortality in Norway

T. Sanner

Department of Environmental and Occupational Cancer
The Norwegian Radium Hospital, Oslo, Norway

Introduction
The number of deaths in Norway caused by cigarette smoking and the economic cost due to morbidity and mortality caused by cigarette smoking have been calculated.

Number of deaths
Since no study on the effect of smoking on the death rates due to different diseases is available in Norway, data from the United States Cancer Prevention Study I (death rates 1959–65) and II (death rates 1982–86) (Surgeon-General, 1989) were used. The relative risks of death from various smoking-related diseases were adjusted for differences in smoking habits in the United States and Norway from the formula:

$$r = (r_{USA} - 1) \times s_{Norway}/s_{USA} + 1$$

where r is the relative risk that a smoker will die of a disease in comparison with a person who has never smoked; r_{USA} is the relative risk found in the American studies, and s_{Norway} and s_{USA} represent the average numbers of cigarettes smoked daily. The average numbers of cigarettes smoked per day were 22.1 by men and 18.6 by women in the United States (Surgeon-General, 1989) and 15.1 and 12.1, respectively, in Norway (personal communication, The Norwegian Council on Tobacco or Health).

The fraction of deaths caused by smoking is calculated from the formula:

$$a = \frac{p(r-1)}{p(r-1) + 1}$$

where p is the fraction of smokers. Since the official death rates are always some years behind, the present calculations are based on the years 1990, 1991 and 1992 (Official Statistics of Norway, 1992, 1993, 1994). At that time, the prevalence of smoking in Norway was 37% for men and 33% for women, and the prevalence of previous smoking was 18.5% for men and 16.5% for women (personal communication, The Norwegian Council on Tobacco or Health).

The number of deaths caused by smoking was calculated from the formula:

$$A = a \times D$$

where D is the total number of deaths caused by the disease. The numbers of deaths caused by cancer, cardiovascular diseases and respiratory diseases are shown in Table 1. The numbers represent the average obtained from the adjusted risk estimates in the two US studies, and this average was used to compensate for the fact that smoking was taken up 25 years later in Norway than in the United States. The risk of dying from smoking in Norway in 1992 thus represents the risk in the United States around 1973. Cardiovascular disease represents the main cause of death due to cigarette smoking in Norway, resulting in more than half of the deaths due to cigarette smoking among both men and women. In the United States, according to the last study of American Cancer Society, about 46% of the smoking-related deaths were caused by cardiovascular disease. According to our calculations, smoking-induced deaths from cancer represent about 27% of all cancer deaths among men and 10% among women. According to the estimates

Table 1. Numbers of deaths in Norway in 1992 due to cigarette smoking

Cause of death	Men		Women		Total	
	No.	%	No.	%	No.	%
Cancer	1447	26.7	460	10.0	1907	19.1
Cardiovascular disease	2629	23.4	1547	15.2	4176	19.5
Respiratory disease	801	39.6	582	26.2	1383	32.6
Total	4877	20.5	2589	12.1	7466	16.5

Numbers represent averages for 1991, 1992 and 1993; percentages are of the total number of deaths in the population.

in the United States, smoking is the cause of approximately 45% of all cancer deaths among men and 21% among women. These differences are probably due to the fact that the average American smoker consumes significantly more cigarettes per day than the average Norwegian smoker, and moreover, that smoking was taken up in the United States many years earlier than in Norway. One third of the cases of respiratory disease resulting in death are caused by smoking.

Of the 7500 deaths caused by cigarette smoking in Norway in 1992, 5600 occurred among current smokers and 1900 among previous smokers. Half of the deaths occurred among persons under 70 years of age. In addition, approximately 500 non-smokers died of passive smoking (Sanner & Dybing, 1996). About 50 deaths are caused by lung cancer, while the remainder are caused by heart disease.

In addition to deaths, smoking causes morbidity resulting in the loss of 1.4 million working days in Norway, and 650 hospital beds are occupied by patients with diseases caused by smoking (Sanner et al., 1993).

Economic costs of smoking in Norway

The economic cost of smoking in Norway was calculated on the basis of the same elements as those used by the Department of Health and Human Services (1990) in their reports to the American Congress. The numbers used in the calculations were obtained from official Norwegian statistics. The results are shown in Table 2. The total cost according to this calculation is about 7.7 million million Norwegian kroner or US$ 1 million million for 1992. Factors such as pain, suffering and personal expenses for patients and their families are not included in the calculation. Expenses related to loss of productivity by smoking, fires in connection with smoking and cleaning are likewise not included.

The costs per death in Norway and the United States are compared in Figure 1. The cost of indirect morbidity is significantly higher in the United States than in Norway due to higher expenses at hospitals. Indirect mortality is higher in Norway than in the United States due to the fact that the age of retirement, and hence the loss of productivity due to smoking-attributable deaths, is higher in Norway. Altogether, the costs in Norway are slightly lower than in the United States.

Table 2. Annual costs due to morbidity and mortality caused by cigarette smoking

Factor	Cost (Norwegian kroner x 10^6)
Direct morbidity	1445
Physician services	292
Hospitalization	921
Medications	232
Indirect morbidity	1720
Indirect mortality	4550
Total	7715

Figure 1. Smoking-attributable costs in Norway and the United States

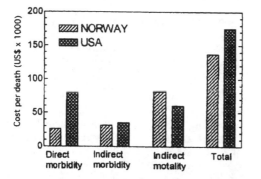

From Department of Health and Human Services (1990)
For the calculation, the smoking-attributable cost was divided by the number of deaths

Per capita, the economic impact was US$ 250 per person for Norway as a whole, while the number in the United States was US$ 220. The difference is due to the fact that the frequency of smoking is much higher in Norway than in the United States.

As pointed out above, these numbers represent only a fraction of the total costs due to smoking. Let us assume that smokers work 15 min less per day than non-smokers because of smoking pauses. In Norway, the gross domestic product shows that we produce goods and services worth about 3 million million kroner per working day. This implies that the extra 15 min per day used by smokers would result in a loss of production and services of 7.5 million million kroner per year, or about the same as that calculated for the costs of smoking due to morbidity and mortality.

Conclusions

The annual number of deaths caused by cigarette smoking has been estimated to be 7500 in Norway. One-half of these deaths occur in people under the age of 70. In addition, the use of cigarettes causes about 500 deaths due to passive smoking. It is calculated that cigarette smoking costs society about 1.2 million million Norwegian kroner per year in direct health care, 1.6 million million kroner in indirect morbidity and 4.2 million million kroner in lost productivity due to premature death.

References

Department of Health and Human Services (1990) *Smoking and Health. A National Status Report to Congress* (DHHS Publication No. CDC 87-8396 (revised 02/90)), Rockville, Maryland
Official Statistics of Norway (1992, 1993, 1994) *Causes of Death 1991, 1992, and 1993*, Oslo
Sanner, T. & Dybing, E. (1996) Health injury from passive smoking. *Tidskr. Nor. Lægefor.*, 116, 617–620 (in Norwegian)
Sanner, T., Juul Andersen, E., Hauknes, A. & Stenmarck, S., eds (1993) *Action Plan for a Tobacco-free Norway, 1994–1988*, Oslo, Department of Health and Social Affairs
Surgeon-General (1989) *Reducing the Health Consequences of Smoking. 25 Years of Progress* (DHHS Publication No. CDC 89-8411), Rockville, Maryland, US Department of Health and Human Services

Effects of smoking on the epidemiology of obstructive lung disease in an older population in the United States

E.A. Frazier[1], W.M. Voller[1], A.D. Hayward[1], S.R. Wilson[2] & A.S. Buist[3]

[1]Center for Health Research, Portland, Oregon; [2]American Institutes for Research, Palo Alto, California, and[3]Oregon Health Sciences University, Portland, Oregon, United States

Although smoking is a well-recognized risk factor for chronic obstructive pulmonary disease, the association between smoking history and asthma has been less well studied, especially among older people with co-existing chronic obstructive pulmonary disease. We have examined how smoking histories correlate with the physiological and personal characteristics of people ≥ 50 years of age with both asthma and chronic obstructive pulmonary disease.

We selected 294 members of a large health maintenance organization on the basis of use of medications or hospitals, who reported medically diagnosed asthma and current symptoms of asthma, for a trial of the efficacy of peak-flow monitoring. They were assessed for lung function, respiratory symptoms, other diseases, use of medication and health care and smoking history.

The smoking histories showed that 37% had never smoked and 63% had ever smoked; of the latter, 5% were current smokers and 58% were ex-smokers. Their mean pack–years was 34. Patients with asthma who had smoked had a significantly lower lung function than those who had never smoked, with a forced expiratory volume in one second of 53 and 69%, respectively, and more dyspnoea as measured by the Borg scale. Both groups showed a significant response to bronchodilators,with the same mean increase (230 ml), indicating that asthmatic patients who have smoked have more fixed, irreversible airflow obstruction than those who have never smoked. Thus, more of those who had smoked used daily inhalations of corticosteroids (87 versus 77%). The use of health care for breathing problems in the previous year did not differ between the two groups overall, but patients who had smoked reported more hospitalizations for breathing problems during their lifetime.

Asthma and chronic obstructive pulmonary disease often co-exist in older persons who have smoked. Recognition of this co-morbidity is important because it affects the degree of airflow obstruction and irreversible disease and probably the costs of care. This finding highlights the importance of targeting smoking cessation or avoidance early in life for individuals with asthma.

Tobacco and cancer

Tobacco-attributable cancer burden: A global review

D.M. Parkin, P. Pisani & E. Masuyer

International Agency for Research on Cancer
Lyon France

In 1990, there were about 9.3 million new cases of cancer worldwide. In this paper, we attempt to estimate what proportion of this total can be ascribed to tobacco smoking. We have not concerned ourselves here with other forms of tobacco use (chewing, snuff) or with the adverse effects of environmental tobacco smoke. First, which cancers are associated with smoking? In fact, epidemiologists have claimed at some time or another to have observed an increased risk for every single cancer type. Since we cannot be sure how much of this is the result of study design or analysis, we decided to include as tobacco-related cancers only those classified as such by the International Agency for Research on Cancer: lung, oral cavity and pharynx; larynx; oesophagus; pharynx; kidney and urinary bladder.

In general, there are two methods for estimating the fraction of disease caused by a particular exposure, such as tobacco. The 'direct' method, in which the difference between observed incidence and the expected incidence (in the absence of exposure) is computed as a proportion (or percentage) of observed incidence:

$$AF = \frac{I - I_o}{I}$$

where I is the actual (observed) incidence and I_o is the incidence in unexposed people. The more usual method is to use the prevalence of the relevant exposure in the population; the relative risk of that exposure is:

$$AF = \frac{P(r-1)}{1 + P(r-1)}$$

where P is the prevalence of exposure and r is the relative risk of exposure

We begin our process of estimation by using the first of these methods for lung cancer. Here, thanks to several cohort studies (Garfinkel, 1985; Doll & Peto, 1976; Hirayama, 1990), we have good information on the rates of mortality from lung cancer by age and sex in non-smokers (i.e. persons who never smoked regularly). In fact, the incidence in non-smokers in these studies (British doctors, Japanese, volunteers in the United States) are quite similar. With these mortality rates and information on survival and case fatality in the same populations, we can readily estimate incidence. The assumptions underlying estimation of the number of cases of lung cancer attributable to tobacco use are, therefore, that (1) lung cancer rates in non-smokers are similar in all populations world-wide, and (2) higher observed rates are the consequence of tobacco smoking in that population.

Proposition (1) is difficult to test for men, since there are no readily available data— even from long ago—on non-smoking male populations around the world (although the similarity of the results from the three cohort studies is reassuring). For women, the data on non-smoking populations worldwide suggest that indeed the non-smoking women in the American cohort did have similar rates to those elsewhere (maybe somewhat higher in fact, possibly because of other exposures such as environmental tobacco smoke). Chinese women, however, have much higher rates of lung cancer, even though they do not smoke. We used the non-smoker rates in the American cohort to estimate how much lung cancer in each world region is due to tobacco. For Chinese women, our best estimate is to suggest that non-smoker rates are some 80% of observed population rates, or that 20% of lung cancer (only) is caused by tobacco. Using these methods, we obtain the results in Table 1. In men in Europe and North America, over 90% of lung cancer is estimated to be attributable to smoking, and only in the lowest incidence areas of East and West Africa are there no attributable cases. The fractions are lower for women, and several areas, including South-Central Asia, have no attributable cases. The highest fractions are in North America (84%), northern Europe (75%) and Australia/New Zealand (71%), where women have been smoking the longest. Overall, this method implies that 87% of lung cancer in men and 45% of lung cancer in women is the consequence of tobacco smoking.

We cannot use this method for the other cancers, for two reasons: we do not know the rates in non-smokers, and the assumption that non-smoker rates are likely to be stable in different populations is untenable. One need think only of the huge regional variations in the incidence of oesophageal cancer and the importance of chemical and biological agents in determining urinary bladder cancer rates, both independent of smoking.

Thus, we must use the prelevance–relative risk method. But the problem is we do not know the prevalence of smoking and the relative risks for various cancers in different parts of the world. What is more, both are changing over time: relative risk is determined by cumulative exposure to tobacco smoke, which can be quite different among current smokers in different countries. For lung cancer, however, we have already estimated attributable fractions in different areas. Using the formula $AF = P(r-1)/1 + P(r-1)$, we can substitute relative risks for lung cancer in smokers from the American cohort to obtain P. This then represents the prevalence of smoking that would have been present if the relative risks seen in the American cohort had been present. So it is an artificial figure; it can be higher or lower than the true smoking prevalence in the population, depending on whether the actual relative risks are greater than, or less than, those in the American cohort.

We can now use this 'artificial prevalence', together with the relative risks associated with smoking for the other cancers in the American cohort, to estimate attributable fractions for these cancers. Table 2 shows the relative risks in the American study and

Table 1. Cases of lung cancer attributable to tobacco smoking by world area

Area	Males		Females	
	Total cases	% Tobacco	Total cases	% Tobacco
East Africa	1 900	1	900	0
Middle Africa	1 500	47	400	0
Northern Africa	8 200	74	2 300	28
Southern Africa	4 500	85	1 100	36
Western Africa	1 200	0	600	0
Caribbean	4 700	84	1 700	55
Central America	5 500	69	2 200	26
South America	29 600	81	6 400	17
North America	123 600	91	71 700	84
China	228 400	89	98 400	20
Japan	31 900	86	11 700	55
Other East Asia	7 100	81	3 100	24
South-east Asia	35 200	80	12 800	43
South-central Asia	74 800	71	12 100	0
Western Asia	24 300	90	4 300	44
Eastern Europe	116 500	92	24 700	46
Northern Europe	40 500	91	17 800	75
Southern Europe	56 900	91	8 800	30
Western Europe	65 300	90	13 200	35
Australia/New Zealand	6 300	89	2 500	71
Other Pacific	150	51	60	34
Total	868 050	87	296 760	45

Table 2. Estimated relative risks for current smokers aged ≥ 35 derived from the American study

Cancer	Male		Female	
Lung				
aged 15–44	6.0		4.5	
aged 45–54	12.7		10.8	
aged 55–64	24.1		14.0	
aged ≥ 65	30.4		12.3	
Oral cavity & pharynx	27.5	[4.5]	5.6	[4.5]
Oesophagus	7.6	[5.0]	10.3	[5.0]
Pancreas	2.1		2.3	
Larynx	10.5	[10.5]	17.8	[10.5]
Urinary bladder	2.9		2.6	
Kidney	3.0		1.4	

From Parkin *et al.* (1994)
Figures in [ ] are those actually used.

the values actually used in the calculations. For cancers of the upper aerodigestive tract, we estimated rather lower values in order to allow for the confounding effects of alcohol (smoking and alcohol drinking go together, and the available relative risks made no adjustment for this).

Table 3 shows the estimated numbers of cases at these sites and the fractions due to tobacco smoking.

Taking these figures together, we can estimate that, in total, some 27% of cancers in men worldwide and some 4% of cancers in women are due to tobacco smoking. These percentages vary considerably by world area, as shown in Table 4, from no attributable cases in either sex in west Africa, up to 41% of cancers in men in eastern Europe and 15% of cancers in women in northern America.

This method of estimation requires several assumptions, as we have seen. Yet estimates of results from national data on relative risk and smoking prevalence seems to give quite similar results. Thus, the US Department of Health and Human Services in 1989 estimated that about 100 000 cancer deaths in men and 40 000 cancer deaths in women in 1985 were due to smoking. Virtually identical results are obtained from the methods used in this paper.

References

Doll, R. & Peto, R. (1976) Mortality in relation to smoking: 20 years' observations on male British doctors. *Br. Med. J.*, **ii**, 1525–1536

Garfinkel, L. (1985) Selection, follow-up and analysis in the American Cancer Society. Prospective studies. *Natl Cancer Inst. Monogr.*, **67**, 49–52

Hirayama, T (1990) *Life Style and Mortality: A Large-scale Census-based Cohort Study in Japan* (Contributions to Epidemiology & Biostatistics, Vol. 6), Framington City, Connecticut, Karger AG

Parkin, D.M., Pisani, P., Lopez, A.D. & Masuyer, E. (1994) At least one in seven cases of cancer is caused by smoking. Global estimates for 1985. *Int. J. Cancer*, **59**, 494–504

Table 3. Other cancers: Cases attributable to smoking in 1990

Cancer site	Males		Females	
	Total cases	% Tobacco	Total cases	% Tobacco
Oral cavity & pharynx	306 000	46	148 000	11
Oesophagus	273 000	55	138 000	10
Pancreas	90 000	30	80 000	14
Larynx	145 000	70	25 000	27
Urinary bladder	223 000	39	66 000	16
Kidney	93 000	40	62 000	5

Table 4. Percentages of all cancer cases in each geographical area attributable to tobacco smoking by sex and cancer site

Area	Total		%	
	Male	Female	Male	Female
Eastern Africa	80 958	79 078	0	0
Middle Africa	37 184	42 797	4	0
Northern Africa	67 031	71 996	22	2
Southern Africa	28 691	25 716	31	4
Western Africa	42 877	50 717	0	0
Caribbean	26 231	24 698	25	6
Central America	54 115	65 026	11	1
Temperate South America	55 710	59 980	23	1
Tropical South America	171 069	161 389	17	1
Northern America	681 843	585 406	26	15
China	1 223 089	1 025 666	30	3
Japan	207 136	152 256	19	6
Other east Asia	53 441	47 781	16	2
South-eastern Asia	189 495	245 487	22	4
South-central Asia	561 195	546 718	23	0
Western Asia	94 984	84 937	37	4
Eastern Europe	401 122	383 342	41	4
Northern Europe	181 625	185 457	30	11
Southern Europe	244 434	197 438	35	2
Western Europe	350 685	324 135	29	2
Australia/New Zealand	39 538	34 700	23	8
Melanesia	2 413	2 430	1	1
Micronesia/Polynesia	364	358	25	5
World	4 795 230	4 397 508	27	4
Developed countries	2 106 383	1 862 734	30	8
Developing countries	2 688 847	2 534 774	25	2
Asia/Pacific	1 715 476	1 508 678	27	4

Smoking and mortality in China: A prospective study of 9351 middle-aged adults in Shanghai, with a 16-year follow-up

Z. Chen[1], Z. Xu[2], R. Collins[1], W.-X. Li[2] & R. Peto[1]

[1]Clinical Trial Service Unit & Epidemiological Studies Unit, University of Oxford, United Kingdom;[2]Department of Epidemiology, Shanghai Medical University, Shanghai, China

Abstract

Background: In recent decades, there has been a rapid, substantial increase in tobacco consumption in China, particularly among men, but little is known from local epidemiological studies about the pattern of smoking-related deaths.

Objective: To assess the current health effects of cigarette smoking in Shanghai, China.

Design: Prospective observational study of mortality in relation to cigarette smoking.

Setting: Eleven factories in urban Shanghai, China.

Subjects: 9351 adults (6494 men and 2857 women) aged 35–64 years at the time of a baseline survey during the 1970s.

Outcome measures: Mortality from all causes and specific causes.

Results: During the average follow-up period of 16 years, 881 men and 207 women died. Of the men, 61% had described themselves as current cigarette smokers at the time of the baseline survey, and their overall mortality rate was significantly greater than that of non-smokers (relative risk, 1.4; 95% confidence interval [CI], 1.2–1.7;

$p < 0.0001$). The excess was almost twice as great (relative risk, 1.8; 95% CI, 1.5–2.2; $p < 0.0001$) among the men who had begun smoking before the age of 25 and was significantly associated with the number of cigarettes smoked ($p < 0.0001$ for trend) after adjustment for other major risk factors. The chief sources of the excess mortality were lung cancer (relative risk, 3.8; 95% CI, 2.1–6.8; $p < 0.001$), oesophageal cancer (3.6; 95% CI, 1.2–10.5; $p < 0.05$), liver cancer (2.0; 95% CI, 1.1–3.7; $p < 0.05$), coronary heart disease (1.8; 95% CI, 1.0–3.2; $p < 0.05$) and chronic obstructive pulmonary disease (2.5; 95% CI, 1.4–4.4; $p < 0.01$). About 20% (95% CI, 12–29%) of all deaths among the men in this Chinese population during the study period could be attributed to cigarette smoking. Of these deaths, one-third were due to lung cancer, one-third to other cancers and one-third to other diseases. Only 7% of the women described themselves as current cigarette smokers at the time of the baseline survey, but they also showed a statistically significant excess of overall mortality (relative risk, 1.7; 95% CI, 1.2–2.5; $p < 0.01$).

Conclusions: Cigarette smoking is already a major cause of death in China, and about 20% of all deaths among middle-aged Shanghai men during the 1980s were due to smoking. The excess was greatest among men who began smoking before the age of 25, about 47% of whom would, at 1987 mortality rates, die at ages 35–69, as compared with only 29% of non-smokers. These estimates reflect the consequences of past smoking patterns. The future effects of current smoking are likely to be larger owing to the recent large increase in cigarette consumption, particularly among the young, in China.

Introduction

In recent decades, there has been a rapid, substantial increase in tobacco consumption in China, particularly among men. On the basis of experience in the west, it has been estimated that, if current smoking patterns persist, tobacco will eventually cause over 2 million deaths each year in China (Peto et al., 1987). Little is known from epidemiological studies, however, about the pattern of tobacco-related deaths and about the evolution of this epidemic in China. This report is of a 16-year prospective study of smoking and mortality in Shanghai.

Methods

The study population consisted of 9351 middle-aged adults (6494 men and 2857 women) from 11 factories surveyed during the 1970s in Shanghai (Chen et al., 1991). Vital status was monitored regularly throughout the factories until 1 January 1993, and the causes of death were sought chiefly from official death certificates, supplemented if necessary by hospital records and by enquiries to family members and factory medical staff. The underlying cause of each death was coded according to ICD-9. During an average of 16 years of follow-up, 389 (4%) individuals were lost to follow-up and 1088 (12%) died. Of these 1088 deaths, 414 (38%) were from neoplastic disease, 384 (35%) were attributed to cardiovascular disease, 93 (9%) were attributed to chronic obstructive pulmonary disease and 180 (17%) to other known causes.

Data for men and women were analysed separately. For men, three categories of smoking at the time of the baseline survey were used: non-smoker, current smoker of 1–19 cigarettes per day and current smoker of ≥ 20 cigarettes per day. As relatively few women were studied and their prevalence of smoking was low, only two categories of smoking were used: non-smoker and current cigarette smoker. The standardized mortality ratio was calculated by the indirect method in a particular smoking category, adjusted for age (five-year groups) and factory. The Cox proportional hazards model was used to estimate relative risks (RRs) and their corresponding 95% confidence intervals (CIs), with simultaneous adjustment for various baseline variables.

Results

Prevalence of cigarette smoking at baseline

At the time of the baseline survey, 61% of the men and 7% of the women were current cigarette smokers. Among the male smokers, 38% had started smoking before the age of 25, and 62% had begun at a later age; the corresponding figures for female smokers were 25 and 75%. Individuals who had started smoking at an early age were particularly likely to be heavy smokers: 56% of men who had started before the age of 25 compared with 41% of those who had started later smoked 20 or more cigarettes daily; the corresponding figures for women were 24 and 8%.

Cancer mortality by smoking habit among men

Among men, cigarette smoking was associated with a 1.8-fold (95% CI, 1.4–2.3; $p < 0.001$) RR for dying from cancer (Table 1), suggesting that about one-third of all deaths from cancer among the men were due to tobacco. The total cancer mortality rates per 100 000 were 231 for non-smokers, 364 for those who smoked 1–19 cigarettes daily and 478 for those who smoked 20 or more cigarettes a day ($p < 0.0001$ for trend). Most of the excess mortality from cancer among male smokers was due to excesses of cancers of the lung (RR, 3.8; $p < 0.001$), oesophagus (RR, 3.6; $p < 0.05$) and liver (RR, 2.0; $p < 0.05$). For cancer of the lung and oesophagus, there was also a strong positive dose–response effect between risk and the number of cigarettes smoked. The risks for lung cancer were particularly large among men who had started before the age of 25; relative to non-smokers, the RRs were 4.3 (95% CI, 2.6–7.2; $p < 0.001$) for those who smoked 1–19 cigarettes daily and 9.2 (95% CI, 6.2–13.5; $p < 0.001$) for those who smoked 20 or more cigarettes daily.

Mortality from vascular disease by smoking habit among men

No significant association was seen among men between cigarette smoking and death from all vascular diseases (RR, 1.1; 95% CI, 0.9–1.4) (Table 1). Of these deaths, only 69 were attributed to coronary heart disease, and they were significantly associated with smoking (RR, 1.8; 95% CI, 1.0–3.2; $p < 0.05$), with a positive dose–response effect between the risk and the number of cigarettes smoked ($p < 0.05$ for trend). The rate of death from stroke was high (23% of total deaths), but there was no apparent association with cigarette smoking. Cigarette smoking was associated with a non-significant twofold increase in the risk for dying from pulmonary heart disease. (This condition should, however, perhaps be considered with chronic obstructive pulmonary disease and not with vascular disease; see below.) Only 16 of the deaths among men were attributed to other vascular diseases, including five from rheumatic heart disease (all in non-smokers) and one from congenital heart disease. The risk of death from other vascular diseases was significantly lower among smokers (RR, 0.3; 95% CI, 0.08–0.83; $p < 0.05$), perhaps because pre-existing rheumatic heart disease prevented smoking.

Mortality from respiratory and other diseases by smoking habit among men

There was a strong positive association between cigarette smoking and the overall risk among men for dying from respiratory disease (Table 1). Most of these deaths were attributed to chronic obstructive pulmonary disease, for which the RR of death among smokers was 2.5 (95% CI, 1.4–4.4; $p < 0.01$). A strong positive dose–response association was also evident between the risk and the number of cigarettes smoked ($p < 0.0001$ for trend). No significant association was seen between cigarette smoking and death from the aggregate of all other causes.

Total mortality rate by smoking habits among men and women

Overall, the number of deaths from all causes was significantly increased among male smokers (RR, 1.4; 95% CI, 1.2–1.7; $p < 0.0001$), with a strong positive dose–response relationship between risk and the number of cigarettes smoked ($p < 0.0001$ for trend) (Table 1). This suggests that about 20% (95% CI, 12–29%) of all deaths in this Chinese male population could be due to cigarette smoking, including 63% of the deaths from lung cancer. Of all the deaths caused by tobacco, however, only one-third were due to lung cancer, about one-third being due to other cancers and one-third involving non-neoplastic diseases. When compared with non-smokers (39% of all men), the RRs for men who started smoking before the age of 25 (23%) and later (38%) were

Table 1. Age-standardized annual mortality rates and relative risks by smoking status at the time of the baseline survey among middle-aged men in Shanghai, China

Cause of death (ICD-9)	Mortality per 100 000 persons (and relative risks[a])					z value for trend[c]
	No. of deaths (51 568[a])	All smokers	Non-smokers (40 381[a])	No. of cigarettss smoked per day		
				1–19 (34 684[a])	≥ 20 (26 884[a])	
Cancer						
Lung (161)	97	128 (3.8)***	36 (1.0)	105 (2.8)**	164 (5.4)****	5.25****
Oesophagus (150)	29	38 (3.6)*	11 (1.0)	30 (2.8)	49 (4.6)**	2.63**
Liver (155)	66	78 (2.0)*	42 (1.0)	77 (2.1)*	80 (1.9)	1.84
Colorectal (153, 154)	22	26 (1.8)	14 (1.0)	22 (1.5)	33 (2.6)	1.51
Stomach (151)	85	87 (1.0)	81 (1.0)	88 (1.1)	84 (0.9)	−0.24
Other neoplastic	51	53 (1.1)	46 (1.0)	43 (0.9)	69 (1.4)	0.83
All (140–239)	351	408 (1.8)****	231 (1.0)	364 (1.6)**	478 (2.1)****	4.82****
Vascular disease						
Coronary heart disease (410–414)	69	76 (1.8)*	52 (1.0)	74 (1.7)	80 (2.0)*	2.05*
Stroke (430–438)	199	192 (1.0)	201 (1.0)	187 (1.0)	200 (1.1)	0.71
Pulmonary heart disease (416)	24	29 (2.0)	14 (1.0)	35 (2.2)	19 (1.5)	0.76
Other vascular	16	7 (0.3)*	31 (1.0)	7 (0.2)*	8 (0.4)	−1.82
All (390–459)	308	305 (1.1)	298 (1.0)	302 (1.1)	309 (1.2)	1.27
Respiratory disease						
Chronic obstructive pulmonary disease (490–496)	82	103 (2.5)**	40 (1.0)	83 (1.9)*	139 (3.7)***	3.95****
Other	12	9 (0.7)	16 (1.0)	6 (0.4)	14 (1.2)	0.09
All (460–519)	94	113 (2.0)**	57 (1.0)	89 (1.5)	152 (3.1)****	3.72***
Other known causes						
Chronic liver disease (571)	25	34 (1.5)	20 (1.0)	30 (1.3)	39 (1.7)	1.07
Trauma (E800–E999)	18	16 (0.6)	21 (1.0)	16 (0.5)	16 (0.5)	−0.83
Other disease	55	57 (1.1)	49 (1.0)	58 (1.1)	54 (1.2)	0.53
All non-cancer, non-vascular non-chronic obstructive pulmonarydiseae	102	106 (1.1)	90 (1.0)	104 (1.1)	109 (1.2)	0.69
Unknown causes	26	24 (1.1)	28 (1.0)	32 (1.5)	9 (0.4)	−0.60
All causes	881	955 (1.4)****	702 (1.0)	890 (1.3)**	1059 (1.6)****	5.23****

[a] Relative risks were estimated in a Cox proportional hazards model, stratified for factories and adjusted for age (years), serum cholesterol (mg/dl) and regular alcohol drinking (yes vs no) at baseline
[b] Observed person–years
[c] Trend test is for non-smokers vs smokers of 1–19 vs smokers of 20 or more cigarettes daily; z values of 1.96, 2.57, 3.29 and 3.89 correspond to two-tailed p values of 0.05, 0.01, 0.001 and 0.0001, respectively, systolic blood pressure (mm Hg), serum
* $p < 0.05$, ** $p < 0.01$, *** $p < 0.001$ and **** $p < 0.0001$ in comparison with non-smokers

1.8 and 1.2, respectively. Assuming the death rates in Shanghai in 1987, the probability that a 35-year-old man will die by age 69 is 36%, which, taken together with present results, suggests that the corresponding probabilities would be 29% for non-smokers and 47% for smokers who began before the age of 25 and 35% for those who began later. Among women, smoking was also associated with a highly significantly increased risk of death from all causes (Table 2). The total mortality rate per 1000 was 393 for non-smokers and 627 for smokers (RR, 1.7; 95% CI 1.2–2.5; $p < 0.01$), with significant excess risks for dying from vascular and respiratory diseases. Hence, in this female population, with a 7% prevalence of smoking, about 5% (95% CI, 1–9%) of the deaths could be attributed to smoking.

Discussion

This study shows that cigarette smoking is a major cause of death in Shanghai, particularly among men. About one-fifth of all deaths among middle-aged men can now be attributed to tobacco, the chief sources of the excess being deaths from lung cancer, oesophageal cancer, coronary heart disease and chronic obstructive pulmonary disease. While far fewer women than men were smokers, there was also a statistically significant excess of overall mortality among female smokers. These results are consistent with recent reports from a shorter prospective study of smoking and mortality among 18 000 middle-aged Shanghai men (Yuan *et al.*, 1996).

In our study, the RR for lung cancer among male smokers was 3.8, and smoking was responsible for about 63% of deaths from lung cancer. This proportion is consistent with the results of other studies in China (Liu, 1992) but much lower than that reported in western populations, where typically a 20-fold increase in risk is seen. This finding may reflect the shorter duration of cigarette smoking and the relatively late age at starting to smoke in China. There may also be a relatively high background rate of lung cancer that is not related to smoking (Mumford *et al.*, 1987; Yuan *et al.*, 1996). As the incidence rate of lung cancer among men in Shanghai during the 1980s was already about two-thirds that in the United States (Yuan *et al.*, 1996), the absolute risk for lung cancer due to smoking in China is already large, even though the RR for lung cancer among Chinese smokers is currently much lower than that among western smokers. Moreover, the mean cigarette consumption of Chinese males increased by more than twofold between 1972 and 1992, from four to 10 per man per day, and there is evidence that smokers are starting at earlier ages (Collaborative Group for Investigating Prevalence of Smoking, 1987). The high background risk among male Chinese non-smokers may be reduced substantially in the future, e.g. by limiting indoor air pollution from cooking

Table 2. Age-standardized annual mortality rates and relative risks by smoking status at the time of the baseline survey among women in Shanghai, China

Cause of death (ICD-9)	No. of deaths	Mortality per 100 000 persons		Relative risk among smokers[a] (and 95% CI)	z value
		Non-smoker at baseline (45 685[b])	Current smoker at baseline (3409[b])		
All neoplastic disease (140–239)	82	170	143	0.9 (0.4–1.9)	–0.26
All vascular disease (390–459)	76	139	255	2.1 (1.2–3.7)	2.47*
All respiratory disease (460–519)	14	14	123	11 (3.4–33)	4.09****
Other causes[c]	35	69	89	1.2 (0.5–3.3)	0.43
All causes	207	393	627	1.7 (1.2–2.5)	2.82**

[a] Relative risks were estimated in a Cox proportional hazards model, stratified for factories and adjusted for age (years), systolic blood pressure (mm Hg), serum cholesterol (mg/dl) and regular alcohol drinking (yes vs no) at baseline.
[b] Observed person–years
[c] Including seven deaths from unknown causes

* $p < 0.05$, ** $p < 0.01$ and **** $p < 0.0001$ in comparison with non-smokers

and heating (Mumford *et al.*, 1987). If they are not, a combination of the high smoking prevalence, the increasing RR due to the effects of more prolonged smoking and the high background rate will mean that tobacco-attributable rates of death from lung cancer in China will soon exceed those now seen in the United States.

Most studies of possible associations between cigarette smoking and liver cancer have been conducted in populations in the west, where the rates of liver cancer are extremely low and alcoholic cirrhosis may be of greater relative importance than in China. Furthermore, the results have been inconsistent. In China, the rate of liver cancer is high and is strongly related to lifelong infection with hepatitis B virus and probably also to exposure to aflatoxins in foodstuffs. In the present study, smoking was associated with a marginally significant, twofold increase in the risk for death from liver cancer, which was independent of alcohol consumption. Similar findings have been reported in other studies in Chinese populations (Yu & Henderson, 1987; Yuan *et al.*, 1996). If this association is causal, it could be of particular public health importance in China, where liver cancer is already a major cause of death.

Cigarette smoking is an important cause of coronary heart disease in western populations, and the present study indicates that cigarette smoking is also a risk factor for these conditions in China, where the mortality rate from the disease is low. By contrast, although smoking has been shown to be a risk factor for stroke in western populations (Yu & Henderson, 1987), particularly in middle-aged people (Neaton *et al.*, 1984), there was no clear association between stroke and cigarette smoking in this or other Chinese populations (Yuan *et al.*, 1996), despite high rates of stroke. About 40% of newly diagnosed cases of stroke in China are due to haemorrhage (Li *et al.*, 1985), which is about three times the proportion reported in many western populations. Haemorrhagic stroke is associated with a higher fatality rate than ischaemic stroke. Therefore, the apparent lack of association between cigarette smoking and mortality from any type of stroke in this Chinese population may be because the association with smoking is mainly for ischaemic stroke (Shinton & Beevers, 1989).

Although the background rates of chronic obstructive pulmonary disease are low in western populations, cigarette smoking still causes large numbers of deaths from the disease, since the RRs are high (10 or more). In China, the background rates among non-smokers are substantial, particularly in rural areas. Thus, although the RR may currently be only twofold, the absolute rate of death from tobacco-related chronic obstructive pulmonary disease is probably already higher in China than in the west.

In summary, our results confirm the reports that cigarette smoking is a major cause of death in China and that about one-fifth of all deaths among middle-aged Shanghai men are caused by the habit. The current health effects of smoking chiefly reflect the consequences of past smoking patterns, however, and the future health effects of current smoking patterns are likely to become much greater, given the recent large increase in cigarette consumption, particularly among the young, in China.

References

Chen, Z.M., Peto, R., Collins, R., MacMahon, S., Lu, J.R. & Li, W.X. (1991) Serum cholesterol concentration and coronary heart disease in population with low cholesterol concentrations. *Br. Med. J.*, **303**, 276–282

Collaborative Group for Investigating Prevalence of Smoking (1987) [Results of national sampling survey on prevalence of smoking.] *Chin. Med. J.*, **67**, 229–232 (in Chinese)

Li, S.C., Schoenberb, B.S., Wang, C.C., Cheng, X.M., Bolis, C.L. & Wang, K.J. (1985) Cerebrovascular disease in the People's Republic of China: Epidemiologic and clinical features. *Neurology*, **35**, 1708–1713

Liu, Z.Y. (1992) Smoking and lung cancer in China: Combined analysis of eight case–control studies. *Int. J. Epidemiol.*, **21**, 197–201

Mumford, J.L., He, X.Z., Chapman, R.S., Cao, S.R., Harris, D.B., Li, X.M., Xian, Y.L., Jiang, W.Z., Xu, C.W., Chuang, J.C., Wilson, W.E. & Cooke, M. (1987) Lung cancer and indoor air pollution in Xuan Wei, China. *Science*, **235**, 217–220

Neaton, J.D., Kuller, L., Wentworth, D. & Borhani, N.O. (1984) Total and cardiovascular mortality in relation to cigarette smoking, serum cholesterol concentration and diastolic blood pressure among black and white men followed five years. *Am. Heart J.*, **109**, 759–770.

Peto, R. (1987) Tobacco-related deaths in China. *Lancet*, **ii**, 211

Shinton, R. & Beevers, G. (1989) Meta-analysis of relation between cigarette smoking and stroke. *Br. Med. J.*, **298**, 789–794
Yu, M.C. & Henderson, B.E. (1987) A case–control study of hepatocellular carcinoma and the hepatitis B virus, cigarette smoking and alcohol consumption. *Cancer Res.*, 47, 654–655
Yuan, J.M., Ross, R.K., Wang, X.L., Gao, Y.T., Henderson, B.E. & Yu, M.C. (1996) Morbidity and mortality in relation to cigarette smoking: A prospective male cohort study in Shanghai, China. *J. Am. Med. Assoc.*, 275, 1646–1650

Smoking and related cancers and other diseases: Results of a 10-year prospective study in Shanghai, China

Y.-T. Gao[1], J. Deng[1], Y.-B. Xiang[1], Z.-X. Ruan[1], Z.-X. Wang[2], B.-Y. Hu[3], M.-R. Guo[4], W.-K. Teng[5], J.-J. Han[6] & Y.-S. Zhang[7]

[1]Shanghai Cancer Institute, [2]Shanghai Anti-tuberculosis, [3]Lu-wan District Centre of Anti-tuberculosis, [4]Hong-kou District Centre of Anti-tuberculosis, [5]Pu-kuo District Centre of Anti-tuberculosis, [6]Shanghai County Centre of Anti-tuberculosis and [7]Feng-xian County Centre of Anti-tuberculosis, Shanghai, China

Abstract

Objective: To explore the relationship between smoking and related diseases among residents of Shanghai.

Methods: A prospective study of smoking and mortality among 213 800 residents aged 20 years and over in urban and rural Shanghai, with over 10 years of follow-up. For subjects aged 40 years and over at the time of the baseline survey in the early 1980s, a Poisson regression model was used to estimate the relative risks for certain diseases among smokers versus non-smokers, after adjustment for age, sex and area.

Results: In urban areas, the relative risks for all causes of death among smokers in relation to non-smokers were 1.5 for men and 1.6 for women; for death from any cancer, the risks were 2.2 for men and 2.0 for women. Smoking was associated with statistically significantly increased risks for cancers of the lung and liver (men and women) and of the oesophagus, stomach, pancreas and urinary bladder (men only). Significantly higher risks were also seen among smokers for cerebrovascular disease, chronic bronchitis and emphysema and pulmonary heart disease. Similar but less extreme results were found in suburban and rural areas. The population attributable risks for death from all causes among men were 21% in urban areas, 19% in suburban areas and 16% in rural areas. For death from any cancers, the population attributable risks were 40, 34 and 34% in the three areas, and those for lung cancer were 72%, 59% and 65%, respectively.

Conclusions: Smoking is a major risk factor for death from cancer, especially for cancers of the lung, urinary bladder, oesophagus, stomach, pancreas and liver. Smoking is also associated with increased risks for dying from cerebrovascular disease, chronic bronchitis and emphysema and pulmonary heart disease.

Introduction

It is well known that tobacco smoking is hazardous to health (Doll, 1986), but there was no comprehensive information on the health effects of tobacco smoking in China until the early 1980s (Gao *et al.*, 1991). In order to explore the relationship between tobacco smoking and cancer and other tobacco-related diseases, a large-scale survey of smoking habits among residents aged 20 years and over in urban and suburban Shanghai and in nearby rural areas was carried out during 1982–83. Subsequently, a prospective follow-up study of the health effects of tobacco smoking was organized for the subjects in the survey. In this paper, we report the results of the first 10 years of follow-up of this cohort.

Materials and methods

Residents aged 20 years and over from urban, suburban and rural areas were selected, and their smoking habits were investigated at the time of the baseline survey during the early 1980s. There were 112 715 subjects in the urban area and 101 582 in the suburban and rural areas, accounting for 94 and 99% of the total population in the corresponding areas. Smokers were defined as people who had smoked one cigarette or more per day for at least one year. All subjects were interviewed at home by trained staff. For quality control of the data, and especially for smoking status, about 5% of all study subjects were re-interviewed (Deng et al., 1985).

The study subjects in the urban area were followed up for 12 years, from January 1983 to December 1994, and those in the suburban and rural areas for 11 years, from January 1984 to December 1994. The causes of death of study subjects were determined annually from official death certificates and were confirmed individually by medical professionals. Persons lost to follow-up were recorded.

The information from the baseline survey was computerized and then updated with the results of several follow-ups conducted before 1995. The last follow-up was carried out in early 1995. In order to estimate the number of person–years at risk for study subjects, record linkage was performed between the updated computer files and the results of the last follow-up which contained information on vital status (alive and still in cohort, deceased, lost to follow-up) and all deaths from cancer among the deceased subjects. Only information on study subjects aged 40 years and over at the start of follow-up was considered in the analysis reported in this paper. Women in suburban and rural areas were not included in the analysis because the prevalence of tobacco smoking was only 3.1 and 1.5%, respectively. Three variables of smoking were used in the statistical analysis: smoking status (yes/no); number of cigarette smoked per day $(0, 1-9, 10-19, \geq 20)$; and age at starting to smoke (non-smoker, ≥ 30, 20–29, < 20 years).

The observed person–years at risk during the period of follow-up were calculated separately by sex, age group, smoking status and study area. The person–years for subjects lost to follow-up were estimated by allowing half a year for the year in which they were lost to follow-up. The software PYTAB was used to calculate person–years (Preston & pierce, 1986). A Poisson regression model was fitted with GLIM(S) (Baker & Nelder, 1985) software and used to estimate the relative risks (RRs) for diseases related to smoking together with 95% confidence intervals (CIs), separately by sex and area, and adjusted for age. Tests were also made for linear trends in RRs with the number of cigarettes smoked and with age at which smoking started. The prevalence of smoking among men and women aged 40 years and over in the three selected study areas was estimated from their smoking status at the beginning of the study (Deng et al., 1985), and the population attributable risks due to smoking (PARs) with 95% CIs for selected causes of death due to smoking were calculated.

Results

The numbers of subjects aged 40 years and over at the beginning of follow-up were 59 685 in urban areas, 38 825 in suburban areas and 53 430 in rural areas, and the proportions of persons lost to follow-up were 4.0, 0.5 and 1.2%, respectively. The numbers of deaths during the interval of follow-up were 6866 among men and 5032 among women in the urban area and 3869 among men and 3985 among women in the suburban and rural areas. The leading causes of death, in order, were cancer, cerebrovascular disease, chronic bronchitis and emphysema, pulmonary heart disease and coronary heart disease for men and women in the urban area, and chronic bronchitis and emphysema and pulmonary heart disease for men in suburban and rural areas.

The relative risks for causes of death that occurred more frequently among smokers than non-smokers are presented in Table 1. Except for oesophageal cancer, liver cancer and pulmonary disease, the relative risks for men were highest in the urban area. The relative risks for urban females were also higher than those for men in suburban and

Table 1. Relative risk estimates[a] for smokers versus non-smokers by cause of death, adjusted for age, in Shanghai, China

Cause of death	Urban		Suburban (male)	Rural (male)
	Male	Female		
All causes	1.5[b-d]	1.6[b-d]	1.3[b-d]	1.2[b-d]
All cancers	2.2[b-d]	2.0[b-d]	1.7[b-d]	1.6[b-d]
Oesophageal cancer	2.6[b-d]	1.9	3.3[b-d]	1.8[b,d]
Stomach cancer	1.9[b-d]	1.2	1.3	1.3
Liver cancer	1.5[b-d]	2.4[b-d]	1.4	1.5[b,c]
Pancreatic cancer	1.7[b,c]	1.5	0.70	1.4
Lung cancer	5.6[b-d]	4.8[b-d]	2.9[b-d]	3.3[b-d]
Urinary bladder cancer	1.9[b]	1.7	0.74	1.6
All non-cancer causes	1.3[b-d]	1.5[b-d]	1.2[b-d]	1.1[b,d]
Cerebrovascular disease	1.4[b-d]	1.2[b]	1.1	0.88
Pulmonary heart disease	1.3[c,d]	3.1[b-d]	1.8[b-d]	1.6[b-d]
Chronic bronchitis and emphysema	1.8[b-d]	3.4[b-d]	1.5[b-d]	1.3[b,d]
Chronic bronchitis and emphysema and pulmonary heart disease	1.7[b-d]	3.4[b-d]	1.6[b-d]	1.5[b-d]

[a] Estimated by use of Poisson regression model adjusted for age
[b] 95% confidence interval of estimates did not include 1.0
[c] Linear trend test for number of cigarettes smoked per day (0, 1–9, 10–19, ≥ 20): $p < 0.05$
[d] Linear trend test for age at which smoking started (non-smoker, ≥ 30, 20–29, < 20): $p < 0.05$

rural areas, except for cancers of the oesophagus and stomach; for chronic bronchitis and emphysema and pulmonary heart disease, urban women had considerably higher relative risks than urban men.

Statistically significant, linear trends with the number of cigarettes smoked and age at starting smoking were observed for most of the diseases in question. Table 2 shows the results for the diseases with the most significant trends: all cancers, lung cancer and chronic obstructive lung disease. The PARs for all causes of death were 21, 19 and 16%, respectively, among urban, suburban and rural men but only 5.8% for urban women. For all cancers, the PARs were 40, 34 and 34% for men in the three areas, and 9.1% for urban women. The highest PARs were observed for lung cancer: 72, 59 and 65% for men in the three areas and 28% for urban women. For oesophageal cancer, the PARs for men were 47, 64 and 40%, respectively. The PARs for cancers of the pancreas and urinary bladder were 28 and 33% for urban men. With respect to the non-cancer causes of death selected in our analysis, the PARs for chronic bronchitis and emphysema were about 20–30% for men in three areas and 19% for urban women. For cerebrovascular disease, the PARs were 17% in urban men and 3.5% in urban women.

Table 2. Linear trend tests of relative risks (RR)[a] for smokers versus non-smokers for selected causes of death, in urban Shanghai, China

Cause of death	Overall RR	No. smoked per day		Age started smoking (years)			
		< 10	10–19	≥ 20	≥ 30	20–29	< 20
All causes	1.5*	1.3*	1.4* $p < 0.001$	1.6*	1.2* $p < 0.001$	1.5*	1.8*
All cancers	2.2*	1.6*	1.9* $p < 0.001$	2.6*	1.7* $p < 0.001$	2.2*	2.8*
Lung cancer	5.6*	2.6*	4.1* $p < 0.001$	7.7*	3.3* $p < 0.001$	5.7*	7.9*
Chronic bronchitis and emphysema	1.8*	1.3	1.8* $p < 0.001$	2.0*	1.2 $p < 0.001$	2.0*	2.2*

[a] Estimated by use of Poisson regression model adjusted for age
[b] 95% confidence interval of RRs did not include 1.0.

The PARs for pulmonary heart disease were 39% for suburban men, 34% for rural men and 18% for urban women.

Discussion

The results of our study convincingly show the deleterious effects of tobacco smoking on health in Shanghai, increasing the risks for death from cancer, chronic bronchitis and emphysema, cerebrovascular disease and pulmonary heart disease. The mortality rate from all causes among smokers was about 50% higher than that among non-smokers in the urban area, and 100% more deaths from cancer occurred among smokers. The risk of dying from lung cancer was five times higher among smokers than non-smokers. Tobacco smoking was also associated with excess risks for other cancers, chronic bronchitis and emphysema and cerebrovascular disease. The significant linear trends with the number of cigarettes smoked and the age at which smoking started in our analysis suggest a causal relationship between tobacco smoking and some diseases. Among Shanghai urban male residents aged 40 and over, 21% of all deaths, 40% of all cancer deaths and 32% of deaths from chronic bronchitis and emphysema are estimated to be caused by tobacco smoking. The relative risks of death from coronary heat disease in smokers are greater than 1.0 for both men and women in the urban area and for suburban men. Although the RRs were not significant, the lower limit of the RRs in the urban area was very close to 1.0. When we combined deaths from chronic bronchitis, emphysema and pulmonary heart diseases for statistical analysis, in order to avoid differences in diagnosis of these diseases between the urban and the other two areas, the combined results showed no difference in statistical significance (Table 1). The results of this study are consistent with those published previously in China and with interim results after five years of follow-up of this cohort (Gao et al., 1991; Deng et al., 1992; Yuan et al., 1996).

Our study has some limitations. First, the smoking status of the subjects in our study was that reported at the time of the baseline interview, and changes during follow-up could not be taken into consideration. However, the rate of smoking cessation was very low in China in the 1980s, and the smoking habits of persons aged 40 years and over tend to be stable with time. Thus, misclassification of smoking status is unlikely to have affected the statistical analysis. Secondly, the delayed effects of tobacco smoking on health should be considered. As the effects of smoking on health depend strongly on smoking habits during early adult life, current mortality rates from tobacco-related diseases in areas where smoking became widespread relatively recently (e.g. suburban and rural) may be underestimates of the eventual magnitude of the tobacco-induced hazard. Last, our analysis did not include any confounding variables associated with tobacco smoking which might affect the outcome of disease. This should be further explored in future studies.

Acknowledgments

We give special thank to the staff of the district centres for anti-tuberculosis in Hong-kou, Pu-tuo and Lu-wan, and of the centres of Shanghai and Feng-xiang counties, for data collection and field management of the cohort. The long-term mortality follow-up was supported by the MRC/ICRF/BHF Clinical Trial Service Unit & Epidemiological Studies Unit in the United Kingdom.

References

Baker, R.J. & Nelder, J.A. (1985) The GLIM System: Release 3.77 Manual, Oxford: Numerical Algorithms Group

Deng, J., Gao, Y.T., Jiao, S.M., et al. (1985) Cross-sectional survey on prevalence of smoking of 110,000 adults in Shanghai urban. Chin. J. Prev. Med., 19, 271–274

Deng, J., Gao, Y.T., Wang, Z.X., et al. (1992) Smoking, air pollution and lung cancer—Results of a prospective study of 210 000 adults in Shanghai, China. Tumor (Shanghai), 12, 258–260

Doll. R. (1986) Tobacco: An overview of health effects. In: IARC Scientific Publications No. 74, Lyon: IARC, pp. 11–22

Gao, Y.T., Zheng, W., Gao, R.N. et al. (1991) Tobacco smoking and its effect on health in China. In: IARC Scientific Publications No. 105, Lyon: LARC, pp. 62–67

Preston, D.L. & Pierce, D.A. (1986) *PYTAB—A Program for Person Year Computations (User's Guide)*,
    Hiroshima: Radiation Effects Research Foundation
Yuan, J.M., Ross, R.K., Wang, X.L., *et al.* (1996) Morbidity and mortality in relation to cigarette smoking
    in Shanghai, China. *J. Am. Med. Assoc.*, 275, 1646–1650 .

A review of case–control studies on smoking and lung cancer in China

T.H. Lam[1] & Y. He[1,2]

[1] *Department of Community Medicine, The University of Hong Kong, China*
[2] *Department of Epidemiology, Fourth Military Medical University, Xi'an, China*

Introduction

Many studies have been carried out on lung cancer and smoking in China; however, because most of the results were published in Chinese in local or national journals, they are not readily available to researchers and people involved in tobacco control in China and internationally. We were requested by the Scientific Committee of the 10th World Conference on Tobacco or Health to review the case–control studies on smoking and lung cancer in China. The aim of this paper is to present our preliminary calculations of pooled odds ratios for lung cancer due to smoking from the available studies in mainland China. We hope that this review covers all of the relevant studies on the subject for easy reference.

Methods

As this review was intended to be comprehensive, we included all reports from case–control studies with data on smoking and lung cancer, published and unpublished. We did not use any criteria to exclude reports at this stage. It is difficult to make a critical appraisal of many of the reported studies because papers written in Chinese and published in Chinese journals are usually brief as compared with papers written in English and published in international journals and do not contain sufficient detail.

We searched Medline and the Chinese Medline for original and review papers on smoking and lung cancer in mainland China. We then checked through the reference lists in the original and review papers. We also searched the proceedings of the Chinese National Symposium on Smoking and Health and relevant international conferences such as the world conferences on tobacco or health. We spoke and wrote to organizations and persons whom we knew to be knowledgeable about such studies in China, such as the Chinese Association on Smoking and Health and Professor Lu Rushan of the Institute of Medical Information, Chinese Academy of Medical Sciences. Studies from Hong Kong and Taiwan and on Chinese elsewhere were excluded, but we intend to include them later. We calculated a pooled odds ratio (OR) from the studies that presented the relevant data, using Mantel-Haenszel's method in the EPI-INFO package.

Results

Up to July 1997, we found 26 papers in Chinese and 18 in English which were relevant. There were 34 published case–control studies, 33 with data available. (Because of limitations of space, the list of 40 references is not given but is available from the authors.) We wrote to the authors of the remaining studies and are awaiting the replies. We also found four unpublished case–control studies with available data. There were three review papers, two of which were the same review (Zhao & Yu, 1993; Yu & Zhao, 1996), which gave pooled ORs (Liu, 1992; Zhao & Yu, 1993; Yu & Zhao, 1996). We also found reports of three cross-sectional studies and six prospective studies, but these are not included in the present review. The large case–control study of Liu *et al.*. and the prospective study of Niu *et al.* are described elsewhere in this volume and were also not included.

Table 1 is a summary of the 33 case–control studies. All showed positive associations between lung cancer and smoking, and all (except for the data on women in one study) showed dose–response relationships. The pooled ORs (95% confidence intervals [CI]) for lung cancer were 3.3 (2.9–3.7) for men (based on 17 studies and 10 897 subjects) and 2.5 (2.2–2.8) for women (13 studies and 6870 subjects). The pooled OR for men and women combined, based on all 33 studies and about 20 000 subjects was 2.7 (2.5–2.9). The pooled OR for the four unpublished studies with data on 914 cases and 914 controls, men and women combined, was 2.3 (1.9–2.8). As the OR from the unpublished data was consistent with that from the published papers, publication bias was unlikely to account for the observed association. On the basis of the pooled OR from the published studies, the attributable risk percentages (95% CI) for lung cancer in smokers were 70 (66–73) for men, 60 (56–64) for women and 63 (60–65) for men and women combined.

The two reviews with pooled ORs were based on 13 published and four unpublished studies. The range of the point estimates of the pooled OR was 3.0–3.1 for men and 2.3 for women.

Analysis of cell types is in progress. The preliminary results show ORs of about 6.0 for squamous carcinoma and 1.6 for adenocarcinoma in men and women combined.

Discussion

Our literature search yielded about 20 more studies than reported in previous reviews. As China is such a huge country, with no comprehensive database, especially for studies carried out earlier in smaller institutions, published in local journals or reported in unpublished reports, we are aware that a few studies might have been missed. We are also aware of the great variation in the methods and the quality of the data and the reports; however, the present review can serve as a starting source of all available data.

Despite the variations, the results were remarkably consistent. Our review showed a higher OR (3.3 in men and 2.5 in women) than previous reviews and that the majority of cases of lung cancer (70% in men and 60% in women) in smokers were attributable to smoking.

At the International Symposium on Lifestyle Factors and Human Lung Cancer in Guangzhou, China, 1996, Wu and Du reviewed the papers presented to that Conference. As the OR for lung cancer due to smoking in China was less than 5, which was lower than that in the West (> 10), they considered that 'recognition and confirmation of lung cancer as a multifactorial disease' was an important issue and stated that 'health effects attributed to cigarette smoking should be evaluated in the context of other coexisting, undesirable lifestyle factors, in order to minimize introducing exaggerated misinterpretations and oversights in scientific studies' (Wu & Du, 1996).

The lower risk estimates than in the west which have been reported in China to date should be interpreted carefully. There are several possible explanations, such as the older age at starting smoking, the smaller quantity smoked and the shorter duration of smoking. These are features of the early stage of the growing tobacco epidemic, as smoking has increased more recently in China than in western countries such as the United Kingdom and the United States. As there is a delay of several decades between the peak of tobacco consumption and the peak of tobacco-related deaths, all the reported case–control studies included here probably yielded underestimates of the risk of lung cancer due to prolonged smoking.

The lower OR observed could also be due to the higher proportion of adenocarcinoma in China than in the west, although the OR for squamous carcinoma in China also appeared to be lower than that in the west. Nevertheless, the OR of about 6 for squamous carcinoma suggests that over 80% of this cell type is already attributable to smoking, even at this early stage of the tobacco epidemic. It would be useful if researchers who describe lung cancer as multifactorial could specify that adenocarcinoma (rather than all lung cancer) is more likely to be multifactorial and could clarify that squamous carcinoma is mainly caused by smoking.

To conclude, it is clear that smoking is already the major cause of lung cancer in China and that the risks are already very high. As the epidemic progresses, with younger

Table 1. Case–control studies on lung cancer and smoking in China

No. of study	First author	Year of publication	Year of study	Location	No. of subjects cases/controls	Odds ratio (95% CI)	Dose–response	Data on cell type
1	Huang GJ	1981	1961–79	Beijing	406/512	M+F: 1.94 (0.89–4.27)	Yes	Yes
2	Liu XY	1981	?	Wuhan	111/111	M+F: 1.91 (1.03–3.58)	Yes	No
3	Xu RH	1983	1981	Tianjin	135/135	M: 5.99 (2.65–13.50); F: 4.02 (1.36–12.20)	Yes	Yes
4	Ren TS	1982	1979–81	Tianjin	216/216	M: 3.58 (1.66–7.82); F: 4.06 (2.07–8.04)	Yes	No
5	Chen XW	1983; 1985	1983	Guangzhou	193/193	M: 4.57 (1.98–10.84); F: 1.67 (0.78–3.61)	Yes	No
6	Wang JS	1985	1980–82	Taiyuan	103/71	M+F: 2.71 (1.71–6.36)	Yes	No
7	Zheng W	1986	1982–84	Shanghai	540/540	M: 3.65 (2.31–5.77); F: 2.09 (1.33–3.29)	Yes	No
8	Jiang MH	1987	1984	Nanchang	125/125	M: 2.72 (1.00–7.66); F: 2.49 (0.64–10.01)	Yes	No
9	Liu Q	1987	1983–84	Guangzhou	203/203	M+F: 3.28 (p < 0.01)	No	No
10	Gao YT; Zhong LJ	1987; 1988; 1991	1984–86	Shanghai	1405/1495	M: 3.9 (2.9–5.4); F: 2.5 (2.0–3.3)	Yes	Yes
11	Hu JF	1988	77–79	Harbin	523/523	M: 3.03 (2.04–4.49); F: 1.88 (1.21–2.91)	Yes	No
12	Wu KG	1989	73–86	Dachang	69/138	M+F: 2.0 (p > 0.05)	Yes	No
13	Xu ZY	1989; 1996	1985–87	Shenyang	1249/1345	M: 2.7 (2.1–3.5)[a]	Yes	No
14	Wu-Williams	1990; 1993	1985–87	Harbin, Shenyang	965/959	M: 2.6 (2.0–3.3)[a]; F: 2.3 (1.9–2.8)[a]	Yes	Adenocarcinoma
15	Sun XW	1990	1985–87	Harbin	140/140	F: 1.22 (0.83–1.80)	Yes	No
16	Liu ZY	1990	1985–86	Xuanwei	110/426	M: 1.20 (0.37–4.39)	Yes	No
17	Zhang HS	1990	1988–89	Jinzhou	100/200	M: 4.00 (1.6–9.9)[a]; F: 3.75 (1.3–10.8)[a]	Yes	No
18	Wang H	1990	1975–87	Baotou	61/122	M: 2.96 (0.90–10.8)	Yes	No
19	Liu P	1991	1983–90	Chongqing	355/350	M: 1.90 (1.05–3.43)	Yes	Yes
20	Yu ZF	1992	1987–88	Harbin	680/680	M+F: 3.50 (2.78–4.40)	Yes	Yes
21	Liu MS	1992	1987–91	Changchun	104/128	M: 4.32 (2.20–8.56); F: 1.67 (0.14–44.48)	Yes	No
22	Fan RL	1992	1990–91	Beijing	403/1151	M: 2.84 (1.90–4.26); F: 3.92 (2.60–5.92)	No	Yes
23	Wang GX	1992	?	Nanjing	154/154	M+F: Association	Yes	No
24	Lubin JH	1992	1984–88	Gejiu	427/1011	M: 2.81 (1.34–6.09)	Yes	No

Table 1 (contd)

No. of study	First author	Year of publication	Year of study	Location	No. of subjects cases/controls	Odds ratio (95% CI)	Dose-response	Data on cell type
25	Huang CY	1992	1990–91	Shichuan	135/135	M+F: 2.00 (1.2–3.4)	Yes	No
26	Liu Q	1993	1983–84	Guangzhou	316/316	M: 4.32 (2.13–8.93) F: 4.26 (2.17–8.41)	Yes	Yes
27	Fu H	1994	1973–89	Dachang	79/188	M: 3.49 (1.8–6.9)	Yes	No
28	Tan AJ	1995	1990–94	Wuhan	156/156	M+F: 1.89 (1.14–3.13) [a]	Yes	No
29	Wang SY	1995 1996	1990–93	Guangzhou	390/390	M: 3.47 (p < 0.01) F: 4.00 (p < 0.01) M+F: 2.88 (1.74–4.77) [a]	Yes Yes	Yes
30	Du YX	1996	1980–85	Guangzhou	849/849	M: 3.54 (2.44–5.11) F: 1.93 (1.30–2.87)	Yes	Yes
31	Lei YX	1996	1986	Guangzhou	792/792	M: 3.68 (2.48–5.48) F: 3.49 (2.28–5.35)	Yes	No
32	Shen XB	1996	1986–93	Nanjing	263/263	Association	Yes	Yes
33	Luo RX	1996	1990–91	Fuzhou	102/306	M+F: 2.7 (1.5–5.0)	Yes	Yes

No. of cases/controls
Pooled OR (95% CI):

M: 4758/6139
3.29 (2.94–3.74)

F: 3266/3604
2.49 (2.25–2.77)

M+F: 1459/1731
2.63 (2.27–3.09)

Total: 9438/11 474
2.72 (2.53–2.89)

Mantel–Haenszel
[based on studies]:

[3–5, 7, 8, 10, 11, 13, 16, 18, 19, 21, 22, 24, 26, 27, 31]

[3–5, 7, 8, 10, 11, 13, 14, 21, 22, 26, 31]

[1, 2, 6, 17, 20, 25, 28, 33]

OR, odds ratio; M, male; F, female
[a] Adjusted OR

people starting to smoke and increasing amounts and duration of smoking, the magnitude of the risk will continue to increase. Tobacco control is the single most important measure in preventing and checking this growing epidemic. Any attempt to divert attention away from smoking, on the basis of the lower risks currently observed, must be examined cautiously.

Acknowledgements
    We wish to thank the University of Hong Kong for the studentship for Dr Y. He, Professor R.S. Lu and Professor S. He of the Chinese Academy of Preventive Medicine and Dr Q.L. Shi of the 4th Military Medical University for their assistance in the literature search and Ms Marie Chi for clerical assistance.

Additional references

Liu, Z.Y. (1992) Smoking and lung cancer in China: Combined analysis of eight case–control studies. *Int. J. Epidemiol.*, **2**, 197–201
Wu, J.M. & Du, Y.X. (1996) Summary of papers and research recommendations presented at the International Symposium on Lifestyle Factors and Human Lung Cancer, Guangzhou, China. *Lung Cancer*, **14** (Suppl. 1), S223–S234
Yu, S.Z. & Zhao, N. (1996) Combined analysis of case–control studies of smoking and lung cancer in China. *Lung Cancer*, **14** (Suppl. 1), S161–S170
Zhao, N. & Yu, S.Z. (1993) Meta-analysis of smoking and lung cancer in China: Combined analysis of fifteen case control studies. *Chung-Hua-Liu-Hsing-Ping-Hsueh-Tsa-Chih*, **14**(6), 350–354

Analysis of the lung cancer epidemic in Taiwan: A crisis?

C.P. Wen, S.P. Tsai & D.D. Yen

University of Texas School of Public Health, Houston, Texas, United States and the John Tung Foundation, Taipei, Taiwan, China

Introduction

The number of deaths from lung cancer in Taiwan has increased fivefold during the past 24 years, and this has become the commonest cancer over the past 15 years. Yet the public and health professionals are not alarmed by this dramatic increase, and hence there is no near-term prospect for a reversal of this trend. We have analysed the causes of this increase and the reasons for the apathy about a situation that is nearing a crisis.

Methods

Standard statistical methods were used, including direct adjustment for age, to mortality data obtained from the Department of Health in Taiwan (Department of Health, 1995).

Results

Figure 1 shows the time trends in age-specific mortality rates from lung cancer among males in Taiwan in 1971–95. The increase was most marked for men > 60, and the increase was almost eightfold by the age of 80. The rates of increase have not slowed down but on the contrary seem to have accelerated recently, most notably in the past five years. In the meantime, the population of Taiwan has increased by 43% and the number of deaths from all causes, by 38%. The age-adjusted mortality rates in males increased by 106%. There were 74% more deaths from lung cancer among males than females in 1971, but by 1995 there were 151% more. When regression lines are fitted, as shown in Figure 2, the total number of deaths from lung cancer is projected to increase to more than 9000 in 2010, from 900 in 1971 and 5200 in 1995. The excess number of deaths from lung cancer in the next 15 years will be 100 000, when compared with 1971, and the excess cost will be US$ 6000 million.

Figure 1. Time trends in age-specific rates of lung cancer per 100 000 males, Taiwan, 1971–95

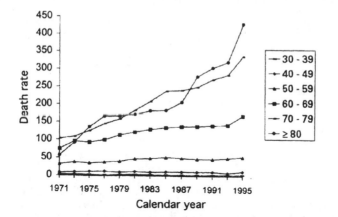

Figure 2. Observed and projected numbers of deaths from lung cancer among males, Taiwan, 1971–2010

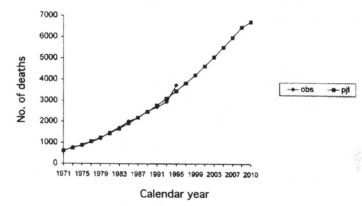

Circles, observed; squares, projected

Discussion

The increase in the rates of lung cancer has been phenomenal. One in eight persons died from all types of cancer in 1971 and one in four in 1995, and the rates for lung cancer during the same period increased from one in nine deaths from cancer to one in five. The increase has accelerated within the past few years, with a fivefold increase among older men. Much of the increase (71%) is real, whereas an increase in the population (8%) and ageing of the population (21%) accounted for the remainder. Smoking was the main cause, accounting for 46% of all deaths from lung cancer, with 66% among males and 9% among females (Tsai et al., this volume). Air pollution, a combination of emissions from the rapidly increasing number of cars and motorcycles and industrial pollution in a booming economy, accounted for as much as 20%, either by itself or in synergistic interaction with smoking.

This increase in the rates of lung cancer meets or exceeds the requirements for an epidemic, but by its magnitude and implications the increase has become a crisis, for the following reasons:

(1) Lung cancer is associated with an extremely high rate of case fatality, and the physical and emotional suffering of both the victims and their families are

beyond description. For society as a whole, the drain on the economy is enormous, with an estimated US$ 60 million a year in direct costs and US$ 260 million in indirect costs. The number of deaths from lung cancer increased fivefold in 24 years, and another fivefold increase will occur in the next 15 years. It has taken only three years to achieve an increase that took 10 years in the 1970s, and it will take only one year to attain that increase in the coming 15 years.

(2) The increase is expected to continue for at least another 20–30 years before any reversal occurs, even if the society were to become smoke-free overnight. This is because carcinogens such as tobacco smoke have a latency of 30 years or more.

(3) The public appears to be unaware of the epidemic and of the urgency to act. They do not know the available options in the battle against smoking-induced cancer. Once stricken by the disease, people cling to the wishful thought that the most advanced treatment available will cure them. The reality is that treatment for lung cancer is disappointing: less than 10% of patients survive for more than five years. Not only are significant resources wasted, but patients suffer both physically and emotionally by going through the treatment process.

(4) The medical profession has been ingrained with the treatment modality and, indeed, has been rewarded for continuing to use curative therapy, whether or not it is effective. As a result, it has little incentive to attack the root of the problem, such as advocating prevention among the healthy population. Given the high prevalence of smoking and the ever-worsening air pollution, the worst is yet to come. This is true particularly because of the insidious nature of the disease, its etiological elusiveness and the exhausting and disappointing treatment. The Government has increased expenditure on medical care but almost exclusively for treatment, which in this case is almost ineffective. As long as the conventional demand for treatment continues, there will be no 'light at the end of the tunnel' in the current 'crisis'.

Conclusion

Unless medical resources are diverted from treatment to prevention, such as anti-smoking campaigns, the increasing trend in deaths from lung cancer will persist for the next 20–30 years, and thousands of millions of US dollars will be wasted. Time is running out. The pending crisis must be publicized. The public must be behind a shift in emphasis in health care.

Reference
Department of Health (1995) *Health Statistics 2. Vital Statistics*, Taipei

Effect of additive interaction between tobacco smoking and domestic radon on the occurrence of lung cancer: A Spanish case–control study

B. Takkouche[1], A. Montes-Martinez[1], A. Barreiro-Carracedo[1] & J. Barros-Dios[1,2]

[1]Department of Preventive Medicine, University of Santiago de Compostela, and
[2]Unit of Preventive Medicine, Complexo Hospitalario Universitario de Santiago, Spain

Introduction

Exposure to residential radon is suspected to be a risk factor for lung cancer, in addition to tobacco smoking, the carcinogenic potential of which is firmly established by more than three decades of evidence (Lubin et al., 1994; Takkouche & Gestal-Otero, 1996). So far, few studies have focused on the effect of joint exposure to tobacco smoking and domestic radon on the occurrence of lung cancer. Such synergy or interaction has been evaluated only as the magnitude of a product term of the individual effects in a regression model in which interaction is defined as a departure from the product of the absolute effects of the two causes. This approach to synergy is uninformative if not clearly misleading. We used Rothman's concept of interaction (Rothman, 1986), defined as a departure from additivity of the individual effects of tobacco smoking and radon, to measure this interaction.

Subjects and methods

In 1992 a case–control study was undertaken in the area of Santiago de Compostela in north-west Spain in order to assess the causal relationship between exposure to radon and lung cancer in a region with high indoor radon concentrations due to the granitic subsoil. The 'cases' were residents of the area of Santiago de Compostela with histologically confirmed, newly-diagnosed primary lung cancer (code 162 of ICD9) who attended the hospital complex of Santiago de Compostela between January 1992 and December 1994. These cases represented all cases of lung cancer that occurred in the area during that time. Only patients who had lived in their current dwelling for five years or more were included in the study. The 'controls' were selected randomly from the 1991 Spanish population census of the Santiago area and were frequency-matched to cases by sex. Only persons older than 35 years were included; those with a previous history of cancer at any site or major respiratory disease were excluded, as were persons with former occupational or therapeutic exposure to radiation.

Interviews were carried out by two staff members trained for this purpose, whenever possible with the selected patient. In some instances, because of the incapacity of the patient, the next-of-kin was interviewed about the patient's habits. The questionnaire included information on the dwelling (location, type, building material, age, alterations), tobacco and alcohol consumption and family antecedents of lung cancer. The interview and radon measurements took place over the same period for cases and controls, and the same schedule was used in both instances. An alpha-track monitor was used for radon measurements, positioned for three to six months.

Logistic regression was used to estimate adjusted odds ratios (ORs) and their 95% confidence intervals. Except for variables that were forced into the model for their biological relevance (age and sex), we used the change-in estimate method to introduce confounding variables (Greenland, 1989). The general fit of the model was assessed by the Hosmer and Lemeshow test (1989). In order to compute the synergy measures explained below, exposure to radon and tobacco consumption were introduced into the model as the dichotomous variables exposed/unexposed and smoker/non-smoker.

The following measures of interaction were computed:

$$\text{Relative excess risk due to interaction} = OR_{radon\ and\ tobacco} - OR_{tobacco} - OR_{radon} + 1$$

$$\text{Attributable proportion due to interaction} = (OR_{radon\ and\ tobacco} - OR_{tobacco} - OR_{radon} + 1) / OR_{radon\ and\ tobacco}$$

$$\text{Synergy index} = (OR_{radon\ and\ tobacco} - 1) / (OR_{tobacco} + OR_{radon} + 2)$$

Results and discussion

At the end of the study, 163 cases of lung cancer and 241 controls were included in the analysis. The odds ratios for exposures to domestic radon, tobacco and the combination are presented in Table 1. Three measures of synergy between the two factors are presented in Table 2 for all cases of lung cancer together and for two histological subgroups: small-cell and epidermoid cancer. The 95% confidence intervals for the odds ratios are wide owing to the small numbers of cases in each category. As

Table 1. Odds ratios for individual and joint exposures to tobacco and domestic radon

Exposure	Odds ratio (95% confidence interval)		
	All cases	Small-cell	Epidermoid
None	1	1	1
Tobacco	9.6 (3.0–30.2)	19.4 (2.6–143)	6.7 (2.5–18.2)
Radon	1.3 (0.3–5.4)	4.9 (0.3-85.5)	0.6 (0.2–16.5)
Tobacco + radon	12.2 (3.5–42.4)	32.9 (3.9–273)	12.1 (3.9–37.4)

Table 2. Measures of synergy between exposures to tobacco and radon

Synergy measure	Histological type		
	All cases	Small-cell	Epidermoid
Relative excess risk	2.3	9.6	5.8
Attributable proportion	19%	29%	48%
Synergy index	1.26	1.43	2.1

expected, tobacco alone was a major risk factor for all types of lung cancer. The odds ratios estimated for radon alone are not conclusive. The effect of the interaction of the two factors is clearer: one-fifth to one-half of the cases of lung cancer among patients exposed to both tobacco smoking and a high concentration of domestic radon are due to the interaction of these two factors. Although further studies are needed, it seems that a public health action on both factors is needed in high-risk populations.

References
Greenland, S. (1989) Modeling and variable selection in epidemiologic analysis. *Am. J. Public Health*, **79**, 340–349
Hosmer, D.W. & Lemeshow, S. (1989) *Applied Logistic Regression*, New York: John Wiley & Sons
Lubin, J.H., Liang, Z., Hrubec, Z., *et al.* (1994) Radon exposure in residences and lung cancer among women: Combined analysis of three studies. *Cancer Causes Control*, **5**, 114–128
Rothman, K.J. (1986) *Modern Epidemiology*, Boston: Little, Brown & Co, pp. 311–326
Takkouche, B. & Gestal-Otero, J.J. (1996) The epidemiology of lung cancer: Review of risk factors and Spanish data. *Eur. J. Epidemiol.*, **12**, 341–349

Tobacco smoking and lung cancer in Viet Nam

N.V. Co, H.L. Phat, D.K. Hung, T.K. Dung & N.V. Nhung

National Institute against Tuberculosis and Redpiratory Diseases, Hanoi, Viet Nam

'Tobacco or health' is an important concept in Viet Nam in view of the relationship with lung cancer. In order to clarify this relationship, we reviewed nine studies published in the medical literature of our country between 1957 and 1995. The results are as follows:

* *Proportion of cases of lung cancers related to tobacco use*: There were 629 cases between 1966 and 1991, before the founding of the national programme against lung cancer in 1993, and 935 cases between 1994 and 1995. The incidence of lung cancer in the population was about 60 per 100 000 inhabitants in 1993.
* *Prevalence of tobacco use*: The prevalence of cigarette smoking was 23%, and that of smoking Laos tobacco in water pipes was 40%, for a combined prevalence of tobacco use of 70–80%.
* *Tobacco use and sex*: The majority of smokers (75–90%) are men; 46% smoke Laos tobacco, 25% smoke cigarettes and 17% smoke both forms.

- *Duration and frequency of tobacco use*: The average duration was 28.9 years for cigarette smoking and 34.1 years for Laos tobacco; the frequency was 17.9 cigarettes per day and 17.2 pipes of Laos tobacco per day.
- *Histological type of lung cancer*: In some studies all types except adenocarcinoma appeared to be related to tobacco use, but the difference was not significant.

Conclusion

The proportion of cases of lung cancer attributable to smoking in Viet Nam is 70–80%, nearly equivalent to that in developed countries (80–90%). Tobacco use in various regions must be surveyed and studies carried out on the relation to different histological types of lung cancer.

Tobacco smoking and hepatocellular carcinoma

C.-J. Chen & M.W. Yu

Graduate Institute of Epidemiology and Department of Public Health, College of Public Health, National Taiwan University, Taipei, Taiwan

Objectives: To review the independent and synergistic interaction between tobacco smoking and other risk factors for hepatocellular carcinoma in Taiwan.

Methods: A series of case–control and cohorts studies have been carried out to assess the effect of tobacco smoking on the development of hepatocellular carcinoma in Taiwan. Histories of tobacco smoking and alcohol consumption were obtained from personal interviews carried out with a structured questionnaire. Serological markers of chronic infection with hepatitis B and C viruses were identified by enzyme-linked immunosorbant assay. Exposure to aflatoxin was assessed from the urinary concentration of aflatoxin metabolites and the serum concentration of aflatoxin-B_1–albumin adducts. Genetic susceptibility markers including cytochrome P450 2E1 and null genotypes for glutathione *S*-transferase M1 and T1 were also tested.

Results: Tobacco smoking is related to an increased risk for hepatocellular carcinoma, acting synergistically with chronic infection with hepatitis B and C viruses, exposure to aflatoxin and alcohol consumption. The effect of tobacco smoking is more striking among people who have the c1/c1 genotype of CYP2E1 than those with c1/c2 or c2/c2 genotypes.

Laryngeal cancer and tobacco smoking

A.N. Zubritsky

Department of Pathology, Taldom Territorial Medical Union Taldom, Russian Federation

Objective: The study reported here was aimed at examining the role of tobacco smoking in the development of laryngeal cancer on the basis of retrospective material in the Cancer Research Centre of the Russian Academy of Medical Sciences in Moscow from 1992 to 1994. The comparison group comprised 50 patients with carcinoma of the skin, 43 of whom were non-smokers.

Results: Out of 31 942 adult patients with malignant neoplasms, 264 cases of neoplastic lesions of the larynx were found, 253 in men and 11 in women, of an average age of 56 ± 3 years. Of the 264 patients, 183 were heavy smokers. Squamous-cell carcinoma was observed in 258 patients, carcinoma *in situ* in two and one case each of adenocystic cancer, carcinoid and embryonal rhabdomyosarcoma and pre-cancer. Most of the cases corresponded to stage 3, and the patients underwent comprehensive treatment before discharge in satisfactory condition to be followed-up by their district oncologist.

Conclusions: Neoplastic laryngeal lesions accounted for 0.83% of cases among 31 942 adult patients with malignant neoplasms treated at the Cancer Research Centre over three years. This cancer was more prevalent in men (96%). Tobacco smoking is the major risk factor for this cancer.

Acknowledgements: Sincere thanks to Professor Ye.G. Matyakin for permission to work in the archives, without which this study would not have been possible.

Naswar (snuff) dipping and oral cancer in north-west Pakistan

S.M. Khan, S. Nasreen & S. Zai

Institute of Radiotherapy and Nuclear Medicine, Peshawar, Pakistan

Aim: Between 1990 and 1996, data on 22 083 cancer patients, 12 548 males and 9353 females, were analysed to determine the frequency of the commonest cancers. This hospital-based study was carried out to ascertain the frequency of oral cancer in north-west Pakistan and its association with use of smokeless tobacco (*naswar*).

Methods: The study was performed at the Institute of Radiotherapy and Nuclear Medicine, which is located in Peshawar, a border town near the Khyber Pass. It is a few kilometers away from Afghanistan and is the only hospital in the region where radiation and nuclear medicine facilities are available under one roof. Most cancer patients are referred to this hospital for treatment. Information including name, age, sex and site and nature of the tumour was coded according to the instructions of the World Health Organization before entry into the computer. Cases with inadequate information were excluded from the study.

Results: Among males, the 10 commonest tumours were skin, lymphoma, oral, urinary bladder, lung, oesophagus, soft tissue, prostate and brain tumours and myeloid leukaemia. Among females, the 10 commonest tumours were of the breast, skin, ovary, oral, cervix and oesophagus, lymphoma (non-Hodgkin and Hodgkin), cancer of the endometrium, myeloid leukaemia and soft-tissue tumours. A total of 15 101 adult patients (excluding Afghan refugees and children) were referred to the Institute with cancer, of whom 869 (5.8%) had oral cancer. The majority of the patients (190) were aged 60–64 years. Oral cancer was seen in 599 men (69%) and 270 women (31%); 478 (55%) used *naswar*, of whom 400 were men (67%) and 78 were women (29%).

Conclusion: Oral cancer is the fourth commonest cancer among adult cancer patients in this province, and 55% patients with this preventable cancer were tobacco users.

Epidemiology of smoking-related cancers in South Africa

F. Sitas[1], H.R.O. Carrara[1], M. Patel[2], M. Hale[3], W. Bezwoda[2], P. Ruff[2], R. Laikier[2], R. Newton[4] & V. Beral[4]

[1]National Cancer Registry; [2]Department of Medicine, University of the Witwatersrand and [3]Department of Anatomical Pathology, Soth African Institute for Medical Research, Johannesburg, South Africa; and [4]Imperial Cancer Research Fund, Oxford, United Kingdom

South Africa has a heterogeneous population of 40 million, and about one-third of all persons over the age of 16 smoke. Information on the local risks of tobacco-attributable disease is sparse, but there is evidence that the incidence of lung cancer is increasing. To study the effects of the tobacco epidemic (and other important risk factors), black patients with a newly diagnosed cancer who are admitted to one of the three major public referral hospitals around Johannesburg are interviewed on an on-going basis. To date, 898 male and 1328 female patients have been interviewed for a case–control study. The controls are patients with cancers not associated with exposure to tobacco.

Among male current smokers, increased age-adjusted odds ratios were observed for lung cancer (odds ratio, 8.4; 95% confidence interval [CI], 3.2–22), oral cancer (7.2; 2.6–20) and oesophageal cancer (5.3; 2.6–11). These risks in relation to smoking are approaching those in developed countries.

For this reason, in order to estimate the impact of tobacco on the rate of premature mortality, the Department of Health has approved the insertion of two questions on the death notification form (reproduced overleaf), which address the smoking habits of the deceased and the next-of-kin (five years before the death). This will allow for the construction of a large case–control study to measure the risk for death overall and due to specific causes in relation to smoking, and will also allow for the follow-up of the next-of-kin in relation to their smoking habits.

BI - 1663

REPUBLIC OF SOUTH AFRICA

NOTIFICATION / REGISTER OF DEATH / STILL BIRTH

in terms of the Births and Deaths Registration Act, 1992
(Act No. 51 of 1992)

Space for Bar Code

* Must be completed in black ink (please tick ✓ where applicable)
* Please refer to instructions

SERIAL No:

FILE No: DATE: **A 00035006**

A PARTICULARS OF DECEASED INDIVIDUAL ☐ / STILLBORN CHILD ☐

Date of birth

Identity number of deceased

Date of death

Age at last birthday   years

Surname

Sex

Maiden Name (If female)

If death occurred within 24 hours after birth

Forenames

No. of hours alive

MARITAL STATUS OF DECEASED   Single ☐   Married ☐   Living as married ☐   Widowed ☐

Religious Law ☐   Divorced ☐   Customary Union ☐

Left thumb print of deceased

PLACE OF BIRTH (municipal district or country if abroad) ————

PLACE OF DEATH (City / Town / Village) ————

PLACE OF REGISTRATION OF DEATH ————

CITIZENSHIP OF DECEASED

B PARTICULARS OF INFORMANT

Identity number

Initials and Surname

Relationship to deceased   Parent ☐   Spouse ☐   Child ☐   Other kin ☐   Other (specify) ☐

Left thumb print of informant

Postal address

Postal Code   Dialling Code

Was the next of kin of the deceased a smoker* during the past five years?   Yes ☐   No ☐   Refuse to answer ☐   Telephone No.

Date ....   Signature ....

C PARTICULARS OF FUNERAL UNDERTAKER

Initials and Surname

Office Stamp of Funeral Undertaker

Designation No.   Place of burial / cremation ————

Date ....   Signature ....

D CERTIFICATE BY ATTENDING MEDICAL PRACTITIONER / PROFESSIONAL NURSE

Postal Address

I, the undersigned, hereby certify that the deceased named in Section A, to the best of my knowledge and belief, died solely and exclusively due to NATURAL CAUSES specified in Section G ☐

I, the undersigned, am not in the position to certify that the deceased died exclusively due to natural causes ☐

Postal Code

SAMDC / SANC Reg. No.

....
INITIALS AND SURNAME   SIGNATURE

Date signed

CERTIFICATE BY DISTRICT SURGEON / FORENSIC PATHOLOGIST

I, the undersigned, hereby certify that a medicolegal post-mortem examination has been conducted on the body of the person whose particulars are given in Section A and that the body is no longer required for the purpose of the Inquest Act, 1959 (Act No. 58 of 1959) and that the cause of death is: Unnatural ☐   Under investigation ☐

Postal Address

Postal Code

Initials and Surname

Place of post-mortem ....   Date

Mortuary Reference ....

Signature ....   Date signed

SAMDC Reg. No.

E FOR OFFICIAL USE ONLY

Initials and Surname of Registrar

Office Stamp ▷

Registration of death approved and burial order issued

Address

Force No. / Designation No.

Persal No.

Date ....   Signature ....

* Someone who smokes tobacco on most days

NOTIFICATION / REGISTER OF DEATH / STILL BIRTH
INFORMATION FOR MEDICAL AND HEALTH USE ONLY
(After completion *seal* to ensure <u>confidentiality</u>)

BI - 1663
Page 2

Space for Bar Code

SERIAL No:

FILE No: DATE: A 0003396

F DEMOGRAPHIC DETAILS

Initials and Surname of deceased

Identity Number

Place of death   1. Hospital: (Inpatient   ER/ Outpatient   DOA   )   2. Nursing Home   3. Home   4. Other (Specify)

FACILITY NAME (If not institution, give street and number)

Usual residential address of deceased #   Suburb

Town / Village

Name of Plot, Farm, etc.   Census Enumerator Area

Street name and number

Magist. Dist.

Deceased's Education (Specify ✓ only highest class completed/achieved)

Postal Code

None	Gr1	Gr2	Gr3	Gr4	Gr5	Gr6	Gr7	Gr8 Form 1	Gr9 Form 2 NTC1	Gr10 Form 3	Gr11 Form 4 NTC2	Gr12 Form 5 NTC3	Univ Tech	CODE

Province

USUAL OCCUPATION OF DECEASED (give type of work done during most of working life. Do not use retired)

Country

TYPE OF BUSINESS / INDUSTRY (e.g. Mining, Farming) refer to instructions

Was the deceased a smoker* five years ago? (✓) :   Yes   No   Do not know   Not applicable (minor)

G MEDICAL CERTIFICATE OF CAUSE OF DEATH

FOR OFFICE USE ONLY

PART 1. Enter the disease, injuries or complications that caused the death. Do not enter the mode of dying, such as cardiac or respiratory arrest, shock, or heart failure. List only one cause on each line.

Approximate interval between onset and Death (Days/Months/Years)

ICD-10

IMMEDIATE CAUSE (Final disease or condition resulting in death)   a.
Due to (or as a consequence of)

Sequentially list conditions, if any, leading to immediate cause. Enter UNDERLYING CAUSE last (Disease or injury that initiated events resulting in death)   b.
Due to (or as a consequence of)

c.
Due to (or as a consequence of)

d.
Due to (or as a consequence of)

PART 2. Other significant conditions contributing to death but not resulting in the underlying cause given in Part 1.

If a female, was she pregnant 42 days prior to death? (✓) :   Yes   No

If stillborn, please write mass in grams

Do you consider the deceased to be: African   White   Indian   Coloured   Other   (Specify)

Method of ascertainment of cause of death:

1. Autopsy   2. Opinion of attending medical practitioner   3. Opinion of attending medical practitioner on duty

4. Opinion of registered professional nurse   5. Interview of family member

6. Other   (Specify)

Where someone lived on most days   * Someone who smokes tobacco on most days

Cardiovascular disease

Cigarette smoking, tar yields and non-fatal myocardial infarct: 14 000 cases and 32 000 controls in the United Kingdom

S. Parish[1], R. Collins[1], R. Peto[1], L. Youngman[1], J. Barton[1], K. Jayne[1], R. Clarke[1],
P. Appleby[1], V. Lyon[1], S. Cederholm-Williams[2], J. Marshall[2], P. Sleight[1] for the
International Studies of Infarct Survival (ISIS) Collaborators

[1]Clinical Trial Service Unit & Epidemiological Studies Unit, University of Oxford,
and [2]Oxford Bio-Research Laboratory, Oxford Science Park, United Kingdom

Heart attacks (myocardial infarcts) are the main way tobacco kills young adults in the United Kingdom, and cigarettes also cause non-fatal heart attacks. In developed countries, about half a million heart attacks occur each year among people who are still only in their thirties or forties, and more than half of these are caused by tobacco.

During the early 1990s, enquiries were made in the United Kingdom of the smoking habits of 14 000 people who had recently had a heart attack ('cases') and of 32 000 who had not ('controls') (Parish et al., 1995). Among people aged 30–49, the rates of myocardial infarct in smokers were about five times those in non-smokers; at ages 50–59, they were three times those in non-smokers, and even at ages 60–79 they were twice as great as in non-smokers (risk ratio, 6.3, 4.7, 3.1, 2.5 and 1.9 at 30–39, 40–49, 50–59, 60–69 and 70–79, respectively; each $2P < 0.00001$). As smoking correlates with alcohol consumption and low body mass index, both of which are somewhat protective against myocardial infarct, standardization for alcohol and body mass index changes these five age-specific ratios to 6.3, 5.3, 3.4, 2.9 and 2.0.

Results for people with no previous history of major neoplastic or vascular disease. Each risk ratio is standardized for sex and for quinquennium of age and is based on a comparison of those using manufactured cigarettes only with those who were not currently using any tobacco and had not been regular cigarette smokers at any time in the past 10 years. The risk ratio is given beside each bar.

After standardization for age, sex and amount smoked, the rate of myocardial infarct was 10% (SD, 5) higher for smokers of medium-tar (risk ratio, 3.2) than smokers of low-tar cigarettes (risk ratio, 2.9; $2P = 0.06$). The difference in risk between cigarette smokers and non-smokers is much larger than the difference between smoking one type of cigarette and another. Even low-tar cigarettes still greatly increase the risk for myocardial infarct, and far more risk is avoided by not smoking than by changing from one type of cigarette to another.

Reference
Parish, S., Collins, R., Peto, R., Youngman, L., Barton, J., Jayne, K., et al. (1995) Cigarette smoking, tar
yields, and non-fatal myocardial infarction: 14 000 cases and 32 000 controls in the United Kingdom.
Br. Med. J., 311, 471–477

Prospective study on the relationship between smoking and death from cardiovascular disease among retired men in Xi'an, China

Q. Shi, L. Li, C. Sun, Y. He & J. Huang

Department of Epidemiology, 4th Military Medical University, Xi'an, China

Introduction
Many epidemiological studies have shown that smoking is one of the most important risk factors for cardiovascular disease in younger populations, but the relationship has

not been defined in the elderly (Philip *et al.*, 1996). Prospective studies performed more than 20 years ago in China showed no significant relationship between smoking and cardiovascular disease among people of all ages (Wu *et al.*, 1991). With the development of the economy, the rate of smoking has increased rapidly. In a national survey of smoking in 1996, the rate of smoking among men over the age of 70 was 38.1%, and the mortality rate due to smoking was increased (China Science and Technology Press, 1997), indicating that smoking is a cause of serious health problems for elderly Chinese men. The objective of this paper was to determine whether smoking is a risk factor for cardiovascular disease among elderly Chinese men.

Subjects and methods

A prospective study on risk factors for cardiovascular disease has been conducted since 1987 among 1268 retired men, who were randomly selected from among all retired men in Xi'an, China. The baseline investigation was perfomed in May–June 1987. The information requested on the questionnaire included demographic characteristics, cigarette smoking (defined by the World Health Organization protocol), alcohol intake, history of hypertension and family history of cardiovascular disease. The height, weight and blood pressure of each man was recorded, and blood samples were taken for laboratory measurement of serum total cholesterol and triglyceride.

During follow-up, each participant was interviewed in person every two years. When a death occurred and was reported, efforts were made to obtain a copy of the death certificate in order to ascertain the recorded primary cause of death. All causes of death were coded by ICD-9.

Relative risks were used as a measure of the strength of the association between cigarette smoking and cardiovascular disease. Cox proportional hazards models were used to control for other variables (David & Micheal, 1993), and 95% confidence intervals (CIs) were calculated for each adjusted relative risk. All analysis were performed with the SPSS software.

Results

The cohort was followed-up over nine years, contributing 11 635 person–years of exposure. Twenty-six men were lost to follow-up. The baseline characteristics of the participants are shown in Table 1. At the time of the baseline investigation, the prevalence of smoking was 34%.

During the follow-up, there were 233 deaths, 76 of which were due to cardiovascular disease. In the baseline investigation, the odds ratios for associations with current smoking were 1.9996 (95% CI, 1.5070–2.6534) for hypertension, 1.0853 (0.8220–1.4324) for hypercholesterolaemia and 1.5996 (1.2643–2.0239) for hypertriglycerid-aemia. The relative risks are shown in Table 2. After adjustment for age, there was no significant association between smoking and cardiovascular disease.

Table 1. Baseline characteristics of study participants

Variable	No.	Mean (SD) or %
Age (years)	1268	63.9 (5.2)
Years of follow-up	1268	9.18 (2.27)
Current smoking	435	34.3%
History of hypertension	329	25.2%
Systolic blood presure (mm Hg)	1268	129 (18.3)
Diastolic blood pressure (mm Hg)	1268	80.0 (11.0)
Serum total cholesterol (mg/dl)	1268	195 (43.7)
Serum total triglyceride (mg/dl)	1268	133 (69.7)
Body mass index (kg/m²)	1268	24.4 (3.09)
Alcohol use	652	51.4%
Exercise	792	62.5%
History of cardiovascular disease	474	37.4%
Family history of cardiovascular disease	340	26.8%

Table 2. Multivariate Cox regression analysis for death froml cardiovascular disease

Variable	B (SE)	Relative risk	95% CI
Current smoking	0.0587 (0.0611)	1.06	0.94–1.20
History of hypertension	0.2409 (0.2895)	1.22	0.69–2.16
Serum total cholesterol (mg/dl)	0.0075 (0.0101)	1.01	0.99–1.03
Serum total triglyceride (mg/dl)	0.0828 (0.0112)	1.09	0.90–1.35
Body mass index (kg/m²)	−0.0041 (0.0097)	0.99	0.97–1.01
Alcohol use	−0.0198 (0.0594)	0.98	0.87–1.10
Exercise	0.0017 (0.0039)	1.00	0.88–1.13
Family history of cardiovascular disease	0.0372 (0.0639)	1.04	0.91–1.18

Discussion

Most case–control studies conducted in China have shown that smoking is an independent risk factor for cardiovascular disease, although one prospective study found different results (Wang *et al.*, 1982). Some researchers have assumed that there are concomitant effects of smoking and other risk factors for cardiovascular disease, especially dyslipidaemia (Wendy *et al.*, 1989). Thus, when the levels of other risk factors are low, the effect of smoking would not be seen. In our study, the levels of serum triglyceride and hypertension at baseline were significantly associated with smoking.

Age is one of the most important factors in cardiovascular disease, and it has been shown that disorders of lipid and carbohydrate metabolism are more common among elderly than younger people (Arnesen, 1992). In our study, the significant effect of smoking disappeared after adjustment for age, indicating that people are affected by smoking before becoming old. Controlling smoking in young people is thus an important means of reducing the rate of death from cardiovascular disease in old people.

References

Arnesen, H. (1992) The metabolic cardiovascular syndrome. *J. Cardiovasc. Pharmacol.*, **20** (Suppl. 8), S1–S4

China Sciuence and Technology Press (1997) *National Prevalence Survey of Smoking Pattern*, Beijing, pp. 22–23

David, C. & Micheal, H. (1993) Cox method for follow-up studies. In: *Statistical Methods in Epidemiology*, Oxford: Oxford University Press, pp. 198–232

Philip, H.F., Barry, R.D., Alfredo, J.B., *et al.* (1996) Cardiovascular disease risk factors in men and women aged 60 years and older. *Circulation*, **94**, 26–34

Wang, J.L., Du, F.C., Wang, H.Y., *et al.* (1982) A five-year cohort study on risk factors of coronary heart disease. *Chin. J. Epidemiol.*, **10**, 81

Wendy, Y.C., Glem, E.P., James, E.H., *et al.* (1989) Cigarette smoking and serum lipid and lipoprotein concentrations: An analysis of published data. *Br. Med. J.*, 784–788

Wu, X.G., Hao, J.S., Wang, J.M., *et al.* (1991) A prospective study about risk factors in the Capital Steel Company in Beijing. *Chin. J. Circulation*, **2**, 127–131

Cigarette smoking and coronary heart disease

J. Huang[1], L. Li[1], D. Xu[1], G. Jia[2], L. Li, Y[2]. He[1] & Q. Shi[1]

[1]Department of Epidemiology and [2]Department of Cardiology of Xijing Hospital, Fourth Military Medical University, Xi'an, China

Introduction

Cigarette smoking has been established as one of the major risk factors for coronary heart disease in many epidemiological studies, although its mechanism of action is not fully understood. The purpose of this hospital-based study was to investigate whether interactions between cigarette smoking and serum lipids might be involved.

Subjects and methods

The participants were in-patients seen in 1991–96 who had undergone coronary angiography and met nationally defined diagnostic criteria for acute myocardial infarct. The case–control study involved 108 patients with coronary heart disease and 45 with other conditions, and the study of serum lipids involved 243 cases of myocardial infarct and 137 cases of coronary heart disease defined by coronary angiography.

All participants responded to a questionnaire designed according to the criteria of the World Health Organization MONICA project, which elicited information on socioeconomic characteristics, smoking habits, history of hypertension and diabetes and other risk factors for coronary heart disease. Serum total cholesterol, triglycerides and high-density lipoproteins were determined.

The variables were compared by t tests for continuous variables and chi-squared tests for categorical variables; logistic regression was used to analyse multiple variables.

Results

The univariate analysis gave an odds ratio for coronary heart disease associated with cigarette smoking of 1.5 (95% confidence interval [CI], 1.1–2.1; $p = 0.12$). There was a significant dose–response relationship with cigarette smoking. Multiple regression analysis indicated that cigarette smoking, age, a fat-rich diet and a family history of coronary heart disease or essential hypertension were risk factors for coronary heart disease (Table 1).

The serum concentrations of total cholesterol and high-density lipoproteins were significantly higher among smokers than among non-smokers (Table 2).

Discussion

Many studies have been conducted on risk factors for coronary heart disease and the interactions between major risk factors, but with varying results (WHO MONICA Project, 1988). In our study, the relationship between cigarette smoking and coronary heart disease was significant in both univariate and multivariate analyses, supporting our previous finding that cigarette smoking is an independent risk factor for coronary heart disease (He et al., 1988; Huang et al., 1993). Since the control group was selected from among in-patients in the same hospital department, the odds ratio may be an underestimate, explaining why it is lower than those in other studies.

In the comparison on serum lipids, inverse relationships were found between cigarette smoking and the serum concentrations of total cholesterol and high-density lipoproteins. A lower high-density lipoprotein concentrations has been reported previously in smokers,

Table 1. Significance of risk factors for coronary heart disease in multivariate logistic regression analysis

Factor	B	SE	OR	95% CI	p
Age	0.80	0.29	2.2	1.2–3.9	0.0061
Cigarette smoking	0.57	0.20	1.8	1.2–2.6	0.0035
Fat-rich diet	0.82	0.41	2.3	1.0–5.1	0.045
Family history of coronary heary disease	2.1	0.80	8.4	1.7–40	0.0080
Family history of hypertension	1.2	0.43	3.3	1.4–7.6	0.0065

Table 2. Serum concentrations of lipids in smokers and non-smokers with cardiovascular disease

Smoking status	No. of cases	Triglycerides	Cholesterol	High-density lipoproteins
Non-smoker	117	1.6 ± 0.85	4.8 ± 1.1	1.2 ± 0.25
Smoker	268	1.7 ± 0.92	4.6 ± 1.0	1.1 ± 0.24
p		0.16	0.015	0.02

but the finding for total cholesterol seems to be in contrast to previous findings (Craig et al., 1989; Hughes et al.). Limitation of the participants to in-patients may also have contributed to this finding.

References

Craig, W.Y., Palomaki, G.E. & Haddow, J.E. (1989) Cigarette smoking and serum lipid and lipoprotein concentrations: An analysis of published data. Br. Med. J., 298, 784

He, Y., Li, L.S., Li, L.S., et al. (1988) A case control study on the relationship between cigarette smoking and coronary heart disease. Chin. Med., 68, 263

Huang, J.Y., Li, L.S., Li, L.S., et al. (1993) A study on role of family history in development of coronary heart disease. Chin. J. Prev. Control Chron. Non-Commun. Dis., B, 158

Hughes, K., Leong, W.P., Thothy, S.P., et al. (?) Relationship between cigarette smoking, blood pressure and serum lipids in the Singapore general population. Int. J. Epidemiol., 22, 637–643

WHO MONICA Project (1988) Geographical variation in the major risk factors of coronary heart disease in men and women aged 35–64 years. World Health Stat. Q., 41, 115–140

Smoking and coronary changes in patients with documented coronary artery disease

J. Majewski & K. Moczurad

Jagiellonian University, Collegium Medicum, Institute of Cardiology, Department of Social Cardiology, Kraków, Poland

Introduction

Cigarette smoking is one of the leading risk factors for coronary heart disease. Population-based studies have demonstrated that smokers have a two- to threefold increase in risk for sudden death from cardiac arrest as compared with non-smokers (Kannel & Thomas, 1982). Unstable angina pectoris is a dramatic clinical manifestation of coronary artery disease associated with the risk for developing myocardial infarct, especially among patients with disease involving many vessels (Freeman et al., 1989). The pathophysiological mechanisms underlying unstable angina pectoris are complex and include progression of atherosclerotic lesions, increased platelet aggregation, coronary thrombus formation and increased vasomotor tone (Brown et al., 1984; Kruskal et al., 1987; Haft et al., 1988), all leading to an imbalance between myocardial oxygen demand and supply.

The purpose of the present study was to analyse the extent of cigarette smoking among patients with unstable angina pectoris and the relationship between smoking and the severity of coronary stenosis.

Material and methods

The study population consisted of 84 consecutive patients with unstable angina pectoris; 70 were men and 14 women, of an average age of 52.2 years (range, 32–71). Of these, 55 patients had a history of myocardial infarct. We analysed the incidence of coronary risk factors and serum lipid profile (total cholesterol, high-density lipoprotein cholesterol, low-density lipoprotein cholesterol and triglycerides). All the patients underwent coronary angiography to assess the severity and incidence of coronary stenosis.

Student's t test and chi-squared test were used to compare the results.

Results

Cigarette smoking was found to be the leading risk factor in the study population. As many as 60 patients were current smokers (Table 1) and had been smoking for a mean of 22.7 years (range, 5–40). Of these, 21 patients smoked > 20 cigarettes per day. The 24 current non-smokers included 11 patients who had never smoked and 13 who had quit smoking after the myocardial infarct. Ofthe 55 patients with a history of myocardial infarct, 42 had continued smoking.

Coronary angiography revealed critical narrowing in one vessel in 33 patients, in two vessels in 24 and in multiple vessels in 27 patients. 'Multi-vessel' disease was found in 22 smokers, significantly more frequently than among non-smokers (Table 2). Single-vessel disease was significantly more frequent among non-smokers.

There was no significant correlation between the number of cigarettes smoked per day and the extent of coronary stenosis among smokers.

Analysis of the serum lipid profile revealed that the concentration of high-density lipoprotein was significantly lower and those of low-density lipoprotein cholesterol and triglycerides higher in smokers than in non-smokers. The total cholesterol concentration was slightly higher in smokers than in non-smokers, the difference being non-significant (Table 3).

Discussion

Cigarette smoking is one of the most important risk factors for coronary artery disease, which in combination with other factors accelerates the atherosclerotic process via various mechanisms. Smoking has a detrimental effect on lipid concentration and a number of haematological parameters that contribute to atherosclerosis (Kannel *et al.*, 1987). The Framingham study demonstrated that cigarette smoking causes a two- to threefold increase in the risk for sudden cardiac death in each subsequent decade in patients between 30 and 59 years of age (Kannel & Thomas, 1982).

Table 1. Risk factors in 84 men and women with unstable angina

Risk factor	No. of patients
Smoking	60
High-density lipoprotein cholesterol < 40 mg%	48
Low-density lipoprotein cholesterol > 155 mg%	37
Family history	35
Hypertension	26
Cholesterol > 250 mg%	24
Triglycerides > 200 mg%	21
Overweight	17
Diabetes	4

Table 2. Coronary changes in smokers and non-smokers

Smoking status	Vessel disease		
	Single	Double	Multiple
Smokers ($n = 60$)	21[a]	17	22[b]
Non-smokers ($n = 24$)	12	7	5

[a] $p < 0.02$
[b] $p < 0.05$

Table 3. Serum lipid concentrations in smokers and non-smokers

Smoking status	LDL (mg%)	HDL (mg%)	Triglycerides (mg%)	Total cholesterol (mg%)
Smokers	151.5 ± 34.7[a]	38.2 ± 8.4[b]	187.5 ± 65.8[a]	226.8 ± 39.2
Non-smokers	146.9 ± 29.8	44.5 ± 12.8	164.4 ± 48.5	225.2 ± 34.8

LDL, low-density lipoprotein; HDL, high-density lipoprotein
[a] $p < 0.05$
[b] $p < 0.02$

It has also been reported that the risk of a second infarct increases significantly with increasing total and low-density lipoprotein cholesterol concentrations in serum. An inverse relationship was observed with respect to high-density lipoprotein cholesterol (Guize & Lion, 1992). In the present study, smokers had a significantly lower high-density lipoprotein cholesterol concentration, and those of low-density lipoprotein cholesterol and triglycerides were higher than in non-smokers. This finding is in accordance with the results of Migas (1988) and Tiwari et al. (1989) in patients who smoked more than 25 cigarettes per day. In 1982, Cabin and Roberts demonstrated that total cholesterol concentration correlated positively with the number of severe stenoses in coronary arteries but not with the extent of narrowing, although there was also a significant relationship between increased triglyceride concentration and degree of coronary stenosis.

In our patients with unstable angina pectoris, multi-vessel disease was significantly more frequent among smokers, whose low-density lipoprotein cholesterol and triglyceride concentrations were increased. In contrast, single-vessel disease was more frequent in non-smokers.

Conclusion

In patients with unstable angina pectoris, there is a significant correlation between smoking and the extent of coronary stenosis. Cigarette smoking has a detrimental effect on the serum lipid profile, in particular by reducing the high-density lipoprotein cholesterol concentration. Smoking cessation would appear to be one of the most important tasks of secondary prevention of coronary artery disease.

References

Brown, B.G., Bolson, E.L. & Dodge, H.T. (1984) Dynamic mechanisms in human coronary stenosis. *Circulation*, **70**, 917

Cabin, H.S. & Roberts W.C. (1982) Relation of serum total cholesterol and triglyceride levels to the amount and extent of coronary arterial narrowing by atherosclerotic plaque in coronary heart disease. Quantitative analysis of 2037 five mm segments of 160 major epicardial coronary arteries in 40 necropsy patients. *Am. J. Med.*, **73**, 227

Freeman, M.R., Williams, A.E., Chisholm, R.J. & Armstrong, P.W. (1989) Intracoronary thrombus and complex morphology in unstable angina. Relation to timing of angiography and in-hospital cardiac events. *Circulation*, **80**, 17

Guize, J. & Ilion, M.C. (1992) Treatment of risk factors of coronary atherosclerosis. *Arch. Mal. Coeur. Vais.*, **85** (Suppl. 11), 1687

Haft, J.I., Haik, B.J., Goldstein, J.E. & Brodyn N.E. (1988) Development of significant coronary artery lesions in areas of minimal disease. A common mechanism for coronary disease progression. *Chest*, **94**, 731

Kannel, W.B. & Thomas, H.E. (1982) Sudden coronary death. The Framingham Study. *Ann. N.Y. Acad. Sci.*, **382**, 3

Kannel, W.B., D'Agostino, R.B. & Belanger, A.J. (1987) Fibrinogen, cigarette smoking and the risk of cardiovascular disease: Insights from Framingham Study. *Am. Heart J.*, **113**, 1006

Kruskal, J.B., Commerford, P.J., Franks, J.J., et al. (1987) Fibrin and fibrinogen related antigens in patients with stable and unstable coronary disease. *N. Engl. J. Med.*, **317**, 1361

Migas, O.D. (1988) The lipid effects of smoking. *Am. Heart J.*, **115**, 272

Tiwari, A.K., Gode, J.D. & Dubey, G.P. (1989) Effect of cigarette smoking on serum total cholesterol and HDL in normal subjects and coronary heart disease patients. *Indian Heart J.*, **41**, 92

EXPERIMENTAL STUDIES ON
EFFECTS OF TOBACCO

Experimental animals

Uterotrophic effect of oestrogens in rats is modified by exposure to cigarette smoke

L.M. Berstein, E.V. Tsyrlina, O.S. Kolesnik, O.G. Krjukova,
S.V. Dzhumasultanova & V.B. Gamajunova

Laboratory of Endocrinology, Professor N.N. Petrov Research Institute of Oncology,
St Petersburg, Russian Federation

Prolonged, uncontrolled treatment with oestrogens or excessive endogenous production over a long period can lead to the development of pathological processes, including neoplastic growth. We proposed earlier that there are two principal types of hormonal carcinogenesis and suggested that there are factors that facilitate a shift from promotional (mitogenic) to genotoxic types (Berstein, 1996a). We consider that tobacco smoking is an important exogenous factor which can modify both the frequency of some malignant tumours and endocrine function (Peto et al., 1992). Women who smoke cigarettes are at increased risk not only of lung cancer but also of osteoporosis and early menopause; decreased risks for endometrial cancer, endometriosis and uterine fibroids have been reported. Although it has been assumed that the mechanism of these decreases is hypo-oestrogenism (Wald & Baron, 1990), that conclusion is not supported by direct studies of blood oestrogen concentrations in smokers. The change in oestrogen production in smokers may be mainly qualitative, with a shift to the powerful genotixicant catechol oestrogens (Liehr & Ricci, 1996), thus reducing the total oestrogenic effect. On the basis of these observations, we assumed that tobacco smoke weakens the specific effect of oestrogens but augments their capacity to damage DNA (Berstein, 1996a; Berstein et al., 1997). The aim of the study reported here was to verify this hypothesis experimentally.

Three-week and three-month studies were conducted on female rats weighing 140–170 g from the Rappolovo animal house of the Russian Academy of Medical Sciences (St Petersburg). The animals were either untreated or were exposed to tobacco smoke, oestrogens or tobacco smoke plus oestrogens. Exposure to cigarette smoke was begun on day 1 of the experiment by placing rats in a sealed 20-L plastic chamber (Balansky et al., 1992), which was filled by means of a 50-ml syringe with 350 ml of mainstream smoke generated by a commercial class Y, filter-tip cigarette ('Prima') with a tar content of 29 mg per cigarette. The chamber was opened after 10 min and, after a 4-min interval to renew the air, was filled again with fresh tobacco smoke six times in the same manner. Sham-exposed animals were kept in a similar chamber for the same times but in the absence of tobacco smoke. After 10 or 79 days, all animals underwent bilateral ovariectomy. Groups of animals then received 1 μg/day of diethylstilboestrol intramuscularly with and without tobacco smoke or tobacco smoke alone. On the last day of the experiment, all the animals were sacrificed by exposure to diethyl ether vapours, and their uteri were separated, weighed and kept in liquid nitrogen until required for assay. The progesterone receptor content was evaluated by dextrane–charcoal radioligand assay; the protein content by the method of Lowry; and alkali-induced DNA winding was examined by fluorimetry (Birnboim & Jevcak, 1981).

The results are shown in Table 1. Irrespective of the duration of the experiment, tobacco smoke by itself did not significantly affect uterine weight or the progesterone receptor content of the uterine tissue of ovariectomized rats. A decrease in body-weight gain was seen in rats exposed to tobacco smoke and oestrogens, separately or in combination, especially during the three-week experiments. In these shorter experiments, diethylstilboestrol did not significantly affect DNA unwinding, and in combination with tobacco smoke actually increased the amount of intact double-stranded DNA. This unexpected stimulation was not seen in the three-month studies, in which diethylstilboestrol had clear DNA-damaging effects. In rats exposed to tobacco smoke for three months, the progesterone receptor-inducing effect of diethylstilboestrol was significantly decreased.

Table 1. Effects of tobacco smoke and oestrogen alone and combined on the uterus of rats

Group	Body-mass gain during experiment (g)	Uterine weight (mg)	Progesterone receptors (fmol/mg protein)	Intact DNA in uterine tissue (%)[a]
Three-week experiment				
Control	+47.8 ± 4/7 (20)	74.7 ± 2.8 (20)	90.4 ± 13.5 (8)	15.7 ± 3.7/100 (4)
Tobacco smoke	+24.9 ± 2.9 (19)[b]	80.2 ± 2.5 (19)	91.0 ± 18.0 (8)	15.7 ± 2.5/100 (4)
Oestrogen	+24.6 ± 2.7 (20)[b]	238.2 ± 6.7 (20)[b]	194.0 ± 23.4 (8)[b]	14.6 ± 1.1/93 (7)
Tobacco smoke plus oestrogen	+20.4 ± 2.9 (20)[b]	237.9 ± 5.7 (20)[b]	182.9 ± 33.5 (8)[b]	20.4 ± 2.3/130 (7)[c]
Three-month experiment				
Control	+76.6 ± 6.6 (12)	136.9 ± 5.4 (12)	77.7 ± 15.0 (3)	37.0 ± 5.0/100 (3)
Tobacco smoke	+63.8 ± 7.0 (12)	141.1 ± 4.1 (12)	98.0 ± 2.0 (3)	35.5 ± 3.5/96 (3)
Oestrogen	+61.6 ± 3.3 (12)[b]	329.5 ± 13.7 (12)[b]	126.5 ± 9.8 (6)[b]	24.5 ± 2.5/66 (3)[b]
Tobacco smoke plus oestrogen	+65.9 ± 6.5 (12)	336.8 ± 20.8 (12)[b]	85.9 ± 7.7 (6)[c]	26.5 ± 6.5/72 (3)[b]

In parentheses, numbers of rats or samples
[a] The data on DNA unwinding are also presented in conditional units, where the control value = 100
[b] Significantly different from controls
[c] Significantly different from those given oestrogen alone

These results indicate that short-term exposure to tobacco smoke does not significantly affect the ueterotrophic action of oestrogens and paradoxically decreases their DNA-damaging action, corresponding to the 'stimulation stage' described by us in young smokers (Berstein, 1996b). The reason for the differences in the percentage of intact DNA in uterine tissue of the control animals in the short and long experiments is unknown but may be due to methodological or seasonal factors; we therefore presented our data in conditional units. The DNA-damaging effect of diethylstilboestrol was more evident in the three-month studies, perhaps because the greater age of the animals made their cellular genome more sensitive to injury.

After three months' exposure to tobacco smoke, one of the most specific effects of oestrogens, i.e. their ability to induce progesterone receptors, was found to be weakened, with an increase in the DNA-damaging effect of oestrogens, similar to the increase in DNA damage induced by the combination of ethanol and oestrogens (Yamagiwa *et al.*, 1994). On this basis, a 'phase structure' of response to tobacco smoke plus oestrogens is suggested. If the exposure to tobacco smoke were extended to a period equivalent to prolonged cigarette smoking in humans or if a more sensitive method, such as the content of oestrogen–DNA adducts in uterine tissue, were used, it is possible that we would find both an effect on oestrogens and an increase in their genotoxicity; however, a decrease in the specific effect of oestrogens can by itself create clinical resistance which, in combination with the reduced hormonal sensitivity of target tissues, might worsen the prognosis of smokers with cancer (Daniell *et al.*, 1993; Berstein *et al.*, 1997).

Acknowledgement
    This study was partly supported by a grant (97-04-48022) from the Russian Foundation for Basic Research.

References
Balansky, R.B., D'Agostini, F., Zanacchia, P. & DeFlora, S. (1992) Protection by N-acetylcysteine of the histopathological and cytogenetic damage produced by exposure of rats to cigarette smoke. *Cancer Lett.*, **64**, 123–131
Berstein, L.M. (1996a) Hormonal carcinogenesis and smoking. *Cancer J.*, **9**, 106–107

Berstein, L.M. (1996b) Age-dependent hormonal–metabolic effects of smoking: Stimulation–depression principle and cancer. In: *Carcinogenesis from Environmental Pollution: Assessment of Human Risk,* Joint conference of the AACR and IARC, Budapest

Berstein, L.M., Tsyrlina, E.V., Semiglazov, V.F., Kovalenko, I.G., Gamayunova, V.B., Evtishenko, T.P. & Ivanova, O.A. (1997) Hormone–metabolic status in moderately smoking breast cancer patients. *Acta Oncol.,* **36,** 137–140

Birnboim, H.C. & Jevcak, J.J. (1981) Fluorometric method for rapid detection of DNA strand breaks in human white blood cells produced by low doses of radiation. *Cancer Res.,* **41,** 1889–1892

Daniell, H.W., Tam, E. & Filice, A. (1993) Larger axillary metastases in obese women and smokers with breast cancer: An influence by host factors on early tumor behaviour. *Breast Cancer Res. Treat.,* **25,** 193–201

Liehr, J.G. & Ricci, M.J. (1996) 4-Hydroxylation of estrogens as marker of human mammary cancer. *Proc. Natl Acad. Sci. USA,* **93,** 3294–3296

Peto, R., Lopez, A.D. & Boreham, J. (1992) Mortality from tobacco in developed countries. *Lancet,* **339,** 1268–1278

Wald, N. & Baron, J., eds (1990) *Smoking and Hormonal-related Disorders,* Oxford: Oxford University Press

Yamagiwa, K., Mizumoto, R., Higashi, S., Kato, H., Tomida, T., Uehara, S., Tanigawa, K., Tanaka, M. & Ishida, N. (1994) Alcohol ingestion enhances hepatocarcinogenesis induced by synthetic estrogen and progestin in the rat. *Cancer Detect. Pre.,* **18,** 103–114

Generation of mammalian cell lines that stably express rat neuronal nicotinic acetylcholine receptor sub-types

Y. Xiao, E.L. Meyer, R.A. Houghtling, J.M. Thompson & K.J. Kellar

Department of Pharmacology, Georgetown University School of Medicine, Washington DC, United States

Introduction

The pharmacological properties of nicotine, including its addictive properties, are mediated by neuronal nicotinic acetylcholine receptors (nAChR). Long-term administration of nicotine increases the number of nicotinic receptor binding sites in rat and mouse brain (Marks & Collins, 1983, Schwartz & Kellar, 1983), suggesting that nicotine can trigger neuronal changes in nicotinic receptors that might be related to or even underlie addiction and/or tolerance. Support for this idea came from studies of autopsied human brain samples, which showed that the density of nicotinic receptors in smokers is markedly higher than in non-smokers (Benwell *et al.*, 1988; Breese *et al.*, 1997).

Neuronal nAChRs are ligand-gated cation channels that are widely distributed in the vertebrate central nervous systems, retina, autonomic ganglia and adrenal gland (Galzi & Changeux, 1995; McGehee & Role, 1995; Albuquerque *et al.*, 1997). Within the central nervous system, some nAChRs are located on axons and cell bodies of dopaminergic, noradrenergic, GABAergic and cholinergic neurons, and it is thought that nicotine influences the release of these neurotransmitters via the nAChRs. In the periphery, the presynaptic cholinergic input to all sympathetic and parasympathetic ganglia and to the adrenal gland is mediated by neuronal nAChRs. Thus, neuronal nAChRs may be involved in widespread functions throughout the central and autonomic nervous systems.

Neuronal nAChRs are composed of two types of membrane spanning sub-units, a and b. Eleven different neuronal nAChR sub-units ($\alpha 2$–$\alpha 9$ and $\beta 2$–$\beta 4$) have been cloned (Sargent, 1993; Lindstrom, 1996; Colquhoun & Patrick, 1997). In view of the existence of many different sub-units and their ability to form functional heteromeric and homomeric nAChRs, the number of neuronal nAChR sub-types could be quite large.

The *Xenopus* oocyte expression system has been the primary means of studying and comparing the properties of potential nAChR sub-types, as defined by their sub-unit composition, although the system may have certain limitations (Colquhoun & Patrick, 1997). Recently, we and others have begun to express nAChR sub-types stably in mammalian cell lines. These new heterologous expression systems should be particularly useful for studying and comparing the pharmacology of neuronal nAChR sub-types. Here we report the preliminary results of our efforts to construct a library of cell lines that are stably transfected with nAChR sub-types and some pharmacological properties of these receptors.

Methods

Eukaryotic expressable rat nAChR sub-unit gene constructs: Plasmids carrying cDNA clones of rat neuronal nAChR sub-unit genes ($\alpha2$, $\alpha3$, $\alpha4$, $\alpha5$, $\beta2$ and $\beta4$) were generously provided by Dr J. Boulter of the Salk Institute. To express the rat neuronal nAChR sub-units constitutively in mammalian cells, cDNA fragments carrying the genes were sub-cloned into the eukaryotic expression vector pcDNA3 (Invitrogen, San Diego, CA).

Stable transfection: Constructs carrying the nAChR sub-unit genes were linearized by restriction digestion within their prokaryotic elements and transfected into human embryonic kidney cells (HEK 293, ATCC CRL 1573) by the calcium phosphate method. The cells were grown in a selection medium containing G418 for three to four weeks before resistant clones were isolated by cloning cylinders.

Results

Stable transfection of HEK 293 cells: The G418-resistant clonal cell lines were initially screened in multiple-probe RNase protection assays to measure the mRNA isolated from each clone. As expected, there was no detectable expression of the mRNA of any of the six nAChR subunit genes in either HEK 293 cells or the cells transfected only with the vector, pcDNA3. The mRNA levels for the appropriate sub-unit genes in cell lines transfected with either one or two nAChR sub-unit genes were, however, quite high (Xiao *et al.*, 1996, 1997).

The clones that expressed the highest levels of the expected nAChR sub-unit mRNA(s) were tested for their ability to bind ^{3}H-($\pm$)epibatidine, a broad-spectrum nicotinic agonist (Houghtling *et al.*, 1995). At a ^{3}H-($\pm$)epibatidine concentration of approximately 3 nmol/L, essentially no specific binding was detected in membrane homogenates from HEK 293 cells, from cells transfected with the pcDNA3 vector only or from cells transfected with only one of the six sub-unit genes ($\alpha2$, $\alpha3$, $\alpha4$, $\alpha5$, $\beta2$ and $\beta4$). In contrast, in membrane homogenates from several cell lines transfected with both α and β genes, specific binding of ^{3}H-($\pm$)epibatidine was quite high, with binding site densities > 100 fmol/mg protein. Five cell lines were selected for further study, and these have been cultured continuously in our laboratory for many generations with no significant change in the levels of expression of the mRNA encoding the sub-units or in the specific binding of ^{3}H-($\pm$)epibatidine.

Saturation analyses of ^{3}H-epibatidine binding to nAChRs in cell membrane homogenates: For each of the five cell lines tested, specific binding of ^{3}H-($\pm$) epibatidine was saturable and represented > 90% of the total binding. Over the concentration range used, ^{3}H-($\pm$)epibatidine binding fit a model for a single site for all of the receptor sub-types expressed in these five cell lines. The K values for ^{3}H-($\pm$) epibatidine binding varied with nAChR sub-type, but all of them were in the picomolar range. The binding site densities ranged from 190 fmol/mg protein for KXa4b2R4 cells to > 8000 fmol/mg protein for KXa34R2 cells. In comparison, the density in rat forebrain (primarily a4/ß2 receptors) in a parallel assay was 72 fmol/mg protein.

Pharmacological characteristics of nAChR binding sites in the transfected cell lines: For the agonists tested, the affinities varied markedly among nAChR sub-types, but the rank order of affinities of agonists at the four receptor sub-types was similar: cytisine > (–)-nicotine > acetylcholine. In contrast, the order of affinities of the antagonists *d*-tubocurarine and DHbE varied at these sub-types.

Up-regulation of ^{3}H-($\pm$)epibatidine binding sites by long-term nicotine treatment in the transfected cells: Prolonged exposure (seven days) of the KXa2b4R1 cells to nicotine markedly increased the density of ^{3}H-(±)epibatidine binding sites in cell membranes in a concentration-dependent manner. The binding site up-regulation was observed with a nicotine concentration as low as 100 nmol/L, and a 14-fold increase was observed at a concentration of 1 mmol/L. Similar increases were observed for the other nAChR sub-types, although the potency of nicotine and its maximal effect to increase the binding sites varied markedly among the nAChR sub-types (Xiao et al., 1996; Meyer et al., 1997).

Discussion

We have generated five HEK 293-derived cell lines that stably express rat α2/β2, α2/β4, α3/β2, α3/β4 and α4/β2 nAChR sub-types, respectively. These cell lines have maintained a high level of receptor expression through continuous culturing for many generations. All five of the nAChR sub-types tested have very high affinity for ^{3}H-(±)epibatidine, although there are clear differences in their K values. In addition, the binding affinities of several other nicotinic drugs vary markedly among these sub-types.

The receptor binding sites in these cell lines, as shown for α4/β2 receptors *in vivo* (Flores et al., 1992), are increased by long-term exposure to nicotine (see also Meyer et al., 1997). The function of the α3/β4 nAChR sub-type expressed in the KXa3b4R2 cell line is being characterized in detail in ^{86}Rb$^+$ efflux assays (Xiao et al., 1997; Meyer et al., 1997) and patch clamp measurements (Zhang et al., 1997).

In conclusion, nAChR sub-types can be expressed in HEK 293 cells to form stable cell lines. A library of such cell lines should be a powerful and convenient new tool for studying the pharmacological and functional diversity of neuronal nAChR sub-types and the molecular bases of the diversity. These studies and studies of native neuronal nAChRs should lead to a better understanding of these receptors, their physiological role and their role in nicotine addiction.

Acknowledgments

This work was supported by National Institutes of Health grants DA06486 and AG09973. ELM was supported by a National Institute of Health predoctoral fellowship grant, DA05739-01.

References

Albuquerque, E.X., Alkondon, M., Pereira, E.F.R., Castro, N.G., Schrattenholz, A., Barbosa, C.T.F., Bonfante-Cabarcas, R., Aracava, Y., Eisenberg, H.M. & Maelicke, A. (1997) Properties of neuronal nicotinic acetylcholine receptors: Pharmacological characterization and modulation of synaptic function. J. Pharmacol. Exp. Ther., 280, 1117–1136

Benwell, M., Balfour, D. & Anderson, J. (1988) Evidence that tobacco smoking increases the density of (-)-[^{3}H]nicotine binding sites in human brain. J. Neurochem., 50, 1243–1247

Breese, C.R., Marks, M.J., Logel, J., Adams, C.E., Sullivan, B., Collins, A.C. & Leonard, S. (1997) Effect of smoking history on [3H]nicotine binding in human postmortem brain. J. Pharmacol. Exp. Ther., 282, 7–13

Colquhoun, L.M. & Patrick, J.W. (1997) Pharmacology of neuronal nicotinic acetylcholine receptor subtypes. Adv. Pharmacol., 39, 191–220

Flores, C.M., Rogers, S.W., Pabreza, L.A., Wolfe, B.B. & Kellar, K.J. (1992) A subtype of nicotinic cholinergic receptor in rat brain is composed of a4 and b2 subunits and is up- regulated by chronic nicotine treatment. Mol. Pharmacol., 41, 31–37

Galzi, J.L. & Changeux, J.P. (1995) Neuronal nicotinic receptors: molecular organization and regulations. Neuropharmacology, 34, 563–582

Houghtling, R.A., Davila-Garcia, M.I. & Kellar, K.J. (1995) Characterization of (±)-[3H]epibatidine binding to nicotinic cholinergic receptors in rat and human brain. Mol. Pharmacol., 48, 280–287

Lindstrom, J. (1996) Neuronal nicotinic acetylcholine receptors. In: Narahashi, ed., Ion Channels, New York: Plenum Press, Vol. 4, pp. 377–449

Marks, M.J. & Collins, A.S. (1983) Effects of chronic nicotine infusion on tolerance development and nicotine receptors. J. Pharmacol. Exp. Ther., 226, 283–291

McGehee, D.S. & Role, L.W. (1995) Physiological diversity of nicotinic acetylcholine receptors expressed by vertebrate neurons. Annu. Rev. Physiol., 57, 521–546

Meyer, E.L., Xiao, Y. & Kellar, K.J. (1997) Pharmacology of the function and regulation of the a3b4 neuronal nicotinic acetylcholine receptor subtype stably expressed in transfected HEK 293 cells. *Soc. Neurosci. Abstracts*, **23**, 385

Sargent, P.B. (1993) The diversity of neuronal nicotinic acetylcholine receptors. *Annu. Rev. Neurosci.*, **16**, 403–443

Schwartz, R.D. & Kellar, K.J. (1983) Nicotinic cholinergic binding sites in the brain: Regulation *in vivo*. *Science*, **220**, 214–220

Xiao, Y., Meyer, E.L., Houghtling, R.A., Thompson, J.M. & Kellar, K.J. (1996) Stable expression of rat nicotinic acetylcholine receptor subtypes in mammalian cells. *Soc. Neurosci. Abstracts*, **22**, 1034

Xiao, Y., Meyer, E.L., Thompson, J.M. & Kellar, K.J. (1997) Generation and characterization of a stably transfected cell line expressing rat a3b4 neuronal nicotinic acetylcholine receptors. *Soc. Neurosci. Abstracts*, **23**, 385

Zhang, J., Xiao, Y., Kellar, K.J. & Morad, M. (1997) Electrophysiological properties of nicotine current in stably transfected HEK 293 cell line expressing a3b4 receptors. *Soc. Neurosci. Abstracts*, **23**, 385

Survival index of offspring of smoking mothers: An animal model

E. Florek[1] & A. Marszalek[2]

[1]*Department of Toxicology and* [2]*Chair of Clinical Pathomorphology, Karol Marcinkowski University School of Medical Sciences, Poznan, Poland*

Introduction

In order to elucidate the hazard that tobacco smoke presents to the developing organism (Florek, 1995; Witschi *et al.*, 1997), we studied the survival index of the offspring of pregnant rats exposed to tobacco smoke.

Materials and methods

We conducted a three-generation study starting with 240 pregnant rats divided into four groups: controls and three groups exposed to tobacco smoke at 500, 1000 or 1500 mg of carbon monoxide equivalent per m^3 of air. Exposure was for 6 h/day on five days per week for 11 weeks: six weeks before mating, two weeks during mating and during three weeks of gestation. Each groups was further divided into two and fed a diet with either a normal level of protein (24%) or a reduced amount (8%).

The numbers of live and dead offsrping were counted, and the numbers of survivors were counted on days 1, 4, 12 and 21 after birth. The results were analysed by Duncan, Student's *t* and Cochran–Cox tests.

The experiment was conducted according to the rules recommended by the World Health Organization and Boyland and Goulding (1968).

Results and discussion

The results are shown in the table. We found decreased survival indices in all groups exposed to tobacco smoke in comparison with the controls. On the day after delivery, the largest difference was found between the controls and animals treated with the lowest concentration of tobacco smoke, with a difference of 9.3% for those on normal diet and 12% for those on the low-protein diet. The survival indices were lower until day 4 after delivery but were significantly reduced only one day after delivery.

It is difficult to determine which component of tobacco smoke affects the developing organism. We suspect that nicotine retarded foetal development either directly or by changing the maternal hormone concentrations (Suzuki *et al.*, 1974); nicotine also affects the circulation. Carbon monoxide concentrations and the formation of carboxy-haemoglobin are known to be increased in smoking mothers (Florek, 1995), and exposure of pregnant rats and rabbits to an elevated concentration of carbon monoxide led to growth retardation of the newborns and greater mortality after delivery (Benowitz, 1988). Further experiments are required to identify the components of tobacco smoke responsible for its effects on perinatal survival.

Table 1. Survival indices of the offspring of pregnant rats exposed to tobacco smoke and the effect of a low-protein diet

Day after birth	Diet	Tobacco smoke	Survival (%)
1	Normal	Control	96.7
		Treated	94.1
	Low-protein	Control	96.7
		Treated	94.1
4	Normal	Control	91.1
		Treated	88.8
	Low-protein	Control	93.4
		Treated	90.1
12	Normal	Control	80.6
		Treated	81.7
	Low-protein	Control	82.4
		Treated	83.0
21	Normal	Control	78.7
		Treated	79.0
	Low-protein	Control	77.3
		Treated	79.4

References

Benowitz, N.L. (1988) Pharmacologic aspects of cigarette smoking and nicotine addiction. *New Engl. J; Med.*, **319**, 1318–1330

Boyland, E. & Goulding, R. (1968) Reproduction test. In: *Modern Trends in Toxicology*, Vol. 1, London: Butterworths, pp. 75–85

Florek, E. (1995) *Toksyczny wplyw dymu tytoniowego i diety na plodnosc, zdolnosc rozrodcza i potomstwo w badaniach eksperymentalnych*, Dissertation, Poznan: Karol Marcinkowski University Press

Suzuki, K., Horiguchi, T., Comas-Urrutia, A.C., Mueller-Heubah, E., Morishma, H.O. & Adamsons, K. (1974) Placental transfer and distribution of nicotine in the pregnant rhesus monkey. *Am. J. Obset. Gynecol.*, **119**, 253–262

Witschi, H., Joad, J.P. & Pinkerton, K.E. (1997) The toxicology of environmental tobacco smoke. *Annu. Rev. Pharmacol. Toxicol.*, **37**, 29–52

Influence of tobacco smoke on gas stabilization in newborn rat lung

A. Marszalek[1], W. Biczysko[1], M. Wasowicz[1] & E. Florek[2]

[1]Chair of Clinical Pathomorphology and [2]Department of Toxicology , Karol Marcinkowski University School of Medical Sciences, Poznan, Poland

Introduction

During gestation, the lungs of the foetus are filled with a fluid produced by differentiating and maturing epithelium, and primary pneumocytes occupy almost the entire terminal lung space. Around day 16–17 of gestation in rats, there is an explosion of differentiation and maturation of secondary pneumocytes, and the production of surfactant begins. The key elements for the stabilization of gases in the newborn lung are the structure of the lung and the action of surfactant. In 1995, we found that surfactant also acts in the drying of the lungs during the first few minutes after delivery (Biczysko *et al.*, 1995). The role of this surface-active material, stored in lamellar bodies, is to enable the transport of fluid from the alveolar lumen into the capillaries (Bland *et al.*, 1989) and allow gas exchange in the lungs after birth. Maternal tobacco smoking has been reported to retard pulmonary development in the foetus. Our aim was to examine ultrastructurally drying of the lung in newborn rats of dams exposed to tobacco smoke.

Material and methods

Groups of pregnant rats ($n = 240$) were exposed to tobacco smoke at 500, 1000 or 1500 mg of carbon monoxide equivalent per m^3 of air or served as controls. Exposure was for 6 h/day on five days per week for 11 weeks: six weeks before mating, two weeks during mating and during three weeks of gestation. Lung tissue was taken from up to two offspring 15 and 30 min after delivery and fixed for routine electron microscopy.

Results

A wide spectrum of changes was seen. In the group with the highest exposure to tobacco smoke, lung development was retarded, being analagous to that on day 17 of gestation. The alveolar septa were thick and covered mainly with primary pneumocytes. The lungs were better developed in the other grioups, with an alveolar appearance. At 15 min after delivery, the lungs of all offspring from treated dams were partially filled with alveolar fluid. Whereas the lungs from animals in the control group were becoming dry by 30 min and the alveolar lumen was well aerated, those from animals exposed to tobacco smoke showed slow evacuation of fluid and most of the alveoli were still filled with fluid after 30 min. Haemaorrhages into the alveolar spaces were observed in the lungs of offspring of dams exposed to the two highest concentrations of tobacco smoke.

Discussion

We found that the formation of the lungs of the offspring of rats exposed to tobacco smoke was retarded: the alveolar epithelium was immature and there were fewer secondary pneumocytes. Furthermore, these cells had fewer, less mature lamellar bodies containing surfactant than those of controls. After birth, many of the lamellar bodies released into the alveolar space did not form a monolayer of surfactant. These changes were accompanied by oedema and haemorrhage into the alveolar space; such complications are common in immature lung. Thus, inhalation of tobacco smoke by pregnant rats led to abnormal lung maturation and reduced formation of surfactant in their offspring, resulting in slower drying of the newborn lung.

References

Biczysko, W., Wasowicz, M., Marszalek, A. & Florek, E. (1995) The entrance of surface active material to pulmonary capillaries in the lungs of newborn rat. *Folia Cytochem. Cytobiol.*, **33**, 25–31
Bland, R.D., Carlton, D.P., Scheerer, R.G., Cummings, J.J. & Chapman, D.L. (1989) Lung fluid balance in lambs before and after premature birth. *J. Clin. Invest.*, **84**, 568–576

Effects of environmental tobacco smoke on eustachian tube surfactant in guinea-pigs

B. Jiang[1], Y. He[2] & L.N. Feng[1]

[1]*Department of Aerospace Clinical Medicine,* [2]*Department of Epidemiology, Fourth Military Medical University, Xi'an, China*

Cigarette smoking has been shown to reduce the amount of pulmonary surfactant and thus damage pulmonary function (Higenbottam, 1985; Mancini *et al.*, 1993). Surface tension-lowering substances are also present in the eustachian tube in canines, rodents and humans. The major function of the eustachian tube is to equalize pressure between the middle ear and the external atmosphere, and surface tension-lowering substances present in the middle-ear cleft facilitate the opening of the eustachian tube. Evidence from studies in experimental animals suggests that substances which lower the surface tension facilitate the opening of the eustachian tube and also allow effective mucociliary clearance (Birken & Brookler, 1972; Jiang & Guo, 1992). It has thus been suggested that a deficiency of auditory surfactant could cause failure of eustachian tube opening and make the ear more susceptible to secretory otitis media. Studies in experimental animals confirmed that the pressure necessary for opening the eustachian tube was increased when effusion was present in the middle ear but was significantly reduced after treatment with artificial surfactant (Kodama & Asakura, 1993). A clinical study showed that clinical symptoms, signs and test results in otorhinolaryngology were improved when adults and children were treated with drugs that facilitated the synthesis of surfactant, with a significant difference between the treated and control groups (Passali & Zavattini, 1987). These results suggest that eustachian tube surfactant plays an important role in its physiological function.

Evidence has been accumulating that cigarette smoke and environmental tobacco smoke affect eustachian tube function. Some epidemiological studies (Strachan et al., 1989; Etzel et al., 1992) have shown that the occurrence of secretory otitis media, a common middle ear disease in children, is associated with paternal cigarette smoking and exposure to environmental tobacco smoke. Zellweger (1991) indicated that long-term passive exposure to tobacco smoke can cause disease in sensitive non-smokers and particularly in children of smoking mothers, who may suffer more frequently from respiratory-tract infections, otitis media and chronic cough as well as exacerbation of pre-existent asthma. Middle ear effusions are also associated with hearing impairments, which may result in abnormalities or retardation in children's hearing, speech and cognition (Reed & Lutz, 1988).

Little is known about the effects of environmental tobacco smoke on eustachian tube surfactant, and the purpose of present study was to investigate those effects.

Material and methods

A standard dose of smoke, from one cigarette three times per day for 10 days, was delivered to 20 guinea-pigs; a further group of 20 animals was unexposed. Tubotympanic washings were collected and analysed with a captive bubble surface tensiometer, the surface tension being calculated from the height and diameter of the bubbles. As these parameters are also changed by pressure and de-pressure, the minimum surface tension and coefficient of stability were determined.

Results

Ten grouped samples were analysed from the exposed and from the control animals. In the exposed group, the mean minimum surface tension was 29.4 ± 6.44, and the mean coefficient of stability was 0.22 ± 0.09; the corresponding values for the control group were 23.8 ± 4.95 and 0.28 ± 0.08 (see table). When these two groups of data were compared, $t = 2.22$ and $p = 0.041$ for mean minimum surface tension, and $t = 2.66$, $p = 0.016$ for the mean coefficient of stability, both significantly higher in the exposed group. Thus, environmental tobacco smoke could affect the eustachian tube surfactant.

Discussion

We found that the mean minimum surface tension in tube washings from guinea-pigs placed in environmental tobacco smoke for a short time was increased significantly, indicating that the ability of surfactant to lower the surface tension was reduced. These results confirm our hypothesis of a relationships between exposure to environmental tobacco smoke, eustachian tube function and secretory otitis media. The Government should thus pass laws limiting cigarette smoking in public and protecting children from passive smoking at home.

References

Birken, E.A. & Brookler, R.H. (1972) Surface-tension lowering substance of the canine eustachian tube. Ann. Otol. Rhinol. Laryngol., 81, 268–271

Etzel, R.A., et al. (1992) Passive smoking and middle ear effusion among children in day care. Pediatrics, 90, 228–232

Higenbottam, T. (1985) Tobacco smoking and the pulmonary surfactant system. Tokai J. Exp. Clin. Med., 10, 465–470

Jiang, B. & Guo, B.L. (1992) Physical characteristics of eustachian tube surfactant. J. Chin. Aerosp. Med., 3, 16–19

Minimum surface tension and coefficient of stability in tubotympanic washings from guinea-pigs exposed to environmental tobacco smoke or unexposed

Exposed		Unexposed		
Minimum surface tension	Coefficient of stability	Minimum surface tension	Coefficient of stability	
30.92	0.23	22.31	0.35	
41.16	0.16	31.56	0.27	
35.23	0.13	30.16	0.22	
32.64	0.16	25.84	0.28	
33.40	0.09	28.30	0.20	
21.68	0.32	17.87	0.32	
21.44	0.36	17.73	0.43	
28.90	0.25	22.09	0.37	
25.39	0.19	21.29	0.37	
23.66	0.32	20.30	0.39	
29.44	0.22	23.75	0.32	Mean

Kodama, H. & Asakura, K. (1993) Role of surface tension lowering substances in the function of normal and diseased eustachian tubes of guinea pigs. *Nippon jibiinkoka Gakkai Kaiho*, **96**, 674–684

Mancini, N.M., *et al.* (1993) Early effects of short time cigarette smoking on the human lung: A study of bronchoalverlar lavage fluids. *Lung*, **171**, 277–291

Passali, D. & Zavattini, G. (1987) Multicenter study on the treatment of secretory otitis media with ambroxol. Importance of a surface-tension lowering substance. *Respiration*, **51** (Suppl. 1), 52–59

Reed, B.D. & Lutz, L.J. (1988) Household smoking exposure—Association with middle ear effusions. *Fam. Med.*, **20**, 426–430

Strachan, D.P., *et al.* (1989) Passive smoking, salivary cotinine concentrations and middle ear effusion in 7 year old children. *Br. Med. J.*, **298**, 1549–1552

Zellweger, J.P. (1991) Passive smoking. *Schweiz. Rundsch. Med. Prax.*, **80**, 492–495

Humans

Inhibition of natural killer cell activity by alveolar macrophages in smokers

M. Takeuchi[1], S. Nagai[2] & T. Izumi[2]

[1]Department of Biotechnology, Kyoto Sangyo University, and
[2]Kyoto University, Kyoto, Japan

Abstract

We investigated the mechanism of the suppressive effect of alveolar macrophages on the activity of natural killer (NK) cells taken from bronchoalveolar lavage fluid and blood from smokers and non-smokers. The activity of NK cells was very low initially in both non-smokers and smokers. After 24 h in culture, the activity increased significantly in non-smokers but not smokers, and the activity of NK cells in the lung was significantly augmented by addition of interleukin-2, also only in non-smokers. Addition of alveolar macrophages from smokers had a significantly greater inhibitory effect on NK cell activity in blood than those from non-smokers. Indomethacin, catalase and thoiurea did not prevent the suppression of NK cell activity by alveolar macrophages, but superoxide dismutase prevented the inhibition. These results suggest that NK cell activity is suppressed in smokers by the release of oxygen radicals from alveolar macrophages.

Introduction

Cigarette smoking is known to inhibit the immune system, and cigarette smokers have decreased helper:suppressor T-cell ratios, decreased serum immunoglobulin concentrations and suppressed NK cell activity (Ferson et al., 1979). NK cells play an important role in immune surveillance against tumours and viral infections in the lung, but many studies have focused on their activity in peripheral blood (Phillips et al., 1985), while little is known about NK cells in the lung (Bordignon et al., 1982). We reported previously that the NK cell activity in the lungs of smokers is lower than that in non-smokers (Takeuchi et al., 1989). Alveolar macrophages play a major role in pulmonary defence mechanisms, and cigarette smoking induces various changes in the metabolism of these cells (Harris et al., 1970). Alveolar macrophages have been shown to inhibit the expression of NK cell activity (Takeuchi et al., 1989), but little is known about this cell-mediated down-regulation. In this study, we investigated the mechanism of the inhibitory effect of alveolar macrophages on NK cell activity in smokers.

Material and methods

The subjects were 10 healthy men, five of whom were non-smokers (mean age, 35.4 years) and five were cigarette smokers (mean age, 34.2 years). The duration of smoking ranged from 4 to 30 years (mean, 13.4), and the consumption was 15–50 cigarettes per day (mean, 27.0) or 4–50 pack–years (mean, 22.8).

Lung effector cells were obtained by bronchoelveolar lavage and purified with Ficoll-Hypaque on a plastic dish and nylon wool column. The alveolar macrophages were purified by E-rosette methods. NK cell activity was assayed by the ^{51}Cr release method after incubation for 4 or 24 h, with K562 as the target cell (E:T = 10). Alveolar macrophages were added at a final concentration of 5–50% to effector cells in the NK cell assay.

To evaluate a possible role of prostaglandins and oxygen radicals produced by alveolar macrophages in the inhibition of NK cell activity, indomethacin and anti-oxidants were added with 25% alveolar macrophages to a final concentration of 2.5×10^{-7} to 2.5×10^{-5} mmol/l of indomethacin, 1.4–1400 U/ml of catalse, 2.5–25 mmol/L of thiourea or 7.5–750 U/ml of superoxide dismutase.

Results
The NK cell activity in lung tissue from smokers showed little cytotoxicity before or after 24 h of incubation. The activity in lung from non-smokers was initially very low (mean, 1.5%) but increased to a mean of 6.1% after 24 h of incubation ($p < 0.05$); the corresponding values for smokers were 1.3% and 2.9%, the difference being non-significant. When interleukin-2 was added to the cultures at a concentration of 50 U/ml, the activity of NK cells in lung was significantly increased in non-smokers but not in smokers.

When alveolar macrophages from smokers were added at a concentration of 5% to autologous blood samples, they significantly inhibited blood NK cell activity, whereas those from non-smokers did not. The 42% inhibition caused by alveolar macrophages from smokers was not inhibited by indomethacin, catalase or thiourea, but was suppressed by superoxide dismutase, the activity returning to the level observed before the addition of alveolar macrophages.

Discussion
Whereas it has been shown previously that heavy smokers have decreased NK cell activity in their blood (Phillips *et al.*, 1985), we have shown that the activity of NK cells in the lungs of smokers is not increased after 24 h in culture, in contrast to those of non-smokers, and no difference is seen between smokers and non-smokers in NK cell activity in the blood. In an earlier study, NK cell activity was augmented by interleukin-2 (Itoh *et al.*, 1985), but the activity in the lungs of smokers in our study was not increased. Our data show that the function of NK cells in the lungs is damaged by smoking. Robinson *et al.* (1984) showed that alveolar macrophages in bronchoalveolar lavage fluid from healthy non-smokers inhibited blood NK cell activity; we have also shown that alveolar macrophages from smokers and non-smokers can inhibit this activity, but we also observed that alveolar macrophages from smokers inhibit blood NK cell activity to a greater extent than those from non-smokers.

Smokers are known to have an increased number of alveolar macrophages, which release more oxygen radicals than macrophages from non-smokers (Richter *et al.*, 1986). Although it is also known that alveolar macrophages can release superoxide anions, other forms of reduced oxygen species and prostaglandins (Hoidal *et al.*, 1979), we found that only superoxide dismutase prevented the inhibition of NK cell activity. These results suggest that the inhibition of NK cell activity mediated by alveolar macrophages is caused by production of oxygen radicals in smokers. The reduced NK cell activity in the lungs of smokers may contribute to the development and progression of lung cancer and cause greater susceptibility to viral infections.

References
Bordignon, C., Villa, F., Vecchi, A., Giavazzi, R., Introna, M. & Avallone (1982) *Clin. Exp. Immunol.*, **47**, 437–444
Ferson, M., Edwards, A., Lint, A., Milton, G.W. & Kersey, P. (1979) *Int. J. Cancer*, **23**, 603–609
Harris, J.O., Swenson, E.W. & Johnson, J.E. (1970) *J. Clin. Invest.*, **49**, 2086–2096
Hoidal, J.R., Beal, G.D. & Repine, J.E. (1979) *Infect. Immunol.*, **26**, 1088–1094
Itoh, K., Shiba, K., Shimizu, Y., Suzuki, R. & Kumagai, K. *J. Immunol.*, **134**, 3124–3129
Phillips, B., Marshall, M.E., Brown, S. & Thompson, J.S. (1985) *Cancer*, **56**, 2789–2792
Richter, A.M., Abboud, R.T., Johal, S.S. & Fera, T.A. (1986) *Lung*, **164**, 233–242
Robinson, B.W.S., Pinkston, P. & Crystal, R.G. (1984) *J. Clin. Invest.*, **74**, 942–950
Takeuchi, M., Nagai, S. & Izumi, T. (1989) *Chest*, **94**, 688–693

Free-radical production in Indian smokers of cigarette, *bidis* and hookah

D. Behera, D. Deva, R. Sharma & K.L. Khanduja

Department of Pulmonary Medicine and Biophysics,
Postgraduate Institute of Medical Education and Research, Chandigarh, India

Tobacco smoking is known to be responsible for a number of pulmonary diseases, including chronic obstructive pulmonary disease and lung cancer. One of the mechanisms associated with disease processes is postulated to be the production of free radicals. In the present study, we determined free-radical production (neutrophil superoxidase) by NBT reduction in 141 smokers in India. The results are shown in the table. All types of smoking products resulted in more free radicals than in controls.

Smoking	Age (years)	TLC (x 1000)	TNC (x 1000)	SO (no PMA)	SO (+ PMA)
Control	38.0 ± 12.8	6.7 ± 1.2	4.1 ± 0.9	1.63 ± 0.72	4.83 ± 0.91
Bidi	42.2 ± 11.8	8.2 ± 1.8	5.7 ± 1.1	10.1 ± 0.16	13.60 ± 1.90
Hookah	54.9 ± 11.6	8.1 ± 5.56	5.5 ± 1.1	3.35 ± 0.81	10.30 ± 2.32
Mixed	42.7 ± 13.4	8.26 ± 1.6	5.6 ± 1.1	5.23 ± 1.28	13.4 ± 1.92
Analysis of variance					
F	5.85	4.69	9.35	65.84	11.75
p	< 0.05	< 0.05	< 0.05	< 0.05	< 0.05

Effect of cigarette smoking on lipid profile: Analysis of mass screening of 29 519 middle-aged Japanese men

W. Chun, A. Sano, H. Nishida, S. Urano & K. Sakagami

Matsushita Health Care Center, Osaka, Japan

We perform annual health check-ups of company employees in order to determine those at high risk for atherosclerosis. The results of blood tests for lipid profile (total cholesterol, high-density lipoprotein cholesterol, triglycerides, fasting blood sugar and uric acid) in men aged ≥ 40 and < 60 were analysed according to the number of cigarettes smoked, divided into non-smokers (13 253 men), light smokers (1–19 cigarettes per day; 6836 men) and heavy smokers (≥ 20 cigarettes per day; 9430 men). The results are shown in the table. The concentration of triglycerides was correlated with smoking, as heavy smokers had a significantly higher concentration than the other two groups, and the concentration of high-density lipoprotein cholesterol was inversely related to smoking, non-smokers having the highest concentration. The concentrations of total cholesterol, fasting blood sugar and uric acid were correlated with body mass index rather than smoking.

Lipid profile	Non-smokers	Light smokers	Heavy smokers
Total cholesterol	212.0 ± 34.6	205.3 ± 34.5	208.0 ± 35.5
High-density lipoprotein cholesterol	58.7 ± 15.4	54.9 ± 14.6	52.1 ± 14.1
Triglycerides	120.9 ± 91.6	130.4 ± 110.4	148.8 ± 117.4
Fasting blood sugar	101.5 ± 18.3	98.7 ± 19.7	99.9 ± 21.1
Uric acid	6.0 ± 1.3	5.8 ± 1.3	5.9 ± 1.3
Body mass index	23.3 ± 2.7	22.7 ± 2.8	23.2 ± 2.9

Effects of smoking on serum lipids and the blood pressure response to a rehabilitation exercise programme for cardiac patients

N. Sarrafzadegan, K.Sadegi, M. Boshtam & N. Mohammadifar

Rehabilitation Unit, Cardiovascular Research Center, Isfahan, Iran

The epidemiological association between cigarette smoking and atherosclerosis is firmly established. Numerous studies have demonstrated that smoking causes dyslipidaemia and increases blood pressure. Cardiac rehabilitation has become an accepted form of treatment for many patients with cardiovascular diseases; the benefits of exercise training have been demonstrated for functional capacity, psychosocial characteristics and lipoprotein patterns of patients. This study provides information on the response of total cholesterol, serum triglycerides, mean systolic blood pressure and mean diastolic blood pressure to a three-month rehabilitation exercise programme according to the smoking habits of the patients. The study group was made up of 20 men and women aged 30–65 years who had a history of acute myocardial infarct, according to the World Health Organization criteria, and were referred to our rehabilitation exercise programme. There were 15 non-smokers and five smokers. A questionnaire eliciting information mainly about the major risk factors, especially smoking status, was completed by each patient. Blood pressure was measured from the right arm in the sitting position according to the World Health Organization standardized protocol, and a fasting blood sample was obtained to measure baseline lipids. These parameters were measured again on the completion of the rehabilitation programme, after three months. During the three months, all the patients exercised two to three times a week for 50–60 min at an intensity of 70–85% of their maximal heart rate.

The mean decrease in serum cholesterol after the exercise programme was 2.3–9.4 mg/dl in smokers and 13.7–15.2 mg/dl among non-smokers ($p < 0.05$). Similar results were were observed for serum triglyceride concentration, with a mean decrease of 15.5–31 mg/dl in smokers and 24–8.6 mg/dl in non-smokers. The mean decrease in systolic blood pressue was 1–9.1 mm Hg in smokers and 19–19.2 mm Hg in non-smokers, and similar findings were reached for diastolic blood pressure. The differences in the changes in systolic and diastolic blood pressure by smoking status were not significant.

The results suggest that smoking can affect the improvement obtained from cardiac rehabilitation exercise programmes by acting on some major factors such as serum lipids and blood pressure.

Effect of smoking on mean systolic and diastolic blood pressure

N. Sarrafzadegan & S. Mostafavi

Cardiovascular Research Centre, University of Medical Sciences, Isfahan, Iran

Smoking has been found not to be a risk factor for hypertension in some epidemiological studies, and the data in fact strongly suggest that smokers have lower blood pressure than non-smokers, whereas the blood pressure of ex-smokers is similar to that of non-smokers. We conducted this study to compare the mean systolic and diastolic blood pressure of smokers and non-smokers by sex and age. This cross-sectional study was carried out on 7870 subjects (4598 women and 3272 men) aged 20–70 years, who were randomly selected from 40 random clusters throughout the city with the main goal of defining the prevalence of smoking in Isfahan. Data were collected by questionnaires and blood pressure measurements according to the World Health

Organization standardized method, from the right in the sitting position. The mean of two measurements was used. The means in different age and smoking status groups were compared by Student's t test.

The mean systolic and diastolic blood pressure in non-smokers, 141.4 ± 29 and 87.4 ± 21, respectively, was significantly higher than that in smokers, 135.8 ± 24 and 85.2 ± 31 ($p < 0.05$), but a sex-specific comparison showed that this difference occurred only in men (see table). Smoking women had significantly higher mean systolic and diastolic blood pressure than non-smoking women ($p < 0.05$). These sex-specific differences were observed in all age groups.

This study supports the earlier finding that smokers have lower blood pressure, but we found this effect only in men. It has been shown that smoking one cigarette increases the heart rate, blood pressure and cardiac index, probably through adrenergic stimulation and catecholamine release. Futhermore, cigarette smoking can increase the risk of coronary artery diseases by many mechanisms, as shown in many previous epidemiological studies.

Sex-specific comparison of mean systolic and diastolic blood pressure in smokers and non-smokers

Sex	Blood pressure	Mean ± standard deviation		p
		Non-smokers	Smokers	
Men	Systolic	138.5 ± 26	135.1 ± 22	0.00
	Diastolic	86.2 ± 12	85.4 ± 32	0.00
Women	Systolic	142.9 ± 31	146 ± 38	0.00
	Diastolic	82.9 ± 18	88 ± 24	0.00

Effects of smoking on the response of blood pressure to exercise and physical activity

N. Sarrafzadegan, S. Mostafavi & M. Boshtam

Cardiovascular Research Centre, University of Medical Sciences, Isfahan, Iran

Clinical studies have shown that direct or indirect exposure to tobacco smoke increases the resting heart rate and systolic and diastolic blood pressure, probably as a consequence of adrenergic stimulation by nicotine. Smoking significantly increases the heart rate (by 34%) and diastolic blood pressure (by 17%). This study was conducted to examine the impact of smoking on the response of the mean systolic and diastolic blood pressure to exercise training in normotensive and hypertensive people.

A total of 8550 men and women were randomly selected from random clusters in Isfahan City, with the main objective of determining the prevalence of hypertension in Isfahan. The questionnaire included questions on smoking status and level of physical activity, which was defined as positive if the participants exercised at least once a week for 30–60 min and negative if otherwise. The questionnaire was completed for each participant and their blood pressure was then measured on the right arm in the sitting position, according to the standardized World Health Organization criteria. The chi-squared test, analysis of variance and unpaired t test were used for statistical analysis.

The results are shown in the table. Smoking was inversely associated with the response of mean systolic and diastolic blood pressure to exercise training in hypertensive men, but a similar effect was not seen in hypertensive women or in normosensive men or women. Smoking cessation is therefore strongly indicated in hypertensive people undergoing exercise training programmes to reduce their blood pressure.

Smoking status	Sex	Blood pressure	With exercise (mean ± SD)	No exercise (mean ± SD)	p value
Normotensive people					
Non-smoker	Male	Systolic	126.9 ± 12.1	128.1 ± 12.3	0.00
Smoker	Male	Systolic	126.9 ± 11.9	133.2 ± 20	0.00
Non-smoker	Male	Diastolic	80.8 ± 7.3	83 ± 12.1	0.00
Non-smoker	Female	Systolic	124.8 ± 14.2	134.7 ± 26.2	0.00
Smoker	Female	Systolic	78.1 ± 9.5	84.1 ± 14.7	0.00
Non-smoker	Female	Diastolic	72 ± 6.2	78.4 ± 16.7	0.00
Hypertensive people					
Non-smoker	Male	Systolic	170.6 ± 3	184.2 ± 17.9	0.00
Smoker	Male	Systolic	174 ± 10.9	170.2 ± 27.1	0.00
Non-smoker	Male	Diastolic	100 ± 13.1	109.5 ± 9.3	0.00
Smoker	Male	Diastolic	108.2 ± 2.5	102.1 ± 17.1	0.00
Non-smoker	Female	Systolic	173.1 ± 26.5	185.3 ± 19.6	0.00
Smoker	Female	Systolic	174 ± 10.9	172.1 ± 28.4	0.43
Non-smoker	Female	Diastolic	101.9 ± 13.3	109.2 ± 10.4	0.00
Smoker	Female	Diastolic	101 ± 2.5	100.5 ± 17,\.1	0.77

Mean values of blood lipids, body mass index and fasting blood glucose in smokers and non-smokers in Isfahan, Iran

M. Boshtam, M. Rafie & N. Sarrafzadegan

Cardiovascular Research Centre, University of Medical Sciences, Isfahan, Iran

Smoking is known to be a risk factor for cardiovascular disease. Because its prevalence is increasing in all countries and as the levels of other risk factors differs between smokers and non-smokers, the mean values for serum lipids, fasting blood glucose and body mass index were determined in the Isfahan population. This study was carried out on samples from a survey of risk factors for cardiovascular disease comprising 2200 participants aged 19–70 years in six age groups. The samples included 277 smokers and 1923 non-smokers and were selected randomly from population clusters in Isfahan. After a standard questionnaire had been completed, we took a 12–14-h fasting blood sample from the subjects. The data were analysed with the t test by SPSS software.

The results are presented in the table. The mean concentrations of low-density lipoproteins and total cholesterol were significantly higher in non-smokers than in smokers. There was no significant difference in the concentrations of other serum lipids, fasting blood glucose or body mass index between smokers and non-smokers. Accordingly, smoking appears to have no negative effect on the factors studied.

Factor	Smoker (mean ± SD)	Non-smoker (mean ± SD)	p
Total cholesterol (mg/dl)	212.26 ± 41.34	224.18 ± 48.46	0.010
Triglycerides (mg/dl)	223.20 ± 134.13	217.10 ± 48.46	0.315
High-density liporotein cholesterol (mg/dl)	34.90 ± 12.00	35.49 ± 7.32	0.438
Low-density liporotein cholesterol (mg/dl)	135.02 ± 36.96	146.73 ± 41.58	0.005
Fasting blood glucose (mg/dl)	100.28 ± 25.55	105.50 ± 37.64	0.116
Body mass index (kg/m²)	24.56 ± 4.04	27.43 ± 16.86	0.073

PASSIVE SMOKING

Passive smoking and the risk for lung cancer

D. Zaridze

*Cancer Research Centre, Russian Academy of Medical Sciences,
Moscow, Russian Federation*

'Passive smoking' is exposure to environmental tobacco smoke, the mixture of effluents directly released into the ambient air between puffs during the burning of tobacco product or re-exhaled by the smoker (Saracci *et al.*, 1992). Exposure to environmental tobacco smoke occurs in the domestic environment, at the worksite and in a variety of other places, including private and public transport, bars, restaurants and offices, wherever active smoking takes place. The ubiquitousness of tobacco smoke makes exposure virtually unavoidable.

The extent of exposure has been documented in several studies: according to different reports, 40–63% of the non-smoking population is exposed to environmental tobacco smoke (Lebowitz *et al.*, 1992). Passive smoking is therefore fundamentally different from active smoking, which is driven by a mixture of personal free choice and social conditioning, while passive smoking, when it entails increased risks of disease, represents an involuntarily incurred hazard. For this class of hazard in the public environment (including the workplace), there is a long-established consensus that regulatory and legislative restrictive measures are a proper method of control (Saracci *et al.*, 1992).

The main component of environmental tobacco smoke is sidestream smoke, which is freely emitted into the air from the smouldering tobacco product in the intervals between puffing a cigarette, cigar or pipe. During puffs, some sidestream smoke escapes directly from the burning tip, while some volatile compounds diffuse through the cigarette paper. Sidestream smoke as found in the environment presents both similarities to and differences from mainstream smoke. More than 3800 individual compounds have been identified in tobacco smoke, and quantitative measurements are available for more than 300 in both mainstream and sidestream smoke. Sidestream smoke contains a number of carcinogens, for six of which there is 'sufficient evidence' of carcinogenicity in humans: 4-aminobiphenyl, arsenic, benzene, chromium compounds, nickel compounds and vinyl chloride (IARC, 1985).

The relationship between passive smoking and cancer and the resulting discussions and debate have largely been concentrated on lung cancer. This is the commonest malignant neoplasm in developed countries, and tobacco smoking is the main cause of this fatal disease, responsible for an estimated 90–95% of cases in men and 80–85% in women (IARC, 1985). Epidemiological studies conducted during the past 15 years have provided evidence of a causal association between exposure to environmental tobacco smoke and lung cancer (Tredaniel *et al.*, 1994).

There have been three large cohort studies on environmental tobacco smoke and lung cancer: one from Japan (Hirayama, 1981) and two from the United States (Garfinkel, 1981; Cardenas *et al.*, 1997). A smaller study was reported in Scotland (Hole *et al.*, 1989). All four studies found an increase in the relative risk (RR) of lung cancer among non-smoking women married to smoking men. In the Japanese cohort, the RRs were 1.4, 1.6 and 1.9 when the husband smoked 1–14, 15–19 and > 20 cigarettes per day, respectively. The increase in the RR for lung cancer of non-smoking women married to smoking men in the American study was small (Garfinkel, 1981). The Scottish study reported an RR for lung cancer of 2.4 for persons with a partner who had ever smoked (Hole *et al.*, 1989). In the recently published American Cancer Society's Cancer Prevention Study II, based on 247 lung cancer deaths, the rate of death from lung cancer adjusted for other factors was 20% higher among women whose husbands had smoked during the current marriage than among those married to 'never smokers' (RR,

1.2; 95% CI, 0.8–1.6). The risk of the women was higher when their husbands smoked ≥ 40 cigarettes per day (RR, 1.9; 95% CI, 1.0–3.6) (Cardenas *et al.*, 1997).

Most of case–control studies have been concentrated on exposure to environmental tobacco smoke due to the spouse's smoking. Typically elevated risks of lung cancer were observed among non-smoking women living with smoking men, the RRs ranging from 1.2 (Brownson *et al.*, 1992; Fontham *et al.*, 1994) to 3.2 (Pershagen *et al.*, 1987). In a case–control study performed in Moscow, Russian Federation, the RR for lung cancer of non-smoking women whose husbands smoked was 1.5 (95% CI, 1.1–2.2) (Zaridze *et al.*, 1998). Increased RRs for lung cancer were observed with increasing pack–years of exposure to the husband's tobacco smoke (Pershagen *et al.*, 1987; Fontham *et al.*, 1994) and number of cigarettes smoked by him per day (Cardenas *et al.*, 1997). The studies suggest that the association between exposure to the husband's smoking and the risk for lung cancer of non-smoking women is somewhat stronger for squamous-cell carcinoma than for adenocarcinoma (Pershagen *et al.*, 1987; Fontham *et al.*, 1994; Zaridze *et al.*, 1998). These results run parallel to the stronger association found between active smoking and squamous-cell lung cancer as compared with adeno-carcinoma (IARC, 1985).

In the case–control study of lung cancer in non-smoking women in Moscow, an association was reported between the type of cigarettes smoked by the husband and the risk for lung cancer among wives. The risk was higher for women whose husbands smoked *papirosy* than for women whose husbands smoked cigarettes. *Papirosy* are cigarettes with a long mouthpiece, which usually contain very high concentrations of tar (> 35 mg/cigarette) and nicotine (> 2.0 mg/cigarette) (Zaridze *et al.*, 1998).

The evidence from the available studies of an association between exposure to environmental tobacco smoke during childhood and the risk for lung cancer is inconsistent, and the data on an effect of exposure to environmental tobacco smoke in the workplace on the risk for lung cancer in Europe suggests no association (Tredaniel *et al.*, 1994), although in some other studies (Fontham *et al.*, 1994), the RR associated with exposure in the workplace was higher than that associated with exposure to husbands' smoking.

In 1986, the Report of the Surgeon General (US Public Health Service, 1986), based on a meta-analysis of the results of the available case–control studies, concluded that the RR for lung cancer of a non-smoking woman living with a smoking man was around 1.4 (95% CI, 1.1–1.5). The overall RR from six studies in Europe was estimated to be 1.45 (95% CI, 1.1–1.9) (Tredaniel *et al.*, 1994). Recently, the Environmental Protection Agency (Department of Health and Human Services, 1993) conducted a pooled analysis of the results of 11 published studies in the United States and estimated that women who had never smoked who were married to smokers had a risk for lung cancer that was 19% higher than that of women married to men who had never smoked (RR, 1.2; 95% CI, 1.0–1.4). The proportion of cases of lung cancer among non-smokers that could be attributed to environmental tobacco smoke in western countries has been estimated to be 20–30% (Vainio & Partanen, 1989). The Environmental Protection Agency (Department of Health and Human Services, 1993) estimated that 3000 lung cancer death per year among non-smokers aged ≥ 35 were attributable to exposure to environmental tobacco smoke.

The causal association between between exposure to environmental tobacco smoke and lung cancer is now clearly established. Even though passive smoking poses a lower risk than active smoking, it yields an appreciable number of deaths because of the large number of potentially exposed individuals. The magnitude of the risk differs from country to country and must be more precisely calculated; however, enough is already known to justify action and the restriction or prohibition of smoking in public places, especially in regions where tobacco consumption is still high.

References

Brownson, R.C., Alavania, M.C.R., Hock, E.T. & Loy, T.S. (1992) Passive smoking and lung cancer in non-smoking women. *Am. J. Publ. Health*, **82**, 1525–1530

Cardenas, V.M., Thun, M.J., Austin, H., Lally, C.A., Clark, W.S., Greenberg, R.S. & Heath, C.W. (1997) Environmental tobacco smoke and lung cancer mortality in the American Cancer Society's Cancer Prevention study II. *Cancer Causes Control*, **8**, 57–64

Department of Health and Human Services (1993) *Respiratory Health Effects of Passive Smoking: Lung Cancer and Other Disorders* (Smoking and Tobacco Control Monograph 4; NIH Publication 93-3605), Washington DC

Fotham, E., Correa, P., Wu-Williams, A., Reynolds, P., Greenberg, R.S., Buffler, P.A., Chen, V.W., Boyd, P., Alterman, T., Austin, D.F., Liff, J. & Greenberg, S.D. (1994) Environmental tobacco smoke and lung cancer in non-smoking women. A multicenter study. *J. Am. Med. Assoc.*, **271**, 1752–1759

Gerfinkel, L. (1981) Time trends in lung cancer mortality among nonsmokers and a note on passive smoking. *J. Natl Cancer Inst.*, **66**, 1061–1066

Hirayama, T. (1981) Nonsmoking wives of heavy smokers have a higher risk of lung cancer. A study from Japan. *Br. Med. J.*, **282**, 183–185

Hole, D.J., Gillis, C.R., Chopra, C. & Hawthorne, V.M. (1989) Passive smoking and cardiorespiratory health in a general population in the west of Scotland. *Br. Med. J.*, **299**, 423–427

IARC (1985) *IARC Monographs on the Evaluation of the Carcinogenic Risk of Chemicals to Humans*, Vol. 38, *Tobacco Smoking*, Lyon

Lebowitz, M.D., Quackenboss, J.J., Krzyzanowski, M., O'Rourke, M.K. & Hayes, C. (1992) Multipollutant exposures and health responses to particulate matter. *Arch. Environ. Health*, **47**, 71–75

Pershagen, G., Hrubec, Z. & Svensson, C. (1987) Passive smoking and lung cancer in Swedish women. *Am. J. Epidemiol.*, **125**, 17–24

Public Health Service (1986) *The Health Consequences of Involuntary Smoking. A Report of the Surgeon General* (DHHS Publication (CDC), 87-8398), Washington DC, US Government Printing Office

Saracci, R., Hill, C., Jarvis, M., Rose, G. & Trichopoulos, D. (1992) Passive smoking and the risk of cancer. In: Zaridze, D. & Bodmer, W., eds, *Cancer Prevention in Europe*, Geneva: Organization of European Cancer Institutes,

Tredaniel, J., Boffetta, P., Saracci, R. & Hirsch, A. (1994) Exposure to environmental tobacco smoke and risk of lung cancer: The epidemiological evidence. *Eur. Respir. J.*, **7**, 1877–1888

Vainio, H. & Partanen, T. (1989) Population burden of lung cancer due to environmental tobacco smoke. *Mutat. Res.*, **222**, 137–140

Zaridze, D., Maximovitch, D., Zemlyanaya, G. & Boffetta, P. (1998) Exposure to environmental tobacco smoke and risk of lung cancer in nonsmoking women from Moscow, Russia. *Int. J. Cancer*, **75**, 335–338

Environmental tobacco smoke, lung cancer and heart disease

P.N. Lee

P.N. Lee Statistics and Computing Ltd, Sutton, Surrey, United Kingdom

Introduction

This paper is a review of the epidemiological evidence on exposure to environmental tobacco smoke and the risks for lung cancer and heart disease, evaluated in meta-analyses. Fuller reviews on the risks for lung cancer and on heart disease, available on request from the author, list the 46 studies of lung cancer and the 23 on heart disease included in the meta-analyses, study-specific relative risks (RRs) and confidence intervals (CIs) for each exposure index and more information on the analyses presented and issues discussed.

Methods

Attention was restricted to lifelong non-smokers in studies published before 1997. Studies with no proper controls or fewer than five cases and which did not separate results for non-smokers were excluded. The studies included match other reviews, e.g. by the Environmental Protection Agency (1992). The RRs and 95% CIs, adjusted for covariates when possible, were extracted for spouses' smoking, and for other indices, such as exposure to environmental tobacco smoke in the workplace and during childhood. The significance of the differences between exposed and unexposed persons and dose-related trends were estimated as required. The study attributes were extracted systematically. In the results on lung cancer, correction was made for misclassification bias by up-to-date methods, to avoid the errors made in earlier attempts (Lee & Forey,

1996). The misclassification rates were based on a review (Lee & Forey, 1995) and recent data for Asia (Lee, 1995; Wewers *et al.*, 1995). The estimated RRs and 95% CIs were combined by fixed-effects meta-analysis. For spouses' smoking, meta-analysis was applied to data subsets to investigate heterogeneity. The likely magnitude of a potential sources of bias was compared with the magnitude of the estimated RRs in order to judge whether any increase in RR could plausibly be attributed to bias.

Results: Lung cancer

Of five prospective and 41 case-control studies, 17 were conducted in the United States, nine in Europe and 20 in Asia. They covered 5480 cases of lung cancer in female non-smokers and 473 in male non-smokers. Common weaknesses of the studies included small sample size (< 100 cases in 28 studies), incomplete histological confirmation (in 25 studies) and use of markedly more interviews with next-of-kin of cases than controls (in five studies). In hardly any of the studies was cotinine used to determine exposure to environmental tobacco smoke or to exclude misclassified current smokers. Other weaknesses were unrepresentative controls, conducting interviews with cases and controls in different situations, incomplete follow-up for mortality and inadequate reporting. In 12 studies of husband's smoking, age was improperly controlled (incorrectly assuming that matching of all cases and controls for age implies age-matching of cases and controls among non-smokers); in over half no adjustment was made for marital status (including unmarried women in the unexposed group), and in almost half no account was taken of confounders at all. Some risk factors were rarely considered.

The overall data for exposure in the workplace (RR, 1.05; 95% CI, 0.96–1.14), based on 16 studies; exposure during childhood (1.01; 0.92–1.11; 16 studies) and social exposure (1.10; 0.94–1.30; 5 studies) show no significant increase with exposure, and no consistent dose–response relationship was seen for these exposure indices. For spouses' exposure, an association was evident. Although this was not significant for wives' smoking (1.24; 0.98–1.57; 15 studies), it was ($p < 0.001$) for husband's smoking (1.16; 1.09–1.25; 42 studies). We now examine the data on husband's smoking more fully.

Husbands' smoking—sources of heterogeneity: The overall RR of 1.16 was highly ($p < 0.001$) heterogeneous. The RRs varied significantly by continent (United States, 1.12; Europe, 1.62; Asia, 1.13; $p_{het} < 0.05$), country in Asia (Japan, 1.30; Hong Kong, 1.45; China, 1.00; $p_{het} < 0.05$), publication date (1981–89, 1.36; 1990–96, 1.06; $p_{het} < 0.001$) and study size (> 100 cases, 1.09; 50–100 cases, 1.43; < 50, 1.24; $p_{het} < 0.05$). The risk was lower ($p < 0.001$) in studies in which confounders were taken into account (1.08 versus 1.46) and in studies in which adjustment or matching was made for age (1.10 versus 1.53). It was higher ($p < 0.01$) in studies in which dose–response data were reported (1.24 versus 1.02). The risk was higher ($p < 0.05$) in studies in which 100% histological confirmation was required of cases. In these studies, there was no consistent evidence of a stronger association with squamous-cell carcinoma than with adenocarcinoma, contrasting with the situation for active smoking.

Husbands' smoking—bias due to confounding: Since there are many risk factors for lung cancer other than smoking, and exposure to environmental tobacco smoke is associated with greater exposure to many such factors (Thornton et al., 1994; Matanoski et al., 1995), and since the association between environmental tobacco smoke and lung cancer is weak, confounding is a real possibility; however, control for confounding was generally poor. Known factors were adjusted for in few studies, e.g. occupation in only six and diet in three, and in many studies there was no adjustment for age or marital status. Although meta-analysis of covariate-adjusted data gave a RR of 1.16, only 0.03 less than that with the unadjusted data, 1.19, the much higher RRs in studies in which confounders were ignored and the *a priori* likelihood of confounding suggest that, had full adjustment for covariates always been conducted, the reduction might have greatly exceeded 0.03.

Husbands' smoking—bias due to misclassification of active smoking status: Since some current or former smokers are misclassified as non-smokers (Lee & Forey, 1995) and the smoking habits of spouses are correlated ((Lee, 1992), estimates of the association between spouses' smoking and lung cancer in non-smokers will be biased (Lee, 1992; Environmental Protection Agency, 1992; Lee & Forey, 1996). The bias depends on the misclassification rate (and how it relates to smoking by the spouse), the between-spouse smoking concordance ratio, the proportions of smokers among subjects and spouses and the risk for lung cancer of misclassified smokers. The misclassification rates seem not to depend on whether the spouse smokes (Lee, 1992; Ogden *et al.*, 1997), but studies in western populations indicate that misclassified 'ever' smokers have smoked less and for a shorter duration than average 'ever' smokers and so would have a lower risk for lung cancer. Reviewing the evidence, Lee and Forey (1995, 1996) estimated that in the west the misclassification rates are equivalent (in their effect on the bias) to denial of smoking by 2.5% of 'ever' smokers with an average risk for lung cancer.

Using a misclassification-adjustment procedure that eliminates earlier errors (e.g. Environmental Protection Agency, 1992; Lee & Forey, 1996), assuming a concordance ratio of 3.0 (Lee, 1992) and basing corrections on data unadjusted for covariates (since the procedures do not work on covariate-adjusted RRs), the RR for the United States is reduced from 1.12 (1.01–1.24) to 1.01 (0.90–1.12) and that for western Europe from 1.19 (0.83–1.72) to 1.12 (0.77–1.63). Two recent studies suggest much higher misclassification rates in Asia. One (Lee, 1995) found that 20.8% of Japanese female smokers (as determined by cotinine) claimed to be non-smokers and had cotinine levels similar to those of self-reported smokers. The other study (Wewers *et al.*, 1995) showed that 62% of Southeast Asian women smokers living in Ohio (United States) denied smoking, although their cotinine values were like those of smokers. Using even a 10% misclassification rate would reduce the RR of 1.20 (1.08–1.34) for Asia to 1.12 (1.00–1.25), while a 20% rate would reduce it to 1.02 (0.90–1.14). Clearly, the biasing effects of misclassification, coupled with uncontrolled confounding, can explain the small elevation in lung cancer risk associated with spouses' smoking.

Husbands' smoking—other possible sources of bias: Studies in which the cases and controls were not matched on vital status, proxy response, hospital and/or place of interview or which had other major weaknesses had higher RRs than other studies (1.24 versus 1.10), suggesting that weaknesses in study design may contribute to the elevated lung cancer risk. Other sources of positive bias include publication bias (RRs being higher in small studies) and recall bias. Inaccurate diagnoses of lung cancer may have led to some negative bias. Negative bias due to misclassification of smoking by the spouse is likely to be much less than positive bias due to misclassification of smoking by the subject (Lee, 1996).

Husbands' smoking—dose–response data: From 28 studies, 40 data sets could be derived on RR by amount smoked, years smoked and/or 'pack-years' of exposure to environmental tobacco smoke. While no data set showed a significant monotonically increasing relationship with trend including and excluding the unexposed group, a dose–response relationship is clearly evident. These data are, however, subject to publication bias, the RRs for exposed versus unexposed being much higher in reports presenting dose–response data (1.24 versus 1.02; $p < 0.01$). Also, the dose–response data are themselves subject to biases due to confounding, smoking misclassification and recall bias.

Relevance of supporting evidence: An autopsy-based study found more 'epithelial, possibly precancerous lesions' in non-smoking women with smoking spouses (Trichopoulos *et al.*, 1992); however, these lesions were no commoner in heavy smokers than in non-smokers. No standard lifetime study in animals exposed by inhalation has been reported. A study (Witschi *et al.*, 1997) in which very high exposure to environmental tobacco smoke increased the risk for lung adenomas in mice not pretreated with carcinogens, but decreased the risk in pretreated mice, is difficult to interpret. A reported association between lung cancer in pet dogs and smoking in the home (Reif *et al.*, 1992) was not statistically significant. None of these observations provides strong evidence that exposure to environmental tobacco smoke causes lung cancer.

Discussion and conclusions: lung cancer

In view of the many common constituents of environmental tobacco smoke and mainstream smoke, some argue that exposure to environmental tobacco smoke must carry some risk for lung cancer (Environmental Protection Agency, 1992); however, differences in the physico-chemical composition of the two types of smoke mean that environmental tobacco smoke cannot simply be viewed as diluted mainstream smoke. Also, since the concentrations of chemicals in environmental tobacco smoke are typically much lower than the permissible limits approved by regulators (Redhead & Rowberg, 1995) and the annual exposure of non-smokers to particles is less than 0.2% that of a typical smoker (Phillips *et al.*, 1994), it cannot necessarily be assumed that environmental tobacco smoke is carcinogenic. It is relevant that most toxicologists do not believe in a zero threshold for carcinogenesis (Kraus *et al.*, 1992). Any effect of environmental tobacco smoke on the risk for lung cancer needs must be shown by epidemiological or experimental evidence; however, the experimental evidence is virtually nonexistent and the epidemiological evidence is unconvincing. An association with the risk for lung cancer risk is seen for only one exposure index, spouses' smoking, and that is subject to various biases. Misclassification of smoking causes major bias and uncontrolled confounding, and publication bias and recall bias are also relevant. Large unexplained variations in RRs by various study characteristics further undermine the validity of any causal inference.

The overall conclusion must be that the data are consistent with no effect of exposure to environmental tobacco smoke on the risk for lung cancer. Although a weak effect may exist, the estimate that 3000 lung cancer deaths a year in the United States are related to exposure to environmental tobacco smoke (Environmental Protection Agency, 1992) is clearly worthless.

Results: Heart disease

Of 10 prospective, 10 case–control and three cross-sectional studies, 13 were conducted in the United States, four in Europe, three in Asia, two in Australasia and one in South America. The numbers of cases varied widely: over half of studies involved < 200 cases, but the three largest studies, all recently published, involved as many as 14 891 (LeVois & Layard, 1995), 3819 (Steenland *et al.*, 1996) and 1389 (Layard, 1995) cases. Owing to incomplete reporting, it is not always possible to identify the weaknesses of these studies. It was clear, however, that nearly all them were based on unconfirmed data from questionnaires to determine non-smoking status and exposure to environmental tobacco smoke. Other weaknesses in a few studies included incomplete follow-up for mortality, obtaining data for cases and controls by completely different methods, use of a highly subjective index of exposure to environmental tobacco smoke and inconsistent reporting of results. In nearly all of the studies adjustment was made for age and marital status. Major risk factors such as blood pressure, cholesterol, social class, education and obesity or weight were each adjusted for in about half the studies.

Twelve sex-specific estimates from seven studies were provided on exposure to environmental tobacco smoke in the workplace; the overall RR (1.07, 0.96-1.19) was nonsignificant. In 21 studies in which 31 estimates were provided for spouses' smoking, the overall RR was significant ($p < 0.01$) for current spouses' smoking (1.08, 1.05–1.12) and for 'ever' spouses' smoking (1.07, 1.03–1.10). The estimates were similar for men and women.

Spouses' smoking—sources of heterogeneity: We shall restrict further attention to 'ever' smoking, as the results for current smoking are similar. The 31 estimates were significantly ($p < 0.01$) heterogeneous, being clearly lower in studies in the United States, in those published recently, in large studies, in studies of fatal heart disease, in those in which dose–response data were available and those published as papers (not abstracts or theses). The heterogeneity was explained by dividing the 23 studies into three groups: three recent, large 'better quality' studies; five other 'better quality' studies; and 14 'worse quality' studies (i.e. studies not published as papers, involving < 100 cases or with evident weaknesses). The RRs varied markedly ($p < 0.001$) between groups (1.02, 0.99–1.06; 1.22, 1.11–1.34; 1.50, 1.30–1.72) but not within groups.

Spouses' smoking—dose–response relationships: Twelve studies provided 22 sets of data, mainly for the number of cigarettes smoked per day. Again, there was a huge difference between the three groups of studies. Of 12 data sets for the last two groups, 11 showed a monotonic increase and eight a significant positive trend. In contrast, no data sets from the first group of studies showed a monotonic increase or a trend.

Spouses' smoking—bias due to misclassification of smoking habits: As the excess risk associated with smoking is much less for heart disease than for lung cancer, it might be thought that there was little misclassification bias for heart disease; however, there are high misclassification rates of patients with diagnosed heart disease who have been advised by their doctor to give up smoking (Lee, 1988), so that people claiming to be non-smokers may include some smokers with a high risk for death from heart disease. The results of a study (Suadicani *et al.*, 1997) in which subjects reported to be non-smokers but who had cotinine levels consistent with those of smokers had a markedly increased RR for death from heart disease (4.01, 1.76–9.13) relative to subjects who admitted smoking, supports this probability. This contrasts with the situation for lung cancer where correction is based on the assumption that misclassified smokers have much lower risks for lung cancer than do subjects who admit to smoking. Misclassification bias may be highly relevant for heart disease.

Spouses' smoking—bias due to confounding: The information provided in studies in which adjustment was made for confounding was insufficient to estimate the effect of the adjustment on the RR, but our analysis suggested that adjustment for age increased the RRs and adjustment for other factors decreased them. The effects of adjustment were often strikingly large, in seven cases by ± 20% (four decreases, three increases). Since in many studies little attention was paid to confounders and the overall RR for spouses' smoking is only 1.07, it is clear that uncontrolled confounding could be an important bias.

Spouses' smoking—other possible sources of bias: The literature has been hugely affected by publication bias: the results on heart disease from the study with by far the most deaths did not appear until 1995, although the results for lung cancer were published in 1981. As some studies were reported years ago only as abstracts or theses and as the literature on heart disease is rather sparse, even though heart disease is much commoner than lung cancer in non-smokers, some publication bias may still exist. Recall bias and diagnostic bias may also be relevant, as evidenced by the results from one study (Tunstall-Pedoe *et al.*, 1995), which showed that angina was associated with self-reported exposure to environmental tobacco smoke but not cotinine, and that cotinine was associated with diagnosed coronary heart disease (on the basis of the subjects' report of a medical diagnosis) but not with undiagnosed coronary heart disease (based on tests carried out at the time of interview).

Relevance of supporting evidence: In our detailed review, my colleague F.J.C. Roe refuted the claim of Glantz and Parmley (1995) that the complex clinical and experimental evidence demonstrates that exposure to environmental tobacco smoke is a risk factor for coronary heart disease.

Discussion and conclusions: Heart disease

In active smokers, lung cancer is usually considered to arise from exposure to the particulate phase of tobacco smoke, while heart disease is often held to result from components of the vapour phase. While passive smokers have relatively greater exposure to vapour than particulate phase components than active smokers, average exposure to environmental tobacco smoke still involves a much lower 'dose' of any smoke constituent than that obtained by average active smoking. This is underlined by reports (Ogden, 1996; Robinson et al., 1996) that heavy smokers receive much greater exposure to environmental tobacco smoke than do passive smokers. Since the risk for heart disease in smokers relative to non-smokers is typically less than 2.0, claims (Glantz & Parmley, 1995) of a RR of 1.3 for exposure to environmental tobacco smoke seem difficult to reconcile with the dosimetry. Recent evidence from three large studies involving 20 000 deaths from heart disease showed little association with spouses' smoking ('ever', 1.02, 0.99–1.06; current, 1.04, 1.00–1.08) and undermines these claims. Anyway, the epidemiological data are subject to various biases, including publication and recall bias and uncontrolled confounding. The much higher rates of death from heart disease among smokers who had denied rather than admitted their habit (Suadicani et al., 1997) suggest that misclassification of smoking status is also an important source of bias.

The reason for some of the increased risks reported remains unclear, but the overall data provide little reason to believe that there is an association between exposure to environmental tobacco smoke and heart disease, let alone a causal relationship. As for lung cancer, the estimate that large annual numbers of deaths from heart disease are due to exposure environmental tobacco must be regarded as scientific nonsense.

Acknowledgements
    I thank B.A. Forey, K.J. Young, F.J.C. Roe, A. Springall and J.S. Fry for considerable assistance in preparing the detailed reviews summarized in this paper, and P. Wassell for typing. I am grateful to various tobacco companies for financial support. I remain responsible for all views expressed.

References
Environmental Protection Agency (1992) *Respiratory Health Effects of Passive Smoking: Lung Cancer and Other Disorders* (EPA/600/6-90/006F), Washington DC
Glantz, S.A. & Parmley, W.W. (1995) *J. Am. Med. Assoc.*, **273**, 1047–1053
Kraus, N., et al. (1992) *Risk Anal.*, **12**, 215–232
Layard, M.W. (1995) *Regul. Toxicol. Pharmacol.*, **21**, 180–183
Lee, P.N. (1988) *Int. Arch. Occup. Environ. Health*, Suppl.
Lee, P. (1992) *Environmental Tobacco Smoke and Mortality*, Basel: Karger
Lee, P. (1995) *Int. Arch. Occup. Environ. Health*, **67**, 287–294
Lee, P. & Forey, B. (1995) *J. Smoking-related Dis.*, **6**, 109–129
Lee, P. & Forey, B. (1996) *Stat. Med.*, **15**, 581–605
LeVois, M.E. & Layard, M.W. (1995) *Regul. Toxicol. Pharmacol.*, **21**, 184–191
Matanoski, G., et al. (1995) *Am. J. Epidemiol.*, **142**, 149–157
Ogden, M.W. (1996) *Anal. Commun.*, **33**, 197–198
Ogden, M.W., et al. (1997) *J. Clin. Epidemiol.*, **50**, 253–263
Phillips, K., et al. (1994) *Environ. Int.*, **20**, 693–712
Redhead, C. & Rowberg, R. (1995) *Environmental Tobacco Smoke and Lung Cancer Risk*, Washington DC: US Congressional Research Service
Reif, J., et al. (1992) *Am. J. Epidemiol.*, **135**, 234–239
Robinson, J.P., et al. (1996) *Am. J. Public Health*, **86**, 1303–1305
Steenland, K., et al. (1996) *Circulation*, **94**, 622–628
Suadicani, P., et al. (1997) *Int. J. Epidemiol.*, **26**, 321–327
Thornton, A., et al. (1994) *J. Clin. Epidemiol.*, **47**, 1143–1162
Trichopoulos, D., et al. (1992) *J. Am. Med. Assoc.*, **268**, 1697–1701
Tunstall-Pedoe, H., et al. (1995) *J. Epidemiol. Commun. Health*, **49**, 139–143
Wewers, M., et al. (1995) *Am. J. Respir. Crit. Care Med.*, **152**, 1917–1921
Witschi, H., et al. (1997) *Carcinogenesis*, **18**, 575–586

Environmental tobacco smoke, air pollution and respiratory symptoms in non-smoking housewives in Hong Kong

C.M. Wong, Z.G. Hu, T.H. Lam, A.J. Hedley & J. Peters

Department of Community Medicine, The University of Hong Kong, Hong Kong SAR, China

Introduction

In Hong Kong, environmental tobacco smoke at home is an important source of air pollution because of the crowded conditions in which most families live. Its effects on the respiratory health of children were shown in a four-year study in 1989–92 (Ong *et al.*, 1991; Peters *et al.*, 1996). The aim of the present study was to examine the effects of environmental tobacco smoke and air pollution on the respiratory health of non-smoking housewives.

In Hong Kong, 97% of women do not smoke (Census and Statistics Department, 1993), and about 50% are housewives (Census and Statistics Department, 1996). The situation provided an opportunity for studying the effects of environmental tobacco smoke in a population free from the effects of active smoking and from occupational exposure.

To date, the effects of environmental tobacco smoke on non-smoking women have been found to be associated with reduced bronchial responsiveness (Jindal *et al.*, 1996), death from cancer in general (Miller, 1990) and lung cancer in particular (Stockwell *et al.*, 1992; Fontham *et al.*, 1994; Cardenas *et al.*, 1997), chronic obstructive pulmonary diseases (Kalandidi *et al.*, 1990), cardiorespiratory signs and symptoms and mortality (Hole *et al.*, 1989), increased numbers of carcinogen–haemoglobin adducts (Hammond *et al.*, 1993), heart disease (Steenland, 1992), impairment of endothelium-dependent dilatation (Celermajer *et al.*, 1996) and increased thickness of the intima media (Howard *et al.*, 1994). The effects on relatively mild symptoms which can affect a large proportion of the population have seldom been studied.

Subjects and methods

The subjects in this study were the mothers of children who had participated in the above-mentioned four-year study on the effects of air pollution in Hong Kong. The study design is depicted in Figure 1. A sub-set of the mothers who were non-smokers and did not work in a full-time job were studied ($n = 2020, 1903, 5754$ and 6224 in the four years).

Six respiratory symptoms, throat problems, cough in the morning, cough in the evening, phlegm in the morning, phlegm day or night and phlegm within three months, were recorded by the subjects in response to a questionnaire brought home by their

Figure 1. Design of questionnaire survey of children in primary (P)-school grades 3–6 over four years in Hong Kong

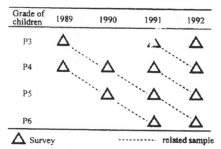

children from school. A variable summarizing whether the subjects had one or more symptoms was defined as the outcome variable for the present study. Exposure to environmental tobacco smoke at home, quantified by the numbers of smokers (father, siblings and other relatives of the children) and whether they lived in a polluted district (compared with a relatively less polluted district) were used as the two main risk factors. Age, housing type (public housing and others), educational attainment (no formal education, primary, lower and upper secondary, tertiary), incense burning, use of mosquito coils and cooking fuel (gas and others) were included as confounding factors.

Logistic regression of any symptom on the two risk factors (environmental tobacco smoke and living in a polluted district) with adjustment for repeated measures (the subjects might have participated in the study one to four times) and adjustment for the potential confounding factors mentioned above was performed by means of the generalized estimating equations procedure (Liang & Zeger, 1986) using the Stata statistical package (StataCorp, 1997).

Results

The crude prevalence of any symptom was generally higher for those living in a polluted district for the four years of the study and was also increased with the level of exposure to environmental tobacco smoke (Table 1). The adjusted prevalence odds ratios for any symptom (95% confidence interval) were 1.13 (1.02–1.26; $p = 0.021$) for living in a polluted district, 1.03 (0.93–1.15; $p = 0.520$) for exposure to one type and 1.16 (0.98–1.39; $p = 0.089$) for exposure to two or more types of smoker at home.

Conclusion

Non-smoking housewives residing in a polluted district were at higher risk of respiratory symptoms than those residing in a less polluted district. The prevalence of any respiratory symptom also increased with increasing exposure to environmental tobacco smoke. The adjusted prevalence odds ratios were about the same as that due to residing in a polluted district.

These results should have a public health implication in formulating smoking cessation programmes targeting smoking at home. Prevention of smoking in the homes of housewives is needed to protect non-smoking women and children from the adverse health effects of environmental tobacco smoke. A housewife who lives in a family with smokers could bring home the message that 'living in a family with a smoker or smokers is like living in a polluted district, as far as the effect on respiratory health is concerned' and could help their husbands and other family members to quit smoking.

Acknowledgements

The authors wish to thank the Environmental Protection Department, Hong Kong Government, Kwai Tsing District Board, Glaxo Hong Kong Limited, The Royal Hong Kong Jockey Club and the Mary Sun Medical Scholarship Fund (Hong Kong–Cambridge Link) for their financial support, and all the schools, head teachers, parents and children for their co-operation and participation in the study.

Table 1. Crude rate of any symptom by district of residence and number of smoker types at home

Variable	1989 (n = 2020)	1990 (n = 1903)	1991 (n = 5754)	1992 (n = 6224)
District of residence				
Less polluted	12.2	10.3	14.0	13.7
Polluted	14.6	11.7	13.3	16.8
No. of smoker types				
None	12.7	10.9	13.1	15.0
1	14.5	11.0	14.0	15.2
2 or more	15.6	12.7	16.9	

References

Cardenas, V.M., Thun, M.J., Austin, H., Lally, C.A., Clark, W.S., Greenberg, R.S. & Heath, C.W., Jr (1997) Environmental tobacco smoke and lung cancer mortality in the American Cancer Society's Cancer Prevention Study II. *Cancer Causes Control*, **8**, 57–64

Celermajer, D.S., Adams, M.R., Clarkson, P., Robinson, J., McCredie, R., Donald, A. & Deanfield, J.E. (1996) Passive smoking and impaired endothelium-dependent arterial dilatation in healthy young adults. *New Engl. J. Med.*, **334**, 150–154

Fontham, E.T., Correa, P., Reynolds, P., Wu Williams, A., Buffler, P.A., Greenberg, R.S., Chen, V.W., Alterman, T., Boyd, P., Austin, D.F., *et al.* (1994) Environmental tobacco smoke and lung cancer in nonsmoking women. *J. Am. Med. Assoc.*, **271**, 1752–1759

Hammond, S.K., Coghlin, J., Gann, P.H., Paul, M., Taghizadeh, K., Skipper, P.L. & Tannenbaum, S.R. (1993) Relationship between environmental tobacco smoke exposure and carcinogen–hemoglobin adduct levels in nonsmokers. *J. Natl Cancer Inst.*, **85**, 474–478

Hole, D.J., Gillis, C.R., Chopra, C. & Hawthorne, V.M. (1989) Passive smoking and cardiorespiratory health in a general population in the west of Scotland. *Br. Med. J.*, **299**, 423–427

Howard, G., Burke, G.L., Szklo, M., Tell, G.S., Eckfeldt, J., Evans, G. & Heiss, G. (1994) Active and passive smoking are associated with increased carotid wall thickness. The Atherosclerosis Risk in Communities Study. *Arch. Intern. Med.*, **154**, 1277–1282

Jindal, S.K., Gupta, D., D'Souza, G.A. & Kalra, S. (1996) Bronchial responsiveness of non-smoking women exposed to environmental tobacco smoke or biomass fuel combusion. *Indian J. Med. Res.*, **104**, 359–364

Kalandidi, A., Trichopoulos, D., Hatzakis, A., Tzannes, S. & Saracci, R. (1990) The effect of involuntary smoking on the occurrence of chronic obstructive pulmonary disease. *Soz. Praeventivmed.*, **35**, 12–16

Liang, K.Y. & Zeger, S.L. (1986) Longitudinal data analysis using generalized linear models. *Biometrika*, **73**, 13–22

Miller, G.H. (1990) The impact of passive smoking: Cancer deaths among nonsmoking women. *Cancer Detect. Prev.*, **14**, 497–503

Ong, S.G., Liu, J., Wong, C.M., Lam, T.H., Tam, A.Y.C., Daniel, L. & Hedley, A.J. Studies on the respiratory health of primary school children in urban communities of Hong Kong. *Sci. Total Environ.*, **106**, 121–135

Peters, J., Hedley, A.J., Wong, C.M., Lam, T.H., Ong, S.G., Liu, J. & Spiegelhalter, D.J. (1996) Effects of an ambient air pollution intervention and environmental tobacco smoke on children's respiratory health in Hong Kong. *Int. J. Epidemiol.*, **25**, 821–828

StataCorp (1997) Stata Statistical Software: Release 5.0, College Station: Stata Corp.

Steenland, K. (1992) Passive smoking and the risk of heart disease. *J. Am. Med. Assoc.*, **267**, 94–99

Stockwell, H.G., Goldman, A.L., Lyman, G.H., Noss, C.I., Armstrong, A.W., Pinkham, P.A., Candelora, E.C. & Brusa, M.R. (1992) Environmental tobacco smoke and lung cancer risk in nonsmoking women. *J. Natl Cancer Inst.*, **84**, 1417–142

Passive smoking from husbands as a risk factor for coronary heart disease in women in Xi'an, China, who have never smoked

Y. He[1,2], T.H. Lam[2], L.S. Li[1], L.S. Li[3], R.Y. Du[3], G.L. Jia[3], J.Y. Huang[1], Q.L. Shi[1] & J.S. Zheng[3]

[1] *Department of Epidemiology, 4th Military Medical University, Xi'an;*
[2] *Department of Community Medicine, The University of Hong Kong, Hong Kong SAR;* [3] *Department of Cardiology, 4th Military Medical University, Xi'an, China*

Up to 1997, 20 epidemiological studies had been conducted on passive smoking and coronary heart disease, and 17 showed an increased risk. On the basis of six review papers with pooled relative risks (RRs), the pooled RR for coronary heart disease associated with passive smoking from a spouse was 1.3 (California Environmental Protection Agency, 1997). In China, the prevalence of smoking in a national survey carried out in 1984 was 61% among men and 7% among women (Weng *et al.*, 1987). Passive smoking at home is a serious health problem for non-smoking women in China. The objective of this paper was to determine whether passive smoking from husbands is a risk factor for coronary heart disease in Chinese women who have never smoked.

Subjects and methods

The subjects were 323 Chinese women who had never smoked who had participated in our two published studies in 1989 (He *et al.*, 1989) and 1994 (He *et al.*, 1994) plus new subjects. Of these women, 115 were confirmed at three teaching hospitals of two medical universities in Xi'an as having coronary heart disease; 37 had myocardial infarct and 78 had coronary stenosis confirmed by coronary arteriography. The 208 controls were derived from three sources: 83 patients with negative findings by coronary arteriography, 35 of whom were originally thought to have coronary heart disease and are referred to as 'misdiagnosed coronary heart disease'; 51 out-patients with no coronary heart disease by WHO criteria and 74 people from a coronary heart disease screening programme in a factory.

A standardized questionnaire was designed to collect information on demographic characteristics (ethnicity, age, educational level, occupation and marital status); past history of hypertension, hyperlipidaemia and diabetes; family history of hypertension, stroke and coronary heart disease; history of smoking and passive smoking from husband; drinking history; physical exercise and psychosocial factors (type A personality, experience of mental trauma and stressful events). A face-to-face interview was conducted by three trained doctors in the wards or in the clinics of the factory hospital. The non-response rate was 4%. The laboratory investigations included total cholesterol, triglycerides, low- and high-density lipoprotein cholesterol. Coronary arteriography was performed by Judkins' technique.

Passive smoking from a husband was defined as having lived with a smoking husband for > 5 years. Single women were considered not to be exposed. The number of cigarettes smoked daily by the husband, the duration of passive smoking and cumulative exposure were defined as the variables of the amount of exposure.

Quality controls included tape-recording of interviews and interviewing the husbands to check the data from the wives. In the single blind interview–reinterview, 68 hospital cases and controls were interviewed at a 20-day interval by a second interviewer who was unaware of the result of the first interview. The 'misdiagnosed coronary heart disease' group was used to check for subjective bias in the interviews

Assuming that the odds ratio for coronary heart disease due to passive smoking at home is 2.0, the proportion of exposure to passive smoking from husbands among the controls was 35%; for a significance of 5% and a power of 80%, 109 cases and 218 controls were required in the study.

The statistical methods used were t and chi-squared tests, the chi-squred test for trend, odds ratio (OR) and 95% confidence interval (CI). Multivariate analysis was performed with an unconditional logistic regression model.

Results

There was no significant difference in the demographic variables or the risk factors between subjects from different sources, so the data for all subjects were combined in the analysis. The cases and controls were of similar age, marital status, occupation and education.

The tape recording of the interview showed that the procedure was objective. The interviews with the husbands and the single blind interview–reinterview all showed good agreement. Use of the 'misdiagnosed coronary heart disease' group suggested that there was no subjective bias in the interviews.

The crude odds ratio for coronary heart disease associated with husbands' smoking (95% CI) was 2.35 (1.41–3.93). Multiple stepwise logistic regression analysis was used to select the final model and to adjust for 18 independent variables. The final model included passive smoking from husbands as the base and age, history of hypertension, family history of coronary heart disease, type A personality, total cholesterol and high-density lipoprotein. The adjusted odds ratio was 1.6 (0.94–2.9). There was no significant interaction between passive smoking from husbands and the major risk factors for coronary heart disease (total cholesterol and high-density lipoprotein) in the final logistic model.

The relationship between the odds ratios and the amount of exposure to passive smoking was examined (Table 1). The crude and adjusted odds ratios showed significant linear trends with the amount smoked daily by the husband, the duration of passive smoking from the husband and cumulative exposure.

Discussion

To avoid potential bias, the subjects from different sources and studies were analysed separately. As the results of the separate analyses were similar, a pooled analysis was justified. The results of the quality control measures for selection of subjects and for the interview suggested that the data were reasonably reliable and free from bias.

Our previous studies (He *et al.*, 1989, 1994) showed a positive association between passive smoking from husbands and coronary heart disease. The result of the present study was consistent with the previous results and suggested that passive smoking from husbands is a likely cause of coronary heart disease in Chinese women who have never smoked. The results of the present study and evidence from Argentina, Australia, Japan, the United Kingdom and the United States support the hypothesis that passive smoking can cause coronary heart disease particularly in women who have never smoked (California Environmental Protection Agency, 1997). Urgent public health measures must be taken to reduce smoking and to protect non-smokers from passive smoking in China.

References

California Environmental Protection Agency (1997) *Health Effects of Exposure to Environmental Tobacco Smoke*, final draft for scientific, public, and SRP review

He, Y., Li, L.S., Wan, Z.H., Li, L.S., Zheng, X.L. & Jia, G.L. (1989) Women's passive smoking and coronary heart disease. *Chung-Hua-Yu-Fang-I-Hsueh-Tsa-Chih*, **23**, 19–22

He, Y., Lam, T.H., Li, L.S., Li, L.S., Du, R.Y., Jia, G.L., Huang, J.Y. & Zheng, J.S. (1994) Passive smoking at work as a risk factor for coronary heart disease in Chinese women who have never smoked. *Br. Med. J.*, **308**, 380–384

Weng, X.Z., Hong, Z.G., Chen, D.Y., Zhang, M., Chen, B.Z. &Tin, B.C. (1987) *A Collection of Data of the 1984 National Smoking Sample Survey*, Beijing: People's Health Publishers

Table 1. **Passive smoking from husbands and odds ratio (OR) (95% CI) for coronary heart disease**

Passive smoking from husband	No. of cases ($n = 115$)	No. of controls ($n = 208$)	Adjusted OR[a] (95% CI)	*p* (linear trend)
No. cigarettes/day				
0	39	113	1.0	
1–10	15	40	0.93 (0.42–2.0)	
11–20	29	35	1.4 (1.3–2.9)	0.006
≥ 21	32	20	3.2 (1.2 7.0)	
Duration of exposure (years)				
0–5 (actually zero)		39	113	1.0
6–15	14	37	0.80 (0.35–1.8)	
16–30	44	41	2.1 (1.1–4.0)	0.012
≥ 31	18	17	2.3 (0.96–5.6)	
Cumulative exposure (cigarettes/day x years)				
0	39	113	1.0	
1–399	33	58	1.2 (0.62–1.4)	
400–799	28	30	1.9 (0.89–4.0)	0.012
≥ 800	15	7	3.6 (1.2–11)	

[a] Adjusted for age, history of hypertension, family history of coronary heart disease, type A personality, total cholesterol and high-density lipoprotein in the final model. The crude odds ratios and their 95% CI are all slightly higher than those of adjusted odds ratios and are not shown.

Lesser known and minor effects of active smoking on non-smokers

M. Whidden

Association for Nonsmokers' Rights, Binfield, Berkshire, United Kingdom

Major reviews of the scientific literature on the effects of passive smoking have tended to focus on the obvious ones or on risks related to its most important effects. For example, the United States Environmental Protection Agency's (1992) review looked at respiratory diseases only. Besides, passive smoking is usually defined as 'breathing in' environmental tobacco smoke; but this is not the only way that non-smokers can be exposed to the harmful constituents of tobacco smoke. For instance, the eyes of non-smokers are exposed to irritating chemicals in smoke even if the non-smokers do not inhale the smoke. The uterine cervix is exposed to harmful constituents of tobacco smoke delivered during sexual intercourse in the semen of a smoking male; his fingers may introduce harmful tobacco-smoke constituents into the vaginal canal during sex. Fœtuses are exposed to high concentrations of tobacco-smoke poisons from maternal smoking during pregnancy. In this presentation, therefore, I shall not just use the term 'passive smoking', but shall also use the broader term, 'forced exposure to the constituents of tobacco smoke' (FECTS). Please note, however, that this term does not include the harm done to non-smokers by the many thousands of fires caused by cigarettes around the world or to the toddlers who are accidentally poisoned when they ingest tobacco, as in cigarette butts.

More comprehensive reviews (Whidden, 1993, updated) reveal that FECTS has been linked to more than 90 adverse physical conditions and diseases in pre-adult humans. Of the lesser-known or minor effects, only some have been shown so far to contribute directly to the well-known, major consequences. For over two decades, we have known that nicotine and cotinine make their way to the female human breast and enter human milk (Fergusson et al., 1976). Some scientists have discussed the possibility that certain minor adverse effects might be suffered by infants who drink contaminated milk (Luck & Nau, 1985; Lebrecque et al., 1989); however, there was a 10-year gap between the time it was known that tobacco-smoke poison entered women's breasts and the first study of FECTS and breast cancer. If the scientific community does finally conclude that passive smoking is a cause of breast cancer, then lessons need to be learned from these circumstances. As it happens, all four studies of FECTS in relation to breast cancer have shown a consistent link between exposure and this major disease in women (Sandler et al., 1986; Hirayama, 1990; Smith et al., 1994; Morabia et al., 1996). This is all the more remarkable because the results of studies on active smoking and breast cancer have been strikingly inconsistent. Most scientists tend to think that the fault must lie in the studies of passive smoking, when instead an obvious flaw exists in the investigations of active smoking and breast cancer: they, in effect, assumed that non-smokers are not exposed to the poisons in tobacco smoke and thus based their extrapolations on incorrect assumptions about their baseline data.

Firstly we should use clues about minor effects that result from FECTS to guide us towards research about possible major effects; secondly we should not allow such a long gap to occur between the time that a clue about tobacco-smoke constituents in non-smokers' bodies is inferred and investigations of the possibility of major effects that might result from these contaminants; and thirdly we should not allow bad science in the active smoking field to get in the way of good science about FECTS.

Discoveries of links between passive smoking by adults and increased risks for certain effects have not been followed up to detect whether a heightened incidence of these same conditions and diseases (or their precursors or early symptoms) occurs in pre-adult humans because of tobacco consumption by adults. In wholly unrelated research, Barker et al (1991) have shown that the lowered birthweight seen in their cohort 'was associated with worse adult lung function' and that infants who suffered bronchitis and pneumonia suffered 'reduced lung function' in later adult life. Of course, maternal smoking during pregnancy is a well-known cause of low birthweight, and passive smoking is a cause of bronchitis and pneumonia in children. Unfortunately, data about maternal smoking during the pregnancies that produced this cohort and during the infancy of the cohort members were not reported. The importance of this unrelated research is obvious: perhaps researchers have not been able to show consistently that passive smoking during adulthood results in reduced lung function because the confounding factors of maternal smoking during pregnancy and passive smoking during infancy have not been taken into account. Again, the pointers for research in passive smoking are obvious.

Some minor effects of pre-adult insults from tobacco smoke may have minor and not-so-minor effects that have not yet been studied. For example, delayed eruption of adult teeth in children exposed to passive smoke (Kieser et al., 1996) may have adverse effects on subsequent dental health. In this instance, a possible further consequence of these children's passive smoking may be that their teeth, once erupted, do not mature as fast as they should, and the children are thus at risk of more tooth decay than they would be otherwise.

Certain effects of passive smoking on children imply that the research must be extended. We have known for some time that passive smoking affects the circulatory system of children, adolescents and young adults (Glantz & Parmley, 1995). More recent research (Glueck et al., 1996) indicates that the risk for Legg-Perthe disease is significantly increased by passive smoking; other circulation-related conditions heretofore not considered as being related to passive smoking should therefore be investigated. 'It has been known for more than 30 years that [passive smoking] and exposure to nontobacco sources of low-level environmental [carbon monoxide] impair exercise performance in normal smokers and non-smokers and promote angina and cardiac arrhythmias in persons with coronary artery disease', and yet 'none of the published studies of the [6-min walk test] have controlled for exposure to these environmental toxins' (Jay, 1997). Indeed, 'the relationship of environmental toxins, such as passive smoke and non-tobacco sources of carbon monoxide, to exercise performance has not been investigated ... in patients with heart failure' (Cahalin et al., 1997). Furthermore, it was about 20 years after this effect was established that the first study of the impact of passive smoking on coronary heart disease was published (Gillis et al., 1984), although I am glad to say that this research was carried out in Scotland. Again, no such gap needs to be allowed to occur between early pointers to 'minor' health effects and research into possible major results of FECTS. A letter in a major medical journal (Bocanegra & Espanoza, 1981), remarkably linking passive smoking anecdotally with Raynaud's phenomenon, was published in 1981, but this lead has still not been followed by further research, and major reviews of the literature on passive smoking and cardiovascular disease have all failed to mention Raynaud's phenomenon.

Pointers to ways forward in research into FECTS are indicated: (i) the major effects on pre-adult humans imply the need to study precursors of those effects; (ii) minor or less well-known effects may point to the aetiology of major effects; (iii) pre-adult exposures may have minor and major effects later in life, and, finally, (iv) conditions linked with passive smoking in adults may point backwards to earlier exposure and its consequences. These early-life effects may be first indicated by minor effects or conditions related to the causation of later important physical results. Unless the minor and contributing effects are given due weight, the identification of other major effects may be delayed.

References

Barker, D.J.P., Godfrey, K.M., Fall, C., Osmond, C., Winter, P.D. & Shaheen, S.O. (1991) Relation of birth weight and childhood respiratory infection to adult lung function and death from chronic obstructive airways disease. *Br. Med. J.*, **303**, 671–675

Bocanegra, T.S. & Espanoza, L.R. (1981) Raynaud's phenomenon in passive smokers. *New Engl. J. Med.*, **303**, 1419

Cahalin, L.P., Semigran, M.J. & Dec, G.W. (1997) Passive smoking and the 6-minute walk test in heart failure (letter). *Chest*, **112**, 289–290

Environmental Protection Agency (1992) *Respiratory Health Effects of Passive Smoking: Lung Cancer and Other Disorders* (EPA/600/6-90/006F). Washington DC: Office of Air and Radiation, Office of Health and Environmental Assessment, Office of Research and Development

Fergusson, B.B., Wilson, D.J. & Schaffner, W. (1976) Determination of nicotine concentrations in human milk. *Am. J. Dis. Child.*, **130**, 837–839

Gillis, C.R., Hole, D.J., Hawthorne, V. & Boyle, P. (1984) The effect of environmental tobacco smoke in two urban communities in the west of Scotland. *Eur. J. Respir. Dis.*, **65** (Suppl. 133), 121–126. See also: Hole, D.J., Gillis, C.R., Chopra, C. & Hawthorne, V.M. (1989) Passive smoking and cardiorespiratory health in a general population in the west of Scotland. *Br. Med. J.*, **299**, 423–427

Glantz, S.A. & Parmley, W.W. (1995) Passive smoking and heart disease: Mechanisms and risk. *J. Am. Med. Assoc.*, **273**, 1047–1053

Glueck, C.J., Freiberg, R., Crawford, A., Roy, D., Tracy, T., Seive-Smith, L. & Wang, P. (1996) Secondhand smoke, hypofibrinolysis, and childhood osteonecrosis of the hip, Legg-Perthes disease. *J. Invest. Med.*, **44**, 357A

Hirayama, T. (1990) Cancer de mama: Avances en diagnostico y tratamiento. In: Diaz-Faes, J., ed., *Epidemiologia y Factores de Riesgo del Cancer de Mama*, Léon: Santiago Garcia, pp. 21–38 (in Spanish)

Jay, S.J. (1997) Passive smoking and the 6-minute walk test in heart failure (letter). *Chest*, **112**, 289

Kieser, J.A., Groeneveld, H.T. & da Silva, P. (1996) Delayed tooth formation in children exposed to tobacco smoke. *J. Clin. Pediatr. Dent.*, **20**, 97–100

Lebrecque, M., Marcoux, S. Weber, J.P., Fabia, J. & Ferron, L. (1989) Feeding and urine cotinine in babies whose mothers smoke. *Pediatrics*, **83**, 93–97

Luck, W. & Nau, H. (1985) Nicotine and cotinine concentrations in serum and urine of infants exposed via passive smoking or milk from smoking mothers. *J. Pediatr.*, **107**, 816–820

Morabia, A., Bernstein, M., Héritier, S. & Khatchatrian, N. (1996) Relation of breast cancer with passive and active exposure to tobacco smoke. *Am. J. Epidemiol.*, **143**, 918–928

Sandler, D.P., Everson, R.B. & Wilcox, A.J. (1986) Cigarette smoking and breast cancer (letter). *Am. J. Epidemiol.*, **123**, 370–371

Smith, S.J., Deacon, J.M., Chilvers, C.E.D. & members of the UK National Case–Control Study Group (1994) Alcohol, smoking, passive smoking and caffeine in relation to breast cancer in young women. *Br. J. Cancer*, **70**, 112–119

Whidden, P. (1993) *Tobacco-smoke Pollution: The Intolerable Poison Tolerated Too Long*, Edinburgh: Association for Nonsmokers' Rights

Whidden, P. (continuously updated) *Update to Tobacco-smoke Pollution: The Intolerable Poison Tolerated Too Long*, Edinburgh: Association for Nonsmokers' Rights

Effects of passive smoking on fibrinogen and lipids

N. Sarrafzadegan, N. Mohammadifard & M. Bagheri

Cardiovascular Research Center, Isfahan University of Medical Sciences, Isfahan, Iran

Passive smoking is considered to be a risk factor for coronary artery disease, possibly as a result of an effect on the concentration of fibrinogen. We investigated the relationship between passive smoking and serum concentrations of fibrinogen and lipids in patients with coronary artery disease and healthy people, by conducting a retrospective case–control study in the university hospitals of Isfahan in 1993. The 168 cases were selected from among patients with acute myocardial infarct, according to the World Health Organization criteria. The control group consisted of 200 people living in the neighbourhood of of the case patients and were matched according to age, sex, socioeconomic status and major risk factors for coronary artery disease. The data were gathered at interviews and by measuring plasma fibrinogen, serum total cholesterol, low-density lipoprotein cholesterol and high-density lipoprotein cholesterol after a fasting period. The data were analysed by the chi-squared and t tests.

The frequency of passive smoking was significantly higher in the case group than the controls, and the risk for acute myocardial infarct among passive smokers was 3.2 times higher than that of non-smokers in the control group ($p < 0.05$). The frequency of a high fibrinogen concentration was significantly higher in passive smokers than in non-smokers, and the risk for increased fibrinogen concentration among passive smokers in the control group was 4.6 times higher than that of non-smokers ($p < 0.05$). A similar difference was not seen in the case group, whereas the mean fibrinogen concentration in passive smokers in the case group was significantly higher than that in passive smokers in the control group ($p < 0.02$). No effects of passive smoking were seen on the lipid profile of the case group, possibly because of the presence of acute myocardial infarct. Hypercholesterolaemia and increased low-density lipoprotein cholesterol were significantly more frequent in passive smokers than non-smokers in the control group ($p < 0.05$).

The results indicate that smoking in public places should to be prohibited, as an important intervention for the prevention of cardiovascular disease.

Measurement of nicotine in indoor air as an indicator of passive smoking

M. Rothberg[1], A. Heloma[2], J. Svinhufvud[1], E. Kähkönen[1] & K. Reijula[1]

[1]Finnish Institute of Occupational Health and [2]Provincial Government of Uusimaa, Helsinki, Finland

The aim of the study was to develop a practical method for determining exposure to environmental tobacco smoke which may spread from designated smoking areas to smoke-free zones. The method should fulfil the following criteria: be sensitive enough to analyse low concentrations, allow analysis of volatile organic compounds and a selected indicator from the same sample and represent a reasonable expense for occupational health units.

The results of laboratory experiments and field tests in smoking areas indicated that nicotine, 3-ethenylpyridine and nicotyrine are unique to tobacco smoke and are not normally present in indoor air. The concentration of nicotine in non-smoking areas in workplaces was low (mean, 1.4 µg/m³), but sufficiently high for analysis. The concentrations of the other components typical of tobacco smoke were too low for reliable results to be obtained. We recommend the collection of nicotine with active sampling as an indicator of exposure to environmental tobacco smoke which spreads from designated smoking areas. Passive sampling can be used for qualitative monitoring only.

Project for public awareness of indoor exposure to tobacco smoke in Hungary

T. Demjén[1], B. Buda[2] & L. Gallay[3]

[1]National Institute for Health Promotion and [2]Semmelweis Medical University, Budapest, Hungary, and [3]University of Penn State, State College, United States

A one-year project financed by the Government of Hungary and the World Bank resulted in an improvement in indoor air and the development of a countrywide tobacco control programme. Public knowledge, skills, attitude and behaviour with regard to passive smoking were improved; there was more knowledge about the principles of passive smoking. The data were collected by opinion polls and by cooperation with other anti-smoking programmes. The project has resulted in a report on a community-based project, with suggestions for countrywide implementation. Further public opinion polls will be conducted and a final report produced. The remaining tasks are the production of media materials, implementation of the programme in different settings with different target groups, monitoring and developing future countrywide strategies.

Effects on children and young people

Exposure of non-smoking pregnant women to environmental tobacco smoke in Guangzhou, China

A. Yuen Loke[1], T.H. Lam[2], C.L. Betson[2], S.C. Pan[3], S.Y. Li[3], X.J. Gao[3], Q.S. Xuan[3] & Y.Y. Song[3]

[1]Department of Nursing and Health Sciences, The Hong Kong Polytechnic University, and [2]Department of Community Medicine, The University of Hong Kong, Hong Kong SAR, China, and [3] Women and Children Health Care Centre of Guangzhou, China

Introduction

Exposure of non-smoking pregnant women to environmental tobacco smoke, or passive smoking, has been shown to be associated with spontaneous abortion, perinatal death, premature delivery and low birthweight. In the west, smoking by pregnant women is a major health problem. In Asia, women smoke much less commonly, but smoking among men is increasing rapidly; therefore, passive smoking by non-smoking women is an increasing problem for maternal and child health.

The 1996 National Prevalence Survey in China (Yang *et al.*, 1997) showed that 70% of men and 4.2% of women were current smokers, with great variations in the prevalence of smoking in different parts of China. The survey also showed that passive smoking was widespread in China; however, passive smoking by non-smoking pregnant women was not studied. There have also been no intervention studies to reduce the exposure of non-smoking pregnant women to environmental tobacco smoke: all of the published intervention studies were targeted at pregnant women who smoked.

In December 1996, we started a baseline survey on smoking and exposure of pregnant women to environmental tobacco smoke and a randomized controlled trial on those who did not smoke and were married to a smoking husband, to test the effectiveness of a health education intervention. The project was still in progress at the time of writing. We present here some preliminary results of the baseline cross-sectional survey.

Methods

There is one Women and Children Health Care Centre in the City of Guangzhou (the largest) and six district centres. All except one district centre participated. A structured standardized questionnaire was designed in order to obtain baseline information on demographic characteristics and the smoking habits of the women, their knowledge, attitudes and actions regarding smoking and passive smoking, their exposure to passive smoking at home, at work and in public places and the smoking habits of their husbands. From December 1996, all pregnant women who made their first prenatal visit to the centres were invited to fill in the questionnaire. The results for 2281 non-smoking pregnant women up to June 1997 are reported below.

Results

Of the 2399 women who completed the questionnaire, 118 or 4.9% (95% confidence interval [CI], 4.0–5.8%) were current smokers or had smoked before and were excluded. Of the 2281 who reported never having smoked, 1626 (71%; 95% CI, 70–72%) were married to smokers, and 655 (29%; 95% CI, 28–30%) were married to non-smoking husbands. About 80% of the women were aged 21–30 years, about 55% were born in Guangzhou, and 60% had an educational level of upper secondary or higher. Table 1 shows that the women with non-smoking husbands (mean age, 27.6; SD, 3.5) and those with smoking husbands (mean age, 27.9; SD, 3.6) were similar in age. The Table also shows that the women with non-smoking husbands had a higher educational level than those whose husbands smoked.

Table 1. Characteristics of pregnant women who had never smoked

Women with non-	Women with smoking husbands ($n = 655$)		Women with smoking husbands ($n = 1626$)		p value
	No.	%	No.	%	
Age (years)					
< 21	1	0.2	1	0.1	
21–25	176	27	433	27	
26–30	368	56	837	52	
31–35	76	12	268	16	
36–40	22	3.3	56	3.4	
41–43	2	0.3	6	0.4	
Not reported	10	1.5	25	1.5	0.13
Birthplace					
Guangzhou	357	54	900	55	
Other parts of Guangdong	201	31	506	31	
Other provinces of China	83	13	189	12	
Not reported	14	2.1	31	1.9	0.89
Educational level					
No formal education	1	0.2	4	0.2	
Primary school	23	3.5	74	4.6	
Lower secondary	200	30	615	38	
Upper secondary	284	43	637	39	
University	144	22	277	17	
Not reported	3	0.5	19	1.2	< 0.001

About one-quarter (25%) of the smoking husbands smoked 1–5 cigarettes per day, 36% smoked 6–15, 14.8% smoked 16–25, and 2.0% smoked ≥ 26 per day; data were missing for 22%. The mean consumption was 11 (95% CI, 10–11) cigarettes per day.

Exposure to passive smoking from family members other than the husbands at home during the last seven days before the prenatal visit was reported by 57% of the women, 70% reported exposure in public places and 34% at work. Among the 1275 working women, 61% reported exposure to passive smoking at work during the last seven days. The women with smoking husbands had significantly longer hours of exposure at all three locations than those with non-smoking husbands (at home, $p < 0.001$; in public places, $p = 0.001$ and at work, $p = 0.005$).

Table 2 shows that 89–95% of the two groups of women could answer the two questions about smoking (lung cancer and smoking in pregnant women) and two questions on passive smoking (children and pregnant women and unborn children) correctly, but only 68–80% could answer a question about smoking and heart disease and one about passive smoking and lung cancer. Almost all (92–93%) had positive attitudes about smoking cessation. No significant difference in knowledge was found between the two groups.

When exposed to environmental tobacco smoke during the last month, about 90% of the women had often or sometimes moved away, about 60% had asked the smoker to move away, and only about half had asked the smoker not to smoke in their homes, but about 95% claimed that they had advised their family, friends or relatives to quit smoking. Table 3 shows these actions in the two groups of women.

Most of the women (80–90%) had experienced discomfort from exposure to passive smoking at home, in public places and at work. Table 4 shows no difference in discomfort from exposure to passive smoking in public places or at work, but, unexpectedly, more women with non-smoking husbands reported discomfort from passive smoking at home than women with smoking husbands. It was possible that some women in the latter group were used to their husbands' tobacco smoke and had become less sensitive. All except two of these 1626 women reported that their husbands were smoking before they married.

Table 2. Proportions of women who agreed with the six knowledge and two attitude statements

	Women with non-smoking husbands (n = 655)	Women with smoking husbands (n = 1626)	p value
Knowledge about cigarette smoking:			
Smoking can cause lung cancer	91.8	89.1	0.07
In pregnant women, smoking can interfere with the normal growth of the foetus	94.8	94.7	1.00
Smoking can cause heart disease	70.8	67.9	0.19
Knowledge about exposure to tobacco smoke:			
Exposure to tobacco smoke can have harmful effects on children	93.9	93.4	0.71
Exposure to tobacco smoke can be harmful to a pregnant woman and her unborn baby	94.7	94.2	0.65
Exposure to someone else's tobacco smoke can cause lung cancer	79.7	76.4	0.10
Attitude towards smoking cessation:			
A person can quit smoking if he/she is determined	93.3	93.4	0.98
Most smokers can benefit from people's support in their effort to quit smoking	92.2	92.6	0.81

Table 3. Actions with regard to exposure to environmental tobacco smoke

	Women with non-smoking husbands (%) (n = 655)	Women with smoking husbands (%) (n = 1626)	p value
At home:			
When my family, friends or relatives were smoking near me, I moved away	90	93	0.04
When my family, friends or relatives were smoking near me, I asked him/her to move away	62	66	0.03
When any person was smoking in my home, I asked him/her not to smoke	54	46	0.03
When I saw my family, friends or relatives smoking, I advised him/her to quit	94	96	0.07
In public places:			
When a stranger was smoking near me in a public place, I moved away	72	72	0.99
When I was exposed to second-hand smoke in a restaurant, I thought of finding another seat to avoid exposure	89	89	0.85
When I was exposed to second-hand smoking in a restaurant, I tried to finish eating as soon as possible and leave	79	79	0.94
When I was exposed to second-hand smoke in a restaurant, I thought of going to another restaurant	59	51	< 0.001

Proportions of women answering 'often' or 'sometimes'

Table 4. Discomfort from exposure to environmental tobacco smoke at home, in public places and at work

Discomfort	Women with nonsmoking husbands ($n = 655$)	Women with smoking husbands ($n = 1626$)	p value
At home:			
Throat irritation	84	78	0.001
Cough (or productive cough)	87	80	< 0.001
Breathing difficulty or problem	86	79	< 0.001
Nose irritation, sneezing and/or runny nose	87	82	0.006
Reduced appetite	86	82	0.014
In public places:			
Throat irritation	82	80	0.39
Cough (or productive cough)	86	85	0.48
Breathing difficulty or problem	83	82	0.80
Nose irritation, sneezing and/or runny nose	85	86	0.89
Reduced appetite	83	84	0.55
At work:	($n = 398$)	($n = 877$)	
Throat irritation	83	84	0.96
Cough (or productive cough)	90	88	0.28
Breathing difficulty or problem	84	84	0.90
Nose irritation, sneezing and/or runny nose	87	88	0.87
Reduced appetite	88	88	0.99

Discussion

In the 1996 Chinese National Prevalence Survey (Yang *et al.*, 1997), 46% of the non-smoking men and 57% of non-smoking women were found to be exposed to passive smoking. A passive smoker was defined as one who inhaled smoke exhaled by a smoker for more than 15 min/day on more than one day per week. For all women, the sources of exposure were home (82%), public places (28%) and the workplace (19%). Although passive smoking by pregnant women was not studied, the highest prevalence of exposure (about 70%) was found for women in the age group 30–39 years.

The present study showed that 71% of the pregnant women were married to a husband who smoked. We found higher proportions of exposure in public places (72%) and at work (34%). Our results suggest that the pregnant women were exposed as much or possibly more than non-pregnant women to passive smoking. Urgent public health measures are needed to protect pregnant women from environmental tobacco smoke in China.

Acknowledgements

We wish to thank the Committee on Research and Conference Grants, The University of Hong Kong for funding this project and Ms S.F. Chung for assistance in data analysis. Participants in this project included doctors from the prenatal clinics at the Guangzhou, Liwan, Bayuan, Yueshou and Dongshan Maternal and Child Health Centres in Guangzhou.

Reference

Yang, G.H., *et al.* (1997) *1996 National Prevalence Survey of Smoking Pattern*, Beijing: China Science and Technology Press

Prenatal exposure to tobacco smoke and maldevelopment of the brain

H. Tanaka

National Institute of Neuroscience, National Center of Neurology and Psychiatry, Kodaira, Tokyo, Japan

Maldevelopment of the brain of offspring whose mothers smoke during pregnancy is being evaluated from data collected in all areas of Japan. As the criteria for the 'foetal tobacco syndrome' do not include maldevelopment of the brain, I proposed the term 'foetal tobacco effects' when the gestational age is < 37 weeks.

Maternal factors during pregnancy, including coffee drinking, use of multiple drugs and disorders such as premature rupture of the membranes or placental abnormalities, were associated at higher frequency with younger foetuses than overall, although the amount of smoking and light drinking during pregnancy were similar for all foetal ages. As an indicator of maldevelopment of the brain, central nervous system involvement was more frequent and severe in younger foetuses than overall. These findings suggest that factors in addition to smoking that reduce the gestational period contribute to central nervous system involvement. Involvement was most frequent in the offspring of women who both smoked and drank heavily during pregnancy.

In conclusion, a causal relationship between prenatal smoking and maldevelopment of the brain of offspring should be investigated, especially with regard to factors that modify the effects of tobacco during pregnancy.

Living with smoking grandparents and upper respiratory symptoms in children aged 3–6 years in Hong Kong

S.F. Chung & T.H. Lam

Department of Community Medicine, The University of Hong Kong, Hong Kong SAR, China

Introduction

In 1992–93, a follow-up study was carried out on a cohort of children who had taken part in a survey on breast-feeding and fertility in Hong Kong in 1988–89 (T.H. Lam et al., unpublished data). The aim of the follow-up was to study the prevalence of acute and chronic respiratory illnesses and associated factors among young children in Hong Kong. One of the major factors studied was passive smoking. Since the prevalence of maternal smoking is low in Hong Kong (2.7% in our study and about 3% among mothers of primary-school children (Hedley et al., 1993)), the power of the study was not great enough to detect any significant statistical difference for maternal smoking. Therefore, we turned our focus to smoking by grandparents. Few studies of the effect of smoking by grandparents on child health can be found in the literature. Nevertheless, a case–control study on passive smoking and childhood hospitalization due to respiratory illness in Hong Kong showed an adjusted odds ratio of 2.4, which was of borderline significance (95% confidence interval, 0.98–6.1), but there was a significant linear trend for mode of exposure (Ching et al., 1995). In a study of primary-school children in Hong Kong, their respiratory symptoms were significantly associated with exposure to passive smoking from family members other than fathers, mothers and siblings ((Hedley et al., 1991). We suspected that most of these other family members were grandparents.

Study design, subjects and methods

This survey was a follow-up study on a cohort of children who had taken part in the survey on breast-feeding and fertility in Hong Kong in 1988-89. The initial cohort consisted of 3230 children who were drawn from a random probabilistic sample of children born between April 1987 and June 1989 in Hong Kong. Between December 1992 and October 1993, when the children were aged 3–6 years, the parents of 2303 children (71% of the initial cohort) were interviewed by telephone.

The main survey instrument was a structured questionnaire written in colloquial Cantonese. The children's mothers were the main respondents to the telephone interview; if the mothers could not be contacted after three or four attempts, responses from another person who was familiar with the health of the children were accepted as a proxy. Since the initial study focused on breast feeding and fertility, a history of passive smoking was not elicited then, and only a few items could be used in the present study. Hence, although a cohort of children was followed-up, the questions about environmental exposures were asked mainly for the present study, which is therefore actually a cross-sectional study.

Results

Of the 2303 children, 56% were boys and 44% were girls. At the time of the interview, they were 3–6 years old: 3% were 3 years old, 41% were 4 years old, 51% were 5 years old and 5% were 6 years old. The mean age was 4.58 years (SD, 0.63). Only two children were not attending an educational institution. Sixty-four children (2.8%) did not live with two parents; of these, 14 lived with their mothers only, six lived with their fathers only, and 44 did not live with either parent. A total of 408 (18%) children lived with one or more grandparents, regardless of whether they lived with their parents or not.

The exposure of the children to environmental tobacco smoke from family members is shown in Table 1. More children were living with one or more smoking grandparents (3.8%) than with smoking mothers (1.4%).

Living with smoking grandparents was associated in the children with 'frequent cough' (adjusted odds ratio (OR), 1.8; 95% confidence interval (CI), 1.1–3.1), 'doctor consultation for frequent cough' (adjusted OR, 1.9; 95% CI, 1.1–3.2) and 'common cold usually lasted for more than six days in one episode' (adjusted OR, 1.6; 95% CI, 1.0–2.6) within the past 12 months. The children who lived with smoking grandparents had also suffered more days from common colds in the previous 12 months (adjusted difference in the number of days, 8; 95% CI, 2–14).

Discussion

Significant associations between living with grandparents who smoked and children's upper respiratory symptoms were found in this study. Children who lived with smoking grandparents may have been exposed to a high dose of environmental tobacco smoke, as grandparents are usually not busy and tend to stay for long hours with their grand-children. There have been few studies on grandparents and child health, but this is a topic worth studying in Asia, where living with grandparents is common. In all societies where extended families are common, health research and health promotion should target all of the persons living with children and not only the parents, particularly on the issue of passive smoking in the family home.

Acknowledgments

We thank the Committee on Research and Conference Grants, The University of Hong Kong for funding this project. We also thank the Department of Health of Hong Kong Government for their assistance, Dr L.Y. Tse and Dr S.F. Tang for their suggestions in the design of the questionnaires, the staff of the maternal and child health centres for answering the enquiry from the parents and helping to retrieve the information.

Table 1. Exposure to environmental tobacco smoke from family members

Family members	Smoking behaviour	No.	%
Mothers	Current smokers	33	1.4
	Ex-smokers[a]	29	1.3
	Never smoked	2231	97
	No. of cigarettes smoked daily:		
	1–10	22	69
	11–20	9	28
	> 20	1	3.1
Fathers	Current smokers	737	32
	Ex-smokers	46	2.0
	No. of cigarettes smoked daily:		
	1–10	178	24
	11–20	538	72
	> 20	32	4.3
Grandparents	Current smokers	78	3.4
who lived with the	Ex-smokers	10	0.4
children	Never smoked/did not live with children	2215	96
	No. of cigarettes smoked daily:		
	1–10	14	19
	11–20	58	77
	> 20	3	4.0
Other family	One or more smokers	37	1.6
members	None had smoked	2266	98
	Total no. of cigarettes smoked daily:		
	1–10	14	38
	11–20	18	49
	> 20	5	14
All family	One or more current smokers	812	35
members	No current smokers and one or more ex-smokers	48	2.0
	None had smoked	1443	63
	Total no. or cigarettes smoked daily:		
	1–10	185	23
	11–20	535	66
	> 20	92	11
	No. of smokers at home		
	1	765	91
	≥ 2	79	9.4

Missing cases excluded
[a] Ever smoked after children were born but had quit

References

Chung, S.F., Lam, T.H., Ng, C.H.V., et al. (1995) A case control study on passive smoking and childhood hospitalization due to respiratory illnesses. In: Proceedings of the Hospital Authority Convention '95, Hong Kong: Hospital Authority, pp. 197–203

Hedley, A.J., Lam, T.H., Ong, S.G., et al. (1991) Studies on Respiratory Health in Hong Kong: Report No. 2, The effects of active and passive smoking on respiratory health of primary school children in Hong Kong. Hong Kong: Department of Community Medicine and Department of Paediatrics, University of Hong Kong

Hedley, A.J., Peters, J., Lam, T.H., et al. (1993) Air Pollution and Respiratory Health in Primary School Children in Hong Kong, 1989–1992, Hong Kong: Department of Community Medicine, The University of Hong Kong

Smoking behaviour of parents of children born in 1990–94 in Agaete, Canary Islands, Spain

J.M. Segura[1], A. López[1], M. López[1], M. Torres[1], J.R. Calvo[1], M.C. Navarro[1], J. Calvo[1], J.C. Orengo[1], M. Marrero[1], S. Flórez[2], A. Ramos[2], O. Rojas[2], S. Solano[2] & C. Jiménez[2]

[1]Universidad de Las Palmas de Gran Canaria, Canary Islands, Spain
[2]Hospital de la Princesa, Madrid, Spain

Introduction

Although there is evidence that passive smoking can cause many of the same diseases as active smoking, a significant percentage of the population continues to smoke. Young adults are more likely to be smokers, probably because they do not feel that the risk applies to them. These include the parents of small children, who thus receive all the dangerous substances from their parents' tobacco smoke, with the associated risks. These children are more likely to have asthma attacks, upper respiratory infections and even sudden death. Furthermore, they receive the message that smoking is normal, and many of them become smokers themselves.

In this survey, we wished to determine the smoking habits of the parents of children born between January 1990 and December 1994 in a rural area of our island, Gran Canaria, Canary Islands, Spain. We also wished to determine their attitudes towards using tobacco during the mothers' pregnancies and around their children.

Subjects and method

We designed a descriptive, cross-sectional survey based on a questionnaire containing 17 questions for data collection. All individuals born between 1990 and 1994 were selected, and a copy of the questionnaire was included in their clinical record. The local paediatrician collaborated by filling in the forms when these children visited the primary health care centre for any reason.

The data were processed and analysed with Epi-Info 6.04. We used the chi-squared non-parametric test to determine differences among fathers and mothers.

Results

Data collection began in April 1995, and we now have data corresponding to 52% of the population with children in that age group, for a total of 136 children. This number of subjects gives us a confidence level of 90–95%. Information was usually obtained from the mothers (59%).

The smoking prevalence was 45% among the mothers and 65% among the fathers. The mothers who used tobacco smoked a mean of 12.8 cigarettes per day (SD, 7.36), and the fathers smoked a mean of 21.1 cigarettes per day (SD, 10.8); 93% of the mothers and 96% of the fathers smoked daily.

Smoking had been continued during the pregnancy by 31% of the mothers and 71% of the fathers; 61% of the smoking mothers and 74% of the smoking fathers used tobacco regardless of the presence of their children.

Conclusions

We can extend our results to the whole population of Agaete, because all of the children of those ages are registered by the paediatrician in the primary care centre and were thus potentially included in the survey. We are reasonably sure that there is no selection bias of children more likely to visit the doctor.

The high percentage of smokers found in our survey is typical of young adults in rural areas. More fathers than mothers smoked (20% more; $p = 0.001$), consistent with other observations; they also smoked more cigarettes per day than the women and were more likely to smoke tobacco daily. The mothers appeared to be more involved in their children's well-being, as a higher percentage of the mothers who smoked did not do so near their children. Many of them did not smoke while pregnant, although > 30% did so.

Greater efforts should be made to convince young parents that their smoking habit could damage their children's health. Health education should also focus on the avoidance of tobacco (and other drugs) during pregnancy, not only by mothers but also by their male partners, whose smoking habit during pregnancy acts as a reinforcing factor, making it more difficult for the women to stop.

Acknowledgements
We wish to thank the local paediatrician, Dr Wilfredo Borges, and the children's nurses, Mrs Dolores Bardaji and Mr Teodoro Almeida, whose collaboration allowed us to carry out this study.

Prevalence of passive smoking among adolescents in relation to the education and socioeconomic status of parents in Isfahan, Iran

N. Sarrafzadegan, S. Mostafavi & F. Tafazzoly

Cardiovascular Research Center, University of Medical Sciences, Isfahan, Iran

Active and passive exposure to tobacco smoke are important causes of mortality, and the American Heart Association has formally concluded that passive smoking is an important risk factor for heart disease in both adults and children. Therefore, we conducted a survey of the prevalence of passive smoking by Isfahan adolescents (14–18 years) and related it to the parent's socioeconomic status, level of education and place of exposure. A total of 860 high-school students were selected randomly from schools which were selected randomly in the city. A questionnaire elicited information on the number of cigarettes smoked at home by the parents, the rooms in which smoking took place, the amount of time the adolescent was exposed to smoking either inside or outside the home and the socioeconomic status and level of education of both parents.

Nearly 60% of the adolescents were passive smokers; 60% were exposed at home, 9% inside cars and 12% in a workplace. Active smoking by fathers was responsible for passive smoking in 97% of cases. The correlation coefficient between passive smoking by the adolescents and their father's job was significant only for unemployed fathers ($r^2 = 0.933$; $p < 0.05$). A nonsignificant inverse correlation was seen between white-collar work and passive smoking by their children ($r^2 = 0.0213$). The relation between passive smoking and the father's level of education showed a significant inverse correlation with 16 years of education or more ($r^2 = -0.0628$; $p < 0.05$) and a nonsignificant positive correlation with 9 years of education or less ($r^2 = 0.0573$; $p < 0.05$). A significant relationship was found between passive smoking by the adolescents and their mother's job. The findings with regard to level of education were similar to those for fathers.

These results show a high prevalence of passive smoking by our adolescents, especially at a lower socioeconomic level (children of unemployed fathers) and a lower level of education. One of the most important tobacco control initiatives in our society must therefore be to target smoking in groups of low socioeconomic status.

Smoking in the home: Changing attitudes and current practices

M.J. Ashley, J. Cohen, R. Ferrence, S.B. Bull, S. Bondy, B. Poland & L.L. Pederson

Ontario Tobacco Research Unit, University of Toronto, Toronto, Canada

Rationale: Exposure to environmental tobacco smoke is causally related to a range of adverse health effects in children. Exposure in the home is an important source, especially for children. Information on public attitudes towards smoking in the home and current practices in the home can help determine the need for programmes and policies and their feasibility.

Methods: Data from a population-based, random-digit dialling, computer-assisted survey of 1764 adults conducted in 1996 in Ontario, Canada, were analysed and compared with data from three earlier provincial surveys. The response rates in these surveys ranged from 63 to 65%.

Findings: Between 1992 and 1996, the percentage of respondents who agreed that parents spending time at home with small children should not smoke increased from 51% to 70%. In 1996, 78% of non-smokers and 43% of smokers agreed with this statement; however, only 34% of the homes surveyed in 1996 were smoke-free. Smoke-free homes were associated with non-smoking respondents, the presence of children and no daily smokers in the home. Only 20% of homes with children and any daily smokers were smoke-free.

Conclusions: Reducing exposure to environmental tobacco smoke in the home should be a public health priority. The trends in attitudes among adults in Ontario suggest that community-based interventions aimed at reducing the exposure of children should be well accepted. Support for informal agreements on smoking in the home, however, may not equate to support for enforceable restrictions imposed by the State.

Passive smoking: Public opinion and behaviour in Victoria, Australia

J. Martin[1], R. Mullins[2] & M. Morand[2]

[1]Victorian Smoking and Health Program and [2]Centre for Behavioural Research in Cancer, Anti-Cancer Council of Victoria, Victoria Australia

The Victorian Smoking and Health Program, also known as Quit, is based in Victoria, a state of Australia which has a population of about 4 million, the majority of whom are based in the city and large regional towns. Legislation to restrict tobacco smoking in public places is *ad hoc*, and many voluntary smoke-free policies have been developed in workplaces and other public places.

For over 10 years the Centre for Behavioural Research in Cancer, on behalf of Quit, has undertaken an annual survey of smoking and health. Some of the questions asked are related to passive smoking. The release of medical information about the health effects of passive smoking and litigation fuelled opinion on the issue in Australia, particularly during the late 1980s. In response, Quit has made passive smoking a central issue in its campaign, capitalizing on publicity and trends illustrated through the research.

Survey

The survey is part of a population survey by a large market research company and involves a representative sample of approximately 2500 Victorians aged ≥ 16. Face-to-face interviews are conducted in the respondents' homes on weekends. This kind of information has been collected since 1985; questions with the same wording have been asked over 10 years, and other questions have been added at different stages.

This paper covers a number of trends illustrated by the research over time, covering: beliefs about the harm of passive smoking; smoking in the presence of children; discouraging visitors from smoking in the house; smoking in restaurants and smoking in gaming clubs, hotels and shopping centres.

Belief that passive smoking is harmful to non-smokers: Over the last 10 years, there has been an increase in the belief that passive smoking is harmful. The greatest change occurred in smokers, from 57% in 1985 to 70 in 1995; the change among ex-smokers was from 76 to 82%, and that among people who had never smoked was from 82 to 89%.

Smoking in the presence of children: Since 1989, the proportion of smokers who said they had not changed their smoking habits around children has fallen from 31 to 22%, and the number of smokers who did not light up at all when with children had increased from 14% in 1989 to 29% in 1994 (Table 1). This trend may be related to a campaign run in 1992 to encourage smokers not to smoke around children. These figures show a positive trend, but it remains disappointing that in 1994 the majority of smokers (45% smoke less + 22% no effect = 67%) continued to smoke around children, albeit at a reduced rate in most cases.

Discouraging visitors from smoking: There is an increasing trend to discourage visitors from smoking in homes. In 1989, only 27% of respondents said they discouraged visitors from smoking, but by 1995 this had risen to 48%. Households in which there were no smokers were the most likely to discourage visitors from smoking.

Smoking in restaurants: The preference for sitting in smoke-free areas in restaurants increased between 1985 and 1995, most of the increase occurring between 1985 and 1988. Increases were seen among people who had never smoked (83 to 91%), ex-smokers (67 to 82%) and smokers (12 to 15%), but only a minority of smokers preferred smoke-free dining, and this has changed little in 10 years. This does not indicate that they would prefer to sit in the smoking area of a restaurant. In fact, the desire for smoking areas was low: in 1994–95, only 12% of Victorians said they would prefer to sit in a smoking zone in a restaurant; even among smokers, less than half (47%) thought that a smoking area would be preferable.

One area in which progress has been made in recent years is the willingness of people who want smoke-free areas to ask for them. In 1992, when we first asked people whether they requested smoke-free areas, only 42% of respondents who wanted it said they always asked. This had increased to 56% by 1995. There is obviously still more room for assertiveness on the part of those who go to restaurants, but the change is encouraging in that the demand may result in more eating establishments providing smoke-free dining.

To make restaurant owners and managers more aware of the widespread support for smoke-free dining, even among smokers, and to encourage diners to ask for smoke-free areas, a promotion was run around World No Tobacco Day 1997, with the theme 'Smokefree Saturday' (Figure 1). The promotion ran throughout the State, including regional areas. Over 4000 restaurants received information on the promotion and the 'Going Smokefree Guide to Implementing a Smokefree Restaurant'. Six hundred restaurants participated in the promotion, declaring their premises smoke free on 31 May, and over 11 000 diners entered a competition on that day. A follow-up telephone survey showed that 24% of the restaurants participating in the promotion that were not

Table 1. Smoking in the presence of children 1989, 1992 and 1994

Smoking	1989 (%) (n = 654)	1992 (%) (n = 606)	1994 (%) (n = 615)
Smoke more	1	2	1
No change	31	22	22
Smoke less	50	51	45
Don't smoke at all	14	23	29
Can't say	4	3	

already smoke free had either changed their policy or intended to as a result of the promotion.

Figure 1. Smoke-free Saturday poster

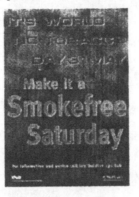

Opinion on smoking in gaming clubs, hotels and shopping centres: The majority of people (55%) believed that smoking should not be allowed at all in indoor shopping centres, although 35% were willing to allow it in special areas only. Very few (7%) believed that smoking should be allowed freely in shopping centres. After the 'Smokefree Saturday' promotions, an increased number of complaints was received from shoppers in shopping centres about the lack of enforcement of smoke-free policies. Fewer people supported a complete ban on smoking in gaming clubs (28%) or hotels (28%); however, the majority believed that smoking should be allowed only in special areas within gaming clubs (63%) or hotels (56%). Very few people believed that smoking should be freely allowed in either gaming clubs (9%) or hotels (16%).

Conclusion
    The results illustrate a great change in awareness about issues associated with passive smoking and an appropriate change in behaviour over the past 10 years. Given the undesirability of regulating what people can do in their own homes, it is reassuring that this change has occurred without the need for regulation. It is also encouraging that more non-smokers are making their desire for smoke-free dining known. Increased assertiveness on the part of the large number of people who would like smoke-free areas or totally smoke-free facilities in places such as hotels and gaming clubs could lead to the provision of such areas, again without the need for regulation.
    The evidence suggests that the efforts of the Quit campaign to increase awareness and change behaviour in regard to passive smoking have been well worthwhile. Charting public opinion on passive smoking has provided Quit with a tool for shaping campaigns to curb smoking in homes, public places and the workplace. It has also helped to inform public policy, thereby reducing the need for Government regulation.

Children's residential exposure to environmental tobacco smoke in the Nordic countries

K.E. Lund[1] & A.R. Helgason[2]

[1]*Norwegian Cancer Society and University of Oslo, Oslo, Norway*
[2]*Tobacco Prevention Center, Stockholm, Sweden*

Five thousand parents of children born in 1992 in Denmark, Finland, Iceland, Norway and Sweden were asked about their smoking behaviour while indoors with their children. The prevalence of daily smoking was 20% among fathers, 15% among married or cohabiting mothers and 47% among single mothers. Both parents reported smoking daily in 7% of the households, while one parent smoked in 22% of the households. The prevalence of smoking varied with social group. Rules to limit smoking indoors had been introduced in 75% of the households, and 82% of the current smokers had tried to change their smoking habits for the sake of their children. Of the parents who had smoked at the beginning of the pregnancy, 77% reported having changed their habits during the pregnancy, but the changes were far less pronounced among expecting fathers than among expecting mothers. In 25% of the households, children were exposed to environmental tobacco smoke at home during the week. In households where at least one parent smoked, 57% reported that children were present when someone smoked.

In spite of the fact that most parents have tried to reduce children's exposure to residential tobacco smoke, about 1 million Nordic children aged 0–12 years are exposed regularly to passive smoking in their homes.

Passive smoking and children: A three-year Nordic intervention and evaluation project

K.E. Lund[1], A.R. Helgason[2], B. Hessulf[2], A.P. Hudtloff[2] & T. Kolset[2]

[1]*Norwegian Cancer Society, Oslo, Norway;* [2]*Nordic Cancer Union*

In 1993, a joint Nordic effort to reduce the prevalence of smoking in the vicinity of children was initiated by the Nordic Cancer Union. The Union established a three-year intervention and evaluation project , headed by the information departments of the five Nordic cancer societies. The objectives of the project are (i) to assess the magnitude of exposure of children to passive smoking in Nordic day-care institutions, with private day-care providers and in private homes; (ii) to monitor the attitudes of the target audiences and their view about restriction of environmental tobacco smoke; (iii) to develop strategies and materials for target audiences in order to alert target groups and reduce children's exposure to environmental tobacco smoke; (iv) to target materials to women in order to reduce overall female smoking and (v) to gain new knowledge as a basis for future interventions in each country.

Knowledge, attitudes and education are independent factors that protect children against environmental tobacco smoke: A population-based survey

Á.R. Helgason[1], A. Skrondal[2] &K.E. Lund[3]

[1]*Tobacco Prevention Centre, Karolinska Institute, Huddinge, Sweden, and Icelandic Cancer Society, Reykjavik, Iceland;* [2]*Section of Medical Statistics, University of Oslo and National Institute of Public Health, and* [3]*Norwegian Cancer Society and Department of Behavioural Sciences in Medicine, University of Oslo, Norway*

The objective of this study was to assess whether attitudes to environmental tobacco smoke and knowledge and beliefs about its potential hazard for children affect whether parents who smoke avoid exposing their children. The study was initiated by the Nordic Cancer Union.

The method used was a cross-sectional suvey. An anonymous questionnaire was sent to a randomly selected sample of 5000 households in the Nordic countries (Denmark, Finland, Iceland, Norway and Sweden) in which a child was born in 1992. The outcome measures included the smoking status of the parents, the prevalence and quantity of weekly exposure to environmental tobacco smoke and knowledge, attitudes and beliefs about the potential hazards of passive smoking.

Parents' attitudes towards children's rights to an environmental tobacco smoke-free environment and the prevalence of definite knowledge and beliefs about the harmful effects of environmental tobacco smoke on children are shown for smokers and non-smokers in Table 1. After multivariate adjustment, level of education, level of knowledge and strong attitudes with regard to environmental tobacco smoke in the vicinity of children appeared to be independent factors related to the prevalence of exposure to environmental tobacco smoke in the home (Table 2).

Although parents who are aware of the potential hazards of passive smoking may expose their children, the present data show that the level of knowledge about the established negative effects of environmental tobacco smoke on children significantly reduce the risk of their exposure in the home.

Table 1. Attitudes and knowledge of parents who smoke and do not smoke with regard to environmental tobacco smoke

Attitudes and knowledge	Smokers (%)	Non-smokers (%)	p value
Parents who 'tend to agree' or 'agree strongly' with statements of attitudes			
Children should have the right to live in a smoke-free home.	87	94	< 0.01
Adults have the right to smoke wherever they want in their own homes.	31	24	NS
An act should be passed forbidding all indoor smoking in the vicinity of children.	53	70	< 0.01
Indoor smoking in the vicinity of children is child abuse.	44	59	< 0.01
Parents who answered 'definitely yes' to statements of knowledge			
Children who are exposed to environmental tobacco smoke are more likely to:			
start to smoke themselves	17	35	< 0.01
have inner ear infections	9	15	NS
develop respiratory disease	28	48	< 0.01
have asthma attacks	36	55	< 0.01

NS, not significant

Table 2. Factors associated with no exposure of children to environmental tobacco smoke in homes where there are one or more daily smokers

Factor	No exposure (%)	Adjusted OR	p value
Family structure			
Single (reference)	32		
Co-habitant	56	2.7	< 0.01
Level of education			
Short (reference)	45		
Medium	53	1.7	< 0.05
Long	60	2.6	< 0.01
Health beliefs and knowledge			
Lowest third (reference)	33		
Middle third	58	2.1	< 0.01
Highest third	64	3.1	< 0.01
Attitudes to environmental tobacco smoke			
Least negative third (reference)	32		
Intermediately negative third	50	1.3	NS
Most negative third	73	2.5	< 0.01

OR, odds ratio; subgroups with higher prevalence of no exposure to environmental tobacco smoke are compared with the reference group.
NS, not significant

TOBACCO AND THE ENVIRONMENT

Damage to the environment: Environmentalism and health

C. Loh

Citizens Party, Hong Kong SAR, China

Introduction

Smoking kills—so the most blunt of the health warnings displayed on cigarette packs remind us. Smoking kills most people with grim regularity, as the statistics recited at this conference demonstrate: the World Health Organization estimates that smoking kills an average of six people every minute, adding up to 3 million per year, and that number is climbing. Smoking, according to the World Health Organization, is emerging as the world's largest single preventable cause of illness and death.

In communities with the will and the resources to fight back, the tobacco industry is under threat. The record settlement made in the United States in 1997, in which American tobacco companies pledged to pay back US$ 368.5 million million and to submit to stringent regulation, is a case in point. So are communities around the world that have banned smoking in public, including 71 Chinese cities to date, from Beijing to Wuhan to Zhuhai. This paper addresses the role of government and local communities in making the transition from a fundamentally unsustainable, artificial way of life to a clean, sustainable, just future.

The challenge

The figures are staggering: 1.1 million million smokers in the world, 75% of them in the developing world. This figure indicates an international health problem of plague-like proportions. There are 300 million smokers in China alone (Reuters, 1997). According to the World Health Organization, smoking kills 500 000 people in mainland China each year and is responsible for 19% of deaths in Hong Kong (Leong, 1997). Nearly all Chinese men smoke, as do more than half of the population of Beijing and other urban areas, and the overall rate is climbing by 2% per year (Anon., 1995). According to the American Medical Association, the number of cases of lung cancer is increasing by almost 5% per year, and the rates are highest in areas where the population has been addicted the longest, such as Shanghai (Anon., 1996a). It was predicted more than 10 years ago that of all of the children under the age of 20 alive at the time, some 50 million, would eventually die from the effects of tobacco; as the author of the study pointed out, that is a particularly powerful statistic for a country with a one-child policy (Peto, 1987). Many people are concerned about the environmental consequences of 1.2 million million Chinese people owning a refrigerator or a car. What about the effect of a population of that size being so thoroughly afflicted by and dependent on tobacco and the tobacco industry?

Smoking also imposes enormous economic costs. An estimate by the World Bank was that tobacco use results in a global net loss of US$ 200 million million per year, half of the losses occurring in developing countries. The costs include direct medical care, absence from work, losses due to fires, reduced productivity and foregone income due to early mortality (Barnum, 1994). An estimate from a study in Hong Kong was that the cost of treating the three diseases directly related to smoking amounted to HK$ 500 million (US$ 64.6 million) per year. If we include productivity losses, the true economic cost of smoking could be as much as HK$ 3 million million (US$ 388 million) every year.

Sustainability

Beyond these millions of lives, smoking poisons the environment. Tobacco cultivation has exhausted the soil and consumed vast quantities of water and trees throughout the world, often at the expense of use of those resources for the cultivation of essential food and often in areas that can least afford to waste their limited resources. The consumption of tobacco results in even more waste, as the visible and seemingly omnipresent debris of cigarette butts and packs litters the globe. Health experts in South Africa estimated that 101 million cigarette butts and 5 million packs are thrown away in their country each day (South Africa Council Against Smoking, 1997). On one 'coastal clean-up' day in the United States in 1995, volunteers collected over 800 000 cigarette butts—by far the most prevalent type of trash—on less than one-tenth of the nation's coastline (Anon., 1996a).

Smoking, or more precisely the international industry built around it, has an even more profound effect on the environment. At the core of environmentalism is the concept of efficient resource use and conservation rather than consumption. Environmentalism is about sustainability, about people respecting the environment that sustains them and recognizing that the resources they use must sustain those who come after them. Beyond the biological costs exacted by tobacco cultivation and consumption, the tobacco industry itself is selling an unsustainable lifestyle, an artificial construct, where poisoning your lungs, your air and your home is depicted as glamorous and cool—and the world is buying.

At the heart of sustainability is health: healthy ecosystems and healthy communities. The tobacco industry, by encouraging the consumption of unhealthy products and targeting the poorest and most vulnerable corners of the globe, is engaging in socially unjust as well as ecologically unsustainable activities.

The tools

Clearly, something must be done. Imperial officials in seventeenth century China, concerned about the effects of tobacco, made the use or distribution of tobacco a crime punishable by decapitation (Anon., 1989). That was perhaps too drastic, but the anomaly today is the law's laxity: even though we know better than before how addictive and how toxic tobacco is, it still remains a legal product rather than a strictly regulated one. In the modern world, however, we also recognize that putting new and better ideas in people's heads is usually a much better option to chopping them off. Our task, then, as people concerned about public health and the environment, is to ensure that fewer are seduced by smoking. The three best tools are:

- legislation, to limit the power and pervasiveness of tobacco advertising;
- fiscal controls, to reflect the real cost of tobacco and encourage users to kick the habit and
- effective public education about the real health consequences of smoking.

Hong Kong enacted tough legislation to curb tobacco smoking advertising in spring 1997. Our laws banned billboards and industry sponsorship of sporting events for two years. Moreover, the law gives the managers of shopping malls and restaurants the right to ban smoking in public; in addition, other public places such as cinemas had already been made smoke-free. The tobacco industry spent HK$ 487 million on advertising and promotion of its products in Hong Kong in 1995 alone (Coopers & Lybrand, 1996) and has managed to sell its message effectively to an ever-younger population. Our hope is that by putting a limit on the industry's most public efforts we can limit the appeal of its products and thus foster the kind of social environment—without the overt symbols of a dangerous habit—necessary for an effective public education campaign.

Legislative measures and greater public awareness have had an effect in Hong Kong, where the population of smokers decreased by almost 10% between 1982 and 1996 (Secretary for Health and Welfare, 1997), and in developed countries, where the overall smoking rate is declining by about 1.5% per year (Nakajima, 1995). Nevertheless, the tobacco industry is expanding at a record pace throughout the developing world. According to independent researchers, Philip Morris has become the biggest source of advertising revenue in China (Anon., 1996c).

Imported cigarettes are more popular and more expensive, and money spent on them is channeled directly out of local communities and into the pockets of multinational corporations abroad. Tobacco is a cheap product: it is cheap to produce and process, stock and ship. Its relatively high proce, short production cycle and suitability for using surplus labour make it attractive to small growers, and its reliable market encourages governments to offer incentives for its production, at the expense of food crops. Thus, beyond the biological opportunity costs and medical expenses resulting from tobacco use, its cultivation and sale impose economic opportunity costs, which the price of the end product should reflect.

Tobacco taxes help the local community keep some of the revenue that would otherwise leave the country. Once appropriated, these all-too-costly tobacco profits can at least be used to benefit local development. More importantly, tobacco taxes discourage smoking, particularly in poorer communities. They are relatively easy to administer and, together with effective controls on advertising, have been proven to decrease consumption.

Any revenue gained by fiscal measures should be put directly towards public health education, with the aim of ensuring that the choice to smoke is made with a full awareness and appreciation of the consequences. It is where that awareness and appreciation have yet to take hold, particularly among youth and women in developing countries, that the tobacco industry is concentrating its efforts—and where we must concentrate ours.

Restructuring the industry

Smoking is an environmental issue, a sustainability issue. We have a moral obligation as well as a practical one to limit its expansion. Despite its shameful history of denial, the tobacco industry is finally being forced to recognize this. One American tobacco executive, quoted after the landmark settlement in the United States, said that his company had agreed to it in order to modify the industry's pariah status. 'We may manufacture a product that's controversial, but it was time to fit back with mainstream America.' (Anon., 1997).

The tobacco industry is likely in time to face similar objections from other communities, although perhaps through other means than American-style litigation. Perhaps, finally, the tobacco industry's own business is as unsustainable as the health and environmental well-being of its customers. As I see it, the tobacco industry has two choices. On the one hand, it may choose to go out with a bang, extracting as much money as it can on the way and leaving an enduring legacy of ill will and ill health wherever it operates. Alternatively, it may choose to begin restructuring itself in order to parlay its strengths—brand-name recognition and a global distribution network—into a business with a future.

As a start, it could perhaps look at alternative uses for tobacco. Tobacco is the most addictive but not the most deadly of the substances that go into a cigarette. Researchers in Kentucky (United States) found that tobacco is one of the easiest plants to engineer genetically and have used it as the basis for a potential vaccine against malaria. A study released by the Southern Technology Council recommends use of tobacco juice as an undercoating on metal to stop corrosion (Associated Press, 1996). (That gives you an idea of its toxicity.)

In the long-term, the industry could build on its non-tobacco goods and companies, such as Kraft and Nabisco, and begin the process of gradually restructuring themselves before they are forced to do so in haste by public outrage, regulation and litigation. They have the choice: leave Marlboro Country b'fore the sun sets, with some small measure of credibility, or be forced out.

At the end of the day, the national economic balance sheet for tobacco is likely to be the main factor in determining whether governments will be sympathetic to implementing domestic tobacco control measures. We must ensure that they get that balance sheet right: that they are not seduced by the well-funded arguments of tobacco lobbyists into believing that this product will do their community good. The bottom line is that smoking constitutes a silent, effective attack on human habitats. Those who care about them—and that should be all of us, including the people making money out of the production and consumption of cigarettes—should do all they can to fight back and to work towards a sustainable lifestyle.

References
Anon. (1989) *Smithsonian*, **20**, 107–109
Anon. (1995) Beijing bans public smoking. *Tobacco News*, 31 December
Anon. (1996a) *Journal of the American Medical Association*, October
Anon. (1996b) 480,437,945,912 cigarette butts unaccounted for. *USA Today*, 3 July
Anon. (1996c) Tobacco industry targets Third World. *St Petersburg Times*, 15 August
Anon. (1997) Tobacco pact calls for strict Federal controls. *Washington Post*, 21 June
Associated Press (1996d) Test aims to use tobacco to make vaccine. 15 April
Barnum, H. (1994) The economic burden of the global trade in tobacco. *Tobacco Control*, **3**
Coopers & Lybrand (1996) A study of the economic impact of a ban on cigarette advertising in Hong Kong.
    Paper prepared for the Association of Accredited Advertising Agencies, 3 June, p. 8
Leong, C.H. (1997) WHO and Hong Kong Department of Health statistics cited in a position paper presented
    to the Legislative Council in connection to the motion debate to introduce a comprehensive ban on direct
    and indirect tobacco advertising, 15 January
Nakajima, H. (1995) Message from the Director-General of the World Health Organization for World No-
    Tobacco Day
Peto, R. (1987) Future mortality from tobacco in China. Paper presented to the Shaghai Symposium on
    Smoking and Health, Shaghai, 14–16 November
Reuters (1997) China chokes on its worst habit. *Soth China Morning Post*, 22 August
Secretary for Health and Welfare (1997) Speech to the Legislative Council of Hong Kong, 15 January
South Africa Council Against Smoking (1997) Press release, 13 February

Tobacco and the environment

S. Parkin

Forum for the Future, London, United Kingdom

Context for concern

Tobacco cultivation occupies a relatively small proportion of the global cropland: 4328 thousand ha, out of a total 1 441 423 thousand ha (0.3%), according to the Food and Agriculture Organization of the United Nations. That may seem unimportant, but before considering the impact of tobacco cultivation on the environment in more detail, the global context for this activity, especially in relation to competition for land use, anticipated population growth, greenhouse gas emissions and climate change, must be considered.

Population soars to 9.5 million million by 2050

Despite a slowing of the annual rate of growth, the world population is expected to rise from 5.6 million million in 1995 to 9.5 million million in 2050: a huge increase in the number of people seeking food, water, shelter, cooking materials, warmth, clothing and personal fulfilment. How are so many people to achieve what the *Human Development Report* (1997) terms the basic opportunities of human development ('to lead a long, healthy, creative life, and to enjoy a decent standard of living, freedom, dignity, self-esteem and the respect of others') 50 years from now, when today 1.3 million million people survive on less than the equivalent of US$ 1 per day, nearly 1 million million are illiterate, well over 1 million million lack access to safe water, 840 million are either hungry or face food insecurity, and nearly a third of people in the least developed countries today (most in sub-Saharan Africa) are unlikely to survive to the age of 40?

Pressures on productive land

Current estimates show that human economic activity of all sorts already uses around 40% of the biological production of the land (terrestrial photosynthesis) each year (Vitosek *et al.*, 1986). While that may sound as if there is plenty of room for manoeuvre, it is important to realize that we use the 40% that is easiest to access and must share it with other people. Further, each year, a significant proportion of that 'take' is rendered unavailable for use in future years, as what were once renewable resources are increasingly being turned into non-renewable ones, for example through loss of topsoil by erosion or land salination. Soaring demand on fresh water supplies for agriculture, industry and municipal use is leading to signs of scarcity, in some cases acute. Twenty-six countries are already described as 'water-scarce': that is, the lack of water is a severe constraint on food production, economic development and protection of natural systems (Postel, 1997).

Marine resources under stress

At the moment, seas and oceans provide about 16% of the protein needs of the world, and around 1 million million people are estimated to depend on fish as their sole source of protein (World Resources Institute, 1994–95). Although a record total catch was recorded in 1995—90.7 million tonnes (80% wild, 20% farmed)—the amount of fish caught *per capita per annum* (15.9 kg) has remained about the same since 1965. Overfishing, the use of trawling techniques which damage the sea-bed and damage to coastal spawning grounds are now raising grave concern about the sustainability of yields in a growing number of fishing areas.

Continuing net losses of forest and woodland cover

In every continent except North and Central America and Europe (where forest cover has increased by 0.3 and 0.9%, respectively), there has been a net loss of forest and woodland cover over the last decade. Globally, the rate of loss is 7.8%, a deeply worrying figure which hides massive local losses. For example, in Malawi the rate of loss over the last decade has been a devastating 22%. The importance of forest and woodland cover to local rainfall, species diversity and soil stability is relatively well known. Plato remarked on and worried about the effects of deforestation, and the deserts of North Africa were once the bread-baskets of the Roman Empire. Known, but less well understood, is the role of forest and woodland cover in ensuring global climate stability. The process of photosynthesis by which trees and plants absorb carbon dioxide and use sunlight to turn it into oxygen and carbohydrates is the stuff of school exams. The intricate and interlinked mechanisms of the ecological systems of the air, land and sea, however, remain matters of some mystery and much computer modeling.

Climate change

Nevertheless, in 1995, the Intergovernmental Panel on Climate Change considered it possible to state that: 'the balance of evidence suggests that there is a discernible human influence on global climate'. This was a historic statement, supported by the majority of the world's climate scientists and backed by a number of clear trends that became apparent through the 'background noise' of climate fluctuations. For example, 1996 was the eighteenth consecutive year in which positive global temperature anomalies were seen since records began in 1860 (World Meteorological Organization, 1997).

While the general trend shows an overall rise in global temperatures —the estimated global mean in 1996 being 0.22 °C above the average for 1961–90—world regions have been affected by unusual extremes of weather: tropical regions have had temperatures above normal, but other areas have experienced above-average rainfall and/or snow cover. In 1996, the trend for above-normal hurricane activity continued, with a near-record two-year total (World Meteorological Organization, 1997).

The arguments of skeptics that global climate change is at best unproven may be countered by major insurance companies. They have experienced a growing number of claims for weather-induced damage, for a total of more than US$ 20 million million per year. Further, personal insurance cover in a number of countries is rising to cover extra claims for flood damage or subsidence damage to property through drought. In France, for example, an increase of 14% has been added to the annual cost of insuring an average house, explicitly to cover 'natural events' (my own insurance company, MATMUT).

Thus, the costs of climate disruption can be traced on a rising line at global level through the annual reports of re-insurance companies and at a local level through a rise in the cost of living due to increased insurance costs. While I am fully conscious that the majority of people in the world, especially those in the most vulnerable areas, are not insured, the importance of this point may be judged by the fact that the global insurance industry is, like the fossil fuel industry, worth roughly US$ 1.6 million million million (Berz, 1992). It is now regretting its passivity when the fossil fuel industry lobbied so effectively to weaken the Climate Convention agreed to at the 1992 Earth Summit. Like the fossil fuel industry, the insurance industry has strong interests in its own survival and fears of what it has called 'capacity problems'—that is, running out of sufficient reserves to meet escalating claims at both international and national level— will hopefully have stimulated it to organize a serious lobby for governments to make a strong agreement at the Third Session of the Conference of the Parties (signatures to the Climate Convention) in Kyoto, Japan, in December 1997.

The weather outlook remains worrying. The notorious El Niño, the irregular upsurging of warm surface water in the Pacific, appeared six months earlier than usual in 1997, the surface water temperatures already being 5 °C above normal in August (Anon., 1997). The last major climatic disruptions associated with El Niño, in 1982–83, caused an estimated US$ 13.6 million million worth of damage to crops and livelihoods. Some climate scientists see a correlation between El Niño and unusual changes in global climate patterns elsewhere. Again, skeptics are advised to check with their commodity brokers. Commodity futures markets are bullish about the potential disruption to supplies of things like palm and fish oil, coffee and cocoa beans and are raising prices and/or buying alternative crops in anticipation. Damage to corn crops in Indonesia, Thailand, Latin America and sub-Saharan Africa could reduce world supplies by up to 1.5% of projected world consumption.

The clinical assessment of the effect of El Niño on the commodity markets masks the reality of its effect on people living where the destructive weather strikes. Commodity brokers will be insured to the eyeballs, as will some of the bigger merchants, but most of the producers won't be. Their crops, communities and in many cases their lives will be lost. In 1982–83, for example, El Niño killed 600 people in floods in southern China and 600 in northern Peru.

Summary

Our concern about the percentage of land devoted to growing tobacco and its impact on local environment and communities should not be viewed in isolation from what are deeply worrying trends now manifesting themselves at a global level. The demands of a growing world population are putting increasing pressure on the life-support services of the land and the sea. In some areas of the world, this pressure has already reached breaking point. It must not be forgotten that the 'discernible human influence on global climate' is due largely to a relatively small percentage of the human population (20%) meeting their needs (and more), by an extraordinarily profligate processing of around 80% of the resources in economies with high energy use during the past 200 years. Poverty degrades the environment, but so does affluence.

Burning fossil fuels that have taken millions of years to lay down in the space of a few hundred years while simultaneously reducing the amount of forest cover and otherwise damaging the functionality of natural pollution handling systems, like wetlands, may be likened to standing in a shower with the tap full on while blocking the plughole with one's toe: eventually, everything flows over, with disastrous consequences.

Tobacco growing and the environment

It is in this context that I turn to tobacco growing, with one question: Does tobacco growing add to the environmental pressures outlined above, or does it play a role in alleviating them? At the outset, it has to be said that any attempt to make an overall evaluation of the impact of tobacco growing on the environment founders almost immediately on the inadequacy or non-independent nature of the information available. A study in 1995 by the United Nations Conference on Trade and Development, based heavily on a study sponsored by the International Tobacco Growers' Association, called for a full economic analysis of tobacco growing to 'take account of any harm to farm workers and environmental costs of deforestation and damage to soil and water resources' (UNCTAD Secretariat, 1995).

What follows here, then, is an attempt to enumerate the environmental features that such an analysis would have to include and to extend them so that they embrace other environmental impacts associated with tobacco growing and use. This is in tune with the current move of industrial sectors, governments and international institutions to develop integrated environmental, social and economic accounting methods (e.g. Serageldin & Steer, undated). The environmental costs to be added to the health costs of growing and smoking tobacco are as follows:

Tobacco seeds
+
4 328 000 hectares of land (FAO, 1995), including opportunity costs
+
US$?000 subsidies (1106 million ECU in 1996 (1 ECU = US$ 1.24, 1996)
+
? tonnes of pesticides and fertilizer
+
? tonnes of coal and wood for curing
+
? net carbon dioxide emissions from growing and curing tobacco
2 600 tonnes per year from smoking (5200 tonnes methane)
+
? soil exhaustion and erosion, water pollution
+
? tonnes of wrapping and packaging (and associated environmental impacts)
+
? tonnes of transport fuel (and associated environmental impacts)
+
environmental costs of marketing
+
US$?000 litter clean-up, fires, room fumigation, etc.

=

5 340 000 000 000 cigarettes per year (1992)

Land use and degradation

In 1992, over 8 million tonnes of tobacco were grown worldwide, over 6 million tonnes of it in developing countries. Tobacco is generally grown on semi-arid land and requires a long growing season: five to six months compared with four months for maize. The water-thirsty seedlings require a three-month growing period before being planted out in fields. It is a greedy crop, requiring significantly more nutrients such as nitrogen, phosphorus and potassium than crops such as coffee, maize and cassava (Table 1). The high demand of tobacco for nutrients requires regular inputs of chemical fertilizers. According to an instruction leaflet given to Kenyan tobacco farmers by British American Tobacco, 16 applications of pesticide are recommended in the seed beds alone. The effect of chemical fertilizers and pesticides on ground and other local water supplies is well known but in the case of tobacco growing poorly chronicled, as is the effect on the health of workers (mostly women) and the children they take to the fields while working. This sort of farming—intensive use of artificial fertilizers and

Table 1. Depletion of soil nutrients by tobacco and other crops

Crop (1 t/ha)	Depletion (kg/ha)		
	Nitrogen	Phosphorus	Potassium
Tobacco	24.4	14.4	46.4
Coffee	15.0	2.5	19.5
Maize	9.8	1.9	6.7
Cassava	2.2	0.4	1.9

From Van Wambeke (1984)

intensive cropping—seriously diminishes the intrinsic fertility of the soil. That and local deforestation associated with tobacco growing speed up soil erosion, already a significant problem in many developing countries.

Some tobacco is sun-dried, but about two-thirds of the global crop, consisting of the most valuable and sought-after leaves, is 'flue-dried' in barns heated to a constant 35 °C by wood, coal or other fuel for 7–10 days. According to a study commissioned by the tobacco industry itself, it can take 2.5–40 kg of wood to cure 1 kg of tobacco, with an average of 7.8 kg (Anon., 1995). Others estimates are much higher. The Ugandan Government and British American Tobacco, for example, admit to use of 100 kg of wood per kilogram of tobacco, although local farmers say they use as much as 130 kg (Muwanga-Bayego, 1994).

Attempts by the tobacco companies to encourage farmers to use some of their land to grow trees for curing have not had significant success, firstly because the favoured tree is the extremely water-greedy eucalyptus and secondly because the price of tobacco is kept low by the tobacco companies, who hold huge stocks. Consequently, many farmers, who may also be indebted to the tobacco company itself for seeds and fertilizers and so on, are already working on very narrow margins. It makes no sense for them to lose tobacco-growing land to trees when they can go on taking wood from the nearest, and still free, forest—even if it is some kilometres away.

Atmospheric pollution

Without a lot more information, it is not possible to arrive at a conclusion on the net contribution of tobacco growing, leaf curing, cigarette manufacture, packaging and distribution to atmospheric pollution. The calculation would have to include carbon dioxide absorbed by the growing plants, of course, but also that released by fertilizer and pesticide manufacture and the fuel used for curing, the absorption capacity lost by felled trees and so on. It is reasonable to assume, however, that the net contribution to atmospheric pollution of 1 kg of tobacco, from the moment the seed is planted to the moment it reaches the lips of the smoker, is considerable.

Once the tobacco is lit, the calculations are easier. Smokers emit an estimated 2.6 million million kg of carbon dioxide and approximately 5.2 million million kg of methane, a more potent greenhouse gas (Whidden, 1991). In Los Angeles (United States), 1–1.3% of the fine particles of its famous smog can be attributed to cigarette smoke: a small contribution to the total perhaps, but one of half a dozen minor sources that together amount for one-quarter of the total pollution, with its consequences on human health and the environment (Anon., 1994).

Such a calculation would also, strictly speaking, include the environmental impacts of fires started by careless smokers and the cost of e.g. 'cleaning' hotel rooms after use by smokers. Scandia Hotels in Sweden, for example, spend over US$ 110 per room. In 1993, 162 deaths from 6200 fires caused by smoking materials were reported by the United Kingdom Fire Service (Home Office, 1995). While we are at it, what about the collection and disposal of smoking-related litter? The 'Tidy Britain Group' estimated that smoking-related litter makes up a huge 40% of the total litter which must be disposed of either by incineration or landfill; both methods of course have significant environmental effects.

An ecological cost–benefit analysis

The case against growing and smoking tobacco has, until recently, rested on the costs and benefits in relation to health. The Canadian economy, for example, is thought to benefit by CAN$ 3 million million from the tobacco industry, but the costs of smoking-related diseases to the health services and to industry from loss of productivity are estimated at CAN$ 3.9 million million. The decision of giant United States tobacco companies to curtail advertising and pay out US$ 368 million million over the next 25 years in part confirms the extent to which state and private health-care systems have been subsidizing tobacco industry profits.

Now the time is more than ripe to argue the environmental and social case against tobacco. I have attempted to make a start at setting the context for how the environmental case should be argued—not only on the basis of the evidence of local environmental degradation but also the evidence of rapidly mounting pressure on the major ecological systems of our Earth. Even on the basis of the jumbled, elderly and partial evidence available, it is impossible to argue that growing and smoking tobacco are environmentally beneficial. Where is the way out?

The trap set for small farmers by tobacco companies—providing loans, seed, fertilizer etc. and guaranteeing to purchase the crop (if not at a guaranteed price)—is similar to those set by other multinational companies dealing in agricultural commodities. But alternative crops to tobacco, such as chilis, potatoes, garlic, cotton and sesame, could be equally if not more profitable to small farmers if similar marketing and other support were available (Karim, 1994), and they would be much less damaging to the environment and to human health, although admittedly they would deliver less value to the controlling corporations. By the same token, the export earnings and tax income of governments dependent on tobacco would be little different if paprika or silk was substituted for tobacco; the transition might be difficult, that is all. Only two countries depend for more than 2.2% of their export earnings on tobacco—Malawi and Zimbabwe—although others contribute more significant proportions to their government's tax coffers. The Tanzanian government receives 10% of its tax revenues from tobacco.

Is it a matter of simply looking for a substitute export crop to tobacco? Or should a careful look be taken at the opportunity costs of other crops in terms of meeting local needs? There are reports of malnutrition in tobacco-growing communities, particularly at harvest and curing time, when the coffers are empty before the passage of the merchants who will buy this year's crop. That, and the balance of imported grain and other commodities might indicate that it would be (i) cheaper, (ii) better for local communities and (iii) better for the environment if meeting local needs took priority over cash crops. For instance, Malawi, a central African country, depends on tobacco for 75% of its export earnings. It is one of the poorest countries in the world in terms of income, and over 45% of its population is classified as poor in human development (low life expectancy, illiteracy, exclusion and lack of material resources) in the *Human Development Report* for 1997. How would the aid agencies feel if they realized that some of the aid they channel into Malawi is subsidizing tobacco companies, which register profits of millions of millions of dollars per year? Thus, the gross national product of Malawi in 1991 was US$ 1.9 million million; 27.2% of that (US$ 49 *per capita*) was provided by overseas development agencies, and Philip Morris' net profits for the year ending April 1997 were US$ 6 million million (Anon., 1997).

After their capitulation to the health case in the United States, the tobacco giants may move to poor countries to grow and sell their products. The trend is already established. A concerted effort by governments, development agencies and health and environment professionals is needed to first remove subsidies from tobacco growing, however indirect they may be, and then oblige the companies to 'internalize' the full cost of their activities, in line with new thinking on integrating environmental and economic accounting.

Some companies may like to use my framework analysis of the environmental life cycle of tobacco growing and, reflecting on what they have had to pay out on health, may calculate that they would be better off setting up an endowment fund to support environmentally-sensitive community development programmes on the 4 328 000 ha they have used for tobacco growing—and I mean in Kentucky as well as in Kenya.

References
Anon. (1994) *New Scientist*, 20 August
Anon. (1995) *Tobacco Reporter*, February
Anon. (1997) *Financial Times*, 28 July
Berz, G.A. (1992) Greenhouse effects on natural catastrophes and insurance. *Geneva Papers Risk Insurance*, 17, 386–392
FAO (1995) *Production*, 49, 176–177
Home Office (1995) *Fire Statistics United Kingdom, 1993*, London
Human Development Report (1997)
Karim, Z. (1994) Bangladesh Agricultural Research Council, Dhaka, quoted in Panoshope, L. *Southern Voices on Environment and Development*, October 1994
Muwanga-Bayego, H. (1994) Tobacco growing in Uganda: The environment and women pay the price. *Tobacco Control*, 3, 255–256
Postel, S. (1997) *The Last Oasis*, W.W. Norton, p. 29
Serageldin, I. & Steer, A., eds (undated) *Making Development Sustainable* (Environmentally Sustainable Development Occasional Paper Series No. 2), Washington DC: World Bank
Vitosek, P.M., Erlich, P.R., Erlich, A.H. & Mateson, P.A. (1986) Human appropriation of photosynthesis. *Bioscience*, 34, 368–373
UNCTAD (United Nations Conference on Trade and Development) Secretariat (1995) Economic Role of Tobacco Producation and Exports on Countries Depending on Tobacco as a Major Source of Income (UNCTAD/CIN/63), 8 May 1995
Van Wambeke (1994) quoted in Goodland, Watson and Ledec, *Environmental Management in Tropical Agriculture*, Westview Press
Whidden, P. (1995) Passive resistance. *Green Magazine*, January
World Meteorological Organization (1997) *World Climate News*, 11
World Resources Institute (1994–95)

Attitudes of smoking and non-smoking Estonian schoolchildren towards the environment

D. Eensoo, A. Saava & K. Pärna

University of Tartu, Tartu, Estonia

Many aspects of human well-being are influenced by the environment, and many diseases can be initiated, sustained or exacerbated by environmental factors. Understanding and controlling people's interactions with their environment is therefore an important component of public health. In its broadest sense, environmental health is the sub-field of public health concerned with assessing and controlling the impacts of the environment on human health. Experts in public health have determined that human well-being if based on health behaviour (including smoking behaviour), about 50%; environment, 20%; genetic factors, 20%; and medicine, 10%. The aim of this study was to compare the attitudes of smoking and non-smoking schoolchildren in Estonia towards the environment and to determine their knowledge about environmental health risks.

Material and methods
    The target group consisted of 3090 schoolchildren in grades 8, 10 and 12, aged 13–18, who were selected randomly from Estonian and Russian secondary schools in Tallinn and from Estonian schools in Tartu and southern Estonian counties. An anonymous, self-completed, multi-choice questionnaire was used to elicit information on knowledge about environmental health risks, attitudes toward the environment, health behaviour, self-image, psycho-social background and the health of the schoolchildren.

The data were analysed with the SAS program, version 6.12. The distribution of answers from smokers and non-smokers was compared by cross-tabulation, and the significance of the differences was evaluated by the chi-squared test. The strength of correlation between characteristics was evaluated by Spearman's test.

Results and discussion

Regular or occasional smoking was reported by 22% of the schoolchildren. Slightly fewer smokers (81%) than non-smokers (88%) worried about their health in relation to pollution of environment ($p = 0.001$); however, 13% of smokers and 8.3% of non-smokers evaluated their health as poor ($p = 0.001$); 46% of smokers and 55% of non-smokers evaluated it as good, and 41% of smokers and 36% of non-smokers evaluated it as average. Smoking may cause poor health, but some of the causes may be psychosocial, as many smokers considered that they had no defined social role. The following correlations were found with the smoking behaviour of the schoolchildren: they did not have fun with their parents ($r = 0.18$); they often considered leaving home ($r = 0.26$); their parents did not understand them ($r = 0.15$); their parents did not consider their feelings ($r = 0.12$); their parents expected too much of them ($r = 0.16$) and their parents were pushing them too hard ($r = 0.16$).

When the schoolchildren were asked questions about global problems, only 44% of the smokers and 50% of the non-smokers ($p = 0.0018$) considered pollution of the environment an important global problem. When the children were given concrete environmental problems, they usually agreed and worried about them. Air pollution was considered the most important problem by both non-smokers and smokers. Other problems they considered of importance were pollution of natural water bodies, preservation of flora and fauna, the increasing amount of waste products and oil spills. The answers of the pupils probably depended on how well known the problem was. The smokers worried less about these problems than the non-smokers.

Both smokers and non-smokers thought that the best way to improve the environment is to change production techniques (30% of smokers and 35% of non-smokers) and to radically change living habits (30% of smokers and non-smokers); however, more smokers (25%) were unable to answer this question than non-smokers (20%), and this is the main reason for the difference in the distribution of answers between smokers and non-smokers ($p = 0.028$). Eight percent of smokers and 8.7% of non-smokers considered that science and technology would solve environmental problems in the future, while 6.9% of smokers and 5.7% of non-smokers thought that they could be solved by international training in environmental issues.

About 90% of the pupils considered that Estonia should produce environmentally friendly products, but more of the smokers (7.9%) were indifferent to the problem than non-smokers (5.7%). The distribution of answers between smokers and non-smokers is significant ($p = 0.001$).

About half of the children preferred protection of the environment to development of the economy, with no difference between smokers and non-smokers, but all found the question difficult to answer.

Conclusion

This study shows that smoking influences young people's attitude towards the environment. Although more smokers evaluated their health as poor, they worried about their health less and they were more indifferent towards environmental problems. In planning health promotion programmes for smokers, the interest of smokers in particular problems must be taken into account.

Carbon dioxide in the expired air of smokers and non-smokers in urban and suburban Mexico City

J. Perez-Neria, L. Martinez-Rossier, R. Quezada-Zambrano, E. Hernandez-Garduno, M. Catalan-Vazquez & J. Villalba-Caloca

National Institute of Respiratory Diseases, Mexico City, Mexico

Introduction

Mexico City is located in the northern part of the Federal District in central Mexico at an altitude of 2240 m. It is characterized by a large, dense population and heavy vehicular traffic. The southern part of the District is suburban and mountainous, with woods and farms.

The two main problems for a large proportion of the inhabitants of Mexico City are smoking and air pollution. The National Council against Addiction in Mexico defines a smoker as a person who smokes more than one cigarette per day. With this criteria, the National Addictions Survey carried out in 1993 in the Mexican Republic by the Ministry of Health showed that 25% of a population sample 16–65 years old were smokers; this percentage increased to 30% for the sample from Mexico City (Tapia-Conyer, 1993). The Automatic Environmental Monitoring Network (RAMA) installed in metropolitan Mexico City has been measuring the concentrations of carbon monoxide, ozone, sulfur dioxide and nitrogen dioxide continuously during the last five years and calculating the mean concentrations every hour; the amounts of total suspended particles and suspended particles < 10 μm in diameter are also measured daily. These measurements showed that the concentrations of these air pollutants exceeded the accepted air quality standards on more than 300 days in a year between 11:00 and 15:00 h (Hernandez-Garduno et al., 1997). Therefore, people of Mexico City who work outdoors are exposed for approximately 4 h/day to high levels of air pollutants.

Analysis of the sources of outdoor air pollutants in Mexico City showed that about 70% originate from combustion of gasoline by motor vehicles, but the main source of individual, voluntary exposure is tobacco smoke. The combustion of both motor vehicle gasoline and tobacco produces carbon monoxide, which, when inhaled, is transported by the haemoglobin in pulmonary capillary blood as carboxyhaemoglobin. A proportion of the carbon monoxide in carboxyhaemoglobin is exhaled, and its concentration can be measured in expired air by means of a carbon monoxide analyser.

Smokers in Mexico City argue that there is no reason to quit smoking because living in Mexico City is the same as smoking two packs of cigarettes daily. We propose that smoking and air pollution have additive or multiplicative effects, increasing exposure to carbon monoxide substantially and therefore augmenting the risks to health. As an initial approach to testing our proposition, we decided to measure the fractional concentration of carbon monoxide in expired air (FECO) of smokers who are outdoors more than 6 h/day, working in the vicinity of heavy traffic in Mexico City. One of the objectives of our study was to determine the effect of adding an acute exposure, motor vehicle exhaust, to a chronic exposure, tobacco smoking, on the FECO and to compare the exposure to carbon monoxide of smokers and non-smokers working in an environment polluted by heavy motor vehicle traffic.

Material and methods

During February and March 1996, we measured the FECO in 892 outdoor workers in six locations in Mexico City by means of a Spirometrics, 3100 CMD/I carbon monoxide analyser. The locations were north-east, north-west, downtown, south-east, south-west and a suburban zone in Milpa Alta County as a control area.

Results

There were 303 smokers and 589 non-smokers, with a mean age of 36 years; 41% were female. The FECO of all participants was higher than the ambient carbon monoxide concentration in metropolitan Mexico City. As the RAMA does not cover the suburban zone of Milpa Alta County, we did not have ambient measurements for this area.

The mean FECO for the non-smokers was lower than that for the smokers in each area. Smokers exposed to heavy vehicular traffic in north-east Mexico City had the highest mean FECO (10.3 ppm), whereas non-smokers in this zone had a FECO of 8.3 ppm ($p < 0.05$). Non-smokers exposed to light vehicular traffic in a suburban area of Mexico City had the lowest mean FECO (3.7 ppm), but smokers in this zone had a significantly higher FECO (6.0 ppm; $p < 0.0001$). When we stratified the data for smokers by years of addiction, there was no effect on the FECO, but when we stratified the data for smokers by daily cigarette consumption, a strong correlation was found (Figure 1). Analysis of the data by multiple regression showed (Table 1) that the best predictors for a high FECO were male sex, daily cigarette consumption, working in the north-east and north-west zones of the City and heavy motor vehicle traffic.

Discussion

The United States Environmental Protection Agency (1979) established a mean of 12 ppm over 8 h as the standard for the outdoor concentration of carbon monoxide; we measured concentrations that surpassed that level. The lack of correlation between FECO and years of smoking and its strong correlation with daily cigarette consumption may be due to the fact that carbon monoxide does not accumulate for long periods in the body, and expired carbon monoxide depends on the persistence of daily inhaled doses.

Figure 1. Fractional concentrations of carbon monoxide (FECO) in expired air of smokers according to number of cigarettes smoked daily

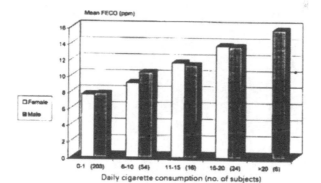

Table 1. Predictors of a high fractional concentration of carbon monoxide in expired air

Variable	Regression coefficient	Standard error	p
Male	0.3869	0.1777	0.0200
North-east	2.6342	0.2516	0.0001
North-west	2.3590	0.2860	0.0001
Daily cigarette smoking	0.3146	0.0165	0.0001
Heavy traffic	3.0456	0.2233	0.0001

   We conclude that measurement of FECO is an alternative, non-invasive method for evaluating the exposure of risk groups, such as smokers and persons who spend most of their time outdoors near heavy motor vehicle traffic (Coultas *et al.*, 1993).

   Smokers exposed to high concentrations of ambient carbon monoxide had a higher FECO than non-smokers. We consider measurement of FECO to be a great importance, because of the role of chronic exposure to carbon monoxide in the genesis of cardiovascular disease in smokers (Jeffrey & Laker, 1992; Penn, 1993; Stanton *et al.*, 1995).

References

Coultas, D.B., Stidley, C.A. & Samet, J.M. (1993) Cigarette yields of tar and nicotine and markers of exposure to tobacco smoke. *Am. Rev. Respir. Dis.*, **148**, 435–440

Environmental Protection Agency (1979) *Air Quality Criteria for Carbon Monoxide* (EPA-600/8-79-022), Washington DC, pp. 6-1, 6-77

Hernandez-Garduno, E., Perez-Neria, J., Paccagnella, A.M., Munguia-Castro, M., Catalan-Vazquez, M. & Rojas-Ramos, M. (1997) Air pollution and respiratory health in Mexico City. *J. Occup. Environ. Med.*, **39**, 299–307

Jeffrey, B. & Laker, D.M. (1992) Smoking and cardiovascular disease. *Am. J. Med.*, **93** (Suppl. 1A), 8S–12S

Penn, A. (1993) Determination of the atherogenic potential of inhaled carbon monoxide. *Res. Resp. Health Eff. Inst.*, **57**, 1–20

Stanton, A., Glantz, P.D. & Parmley, W.W. (1995) Passive smoking and heart disease. Mechanisms and risk. *J. Am. Med. Assoc.*, **272**, 1047–1053

Tapia-Conyer, R. (1993) Encuesta Nacional de Adicciones, Vol. II, Tabaco, Mexico, SSA

TOBACCO ADDICTION

Consumption of cigarettes, nicotine dependence and health status

H. Sovinová[1] & L. Csémy[2]

[1]National Institute of Public Health, and [2]Prague Psychiatric Centre,
Prague, Czech Republic

Abstract

We describe the prevalence of smoking among the adult population of the Czech Republic and associations between health status and smoking. The data were derived from a cross-sectional health survey of a sample of 1397 residents aged 18–64. Almost one-third of the respondents were current smokers, and 25% reported smoking on a daily basis. The mean consumption of daily smokers was 15 cigarettes per day for men and 12 for women. Indicators of subjective and objective health status were examined in relation to the level of tobacco consumption and to the score in the Fagerström test of nicotine dependence. The differences in indicators of health status suggest more health problems among smokers with a mean daily consumption of > 10 cigarettes. Similarly, smokers with mild nicotine dependence reported fewer days off work during the previous 12 months than smokers who were moderately or severely dependent on nicotine.

Introduction

At the end of 1996, the National Institute of Public Health conducted an extensive study among the general adult population of the Czech Republic to identify the extent and context of various forms of addictive behaviour, covering tobacco smoking, alcohol consumption and use of psychoactive pharmaceuticals and illicit drugs. In this paper, we concentrate on the prevalence of the smoking and patterns of cigarette consumption in adults and examine the relationship between nicotine dependence and health status.

Methods

We used a probability sampling procedure with quotas. The studied sample corresponded fairly well to the whole population with regard to major demographic characteristics such as sex, age, level of education and region of residence. The analyses are based on face-to-face interviews performed by trained interviewers at the end of 1996, with 1397 residents of the Czech Republic aged 18–64 (mean, 39.2 years; SD, 13.2). Men represented 49% of the sample.

The questionnaire elicited information about use or misuse of alcoholic beverages, tobacco, psychoactive pharmaceuticals and illicit substances. Three indicators of health status were taken into account: a subjective estimate of the respondent's health status on the Likert scale, where 1 indicates very good health and 5 very poor health, and two objective indicators, one being the number of episodes of illness during the previous 12 months and the other time off work because of illness during the previous 12 months.

Results

The prevalence of smoking is shown in Table 1. The overall prevalence of current smoking in the adult population was about 26%, with 29% of men and 22% of women reporting daily smoking; 16% were ex-smokers. The percentage of lifetime non-smokers was much higher among women (62%) than men (47%). We focused our attention on the daily smokers.

The mean number of cigarettes smoked per day varied significantly with sex: 15 per day for men and < 12 for women. Table 2 shows the distribution of smokers according to cigarette consumption. Most men smoked 16–20 cigarettes per day, and most women 6–10 per day. We found no significant association between daily smoking and age, but

Table 1. Smoking status by sex

Smoking status	Men	Women
Daily smokers	28.6	21.7
Irregular smokers	3.1	5.0
Ex-smokers	21.8	11.1
Non-smokers	46.5	62.2

there was a clear inverse relationship between smoking and the level of education ($\chi^2 =$ 42.67; degrees of freedom = 12; $p < 0.001$ for men and $\chi^2 = 22.55$; degrees of freedom = 12; $p < 0.05$ for women).

The mean values for the three indicators of health status are given in Table 2 according to daily cigarette consumption. Values indicative of poorer health were recorded for a consumption of > 10 cigarettes per day. One-way analysis of variance to test the differences in group means gave an F probability of < 0.05 in all three comparisons. When the same indicators of health status were examined in relation to the score in the Fagerström test of nicotine dependence, smokers reporting weak dependence (about 40% of all daily smokers) had better health than smokers with moderate or severe nicotine dependence. While smokers who were weakly dependent reported taking only 10 days off work in the preceding year, those with higher scores had taken ≥ 20 days off work (Table 3).

Discussion and conclusion

In concordance with the results of many epidemiological studies, we found that the prevalence of regular and heavy smoking was higher among persons with less education. We found almost identical smoking patterns among men and women with a university level of education, while the differences gradually increased with lower levels of education. One possible explanation is the greater convergence of the social roles of men and women with more education.

The associations between cigarette consumption, degree of nicotine dependence and indicators of health status should be interpreted with caution, since many other

Table 2. Objective and subjective indicators of health status by average daily consumption of cigarettes

Health indicator	Average no. of cigarettes per day				
	1–5	6–10	11–15	16–20	≥ 21
Subjective health status (average score)	2.3	2.3	2.6	2.6	3.0
Average no. of episodes of illness (past 12 months)	1.9	1.7	2.0	1.9	3.1
Average no. of days off work (past 12 months)	12.2	14.1	22.1	16.7	37.4

Table 3. Objective and subjective indicators of health status and strengths of dependence measured by Fagerström test of nicotine dependence

Health indicator	Score (% of daily smokers)			
	0–1 (weak) (40%)	2–3 (moderate) (25.3%)	4–6 (severe) (27.8%)	7–10 (very severe) (6.3%)
Subjective health status (average score)	2.2	2.6	2.8	2.4
Average no. of episodes of illness (past 12 months)	1.5	2.1	2.0	2.6
Average no. of days off work (past 12 months)	10.6	21.2	22.6	22.3

factors that may affect health could not be controlled for in this survey. Nevertheless, regular heavy smoking affected the health status of the population.

Our major findings are that:
- approximately 25% of the adult Czech population smokes cigarettes daily;
- more men than women smoke tobacco regularly and heavily;
- an inverse relationship between smoking and level of education was confirmed for men;
- heavier cigarette consumption was associated with poorer scores for indicators of health status;
- people with moderate and severe nicotine dependence reported more episodes of illness and more days off work than those with a low score.

The future of nicotine delivery: Technology, policy and public health

K.E. Warner[1], J. Slade[2] & D.T. Sweanor[3]

[1]University of Michigan, Ann Arbor, Michigan; [2]Robert Wood Johnson Medical School, New Brunswick, New Jersey, United States; [3]Nonsmokers' Rights Association, Ottawa, Ontario, Canada

In developed countries, concerns about the health effects of smoking have led to the introduction of new methods of delivering nicotine. The tobacco industry is producing devices made to look like cigarettes in which radically different techniques are used to deliver nicotine to smokers and which reduce smokers' exposure to some of the poisons in conventional cigarette smoke. The industry's intent is to keep smokers dependent on nicotine and the industry's products. In contrast, the pharmaceutical industry has developed nicotine replacement products with the purpose of helping smokers to wean themselves off nicotine altogether. Given a potentially enormous market for less hazardous cigarette substitutes, however, it is possible that an aggressive competition might soon develop between the tobacco and pharmaceutical industries to serve a large population of long-term nicotine addicts. In this paper, we describe some of the new techniques, discuss policy issues raised by this newly emerging market and consider implications for public health.

Techniques

The tobacco industry's new devices are intended to serve two purposes: to give consumers an alternative to quitting smoking that they believe is less dangerous than smoking and to offer smokers products that, by creating less foul-smelling smoke or less smoke altogether, will be more acceptable to non-smokers around them.

The most technologically radical of these devices were introduced during the past decade. In 1988, R.J. Reynolds test-marketed Premier, a device that looked like a cigarette on the outside but bore no resemblance to one on the inside. Once its carbon fuel element was ignited, Premier produced an aerosol from glycerine and a tobacco extract adsorbed onto alumina beads proximal to the fuel element. The product yielded normal concentrations of nicotine and carbon monoxide but very little of the particulate matter commonly referred to as 'tar' (R.J. Reynolds Tobacco Co., 1988). According to its patent, the small amount of processed tobacco found in the device was optional. It served no biological or structural function. Rather, it is conjectured, it may have served a *legal* function: by including tobacco particles in a device that looked like a cigarette, the Company may have thought that the United States Food and Drug Administration would choose not to evaluate the product as a drug delivery device, treating it instead as a tobacco product, which the agency had not yet regulated (Department of Health and Human Services, 1989). Premier failed its tests and was taken off the market. Recently, R.J. Reynolds introduced a slightly less radical but still remarkably innovative product, Eclipse, in test markets in four countries (Pauly *et al.*, 1995). Like Premier, Eclipse burns no tobacco. Rather, it heats tobacco at very high temperatures, again relying on a heating element at the front end. It, too, produces normal levels of nicotine, fairly high levels of carbon monoxide and very little tar. The Food and Drug Administration has been petitioned to regulate Eclipse as a drug delivery system.

Premier and Eclipse would appear to represent only the tip of the technological iceberg. There are dozens of patents outstanding for novel nicotine delivery devices, including a Philip Morris product that has an electrical heating coil in the shaft of the 'cigarette' (Davis & Slade, 1993).

On the other side of today's nicotine marketplace, the pharmaceutical industry is producing nicotine replacement products, including nicotine chewing-gum, the patch and, most recently, a nasal spray and an inhaler. In the United States, the first two of these are available over-the-counter, while the latter two are available only by prescription. More nicotine replacement products wait in the wings, including a nicotine 'lollipop' (Leischow *et al.*, 1996).

The apparent desire of many smokers to reduce their risks but their inability or unwillingness to quit smoking suggest that many smokers will seek ways of satisfying their nicotine needs without exposing themselves to the enormous risk associated with smoking conventional cigarettes. Until now, smokers have not had truly less dangerous products with which to satisfy their nicotine addiction. Today, they have a few alternatives, such as patches and chewing-gum, but these must be considered primitive in comparison with what might be forthcoming.

Policy

We believe that it is essential for the public health community to consider what kind of nicotine maintenance market should be permitted in the coming years. Today, the tobacco industry has a huge advantage over the pharmaceutical industry in catering to this new market. Tobacco products are essentially unregulated. New cigarettes, even totally new devices like Eclipse, can be introduced at the whim of the companies, with no requirement that a lower risk be demonstrated. In contrast, pharmaceutical innovations are subject to long, costly, scientifically exacting review processes to establish their safety. This greatly delays the pharmaceutical companies' ability to get the products onto the market and forces them to charge high prices to recover the expensive research and development.

This situation is exactly the opposite of that which logic would recommend. The most dangerous nicotine-delivery system ever developed, the cigarette, is freely introduced and widely available. The safest nicotine-delivery systems ever developed, nicotine replacement products, are severely constrained by an expensive regulatory system. Governmental health authorities ought to consider reversing the favouritism granted to tobacco products. They could regulate *all* nicotine-delivery products in a balanced manner, allowing the least hazardous ready access to the market—through fewer advertising restrictions, lower taxes and so on—while imposing marketing and sales restrictions and high taxes on the relatively more dangerous nicotine innovations (Warner *et al.*, 1997).

Implications for health

If the creativity of the tobacco and pharmaceutical industries were harnessed, new, consumer-friendly products could be marketed to displace some of the massive market for cigarettes. By doing so, they could begin to reduce the tragic toll of disease and death produced by cigarettes.

We want to close with a caution, however. The current generation of ostensibly less hazardous products is not the tobacco industry's first attempt to address smokers' health concerns. Previous generations of purportedly 'safer' products included filtered cigarettes, introduced in the 1950s in response to the first major public 'scare' about smoking and lung cancer, and low-tar and -nicotine cigarettes, introduced in the late 1960s with much the same reasoning (Slade, 1989; Warner *et al.*, 1997). In both cases, these new products gave worried smokers what they perceived to be a means of reducing their risk—switching to the new products without having to take the far more difficult step of quitting smoking altogether. Evidence suggests that they have reduced their risk little if at all, in part because smokers have learnt to compensate for the products' lower nicotine yields by smoking more cigarettes, inhaling more deeply and so on (Kozlowski & Pillitteri, 1996). It is therefore possible that the introduction of both filtered cigarettes and low-tar and -nicotine cigarettes has *increased* the aggregate damage done by cigarettes, by encouraging more people to continue smoking than would have in the absence of these innovations (Department of Health and Human Services, 1989). Given this history, we are concerned that any new alternatives to traditional cigarettes will pose a risk to health, even if they are truly less dangerous for the smoker who switches to them and would otherwise have quit.

This said, we also believe that the market for long-term nicotine maintenance is coming, whether we like it or not. Further, we believe that, properly managed through regulation that covers people's simultaneous desires to consume nicotine and to be safe, this new market could represent a turning point in the decades-old battle against tobacco-produced disease. The availability of consumer-acceptable nicotine-only products might permit the adoption of a policy of phasing nicotine out of conventional tobacco products (Benowitz & Henningfield, 1994), without necessarily exposing nicotine-dependent smokers to higher concentrations of other poisons. The latter might occur in the absence of acceptable nicotine substitutes, as smokers consume more cigarettes in order to achieve 'adequate' concentrations of nicotine.

Creative strategies to prevent the initiation of nicotine addiction can augur a brighter future in the tobacco-and-health arena. For the foreseeable future, however, the projected millions of tobacco-attributable deaths can be reduced only by encouraging smokers to quit smoking. For many people, renouncing nicotine is simply too difficult, as is reflected in the dismally low rates of success in quitting smoking. The emergence of consumer-acceptable nicotine-only products, available at low cost without prescription, could conceivably help such people to be tobacco-free, if not nicotine-free. Although nicotine itself carries some risk (Benowitz & Gourlay, 1997), that risk pales in comparison with the dangers of smoking. The market for long-term nicotine maintenance is coming. We choose to view this development with cautious optimism.

References

Benowitz, N.L. & Gourlay, S.G. (1997) Cardiovascular toxicity of nicotine: Implications for nicotine replacement therapy. *J. Am. Coll. Cardiol.*, **29**, 1422–1431

Benowitz, N.L. & Henningfield, J.E. (1994) Establishing a nicotine threshold for addiction. *New Engl. J. Med.*, **331**, 123–125

Davis, R.M. & Slade, J. (1993) Back to the future—with electrically powered cigarettes. *Tobacco Control*, **2**, 11–12

Department of Health and Human Services (1989) *Reducing the Health Consequences of Smoking: 25 Years of Progress. A Report of the Surgeon General* (DHHS Publication No. (CDC) 89-8411), Public Health Service, Centers for Disease Control, Center for Chronic Disease Prevention and Health Promotion, Office on Smoking and Health. Washington DC: Government Printing Office

Kozlowski, L.T. & Pillitteri, J.L. (1996) Compensation for nicotine by smokers of lower yield cigarettes. In: US Department of Health and Human Services, *The FTC Cigarette Test Method for Determining Tar, Nicotine, and Carbon Monoxide Yields of US Cigarettes. Report of the NCI Expert Committee* (NIH Publication No. 96-4028), Public Health Service, National Institutes of Health. Bethesda, Maryland: National Cancer Institute, pp. 161–172

Leischow, S.J., Stine, C.M., Nordbrock, J., Marriott, J. & Zobrist, R.H. (1996) One week trial of oral transmucosal nicotine for smoking cessation (Abstract). *J Addictive Dis.*, **15**, 146

Pauly, J.L., Streck, R.J. & Cummings, K.M. (1995) US patents shed light on *Eclipse* and future cigarettes. *Tobacco Control*, **4**, 261–265

R.J. Reynolds Tobacco Company (1988) *Chemical and Biological Studies of New Cigarette Prototypes that Heat Instead of Burn Tobacco*, Winston-Salem, North Carolina

Slade, J. (1989) The tobacco epidemic: Lessons from history. *J. Psychoactive Drugs*, **21**, 281–291

Warner, K.E., Slade, J. & Sweanor, D.T. (1997) The emerging market for long-term nicotine maintenance. *J. Am. Med. Assoc.*, **278** (in press)

Reflection on alternative nicotine delivery systems

M.C. Taylor

Physicians for a Smoke-Free Canada, Ottawa, Ontario, Canada

There has been a recent trend in part of the tobacco-control community to advocate the development and promotion of alternative nicotine delivery systems, as exemplified by a conference held in Toronto in early 1997 ('Alternative Nicotine Delivery Systems. Harm Reduction and Public Health', held jointly by the Addiction Research Foundation, the Ontario Tobacco Research Unit and the American Society of Addiction Medicine). The underlying premise of many advocates of alternative nicotine delivery systems is that only a fraction of the very large number of nicotine addicts who receive their dose of nicotine through tobacco products will be able to quit smoking. A further assumption of this harm-reduction approach is that providing nicotine to these addicts in a vehicle which does not involve ingesting tobacco could dramatically reduce the aggregate health consequences of tobacco use. One proponent of alternative nicotine delivery systems cautioned at the conference held in Toronto: 'unless we establish an aggressive harm reduction strategy that promotes the use of alternative nicotine delivery products our campaign may not achieve our goal of reducing [smoking] prevalence to 15%' (G.N. Connolly, 'Closing the gaps: A public health agenda for nicotine harm reduction').

Proponents of alternative nicotine delivery systems suggest that a market-driven solution to tobacco use could be found in the introduction of new and safer nicotine products to consumers. To expand the availability of new delivery systems for nicotine they are suggesting changes by government regulators, nicotine product manufacturers, advertisers and retailers. Governments are urged to reduce the red-tape faced by pharmaceutical companies: 'Society poorly regulates the cigarette and over regulates nicotine gum. The proper regulatory response is to implement a strategy that levels the regulatory playing field between the cigarette and AND [alternative nicotine delivery] products' (G.N. Connolly, as above). Pharmaceutical companies are urged to be more aggressive marketers: 'I think it important that drug manufacturers, who will profit from less cigarette sales, pursue this in their advertising and that they lift any voluntary restraints they have from directly competing with tobacco products and attacking the tobacco industry' (G.N. Connolly, as above). 'We can give consumers a choice, and manufacturers an incentive to compete for the nicotine market…we can allow private enterprise to unleash its creativity in order to address our leading cause of preventable death' (D. Sweanor, 'Alternative nicotine delivery as a harm reduction strategy—getting rid of the dirty syringe'. Adapted from a paper used at a panel discussion at the American Society of Addiction Medicine Conference, Toronto, 1995). The prospect of nicotine products being 'widely available, at least in a basic maintenance dose, in such places as overnight convenience stores' (R. Room, 'Control systems for pyschoactive substances'. Paper presented at the Conference on Alternative Nicotine Delivery Systems, Toronto, 1997) is suggested as a progressive step. Advertisers of new nicotine products are reminded that the 'successful alternative nicotine delivery systems product will not forget pleasure' (L. Kozlowski, '"Better, smoother and not a cough in a carload'. Lessons from cigarette advertising and attempts to control it in the United States from 1900 to 1965 with a selective, brief history of earlier tobacco use'. Paper presented at the Conference on Alternative Nicotine Delivery Systems, Toronto, 1997).

Smokers may be less convinced than these theorists that today's alternative nicotine products are satisfactory substitutes for cigarettes. Currently, there is no widely available delivery system which provides nicotine to the drug user in ways which approximate cigarette smoke. Chewing-gums and nicotine patches do not provide the dramatic peak in serum nicotine levels which the smoker's brain has come to crave. To develop and test such systems and to establish their safety and efficacy as part of a strategy of alternative nicotine delivery systems will require considerable resources. Subsequently, extensive marketing will be necessary to convince smokers to switch to the new systems.

The economic investment required to launch such a strategy would 'eclipse' the current investment by western governments in preventing nicotine use. Not surprisingly, the resources needed to launch alternative nicotine products are possessed by the tobacco industry, which has already taken dramatic moves in this direction in the development of the Eclipse cigarette by R.J. Reynolds.

A number of very serious issues must be considered before the tobacco control community embraces an alternative nicotine delivery strategy. Until now, we have operated on the premise that nicotine addiction is a disease that young people develop as a result of a number of external influences. The tobacco industry has worked very hard to addict children through aggressive advertising. We have told governments that the industry must be kept away from children, through total bans on advertising and sponsorship. The industry has been discredited as merchants of death, a reputation richly deserved. In industrialized societies, tobacco use has been eliminated from an ever-expanding list of public places, and the effect is that the exposure of children has been reduced. A major emphasis on alternative nicotine delivery will require a complete reversal of our thinking. We would have to accept that nicotine addiction, rather than being a preventable disease, is a fundamental human characteristic which we are powerless to change. The role of the health community will be shifted from curing or preventing nicotine addiction to ensuring that it is satisfied in the least toxic form possible.

As such alternative nicotine products are now and will increasingly be provided by tobacco companies, we will have to develop a new understanding of the social and economic role of this industry. We will have to accept tobacco companies as legitimate businesses and their managers as honest business people. We will have to trust their actions and be at least passive partners in the research, development and marketing of new tobacco products. The spectre of the health community approaching government arm in arm with the tobacco industry is one which I find profoundly disturbing, even though I know that it has already happened in Canada in connection with the Eclipse cigarette.

Nicotine is, of course, one of the reasons people smoke. In the process of receiving their dose of nicotine, addicts are exposed to thousands of toxic compounds produced from burning tobacco leaves. Nicotine is probably not directly responsible for the cancers which tobacco causes, or the respiratory diseases, but there is evidence that nicotine is directly responsible for some of the cardiovascular consequences of tobacco use. While decidedly preferable to tobacco smoking, pure nicotine ingestion cannot be considered innocuous. Those products developed by the pharmaceutical industry, including nicotine chewing-gum and patches, provide nicotine in what is probably the safest possible form, and some addicts rely on these products for very extended periods; however, for the majority of smokers, the nicotine is not produced in a satisfactory format, since the 'hit' of nicotine supplied by smoking is not mimicked by these products.

The product furthest along in development to achieve the objectives of satisfactory nicotine delivery and harm reduction is R.J. Reynold's Eclipse system, currently under development in many countries, including Canada. This product is similar in appearance to a cigarette but heats the tobacco instead of burning it. The result is the delivery of nicotine in aerosol form to the smoker, with very little production of smoke. The nicotine delivery is the same as with cigarettes, including the sudden surges in serum level which many smokers require. The concentration of many toxic compounds is lower than in conventional cigarettes, but the concentration of carbon monoxide is higher.

The health advantages of the Eclipse system are far from proven. A detailed search of the medical literature from January 1994 to July 1997 turned up only one paper on the subject of tobacco-heating cigarettes. Interestingly, the paper was from the R.J. Reynolds Tobacco Company and reported a comparison of the mutagenicity of the urine of smokers of regular cigarettes with that of smokers of a tobacco-heating cigarette (Smith *et al.*, 1996). While the urine of the group smoking Eclipse contained lower concentrations of cancer-causing chemicals than the urine of regular smokers, these chemicals were still present in significant quantities. There is no evidence whatsoever that tobacco-heating cigarettes are any safer than regular cigarettes. The tobacco industry may have data on this question, but until methodologically sound studies are published in peer-reviewed journals, we have no way of assessing the evidence.

There are high risks associated with introducing such a product to the market:

- Pregnant women might switch to Eclipse rather than quitting altogether. New research shows that nicotine and its metabolites cross the placenta and are excreted in breast milk, suggesting that this may result in the addiction of infants at the very beginning of life and predispose children to smoking or other forms of nicotine addiction.
- If the tobacco industry is allowed to market new alternative nicotine devices, there is good historical reason to believe that it would do so in a way that recruits children and youth. Such recruitment of a new generation would needlessly extend the pandemic of tobacco use well into the next millenium.
- Smokers may be discouraged from quitting, since they could switch to a 'safer' product.
- Former smokers could be recruited back to nicotine addiction in the belief that they could smoke with impunity.
- Initiatives to reduce smoking through bans on smoking in public and work places could be stalled.
- Smokers could be encouraged to continue smoking in their home, increasing their own tobacco consumption and providing role models for smoking to their children.
- The de-legitimization of tobacco and smoking could be stalled.
- A new smoking 'fad' could emerge.

Similarly, alternative nicotine products developed by the pharmaceutical industry cannot be assumed to be benign, in either their current or future forms. Whether delivered through patch, chewing-gum, inhaler or lollipop, nicotine is a powerful and toxic substance. The probability that large segments of the population will become addicted to nicotine, underestimate the health consequences of its use and hold strong beliefs about the benefits of its consumption (i.e. physical and mental alertness, weight loss) has already been established. There is an established reluctance of governments to adequately regulate and control nicotine. There is no *prima facie* reason to believe that pharmaceutical companies will continue to resist use of lifestyle advertising and other promotional strategies to encourage non-therapeutic long-term use of nicotine products.

A number of conditions should be met before the health community invests further time and resources in proposals for alternative nicotine delivery systems. First, there must be sound scientific evidence that the products being promoted are safer: there must be a soundly predictable reduction in morbidity and mortality. Reliable estimates are needed of the number of smokers who can be moved to alternative nicotine systems. The economic cost of this market shift and the impact on cessation should also be measured. Most importantly, reliable measures are needed of the lives saved by shifting smokers to new nicotine delivery systems. These estimates must be compared with the number of lives that could be saved by a comprehensive strategy of reducing tobacco use by established policy tools (total advertising ban, dramatic price increases, access restrictions and effective education) and by developing new policy tools (changed legal status of tobacco and reduced availability of tobacco products).

In addition to epidemiological concerns, there are economic considerations that should weigh against the early adoption of an alternative stratgey of nicotine delivery systems. Shifting smokers to new nicotine products will divert funds that are theoretically available to campaigns to reduce tobacco use into a for-profit market of alternative products. It is impossible at this point to predict the economic impact of a successful market of alternative nicotine delivery systems; however, shifting the expenditure of only 1% of the Canadian smoking population to alternative nicotine products would involve a far greater private expenditure on maintaining nicotine addiction (approximately CAN$ 80 million per year) than is currently allocated by public funds to reducing smoking or curing nicotine addiction (CAN$ 10 million in Federal expenditures in 1997–98).

Lessons on the market potential for—or consumer vulnerability to—new nicotine products may be found in the early Canadian experience with the nicotine patch. Between 1991 and 1993, new prescriptions for nicotine patches rose from 0 to over 600 000 (R.

Ferrence, Ontario Tobacco Reduction Unit, Toronto, personal communication). That is, almost 10% of Canadian smokers were recruited to try the patch in the second year of its marketing. Pharmaceutical manufacturers could not advertise the patch directly to consumers, although it was directly advertised to physicians and promoted to the general public through news and information media. In both direct and indirect promotion, the patch was represented as a therapeutic aid to smoking cessation. The boom market did not last long (by 1994, new prescriptions had fallen to 200 000), but one patch manufacturer was penalized for charging excessive prices for the product. (On 18 October 1994, the Patented Medicine Prices Review Board obtained a 'voluntary compliance undertaking' from CIBA Geigy Canada Ltd to offset excess revenues of CAN$ 3.6 million, including a payment to the Government of Canada of CAN$ 2.9 million. This is one of only three cases in which the Board has used its quasi-judicial powers.) If 10% of all smokers could be shifted without direct advertising to try an expensive product designed to help them quit, when only 48% of smokers declared themselves to be contemplating or preparing to quit (Health Canada, 1994), how much larger is the potential market for substitute nicotine products that are advertised, affordable and accessible? What is the market for products that better satisfy the symptoms of nicotine addiction? What is the potential market for nicotine manufacturers if their products are not used therapeutically for short periods but become part of a long-term drug use pattern?

A market-driven for-profit solution to tobacco use has no inherent economic superiority over a publicly funded not-for-profit solution to nicotine addiction. The investment of transnational companies in a 'harm reduction' strategy which also builds a lasting commercial market for an addictive substance cannot, on health or economic grounds, be viewed as inherently superior to public investments in reducing smoking. The development and particularly the marketing of new nicotine products must be taken out of the hands of the tobacco industry. This industry has proven itself incapable of restraining its activities, particularly in the recruitment of non-smoking populations, such as children. There is no reason to believe that R.J. Reynolds will market Eclipse with any greater respect for public health than it has marketed Camel cigarettes.

Changing the emphasis from the initiation and prevention of tobacco use to alternative nicotine delivery systems would require significant rethinking of our activities on tobacco control and reallocation of resources and expertise. Until convincing evidence is available that these products are indeed safer and until control of their marketing and development has been taken out of the hands of the tobacco industry, this approach cannot be recommended. Nicotine addiction is not a fundamental human characteristic but a tragic childhood disease that we should continue to work hard to prevent.

References

Health Canada (1994) *Survey on Smoking in Canada, Cycle Three, Fact sheet No. 6, Readiness to Quit Smoking*

Smith, C.J., et al. (1996) Human urine mutagenicity study comparing cigarettes which burn or primarily heat cigarettes. *Mutat. Res.*, **361**, 1–9

Context stimuli can modify the craving generated by smoking-related cues

B. Willems[1], M. Dols[1], R. Bittoun[2], M. van den Hout[1] & H. Adriaanse[1]

[1]University of Maastricht, Maastricht, Netherlands; [2]University of Sydney, Sydney, New South Wales, Australia

Summary

The experiment reported here was designed to test whether the craving generated by smoking-related cues is caused mainly by signals indicating the possibility or lack of possibility of smoking. Forty smokers participated in the experiment. Smoking-related cues were presented in two contexts: one that predicted 'smoking' and the other that predicted 'no smoking'. The dependent variable in this research was the urge to smoke (craving), measured on a VAS scale. The expectation was that the craving due to exposure to relevant cues would be greater in a context that predicted smoking than in a context that predicted no smoking. The results corroborated this expectation; when a cue predicted smoking and therefore the participants expected to smoke, the self-reported urge to smoke was significantly greater than when a cue predicted no smoking. Furthermore the results suggest that the contexts interfered with the craving generated by smoking-related cues, which appeared to be inhibited by the no-smoking context. The results suggest that the cue-induced urge to smoke can be modified by changing the smoker's expectancy about smoking.

Introduction

Smoking can be seen as a learnt phenomenon. Sensory and environmental stimuli can become powerful conditioned reinforcers and also serve as cues for conditioning craving and other withdrawal effects (Russell, 1990). Interpretations of the cue reactivity paradigm are derived primarily from the framework of classical conditioning. During a history of smoking, certain stimuli, like environmental contexts and paraphernalia reliably accompany drug administration. These stimuli are assumed to become conditioned by pairing with the unconditioned stimuli for the drug, which can elicit conditioned responses. In cue reactivity studies, addicts' reactions to representations of drug-paired stimuli are considered to be conditioned responses. Several studies have shown that exposure to smoking-related cues elicits greater reactivity across a number of response domains than does exposure to neutral cues (Sayette & Hufford, 1994; Drummond et al., 1995). Cue reactivity and relapse have been shown to be connected to both smoking and alcohol use (Drummond et al., 1995). Urges and cravings have been related theoretically and empirically to the maintenance of cigarette smoking and have been posited to play a major role in the high rates of relapse frequently encountered in treatment programmes for cigarette smokers (Tiffany & Drobes, 1990).

Thus, certain conditioned (smoking-related) stimuli can elicit a motivational state (craving) which enhances the risk for relapse. An important question is the role of smokers' expectancies in these craving experiences, as they may play an important role in learning new associations. For example, Marlatt (1990) showed that outcome expectancies were more important for drinkers' feelings than were the physiological effects of alcohol. Marlatt also found that people showed no craving when they were not allowed to smoke but that their craving increased enormously when they were aware that they were allowed to smoke.

These findings were of great relevance for the present study, which was designed to test whether a cue (context) that predicts the possibility or impossibility of smoking affects cue-induced craving. In many treatments for addictive behaviour, attention has been concentrated on 'unlearning'. For example, the goal in cue exposure therapy is to extinguish the conditional response by confrontation with a conditioned stimulus and prevention of unconditioned stimuli. The central element is the breaking of the conditioned stimulus–unconditioned stimulus bond. Instead of breaking a learnt association between stimuli and drug responses, it may be more appropriate to recondition an association: learning new associations instead of breaking old ones.

In learning, context may play an essential role. We presented two contexts predictive of the conditioned stimulus–unconditioned stimulus relationship and proposed that the craving would be altered by learning new associations between the context and the behaviour. New cues may become predictors of the possibility or impossibility of smoking and may influence the craving to smoke.

The following hypotheses were formulated in this research:

1. A context that predicts the possibility of smoking increases the urge to smoke, while a context that predicts the impossibility of smoking does not.

2. If a context stimulus is offered that predicts that smoking-related cues will not be followed by smoking, the craving-increasing effect (difference in craving between urge ratings before and during exposure) of relevant cues will be inhibited.
3. The craving generated by a cue is due mainly to its predictivity for the possibility or impossibility of smoking.

Method

The participants were 40 heavy smokers (> 20 cigarettes per day) who were familiar with the sensation of craving. A within-subject design was used. The dependent variable was subjective craving, measured on a 100 mm VAS scale, accompanied by the question: 'How strong is your urge to smoke?'. The scale ranked from 'none' (0) to 'extreme' (100). During each session, craving was measured 24 times by asking the participants to rank their urge to smoke on the VAS scale at that particular moment. The independent variables were the smoking and non-smoking contexts, designated by coloured cards. At the second context presentation, the card was accompanied by conditioned cues: the smoker's favourite brand of cigarettes, a lighter and an ashtray.

All participants received both contexts. Half of all subjects received a blue card designating non-smoking and a yellow card designating smoking, and the other half received the cards designating the opposite contexts. In the non-smoking context, the conditioned cues were not followed by smoking; in the smoking context, the conditioned cues were followed by smoking and subsequent nicotine uptake. Before the start of the test, the participants were told which colour meant 'allowed to smoke' and which one meant 'not allowed to smoke'. They received 12 cards, although the number was not mentioned. In both contexts, the procedure started with presentation of a card, followed by the first craving assessment. After the first assessment, the same card was presented again, together with the conditioned stimuli (cigarettes, lighter and ashtray), directly followed by the second craving assessment. Each context presentation finished with the absence or presence of the unconditioned stimulus, which was one puff of a cigarette. There was a 2-min break between each context presentation.

During the sessions, the subject could see the smoking-related cues only when the conditioned stimuli were presented; otherwise, exposure to these cues would have continued, which might have influence the results of the study. Furthermore, no smoke was allowed in the room, to ensure that the smoke itself was not a continuing conditioned stimulus. Subjects therefore were asked to to exhale the smoke through a window, to put out the cigarette immediately after inhaling and to cut the end off the cigarette so that no smoke could escape from the butt.

Results

The increasing effect of a smoking predicting context compared with a non-smoking predicting context on subjective urge ratings (hypothesis 1) was studied with a 2 x 2 x 6 MANOVA. A significant effect was found for context [$F_{1,39}$ = 32.53; $p < 0.001$]. As the effect of context during exposure could be different from that during non-exposure, a new MANOVA was performed to measure the difference in craving between the smoking and non-smoking contexts in the absence of exposure to relevant cues. The urge to smoke during non-exposure was significantly higher in the smoking context than in the non-smoking context [$F_{1,39}$ = 29.45; $p < 0.001$]. Similar effects were found for the effect of context during non-exposure: the context had a clear effect on the urge to smoke [$F_{1,39}$ = 32.57; $p < 0.001$] when cigarettes, lighter and ashtray were presented. These results support hypothesis 1.

Another important question is whether the craving-increasing effect of relevant cues is inhibited when a context stimulus is offered that predicts that the conditioned stimulus will not be followed by the unconditioned stimulus (hypothesis 2). We found that exposure to smoking-related cues influences the urge to smoke in both the smoking context [$F_{1,39}$ = 19.34; $p < 0.001$] and the non-smoking context [$F_{1,39}$ = 4.14; $p < 0.049$]. Furthermore, the interaction between the effect of context and the effect of exposure was significant [$F_{1,39}$ = 10.01; $p < 0.003$]. Exposure to cues (the difference between exposure and non-exposure) had less effect in the smoking than in the non-smoking context. We found a larger difference between exposure and non-exposure in the smoking than in the non-smoking context, indicating that exposure to salient cues has less effect on the urge to smoke in a context that predicts the absence of smoking. These findings support hypothesis 2.

The last question was whether the craving generated by a cue is due mainly to its predictivity for the unconditioned stimulus (hypothesis 3). The above results suggest that the contexts and their predictivity for the unconditioned stimulus influence craving. Both the predictivity and relevance or conditioning history of cues seem to influence people's craving. To test the importance of the two factors in generating craving, that experienced during non-exposure in the smoking context was compared with craving during exposure in the non-smoking context. Hypothesis 3 suggests that the predictivity of a cue for the unconditioned stimulus will be more influential in generating craving than the relevance or conditioning history of a cue; craving during non-exposure in the smoking context will be greater than that after exposure in the non-smoking context. Another MANOVA showed a significant difference between the effect of predictivity for an unconditioned stimulus and the effect of cue relevance [$F_{1,39} = 20.41$; $p < 0.001$], indicating that a neutral cue predicting smoking has more effect than presentation of a relevant cue predicting no smoking. In other words, the craving generated by smoking-related cues is due mainly to their predictivity for unconditioned stimuli and less to their history of conditioning history with the unconditioned stimuli. These findings support hypothesis 3.

We also tested whether the trial influenced the results. The results of the study show a general decline in craving over time in both contexts, both during non-exposure and exposure; however, no significant effect of 'trial' was found [$F_{5,195} = 2.00$; $p = 0.081$]. It can be concluded that the participants' urge to smoke did not change significantly during the session, and the observed decline in craving could be due to coincidence.

Discussion and implications

One of the findings presented showed that smokers had greater craving when they expected to smoke in a short while than when they expected not to smoke soon. Their expectations about smoking were manipulated by the two cards representing the two contexts. Before the experiment, the cards had no relevance and did not induce conditioning in connection with smoking; they then became conditioned stimuli, capable of eliciting a conditioned craving response. Predictivity for smoking appears to be relevant in turning neutral stimuli (blue and yellow cards) into conditioned stimuli.

Cue reactivity was not totally conditional on actual smoking. Even if the salient cues did not predict smoking , exposure to the cues increased the urge to smoke. Thus, conditioning history and relevance still seemed to play a role. The large number of pairings between salient cues and smoking may have made the association between these cues and smoking very powerful and hard to break. The results also showed that the craving generated by a cue is due mainly to its predictivity for smoking. The main explanation for these findings might be that predictivity for smoking influences subjective urge more than the relevance or conditioning history of a cue. The cards (and therefore the contexts) have become more powerful predictors of being allowed to smoke than the cigarettes, lighter and ashtray. Another explanation could be the interaction between the effect of the contexts and the effect of exposure to salient cues. Expecting to smoke or not to smoke might influence the relevance or conditioning history of cues and thus decrease the influence of the conditioning history of a cue in generating craving. Expectancy in regard to smoking might elicit or suppress pleasant memories or feelings accompanying smoking.

By creating an environment in which no smoking is allowed, policy-makers can influence smokers' urge to smoke and make it easier for them to stop smoking. It is not the actual availability of reinforcers (cigarettes and other salient cues) that is important in helping people stop smoking, but the expectancy that these cues can be realized. A smoker may sometimes expect to be able to smoke in a non-smoking environment and not to smoke in a smoking context. Smokers who want to quit might be helped to do so by methods based on this experiment which control their expectancies about smoking. By asking smokers to create smoking and non-smoking contexts themselves, with the aid of two distinctive cards, they could be taught that they can influence their smoking behaviour. By slowly replacing the cards by cognitive statements and by creating more non-smoking contexts, smokers could be helped to quit their compulsive behaviour.

The findings of our study can be used to teach smokers that the relationship between craving and smoking is not uni-directional. Craving or the urge to smoke is often seen as a cause of smoking and relapse. The results of this study show that the relationship between craving and smoking may also be the reverse: smoking or expectancy in regard to smoking influence craving. Thus, craving is due to smoking instead of smoking being due to craving.

References

Drummond, D.C., Tiffany, S.T., Glauting, S. & Remington, B. (1995) Cue exposure in understanding and treating addictive behaviours. In: Drummond, D.C., *et al.*, eds, *Addictive Behaviour: Cue Exposure, Theory and Practice*, New York: Wiley

Marlatt, G.A. (1990) Cue exposure and relapse prevention in the treatment of addictive behaviours. *Addictive Behav.*, 15, 395–399

Russell, M.A.H. (1990) Nicotine and its control over smoking. In: Wonnacott, S., Russell, M.A.H. & Stolerman, J.P., eds, *Nicotine Psychofarmacology; Molecular, Cellular and Behavioural Aspects*, Oxford: Oxford University Press, p. 374

Sayette, M.A. & Hufford, M.R. (1994) Effects of cue exposure and deprivation on cognitive resources in smokers. *J. Abnorm. Psychol.*, 103, 812–818

Tiffany, S.T. & Drobes, D.J. (1990) Imagery and smoking urges: The manipulation of effective content. *Addictive Behav.*, 15, 531–539

Tobacco manufacturers manipulate nicotine content of cigarettes to cause and sustain addiction

C.E. Douglas

Tobacco Control Law & Policy Consulting, Ann Arbor, Michigan, United States

Virtually all mass-marketed cigarettes are designed by their manufacturers to cause and sustain a powerful addiction to their use. It has been shown that 77–92% of smokers are physically dependent on nicotine in cigarettes, and consumers use these products almost exclusively for pharmacological purposes (Centers for Disease Control and Prevention, 1994). Cigarettes deliver into the body pharmacologically active doses of nicotine which exert psychoactive effects on the brain that motivate repeated, compulsive use of the drug. The pharmacological processes that cause addiction to nicotine are similar to those that cause addiction to heroin and cocaine, a conclusion reached by Government health authorities and the tobacco industry. All leading experts and public health organizations with expertise in tobacco or drug addiction recognize that nicotine is addictive (e.g. Department of Health and Human Services, 1988; World Health Organization, 1992).

Despite the desire of most smokers to quit smoking, fewer than 3% succeed each year (Centers for Disease Control and Prevention, 1994). After an extensive investigation in 1994–96, the Food and Drug Administration concluded that "the cigarette manufacturers have consistently focused their product research and development efforts on developing methods to maintain or enhance nicotine deliveries. These activities are remarkable for their sustained duration and for the fact that each cigarette manufacturer independently acquired similar capabilities to manipulate and control nicotine deliveries." Indeed, as one cigarette company official put it, the tobacco industry is "a specialized ... segment of the pharmaceutical industry," which manufactures products designed to deliver nicotine to the user (Teague, 1972; Department of Health and Human Services, 1996).

It is now beyond dispute that the delivery of nicotine to tobacco users is responsible for widespread addiction. Few consumers engage in long-term tobacco use in the absence of addiction. The tobacco manufacturers' deliberate control of nicotine is therefore directly responsible for the modern pandemic of lung cancer, heart disease and other tobacco-caused illnesses. Tobacco products do not exist commercially without nicotine. Tobacco manufacturers argue publicly that taste is an independent reason for tobacco use, but they have failed in their attempts to sell non-addictive, low-nicotine products that provide tobacco 'taste'. Three decades of documents and other evidence from the major cigarette manufacturers establish that they intend their products to have, and to be used for, their drug effects (Department of Health and Human Services, 1996). The evidence further establishes that the major cigarette manufacturers have conducted extensive research to understand precisely how nicotine affects the brain, the central nervous system and other systems of the body. In 1969, the vice-president for research and development at Philip Morris reported to the Board of Directors that "the ultimate explanation for the perpetuated cigaret habit resides in the pharmacological effect of smoke upon the body of the smoker". Smokers' craving for cigarettes is so strong, he added, that "the cigaret will even preempt food in times of scarcity". Likewise, in 1972, the assistant director of research at R.J. Reynolds Tobacco Company, who was later promoted to director of corporate research, wrote that nicotine is "a potent drug with a variety of physiological effects" and "a habit-forming alkaloid" (Wakeham, 1969; Teague, 1972; Department of Health and Human Services, 1996).

Cigarette manufacturers employ a variety of methods to control nicotine delivery with space-age precision. Some of the methods used include: using high-nicotine tobaccos to raise the nicotine concentration in lower-tar cigarettes; adding extraneous nicotine in the production of 'reconstituted tobacco', which is used in many cigarette brands; adding ammonia compounds to increase the delivery of 'free' nicotine by raising the alkalinity or pH of tobacco smoke; using filter and ventilation systems to remove a higher percentage of tar than nicotine; genetically engineering tobacco plants to increase their nicotine content; using chemicals that act synergistically to strengthen the pharmacological effects of nicotine; and developing nicotine analogues that retain its reinforcing characteristics (British American Tobacco Co., 1968; Irby, 1974; Spears & Jones, 1981; British American Tobacco Co., 1982; DeNoble, 1982; Brown & Williamson Tobacco Corp., 1991; Fisher et al., 1991; Brown & Williamson Tobacco Corp., 1994; DeNoble, 1994; Martin & Bogdanich, 1995; Farone, 1996; Wittes, 1996).

The inevitable consequence of the tobacco industry's manipulation and control of nicotine is to keep consumers using cigarettes, by causing and sustaining their addiction to nicotine. The addiction to tobacco now being experienced by hundreds of millions of human beings around the world cannot be reduced significantly unless and until the manipulation and control of nicotine and other drug-enhancing substances by tobacco manufacturers is strictly regulated by appropriate government health authorities.

References

British American Tobacco Co. (1968) Minutes of BATCO Research Conference at Hilton Head, South Carolina, 24–30 September

British American Tobacco Co. (1982) Minutes of BATCO Research Conference at Montebello, Canada, 30 August–3 Sept.ember

Brown & Williamson Tobacco Corp. (1991) Handbook for Leaf Blenders and Product Developers

Brown & Williamson Tobacco Corp. (1994) Transcript of meeting with Food and Drug Administration, 17 June

Centers for Disease Control and Prevention (1994) Cigarette smoking among adults—United States, 1993. Morbid. Mortal. Wkly Rep., 43, 925–930

DeNoble, V.J. (1982) Project Number 1610 (Behavioral Pharmacology) Objectives and Plans - 1982–1983, Philip Morris Inc., 20 July

DeNoble, V.J. (1994) Hearings Before the Subcommittee on Health and the Environment of the Committee on Energy and Commerce, US House of Representatives, 103rd Congress, 2nd Session 33, 28 April

Department of Health and Human Services (1988) The Health Consequences of Smoking: Nicotine Addiction, A Report of the Surgeon General, Washington DC: Government printing Office

Department of Health and Human Services (1996) Nicotine in cigarettes and smokeless tobacco is a drug and these products are nicotine delivery devices under the Federal Food, Drug, and Cosmetic Act: Jurisdictional determination. *Fed. Reg.*, **61/168**, 44944, 44824–44825

Farone, W.A. (1996) *The Manipulation and Control of Nicotine and Tar in the Design and Manufacture of Cigarettes: A Scientific Perspective* (FDA affidavit), 8 March

Fisher, P.R., *et al.* (1991) *New Variety of Tobacco Plant*, US patent application, assigned to Brown & Williamson Tobacco Corp.

Irby, R.M., Jr (1974) *Nicotine Content of Reconstituted Tobacco*, American Tobacco

Martin, J. & Bogdanich, W. (1995) *Defendants' Memorandum in Support of Summary Judgment*. In: *Philip Morris Companies Inc. v. American Broadcasting Companies, Inc.*

Spears, A.W. & Jones, S.T. (1981) Chemical and physical criteria for tobacco leaf of modern day cigarettes. *Recent Adv. Tobacco Sci.*, **7**, 19–39

Teague, C.E. (1972) *Research Planning Memorandum on the Nature of the Tobacco Business and the Crucial Role of Nicotine Therein*, R.J. Reynolds Tobacco Co.

Wakeham, H. (1969) *Smoker Psychology Research*. Presented to Philip Morris Board of Directors, 26 November

Wittes, B. (1996) Philip Morris v. ABC: The Case ABC Never Made. *Legal Times*, 15 January

World Health Organization (1992) *The ICD-10 Classification of Mental and Behavioural Disorders: Clinical Descriptions and Diagnostic Guidelines*, Geneva

Super tobacco cultivated in southern Brazil

J.E. Murad

Chamber of Deputies, Brasilia, Brazil

Interest in obtaining a tobacco plant with a high percentage of nicotine was expressed many years ago. Dr James F. Chaplin from the United States Department of Agriculture noted in 1977 that although producers have the means to reduce tar levels almost all of the methods also reduce the levels of nicotine and other substances. He stated that '...it may be more desirable to increase the levels of nicotine so that when there is any reduction there may be still enough nicotine to satisfy the smoker'.

Dr David A. Kessler of the United States Food and Drug Administration in June 1994 made a number of comments about the manipulation of the nicotine concentration in certain varieties of tobacco. He noted that any substance or product that is absorbed by the organism and provokes changes in one or more functions is considered to be a 'drug', and those criteria apply to nicotine. He noted further that nicotine should be classified as a drug that causes dependence, characterized by craving, tolerance and withdrawal symptoms.

In 1994, the Brazilian Congress was informed that Souza Cruz, a multinational tobacco processing company, would be supplying farmers in southern Brazil with seeds of a special, genetically manipulated tobacco, known as Y-1, which was to be cultivated with special fertilizers. This variety contains approximately 6% nicotine—twice the percentage found in ordinary tobacco. It is therefore more addictive and thus more profitable for the producing company. We asked that a parliamentary commission be constituted to investigate the new product impartially. We also contacted the Ministry of Health, which informed us that Souza Cruz had confirmed the production of 3.5 tonnes of Y-1 tobacco in southern Brazil but had noted that it had never been commercialized in Brazil or in any other country, principally because the United States authorities had denied a patent for the product. The Ministry of Health noted, however, that no proof was provided to support these statements.

In December 1992, Brown & Williamson Tobacco Corp., a multinational tobacco company in the United States, filed a patent for Y-1 tobacco with the Institute of Industrial Property of the Ministry of Industry and Commerce of Brazil; however, the company withdrew its request in March 1994, before any tests had been carried out, at about the time Dr Kessler made his comments about nicotine dependence.

Y-1 tobacco is a new variety of 'hardened' tobacco, which combines a high percentage of nicotine with good agricultural and morphological characteristics. The percentage of nicotine is generally even greater than 6%, on the basis of the dry weight of the leaves. This variety was obtained by complex genetic manipulation. It closely resembles a variety known as SC 58 but with a higher nicotine content. There is evidence that Y-1 tobacco was planted in Brazil through a contract with Souza Cruz Overseas (Brown & Williamson in Brazil) and that 1000 lbs (450 kg) were sent to an American cigarette producer. That producer reported that 3.5–4 million pounds (1.6–1.8 million kg) of tobacco containing 10% Y-1 tobacco were stored in the United States for use in several brands.

Nobody admitted responsibility for sending the seeds of Y-1 tobacco to be cultivated in Brazil. The Brown & Williams Company and the company that undertook the genetic manipulation both placed the blame on Souza Cruz. The outcome is nevertheless that a multinational tobacco company sent tobacco seeds with a high nicotine content to be cultivated in Venancio Aires, Rio Grande do Sul, and that these seeds probably entered Brazil illegally.

The family as a cornerstone of tobacco addiction

J. van Reek, H. Adriaanse & F. Vergeer

University of Maastricht, Maastricht, Netherlands

In a World Health Organization cross-sectional survey of weekly smoking by 1226 schoolchildren in the fourth class of secondary school (mean age, 16) in The Netherlands at the end of 1991 and beginning of 1992, the prevalence was 29%. An analysis was performed to find the explanatory variables for this behaviour. Weekly smoking was entered as the dependent variable in a stepwise logistic regression with three family-related and five other independent variables (Table 1). Using a classification table of observed and predicted smoking, we could predict 70% of the weekly smokers. Only the family-related variables are potential long-term influences, as e.g. relationships with best friends are highly changeable at this age. When the family variables were entered into the logistic regression model, however, only 22% of the observed smokers were predicted correctly. We investigated the accuracy of classification by these variables over a period of two years (van Reek et al., 1995) and found that we could classify 68% of weekly smokers correctly cross-sectionally and 23% longitudinally, on the basis of smoking by peers, smoking by parents, tobacco available from parents, self-efficiency, beliefs and age. These studies indicate that weekly smoking by schoolchildren cannot be predicted accurately.

Table 1. Zero-order correlation coefficients for weekly smoking and eight explanatory variables

Variable	Correlation coefficient
Family-related	
No. of smokers among older siblings	0.26
No. of smokers among parents	0.20
Pocket money	0.13
Other	
No. of smokers among best friends	0.64
Alcohol drinking	0.35
Gambling	0.15
Church-going	0.16
Age	0.16

All correlations significant at $p < 0.01$

When the development of smoking behaviour was followed up in a study in Derbyshire, United Kingdom, for 10 years (Swan et al., 1990), it was found that the risk for becoming a smoker was increased when the child had siblings who smoked, had friends of the opposite sex or was susceptible to peer pressure. In a study in the United States of the influence of parental behaviour, a first phase of living in a disharmonious family and a second phase of disruptive behaviour were found to precede the onset of smoking (Cohen et al., 1994). Harmonization of families is an unrealistic goal, but health education in the classroom has been found to postpone the onset of smoking (Laugesen, 1995).

The prevalence of smoking among schoolchildren can also be investigated at the regional level. In the North Karelia Youth Project, a lasting effect of health education in the classroom was found only in conjunction with an overall community programme (Vartiainen et al., 1990).

At the national level, publicity campaigns and legislative measures such as advertising bans, price increases and reduced sales to minors can lower the prevalence of smoking among adolescents (Laugesen, 1995), but the specific effects and mechanisms of the interventions are difficult to investigate.

Thus, smoking among adolescents can be explained but not be predicted at the individual level and can be predicted but not explained at the national level. Intervention at the national level would therefore appear to be the most effective approach.

References

Cohen, D.A., Richardson, J. & LaBree, L. (1994) Parenting behaviors and the onset of smoking and alcohol use: A longitudinal study. Pediatrics, 94, 368–375

Laugesen, M. (1995) The impact of tobacco policies on trends in tobacco consumption. In: Slama, K., ed., Tobacco and Health, New York: Plenum Press, pp. 151–155

van Reek, J., Knibbe, R. 7 Engels, R. (1995) Predictors of smoking behaviour. In: Slama, K., ed., Tobacco and Health, New York: Plenum Press, pp. 387–389

Swan, A.V., Creeser, R. & Murray, M. (1990) When and why children first start to smoke. Int. J. Epidemiol., 19, 323–330

Vartiainen, E., Fallonen, U., McAlister, A.L. & Puska, P. (1990) Eight-year follow-up results of an adolescent smoking prevention program: The North Karelia Youth Project. Am. J. Public Health, 80, 78–79

Are the smoking habits and nicotine dependence of psychiatric patients related to medication or diagnosis?

A. Batra, I. Hehl, I. Garfami, G. Farger & G. Buchkremer

Department of Psychiatry and Psychotherapy, University of Tübingen, Germany

Introduction

A higher prevalence of smoking is found among psychiatric patients than in the general population: e.g. > 80% among schizophrenic patients (e.g. Hughes et al., 1986) and about 60% among patients with affective psychosis (Breslau et al., 1993). Alcoholic and drug-dependent patients have smoking rates > 80% (Hurt et al., 1995). The reasons proposed are boredom, use of nicotine for activation, reduction of the side-effects of neuroleptics and neurobiological mechanisms.

The objectives of this study were to determine whether there is a higher prevalence of smoking among psychiatric in-patients than in the general population; whether the smoking status, number of cigarettes per day and degree of nicotine dependence are related to diagnosis or medication; and whether serum cotinine concentrations correlate with daily dose of neuroleptics, dependence score or number of cigarettes smoked per day.

Methods

We interviewed 368 psychiatric patients in a standardized interview and recorded sex, age, number of cigarettes smoked per day, score in Fagerström's test for nicotine dependence and medication. The disorders of the patients were diagnosed according to the criteria of ICD-10. Blood samples were collected for determination of serum cotinine from 29 patients after abstinence from tobacco for at least 6 h.

Results

The prevalence of smoking was 56% for the whole population, with a rate of 65% among men and 48% among women. The mean age of the smokers was 36.9 years (SD, 10.9), while that of the overall population was 43.2 years (SD, 16.9). Cigarette smoking was significantly related to a diagnosis of drug dependence (94%), alcoholism (76%) or schizophrenia or schizoaffective disorder (64%; χ^2, 66.7; $p < 0.0001$).

Significant correlations were found between smoking and age (−0.29), sex (−0.18) and diagnosis (−0.13); between nicotine dependence score and diagnosis (−0.12); and between cigarettes per day and sex (−0.13), diagnosis (−0.17) and chlorpromazine equivalents (as a measure of medication; 0.22). No correlation was found between medication and smoking or nicotine dependence score or between any parameter and serum cotinine concentration. As the metabolism of cotinine may be affected by neuroleptics, this compound may not be suitable for measuring tobacco consumption in this situation.

Discussion

Some of the reasons proposed for the high prevalence of smoking among schizophrenic patients are boredom, stimulation of the reward system by increased release of dopaminergic substances in the nucleus accumbens after nicotine intake and minimization of the extra-pyramidal side-effects of neuroleptics after induction of hepatic enzymes. The large differences in prevalence among patients with different diagnoses make boredom an unlikely explanation. Stimulation of the reward system might explain the very high prevalence among drug-dependent and alcoholic patients. As the intensity of smoking is related to chlorpromazine concentration, schizophrenic patients may smoke to minimize the side-effects of neuroleptics.

References

Breslau, N., Kilbey, M.M. & Andreski, P. (1993) Nicotine dependence and major depression. *Arch. Gen. Psychiatr.*, **50**, 31–35

Hughes, J.R., Hatsukami, D.K., :itchell, J.E. & Dahlgren, L.A. (1986) Prevalence of smoking among psychiatric outpatients. *Am. J. Psychiatr.*, **143**, 993–997

Hurt, R.D., Dale, L.C., Offord, K.P., Croghan, I.T., Hays, J.T. & Gomez-Dahgl, L. (1995) Nicotine patch therapy for smoking cessation in recovering alcoholics. *Addiction*, **90**, 1541–1546

Smoking: A predictor or even a promoter of opiate dependence?

P.M. Liebmann, M. Lehofer, M. Moser, T. Legl, G. Pernhaupt & K. Schauenstein

Department of General and Experimental Pathology, University of Graz, Austria

Introduction

Although it is frequently observed clinically that former opiate addicts are usually smokers and that smoking may be the first step to heroin dependence, a possible association between smoking and heroin dependence has not yet been formally investigated. The aim of this study was to determine the ages at which smokers began regular smoking and using illicit drugs in comparison with smokers who did not use such drugs.

Materials and methods

Seventy clinically well-characterized, unmedicated, detoxified opiate addicts who were participating in a two-year rehabilitation programme in a therapeutic community were included in the study; 70% were men, the mean age was 27.1 years (SE, 0.87), the length of heroin dependence was 12 ± 1 years and the length of rehabilitation was 10.6 ± 1.2 months. The ages at which regular smoking and illicit drug use had begun were recorded retrospectively. Data on sex- and age-matched people in the general population were used as a control and were derived from national surveys of smoking behaviour among more than 5.3 million Austrian citizens (Österreichisches Statistisches Zentralamt, 1987, 1994).

Results

As shown in Figure 1, the heroin addicts had started smoking an average of four years earlier than normal smokers, implying that, for example, 40% of heroin addicts or future heroin addicts are regular smokers at the age of 13, while only 0.6% of the normal population smoke at that age. Regular use of illicit drugs was begun more than two years before regular smoking begins in the general population.

Figure 1. Age of onset of smoking and use of illicit drugs in subsequent opiate addicts in comparison with sex-matched normal smokers

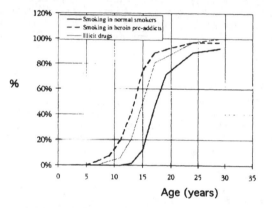

Discussion

The results suggest that future heroin addicts find addictive drugs highly attractive in general. Apart from the psychosocial reasons reported by the addicts, a deficient response of the endogenous opioid system may be involved in this early affinity for nicotine and heroin. This conclusion is corroborated by experimental data from our group (Liebmann et al., 1994; Lehofer et al., 1997; Liebmann et al., 1997). The attraction of nicotine for future heroin addicts may reflect an initial attempt to compensate this deficiency with easily available drugs. A further possible explanation is a combination of psychosocial and physiological factors. During puberty, the neuroendocrine and the endogenous opioid system undergo fundamental rearrangements (Mauras et al., 1986). Early nicotine intake might interfere with these events and thus, in line with the proposal of Kandel et al. (1992), might even initiate the development of heroin dependence. Our results demonstrate a possible predictive or even a promoting role of early smoking in future heroin dependence.

References

Kandel, D.B., Yamaguchi, K. & Chen, K. (1992) J. Stud. Alcohol, 53, 447–457
Lehofer, M., Liebmann, P.M., Moser, M., et al. (1997) Addiction, 92, 163–166
Liebmann, P.M., Lehofer, M., Schönauer-Cejpek, M., et al. (1994) Lancet, 344, 1031–1032
Liebmann, P.M., Lehofer, M., Moser, M., et al. (1997) Biol. Psychiatr., 42, 962–964
Mauras, N., Veldhuis, J.D. & Rogel, A.D. (1986) J. Clin. Endocrinol. Metab., 62, 1256–1263
Österreichisches Statistisches Zentralamt (1987) Statistische-Nachrichten, 42, 328–332
Österreichisches Statistisches Zentralamt (1987) Statistische-Nachrichten, 49, 479–489

Potentiating effect of heroin on smoking rates

M. Lehofer, P.M. Liebmann, M. Moser, T. Legl, G. Pernhaupt & H.G. Zapotoczky

Department of General and Experimental Pathology, University of Graz, Austria

Introduction

The results of studies in experimental animals indicate that some effects of nicotine are mediated through endogenous opioids (Davenport *et al.*, 1990), suggesting a common neurophysiological pathway of nicotine and heroin dependence. It was the aim of the present study to investigate changes in smoking behaviour during the evolution from pre-dependence to dependence, detoxification and rehabilitation.

Materials and methods

Seventy clinically well-characterized, unmedicated, detoxified opiate addicts who were participating in a two-year rehabilitation programme in a therapeutic community were included in the study; 70% were men, the mean age was 27.1 years (SE, 0.87), the length of heroin dependence was 12 ± 1 years and the length of rehabilitation was 10.6 ± 1.2 months. The subjects were asked to quantify their smoking rate before and during opiate dependence, during detoxification and currently, when free of opiates.

Results

As shown in Figure 1, 60% of the age- and sex-matched healthy population were non-smokers, whereas only 13% of the future addicts were non-smokers before heroin dependence. The proportion of heavy smokers (> 20 cigarettes per day) was similar among future addicts (18%) and among normal smokers (20%). During heroin dependence, the proportion of heavy smokers increased markedly, to 82%. During detoxification, the frequency of smoking generally decreased, and the proportion of heavy smokers decreased to 41%. During rehabilitation, the pre-dependence distribution was re-established.

Discussion

These results suggest an association between tobacco smoking and heroin dependence. Since cigarette smoking precedes opiate dependence in most heroin addicts (P.M. Liebmann *et al.*, this volume), the heroin abuse is not responsible for the initiation of tobacco smoking; however, heroin intake markedly intensifies smoking, suggesting a reinforcing effect of opiates on nicotine intake, which is in line with other reports (Mello *et al.*, 1980; Schmitz *et al.*, 1994). Our results demonstrate a reversible potentiating effect of heroin on nicotine consumption.

Figure 1. Cumulated frequency distribution of smoking behaviour among ex-addicts and healthy controls

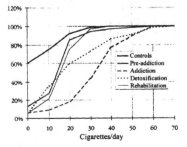

References
Davenport, K.E., Houdi, A.A. & Van Loon, G.R. (1990) *Neurosci. Lett.*, 113, 40–46
Mello, N.K., Mendelson, J.H., Sellers, M.L. & Kuehnle, J.C. (1980) *Psychopharmacol. Berlin*, 67, 45–52
Schmitz, J.M., Grabowski, J. & Rhoades, H. (1994) *Drug Alcohol Depend.*, 34, 237–242

Smoking is associated with other types of risk behaviour

D. Hrubá, E. Nová & P. Kachlík

Faculty of Ledicine, Masaryk University, Brno, Regional Hygiene Office, Klatovy, Czech Republic

At the Department of Preventive Medicine, we have developed several educational anti-smoking programmes for various groups of the population and have used them in intervention studies with the participation of co-workers at regional offices for hygiene and preventive medicine.

One group consisted of children at almost 100 primary schools, who were involved in a programme known as 'Smoking and me' as part of a school-based programme in which facts about smoking, alcohol, drugs and gambling were presented and skills for saying 'No' were taught in 24 lessons over four years. The aim of the programme is to direct children's attitudes to a healthy lifestyle and help them decide not to accept risk behaviour. The effect of the intervention is evaluated each school year from the anonymous answers to a questionnaire. The answers showed clearly that children who were current or occasional smokers during the summer holidays drank significantly more alcoholic beverages regularly, were more often drunk at school, used illegal drugs, did not exercise in their leisure time and did not like to read.

Another target population was adolescents at secondary schools and in apprentice homes; students at high-schools for nurses were also involved. In this group also, occasional and current cigarette smoking were significantly associated with drinking and abuse of alcoholic beverages, use of illegal drugs, bad nutrition (i.e. an inadequate intake of vegetables and excessive intake of sugar, salted nuts, chips and hamburgers), refusal to use safety belts in cars, getting lifts with drunk or unknown drivers and spending leisure time in sedentary activities to the detriment of exercise.

A third anti-smoking intervention programme concerned women. To obtain data on the effect of various environmental factors on reproductive function in women, we administered questionnaires to teachers at primary schools in seven Czech regions with significantly different prevalences of toxicity during pregnancy and early childhood. No geographical differences were seen in the reproductive function of this homogeneous group of university-educated women, but some differences were found in relation to smoking status. All of the women who smoked > 20 cigarettes per day but only 30% of the non-smokers had had a previous abortion. Furthermore, the teachers who smoked drank more coffee; we did not include questions about alcohol and drug use because we did not expect that we would receive reliable answers.

Smoking thus appears to be associated with other types of risk behaviour. Some indication of the reason for the association might be provided by the results of genetic research showing individual predisposition to susceptibility to drug dependence. Thus, chromosome 11 containes the D2 gene which codes for the receptors for dopamine, the primary mediator of feelings of pleasure. DNA containing significantly more of the allele coding for aberrant dopamine receptors that result in lower dopamine activity has been found in the brains of alcoholic patients and in the genotypes of heavy smokers, obese patients with bulimia and gamblers. Thus, these people naturally receive less pleasure than others and cope by abusing alcohol, nicotine, drugs and chocolate.

The epidemiology of nicotine dependence

K. Fagerstrom

Pharmacia & Upjohn, Helsingbotg, Sweden

Caffeine in tea and coffee is probably the world's most heavily used drug, but it is followed by nicotine and alcohol. If one looks at dependence instead of prevalence, nicotine may addict more users than any other drug. The lifetime dependency on nicotine is approximately 24% in China and 14% in the United States. Approximately 75% of the smokers in the western world can be classified as dependent.

In countries where the prevalence of smoking has declined, there is some evidence that less dependent smokers give up first and the remaining smokers become more dependent. Unfortunately, the stronger the dependence, the more difficult it is to give up. Co-morbidity between smoking and e.g. depression and attention deficit syndrome also seems to be more common where the prevalence of smoking has declined. This adds to the difficulties that smokers encounter when trying to give up.

Sweden is the industrialized country with the lowest prevalence of smoking: 19% of the adult population. Logically, Sweden should also enjoy less tobacco-related harm than other countries; however, tobacco dependence is more common, since about 9% of the population uses smokeless tobacco (*snus*) daily.

In programmes to control tobacco use, it is important to change not only prevalence but also dependence, since tobacco-related diseases occur more frequently among more dependent smokers.

Tobacco dependence and other drug dependences: Similarities and differences

S. Shiffman[1] & J. Henningfield[2]

[1]*University of Pittsburgh, Pittsburgh, Pennsylvania, and* [2]*Pinney Associates, Bethesda, Maryland, United States*

Tobacco control policy has developed independently of drug policy, and tobacco use is seldom construed as a drug problem. Yet, scientific studies have shown that tobacco use is largely driven by nicotine dependence. In this paper, we consider the ways in which tobacco use resembles and differs from use of other abused drugs. In particular, we consider similarities and differences between tobacco and opiates and cocaine, which are widely abused illicit drugs, and also alcohol, another licit drug in widespread use in most countries. In our comparisons, we consider domains ranging from the medical and social consequences of use, pharmacological and behavioural aspects of use through social attitudes and policies applying to use of tobacco and other drugs. Table 1 summarizes the comparisons, which are briefly outlined in the text. Detailed comparisons and documentation are beyond the scope of this paper. Two references are especially appropriate for those desiring more information: US Department of Health and Human Services (1988) and Henningfield *et al.* (1995).

Drug-related harm

As Table 1 shows, tobacco use causes far more medical harm than other abused drugs. Indeed, in the United States, for example, the annual number of deaths due to tobacco far exceeds that due to all other abused drugs combined. It is also striking that smoking seems to be harmful even at very low levels, whereas casual use of other substances appears to be associated with relatively little direct harm, the main risk being progression to higher levels of use. Tobacco also directly harms the health of others, through exposure to sidestream smoke. This is much less true of other drug use. In contrast, other forms of drug use are more closely associated with many forms of individual and social pathology. These in turn may cause the behaviour of users to put at risk the health of non-users; such behaviour includes poor driving resulting in traffic accidents and crime associated with drug trafficking. More broadly, the use of other drugs causes more social harm to non-users, because the user does not fulfil his or her social roles as, for instance, spouse, parent, bread-winner and co-worker,. Because of the different nature of the harm due to tobacco and to other drugs, the consequences of use follow very different time-courses. The medical harm due to tobacco use takes decades to become evident, even after very heavy use, whereas the psychological and social harm due to other drug use is often evident very soon after heavy use.

Pharmacology

Although the four drugs under consideration differ in their pharmacological actions, they have much in common. All of them target receptor mechanisms in the brain and result in measurable changes in brain activity. In the case of all except alcohol, specific receptor complexes have been identified. All have been shown to have some effects on the dopaminergic neuronal tracts associated with the experience of reward and reinforcement. In each case, the effects of the drug are dependent on the speed of administration as well as the absolute dose. In the case of tobacco and cocaine in particular, smoking can be used to deliver the drug very rapidly to the brain, which appears to result in a magnification of its effects or in qualitatively different effects. In the case of nicotine, this helps explain why smoking tobacco can be so addictive, while nicotine medications—which provide nicotine more slowly—have little potential for abuse or addiction. Organisms develop tolerance to all of the drugs in question. i.e. with exposure, more drug is needed to achieve the same effect. Each of the drugs also leads to the development of withdrawal symptoms and craving when it is discontinued. Thus, pharmacologically, tobacco smoke resembles other abused and addictive drugs. It should be noted, however, that the different drugs have different effects on psychomotor and cognitive performance. Alcohol and opiates (classically 'depressant' drugs) clearly can interfere with performance in decision-making, attention and learning. In contrast, nicotine and cocaine may actually enhance some performance measures. This is highly relevant to how the drugs are regarded in social policy.

Behavioural effects

Owing to their actions in the brain, all four drugs have subjective effects that are discernible and differentiated by humans and lower animals. All of the drugs show potential for abuse in standardized tests, demonstrating their reinforcement potential. Under the appropriate circumstances (which differ by drug), animals will self-administer each of the four drugs, again demonstrating the ability of the drugs to control behaviour. Humans continue to use all of these drugs, despite harm to the individual. This partly explains the priority that drug use comes to acquire: the person acts as though the drug were very valuable, despite its lack of biological survival value. While all of these factors indicate the drug's ability to promote use and to exert control over the user's behaviour, all of the drugs are subject to price sensitivity, with use dropping if price increases. This shows that drug use is not immune from other influences.

Patterns of use

Despite the many similarities of nicotine to the other drugs, the pattern of use is very different. At least in the west, where such smoking habits are affordable, users typically self-administer 10–60 unit doses per day, often averaging 15–20 per day (considering a cigarette as a dose). In contrast, the other drugs are used at much lower frequencies, even by abusers or addicted users, although this reflects in part the disabling effects of the other drugs at high doses. Tobacco also titrates blood nicotine levels;

Table 1. Comparison of tobacco smoking with alcohol, cocaine and opiate use

	Tobacco	Alcohol	Cocaine	Opiates
Drug-related harm				
Deaths due to use (United States, annual)	434 000	85 000	81 000	6500
Harm from low-level use	Yes	No	No	No
Medical harm to non-users	Yes	No	No	No
Social pathology	No	Yes	Yes	Yes
Social harm to non-users	No	Yes	Yes	Yes
Long-delayed harm	Yes	No	No	No
Pharmacology				
Central nervous system receptor mechanisms	Yes	Yes	Yes	Yes
Effects on brain	Yes	Yes	Yes	Yes
Affect on brain 'reward' system	Yes	Yes	Yes	Yes
Effects influenced by pharmacokinetics	Yes	Yes	Yes	Yes
Rapid delivery to brain	Smoking	No	Crack	No
Tolerance	Yes	Yes	Yes	Yes
Withdrawal	Yes	Yes	Yes	Yes
Craving	Yes	Yes	Yes	Yes
Use impairs performance	No	Yes	Yes	Yes
Behavioural effects				
Subjective effects	Yes	Yes	Yes	Yes
Abuse liability	Yes	Yes	Yes	Yes
Animal self-administration	Yes	Yes	Yes	Yes
Use despite harm	Yes	Yes	Yes	Yes
Drug acquires priority	Yes	Yes	Yes	Yes
Use is price-sensitive	Yes	Yes	Yes	Yes
Patterns of use				
Daily frequency	10-60	1-20	1-5	1-4
Drug titration	Yes	No	No	No
Addiction after any use (%)	32	15	17	8
Situational use prevalent	No	Yes	Yes	Yes
Associated with other drug use	Yes	Yes	Yes	Yes
Social policy				
Legal	Yes	Yes	No	No
Use unrestricted	No/Yes	No	No	No
Age restrictions	No/Yes	Yes	Yes	Yes
Use of price to deter use	No/Yes	Yes	Yes	Yes
Promoted and advertised	Yes	Yes	No	No
Cessation and treatment				
Cessation promoted	Yes	Yes	Yes	Yes
Low success rates	Yes	Yes	Yes	Yes
High relapse rates	Yes	Yes	Yes	Yes
Behavioural therapy	Yes	Yes	Yes	Yes
Pharmacological therapy	Yes	Yes	No	Yes
'Success' = total abstinence	Yes	No	No	No
Harm reduction as treatment goal	No	Yes	Yes	Yes

although the regulation is imprecise, users react to changes in nicotine delivery so as to preserve a certain level of nicotine in their bloodstream. Titration is also evident among users of other drugs, but much less so. Use of the other drugs is more often marked by episodic patterns, including bingeing. At least in the United States, a high proportion of people who try tobacco smoking, even once, progress to diagnosable nicotine dependence. The proportion is much lower for the other drugs. Indeed, while heavy and addicted use is the prevalent pattern of tobacco smoking (although there are exceptions), intermittent and non-addictive use is the predominant pattern for the other drugs. Each of the drugs is also associated with other drug use; poly-drug abuse has become the predominant pattern of drug use.

Social policy

The various drugs differ in their legal status in most countries: tobacco and alcohol can typically be sold, bought and consumed legally, with some exceptions for alcohol, whereas cocaine and opiates are illegal almost everywhere. Other social constraints differ. Even in places where alcohol is legal, there are typically restrictions on its use. Restrictions on tobacco use are relatively recent developments and are not yet global. Interestingly, limitations on use in certain places are based on prevention of incidental harm to others only in the case of smoking. Of course, use of illicit drugs and access to them by youth is restricted by their illegal status. Even though alcohol is legal in most places, access is typically restricted by age. Such restrictions are only now being applied to tobacco, and age-restriction policies vary widely across the world. The implicit or explicit use of price as an instrument of policy to discourage use varies with drugs. The illicit status of cocaine and opiates makes them more expensive and harder to obtain. Taxation of alcohol is frequently used as a means of deterring excessive use and access by youth. Such policies are only now being applied to tobacco, and their application is uneven.

Cessation and treatment

Abusers of each of the drugs are encouraged to cease use as a matter of policy. Unfortunately, the rates of cessation of use of all of the drugs are poor, and high rates of relapse are seen once cessation has begun. Behavioural treatments are available to promote withdrawal from each drug; indeed, the treatment approaches tend to be very similar, reflecting the common underlying process of addiction. Proven pharmacological treatments are available for opiates, alcohol and tobacco smoking. In the case of opiates and tobacco, the predominant approach is agonist substitution, in which the user is temporarily given the very drug they have used in order to blunt the emergence of craving and withdrawal. Treatment of alcohol abuse more often involves treatment with an antagonist. While a pharmacological treatment for cocaine addiction has long been sought, no proven treatment is yet available. Policy-makers have advocated treatment for alcohol, cocaine and opiate abusers; however, promotion of treatment for smoking is a recent, weak and spotty phenomenon. Despite evidence that treatment works and may be necessary for some smokers, policy-makers have overwhelmingly relied on the presumed ability of smokers to quit on their own, by means of 'willpower' or informal methods. This situation has changed only recently in a few countries, notably the United Kingdom and the United States. Finally, it is striking that the goals of treatment and the means by which treatment is evaluated differ across drugs. Only in the case of smoking is absolute abstinence (literally, 'not even a puff') for a prolonged period (often six months or more) regarded as the sole measure of treatment efficacy. In the case of the other drugs, partial desistance or reduction of use is regarded as a positive outcome and is reflected in outcome measures such as days of use and amount of use. Similarly, changes in the amount of use (e.g. 'controlled drinking') or patterns of use (e.g. use of clean needles, not driving while drinking) that reduce the harm due to use are regarded as legitimate targets of treatment. For smoking, despite evidence that the harm is dose-related, harm reduction has not been accepted as part of the predominant treatment strategy.

Conclusions

Enumeration of the differences and similarities between tobacco smoking and use of other licit and illicit drugs is a useful analytical exercise. It shows that tobacco smoking is in many important ways like other forms of drug abuse and addiction. At the same time, it reveals that we have not taken tobacco use seriously as a form of harmful substance abuse. Even though tobacco use causes far graver health consequences than other forms of drug abuse, societies have generally put much more energy and resources into combatting those other forms. This is probably because the harm brought about by tobacco use is distant, and also because tobacco use does not interfere with the users' ability to fulfil their immediate social obligations to their family, employer and community—at least until they fall ill and die. Perhaps, as a result, tobacco use does not elicit the same intense moral judgement that is evoked by abuse of the other drugs. Consequently, we have not, until recently, applied serious policy leverage to reducing tobacco use. Even now, the application of policy instruments such as age restrictions, barriers to access, pricing policy and restraints on advertising and promotion are in their infancy and are by no means global. In the same vein, the lack of emphasis on treatment as an avenue for tobacco control is evident. Tobacco control policy has relied almost exclusively on media and school campaigns to prevent the onset of tobacco use by youth. Only recently and in a few places are policies beginning to include the essential role of treatment for adult tobacco smokers who want to stop smoking but need help to do so. Even less attention has been paid to the potential to reduce the tobacco-related harm among people who will continue to smoke. Drug control policy is not always a model of successful policy, and we are not arguing that its approach ought to be adopted wholesale for tobacco control; however, we must recognize tobacco smoking as a dangerous form of drug abuse that causes far more harm to health than other forms of drug abuse. It is urgent that we apply to tobacco control the energy and focus that is often restricted to control of other drugs.

References
Henningfield, J.E., Schuh, L.M. & Heishman, S.J. (1995) Pharmacological determinants of cigarette smoking. In: Clarke, P.B.S., Quik, M., Adlkofer, F.X., & Thurau, K., eds, *Effects of Nicotine on Biological Systems II*, Basel: Birkhauser Verlag, pp. 247–256
US Department of Health and Human Services (1988) *The Health Consequences of Smoking: Nicotine Addiction. A Report of the US Surgeon General*, Washington, DC: US Government Printing Office

WOMEN AND TOBACCO

Prevalence and attitudes

Changes in smoking behaviour among pregnant women in England, 1992–97

L. Owen & A. McNeill

Health Education Authority, London, United Kingdom

We report some key findings from national surveys conducted by the Health Education Authority among pregnant women to monitor their knowledge, attitudes and behaviour in relation to smoking during pregnancy.

The health consequences of smoking include premature death from lung cancer, cardiovascular disease, bronchitis and emphysema. Women who smoke during pregnancy incur additional risks to themselves and their babies, including a doubling of the risk for an ectopic pregnancy, an increased risk for miscarriage, a reduced supply of oxygen to the foetus, a greater likelihood of lowering the birth weight to a level associated with infant mortality and an increased risk for perinatal death. The health of the newborn child is also at risk. Many studies have shown that smoking during pregnancy increases the risk for sudden infant death syndrome. Respiratory problems such as chronic cough, phlegm and wheeze and 'glue ear' are associated with exposure to smoky atmospheres. Passive smoking is also believed to exacerbate the symptoms of asthma in children. This list is not exhaustive but illustrates the clear health gains of encouarging pregnant women to stop smoking.

Since 1992, the Health Education Authority in England has carried out seven surveys of pregnant women. The first three covered 500–625 women, while the four most recent surveys involved interviewing about 1000 women at various stages of their pregnancy. The increase in the sample size from 1994 onwards was made possible by increased funding. Quota sampling was chosen as the most cost–effective means of obtaining a representative sample of pregnant women, even though it is not as rigorous as random sampling. Interviewing at home was adopted in preference to contact through, for example, antenatal clinics, to prevent bias in the resulting sample. Quota controls were set for age and socioeconomic groups.

The surveys are designed to monitor:

- the smoking prevalence among pregnant women and how it changes with time;
- the changes that pregnant women make in their smoking habits during pregnancy;
- what pregnant women know about the risks of smoking during pregnancy and of passive smoking;
- the nature of the interventions of health professionals as reported by pregnant women
- pregnant women's reports of the smoking habits of their partners and whether they changed.

Results

Figure 1 shows the overall prevalence of smoking among pregnant women divided into two broad socioeconomic groups: (i) professional and skilled non-manual workers and (ii) skilled and unskilled manual workers and unemployed women. In 1997, 27% of pregnant women smoked—the same as in January 1992. The prevalence of smoking in the group of lower socioeconomic status was almost double that in pregnant women in the higher category, the highest prevalence rates beng found among women aged 16–24.

Other factors that have been linked to a high prevalence of smoking are low educational attainment, low income, poor housing and having an unplanned pregnancy. In the 1997 survey, pregnant women whose partners smoked were four times as likely to smoke as those whose partners did not smoke (44 vs 11%).

Figure 1. Prevalence of smoking among pregant women by social class, England, 1992–97

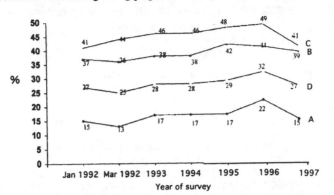

A, Professional and skilled non-manual workers; B, skilled and unskilled manual workers and unemployed women; C, as B, but ages 16–24; C, all

As part of the previous Government's commitment to improving the health of the nation, targets were set to reduce the smoking rates in the population; one that was set was for one-third of pregnant women to stop smoking at the start of their pregnancy by the year 2000. Although a significant proportion of pregnant women do give up when they become pregnant, about one-third continue to smoke. In 1997, 42% of pregnant women had smoked in the 12 months before their pregnancy, but only 26% during the pregnancy. Similar figures were seen in the other surveys. Even if all women do not give up smoking when they become pregnant, many do change their smoking behaviour. Thus, 11–18% changed their behaviour before the pregnancy and 53–67% did so during the pregnancy. The main change is to reduce the number of cigarettes smoked per day. In 1997, 34% of pregnant women who had smoked in the 12 months before becoming pregnant reported cutting down, while 29% reported giving up altogether. A further 28% said that they had not changed their behaviour; 4% had managed to stop smoking altogether but had started again before the pregnancy had gone to full term.

Making a positive change in smoking habits was related to social class, those in the higher category being more likely to make a change. Among women in the 1997 survey who changed immediately before or during their pregnancy, smokers in the higher social class were nearly twice as likely to have given up altogether than women in the lower category (56 and 32%, respectively).

In the 1997 survey, 17% of the women gave up smoking during pregnancy. Our analysis is focused on those who quit in the third trimester of pregnancy, since a woman in the first trimester of pregnancy cannot have stopped in the second or third trimester, whereas a woman in the third trimester could have stopped in the first, second or third trimester. Looking only at women in the third trimester of pregnancy, 16% of smokers quit in the first trimester, 3% in the second and 2% in the third.

The other main findings of the surveys were that pregnant women who smoke are more moderate in their views of the dangers of smoking than non-smokers. They are less likely, for example, to think that smoking is very dangerous, either to themselves or their baby, and are less likely to think that passive smoking is very dangerous to unborn or newborn babies. Smokers were less likely to agree that stopping or cutting down on smoking during pregnancy is important, and they attached greater importance to alcohol consumption and stress.

The habitual nature of smoking can be judged by how soon after waking up people smoke their first cigarette: 20% of the pregnant women claimed to have smoked their first cigarette within 5 min of waking, 13% within 15 min and 17% within 30 min. Among the main reasons given for smoking during pregnancy, 56% cited habit and

36% cited addiction. The other main reasons were stress relief (32%), enjoyment (22%), relaxation (14%) and boredom (14%).

What can be done?

These findings show that the prevalence of smoking during pregnancy is still worryingly high, particularly among young, pregnant, skilled and unskilled manual workers and the unemployed. The organizations, institutions and social structures in the communities in which these women live must therefore be addressed.

As the surveys indicate that pregnant women who smoke are more likely to have partners who smoke, interventions aimed at pregnant women should include components relevant to their partners so that they will be convinced to give up smoking.

The finding that although large numbers of pregnant women do change their smoking behaviour most cut down rather than quitting goes against the best available advice, since smokers who cut down often compensate by inhaling more. Furthermore, recent research by the Health Education Authority suggests that cutting down has little beneficial effect on the outcome of pregnancy.

Disappointingly, a proportion of women who managed to quit during pregnancy relapsed before the baby was born. In one study in the United States, 56% of pregnant women who quit smoking during pregnancy relapsed within 30 days of the birth of the baby. Interventions aimed at encouraging pregnant women to quit should obviously include components aimed at discouraging relapse. Efficacious interventions have been identified, and appropriate professionals should be trained to deliver them.

We found that pregnant smokers are less likely to believe that either active or passive smoking is very dangerous; some believed that smoking has certain benefits, like stress relief and relaxation. Knowledge about the health consequences of smoking must therefore be improved by a continuing programme of health education delivered through the media and through professionals and community-based organizations.

Finally, large numbers of pregnant women say that they smoke from habit or due to addiction. The use of nicotine replecement products in pregnancy is counter-indicated, but some medical practitioners argue that nicotine delivered by alternative routes is safer than nicotine delivered through cigarettes. More research is needed to determine the risks and benefits of nicotine replacement therapy during pregnancy.

Smoking among pregnant women: Epidemiology and cessation

A. Batra, V. Heuer-Jung, P.E. Schupp, B. Eckert & G. Buchkremer

Department of Psychiatry and Psychotherapy, University of Tübingen, Germany

Introduction

The National Department of Statistics in Germany regularly investigates health beliefs and health behaviour in Germany. In 1995; it investigated the smoking habits of persons > 15 years of age. About 33% of all men and 20% of all women in Germany are smokers; the prevalence is highest in the age group 20–40, with prevalences of 46% among men and 35% among women. The smoking behaviour of these young to middle-aged women is important for their fertility, their pregnancy and their children, as the risks for infertility and complications during pregnancy, the correlation between the number of cigarettes smoked daily and the body weight of newborn children and the increased risks for respiratory diseases and sudden infant death syndrome are well documented (Cnattingius *et al.*, 1988; Laurent *et al.*, 1992). Nevertheless, only 35% of women give up smoking when they learn that they are pregnant; about 32% reduce their cigarette consumption and another 33% do not change their smoking habits (Windsor & Orleans, 1986).

In order to determine the smoking behaviour of pregnant women, we interviewed 80 women the day after they were delivered. We asked for socioeconomic data and smoking habits, including daily cigarette consumption, any change in smoking habits with the onset of pregnancy and beliefs about health and smoking. We also recorded the weight and height of the newborn babies. We furthermore developed a smoking cessation programme (Heuer-Jung et al., 1996) tailored to pregnant women and women with tobacco-related problems such as infertility or risk factors such as use of oral contraceptives. We used a behavioural treatment programme, adding information about the risks of smoking during pregnancy and instructions for a healthy diet; nicotine replacement therapy was not prescribed, although nicotine patches had to be prescribed in one case after many previous frustrating attempts to quit. The participants attended therapy sessions once a week for six weeks.

We compared the therapy outcome and abstinence rates after six months in 10 pregnant women and 57 other women, some with one of the risk factors, and compared these data with those for 72 women who had participated in a standard behavioural treatment programme combined with nicotine replacement therapy and 36 women who had merely been advised by their physician to stop smoking.

Results

Of the 34% of women who smoked at the beginning of pregnancy, 44% quit smoking, 33% reduced their daily consumption of cigarettes and 22% did not change their smoking behaviour. Of these smokers, 53% had smoked during their previous pregnancy, 60% admitted that they wanted to keep on smoking or start smoking again after their child was delivered, and 60% were convinced that smoking harms both the mother and the child. Although 76% recalled having been asked about their smoking status by their gynaecologist, only 44% reported that they had been advised to stop. None had participated in any treatment for smoking cessation. There was a clear correlation between the body weight and the length of the newborns and the number of cigarettes smoked during the pregnancy.

After completing the therapy, 70% of the pregnant women remained abstinent; 58% of those participating in the modified cessation programme quit, whereas 42% of the women on the standard behavioural programme had been able to quit. If no support was given, only 5.5% stopped smoking. Six months later, 30% of the pregnant women were still abstinent, in comparison with 19% in the other groups and 3% of controls.

Conclusion

Smoking during pregnancy clearly harms the child. As giving up smoking at the onset of pregnancy appears to be even more important than reducing cigarette consumption during pregnancy, better health education should be given to pregnant women. Because some pregnant women clearly cannot stop smoking in response to their physician's advice, treatment programmes are needed that are tailored to their needs. Increasing the appeal of such programmes by adding specific information and motivational factors might improve compliance and treatment outcome. Our preliminary results confirm the increased efficaciousness of tailored behavioural therapy programmes even in the absence of nicotine replacement therapy; the rates of abstinence might increase even further if the latter is included as well. Further investigations should concentrate on this aspect.

References

Cnattingius, S., Haglund, B. & Meirik, O. (1988) Cigarette smoking as a risk factor for late fetal and early neonatal death. Br. Med. J., 297, 258–261
Heuer-Jung, V., Batra, A. & Buchkremer, G. (1996) Raucherentwöhnung bei speziellen Risikogruppen: Schwangere Frauen und Raucherinnen mit Kontrazeptivaeinnahme. Prax. Klin. Verhaltensmed. Rehabil., 34, 114–117
Laurent, S.L., Thompson, S.J., Addy, C., Garrison, C.Z. & Moore, E.E. (1992) An epidemiological study of smoking and primary infertility in women. Fertil. Steril., 57, 565–572
Windsor, R.A. & Orleans, C.T. (1986) Guidelines and methodological standards for smoking cessation intervention research among pregnant women: Improving the science and the art. Health Educ. Q., 13, 131–161

Tobacco and the Indian woman

M.B. Aghi

Tata Institute of Fundamental Research, Mumbai, India

A casual study of the figures for the consumption of tobacco in India may give the impression that smoking in this part of the world does not qualify as a public health problem. For instance, the annual consumption of cigarettes per adult in India works out to just 160; the corresponding figures are about 4000 for the United States, 3050 for the United Kingdom and 2810 for Japan. But these figures must be viewed in the light of the fact that most of the Indian population lives in villages where tobacco is consumed not in the form of cigarettes but in the form of *bidis* and chewing tobacco, by itself or with betel leaf, lime and areca nut. Cigarette smoking is common mainly in urban India. Indian women by and large do not smoke, as yet. A number of surveys conducted among university students have indicated that no more than 2–5% of women had ever smoked. No figures are available for the total urban population, but the prevalence is less than 10%, if that high. Today's trend in cigarette smoking is seen among girls who work for multinational companies, airlines or in mass media like television and films, because these young ladies identify themselves with their counterparts in the western world. Fortunately, this number is negligible. It is not yet acceptable in the Indian lifestyle for daughters and daughters-in-law to smoke, although men may smoke.

There are well-defined pockets of tobacco use all over India where men, women and even children use tobacco. The tobacco profile of women in rural India is indeed very colourful: they chew *pan* (betel leaf) with tobacco and lime, as in Kerala (20%); they smoke *bidis* (small indigenous cigars) and hookahs, as in Bihar (22%) and parts of Punjab and Haryana; they smoke *dhumti* in Goa (3%); they rub and plug burnt powdered tobacco inside the cheek or under the lip in Maharashtra (22%), Gujarat and Bihar. In Andhra, they smoke cheroot-like products called *chutta* in reverse (28%), i.e. when the cheroot is well lit, they put the lighted end inside their mouths. Women in rural India who indulge in tobacco habits are equal to the men, with a similar distribution. The prevalence of smoking among women in various areas of India is shown in Table 1; the various types of tobacco use are listed in Table 2.

Let us dwell a bit more on the profile of women in Andhra Pradesh and Kerala. Women in Kerala chew tobacco with betel leaf and areca nut. They are full-time housewives and also work in the field, growing, tending and harvesting paddy. The literacy rate in Kerala is higher than in most other parts of India; in addition, the women are alert, independent and individualistic. They have their private supplies of chewing material and use it whenever they want. Their counterparts in Andhra are less literate, have more children, seem poorer and may or may not chew tobacco but smoke the *chutta*. They smoke it in reverse because they consider that it is not feminine to smoke the conventional way. The women in Kerala suffer from precancerous lesions of the buccal mucosa and buccal groove on or under the tongue, and women in Andhra also end up with lesions on the palate. None of them is aware of the ill effects of tobacco. On the contrary, they have many reasons for practising the habit. Women in Maharashtra smoke to postpone hunger.

How do they learn to these habits and what do they know about them? They take to them innocently and unknowingly. The mother in Andhra asks her small daughter (4–5 years or more) to light her *chutta*; often, the daughter will have to take a puff to see if it is well lit. This develops into a habit. She reasons, 'There cannot be anything wrong with the habit since my mother has it'. If she goes through childhood without taking up the habit, she takes to it during adolescence, as all her friends do it. She is often advised to take up the habit as a cure for minor (constipation, gas) and some major (anaemia, rheumatism) ailments. The dynamics are the same for other modes of smoking, whether

Table 1. Prevalence of tobacco use among women in
India in population-based house-to-house surveys

Area	Sample size	Tobacco users (%)	
		Women	All
Bhavnagar	10 071	15	44
Ernakulam	10 287	39	59
Srikakulum	10 169	67	74
Singbhum	10 048	33	56
Darbhanga	10 340	51	64
Pune	101761	49	64
Mainpuri	34 997	21	57

Table 2. Types of tobacco use among women in India

Area	Chewing (%)	Smoking (%)	Mixed (%)
Bhavnagar	15		
Ernakulam	38	1	1
Srikakulum	3	64	–
Singbhum	26	5	2
Darbhanga	7	41	4
Pune	49	–	–
Mainpure	9	11	1

it be *bidi, hookah* or *dhumti*. Women start chewing *pan* with tobacco because it is the way of life in the part of the country in which they live. The same applies to rubbing and plugging tobacco.

The rural Indian's attitude to smoking is almost always one of benign tolerance, verging on acceptance and very often inclining towards recommendation and prescription. Unlike packs of cigarettes, those of *bidis* have no warning on them; even if they did, few could read them. As if this were not enough, women have attributed many magical and medicinal properties to tobacco. If it cures toothache for women in Kerala, it helps women in Maharashtra to keep their mouths clean. Women in Andhra can get rid of the foul smell in their mouths in the morning, control morning sickness when pregnant and bear labour pains during delivery. And of course, it always helps to have a little fun, relax, socialize and enjoy a dull existence. What has research to say about these reasons for tobacco habits?

Oral cancer is one of the most frequent cancers in India. It is almost invariably found where tobacco habits exist. In our study, in which we examined almost 100 000 people, oral cancer was systematically associated with tobacco use. In our 10-year follow-up study of the incidence rates of oral cancer and the natural history of precancerous lesions in Indian villagers, we found the overall crude annual incidence rate of oral cancer to be 16 per 100 000 in Kerala and 14 per 100 000 in Andhra. The incidence in the older age group was six times that in the middle-aged group. In Andhra, the older age group had an incidence of oral cancer of 93 per 100 000. The tobacco habits described in this paper have been shown to be high-risk factors for many other types of cancer, like those of the pharynx, oesophagus and lung. It has also been shown that, just like cigarette smoking, *bidi* smoking causes chronic bronchitis. The overall health effects of the various tobacco habits have not, however, been studied so far. A 10-year follow-up study of mortality in relation to tobacco chewing and smoking at our institute revealed that the crude relative risk was 3.4 for females tobacco users and 2.3 for male users.

Other studies have shown the effects of chewing tobacco on reproduction: the rate of stillbirth was three times higher in chewers (50 out of 1000 pregnancies) than non-chewers (17.1 out of 1000 pregnancies), the birthweight of infants of chewers was

100–200 g less than those of non-chewers, and there was greater loss of male foetuses by chewers than non-chewers.

An intervention was launched to persuade people to give up their tobacco habits. The strategies combined personal interaction with films, folk drama, radio slogans, plays, newspaper articles, posters and slide projections in movie theatres. Personal interaction is considered to have the greatest impact. The intervention was more successful with females than males in Kerala, and 13% of women and 5% of males have given up tobacco use.

The findings in the west are contrary to what we have found. Bobbie Jockobson in her book *Lady Killers* demonstrated that it is very hard for women to give up smoking, and anyone reading the book will wonder how a woman in the west could ever give up the habit when the whole world is working against it. The situation is no different in India, and poverty is added to all of the other pressures; the burdens of women in India are heavy. What is the difference then? I conducted 10 case studies of women who had given up their habit. One glaring commonality in the results was, 'You talked to me, convinced me, I tried, found truth in what you said; I was determined, and so I gave up'. It would seem to be important to interact with users on a personal basis, to convince them, to support them and to show them how to quit. It is not enough to advise. Women are more open in one-to-one situations than men. They reveal their weaknesses and have less ego hang-up. The second commonality of the results is that, despite all the miseries, pressures and discomforts of life, women in villages in India are usually emotionally very secure. There is hardly any threat to wifehood. They have the comfort and peace of mind that their husbands will always be theirs; whatever the husbands have belongs to their wives. They also have security and the support of their children, especially if they are in early adolescence and going to school. They can influence the women through their knowledge and tender love. I have no scientific data to support this idea except to show you the lifestyle of the rural Indian woman.

Tobacco dependence: Issues and concerns of women, children and families in south Asia

M.B. Aghi

Tata Institute of Fundamental Research, Mumbai, India

The objective of this study was to show that tobacco use is a serious problem in south Asia. The tobacco issues and tobacco habits in this part of the world are different from those elsewhere, as tobacco is not only smoked but also chewed, rubbed on the teeth and plugged in the mouth. The method used was review and critical analysis of various studies to identify commonalities and differences, so that interventions and prevention can be planned and carried out. As no statistics were available on any country as a whole, sample surveys were performed at different intensities. The conclusions are based on sparse but very compelling data which point to strong commonalities and some country-specific differences.

The consumption figures are shown in Table 1, with those in certain developed countries for comparison. They appear to be very low. The alarming factor is that south Asians also smoke indigenous cigarettes (*bidis*) and chew tobacco by itself or with betel leaf, lime and areca nut. These increase the risk. Smoking of cigarettes is common in urban areas, mostly among men. Women in urban areas are beginning to smoke, although the rate is still no more than 10% at the most and is much lower in Pakistan and Bangladesh. The increase is seen mostly among college girls and women who work in advertising or the electronic media and for multinational companies. Women

Table 1. Annual consumption of cigarettes
by adults in south Asia and selected developed
countries

Country	Consumption (no. of cigarettes/year)
Bangladesh	270
India	160
Nepal	150
Pakistan	670
Sri Lanka	500
Japan	2810
United Kingdom	3050
United States	4000

in so-called 'modern households' also smoke cigarettes, peer pressure being the dynamic in this group. Another factor that leads to such behaviour is defiance. The reasons reported are anxiety reduction, socializing, appearing independent or daring and showing an attitude of 'Who cares?'.

Large slums are found throughout south Asia, and children (especially boys) in these areas smoke cigarettes, not because of peer pressure or adult modelling but mainly to imitate movie stars. Life is dull, dangerous and devoid of any direction. Going to the movies and looking at movie posters are an escape, and they pretend to be movie stars. Rural south Asia presents a different picture. Much less uniformity is seen than in urban areas. In some villages, tobacco use is almost universal. Men, women and children, both boys and girls, consume tobacco in various forms: men mostly smoke and women mainly chew, although some men chew and some women smoke *bidis*. Almost all will tell you that they use tobacco to pass the time, to socialize, to relax and to enjoy their dull existence.

The crude relative risks for male and female tobacco users are similar in all the countries of south Asia. The level of awareness is also almost identical, with more awareness in urban areas and among educated people; however, this seems to make little difference, because the urban groups who are aware also seem to rationalize. Unlike in the developed world, this awareness does not seem to incite people to seek guidance to give up tobacco. In the rural areas, not only is there lack of awareness but villagers and especially women believe that tobacco has many medicinal and magical properties: that it purifies the breath (both men and women but mostly women), that it alleviates toothache (all), that it wards off hunger (poor people), that it keeps one awake (policemen and night guards), that it helps to eliminate morning sickness and labour pains (women), that it makes you confident (young rural men) and that it makes you look smart and modern (young rural men).

The implications of these findings are that there is a great need to educate people about health. Health education should start with the necessary information. Strategies should be so designed that they are understood, liked and are relevant to the lifestyle.

Influence of sex on smoking behaviour in Turkey

N. Bilir, B. Güçiz Doðan & A.N. Yyldyz

Department of Public Health, Hacettepe University, Ankara, Turkey

The aim of this study was to investigate the possible effect of sex on smoking behaviour in children and various professional groups. This descriptive study was conducted in Ankara, the capital of Turkey. Representative samples were selected from various professional groups, comprising 552 high-school students, 512 secondary-school students, 254 teachers, 237 physicians, 109 journalists, 149 sportsmen and 130 artists. The data were collected between April and December 1996 with a pre-tested questionnaire developed for this study. SPSS 5.0 statistical software was used for analysis.

All of the adults who participated in the study were in their 30s, except for the sportsmen, whose mean age was 23.7 years; that of high-school students was 16.5 and that of secondary-school students was 13.7. Approximately equal numbers of females and males were found among the journalists, artists and physicians, whereas males represented 62% of the high-school students, 54% of the secondary-school students, 41% of the teachers and 88% of the sportsmen. About two out of three teachers had smoked previously or smoked currently, with a higher percentage of current smokers among female teachers (54%) than male teachers (46%). The prevalence of smoking was highest among the journalists (64%) in both men and women. While 36% of the sportsmen interviewed smoked, the percentage dropped to 28% for sportswomen. Forty percent of the female artists, who constituted 54% of the artists' group, said that they smoked; the percentage was 53% among male artists. The percentage of female physicians who had never smoked was 54%, while only 24% of male physicians were non-smokers. Among secondary- and high-school students, the percentages of girls who smoked (2.6 and 20%, respectively) were approximately half that of boys, and the percentage who had never smoked was higher among girls than boys. The prevalence of smoking increased steadily with age in all groups, independently of sex. The mean number of cigarettes smoked per day was smaller among females than males in all groups. The results of logistic regression analysis showed that sex, education, age and sibling smoking increased the smoking prevalence, while having children affected it inversely.

The smoking rate is thus higher among males, except among teachers; however, when ex-smokers are included, the rate of smoking is still higher among male teachers. In all groups, the males smoked more cigarettes per day than females. Thus, not only level of education, age, sibling smoking and having children but also sex significantly affects smoking behaviour.

Attitudes towards cigarette smoking among women of child-bearing age in Poland

J. Szymborski, B. Chazan, W. Zatonski, M. Komar-Szymborska, J. Niezurawski & T. Kowalczyk

National Research Institute of Mother and Child, Warsaw, Poland

The aim of this study was to evaluate women's attitudes towards cigarette smoking and to determine their preferences and socioeconomic characteristics. The participants were a representative group of 1385 women aged 15–49 in three areas of Poland. Each woman filled in a standardized questionnaire in the presence of the interviewer.

The prevalence of smoking in this group was 31%, with 3.3% among those aged 15–18, 12% aged 19–25, 21% aged 26–32, 33 aged 33–39 and 31% aged ≥ 40. The majority of the women who smoked had children and were older than those who did not have children. The prevalence of smoking among pregnant women was 12%.

When asked about the numbers of cigarettes smoked daily, 46% said they smoked 10 per day, 47% smoked 11–20 cigarettes per day, 2.3% smoked ≥ 21 and 3.5% did not know. The questionnaires also revealed that the women who smoked took advantage of the gynaecological services at community health centres more frequently than non-smokers. Other factors that increased the frequency of cigarette smoking were a lower frequency of religious practice, lack of employment, living in cities, a low level of education and alcohol drinking.

Tobacco habits among Bajau and Kadazan women in Sabah, Malaysia

C.-Y. Gan

Department of Social and Preventive Medicine, University of Malaya, Kuala Lumpur, Malaysia

Two cross-sectional surveys were conducted to document the prevalence and practice of tobacco habits among the indigenous people of Sabah State. The sample size was estimated, and multistage sampling was carried out in the two selected districts. A questionnaire designed for a structured interview was used. A total of 431 rural Bajau women and 472 rural Kadazan women responded. The prevalence of smokeless tobacco use among rural Bajau women in Kota Belud district was 77%, and that among rural Kadazan women in Tambunan district was 60%. In both ethnic groups, tobacco was seldom chewed by itself but was used as an ingredient in the ritual of betel chewing. In betel chewing, a number of products in various combinations are chewed: areca nut (seed of *Areca catechu* L.), the leaf of *Piper betle* L., lime from boiled sea-shells, *gambir* (a preparation from the leaves and twigs of the shrub *Uncaria gambir*) and tobacco. The use of smokeless tobacco was common among women, but the prevalence was low among men; however, the prevalence of smoking among the women was low. The prevalence of smoking was only 3.3% among Bajau women and 11% among Kadazan women. Both hand-rolled and manufactured cigarettes were smoked. Factors that influenced tobacco use among women included easy access to locally grown tobacco, low educational status and the cultural and social acceptance of tobacco use. Preventive and control measures against tobacco use are required in these communities.

Hubble-bubble (*narguileh*): A female pattern of smoking

Y. Mohammad

Syrian Thoracic Association, Lattakia, Syria

In the eastern Mediterranean coastal region, women traditionally smoke 'hubble-bubble' (water pipes or *narguileh*) during their daily or weekly gatherings, with their children playing nearby. The hubble-bubble pipe consists of a narrow-necked glass container, a hose and firebrands. The container is half-filled with water, and a vertical tube leads from the water to a wad of tobacco at the narrow opening, which is lit with brands. The hose is inserted into the air space above the water, and smoke is drawn out.

We studied the chronic respiratory effects of this habit in 100 women (active smokers) and 100 children aged 0–8 years (passive smokers). The women were examined for the prevalence of chronic cough, sputum, dyspnoea and wheeze and for forced expiratory volume in one second (FEV_1) and alterations in small airways diameter (MMEF) in relation to the duration of smoking and the cumulative amount smoked. The children were examined for chronic cough, dyspnoea and wheeze.

The women were found to have a high prevalence of chronic bronchitis (35–85% depending on the cumulative quantity and duration of smoking). Dyspnoea was found in 26% and wheeze in 12%. The MMEF was reduced to < 20% of the predicted value in 98% of the women, regardless of the quantity or duration of hubble-bubble smoking. FEV_1 was reduced in 35%, and the reduction was quasi-linear with the cumulative amount smoked. Examination of the children showed that 35% had recurrent cough, the percentage increasing with the duration of exposure, and 26% had dyspnoea; only 12% of control children coughed recurrently and 6% had dyspnoea.

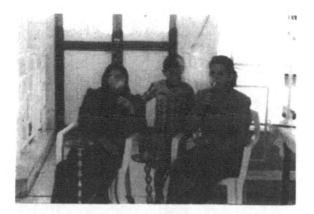

Health effects

Risk for multiple prior miscarriages among middle-aged women who smoke

M. Schofield[1], G. Mishra[2] & A. Dobson[2]

[1]*School of Health, University of New England, Armidale, and*
[2]*Department of Statistics, University of Newcastle, Australia*

Abstract

We present retrospective self-reported data from the baseline survey of the Australian Longitudinal Study on Women's Health on the relationship between smoking and history of miscarriages among 14 200 women aged 45–49 at the time of the survey. The sampling frame was the database of the national health insurance system. Participants were randomly selected, with over-sampling from rural and remote areas, and are broadly representative of Australian women in this age group. Polychotomous logistic regression analyses were used to test the hypotheses that current smoking status and age at starting to smoke are associated with the number of miscarriages reported. There was a strong positive relationship between smoking status and the number of reported miscarriages. Ex-smokers were 1.25 times more likely to have had two or more miscarriages, light smokers (1–19 cigarettes per day) were 1.39 times more likely, and women who smoked 20 or more per day were 1.78 times more likely compared with women who had never smoked. An inverse relationship was also found between age at starting to smoke and a history of miscarriages. The findings provide strong evidence of a link between smoking and miscarriages and suggest that new initiatives are needed to prevent smoking among women of child-bearing age.

Introduction

It is well known that tobacco smoking by pregnant women is associated with poor pregnancy outcomes, such as low birth weight of children and reduced fecundity (Poswillo & Alberman, 1992; Tzonou *et al.*, 1993). A relationship between smoking and miscarriage has not been found consistently, however (Kline *et al.*, 1995). In one study of nearly 18 000 pregnant women tested by ultrasound, early pregnancy failure was not associated with smoking (Pandya *et al.*, 1996). A case–control study involving 94 women who had had two or more unexplained miscarriages and 176 normal pregnancies gave a 40% increased risk for miscarriage among current smokers relative to women who had never smoked, and the risk was found to increase with the number of cigarettes smoked per day (Parazzini *et al.*, 1991). A study of 650 women in assisted fertility programmes showed that smokers produced fewer oocytes and had a pregnancy rate less than half that of non-smokers; smokers who did become pregnant had an increased rate of miscarriages (Harrison *et al.*, 1990). The inconsistent findings may be due to confounding by other exposures such as alcohol use, or may reflect the lack of a true association (Kline *et al.*, 1995). Further research into a wide range of potential confounders is needed to clarify whether a true relationship exists.

The aim of the Australian Longitudinal Study on Women's Health is to examine the relationships between biological, psychological, social and lifestyle factors and women's physical and emotional health over 20 years. The national baseline survey of 14 200 women aged 45–49 years (middle-aged group) was used to examine the relationship between cigarette smoking and the frequency of miscarriage. Two hypotheses were investigated: the first that women who have never smoked have a lower risk for multiple miscarriages than ex- or current smokers and secondly that the earlier a woman starts to smoke the higher her risk for multiple miscarriages.

Methods

The mailed baseline questionnaire contained questions about current smoking status: 'never' smoker, ex-smoker, smokes < 20 per day, smokes ≥ 20 cigarettes per day. Ex-smokers were also asked about the quantities they used to smoke per day and the time (in years) since they had stopped cigarette smoking. Both smokers and ex-smokers were asked the age at which they had started smoking.

The answers to questions about alcohol consumption were categorized by quantity and frequency as: non-drinker, occasional drinker and regular drinker (≤ 1 standard drink per day). Area of residence was categorized as 'urban', 'rural' or 'remote'. Level of education was categorized as 'no formal qualification', 'completed school education' (10–13 years of school) and 'tertiary qualified' (trade, apprenticeship, diploma or university degree). Marital status was categorized as 'married/de facto', 'divorced/separated/widowed' or 'single'. The number of live births and the number of terminations were included in the analysis.

Polychotomous logistic regression models (Begg & Gray, 1984) were used to estimate the association between the number of miscarriages and smoking status, with adjustment for area of residence, marital status, educational level, alcohol consumption and numbers of births and terminations, as well as the joint effects of the last two variables. Polychotomous logistic regression was also used to examine the relationship between age at starting to smoke and the number of miscarriages experienced.

Results

Univariate analyses (not shown here) suggested a clear dose–response relationship between a history of multiple miscarriages and the amount smoked, with heavy smokers having double the risk of women who had never smoked. Similarly, there was an inverse gradient between age at starting to smoke and the risk for miscarriage. Other variables significantly related to miscarriage in the univariate analyses included the number of live births and terminations, the joint effect of births and terminations, alcohol consumption, education, marital status and area of residence.

Table 1 shows the adjusted odds ratios for the three categories of smoking status relative to the reference category of 'never smoked' for a single miscarriage and for two or more miscarriages. The risk for a single miscarriage was significantly greater for ex-smokers and smokers of ≥ 20 cigarettes a day. The risk for multiple miscarriages increased with the number of cigarettes smoked each day, to a maximum risk for those smoking ≥ 20 cigarettes per day. Women who started after the age of 18 had a significantly lower risk of having multiple miscarriages.

Discussion

We examined retrospectively reported lifetime histories of miscarriages among women aged 45–49 years in 1996. Self-reported histories of miscarriages were found to have a strong dose–response relationship with current smoking status and age at starting to smoke. Interpretation of this finding is somewhat limited by the failure to

Table 1. Adjusted odds ratios (OR) and 95% confidence intervals (CIs) for smoking status in relation to a history of single and multiple miscarriages

Smoking status	No. of miscarriages ($n = 11\ 384$)			
	1		≥ 2	
	OR	95% CI	OR	95% CI
Never	1.00	–	1.00	–
Ex-smoker	1.22*	1.08–1.37	1.25*	1.06–1.48
< 20/day	1.08	0.88–1.33	1.39*	1.07–1.81
≥ 20/day	1.24*	1.04–1.47	1.78*	1.43–2.21

establish the temporal order of the occurrence of miscarriage in relation to variables such as age at starting to smoke, age at quitting for ex-smokers and events such as live births and terminations. Against this limitation, however, the strength and consistency of the relationship provides confidence. Furthermore, since most women smokers in Australia start smoking by the age of 15 and most pregnancies occur after the age of 15, it is reasonable to assume that smoking preceded miscarriages in the majority of cases.

A strength of this study was the large sample size, which allowed us to adjust for several established confounders, other factors found to be significantly related to miscarriage, such as area of residence and the complex associations between miscarriages, births and terminations. A second strength is that the sample, randomly selected from the national Medicare database, is largely representative of Australian women. Third, the narrow age range selected provides good control of potential cohort effects such as changing patterns of smoking and contraceptive use over time. Fourth, the data can be considered to represent lifetime risk of multiple miscarriages.

In conclusion, the study provides strong evidence of serious health risks for women during child-bearing years, which may provide more immediate and personal incentives for women to refrain from smoking. These results could assist the development of anti-smoking campaigns aimed at younger women, a target group of high priority for anti-smoking messages.

Acknowledgements
The research on which this paper is based was conducted as part of the Australian Longitudinal Study on Women's Health (University of Newcastle and University of Queensland). We are grateful to the Department of Health and Family Services (Australian Commonwealth Government) for funding.

References
Begg, C. & Gray, R. (1984) Calculation of polychotomous logistic regression parameters using individualized regressions. *Biometrika*, 71, 11–18
Harrison, K.L., Breen, T.M. & Hennessey, J.F. (1990) The effect of patient smoking habit on the outcome of IVF and GIFT treatment. *Aust. NZ J. Obstet. Gynaecol.*, 30, 340–342
Kline, J., Levin, B., Kinney, A., Stein, Z., Susser, M. & Warburton, D. (1995) Cigarette smoking and spontaneous abortion of known karyotype: Precise data but uncertain inferences. *Am. J. Epidemiol.*, 141, 417–427
Pandya, P.P., Snijders, R.J., Psara, N., Hilbert, L. & Nicolaides, K.H. (1996) The prevalence of non-viable pregnancy at 10–13 weeks of gestation. *Ultrasound Obstet .Gynecol.*, 7, 170–173
Parazzini, F., Bocciolone, L., Fedele, L., Negri, E., La Vecchia, C. & Acaia, B. (1991) Risk factors for spontaneous abortion. *Int. J. Epidemiol.*, 20, 157–161
Poswillo, D. & Alberman, E. (1992) *Effects of Smoking on the Fetus, Neonate and Child*, New York: Oxford University Press
Tzonou, A., Hsieh, C.C., Trichopoulos, D., Aravandinos, D., Kalandidi, A., Margaris, D., Goldman, M. & Toupadaki, N. (1993) Induced abortions, miscarriages, and tobacco smoking as risk factors for secondary infertility. *J. Epidemiol. Commun. Health*, 47, 36–39

Risk for early menopause among Australian women who smoke

M.Schofield[1], G. Mishra[2] & A. Dobson[2]

[1] *School of Health, University of New England, Armidale, and* [2] *Department of Statistics, University of Newcastle, Australia*

Abstract
We examined the relationship between smoking status and self-reported natural menopause among 14 200 women aged 45–49 years in the Australian Longitudinal Study on Women's Health. The sampling frame was the database of the national health insurance system. Participants were randomly selected, with over-sampling from rural and remote areas and are broadly representative of Australian women in this age group.

Polychotomous logistic regression analyses were used to estimate the association between current smoking status and early menopause and peri-menopausal status after adjustment for potentially confounding factors. Smokers of 1–19 cigarettes per day were 1.48 times more likely to be peri-menopausal, and women who smoked ≥ 20 per day were 1.74 times more likely to be peri-menopausal than those who had never smoked. Both groups of smokers were 1.8 times more likely to report post-menopausal status than women who had never smoked. For ex-smokers, the risk for earlier onset of menopause declined rapidly after quitting. The results extend earlier evidence of a link between smoking and early menopause by estimating the effects of quitting and by controlling for a wide range of potential confounders.

Introduction

Early menopause has been associated with age, parity, smoking and social class (Vermeulen, 1993; Torgerson *et al.*, 1994; Cramer *et al.*, 1995a), age at menarche and family history (Torgerson *et al.*, 1994; Cramer *et al.*, 1995b), cycle length (Cramer *et al.*, 1995c), oral contraceptive use (Vermeulen, 1993), alcohol consumption (Torgerson *et al.*, 1994) and weight Cramer *et al.*, 1995b,c). International research has consistently found a strong dose–response relationship between smoking and early menopause (Vermeulen, 1993; Torgerson *et al.*, 1994, Cramer *et al.*, 1995a,b,c), as did an Australian study in the early 1980s (Adena & Gallagher, 1982). Different studies have controlled for different factors, however, and some have not controlled for any potential confounders. In the current study, we aimed to determine the strength of the relationship between smoking and early menopause among a large group of Australian women, with control for known confounders. We examined the risk for early menopause among current smokers and ex-smokers relative to 'never' smokers after control for a range of demographic and behavioural risk factors, including age, marital status, level of education, area of residence, country of birth, number of pregnancies, alcohol consumption and weight.

Methods

The sampling frame of the Australian Longitudinal Study on Women's Health was the database of Medicare, the national health insurance system. Women aged 45–49 years were randomly selected, with over-sampling from rural and remote areas, and are broadly representative of Australian women in this age group. A total of 14 200 (53%) women responded. The longitudinal study began with a mailed baseline survey in 1996. Current smoking status was categorized as: 'never' smoker, ex-smoker, smokes < 20 per day or smokes ≥ 20 cigarettes a day. Ex-smokers were asked about the quantities they used to smoke per day and the time (in years) since quitting. Natural menopause was assessed by asking women whether they had had any menstrual bleeding within the last 12 months; those who said 'no' were categorized as post-menopausal; those who reported menstrual bleeding in the previous 12 months but not in the previous three months were categorized as peri-menopausal. Women who had had a hysterectomy or were on hormone replacement therapy were excluded from the present analyses. Marital status was categorized as 'married/de facto', 'divorced/separated/widowed' or 'single'. Level of education was categorized as 'no formal qualification', 'completed school education' (10–13 years of school) and 'tertiary qualified' (trade, apprenticeship, diploma or university degree). Area of residence was categorized as 'urban', 'rural' or 'remote'. The answers to questions about alcohol consumption were categorized by quantity and frequency as non-drinker, occasional drinker and regular drinker (one or more standard drinks per day). There were also questions about the number of pregnancies and use of oral contraceptives. Weight and height were reported and the results used to estimate body mass index.

A polychotomous logistic regression model (Begg & Gray, 1984) was used to estimate the association between menopausal status and smoking status, with adjustment for significant variables from the univariate analyses: number of pregnancies, alcohol consumption, age, body mass index, country of birth and educational level.

Polychotomous logistic regression was also used to examine the relationship between menopausal status and time since quitting smoking, with adjustment for number of pregnancies, alcohol consumption, age, body mass index, country of birth, education and marital status.

Results

Table 1 shows the adjusted odds ratios for peri-menopause and post-menopause for smokers relative to 'never' smokers. The relative risk for peri-menopause was 1.5 (95% confidence interval (CI), 1.2–1.8) for smokers of 1–19 cigarettes per day and 1.7 (95% CI, 1.4–2.1) for women who smoked ≥ 20 cigarettes per day relative to 'never 'smokers. Both groups of smokers were 1.8 times more likely to be post-menopausal than women who had never smoked. Women who had quit smoking within the last two years had 1.5 times (95% CI, 1.1–2.0) the risk for being peri-menopausal when compared with 'never' smokers. But for women who had quit a longer time before, there was no evidence of continuing risk.

Discussion

The results confirm the hypothesis that menopausal status, measured by time from cessation of menstrual periods, is related to current smoking. The study extends previous research by including a wide range of potential confounders and by examining the possible effect of time since quitting smoking. Although interpretation of the findings may be somewhat limited by reliance on women's self-reporting of menstrual history, this method is the only one feasible for determining menopausal status in the context of a large postal survey. One strength of this study is the large sample size, which allowed us to adjust for several established confounders and other factors. Another is that the sample, randomly selected from the national Medicare database, is largely representative of Australian women. Thirdly, the narrow age range selected provides good control of potential cohort effects such as changing patterns of smoking and contraceptive use over time. Of potential relevance to health promotion is the evidence that the risk for early menopause (and the associated premature hormonal changes) declines rapidly when women give up smoking, as only those who had quit within the past two years were at increased risk of being peri-menopausal.

Acknowledgements

The research on which this paper is based was conducted as part of the Australian Longitudinal Study on Women's Health (University of Newcastle and University of Queensland). We are grateful to the Department of Health and Family Services (Australian Commonwealth Government) for funding.

Table 1. Adjusted odds ratios (ORs) and 95% confidence intervals (CIs) for smoking status and time since quitting for early peri-menopause and early natural menopause

Smoking variable	Peri-menopause		Post-menopause	
	OR	95% CI	OR	95% CI
Smoking status (*n* = 7527)				
Never	1.00	–	1.00	–
Ex-smoker	1.08	0.95–1.22	0.99	0.81–1.21
< 20 per day	1.48	1.20–1.83	1.79	1.30–2.46
≥ 20 per day	1.74	1.44–2.11	1.84	1.38–2.47
Quit smoking timeframe (*n* = 7432)				
Never	1.00	–	1.00	–
Current smoker	1.64	1.41–1.91	1.79	1.42–2.26
Quit 0–2 years	1.48	1.08–2.04	1.34	0.80–2.25
Quit 3–5 years	0.69	0.49–0.96	1.00	0.62–1.63
Quit 6–9 years	1.30	0.96–1.76	1.30	0.79–2.14
Quit 10–14 years	1.09	0.86–1.37	0.85	0.56–1.13
Quit 15–24 years	1.00	0.84–1.20	0.80	0.58–1.12
Quit 25–35 years	1.03	0.79–1.34	0.99	0.63–1.56

References
Adena, M.A. & Gallagher, H.G. (1982) Cigarette smoking and the age at menopause. *Ann. Hum. Biol.*, **9**, 121–130
Begg, C. & Gray, R. (1984) Calculation of polychotomous logistic regression parameters using individualised regressions. *Biometrika*, **71**, 11–18
Cramer, D.W., Harlow, B.L., Xu, H., Fraer, C. & Barbieri, R. (1995a) Cross-sectional and case-controlled analyses of the association between smoking and early menopause. *Maturitas*, **22**, 79–87
Cramer, D.W., Xu, H. & Harlow, B.L. (1995b) Family history as a predictor of early menopause. *Fertil. Steril.*, **64**, 740–745
Cramer, D.W., Xu, H. & Harlow, B.L. (1995c) Does 'incessant' ovulation increase risk for early menopause? *Am. J. Obstet. Gynecol.*, **172**, 568–573
Torgerson, D.J., Avenell, A., Russell, I.T. & Reid, D.M. (1994) Factors associated with onset of menopause in women aged 45–49. *Maturitas*, **19**, 83–92
Vermeulen, A. (1993) Environment, human reproduction, menopause, and andropause. *Environ. Health Perspectives*, *101* (Suppl. 2), 91–100

Tobacco and the health of women

M.A. Pope[1,3], M.J. Ashley[1,2] & R. Ferrence[1-3]

[1]*Ontario Tobacco Research Unit,* [2]*University of Toronto,* [3]*Addiction Research Foundation, Ontario, Canada*

Background and objectives: Tobacco is the leading, preventable cause of premature death and disability among women in many developed countries, yet tobacco continues to be marketed to women worldwide. This paper documents the impact of tobacco on the health of Canadian women, summarizes findings of particular relevance to women and reviews evidence that women may be more susceptible to some consequences of use.

Methods: Original research and review articles identified through Medline and the Smoking and Health database were assessed, as were pertinent reports and recent meta-analyses.

Findings: At least 10 500 deaths among Canadian women each year are attributable to smoking, and this rate will continue to increase. Lung cancer, ischaemic heart disease, chronic obstructive lung disease and stroke are the leading causes of these smoking-related deaths; lung cancer now exceeds breast cancer as the leading cause of death from cancer in this group. Women who smoke also have sex-specific risks and may be more susceptible to the effects of smoking on the lung and, possibly, ischaemic heart disease.

Conclusions: Policies and programmes aimed at prevention and cessation of smoking among women must continue to be public health priorities.

Smoking in pregnancy

I. Nerin, L. Sanchez Agudo, D. Guillén, M.J. Ruiz, R. Vicente & C. Toyas

Faculty of Medicine, University of Zaragoza, Spain

Objectives: To determine the prevalence of smoking in a group of pregnant women and to evaluate changes in tobacco habits and the response to medical advice during pregnancy.

Methods: We designed a questionnaire which was given at a personal interview immediately after delivery to women admitted to the obstetric services of the Red Cross Hospital in Barcelona, the university clinic and the Miguel Servet Hospital in Zaragoza over a period of two months. Women who had quit smoking during their pregnancy were telephoned after one year to evaluate the relapse rate.

Results: A total of 409 women were interviewed, 127 (31%) in the Red Cross Hospital, 110 (27%) in the university clinic and 172 (42%) in the Miguel Servet Hospital. The mean age of the women was 29.6 years (SD, 5.2). The important results are shown in Table 1.

Conclusions: The prevalence of smoking before pregnancy was 58%. Only 19% of the smokers quit smoking while pregnant on their own initiative, and many relapsed in the first year (47%). The results indicate the need to improve the information that pregnant women receive about tobacco and show that pregnancy and the post-partum period are the right time to carry out interventions against smoking.

Table 1. Smoking prevalence and control measures among pregnant women in three hospitals in Spain

Parameter	Red Cross Hospital		University clinic		Miguel Servet Hospital		Total	
	No.	%	No.	%	No.	%	No.	%
Prevalence of smoking during prior pregnancy	66	51.9	71	64.5	100	58.1	237	57.9
Medical advice given	54	42.5	52	47.2	73	42.5	179	43.8
Quitting rate	19	28.8	26	36.6	34	34	79	33.3
Relapses after one year	8	42.1	11	42.3	19	55.9	37	46.8

YOUTH AND TOBACCO

Prevalence

Tobacco use among French children

A.J. Sasco[1], M. Poncet, I. Gendre, R. Ah-Song, V. Benhaïm-Luzon

Unit of Epidemiology for Cancer Prevention
International Agency for Research on Cancer, Lyon, France

[1]Director of research at the Institut National de la Santé et de la Recherche Médicale, France. At the time of the conference, Dr Sasco was also Acting Chief, Programme for Cancer Control, World Health Organization.

Introduction

Health behaviour is often acquired in childhood or adolescence. As children who start to smoke at an early age have an increased risk of developing tobacco-related diseases while still young, tobacco smoking in this age group is a real public health problem. One way to fight this plague is to identify the risk factors for such addictive behaviour; indeed, the key to successful health promotion may be efficient, adequate education starting at a young age. In order to achieve long-term results and a healthy population in the years to come, it is crucial to concentrate our efforts on school-age children. The objectives of this study were, first, to quantify pupils' smoking habits and knowledge about tobacco and secondly to evaluate the population in one region of France at risk of becoming smokers.

Material and methods

The survey was conducted in the Loire region of France with an anonymous, self-administered questionnaire and involved a randomly selected, representative sample of 5% of schools, stratified on public or private and urban or rural. The study population comprised 92 classes with five grades in 32 schools. All necessary authorizations were obtained as well as the agreement of the school directors, teachers and parents.

The questionnaire is derived from an American model which was designed to evaluate the health habits and knowledge of pupils in the 'First National Child Survey' and prepared for that study by the American Health Foundation. It was translated and adapted to the European context, and errors and inconsistencies were checked by a reverse translation from French to English. The questionnaire was tested in a pilot study carried out in a school in Lyon, France (Sasco *et al.*, 1997). Two forms were used, one for grades CE1–CE2 (mostly children aged 7–9) and one for grades CM1–CLIS (children aged 10–12). The two questionnaires contained 60 and 71 questions, respectively, about behaviour and knowledge with regard to diet, safety measures, health habits and prevention. Questions about tobacco and alcohol consumption were included only for the higher grades.

The survey was conducted from April to June 1996. All the children present at the hours of the data collection were included. The questionnaires were filled in during school time under the joint supervision of teachers and ourselves (M.P., R.A.S.). The data were analysed with the SAS and EGRET programs.

Results

Out of a total population of 2057 pupils, eight were excluded: six by the teachers, one by the parents and one by the pupil. Thus, 2049 questionnaires were collected, 1069 in the lower grades and 980 in the higher grades. Our sample comprised 81% pupils from urban areas and 19% in rural areas. The survey on tobacco included the 980 pupils in the higher grades, of whom 50% were boys and 50% girls; only one child did not state her or his sex. The pupils were aged 8–13 years with a median of 11. The ethnic distribution showed a majority of Europeans (79%), with 11% Arabs, 1.8% Asians, 1.4% black Africans, 7.1% others and 0.4% unknown. The pupils most often lived with both parents (82%), but 13% lived with the mother only, 1.8% with the father only and 1.2% with other persons; 2% did not answer this question. Social class was variable, with 44% upper class, 35% median class and 17% lower class; data were not available for 4%. Practising one sport was reported by 71% of the pupils, while 28% had no regular physical exercise outside school hours.

Three questions in the questionnaire concerned tobacco: two about past history of smoking and one about intention to smoke. The results show that 12% of the children had already smoked at some time in the past, 4.3% during the month preceding the survey, and 13% planned to become smokers. Most children were aware of the health problems associated with tobacco use, particularly concerning lung disease. Indeed, most of them were aware of a causal link between smoking and diseases of the lung (90%) and heart (46%). Over 88% agreed that it is difficult to stop smoking.

The population of children who had ever smoked showed several particularities. They were usually boys (odds ratio [OR], 1.9; 95% confidence interval [CI], 1.3–2.9) and European (OR, 2.2; 95% CI, 1.2–4.3). They were fractionally older than the non-smokers, with a mean age of 10.7 *versus* 10.6 years. They more often lived with only one parent (OR, 1.7; 95% CI, 0.69–2.0) or with persons other than their parents (OR, 2.8; 95% CI, 0.74–11). The type of school and the area did not appear to be important (OR, 1.2; 95% CI, 0.74–1.9 for private school and 1.1, 0.65–1.9 for urban area), and socio-economic level played no large role (OR, 1.1; 95% CI, 0.69–1.7 for high level). The smokers had more often already tried alcohol (OR, 4.0; 95% CI, 1.9–8.5) than the non-smokers. The pupils who had ever smoked not only intended to smoke in the future (OR, 3.9; 95% CI, 2.4–6.6) but also intended to drink alcohol (OR, 1.9; 95% CI, 1.2–3.0). The absence of physical exercise decreased the risk (OR, 0.68; 95% CI, 0.41–1.1), while the absence of intention to graduate increased it (OR, 1.4; 95% CI, 0.66–2.8). The determinants of intending to smoke when adult were similar for those who had already smoked and those who not yet started. The main determinants were sex (OR, 1.9; 95% CI, 1.3–2.9 for boys), ethnic origin (OR, 2.2; 95% CI, 1.2–4.3 for European) and intention to drink alcohol (OR, 3.4; 95% CI, 2.1–5.6). Similar results were observed in a multivariate analysis, which is summarized in Table 1.

Discussion

Our study was well received, both by the children who filled in the questionnaire and by the school authorities. Only one child and one family refused to participate in the survey. Our sample covered 0.5% of the child population of the Loire region, and the results can be extrapolated to all children living in the area. Similar results have been obtained in other studies carried out in France and elsewhere. This survey demonstrates an association between children's smoking experience and intention to smoke and their ethnic origin, alcohol use and sex. These results show the importance of informing children at an early age about the risks to health associated with tobacco use, but much more than school-based information is needed to achieve conscious, responsible management of health.

Acknowledgments
We express our most sincere thanks to the pupils, teachers and directors of the schools who kindly participated in this study. Our thanks also go to the Ligue Nationale contre le Cancer, Comité de la Loire, for their generous support of the Aventure-Santé project. Dr Roland Ah-Song and Isabelle Gendre received Special Training Awards from the Unit of Epidemiology for Cancer Prevention of the International Agency for Research on Cancer.

Reference
Sasco, A.J., Marsot, M. & Gendre, I. (1997) [Health promotion: Knowledge and health habits of French primary school children: A pilot study] *Rev. Epidémiol. Santé Publ.*, **45**, S75–S76 (in French)

Table 1. Determinants of tobacco use

Determinant	Univariate		Multivariate	
	OR	95% CI	OR	95% CI
Sex				
Girl (reference)	1			
Boy	2.0	1.3–3.0	1.7	1.1–2.7
Age (years)				
< 10 (reference)	1			
10	4.4	0.58–32	4.9	0.65–38
11	6.0	0.80–44	6.6	0.87–50
≥ 12	7.6	0.97–59	9.4	1.5–76
Ethnic origin				
Non-European (reference)	1			
European	1.9	1.0–3.4	1.3	0.26–6.9
Family				
Both parents (reference)	1			
Only one parent	1.7	0.69–2.0	1.2	0.67–2.0
Other	2.8	0.74–11	2.2	0.54–9.0
School				
Private (reference)	1			
Public	1.2	0.74–1.9	1.2	0.72–2.1
Area				
Rural (reference)	1			
Urban	1.1	0.65–1.9	1.4	0.78–2.4
Socioeconomic level				
High	1.1	0.69–1.7	0.97	0.61–10
Median (reference)	1			
Low	0.48	0.23–1.0	0.42	0.20–0.89
Practice of sport				
Yes (reference)	1			
No	0.68	0.41–1.1	0.77	0.46–1.3
Alcohol use				
No (reference)	1			
Yes	4.0	1.9–8.5	3.9	1.8–8.3
Intention to graduate				
Yes (reference)	1			
No	1.4	0.66–2.8	1.3	0.60–2.6
Intention to smoke				
No (reference)	1			
Yes	3.9	2.4–6.6		
Drink alcohol				
No (reference)	1			
Yes	1.9	1.2–3.0		

Smoking habits of eighth- and ninth-grade schoolchildren in Halland County, Sweden

A. Baigi[1] & T. Melin[2]

[1]Research and Development Unit, Halland County Council, and
[2]School Health Services, Halmstad, Halland County, Sweden

Introduction

Most adult smoking habits have already been adopted before the age of 20. There is a very rapid increase in the numbers of new smokers among senior-school students— that is to say, grades 7–9 of the Swedish school system. In grade 7, although at least half of the students, both boys and girls, have experimented with smoking, habitual (daily) smoking is still rare. Two years later, however, by the age of 16, not only are many ninth graders regular smokers, but many of the remainder are occasional smokers, at risk of lasting nicotine dependence.

Smoking habits are known to differ between girls and boys. During the past two decades, the prevalence of smoking has increased markedly among girls, and now exceeds that among boys. In Sweden, however, many boys use snuff instead. Not only has the World Health Organization's goal of reducing tobacco use among young people not been achieved, but a recent European Community survey has shown smoking to be very prevalent among the young.

The reasons why young people use tobacco are complex. Nonetheless, they need to be clarified, as they are of crucial importance in planning preventive initiatives. One way of obtaining such information is to ask young people themselves, as was done in the present study. In an earlier study of lifestyle factors among people aged 18–74 in the County of Halland, in Sweden, a high prevalence of tobacco use was found among adolescents. At the same time, information from teachers, school medical officers, school nurses and information officers suggested that habitual smoking by teenagers had become prevalent even earlier, reaching a peak in grades 8 and 9. It was therefore decided that the patterns of tobacco use among young people merited further study.

The purpose of the present study was to trace the origins of habitual smoking and snuff use among the young, in order to provide a basis for planning future preventive measures.

Methods

The study was designed as a joint initiative by the public health department of Halland County Council and all six municipalities in the County. A working group was formed of one representative from each local authority to design a study of smoking habits at the senior-school level in all schools in the municipalities concerned. It was intended to include all eighth and ninth graders, a total of 6600 students. A questionnaire comprising relevant items concerning smoking habits was constructed.

During March 1994, questionnaires were sent to all eighth- and ninth-grade students in the County. Of these 6600 questionnaires, 5310 (80%) reached the students as intended. Of those who received the questionnaires, 5257 duly filled them in—a response rate of 99%. To facilitate comparison of the two grades, the data were sorted; to facilitate comparison with Sweden as a whole, the questionnaire items were designed to be comparable to the smoking-related items on the national substance-abuse questionnaire designed by the National Association for Information on Alcohol and Drugs.

Student's t test was used to determine the significance of differences between the sexes and between the eighth and ninth grades, both in the County as a whole and in Halmstad, the County town. As a complement to the strictly statistical analysis, the students' comments on smoking habits and the causes of nicotine dependence were also reviewed.

Results

The prevalence of smoking among eighth and ninth graders in the County of Halland was 18%. Daily smoking was more prevalent among girls than among boys, the respective figures being 21 and 16%, but actual daily consumption may in fact have been higher among boys, as 22% of the boys smoked > 10 cigarettes a day, as compared with 20% of the girls. The various municipalities in the County differed significantly in tobacco use by students, the prevalence being higher in the municipalities of Halmstad and Kungsbacka, which are the largest towns in the County. Comparison of the prevalence of smoking among ninth graders in Halland (17% for boys and 23% for girls) with corresponding figures for the country as a whole (20% for boys and 26% for girls) showed the rate to be lower in Halland.

In Halland, 11% of the boys and 12% of the girls in the two grades were daily smokers, although here too the rates were lower than the corresponding figures for the country as a whole. In Halland, the prevalence of smoking increased from 16% in grade 8 to 20% in grade 9. Thus, the bulk of the smokers were to be found in the 9th grade. Of boys in the two grades in Halland, 14% (approximately 700) used snuff, as compared to only 1.1% of the girls.

The questionnaire item 'Why do you smoke?' yielded abundant information on the risk factors involved. Response to this item was keen, which suggests that the teenagers were concerned about their health. A review of the answers showed that the predominant causes of smoking were fairly evenly distributed among both the municipalities and the various schools in the County. The predominant reasons given were: peer pressure, to be 'tough' and to feel grown up. These were followed by less prevalent contributory factors, some of the other reasons given being the example set by parents, 'It tastes good' (i.e. after having become nicotine-dependent), curiosity, 'It's thrilling' and 'It's relaxing'. Thus, progression to habitual smoking could be divided into three phases. The first is characterized by a need to appear trendy and grown-up and to be accepted by the peer group. Then follows discovery of what the children described as the positive attributes of smoking: that it 'tastes good' and that 'it is relaxing'. The final phase is characterized by second thoughts and a desire to reduce smoking or quit completely.

Discussion

Of the adult population of Halland, 22% are habitual smokers (Baigi, 1993). The figure is the same for men and women and almost the same as the prevalence among ninth graders. This suggests that most adult smokers become regular smokers by 15–16 years of age. Owing to the manifest addictive effect of nicotine, even occasional smokers generally become regular smokers. In the present study, the prevalence of smoking was found to increase from 16% in the eighth grade to 20% in the ninth grade. Although it is known that approximately 50% of young people have experimented with smoking by the age of 13.5, there are few smokers of this age in the sixth and seventh grades. Thus, the main increase in the numbers of smokers would seem to occur between the seventh and eighth grades.

Nicotine is the most addictive toxic constituent of tobacco.; it is also a harmful component. The prevalence of habitual smoking was almost the same among boys and girls, but if those who used at least one carton of snuff a week are included, the prevalence of daily nicotine consumption among boys increases strikingly. In most cases, consumption of one carton of snuff a week means that it is used daily. A very small proportion both smoke and take snuff on a daily basis. While there is every reason for concern over the marked increase in smoking among girls, it should be borne in mind that nicotine consumption is nevertheless very heavy among Swedish boys.

Owing to the spread of tobacco consumption among young people and the serious consequences of smoking, even passive smoking, Halland County Council has launched a comprehensive preventive programme. A secondary purpose of this programme is to reduce the incidence and severity of certain basic categories of disease such as asthma, lung cancer and cardiovascular diseases. To this end, the following specific aims have been set up:

- to stimulate public demand for a smoke-free environment;
- to promote the Tobacco-free School project, at least one health information officer is to be appointed in each municipality, whose principal task is to prevent incipient tobacco use;
- to establish a think-tank to evolve fresh ideas and suggest subjects for health education to be presented in an interesting and attractive manner;
- to combine the efforts of local education authorities and headmasters to solve the practical aspects of the preventive campaign;
- with the help of health information officers, arrange parent meetings outside the school;
- to launch continual questionnaire studies of tobacco usage (both smoking and snuff-taking) among young people;
- to increase awareness and knowledge of the harmful effects of tobacco, e.g. by means of information campaigns and education;
- to provide all those in the County who are engaged in anti-smoking initiatives with the necessary resources, e.g. videofilms, tape cassettes, brochures and exhibition material;
- to train supervisors who can run smoking cessation groups;
- to promote awareness among students and staff about the school policy on tobacco, with clearly defined goals and a realistic plan of action for their achievement;

- to promote self-confidence and self-image enhancement among students by appropriate training and attitude evaluation;
- liberal use of posters, visual aids and information campaigns;
- to run smoking cessation programmes among students and staff;
- to give certain students extra training about tobacco use to enable them to disseminate such knowledge among their classmates.

It is intended that these measures will constitute an overall campaign in which the school, parents and students form a tripartite coalition to work actively in a common preventive endeavour. As a complement, an epidemiological monitoring system has been planned for the surveillance of all schools in the County. Eventually, these endeavours will be combined with initiatives focused on alcohol consumption and other forms of substance abuse and dependence.

Reference
Baigi, A. (1993) H‰lsoprofiler i Halland 1982–91, FolkhÂlsosektion, Landstinget Halland 1991 [Health profiles in Halland County] (in Swedish)

Smoking trends among young adults in the United Kingdom

L. Owen & K. Bolling

Health Education Authority, London, United Kingdom

Despite a general decline in the prevalence of regular smoking among adults, recent surveys commissioned by the Health Education Authority for England have shown no evidence of any decline among persons aged 16–24. Indeed, among young women, the prevalence of smoking increased between 1994 and 1996. This rise is attributable solely to an increase among young women in manual occupations, as young women in non-manual occupations showed no change in prevalence.

We describe the smoking prevalence among all adults and adolescents and then show how the prevalence and trends differ for the young adults. We conclude with a consideration of communication strategies aimed at young adults who smoke. The data for adults are taken from the General Household Survey of the Office of Population Censuses and Surveys, and those for adolescents from a survey of secondary schools by the same Office. data on young adults in 1994–96 are extracted from the Health Education Authority's adult tracking survey.

Over the last 20 years, there has been a steady decline in cigarette smoking in the United Kingdom (Figure 1). Among men, the prevalence declined from 51% in 1974 to 28% in 1994. Among women, the decline in smoking over the same period was from 41 to 26%. For the most part, the prevalence has been significantly higher in men than in women, although it is worth noting that the gap between the two has narrowed over the years.

The prevalence of smoking among adolescents (aged 11–15), however, is very different (Figure 2): it has remained high over the last 15 years and has risen steadily over the last four years. Thus, in 1990, 10% of 11–15-year-olds were regular smokers, and this had risen to 13% by 1996. Direct comparisons of the smoking prevalences of adults and adolescents are complicated by the fact that the definitions of 'regular smoking' differ for the two groups: ≥ 1 cigarettes per day for persons aged ≥ 16 and ≥ 1 cigarettes per week for those aged 11–15. Figure 2 also shows that the smoking prevalence among adolescent girls is significantly higher than than that among boys, and, if anything, the gap appears to be widening. Thus, in 1996, 15% of adolescent girls and 11% of boys were regular smokers. The prevalence is strongly related to age, such that only 4% of 12-year-old girls are regular smokers compared with 33% of

Figure 1. Prevalence of cigarette smoking by sex among persons aged ≥ 16, England, 1974–94

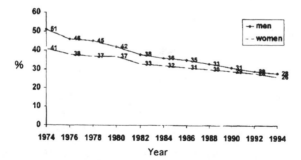

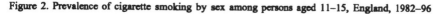

Figure 2. Prevalence of cigarette smoking by sex among persons aged 11–15, England, 1982–96

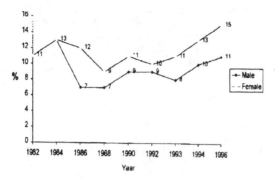

those aged 15. The figures for regular smoking among boys are 2% for 12-year-olds and 28% for 15-year-olds.

The smoking behaviour of young adults aged 16–24 has been relatively neglected, as they fall almost half-way between adults and adolescents. Figure 3 shows the trends over the past 20 years and illustrates the differences from the overall picture. The prevalence among males in this group fell from 47% in 1974 to 35% in 1994.; however, the decline with time was less than that for all males, and the steady downward trend seen for all males is not found in this age group. In fact, although the figures fluctuate slightly, the prevalence among 16–24-year-old males was exactly the same in 1984 and 1994: 35%. Over the same period, the rates for males of all ages fell by 8%. The trends for 16–24-year-old females show an almost identical picture: a decline from 41 to 34% over the 20-year period, which is slower than that for females of all ages, and no decline over the last 10 years (34% in both 1984 and 1994). In many ways, the trends in smoking in this group appear to have more in common with those of adolescents than those of adults. Interestingly, however, the male and female prevalences are almost the same, which is unlike the figures for adolescents, in which the prevalence among girls is significantly higher than that among boys.

The most recent figures on smoking among young adults are provided by the national tracking survey of the Health Education Authority, which is based on a sample of 17 000 adults per year. This survey shows that between 1994 and 1996 the prevalence of smoking was broadly static, with an overall prevalence of about 26%. This static situation is seen in all age groups except 16–24. In this group, the prevalence rose by 2% between 1994 and 1996, from 32 to 34%. There was an even more noticeable shift among 16–24-year-old females, with an increase of 5% between 1994 and 1996, from 28 to 33%, over a period when the prevalence in all other age groups showed little change. These limited data suggest that smoking in this age group is on the rise.

Figure 3. Prevalence of cigarette smoking by sex among persons aged 16–24, England, 1974–94

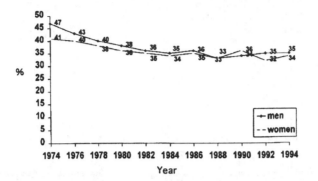

In the United Kingdom, smoking education campaigns aimed at adults have traditionally been centred around cessation, while adolescent smoking campaigns have focused on preventing uptake. The surveys show, however, that although 60% of young adult smokers take up smoking before the age of 16, a sizeable minority—40%—is actually taking up smoking at the age of ≥ 16. The presence of what we might call these 'late starters' suggests that amoking education campaigns for young adults should address both cessation and prevention of uptake.

Although the trends among young adults have shown signs of rising, there are reasons to believe that this age group may be responsive to health education campaigns that are appropriately targeted. For example, in the Health Education Authority's surveys, 60% of young adult smokers expressed a desire to quit, and 21% were currently trying to quit. There is also some evidence that young adult smokers are less dependent on nicotine than older smokers; in particular, young adult smokers have consumption levels lower than the average. Thus, in our recent survey, 31% of smokers aged 16–19 and 22% of all smokers smoked < 10 cigarettes per day. The cessation rates of such 'light' smokers do not differ from those of 'heavier' smokers, however, and in some respects they may be harder to influence if they do not identify themselves as addicted or habitual smokers.

It is important that any communication to this age group be appropriately targeted. Communications research at the Health Education Authority suggests that there is no universal strategy that is likely to meet the needs of such a heterogeneous group: 16–24-year-olds encompass those in the pre-family and family life stages; those who are still living in the parental home and those who are living independently; and people in a variety of social settings, including work, school, higher education and unemployment. Each of these sub-groups would ideally benefit from a customized communication strategy that reflects their social circumstances and predisposition to give up. Finally, any communication strategy that is designed to encourage smokers to quit must be backed up by the provision of smoking cessation support.

Smoking in transition: A longitudinal study of Scottish adolescents

S. Pavis, R. Bell, A. Amos &S. Cunningham-Burley

Department of Public Health Sciences and RUHBC,
University of Edinburgh, Medical School, Edinburgh, Scotland

The period of transition from school to work, occupational training or further education is of major importance in shaping young people's attitudes, values and behaviour. Few studies have looked at how changes in young people's lives over this period influence smoking behaviour. In this study, we followed-up 106 15-year-olds for 18 months. A mixture of qualitative and quantitative methods was used to map changes that occurred over this period in their lives, to contextualize their cigarette consumption and to provide insights into the meanings that they attach to their behaviour.

The study was designed to address two questions:

- What are the main patterns of smoking among young people in their final compulsory year at school (15- and 16-year-olds), and how do these relate to attitudes about smoking, sex, social and family relationships and occupational and educational aspirations?

- What is the immediate and longer-term direct and indirect impact of the transition from school to further education, training, employment or unemployment on smoking patterns and consumption and on its perceived function and role?

Design and method

The study cohort was recruited through two state comprehensive schools on the east coast of Scotland. The schools were co-educational, with exam results similar to the national average, in a catchment area that covered a range of socioeconomic groupings, both rural and urban. The sample size at first interview was 106 (Table 1). This cohort was large enough to allow statistical analysis of a range of health-related behavioural and occupational and educational destinations, while small enough to allow qualitative data collection and analysis. The sample appeared to be slightly skewed towards higher academic achievers but nonetheless included pupils with a wide range of academic destinations.

Respondents were interviewed three times over 18 months. A structured questionnaire and an in-depth semi-structured interview were used in each round. The questionnaire sought quantitative data on occupation (school, work, training, further education), academic achievement, future plans, income, leisure and social activities, health-related behaviour (smoking, alcohol, exercise) and the home situation. The interviews covered topics and issues raised in the questionnaire in greater depth to gain a deeper understanding of the respondents' lives and to locate their health-related behaviour within their social and cultural contexts. All interviews were tape-recorded and took 30–70 min to complete.

Key findings

The 18 months after the end of compulsory schooling were marked by significant changes in occupational status. Two patterns were discernable which reflect wider trends in Scotland: young people are staying on at school longer than before, and girls are more likely to stay on at school and less likely to enter training than boys. By round 3, 50% of girls and only 15% of boys were still at school.

The proportion of regular smokers (≥ 1 cigarettes per week) increased at each round among both males and females (Table 2). This increase was greater among young men, rising from 14% at round 1 to 47% at round 3, than among young women: 18% at round 1 to 33% at round 3.

Examination of the patterns and trends in individual pathways revealed considerable continuity and change in smoking behaviour over this period, many respondents moving backwards and forwards between different categories of smoking. For example, a notable sex difference is seen among the 76 respondents who at round 1 had never tried smoking or had tried it once: 75% of the female 'never' smokers in round 1 were still 'never' smokers by round 3, but only 41% of the males were still 'never' smokers in round 3.

Table 1. Numbers of pupils interviewed at each round by sex

Round	Male	Female	All	Response rate (%)
1	57	49	106	–
2	52	46	98	92
3	47	42	89	84

Table 2. Changing patterns of smoking status by sex (%)

Smoking status	Round 1 ($n = 106$)		Round 2 ($n = 98$)		Round 3 ($n = 89$)	
	Male	Female	Male	Female	Male	Female
Never/once	68	57	51	50	36	50
Used to	11	18	2	9	13	5
Sometimes	7	6	13	11	4	2
Regularly (> 1 per week)	14	18	33	30	47	33

Regular smoking among young people is usually defined as smoking ≥ 1 cigarette per week. In our study, this category comprised three sub-groups: (i) those who smoked solely with one group of friends and in one social setting: they described their behaviour as being 'sociable' or 'part of a group', and tended to smoke the least; (ii) those who smoked with various friends and in different social settings: they still talked of smoking as a social activity but tended to smoke more heavily; (iii) those who smoked with friends and on their own, at regular intervals and to punctuate the day: they tended to smoke the most heavily. Movement between these three types of regular smoking over the three rounds was not always progressive or unidirectional.

In round 1, all but one of the regular smokers smoked Kensitas Regal brand. At subsequent rounds, Regal remained the most popular brand but other brands became more popular, accounting for 29% at round 2 and 39% at round 3.

At each round, over two-thirds of regular smokers, both male and female, reported that the majority of their close friends were smokers. This finding supports the qualitative report that many regular smokers saw smoking as a social activity.

The qualitative part of the interviews revealed that this period of young people's lives is marked not only by occupational transitions but also by changes in friendship groups and social activities. The interviewees commented on changes in friendship groups which were associated with changes in smoking and other health-related behaviour. These changes were not restricted to persons who had left school and met new people; school attenders commented that changing classes often resulted in the formation of new friendships. Leisure patterns also changed, for example, the frequency and location of drinking alcohol. In rounds 1 and 2, alcohol was drunk, particularly by young men, in streets or parks or illicitly at home. By round 3, young people were more likely to drink in pubs and at discos, albeit still illegally. Changes in occupational status also appeared to influence alcohol consumption, the amount being consumed, particularly during the week, being controlled because of concern about the possible impact on performance at work or school. This was also a period of a marked increase in experimentation with illegal drugs, particularly cannabis, though few had become regular users.

Discussion

Most longitudinal studies on smoking among young people have focused on collecting quantitative data, and any qualitative data have tended to be limited in scope and depth and have been analysed within a quantitative paradigm. Our study is novel, in that detailed in-depth qualitative data were collected at each of the three rounds of interviews. These data therefore enabled us to explore continuity and changes in smoking over this period and the meaning that young people attached to them, and thus to investigate changes in smoking in the context of their experiences of the transition to adulthood.

Developing an appropriate method for analysing such a large, complex data set posed new and significant challenges. We adopted a case study approach in which individual biographies were analysed three times for links between the processes involved in becoming or not becoming a smoker and other transitional processes in their lives. This analysis is ongoing. We believe that a case study approach provides a depth of understanding individual biographies in the context of social transitions which is not captured in more traditional forms of longitudinal analysis. This can further our understanding of important social processes and their relationship to health-related behaviour.

The period between 15 and 17 years is marked by significant transitions in all aspects of young people's lives: social, economic and occupational. The process involved in whether or not a young person becomes a smoker is inextricably linked with these other aspects of their lives, in particular their friendship groups and social activities, including use of alcohol and illegal drugs. Previous research with younger adolescents has shown that becoming a smoker is not a straightforward, unidirectional process. This study indicates that this dynamic process continues into and beyond the mid-teens. This can be most 'richly' explored through in-depth analysis of individual biographical cases combined with aggregated data to identify trends, thereby giving insight into the operation of both social structure and individual agency in smoking uptake and maintenance.

Tobacco use among adolescents aged 10–16 in Gran Canaria, Canary Islands, Spain

J.M. Segura[1], J.R. Calvo[1], M.C. Navarro[1], M. Torres[1], M. López[1], A. López[1], J.C. Orengo[1], J. Calvo[1], M. Marrero[1], S. Flórez[2], A. Ramos[2], O. Rajas[2], S. Solano[2] & C. Jiménez[2]

[1] *University of Las Palmas de Gran Canaria, Canary Islands, and* [2] *Hospital de la Princesa, Madrid, Spain*

Objectives

In this survey, we tried to assess tobacco consumption among adolescents aged 10–16 on the island of Gran Canaria (Canary Islands, Spain). We also determined other characteristics related to their smoking behaviour, such as its frequency and quantity, and the ways they start smoking. We also explored their thoughts about tobacco as a risk factor for health.

Subjects and method

We carried out a descriptive, cross-sectional survey using cluster sampling, in which the clusters were groups of pupils in a classroom in a certain school. We divided our island into five geographic areas (north, south, centre, city and ouskirts of the main city). In each of them except for the city, we randomized a town, and in the selected town we randomized a primary and a secondary school for sampling. At least 25 pupils per age group and area were needed in order to ensure a 95% confidence level. In fact, we took more individuals per group because of the sampling method used.

A questionnaire was designed, consisting of 12 items, and the adolescents were asked to fill it in themselves anonymously, in the absence of the teacher but in the presence of one of a team of six interviewers who had been trained in conducting such work, in order to avoid conditioned answering. The data were processed with dBASE 5.0 and further analysed using Epi-Info 6.04 (Spanish version) by an epidemiologist.

Results

We rejected 13 questionnaires because of defective completion. Two pupils refused to take part in the survey. The smoking habits of the remaining participants are shown in Table 1. The age at starting to smoke was < 9 years for 17% of the boys and 10% of the girls; at 9–11 years for 24% of the boys and 20% of the girls; at 12–14 years for 46% of the boys and 56% of the girls and at ≥ 15 years for 12% of the boys and 13% of the girls. Among the smokers, 32% of the boys and 38% of the girls used tobacco daily, while 12 and 12% smoked only on weekends; 55% of the boys and 50% of the girls

Table 1. Smoking habits among adolescents aged 10–16 in the Canary Islands

Age (years)	No.		Smoking (%)									
			No response		None		Once		More than once		Regularly	
	Boys	Girls	Boys	Girls	Boys	Girls	Boys	Girls	Boys	Girls	Boys	Girls
10	90	98	3.3	5.1	83.3	88.8	5.6	4.1	5.6	1.0	2.2	1.0
11	120	98	1.7	4.1	80.0	84.7	8.3	6.1	9.2	3.1	0.83	2.0
12	118	103	1.7	0	76.3	82.5	11.7	12.6	8.5	3.9	1.7	0.97
13	109	107	1.8	2.8	44.0	48.6	22.9	14.0	17.4	17.8	13.8	16.8
14	81	100	0	0	43.2	25.0	19.8	26.0	22.2	29.0	14.8	20.0
15	83	88	1.2	0	45.8	25.0	19.3	21.6	21.7	31.8	12.0	21.6
16	82	92	0	1.1	32.9	27.2	18.3	23.9	26.8	25.0	22.0	22.8

smoked only occasionally. The number of cigarettes used weekly was ≤ 10 for 49% of boys and 45% of girls, but 17% of boys and 21% of girls reported smoking > 40 cigarettes per week. A large number of adolescents managed to buy cigarettes themselves; 43% bought cartons of 20 packs, and 20% bought single cigarettes.

Sixty-seven percent of boys and 66% of girls thought tobacco use was very harmful to their health, while 25% of the boys and 29% of the girls considered that it was bad for them. Only 1.5 and 0.4% considered that smoking was not harmful to health.

Conclusions

We focused on adolescents at school because of the difficulty of reaching those who do not go to school and because the aim of our study is to be the basis of future actions in health promotion and education, which will probably be developed in schools.

Our data show that a significant number of adolescents smoke. As the age at first contact with tobacco seems to be very low, our efforts in preventing young people from becoming smokers should address pupils in elementary school as well. We also found that a large percentage of adolescents manage to buy tobacco, and this finding should be taken into account by our Goverment. The fact that it is possible to buy single cigarettes in our country makes it easier for young people with very low incomes to accede to tobacco.

Although most of the adolescents interviewed knew that tobacco is harmful, this did not appear to affect them, and the knowledge had no influence on their habit. This finding and the fact that use of tobacco in our sample was more often daily than at weekends should be taken into consideration in health promotion campaigns.

Acknowledgements
This survey was supported by the Fundación Universitaria de Las Palmas and the Servicio Canario de Salud.

Incidence of tobacco smoking among students in Slovenian secondary schools

E. Stergar[1] & M.Tomori[2]

[1]Institute of Public Health of the Republic of Slovenia, and [2]School of Medicine, University of Ljubljana, Ljubljana, Slovenia

Background

The purpose of this paper is to present the incidence and prevalence of smoking among Slovenian students in secondary school (15–18 years old) and their attitudes towards cigarette smoking, the perceived health consequences of smoking and protective and risk factors for smoking. Two surveys were conducted, in 1995 and 1996. The study in 1995 was conducted under the aegis of the European School Survey Project on Alcohol and Other Drugs simultaneously in 26 European countries, all participants using the same methods. In the 1996 survey, 4706 students in 94 Slovenian secondary schools were studied.

Methods

For both surveys, random samples were drawn from lists of all enrolled students. The first survey covered 3600 first-year students; the answers of 2420 students born in 1979 were analysed. In the second survey, the answers of 4706 first- to fourth-year students were analysed. The individuals selected represented the 'key persons' in a classroom comprising up to 36 pupils. The mean age was 15 years and 9 months in the first survey and 17 years and 3 months in the second.

In both studies, the students were asked to complete a questionnaire. The questionnaire used in the first survey had 41 questions focused on use of alcohol, tobacco and illegal drugs during lifetime, last year and last month; questions on attitudes towards drug use, health risks of drug use and school performance were added. The questionnaire used in the second survey had 117 questions; part of the questionnaire was focused on the problem of suicide and self-destructive behaviour. Questions on the family, social support, health-related habits, sexual behaviour and attitudes to health were added for the Slovenian study.

The questionnaires were filled in anonymously in the presence of school counsellors during regular lessons but in the absence of teachers. The information obtained in both studies was kept strictly confidential.

Data were processed with the SPSS computer package (1995 study) and Statistica W (1996 study).

Results

In 1995, 41% of the first-year students reported never having smoked cigarettes. Nearly one third of the respondents who reported use of tobacco had smoked their first cigarette at the age of ≤ 11 years; the difference between boys and girls was significant at $p < 0.001$, more boys than girls having smoked their first cigarette at those ages. Most of the regular cigarette smokers had begun smoking on a daily basis when ≥ 14 years old, and, again, a larger percentage of boys had begun at those ages. With regard to frequency, 73% of the respondents said that they had not used tobacco during the 30 days preceding the survey, while 7.7% smoked < 1 cigarette per week. Of those who used tobacco weekly or daily, 81% smoked ≤ 10 cigarettes, with no difference in the number of cigarettes smoked by boys and girls. Occasional smoking was reported by 83% of students and regular cigarette smoking by 56%. They underestimated the harmful effects on health of occasional and daily tobacco use.

In the 1996 survey, 73% of the respondents said they were not smokers. Significant differences were seen between boys and girls ($p < 0.0000$; contingency coefficient [C], 0.08): girls were more often non-smokers or smoked 1–10 cigarettes per day, while boys were more often moderate or heavy smokers. Significant differences ($p < 0.0000$) were seen for both boys and girls according to the year of schooling: the higher the year the greater the proportion of smokers. Analyses of groupings of non-smokers, light smokers and other smokers revealed certain protective factors. The contingency coefficients for attitudes to health promotion were 0.36 for avoiding tobacco smoking, 0.22 for not drinking alcohol, 0.23 for not using illicit drugs; pupils who agreed strongly or very strongly with these attitudes were more often non-smokers. More non-smokers assessed their lifestyle as healthy or very healthy ($C = 0.31$) or felt optimistic about their future ($C = 0.10$), had grown up in stable families with emotional support from their parents and friends ($C = 0.13$) and who showed no or little depression on Zung's scale ($C = 0.12$). Non-smokers more often engaged in 'positive' spare-time activities, such as athletics ($C = 0.16$) and hobbies such as writing, drawing ($C = 0.11$), reading books ($C = 0.11$) and playing a musical instrument ($C = 0.08$). Pupils who smoked were more likely to use legal and illegal drugs, to engage in 'negative' leisure time activities (frequently going to a disco, hanging around, dancing wildly or playing slot machines) and to date.

The results of the two surveys are complementary. They reveal the prevalence of smoking among secondary-school students, the determinants of adolescent smoking, protective and risk factors and changes in smoking behaviour during schooling. The information should be used as a solid basis for planning preventive programmes for schoolchildren and young people. A comparison of the data for students in the first class in 1995 and 1996 shows minimal changes in smoking prevalence, but comparison with data for 1990, when the first survey of secondary-school students was performed in Slovenia, shows a decrease of nearly 10% in non-smokers, especially among girls.

Prevalence of smoking among Moscow schoolchildren and approaches to prevention

A.A. Alexandrov, V.Yu. Alexandrova & E.1. Ivanova

National Research Centre for Preventive Medicine, Moscow, Russian Federation

The danger of smoking is well known; data from our centre show that smoking even three to four cigarettes per day shortens the mean life span by one year. Yet, there are more than 18 million male and 5 million female smokers aged 25–64 in Russia, most of whom acquire the habit at an early age. Our goal was to evaluate the prevalence of smoking among Moscow schoolchildren and to study means for prevention.

Surveys

Since 1986, we have performed annual suveys among schoolchildren, obtaining information on smoking status from 'form leaders'. Thus, two children in each form fill in a questionnaire on the number of smokers and the extent of smoking among their classmates. The answers usually correspond, at least for an entire school. The answers of the form leaders compare well with those to anonymous questioning, so that it is relatively easy to acquire data. Our annual questioning of 220–318 adolescents thus provided information on 3000–5000 schoolchildren.

This method was applied in one Moscow district, where the questioning of 220 persons provided the smoking status of 3062 schoolchildren. In 1995, 30% of boys and 18% of girls aged 11–17 were smokers. The prevalence increased from 8.9% in boys and 1.8% in girls in the fifth grade to 52% and 43% in the 11th grade (Figure 1). The sharp rise in smoking prevalence among boys in the sixth form and in girls in the seventh form indicate the necessity of preventive measures for 11–12-year olds.

The prevalence of smoking among schoolboys has been stable over the last decade, at 28–32%, except in 1993 when there was sharp decline in regular smoking. The prevalence of regular smoking among girls increased from 5.4% in 1986 to 12% in 1996, with the same sharp decline in 1993. The prevalence among all girls increased during the decade, from 12 to 18%. We attribute the sharp decline in 1993 to the beginning of economic reforms in our country, when a drastic rise in cigarette prices made it impossible for most schoolchildren to purchase cigarettes. Comparative stabilization of the economy resulted in an increase in the number of regular smokers to the previous level. Tobacco advertising, which began in 1992–93, has not significantly affected the prevalence, although its contribution is clear and its prohibition necessary.

In a survey of 15-year-old students at three vocational training schools with Fagerström's questionnaire, one of every 10 students showed marked tobacco dependency. In only 15% of cases, the adolescent's immediate milieu had negative reactions and made efforts to stop the child from smoking; 20% were indifferent.

Figure 1. Prevalence of smoking among schoolchildren in forms 5–11, Moscow, 1995

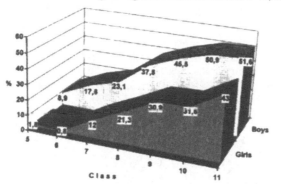

Prevention

Within a programme for the prevention of precursors of atherosclerosis, we examined a random sample of 12-year-old schoolboys, comprising 477 pupils at seven of 44 schools in one district (intervention group) and 528 boys at 16 of 30 schools in a second district (control group). They were examined every year until graduation and then once again five to six years after graduation. The preventive measures were aimed at disturbances of the lipid spectrum, elevated blood pressure, obesity and smoking, and included individual and group sessions with children and their parents and distribution of written medical information.

The initial smoking rate was found to be 0.5% in the intervention district and 0.0% in the control district; the corresponding rates were 6.3 and 1.0% in 13-year-olds and 15 and 25% in 15-year-olds, the difference being significant. There was no significant difference in the rates for 17-year-olds (39 and 43%). When the population was examined again five years after the end of the intervention, there were 58% smokers in the intervention district and 60% in the control district. Preventive measures must therefore be continuous, and anti-tobacco programmes are necessary for adolescents transiting from school to adult life.

The results of this programme are comparable to those of another intervention programme involving 1121 and 1963 children of a similar age group aimed only at smoking prevention. The measures included individual and group talks, lectures on various aspects of smoking abuse, visual demonstration of the immediate harmful effects of tobacco, slides, films and posters, anti-smoking contests and the development of psychological skills for resisting smoking. There were 10% fewer new smokers in the intervention group than in the control group, even three years after the end of the preventive measure. The mono-factorial prevention programme addressed the whole population, while the multi-factorial programme described above was more individual and addressed not only the schoolchildren but also their parents.

On the basis of this experience, we have designed a school course on smoking prevention for the first to the eleventh grades, consisting of 15 lessons, and have begun teachers' training. This is part of the State programme on smoking prevention. Some difficulties that we have encountered are the small number of trained teachers, inadequate financing and reluctance of school administrators to assign enough time for health education. The course is based on developmental psychology. Information on the harmfulness of smoking is given to junior schoolchildren in the form of fairy tales; adolescents are trained to make their own decisions and to oppose undesirable influences of their peers; the role and importance of advertising are discussed. The schoolchildren participate in plays, such as 'Court-room session: Mankind versus the cigarette' and in poster competitions. Consultations are available for parents whose children smoke. Senior students take part in discussions, competitions and plays in order to reinforce their anti-tobacco positions.

We have begun by a course of 18 lessons for fifth and sixth graders in one Moscow district and a supporting course for sixth and seventh graders consisting of 10 lessons.

Conclusions

The smoking rates in children and adults indicate the existence of a smoking epidemic. The widespread habit of smoking among Moscow schoolchildren shows the necessity for State preventive programmes. Multifactorial and monofactorial prevention reduces the prevalence of smoking, but the effect ends with termination of the intervention.

Patterns of tobacco use among Russian students

M.R. Torabi & J.W. Crowe

Department of Applied Health Science, HPER School, Indiana University, Bloomington, Indiana, United States

Tobacco use is the most readily preventable cause of premature death; it is a worldwide problem, with a significant impact on health and well-being (Melia & Swan, 1986; Aoki *et al.*, 1988; Torabi, 1989–90; Crowe *et al.*, 1994; Johnston *et al.*, 1994; Indiana Prevention Resource Center, 1995). In order to design an effective tobacco education programme, it is important to understand smoking patterns and the underlying factors associated with smoking in different cultures. The purpose of this study was to examine the prevalence and pattern of tobacco use among a sample of seventh- to ninth-grade students in the Russian Federation.

Method

A questionnaire containing 11 closed and open-ended questions, adapted from a study of youth risk behaviour by the Centers for Disease Control and Prevention in the United States, was tested among a sample of 210 Russian students, and the questions were slightly modified as a result. A cluster sampling technique was used to select 1118 seventh- to ninth-grade students in urban and rural schools in the district of St Petersburg. The data were analysed by descriptive methods and chi-squared testing of statistical significance. The descriptive findings were also compared with current data on tobacco use among American students in the same age range.

Results

Of the 1118 students who participated in the study, 46% were girls and 54% were boys; 16% were 13 years old, 52% were 14, and 32% were ≥ 15. About 3.7% had ever used smokeless tobacco, as compared with 13% of American students. All cigarette smoking during their lifetime was reported by 50% of Russian students aged 13, 56% of those aged 14 and 62% of those aged ≥ 15; this gradual increase was significant ($\chi^2 = 9.01$; $p < 0.01$). Regular smoking was reported by 22% aged ≤ 13, 32% aged 14 and 37% aged ≥ 15 ($\chi^2 = 16.05$; $p < 0.01$).

The ages at which smoking started are shown in Table 1. Younger students were more likely to have started smoking early than older students ($\chi^2 = 45.5$; $p < 0.01$). Smoking of cigarettes at school during the previous 30 days was reported by 10% aged ≤ 13, 19% aged 14 and 23% aged ≥ 15 ($\chi^2 = 15.82$; $p < 0.01$).

All smoking during their lifetime was reported by 64% of the girls and 52% of the boys ($\chi^2 = 18.2$; $p < 0.01$); the difference between girls and boys with regard to the age at which they smoked a whole cigarette for the first time (Table 2) was also significant ($\chi^2 = 86.0$; $p < 0.01$). Furthermore, a higher percentage of girls (37%) than boys (28%) had ever smoked regularly ($\chi^2 = 13.5$; $p < 0.01$), and the girls were younger when they had started to do so (Table 2). The percentage that had smoked during the previous 30

Table 1. Ages of 1118 students at starting to smoke, Russia

Age group (years)	Age at starting to smoke (%)			
	< 9	9–10	11–12	≥ 13
≤ 13	1.8	2.5	8.2	4.5
14	1.9	2.5	6.5	17.0
≥ 15	2.1	3.1	4.0	24.5

Table 2. Smoking behaviour of 1118 students by sex, Russia

Age group (years)	Smoking behaviour (%)			
	First smoked a whole cigarette		Started smoking regularly	
	Boys	Girls	Boys	Girls
< 9	3.6	10.2	1.4	2.6
9–10	1.6	9.6	4.3	7.9
11–12	11.2	18.0	4.3	7.9
≥ 15	26.2	11.6	17.2	17.5

days was 31% for girls and 24% for boys ($\chi^2 = 9.99$; $p < 0.01$), and a higher percenatage of girls (23%) than boys (15%) had smoked at school during the previous 30 days ($\chi^2 = 13.5$; $p < 0.01$). The girls also smoked more cigarettes per day than boys (Table 3; $\chi^2 = 14.6$; $p < 0.01$).

Discussion

Smoking is thus very prevalent among seventh to ninth graders in Russia, and a small percentage have tried smokeless tobacco. More girls than boys smoked cigarettes; they started smoking at an earlier age, smoked more cigarettes and were more likely to smoke at school than boys. The younger students started smoking earlier, indicating a trend towards a higher smoking prevalence. Educational programmes are therefore essential and should be begun at an early age, both at home and at school. Advertising and promotional activities of tobacco companies, which glamourize this destructuve behaviour must be banned completely.

References

Aoki, M., Hisamichi, S. & Tominaga, S. (1988) *Smoking and Health 1987*, New York. Excerpta Medica
Crowe, J.W., Torabi, M.R. & Nakurnkhet, N. (1994) A cross-cultural study of samples of adolescents' attitudes, knowledge, and behavior related of smoking. *Psychol. Rep.*, **75**, 1155–1161
Indiana Prevention Resource Center (1995) *Alcohol, Tobacco, and Other Drug Use by Indiana Children and Adolescents—1995*, Bloomington
Johnston, L.D., O'Malley, P.M. & Bachman, J.G. (1994) *National Survey Results on Drug Use from the Monitoring the Future Study, 1975–1993*, Vol. 1, *Secondary School Students*, Rockville, Maryland: National Institute on Drug Abuse

Table 3. Numbers of cigarettes smoked per day during the previous 30 days among 1118 students, by sex

No. of cigarettes	Boys (%)	Girls (%)
1–5	15.1	19.3
6–10	4	6.6
11–20	2.2	3.1
> 20	1.4	2.6

Melia, R.J.W. & Swan, A.V. (1986) International trends in mortality rates for bronchitis, emphysema, and asthma during the period 1971–1980. *World Health Stat. Q.*, **39**, 206–217

Torabi, M.R. (1989–90) Tobacco use by samples of American and Turkish students: A cross-cultural study. *Int. Q. Commun. Health Educ.*, **10**, 241–251

Prevalence and trends of cigarette smoking among children and adolescents in Siberia

D. Denisova

Institute of Internal Medicine, Novosibirsk, Russian Federation

Introduction

Tobacco use accounts for nearly 3 million deaths each year and has been identified as the leading cause of preventable death in the developed world. The results of the World Health Organization MONICA Project show that the mortality and morbidity rates from cardiovascular disease in western Siberia (Novosibirsk) are higher than in other European coutries. The purpose of this study was to investigate the prevalence of and trends in cigarette smoking among schoolchildren in various parts of Siberia.

Materials and methods

A sample of 1318 children, 660 boys and 658 girls aged 10–14 were studied in Novosibirsk in 1984–85. In 1989–90, 662 of the same children (317 boys and 345 girls) were studied again, when they had reached the age of 15–17; 619 (319 boys and 300 girls) were monitored at the age of 15–17 in 1994. In Chukotka, the far north region of Russia, a cross-sectional study of 322 native and non-native adolescents (165 boys and 157 girls) was conducted under expedition conditions in 1990. The surveys were carried out with standardized methods according to World Health Organization recommendations. The studies included an interview with a standardized questionnaire to elicit information about smoking, physical activity, alcohol consumption; anthropometry (weight, height, body mass index); double measurement of arterial blood pressure; biochemical analysis of blood (total cholesterol, triglicerides, high-density lipoprotein cholesterol, thiocyanate) and 24-h dietary recall. The parents received a questionnaire by mail. Subjects were considered to be smokers if they smoked ≥ 1 cigarette per week.

Results

The prevalence of smoking among Novosibirsk schoolboys aged 10–14 was 15%; 43% of them smoked weekly, and the peak of smoking onset was at the age of 11–12. The prevalence of smoking among schoolgirls aged 10–14 was not determined. In the repeated survey of the same children after five years, the prevalence of smoking among boys had increased from 12% at the age 10–12 to 45% at the age of 15–17, and 19% of 15–17-year-old girls were smokers. Most of the smokers (42% of the boys and 13% of the girls) smoked every day. The prevalence of smoking among the young in Chukotka was the same among natives and non-native boys: 40–41%; among girls, the percentage of smokers was higher in natives (23% versus 13%). The study of adolescents in the next five-year period in Novosibirsk showed some decrease in the weekly smoking rate in boys, from 45 to 34%, and the percent of daily smokers decreased significantly, from 42% in 1990 to 25% in 1994. A negative association between cigarette smoking and blood high-density lipoprotein cholesterol concentration was seen in the adolescents. The serum thiocyanate concentrations were correlated positively with the smoking rate and negatively with the concentrations of blood high-density lipoprotein cholesterol. The mean concentrations of serum thiocyanate were 36.6 among daily smokers and 23.5 in non-smokers.

Conclusions

A high prevalence of smoking was seen among adolescents in Siberia, with no significant difference between those in Novosibirsk and Chukotka. Girls began to smoke later than boys. Regular smoking had a negative effect on the blood high-density lipoprotein cholesterol concentration. The prevalence of cigarette smoking among Siberian adolescents is similar to that in the Siberian adult population according to data from the MONICA Project in Novosibirsk.

Smoking among secondary-school students in Bangladesh

N. Islam

ADHUNIK, Dhaka, Bangladesh

Introduction

Smoking is very prevalent in Bangladesh, but the only systematic survey that has been carried out among secondary-school children is the one by myself and S. Alam in 1994, supported by BMRC and the World Bank, which involved 7402 students. We therefore decided to conduct a survey in 30 secondary schools in the capital city of Dhaka and in the port city of Chittagong, which is the second largest city in the country, situated 340 km from Dhaka. Communication between the two cities is excellent, and there is a free flow of people of all ages and categories. As Dhaka is the capital, students come from all outlying districts; in Chittagong, most of the students are local.

Materials and methods

A baseline prevalence survey of tobacco habits was conducted among 13 887 students in 30 schools, which were chosen randomly in the two cities, with 7825 in Dhaka and 6062 in Chittagong. The students were interviewed and given a structured questionnaire with questions that could be answered easily by children aged ≥ 10 years, requesting information on age, class, religion, place of residence, family background, economic conditions and the reasons for smoking, how it was initiated, age at starting, daily consumption, reasons for quitting and their knowledge about the hazards of smoking. None had been exposed to an anti-tobacco campaign. Before the questionnaire was distributed, the study was described briefly and instructions were given on how to fill it in. The questionnaires were anonymous, and the students were assured of the confidentiality of the information. All of the students filled in the questionnaire.

Results

Most of the students in Dhaka (53%) were in the age group 13–14. Most (96%) lived with their parents, while 2.7% lived with relatives and a few in hostels. In Chittagong, 46% of the students were aged 13–14, and 96% lived with their parents.

Of the 7825 students interviewed in Dhaka, 873 (11%) were current smokers, 6534 (84%) had never smoked, and 336 (4.3%) were ex-smokers. The prevalence of smoking was 2.3% among 11–12-year-olds but 35% among 13–14-year-olds; by the age of 15–16, it had reached 63%. In Chittagong, the prevalence of smoking was 14%, 85% had never smoked, and 1% were past smokers. The prevalence in the age group 11–12 was 9.7% but was 37% at 13–14 and 53% at 15–16.

In Dhaka, 383 of the smokers (44%) had started to smoke at the age of 13–14, 21% at 10 years of age, 21% at 11–12 and 13% had started at the age of 15. In Chittagong, 71% of the students had started to smoke at 13–14, 18% at 11–12, 7.2% at the age of 10 and 3.8% at 15 years of age. The consumption was ≤ 5 cigarettes per day for 80% of the students, 6–10 by 14% and > 10 by 5.5% in Dhaka and ≤ 5 cigarettes per day for 78%, 6–10 by 18% and > 10 by 3.8% of students in Chittagong.

In Dhaka, 73% of the students started to smoke because of the influence of their friends, and 4.2% acquired the habit at home, while 19% did not admit to any influence.

The corresponding figures in Chittagong were 66, 12 and 21%, respectively.

Discussion

The first survey of the prevalence of smoking among schoolchildren carried out among 7402 students by ourselves in 1994 showed prevalence rates of 5% in Dhaka and 6% in Chittagong. The present study involved 13 887 students and showed rates of about 35–37% among 13–14-year-olds and 53–63% at age 15–16. The similarity of the observations in the two cities indicates that the findings are representative of the whole country.

A study in urban Delhi, India, among children aged 12–19 in six schools in 1978 showed that 9.8% smoked, the frequency increasing to 5.4% at age 14 and 27% at age 19. Of the 102 students who smoked, only 35% did so regularly (Babu et al., 1978). Thus, the rates in Bangladesh are almost double those in Delhi. Yen et al. (1990) in Taipei found an average smoking rate of 33% among students in grades 7–9, the rate increasing with grade (21, 33 and 46%). The children had started smoking around the age of 10. These findings are similar to ours.

Various factors can contribute to smoking. The striking feature of our survey is that the major contributing factor was not parental smoking but peer influence. The anti-tobacco movement must pay greater attention to children at secondary-school level. Educational programmes should be designed to propagate knowledge about the hazards of tobacco to students.

References

Babu, S.D., Chuttani, C.S. & Murty, N.S. (1978) Some epidemiological factors related to smoking among secondary school children of Delhi urban area. Int. J. Epidemiol., 2, 183

Yen, D.D. et al. (1990) E Research about the Taipei Junior High School Students Smoking Behaviour, Taipei, John Tung Foundation

Smoking: A rising ill among Malaysian youth

M.A. Kolandai

Consumers Association of Penang, Malaysia

Introduction

Adolescents in Malaysia have been a concern to society and have occupied much media attention over the past two years. The web of social ills in which they have been caught includes smoking, drug abuse, loafing, gangsterism and baby dumping. I wish to describe here the conflicts and contradictions confronting young people, which are encouraging them to smoke.

Malaysia is a multi-ethnic society where Islam is the official religion. It has a population of about 20 million; 45% of the population is under the age of 20, and 20% is between the ages of 10 and 20. It is the latest target of the cigarette companies, and the prevalence of smoking is growing at a rate of about 3% per annum. Some key anti-smoking actions have been taken by the authorities which are relevant to the young, but there are some obvious contradictions in their implementation:

• Although cigarette advertisements in the media are banned, advertisements are allowed at the point of sale and indirect cigarette advertisements appear in the media, with aggressive brand-name advertising.

• A religious *fatwa* issued by the National Islamic Council forbidding smoking for Muslims is not gazetted or implemented at State level.

• While people under the age of 18 are forbidden to smoke or buy cigarettes and there is a ban on cigarette vending machines, major international and local sports events are sponsored by tobacco companies and top Government officials officiate at and endorse activities sponsored by these companies.

Smoking among Malaysian youth

The prevalence of smoking is increasing among young Malaysians. In a survey conducted in 1994 involving 1000 teenagers around Kuala Lumpur, 71% smoked, whereas in a study in 1985 of 4106 schoolchildren in the same area, only 9.8% smoked (Thambypillai, 1985). In a survey conducted among 16-year-olds in a school in the State of Penang in 1993, 41% of the boys smoked. In a survey among 4347 youths aged 13–25 in 1996, the reasons given for smoking included relieving stress, getting 'a high', for the taste, for a 'macho' image, for satisfaction and for inspiration. The largest percentage of teenagers who smoked (72%) came from poor families, as among adults (Chapman & Wong, 1990).

As mentioned above, multinational tobacco companies are notorious for getting round the ban on direct advertising, by selling cigarette-brand-related products, sponsoring activities that are appealing to young people, such as rock concerts, music shows on television, dance competitions and all major international and local sports tournaments, including the last Olympic Games. The Malaysian Tobacco Company, a local subsidiary of British–American Tobacco, organizes special events for young people, such as 'freak-outs' and 'bunjee jumping'. Some companies have television programmes featuring, for example, daring sports and feature films.

Not only is the ban on direct cigarette advertising in Malaysia a farce, but indirect advertising appears to be more insidious and effective. In a survey conducted in July 1997 involving 32 boys and 38 girls aged 14–17, 45% identified the indirect advertisements on television as cigarette advertisements, as the companies wish them to do. When asked to describe the advertisements, 58% found them appealing, 15% found them interesting and 12% found them stylish. When asked to describe smoking, 14% said it gave them inspiration, 10% said it was adult, 7% said it was stylish, 7% said it was macho and 6% said it was fun.

There has been a long-standing disagreement within Muslim circles about whether smoking is *haram* (forbidden) or whether it is *makruh* (discouraged). In March 1995, the National Religious Council determined that it was *haram* for Muslims. This has serious consequences, since Muslims form the largest ethnic group of smokers, 24%, the majority of tobacco growers are Muslims, and many Muslims are involved with the tobacco companies. Many are unaware of the *fatwa*, and some are still confused about whether smoking is *haram* or *makruh*. In our survey, 74% of the students said smoking was *haram* and 26% of them said it was *makruh*. If most Muslim youths believe that smoking is *haram*, it is confusing for them to see adult Muslims smoking, engaging in tobacco cultivation and promoting and selling cigarettes. In our modern, materialistic, urban lifestyle, however, the young people know that on many occasions public health and well-being take second place to economic concerns.

One of the reasons why Malay youths are susceptible to smoking is their rural roots, where for generations they have been exposed to a traditional culture of smoking. Furthermore, with rural–urban migration, Malay youth may have difficulty in adjusting to the fast-paced, competitive, materialistic lifestyle in nuclear families, which is in sharp contrast to their slow-paced, cooperative and community lifestyle in extended families. In their search for a new identity and friends, smoking appears to provide quick 'status' and 'maturity' and a new identity. They also believe that if the product were bad, the Government would have banned it. The Government is viewed as the guardian, protector and provider for the people. When young people were asked what action the Government should take if smoking is dangerous for health, 67% said cigarettes should be banned, 34% said tobacco cultivation should be banned, and 51% suggested a ban on cigarette advertisements on television.

Conclusions

A comprehensive national policy on tobacco control is needed, which is respected by all sectors of society. We must stop paying lip service and take concrete action. Some of the suggestions made by young people are:

- to ban all forms of cigarette advertisement and promotion, including the sponsorship of sports events;
- to phase out tobacco cultivation;
- to implement the *fatwa* on smoking;
- to increase taxes on tobacco and increase the price of cigarettes substantially so that young people cannot afford to buy them;
- to make the warning on cigarette packs more serious and larger and
- to extend no-smoking zones to more public areas and all places of worship.

Reference
Thambypillai, V. (1985) Smoking among urban Malysian school children. *Soc. Sci. Med.*

Smoking behaviour of Taiwanese adolescents: A case study of a senior technical high school

N.-Y. Chiu, L.-Y. Hsieh & S. Mo

Departement of Psychiatry, Changhua Christian Hospital, Changhua, Taiwan

Although the harmful effects of smoking are well known, there are still many smokers in Taiwan. Previous reports from the Executive Yuan showed that the prevalence of smoking among young people aged 15–19 was 6.0%. Understanding the patterns of tobacco use among adolescents and their knowledge, attitudes and perceptions is crucial to the effort of reducing tobacco-related morbidity and mortality by smoking prevention and interventions. We conducted a survey in a senior high school.

Materials and methods

The subjects were 1188 students in 25 classes in a public senior technical high school in a rural area of Taiwan. The students completed a questionnaire requesting information on smoking behaviour, willingness to quit smoking, anti-smoking attitudes and knowledge about the harmful effects of smoking. The students answered the questionnaire anonymously in the absence of teachers. Properly completed questionnaires were obtained from 1119 students comprising 1022 boys and 97 girls. The data were analysed by analysis of variance with the SPSS program.

Results

Overall, 7.3% of the students, 7.8% of the boys and 1.1% of the girls were current smokers, i.e. had smoked within the past 30 days; 13% had ever tried a cigarette. The prevalence was thus higher among boys than girls, but no significant difference was found with regard to grade or family background. The average age at starting smoking was earlier than reported previously. Frequent smoking ($\geq$ 20 cigarettes during the previous 30 days) was also begun earlier, usually in junior high-school. The latency between initiation and frequent smoking was about 1.5 years. Initiation usually occurred at school at the invitation of classmates, from curiosity or for fun.

The reasons given by frequent smokers for their habit were to alleviate depression and to release tension. They usually smoked in entertainment establishments and at school while meeting with friends during leisure time. Most of them smoked 6–10 imported cigarettes per day, a larger number than in previous studies; 69% had low nicotine dependence.

Most of the students, including the smokers, were aware of the harmful effects of smoking, although non-smokers were better informed than smokers. The media were the main source of information about tobacco. The main reasons for failing to give up smoking were unhappiness and boredom; few smokers had sought help from others. Although many of the students' parents smoked, most disapproved of smoking by adolescents.

Suggestions

Because of the trend towards an earlier age at starting smoking, anti-smoking education should begin in primary school. The influence of peers on adolescents should be taken into account in anti-smoking programmes. As there is a close relationship between emotion and adolescent smoking behaviour, proper management of their emotional problems is crucial. Anti-smoking education should be conducted in cooperation with parents, and schools should have comprehensive anti-smoking projects and additional education for smokers. The media, social, medical and public welfare organizations and the Government should enhance their anti-smoking efforts. Other aspects, such as family status, the attitudes of parents, the characteristics of the students, social adaptability and scholastic achievement should also be explored.

Tobacco use among adolescents in Mongolia

Ts. Sodnompil, Sh. Oyunbileg & D. Lhkaijav

Health Management, Information and Education Centre, Ulaanbaatar, Mongolia

Background

The objective of this study was to evaluate current tobacco use and trends among adolescents, its causes, and directions for future action. We conducted a descriptive study in autumn 1996 based on answers to a questionnaire comprising 120 questions, using probability sampling methods, simple random sampling and cluster sampling. The survey covered 2040 young people aged 10–20 (1% of all those in the country), 80% of whom were schoolchildren and students, 10% of whom were unemployed street children and 10% of whom were children working as herders or in other occupations. The survey was carried out in four *aimags* differing in natural, climatic and socioeconomic characteristics and in six districts of the capital city. A database was created in two files by means of the DBase III Plus program in DOS. We calculated the standard division and dependent and independent variables using the Epi Info 6 program.

The results of the survey will form the basis of a national programme on the health of pupils and adolescents to be implemented by the Government in 1997–2000.

Findings

Of the 2040 adolescents involved in the survey, 49.7% were male and 50.3% female; 38% were aged 10–13, 27% were aged 14–16 and 35% aged 17–20. With regard to level of education, 35% had primary education, 57% had secondary education and 5.5% were uneducated. Schoolchildren represented 64%, 12% were students, 6.7% were workers, 0.9% were officers, 2.6% were herders and 5.0% were street children; 8.6% were unemployed and not enrolled in school. The place of residence was in the city for 65% and in the countryside for 35%; 74% lived in families of four to six people, and 26% lived in families consisting of more than seven members.

Two children out of three (66%) lived in a family with one or more smokers; 79% had fathers who smoked, 13% had brothers who smoked, and 8.0% had mothers who smoked. About 19% of the young people had sufficient knowledge about the ill effects of smoking, 49% had satisfactory knowledge, 12% had insufficient knowledge and 19% had no idea, indicating that these teenagers had inadequate knowledge about the hazard ($p < 0.005$).

Nearly 16% of the respondents smoked and had started smoking at an average age of 16.7 ± 2.5 years; males had started at 16.8 ± 2.5 years and females at 17.2 ± 2.1 years ($p = 0.03$). The number of smokers increased with age, while the difference between the sexes decreased (Table 1). Nearly 3% used other kinds of tobacco, mainly snuff. Among the smokers, there was a higher percentage who lived in the city; 79% lived in families with other smokers, which was three times more than those who lived in non-smoking families ($p = 0.005$). Cigarette consumption was 1–2 cigarettes per day by

Table 1. Smoking status by age
and sex, Mongolia, 1996

Age group (years)	Smokers (%)	
	Male	Female
10–13	14.6	5.5
14–16	30.6	38.3
17–20	54.8	56.2

33%, 3–5 cigarettes per day by 42% and almost a pack of cigarettes per day by 6.3%; 65% smoked a whole cigarette at the same time. Younger teenagers reported that they smoked in doorways or on the street, while those aged 17–20 said they smoked 'everywhere'. About 45% of the smokers purchased their own cigarettes, and 64% bought them for somebody else. Although one third of the smokers are only 10–13 years of age, most of them bought cigarettes from a shop or a street vendor, and 98% were not questioned about their age.

About two thirds of the smokers said they wanted to quit smoking. Twice as many males aged 17–20 wanted to quit as those aged 14–16, and 2.5 times as many males as females aged 17–20 wanted to quit ($p = 0.005$). About 55% of the smokers who wanted to quit did so because cigarettes are harmful, 22% because of the price and 14% because their parents urged them to. The percentages of smokers (82%) and all adolescents (96%) who drank alcohol began to increase at the age of 13–15 (Table 2). One third of the young people who smoked and drank alcohol said that they were not healthy ($p < 0.002$).

Discussion

In 1989, the World Health Organization developed its 'Tobacco or health' programme, and countries of the Western Pacific Region are working to achieve bans on tobacco advertising. The Mongolian Parliament adopted an anti-tobacco law in 1994, and national anti-tobacco conferences have been held; however, the recommendations made have not yet been completely implemented.

In a study in 1991, N. Chagnaa found that 31% of boys and 1% of girls were smokers, and a survey in 1993 by G. Tserenjigmed showed rates of 24% among boys and 53% among girls. We found rates of 12% for boys and 20% for girls. Thus, tobacco use in this age group appears to have increased between 1991 and 1993 and then declined. G. Tserenjigmed found, however, that 71% of smokers smoked 1–2 cigarettes per day and 21% smoked 4–6 per day, whereas we found that 33% smoked 1–2 cigarettes per day and 42% smoked 3–5 per day. Comparison of the results of the 1993 survey with ours also shows that, despite a reduction in smoking prevalence among adolescents, they are starting to smoke earlier (10–13 years) and smoke more cigarettes per day.

Although two of the main recommendations of the second national conference on tobacco were to prohibit the sale of tobacco products to minors and to ban smoking around children, most of the children were not asked their age when they bought cigarettes on the street, and two-thirds of them lived in families with smokers.

Anti-tobacco advocacy, information and the price of cigarettes are important factors for preventing the onset of smoking and for quitting. Many adolescent smokers want to give up smoking, indicating that they know about its harmful effects.

Table 2. Average age at beginning to smoke
and drink alcohol, Mongolia, 1996

Age group (years)	First smoking (%)	First drinking alcohol (%)
< 9	5.1	0.3
10–12	13.2	4.1
13–15	39.2	26.6
≥ 16	42.5	69

Comparative survey among smoking and non-smoking students in Mongolia

G. Dashzeveg, G. Sukhbat & N. Khurelbaatar

Ministry of Health and Social Welfare, Ulaanbaatar, Mongolia

Mongolia has a large population of young people: more than 50% are children and adolescents, who are the most susceptible to tobacco advertising. Smoking is the main cause of death in the country, causing two-thirds of all deaths among people over the age of 40. We have therefore undertaken a broad programme of research to determine attitudes to smoking and to identify target groups for tobacco control. The main purposes of this study were to conduct surveillance among young people to obtain baseline data, to study the conditions leading to smoking, to establish the main causes of smoking among students and to study the main diseases in smokers and non-smokers.

The survey was conducted among 1170 students, 655 male and 515 female, at Mongolian universities and among 230 smoking and 230 non-smoking students. The percentages of smokers were 24 ± 2.0 overall, with 38 ± 2.2% among male students and 9.1 ± 0.34% among female students. Of the 230 smokers, 30 (13%) had begun at the age of 8–11, 27 (12%) at 12–15 years, 128 (55%) at 16–19 years and 45 (20%) at ≥ 20 years of age. Their cigarette consumption is shown in Table 1.

None of the smokers but 36% of the non-smokers lived in non-smoking families; 40% of the smokers had one family member who smoked, 38% had two, 17% had three, 2.6% had four and 2.4% had five smokers in the family. Fifty percent of smokers and 30% of non-smokers agreed to smoking by their relatives. When asked why they had begun to smoke, 53% said it had been out of curiosity, 19% to make friends, 13% because of stress and 11% did not know. The conditions that led to smoking were: after eating (31%), emotional stress (30%), fatigue (23%), overwork (3%) and in order to have more free time (4%).

Forty percent of the smokers and 30% of the non-smokers had some health problem. Diseases of the respiratory system were found in 11% of smokers and 4.1% of non-smokers, cardiovascular disease in 9.1% of smokers and 8.2% of non-smokers, digestive disorders in 8.3% of smokers and 9% of non-smokers and other diseases in 12% of smokers and 8.7% of non-smokers.

Conclusions

Smokers are at greater risk for respiratory disease than non-smokers. More than half of the smokers agree to smoking by their relatives, so that more members of their families smoke. The main reasons for starting to smoke are curiosity and to make friends, and most started at the age of 16–19. Most of the smokers, however, wished to stop smoking for themselves and their family members, and effective public health activities should therefore be organized to assist cessation.

Table 1. Numbers of cigarettes smoked, Mongolia

No. of cigarettes	Smokers	
	No.	%
2–4 per week	51	22 ± 2.7
2–4 per day	60	26 ± 2.9
3–5 per day	68	30 ± 3.0
6–10 per day	39	16.9 ± 2.5
11–15 per day	6	2.6 ± 1.1
16–20 per day	2	0.8 ± 0.6
≥ 21 per day	4	1.7 ± 0.85

Frequency of tobacco and alcohol use among first-year university students in the United States, 1996

J. Lee[1], S. Parrott[2], W. Feigelman[3], R. Wu[4] & M. Forouzesh[1]

[1]California State University, Long Beachn California, [2]University of California, Los Angeles, California, [3]Nassau Community College, Garden City, United States; and [4]Suzhou University, Suzhou, China

Objectives: As tobacco and alcohol use often coincide, so that people who smoke frequently also drink frequently, we examined the frequency of tobacco and alcohol use among students entering their first year of university.

Methods: Data were obtained by sex, ethnic group and socioeconomic status from the Higher Education Research Institute at the University of California at Los Angeles. Socioeconomic status was determined on the basis of the type of higher educational establishment. A total of 354 853 students were asked if they smoked cigarettes and drank beer, wine or spirits frequently, occasionally or not at all. The data were weighted to reflect the population of first-year university students in the United States.

Results: The most frequent patterns of tobacco and alcohol use were use of neither, no smoking but occasional drinking, occasional drinking and frequent smoking and frequent smoking and drinking. The association between alcohol and tobacco appeared to be stronger among women than among men, as measured by the proportion of wine or spirit drinkers who smoked (61% versus 48%). The correlation coefficients for tobacco and alcohol use ranged from 0.29 for blacks, who had the lowest use of tobacco and alcohol, to 0.58 for Asians. Two-year colleges had the highest proportions of smokers (40%) and frequent smokers (21%), and universities had the highest proportion of frequent smokers who drank frequently (51%).

Conclusions: The close association between tobacco and alcohol use in this population suggests that preventive interventions for tobacco should also target alcohol use.

Prevalence of current smoking among Iranian adolescents estimated from plasma cotinine

N. Sarrafzadegan, M. Boshtam, G.R. Naderi, S. Asgari & F. Tafazoli

Cardiovascular Research Center, University of Medical Sciences, Isfahan, Iran

In the industrialized world, about one third of all men smoke cigarettes. In the developing world, about one half smoke. The figures for adolescents and women are slightly lower, but the numbers are rising rapidly. Self-reported smoking rates are likely to give a substantial underestimate of the prevalence of smoking. We report here a study in which the prevalence of smoking among adolescents was estimated from plasma cotinine, a biochemical marker of tobacco smoking.

The subjects were 860 high-school children, 470 boys and 390 girls, aged 14–18, who were randomly selected from high-schools. They were asked to fill in a questionnaire giving details of smoking habits and passive smoking and to provide samples of blood for assessment of plasma cotinine. The concentration of plasma cotinine was determined by high-performance liquid chromatography. The plasma cotinine cut-off value used to discriminate true smoking was 13 ng/ml. All the children claimed to be non-smokers, but 59 samples (7%) were classified as from smokers, with a plasma cotinine concentration > 13 ng/ml. The mean values for plasma cotinine were 2 ± 3.2 ng/ml in true non-smokers and 220 ± 98 ng/dl in smokers. Since nicotine and cotinine are specific to tobacco, and passive smoking has been found to induce only a small increase in concentrations, there was some denial of active smoking, which results in underestimation of the true prevalence of smoking among adolescents in Isfahan.

Attitudes

Why they smoke: A qualitative study among Taiwanese university students

S.-J. Huang

Department of Health Education, National Taiwan Normal University, Taipei,
Taiwan

Introduction

The aim of this study was to collect data from in-depth interviews with university students and to explore the reasons for smoking in order to design an effective intervention campaign. Smoking is highly detrimental to the health situation in Taiwan, with 19 072 deaths attributable to smoking, representing 19% of all deaths in 1989 (Wen *et al.*, 1992). The smoking rate is high among males (55%) and moderate among females (3.2%) (Li, 1995). The prevalence of smoking among young people is also high, at 30% among male college students and 2.9% among female students (Huang *et al.*, 1988). In this study, we examined the influences of cognitive factors and the social environment (Janz & Becker, 1974; Langlie, 1977; Mermelstein *et al.*, 1983) on the smoking behaviour of university students.

Methods

The students who participated in this study were in the 1993 academic years at a national university; 20 students were selected randomly according to smoking status, and 13 (seven male and six female) completed the in-depth interview. There were four who had never smoked, all female; three current smokers, who had smoked every day or from time to time during the previous six months, all males; and six experimental smokers, who had experimented with smoking but had never smoked for a long time, two of them female and four male.

A semi-structured questionnaire was designed to elicit information on their background, current smoking behaviour and their close family, how they viewed their current and future health status, knowledge about smoking and health and their attitude towards smoking. An open interview was then conducted to see how they coped with pressure. The questions were designed by the researcher and posed by an experienced reearch assistant who had received training in psychiatric clinics. The interview was tape-recorded with the permission of the students, and the tapes were transcribed for further analysis, to develop categories and themes and to arrive at a conclusion.

Results

The interview showed that smokers considered they had greater physical resistance to cigarettes, had friends who smoked, perceived fewer harmful effects of cigarettes and had less self-confidence. Non-smokers tended to be more effective, more resistant to invitations to smoke and have a greater perceived susceptibility to chronic disease. These results are similar to those of Huang *et al.* (1991), who found that students at junior and senior high-schools and vocational schools smoked because they were bored and felt pressure in connection with their studies. Smoking was considered to be a mechanism for coping with pressure and filling a blank life. Another study showed that smokers had worse scholastic results and less expectation of higher education (Huang, 1982). The female students considered that it was unfeminine to smoke and associated the habit with prostitution. This attitude reflects the association of smoking with promiscuity in the United States in the early twentieth century, in Japan in the mid-1990s and in Africa recently (Waldron *et al.*, 1988).

Smoking is therefore not only a physical problem but is also related to mental and social maladjustment. Does this mean that smokers are failures? The problem is worth exploring. Older, but not younger, students indicated that they smoked for sociability, and that was used as an excuse to smoke. The finding that young people were more likely to smoke if they had friends who smoked indicates that it would be worthwhile investigating whether social networks could help them cope with daily life.

Implications

Several important implications of these findings should be highlighted. As the female students smoke less than the males, anti-smoking education should focus on males. Not only information about the harmful effects of cigarettes but also ways of coping with pressure and life skills should be taught and practised in class.

The content of anti-smoking education programmes should focus on both the short-term and the long-term effects of smoking. Students could be instructed to record their family history of chronic diseases to raise their perception of susceptibility to the effects and to their severity. Personal case reports or testimonies could be given in the mass media. Group counselling or paired teaching with peers and girl friends could also be organized to increase effectiveness. The anti-smoking message could be integrated in the feminist movement in Taiwan, which has had a high profile recently. As not smoking is regarded as a traditional female virtue, females should be shown as healthy and empowered by the knowledge that they should not smoke.

The result of the qualitative study with regard to the relationship between smoking, pressure and academic achievement could be applied in designing a quantitative study, and the use of a larger sample from various settings might be considered.

References

Huang, S. (1982) The incentives and modeling of the smoking behavior of the male students in junior high schools. *J. Health Educ.*, 1, 14–33

Huang, W., Tan, W., Chu, J. & Wu, J. (1988) The attitude and practice of smoking behavior and the related influential factors. *Health Educ. J.*, 9, 35–51

Huang, S., Chen, C. & Lai, S. (1991) *The Smoking Behavior of the Youth in Taiwan*, Taipei, Department of Health

Janz, N.K. & Becker, M.H. (1974) The health belief model: A decade later. *Health Educ. Q.*, 11, 1–47

Langlie, J.K. (1997) Social networks, health beliefs and preventive health behavior. *J. Health Soc. Behav.*, 18, 244–260

Li, Y.C. (1995) Preventing the risk factor—smoking. *Health Rep.*, 51, 35–44

Mermelstein, R., Lichetin, E., McIntyre, K. & Partener, K. (1983) Support and relapse in smoking cessation program. *J. Consult. Lin. Psychol.*, 51, 463–466

Waldron, I., Bratelli, G., Garriker, L., Sung, W.C., Vogeli, C. & Waldman, E. (1988) Gender differences in tobacco use in Africa, Asia, the Pacific, and Latin America. *Soc. Sci. Med.*, 27, 1269–1275

Wen, C.P., Tsai, S., Yen, D.D., Lin, S.H., Chen, H.L. & Tsai, S.F. (1992) Risk assessment of active and passive smoking in Taiwan—Smoking attributable mortality. In: Eighth World Conference on Smoking or Health, Buenos Aires, Argentina

Smoking behaviour and mental health status among senior high-school and vocational high-school students in Taiwan metropolitan areas

D.D. Yen, S.-Y. Huang, A.-P. Ma, H.-H. Chou, M.-H. Yang & T.-P. Lo

John Tung Foundation, Taipei, Taiwan

Objectives and process

The main purpose of this study was to explore the distribution, relativity, correlation, diversity and predictivity of smoking behaviour and mental status among senior high-school and vocational high-school students in Taiwan metropolitan areas. All of such students in Taipei, Taichung and Kaoshiung enrolled during the 1995 academic year were included. The sample was selected by the 'PPS' method, and a questionnaire was developed. A total of 3025 students were selected from 22 schools.

Main findings

The prevalence of smoking was 19% among the students, 55% among their fathers, 4.4% among their mothers and 19% among their best friends. Most of the students smoked when they felt sad or in amusement places with their classmates and friends. Most bought cigarettes at 24-h service shops, had smoked for < 1 year, smoked < 5 cigarettes per week, had smoked their first cigarette at school, liked to smoke on holidays, had started smoking in the ninth grade and favoured foreign cigarettes. They had insufficient knowledge about the hazards of smoking, did not accept smoking behaviour and tended to be in good mental health.

There were significant differences between smokers and non-smokers in their attitudes to smoking, the smoking habits of their social reference group, five sociodemographic variables, their knowledge about the hazards of smoking and their mental health status (Table 1). Twelve variables can be used to predict 45% of the variations in students' smoking habits.

Recommendations

The information on the smoking behaviour of these students, including when and where they smoke and with whom, the sources of cigarettes, how long they have smoked, how many cigarettes they smoked per week, where and when they began smoking and their tobacco preference, is important for planning, implementing and evaluating smoking education programmes. Students at senior high-schools and vocational high-schools must understand that their mental health is easily affected by a high degree of urbanization, with a stressful lifestyle and keen competition. There are many ways of confronting these challenges, and smoking should not be regarded as one of them. Since adolescents are readily influenced by their environment and especially by peer groups, peer pressure should be taken into account in anti-smoking education programmes. As families still play an important role in the smoking behaviour of adolescents, parents should take more responsibility in preventing their children from smoking.

Smoking should be an integral part of a comprehensive health education curriculum. At present, there is no obligatory health education programme in senior high-schools and vocational high-schools in Taiwan. This should be changed as soon as possible. A Tobacco Hazards Control Act has been in effect since 19 September 1997. It should be reinforced to protect the public from the hazards of tobacco and promote health.

The psychological traits and the subculture of adolescents are major factors in their knowledge, attitudes and practices with regard to tobacco. In order that anti-smoking programmes be effective, more studies should be carried out on the inner world of adolescents.

Table 1. Multiple stepwise regression analysis of the smoking habits of 2413 students

Variable	Multiple R	R^2	Added R2	Beta	F value[a]
Attitude towards smoking	.58171	.33839	.33839	.44187	1233.1352
Smoking behaviour of best friend	.64192	.41206	.07367	.25742	844.54576
Location of school	.64828	.42027	.00821	-.07270	582.12191
Sex	.65292	.42630	.00603	.10486	447.32687
Type of school	.65708	.43175	.00545	-.08955	365.76778
Sensitivity score	.66069	.43651	.00476	-.04240	310.63722
Non-adjustment score	.66349	.44022	.00371	.11181	270.18755
Overall mental health score	.66503	.44226	.00204	-.09339	238.28541
Birth preference	.66645	.44416	.00190	-.04638	213.35128
Degree of urbanization of residence	.66766	.44577	.00161	-.04273	193.19343
Mothers' occupation	.66886	.44738	.00161	.04048	176.70392
Knowledge about smoking score	.66991	.44878	.00140	-.03841	162.83355

[a] All $p < 0.001$

Smoking behaviour of schoolteachers in Mie Prefecture, Japan

Y. Osaki, T. Ohida & M. Minowa

Department of Epidemiology, National Institute of Public Health, Tokyo, Japan

Introduction

As it has been reported in many studies that smoking behaviour is established during adolescence, anti-smoking education in school, provided by teachers, is important for preventing smoking. We conducted a survey on the smoking status and attitudes toward anti-smoking education at school among teachers in Mie Prefecture, located in the middle of Honshu Island near Nagoya, which includes some urban areas.

Methods

We surveyed about 90% of all teachers in public kindergartens and elementary, junior high- and senior high-schools in this prefecture. Anonymous questionnaires were distributed to about 14 000 teachers and 2000 other staff and were collected by the person responsible for this survey at each school. After completing the questionnaires, the teachers put them into envelopes and returned them to the responsible person. A total of 13 998 questionnaires were returned; after exclusion of incomplete questionnaires and those completed by other staff, 12 198 were analysed. The response rates were 98% for elementary-school teachers, 88% for junior high-school teachers and 75% for senior high-school teachers.

Results and discussion

The smoking rates were 45% among male teachers and 3.1% among female teachers; both these figures are lower than those in the general population (Table 1). Surprisingly, 88% of the male teachers smoked at school, mainly in the teachers' room; female teachers were are less likely to smoke at school (Table 2).

Table 1. Prevalence of smoking among teachers (6133 men and 6060 women) and in the general population of Japan, by age and sex, 1995

Age group (years)	Prevalence (%)			
	Teachers		General population	
	Male	Female	Male	Female
20–29	47	3	65	23
30–39	46	3	66	19
40–49	46	4	62	14
50–59	39	1	58	13

Table 2. Where teachers smoke, by sex

Place	Smokers (%)	
	Male ($n = 2747$)	Female ($n = 192$)
Teachers' room	70	8
Smoking room	25	6
Meetings	20	1
Own room	33	20
At school	88	29
At home	74	72

When asked about school regulations on teachers smoking, approximately half of the respondents replied that they were not allowed to smoke in the classroom and corridors, but only 19% of male and 14% of female teachers reported they were not allowed to smoke in the teachers' room. Men were more likely to report that they were not permitted to smoke at school. When smoking was restricted to the teachers' room, most men smoked there, but some of them smoked in school even when they were not allowed to smoke in the teachers' room.

About 60% of the smokers wanted to quit smoking, and 50–60% had tried to do so. Providing smoking cessation programmes for teachers is thus an important strategy for smoking control in schools. Most of the teachers, whether they smoked or not, agreed that there should be some ban on smoking by teachers in school, although the male smokers were less likely to support a complete ban. Most of the teachers agreed that anti-smoking education for students is necessary in school, and about 70% agreed that teachers were responsible for this. About 36% of male and 21% of female teachers had had experience of anti-smoking education. This was not related to smoking status, but only 14% of the male and 8% of the female teachers were confident about their ability to supply anti-smoking education. In spite of the responsibility they bear for anti-smoking education, < 50% of the teachers knew about the health hazards of smoking.

In conclusion, schoolteachers must learn about smoking and health, including medical knowledge and educational techniques and skills. They must be encouraged to quit smoking: many want to quit, and their smoking status is related to their attitude to promoting anti-smoking in school. Teachers' smoking in school must be restricted because schools are public places and their smoking habit may influence that of their students.

Factors that contribute to adolescent smoking

K. Pärna, A. Saava & D. Eensoo

University of Tartu, Estonia

Childhood and adolescent development includes the establishment of attitudes and behaviour that directly and indirectly influence their health (Jessor, 1984; Maxey et al., 1992). Decisions about the use of tobacco are among the most important health-related choices that individuals can make. Largely because of the long delay between cause and full effect, people tend to misjudge the hazards of tobacco (World Bank, 1993). Tobacco is frequently used for the first time before school graduation, indicating that if schoolchildren and adolescents could be kept away from tobacco, most of them would not smoke in adulthood (Elders et al., 1994).

The aim of this study was to assess the prevalence and patterns of tobacco smoking and, using the PRECEDE (predisposing, reinforcing and enabling constructs in educational/environmental diagnosis and evaluation) framework (Figure 1), to explore the factors that contribute to smoking among adolescents in Estonia.

Material and methods

The primary sampling unit was a school. As about 50% of the population of Tallinn is not Estonian, the sampling was stratified by nationality. The schools were chosen randomly from telephone books, excluding special schools. The second stage of the sampling was by grade. We chose grades 8, 10 and 12, with children aged mostly 13–14, 15–16 and 17–18, respectively. The sample represented 20% ($n = 1269$) of Estonian and 17% ($n = 901$) of non-Estonian schoolchildren, for a total of 18% ($n = 2170$) of the schoolchildren in these grades in Tallinn.

Data were collected from questionnaires consisting mainly of structured multiple-choice and a few open questions. The 20 questions used in this study were intended to provide an estimate of the prevalence of smoking and to elicit information on factors that presumably predispose to, enable or reinforce consumption of tobacco among adolescents. These included personal (age, sex, nationality, religion, education of father, occupation of father, occupation of mother, number of children in family, knowledge, attitudes), inter-personal (smoking by mothers, fathers, siblings and friends) and environmental (passive smoking, permission to smoke at school, supervision of smoking limitations at school) factors.

Ten Estonian and seven Russian secondary schools in Tallinn participated in the study. The data were collected in classrooms during September–November 1995, when all pupils who were present participated; one to five pupils of each classroom were absent at the time of the survey. The pupils were assured of the anonymity and confidentiality of their responses. To prevent the dissemination of information, the survey was carried out during the same day in all the schools.

The data were analysed with SPSS statistical software. Chi-squared tests were used to evaluate the differences between groups. Stepwise logistic regression was used to analyse the combination of significant contributing factors (Hosmer & Lemeshow, 1989; Engelman, 1990).

Results and discussion

Of the adolescents studied, 16% had smoked every now and then, 10% smoked regularly, 38% had tried but did not smoke any more and 36% had never tried. The reported ages at the time of first smoking ranged from 5 to 17 years (mean, 13.4 years; SD, 2.1; mode, 14.0). Multivariate stepwise logistic regression analysis showed that the prevalence of smoking increased with age. The rate was higher among non-Estonian than among Estonian girls and lower among non-Estonian than among Estonian boys. The most prevalent predisposing factor for girls was the occupation of the father, and girls whose fathers were unemployed, dead, retired or had an unknown occupation were more likely smoke. The most important predisposing factor for boys was the type of family: boys who lived with both their parents were less like to smoke than boys living with a mother and a stepfather or a father and a stepmother. No relationship was found between other family factors such as occupation of mother, education of father, number of children in the family, religion, knowledge about adverse effect of tobacco on health or smoking habits.

Friends' smoking was a common reinforcing factor on the smoking habits of both girls and boys. The prevalence was higher among boys if their siblings smoked. Contrary to other reports (Friedman *et al.*, 1985; Bandura, 1986; World Health Organization, 1986), smoking among boys tended to decrease if their fathers smoked. This may be due to the fact that a cross-sectional study cannot account for temporal changes in behaviour or because the behaviour was experimental and transient.

Figure 1. Phases of the PRECEDE framework

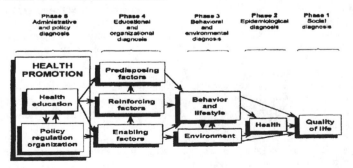

From Green & Kreuter (1991)

Passive smoking was associated with a higher prevalence of smoking. It is difficult to determine whether passive smoking is only an enabling factor for smoking or also a reinforcing factor. Tobacco smoke in the environment could be strongly linked to smoking of parents at home, where schoolchildren spend most of their time. This possibility was analysed by removing passive smoking from the final model. In this model, mothers' smoking was statistically significantly associated with smoking among boys. Other environmental factors, such as permission to smoke in certain places at school were considered by the girls to be associated with smoking. The higher prevalence of smoking among the girls who agreed that smoking should be allowed in certain places at school may simply reflect the opinion of girls who smoked and not be a characteristic of the school. After the schools were grouped by the odds ratio for permission to smoke (< 1, 1–3, > 3), this factor did not contribute to smoking among girls and therefore cannot be overestimated as enabling in the final model. The PRECEDE model of factors contributing to smoking indicated similar results for girls and boys in this study.

Conclusion

The findings of this study show that every fourth adolescent in Tallinn is either an occasional or a regular smoker. This behaviour seems to start in early adolescence. The predisposing factors include age, sex and nationality. An unstable family situation appears to affect the smoking habits of adolescents. Reinforcing factors, such as friends who smoke, were strongly associated with smoking among girls and boys. Siblings' smoking affected smoking among boys, but boys were less like to smoke if their fathers were smokers.

Passive smoking was found to be an enabling factor for smoking: longer exposure to tobacco was associated with larger numbers of smokers. Smoking among girls was also associated with their opinion about permission to smoke in certain places at school.

The need for prevention of smoking among adolescents in Estonia is evident, at the individual, community and policy levels.

Acknowledgement
This study was supported by the Estonian Science Foundation.

References

Bandura, A. (1986) Social Foundations of Thought and Action. A Social Cognitive Theory, New Jersey: Prentice-Hall, pp. 47–105, 142–181

Elders, M.J., Perry, C.L., Eriksen, M.P. & Giovino, G.A. (1994) The report of the Surgeon General: Preventing tobacco use among young people. *Am. J. Public Health*, **84**, 543–547

Engelman, L. (1990) Stepwise logistic regression. In: Dixon, W.J., Brown, M.B., Engelman, L., *et al.*, eds, *BMDP Statistical Software Manual*, Vol. 2, Los Angeles: University of California Press, pp. 1013–1045

Friedman, L.S., Lichtenstein, E. & Biglan, A (1985) Smoking onset among teens: An empirical analysis of initial situations. *Addict. Behav.*, **10**, 1–13

Green, L.W. & Kreuter, M.W. (1991) *Health Promotion Planning: An Educational and Environmental Approach*, Moutain View: Mayfield Publishing Co., pp. 44–187

Hosmer, D.W. & Lemeshow, S. (1989) Applied Logistic Regression, New York: John Wiley & Sons, pp. 1–75

Jessor, R. (1984) Adolescent development and behavioral health. In: Matarazzo, J.D., Weiss, S.M., Herd, J.A., *et al.*, eds, *Behavioral Health: A Handbook of Health Enhancement and Disease Prevention*, New York: John Wiley & Sons, pp. 69–90

Maxcy, Rosenau & Last (1992) *Public Health and Preventive Medicine*, 13th Ed., Prentice Hall International Inc

World Health Organization (1986) Young people's health—A challenge for society. Report of a WHO study group on young people and 'Health for all by the year 2000' (WHO Technical Report Series 731), Geneva, pp. 1–117

World Bank (1993) *Investing in Health: World Development Indicators*, Oxford: Oxford University Press

An adolescent's perspective on adolescent smoking

K. Koplan

Yale University, New Haven, Connecticut, United States

In an effort to replace the thousands of adult smokers who die every day from tobacco use, tobacco companies are aiming intensive advertising campaigns at adolescents worldwide. A particular target of these companies is adolescent girls in both developed and developing countries. Adolescents are also the key target of counter-marketing attempts by public health professionals whose aim is to discourage smoking uptake. While the tobacco companies have been hugely successful in their marketing efforts, public health professional all over the world often miss their target, and the rates of adolescent smoking are stable in many countries and are increasing in others. Public health campaigns have been largely misdirected and ineffective.

It is more behaviour- and cost-effective to prevent young people from smoking than to encourage smokers to quit once they have begun. Most people begin smoking in adolescence, before the age of 20. Restricting the access of young people by policy reform, such as regulations with regard to sales to minors and heavy taxation, is of great value, but I focus on health education campaigns directed to teenagers: an adolescent's view of what constitutes an effective programme to prevent adolescents from becoming smokers. Three aspects of anti-smoking programmes are vulnerable to crucial errors that undermine their effectiveness: the age at which anti-smoking education begins, the content of the message and the messenger.

The idea that young children should not be told about smoking, alcohol, sex or drugs is erroneous. An intervention aimed at teenagers should begin earlier, since by adolescence many views and attitudes have already been shaped by culural influences and the media, often with no thoughtful or effective health education. A more effective campaign would begin during the first years of school, at the ages of four to six. A corollary to an earlier campaign would be age-specific material to appeal to children with different values and motivations. For example, the concepts of 'smelly', 'disgusting' and 'causing bad breath' are particularly effective at this age, because young children are attuned to the sensory aspects of life and are less influenced by social mores. The idea of black lungs, yellow fingers and smelly breath and clothes disgusted me at that age, and I began to view smokers as unattractive and thoughtless. The idea that smoking 'stinks' and is an unattractive habit should be enforced early, repeatedly and colourfully.

The focus on young children can have a broader effect on family health. Evidence has shown that parents' smoking influences children to smoke. As stated by Dr Mochizuki-Kobayashi (this volume), however, children can influence their parents. A study in Shanghai showed that more than 90% of men who smoked knew that smoking was bad for their health; to move beyond knowledge to a behavioural response, children in many communities in China have been encouraged to write letters to their fathers, encouraging them to quit smoking. Children follow by example, not by verbal reminders with no basis in action.

The content of an anti-smoking message cannot be the information derived from the hundreds of papers on the health hazards of tobacco use. Young people think that contracting long-term health effects like cancer, heart disease, stroke and emphysema does not apply to them; but bad breath, smelly clothes and yellow teeth affect them, as they are very conscious of their image. Health arguments can never compete with a glamorous lifestyle: cowboys are more effective than doctors in suggesting an attractive lifestyle. Adolescents need something concrete, visible or physical: young teenagers may be influenced by yellow teeth, bad breath and reduced athletic performance, while older ones are more influenced by sophistication and attractiveness to the opposite sex. Youth in developing countries may find that smoking is sophisticated and western, which are deemed to be desirable. The message must be passed that smoking is neither sophsiticated nor western. Many teenage smokers who are perfectly aware of the full health effects of smoking will nevertheless smoke in a social situation, using it to overcome their self-consciousness or their need for acceptance or comfort. This aspect of smoking is hard to combat, partially because there is no replacement; but we must attempt to remove the cigarette as a tool for easing the entry of adolescents into a more 'adult' or at least more complex social atmosphere.

The least effective way of delivering an anti-smoking message is through an older authority figure such as a physician: they are not the people to whom adolescents listen. Adolescents are rebellious, not obedient, and are not afraid of dying or of consequences to their health. Also, they don't want to be lectured to or patronized; they want to be treated as adults and be spoken to as such. The most effective provider of an anti-smoking message would be peer leaders: adolescents are more likely to listen to each other than to adults. Peer pressure can influence both healthy and unhealthy behaviour. We should create an environment in which there are more young people advocating a healthy lifestyle and influencing their peers.

Counter-advertising is another useful tool for combating adolescent smoking, when an appropriate spokesperson is used, who should be someone teenagers think is sophisticated and whom they want to emulate. People like the rock and movie star Madonna, Chris O'Donnell, the star of 'Batman and Robin', the actress Sandra Bullock and the actor Will Smith are examples of appropriate spokespeople for my age group in my country. If you are from North America and these names don't sound familiar to you, that should impress upon you the importance of talking to teenagers to find out who they think is 'cool'. Those of you from other countries will find that there are teenage idols everywhere; however, many of them smoke. This is a significant problem, as these people are very visible and influential. Countless celebrities in films, television and music in Hollywood, New York, London, Hong Kong, Shanghai and Mumbai who are seen smoking in movies, concerts and in real life undo many health promotion and education efforts in a split second.

I urge anti-smoking health professionals to seek out adolescents in their own countries to gain the information necessary to create effective programmes; even unstructured interviews with randomly chosen adolescents are better than leaving the decisions to health professionals. My views may reflect only one part of the world, but in many ways important for anti-smoking campaigns, teenagers in Brazil, China, Germany, Turkey and the United States have more in common with each other than with middle-aged health workers in their own countries.

Why young people in Switzerland smoke

H. Krebs, D. Hänggi & V. El Fehri

Swiss Association for Smoking Prevention, Bern, Switzerland

We submit the results of a representative survey among 617 young people aged 13–19. The aim of the survey was to acquire more knowledge concerning the attitudes and opinions of young people about smoking. The results may help to optimize campaigns and actions designed to dissuade youngsters from smoking. The intention is that the survey be conducted every three to five years in the future, so as to identify tendencies and adapt strategies accordingly. The survey was based on telephone interviews conducted in May–July 1997. The questions were drawn up for 10 focus groups, divided into smokers and non-smokers and according to the linguistic regions of Switzerland (German and French). The participants were grouped into non-smokers who had never smoked, non-smokers who had smoked previously, smokers who smoked a maximum of 5 cigarettes per day and smokers who smoked > 5 cigarettes per day.

Results of the survey

More than three-quarters of those surveyed were non-smokers, and the difference among girls and boys was minimal. One-third of those questioned in every age group had never smoked cigarettes, but 21% of those surveyed were smokers. The smoking habits varied according to age, with a prevalence of 4% among 13–14-year-olds, 23% among 15–16-year-olds and 33% among 17–19-year-olds.

When asked if they thought they would still be smoking in two years, 15% of the smokers and only 3% of the non-smokers thought that they would definitely still be smoking, and 37% of the smokers and only 3% of the non-smokers thought that they would probably still be smoking. Two-thirds of the non-smokers were sure that they would remain non-smokers, while only 7% of the smokers felt that they would definitely be non-smokers by that time. The responses were somewhat over-optimistic and indicate that young people underestimate the potential for addiction.

Most of the youngsters questioned (52%) had had their first experience of smoking cigarettes in the company of friends and colleagues, often (27%) at parties and only rarely alone in secret (7%) or at home (5%).

An above-average number of young people who smoked lived in households where their parents smoked. Their friends were also more often smokers than were the friends of non-smokers. More than half of the friends of smokers who smoked > 5 cigarettes per day were also smokers. Young people of each sex aged 17–19 were more likely than 13–16-year olds to have friends who smoked.

The eight commonest reasons for smoking were: for enjoyment or pleasure ('because I like the taste; 40%), because friends or colleagues smoke (24%), from force of habit (20%), to ease stress, problems or frustration (19%), for a calming or relaxing effect (18%), dependency or addiction ('because I cannot give up') (14%), out of boredom or insecurity (11%) or because smoking is 'cool' (8%). The predominant feature is the difference according to age and the number of cigarettes smoked daily. Conclusive indications of potential addiction emerged. As the qualitative section of the study shows, the young people themselves frequently underestimated this aspect. Younger smokers or consumers of ≤ 5 cigarettes per day (including many occasional smokers) often lit up because friends and colleagues were also smoking. Older and more frequent smokers (> 5 cigarettes per day) said they did so from force of habit, because of the calming, relaxing effects or due to dependency or addiction.

Around 60% of the smokers aged 17–19 but only 20% of younger smokers felt that giving up smoking was difficult. Consequently, the more they smoke, the more difficult it becomes for them to give up. These are unmistakable signs of potential addiction to smoking. Six out of 10 smokers had recently thought about giving up, and four out of 10 had already tried (50% of 17–19-year-olds but only 28% of 13–16-year-olds).

The most frequently cited reason for wanting to give up smoking was health (61%), followed by cost (26% said that cigarettes were too expensive), fitness or sport (12%) and the desire not to become addicted (12%). The commonest reason for having given up smoking was health, while the second commonest was the cost of cigarettes, although the gap between these two answers was substantial. The six commonest reasons given for not smoking were because it is not healthy (66%), because I don't particularly like the taste (27%), because cigarettes are too expensive and the money can be put to better use (22%), because of fitness or sport (12%), because I don't want to become dependent on or addicted to cigarettes (8%) and because I find smokers repulsive (8%). Cost was given as a reason particularly by 17–19-year olds, who presumably realized how much money their colleagues who smoked spent on cigarettes.

Smoking bans

The lower the age of those surveyed, the more likely they were to encounter smoking bans. This applies to school playgrounds, the home and, of course, the workplace. In general, smoking is not allowed at school in Switzerland among pupils under the age of 16. There are considerable differences among the age groups: nine out of 10 children under the age of 14 are not allowed to smoke on the school premises. Among 17–19-

year olds, only four out of 10 were not allowed to smoke at school; 58% of 13–14-year olds but only 39% of 17–19-year olds were banned from smoking at home; 47% of 17–19-year olds reported that smoking was forbidden at their workplace.

Acceptance of smoking bans depends to a large extent on the age of the young people and on their smoking habits. Smoking bans are most widely accepted in restaurants (except smoking zones), with 78% of the smokers and 58% of the non-smokers in agreement with the bans. Resistance to smoking bans is encountered in discotheques, particularly on the part of 17–19-year-olds; a clear majority of non-smokers was also against smoking bans there.

Acknowledgements

The survey was commissioned by the Swiss Association for Smoking Prevention, Swiss Federal Health Ministry. Two agencies were involved, the Institute and LINK Marketing Research, Kommunikation und Publikumsforschung Hans Krebs.

School education, smoking habits of parents and children and childrens' attitudes to future smoking: Results of the Heidelberg Children Study

M. Pötschke-Langer, L.R. Pilz & L. Edler

Deutsches Krebsforschungszentrum, Heidelberg, Germany

Introduction

As in many countries, the prevalence of smoking among young people aged 14–19 of each sex in western Germany increased after the 1950s, but there was a sudden decline following the highest prevalence of about 45% in 1975. The decline is believed to be due to governmental prevention strategies, with health promotion programmes in the school curricula and mass media campaigns. The prevalence of smoking among young people now appears to be stabilizing at about 25%, which, however, is still too high in view of the serious consequences of tobacco consumption for human health. Further care must therefore be taken to educate young people in this public health field.

Design of the Heidelberg Children Study

The Heidelberg Children Study, initiated by Ernst Wynder, President of the American Health Foundation, was designed as a survey of the health and behaviour of children in the fourth and fifth grades in all public schools in Heidelberg and in selected schools in the county. The answers to a comprehensive questionnaire (to be published elsewhere) and a well-planned interrogation by trained interviewers provides a database for investigation of the current prevalence of smoking in these age groups and the related factors.

Letters were sent to all primary schools (*Grundschulen*) and all secondary schools (*Hauptschulen*, with the lowest educational level), *Realschulen* (intermediate educational level) and *Gymnasien* (highest educational level). With one exception, all of the schools contacted took part in the study. Teachers and parents were not informed about the content of the questionnaire. A team of seven interviewers was sent to the schools, and the questionnaires were filled in during one school period (45 min). Special topics of interest in the study were attitudes, beliefs, behaviour and knowledge about tobacco and alcohol use, exercise and leisure-time activities, dietary habits, dental care, body image, general health, physical ailments, use of medication and psychosocial adjustment. The coded answers were analysed by standard statistical methods for frequencies and associations.

Among the 4252 children aged 9–11 who were eligible, 3828 children (90%) participated in the study, comprising 1856 girls (48%) and 1951 boys (52%).

Results and discussion

We found no marked differences between the city of Heidelberg and small towns and villages in Rhein-Neckar County with regard to the smoking behaviour of the children and parents surveyed. In this report, we concentrate on the type of school and sex-specific differences.

The overall prevalence of smoking among the children in this study was 10%. There was a clear difference by sex, fewer girls (5.2%) than boys 9.5%) answering 'Yes' to the question 'Have you ever smoked?'. The prevalence of smoking was significantly lower among boys aged 9–10 years in the *Grundschulen* (9.5%) than in the *Hauptschulen* (20%), *Realschulen* (15%) or the *Gymnasien* (13%). A similar picture was observed for girls in the *Grundschulen* (5.2%), *Hauptschulen* (16%), *Realschulen* (9.5%) and *Gymnasien* (2.6%). The prevalence of regular smoking (every day during the past week) was, however, very low (none in the *Grundschulen*, 2.1% of boys in the *Hauptschulen*, 1.1% in the *Realschulen* and 0.32% in the *Gymnasien* among boys and under 1% in all schools for girls); in the *Hauptschulen*, however, 6.5% of the boys and 8.8% of the girls said they had smoked on at least 1–3 days of the previous week, in contrast to 1.6% of boys and 0.6% of girls in the *Gymnasien*.

When asked 'Do you intend to smoke some day?', the majority of the children answered 'No' or 'Probably not', ranging from 74–90% for girls and 62–84% for boys, depending on the type of school (Figure 1). One group likely to become smokers are the boys (9.2%) and girls (7.8%) in the *Hauptschulen* and the boys (7.6%) in the *Realschulen*. In addition, boys at the lowest educational level were uncertain: 10% of boys in the *Hauptschulen* answered 'Perhaps', and 12% gave no answer. No equivalent behaviour was observed for the girls.

The smoking behaviour of the parents, shown in Figure 2, reveals notable differences between school types: Most remarkable is the difference between families with children in *Hauptschulen*, in which 58% of the fathers and 46% of the mothers were smokers, and families with children in *Gymnasien*, in which 30% of fathers and 20% of mothers were smokers. The children of non-smoking parents, independently of school type, have a good chance of not becoming smokers. The relationship between children's attitudes to future smoking and the present smoking of their parents is remarkable, as children of non-smoking parents are much more likely to intend not to smoke: 65% in *Hauptschulen*, 76% in *Realschulen* and 78% in *Gymnasien*. Only about 54% of the children in *Hauptschulen*, 64% in *Realschulen* and 68% in *Gymnasien* said they did not intend to smoke in the future. This is in contrast to children with one parental smoker and children whose two parents smoked.

We analysed alcohol consumption, security behaviour and watching television or videos as indicators of a risk-taking attitude and observed very similar results, pointing to a riskier attitude and behaviour among children in the lower-level educational section.

Conclusions

Most children in this age group have never tried smoking and do not express any intention to do so. The level of education is an important factor in determining who becomes a smoker, and it seems likely that parental smoking provokes smoking in their children. Efforts to lower the smoking prevalence among young people should start before the age of 10 years in elementary schools (*Grundschulen*) in Germany, or even in kindergartens. Targeting families with low educational and social levels is strongly indicated. The relationship of these areas with other social factors (e.g. income) needs further investigation.

Figure 1. Intention to smoke in the future among 3601 children aged 9–11 in the Heidelberg Children Study

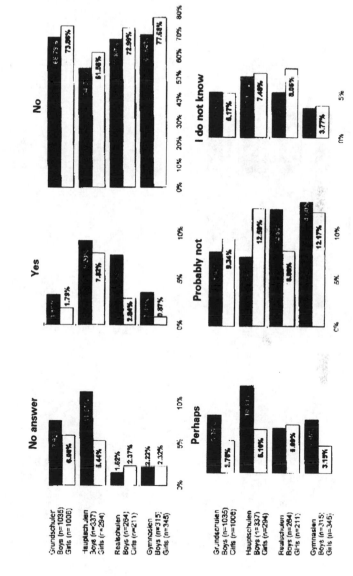

Figure 2. Smoking behaviour of parents reported by their children in the Heidelberg Children Study

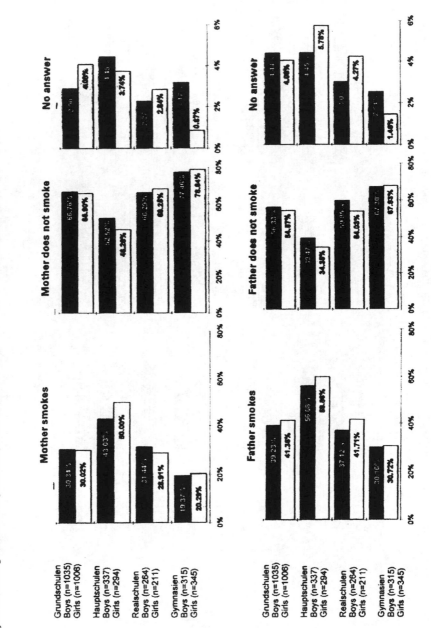

Speculations on cigarette smoking among youngsters in Greece

K. Athanasiou

School of Education, Aristotelian University of Thessaloniki, Thessaloniki, Greece

Greek society is a very interesting case from the point of view of smoking, since Greece now has the highest per capita consumption of cigarettes among the countries of the European Union (Figure 1). This unfortunate fact emphasizes the necessity of anti-smoking campaigns based on serious studies of the smoking habits and attitudes of various population groups. The situation is clear, since the rate of death from lung cancer has shown a continuous increase over the past few decades (Figure 2), and Greece is one of the few developed countries in which there has been an increase in mortality from coronary heart disease during recent years (Uemura & Pisa, 1988). One interesting aspect of the situation of smoking in Greece is that although it has had the highest consumption of cigarettes in Europe for at least the past 15 years, it does not have the worst rate of lung cancer (Figure 3).

Figure 1. Annual per capita cigarette consumption in the countries of the European Union, 1985–94

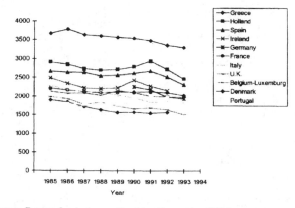

From European Bureau for Action on Smoking Prevention (1994)

Figure 2. Annual per capita consumption of cigarettes in Greece in relation to rates of death from lung cancer 20 years later

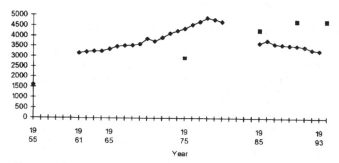

From Trichopoulos *et al.* (1987)

Figure 3. Cigarette consumption and rates of lung cancer in the European Union

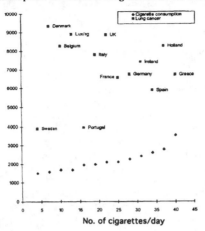

No. of cigarettes/day

From Peto *et al.* (1994)

There are various possible explanations of this discrepancy.

One explanation could be the fact that smokers in Greece have not passed the gap of 20–25 years that is necessary for this negative record of lung cancer mortality. This does not seem to be the case, however, since data on smoking in Greece over the last 47 years show that the annual per capita cigarette consumption reached its peak during the years 1977, 1978 and 1979, to almost 5000 cigarettes per capita per year, while in 1985 (the first year of the comparative study shown in Figure 1), the curve for cigarette smoking had already reached a low plateau (Figure 2).

A second possible explanation might be that, for several years, this country has had the highest per capita consumption of fruit and vegetables of all the countries in the world. Numerous data now suggest a protective role of fruits and vegetables against lung cancer (Davis, 1989). For example, phenethyl isothiocyanate, which occurs in broccoli and cabbage, inhibits covalent DNA binding of tobacco-specific nitrosamines. Ellagic acid, which occurs in various fruits, nuts, berries, seeds and vegetables, has been shown to protect against the carcinogenic effects of benzo[*a*]pyrene. Flavonoids inhibit initiation by benzo[*a*]pyrene and aflatoxins and have other anti-carcinogenic activity. β-Carotene and other carotenoids are important antioxidants in the diet that could protect the body fat and lipid membranes against oxidation. Carotenoids have been shown to be anti-carcinogens in rats and mice and may be anti-carcinogens in humans. Their protective effects in smokers might be related to the high level of oxidants in both cigarette smoke and tar. Vitamin E (tocopherol), dietary ascorbic acid (vitamin C) and selenium are all important antioxidants.

A third explanation has to do with the fact that, although Greeks are heavy smokers on the average, they generally start smoking quite late in life, owing to social factors related mainly to the structure of the Greek family. Thus, only 10% of all smokers in Greece are under 17 years of age. Previous data have shown that the probability of dying of lung cancer is closely related to the age of smoking initiation: the annual death rate from lung cancer among people aged 55–64 is about three times higher for those who started smoking at age 15 than for those who started at age 20 or 25, for smokers of 21–39 cigarettes per day (Tomatis *et al.*, 1990).

In Greece, two of the most typical reasons for starting to smoke seem to be enrolment in university and recruitment into the army. In a recent study of 1136 university students, 23% were regular smokers and 12% were occasional smokers. A substantial percentage had started smoking after enrolment in the university (Athansiou & Macris, 1994). In that study, 16% of the smokers had begun smoking during the previous three months,

27% during the previous six months and 29% within the past 1–2 years. This means that the majority became smokers after entering university, indicating that anti-smoking campaigns should be addressed to first-year university students, who are very vulnerable to various pressures to start smoking at this turning-point of their lives. The case of Greek youngsters indicates the importance of specific characteristics of each society in the development of attitudes to such matters as smoking and the importance of taking them into consideration when developing preventive strategies.

References

Athanasiou, K. & Macris, G. (1994) Smoking and cancer: Exploring the level of knowledge and attitudes of Greek youngsters and parents. In: 9th World Conference on Tobacco and Health, Paris, 10–14 October 1994

Davis, D.E. (1989) Natural anticarcinogens and changing patterns in cancer: Some speculation. *Environ. Res.*, **50**, 322–340

European Bureau for Action on Smoking Prevention (1994) *Tobacco and Health in the EU: An Overview*, Brussels

Peto, R., Lopez, A. D., Boreham, J., Thun, M. & Heath, C., Jr (1994) *Mortality from Smoking in Developed Countries 1950–2000*, Oxford: Oxford University Press

Tomatis, L., *et al.* (1990) *Cancer: Causes, Occurrence and Control* (IARC Scientific Publications No. 100), Lyon, International Agency for Research on Cancer, p. 173.

Trichopoulos, D., Hatzakis, A., Wynder, E., Katsouyanni, K. & Kalandidi, A. (1987) *Environ. Res.*, **44**, 169–178

Uemura, K. & Pisa, Z. (1988) Trends in cardiovascular disease mortality in industrialized countries since 1950. *World Health Stat. Q.*, **41**, 155–178

Influence of youth culture on smoking: Two surveys in Ostrobothnia, Finland

P. Rautama

Provincial State Office of Western Finland, Department of Education and Culture, Service Unit of Vaasa, Vaasa, Finland

Introduction

Smoking among pupils and young people in Finland is a serious health problem. The new *Tobacco Act (1995)* will set new restrictions on the availability and advertising of tobacco products and also on smoking in school premises. According to Piispa (1997), the tobacco policy is primarily aimed at controlling smoking as an activity in itself rather than tobacco sales. Because health education alone has not been able to diminish the prevalence of smoking among youngsters in the intended way, it has been necessary to introduce restrictions.

Local and regional surveys conducted in the three Ostrobothnian provinces indicate that even though the prevalence of smoking among pupils in this region is still quite low, it must be reduced if the pattern of the rest of the country is to be avoided. One of the tasks of the Provincial State Office is to steer and monitor the impact of the *Tobacco Act*. Effective steering requires that the Office develop it assessment and evaluation mechanisms in the field and produce new tools for health education in schools. The surveys described below were carried out by the Provincial State Office of Western Finland with a view to fulfilling this intention.

The cultural meaning of smoking

At the time of puberty, young people live within the sphere of influence of three cultures. The influence of the home is decreasing, in some cases through crises, but it is maintained in the deepest strata of the personality. The influence of friends in influencing daily action increases. The significance of school is greatest in the lower stages of comprehensive schooling but decreases, at least momentarily, when the pupil moves on to the upper stage. Children's paths to youth are determined in advance by their origin and cultural background, although incident and free will also affect it (e.g. Kivirauma, 1997).

One of the tasks of schools is to promote healthy growth and health promoting behaviour. Implementation of this task often collides with the dilemma brought about by the clash between the values of youth culture and those of the school. Schools should be able to assimilate the values of the youth subculture as widely as possible. The task presupposes more modern media publicity and discussions as well as projects targeted to changing the cultural climate (Piispa, 1995).

Health education project: 'A smoke-free culture: the non-smoking pupil'

The former Provincial State Office of Vaasa (since 1 September 1997, this region has been part of the Province of Western Finland) established a three-year, multi-disciplinary project in the autumn of 1994 to increase knowledge about the cultures in which smoking originates and to make use of that knowledge in health education in schools.

In the first stage of the project in January 1995, a sample study was carried out in all comprehensive schools in three provinces of Ostrobothnia (formerly the Province of Vaasa), targeting over 2000 13-year-old pupils, in order to determine their smoking behaviour. The results showed that 4.2% smoked daily, boys more frequently than girls and Finnish pupils more than Swedish ones, while 76% did not smoke. The project was widely advertised in the press. An important finding was that the smoking habits of the parents influence the children's habits. In particular, a non-smoking father often leads to a non-smoking child, and daily smoking by the mother is associated with daily smoking by the child.

In the second stage of the project, at the end of 1995, a sample study was implemented in five Finnish and four Swedish comprehensive schools. The aim of the study was to determine in greater detail the reasons for smoking among pupils over the age of 14 and the place of smoking in youth culture. The proportion of those who smoked daily had increased from 4.2 to 11% and the proportion of non-smokers had decreased from 76 to 73%. Curiosity was the most common reason for experimenting with smoking, and the great majority began to smoke together with their friends. Smoking was continued because friends smoked, 'smoking calms' and it is believed to be popular.

The third stage of the project began in May 1996. Its purpose was to develop efficient new tools for health education. An intervention based on the earlier studies was implemented in three schools targeting pupils, homes and reference groups. Each school was responsible autonomously for the design of the project, following guidelines laid down by the steering group. The Provincial State Office granted each school a share of the costs of the project. The campaigns therefore differed from school to school, but were integrated into school subjects, especially expression and art. In addition, the schools tested how easy it was to buy cigarettes in stores and arranged parents' meetings, plays and radio programmes. The school dentist made a mini-intervention in each school. Despite the intentions, no group of pupils who wished to quit smoking was formed.

The action was productive, because the proportion of non-smokers increased in one school and decreased more slowly in two others in comparison with the control schools. Although the proportion of those who smoked daily increased, the increase was less than in control schools. The onset of smoking was postponed in all schools. Because the actions were directed towards younger age groups as well, the long-term results of the intervention are not yet known, but the results indicate that such education should be continued. Homes must also be linked to this programme more closely than before.

The youth survey in Ostrobothnia, 1997

It made sense, both chronologically and as a follow-up to the project described above, to set up a youth survey in Ostrobothnia in 1997. The aim of the survey was to clarify the attitudes and ethical values of adolescents aged 15–24. The survey is based on the survey of the British newspaper, The Daily Mirror, in autumn 1996, which was designed to support the 'Build a better Britain crusade' to restore British civic values. The Ostrobothnian survey involved 3754 young persons in 15 municipalities and counties, 1000 of whom were selected to participate at regular intervals. The outcomes relating to smoking and its place in youth culture are described here. Thus, 23% of the young people considered that it was wrong to smoke. Anti-smoking Ostrobothnian youth had the most serious attitudes to the ethical education received at school and were rarely absent from school.

Conclusions

The Finnish *Tobacco Act*, a relatively restrictive law in the European frame of reference, has not yet affected the smoking habits of the young. Although the restrictions are well accepted by young people, the failures of enforcement must be recognized. The *Act* could be strengthened in several ways: for example, in one case, the pupils disapproved of their school-bus driver smoking. The results of the survey indicate that the example of parents in smoking is very important for their children. Furthermore, pupils who take school seriously adopt the ethical values of the school more easily than other pupils.

Tobacco seems to be a common fetish of the male culture for pupils who have a negative attitude to school, are poor achievers and are searching for an identity from values other than those that the school provides. This kind of subculture rejects the school values actively and constructs its own values in opposition. In this case, the school is unable to affect the cultural factors behind the pupils' smoking, including socioeconomic status, self-confidence, friends and hobbies of the young person.

Any project that seeks to alter the cultural climate, make it more positive to restrictions, render it more difficult to obtain tobacco and reduce its popularity in common life is positive. This could be one way to sustainable health education that could make the smoking lifestyle something for museums, existing only in French and American movies.

References

Piispa, M. (1995) *The Cultural Significances of Tobacco and Affecting on Them* (Publications Series 87/1995), University of Tampere, Department of Journalism and Mass Communication

Piispa, M. (1997 Popular education, paternalism, protection. Public discourse on alcohol policy and tobacco policy in Finland. *Acta Univ. Tamperensis,* **564**

Kivirauma, J. (1997) Social background and gender in comprehensive school, and the effect of schooling. In: Raivola, R., Valtonen, P. & Vuorensyrjä, M., eds, *Koulutus, Yhteiskunta, Menestys* (Suomen Akatemian julkaisuja 7/97), Helsinki: Suomen Akatemian Koulutuksen vaikuttavuusohjelman tutkimuksia

Smoking behaviour of ninth-form pupils in Pitkäranta (Russian Federation) and in North Karelia (Finland)

K. Tossavainen[1], U. Kemppainen[1], E. Vartiainen[2], V. Pantelejev[3] & P. Puska[2]

[1]*University of Kuopio and* [2]*Institute of Public Health, Finland;* [3]*Central Hospital, Pitkäranta, Russian Federation*

Background

With regard to the health of future generations, it is very important to fight against smoking and defend young people's right to make informed choices without the false images created by the tobacco industry. Many new trials based on social influence, unlike traditional models of health education, have been promising in this area. The North Karelia Youth Project (1984–88) in eastern Finland and its follow-up (1995) is a Finnish model of this approach to promote young people's health. The study was further extended to 10 schools in Pitkäranta in the Karelian Republic of the Russian Federation. Cigarette smoking was estimated from a broad self-administered questionnaire. The population consisted of 371 ninth-form pupils in the district of Pitkäranta in Russian Karelia and 1949 pupils in eastern Finland. All of the pupils were 15 years of age.

The aim of this paper is to give preliminary quantitative data on the smoking behaviour of these pupils. The prevalence of smoking is presented as percentages with chi-squared tests. Logistic regression analysis was used to examine how the smoking behaviour of the family and friends, non-smoking skills, functional meanings of smoking and social normative beliefs are related to the onset of young people's smoking.

Results

The smoking behaviour of girls and boys differed significantly in both countries. Of the boys, 33% in Pitkäranta and 24% in eastern Finland were regular smokers (daily or 1–2 times per week); of the girls, 9% in Pitkäranta and 27% in eastern Finland were regular smokers. The sex difference was greatest in Pitkäranta ($p < 0.001$); in eastern Finland, the difference was not statistically significant. Occasional smoking (1–2 times per month or less often) was more common among the Finnish boys (12%) than the Russian boys (3%) and among the girls (6% were occasional smokers in Pitkäranta and 17% in eastern Finland). Thus, 64% of the boys in both Pitkäranta and in eastern Finland were non-smokers, and 85% of the girls were non-smokers in Pitkäranta and 56% in eastern Finland.

Having a best friend who smoked was the main factor affecting regular smoking in both countries. This variable was the only predictor in the Pitkäranta model. Having a best friend who smoked meant that the young person's own probability of smoking in Pitkäranta was 15-fold and in eastern Finland, 16-fold, compared to having a best friend who did not smoke. Having a best friend who smoked explained 29% of the variation in regular smoking in Pitkäranta and 39% of the variation in eastern Finland. Having a smoking sibling (in eastern Finland) added only 2% to the explanatory degree.

Non-smoking skills were investigated on the basis of agreement or disagreement with six statements. In Pitkäranta, the only predictor that passed the criterion for the model was the opinion 'It's not dangerous to smoke a few cigarettes with friends'. This alone explained 38% of the variation in smoking in Pitkäranta. The opinion 'It's hard for me to refuse a cigarette offered by a peer' was the most important predictor in eastern Finland (explanatory degree, 47%). Five refusal skills together explained 59% of the smoking among ninth-form pupils in eastern Finland.

The functional meaning of smoking was measured on the basis of affirmation or disagreement with eight claims. The statement 'Smokers are more adult' as the only predictor passed the criterion for the model in Pitkäranta and explained 11% of smoking. In eastern Finland, the first variable to pass the criterion was the statement 'Smoking is fun', which explained 17% of smoking. Two variables that met the model explained 25% of the variation in regular smoking in eastern Finland.

Social normative beliefs were studied by agreement or disagreement with five statements related to smoking restrictions. Smokers had more negative attitudes to smoking restrictions than non-smokers. In Pitkäranta, regular smoking was linked with the concept 'Smoking should be allowed on school premises'. This variable explained 16% of the variation in smoking. The second predictor in Pitkäranta was that smokers do not want smoking to be forbidden in public places. These factors together explained about 19% of the variation in regular smoking. In eastern Finland, regular smoking was also associated with the claim that smoking should be allowed on school premises. This variable alone explained 47% of the variation in regular smoking. Non-smokers had a more negative attitude towards smoking in public places and at home. This model explained 60% of the variation in regular smoking.

Discussion

In Finland, recommendations for the promotion of young people's health and non-smoking behaviour were published by an expert group in 1996. The five main principles would be valuable in Russian health promotion, too. The first two are the legislation on cigarettes and how the authorities enforce the legislation. The legislation has to be made more effective by focusing on the restrictions, by using various sanctions and especially by making control of cigarette sale and marketing more effective. Selling tobacco to under-18-year-olds must be forbidden. New resources have to be found and economic resources have to be used more effectively on promoting non-smoking behaviour. The municipal authorities and the State should develop new, concrete health policy strategies. It is also important to develop the competency of health educators. It is essential to develop education on smoking behaviour and non-smoking behaviour in the fields of health, social care and teaching. Professional health-care and educational personnel have an important role in influencing opinions about health promotion. Parents, too, need support in their educational work and in changing their own behaviour.

Since peer pressure is the crucial factor in smoking among young people, the aim of health education should be to teach young people how to identify and resist these pressures. They should be given a positive understanding of health and its prerequisites in the social environment. Thus, young people may be trained to control health matters in their own lives. They must be given the possibility to develop a positive self-image and self-esteem as apart of every-day life and education. Teachers and health-care personnel should work together in this way.

Psychosocial aspects of acquisition and cessation of tobacco habits in India

M.B. Aghi

Tata Institute of Fundamental Research, Mumbai, India

Objective

To examine the dynamics of how and why people take up tobacco and why some give it up. Although the consensus is that tobacco use is a learnt behaviour, acquired through the influence of peers and adult and media role models, there is little agreement on why some people take up the habit and others do not. Scientists view tobacco use as an addiction. While tobacco use certainly has features of classical dependence, such as withdrawal syndrome and dose–response effects, many people do not show all such effects. Nor is the concept of addiction helpful in explaining the phenomenon of cessation, since millions of people worldwide have given up tobacco.

Tobacco seems to act as a mild stimulant, and most smokers find smoking highly pleasurable. Except for this explanation, the solace that habitual smokers get from nicotine is not obvious. Still less is known about tobacco chewing. Villagers in india who use tobacco report that it helps to banish 'vacancy of mind' and boredom, leaving an impression of slight narcosis or temporary elation.

Much information is available about the initiation of smoking among children in developed countries, including peer pressure and parental smoking. Little is known about the smoking behaviour of children in South Asia, although many more children in rural than in urban areas can be seen smoking. In India, few formal data have been accumulated, owing to financial constraints. This presentation is based on personal research in the area of acquisition and cessation of tobacco habits.

Urban smoking patterns

In urban areas of India, the dynamics of smoking are similar to those in the developed world, where young people smoke because their peers smoke. Urban areas of India have great economic diversity, however, and peer pressure varies with economic class. A middle-class boy is unlikely to respond to pressure from his rich friends to smoke, because he may not be able to afford the habit. Among the very wealthy, only men and women who consider themselves 'ultra-modern' smoke, but their number is negligible.

Moreover, a significant number of middle-class families have traditional values. The men in such families rarely smoke and the mothers almost never. Although it is acceptable for men to smoke in South Asia, it is not yet acceptable for women and girls or for young boys, although this number is increasing.

The real tobacco problem is found among the large number of urban poor. Many boys below the age of 15 smoke, and even those as young as five and six. They smoke not because of peer pressure or adult example but because their heroes in the movies or the media smoke.

The rural scene

Villagers are unaware of the health hazards of smoking. They lack education, cigarette advertisements (which, though not very impressively, do include a warning on smoking) are not found in villages, and the warning label on bundles of bidis— cheap products consisting of 2 g of coarse tobacco rolled in a piece of dried tembumi leaf—has little effect because most villagers are illiterate.

Villagers believe that tobacco has medicinal and even magical properties. For some it is a panacea for toothache, bad breath and gastric ailments and is used to postpone hunger and to keep awake. Young boys see their fathers smoke and are often sent by their fathers to buy bidis; they may take a few from the bundle without their fathers' knowlege. Bidi advertisements often have photos of movie stars. Young boys work in the fields, where the atmosphere is conducive to smoking. Many local employers (tea shop or village grocery store owners, for example) give free bidis to boys to encourage and attract them to their work. Since village life is rather dull, much of the leisure time is spent getting together to gossip, which is also conducive to taking up tobacco. Young boys believe that if they want to go to the city to work, they must learn to smoke.

Interventions

A realistic approach to breaking the tobacco habit involves eliminating the old response and acquiring a new one. Therapists in the primary health structure should help tobacco users to develop a series of graded tasks leading to a tobacco-free life, remembering that people should not be looked down on because they have a bad habit: the habit must be regarded as a health, not a moral, problem. Medication should be administered only to relieve discomfort or pain from minor tobacco-related complaints. Understanding, encouragement and support should be given, and planned activities should involve the user completely.

We carried out an intervention project to prevent oral cancer in three rural areas where independent studies had shown that uptake of the tobacco habit was influenced largely by parents, peers and neighbours and that the rationale for initiating and continuing tobacco use was its perceived medical value. There was little awareness of any ill effects of tobacco use. A sequential programme of intervention was devised. Individuals were made aware of the structures within the oral cavity and the concept of oral health. The link between tobacco habits and oral cancer was explained. Possible ways of giving up tobacco were then discussed. Withdrawal symptoms were explained as real but temporary phenomena. The financial, health and aesthetic benefits of giving up tobacco were pointed out. Support and encouragement were given to those who attempted and failed to give up their habit. Reinforcement was provided to those who had succeeded, and a model and leadership role was suggested.

This intervention programme involved two approaches: personal communication and the mass media. Once a year, participants received a diagnosis from a dentist and were then seen by a social scientist. Most of the subjects also participated annually in a group situation. The mass media used for the intervention included films, radio broadcasts and newspaper articles. A documentary film made for the study detailed the relationship between tobacco use and oral cancer. Posters were placed in villages as reminders of the intervention. The radio in India is Government-operated, and radio broadcasts helped to increase the credibility of the intervention messages. Where radio was not available, folk drama was used to eradicate existing misconceptions. Newspaper articles were written specifically for this project and published in the local-language newspapers. The format and content of each intervention strategy were pre-tested and implemented on that basis. For example, we found that the optimal way of screening the film would be to show it to groups of about 25 and then to invite comments from viewers, emphasizing its salient points. The film was then shown again to reinforce the message.

As an incentive and aid to intervention, medicines for common ailments were distributed, dental extractions were performed in field clinics, and the visit to the clinic was used to reinforce the intervention message. The programme was evaluated from feedback and restructured each year before a new follow-up began.

The feasibility of organizing cessation camps in the village was tested and seemed promising. We worked with the villagers for three days, preparing individualized schedules for each villager to follow in order to give up the habit; 18 out of 23 of those who participated were able to give up tobacco. How many actually quit permanently will be judged when we go for our regular follow-up.

Exploring children's perceptions of smoking with the 'draw and write' investigative technique

L. Porcellato, L. Dugdill, J. Springett & F. Sanderson

Liverpool John Moores University, Institute for Health, Liverpool, United Kingdom

Introduction

There is a paucity of research on smoking among young children, even though it is known that the developmental process that leads to smoking begins in early childhood through the mechanism of primary socialization, when exposure to the habit fosters children's attitudes, beliefs and perceptions about tobacco smoke (Royal College of Physicians, 1992). This scarcity has resulted in a lack of awareness of the thinking of young children about smoking and the extent to which they smoke. This has implications for the development of appropriate interventions for school health education, as effective methods are based on the thinking of target groups. It is therefore imperative to determine the depth and breadth of children's understanding and knowledge about smoking, in order to ensure a relevant strategy. The purpose of this study was to examine the perceptions that make up the attitudes and beliefs about smoking of children at the age of 6. The findings will help to fill the significant gap in the literature on young children and smoking and assist in the development of pro-active health promotion.

Method

The dearth of research on smoking and the young has been exacerbated by the lack of appropriate methods of data collection from children this age. Despite the myriad available instruments for adults, few are suitable for children and even fewer are child-centred: the tools that allow children to play an active role in research, thus acknowledging that they are a valuable source of information.

One qualitative method that has proved to be viable for investigating children's perceptions of health and illness is drawing (Williams *et al.*, 1989; Shaver *et al.*, 1993; Oakley *et al.*, 1995). The 'draw and write' investigative technique (Wetton, 1990) requires children to draw pictures and write responses to questions read aloud by the researcher. Scribes are provided to assist children who write with difficulty. The written responses are coded to determine the frequency of specific responses, allowing evaluation of perceptions. The method (Somerset Health Education Authority and Somerset Education Consultants with the Best of Health Project, 1994) was used with a representative sample of 216 primary schoolchildren aged 6 (107 boys and 109 girls) in the City of Liverpool.

Results

During the first enquiry, the children were asked to draw someone who smokes and to write how thay thought that person felt and where they thought the smoke goes. Negative comments were expressed about smokers by 65% of boys and 68% of girls and positive comments by 29 and 31%, respectively. Most of the children (70%) thought that the smoke went generally into the body; six children specified the lungs and two the heart, and one child mentioned asthma.

The children were also asked to draw a young person who had just started to smoke and to write answers to the questions, 'Why does your person wants to smoke?' (Figure 1) and 'Where did they learn to smoke?' (Figure 2). Imitation was mentioned by at least 50% of the children, and curiosity and the desire to try smoking were cited by 32%. Girls in particular noted parental smoking (23%) and the image of smoking as being 'big', 'good' or 'cool' as the rationale for young people taking up the habit. In the answers to the second question, familial references (parents, home, siblings and relatives) accounted for almost 50% of all responses. Interestingly, the boys cited mothers and fathers with equal frequency (13%), whereas girls tended to use the generic term 'parents' (16%). Other people were seen as sources of learning by boys in particular (25%), and many of the children thought that friends and places such as the shop, the street and the park were places where one could learn to smoke. The fact that television was mentioned by only two children indicates that the advertising ban has been effective and lends credence to those who advocate a complete ban of all tobacco advertising.

Conclusion

The overall findings of this study suggest that local primary schoolchildren aged 6 generally have a negative attitude to tobacco and have a broad understanding of the nature of smoking. Most are aware that some health risk is involved in taking up the habit, they have well-formulated ideas about how the habit is acquired, and they acknowledge the significant influence of the family in the acquisition. The results highlight the fact that young children have well-defined perceptions about smoking. This insight into their thinking about the habit will provide the foundation on which to build an effective smoking prevention model for health promotion.

Figure 1. Examples of responses to the questions 'How does the person feel?' and 'Where does the smoke go?'

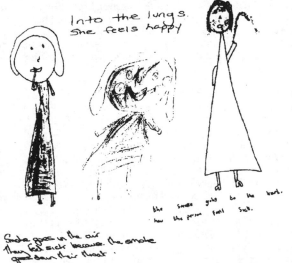

Figure 2. Examples of responses to the questions, 'Why does your person want to smoke?' and 'Where did they learn to smoke?'

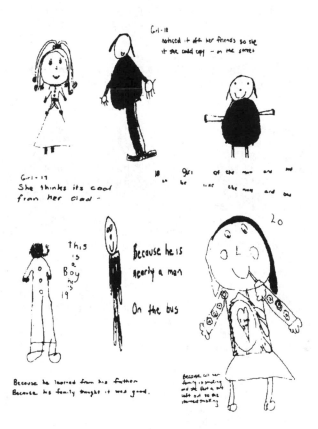

Acknowledgement

The research study was funded by The Roy Castle Lung Cancer Foundation.

References

Oakley, A., Bendelow, G., Barnes, J., Buchanan, M. & Husain, N. (1995) Health and cancer prevention: Knowledge and beliefs of children and young people. Br. Med. J., 310, 1029–1033

Royal College of Physicians (1992) Smoking and the Young, London

Shaver, T., Francis, V. & Barnett, L. (1993) Drawing as Dialogue (ERG Technical Notes Series No. 2), Liverpool: Education Resource Group, Liverpool School of Tropical Medicine

Somerset Health Education Authority and Somerset Education Consultants with the Best of Health Project (1994) The Draw and Write Technique for the Primary School into Children's Changing Perceptions of Cigarette Smoke, Cigarette Smokers and Cigarette Smoking, Southampton: Health Education Unit, School of Education, University of Southampton

Wetton, N.M. (1990) Draw and Write Technique, Southampton: Health Education Unit, School of Education, University of Southampton

Williams, T., Wetton, N. & Moon, A. (1989) A Picture of Health: What Do You Do that Makes You Healthy and Keeps You Healthy? London: Health Education Authority

Do parents and children know each other's smoking experience and attitudes towards children's smoking?

S.F. Chung[1], Z.M. Wat[2], S.H. Tong[2], S.L. Tsang[2], Y.H. Tsang[2], C.H. Wong[2], C.Y. Wong[2], H.S. Wong[2], H. Wong[2], K.C. Wong[2], M.K. Wong[2], S.T. Wong[2], S.H. Wong[2] & W.Y. Wong[2]

[1]*Department of Community Medicine and* [2]*Medical Students in the Health Behaviour and Medical Care Programme 1994–95, Department of Community Medicine, The University of Hong Kong, Hong Kong SAR, China*

Introduction

In 1994, a survey on youth smoking and health in Hong Kong showed that 29% of junior secondary-school students (mostly aged 12–15 years) had ever smoked cigarettes. More than half had smoked their first cigarette when they were in primary school or before, i.e. at the age of ≤ 11 years., and about 3% had smoked their first cigarette when they were ≤ 6 years old (Lam *et al.*, 1994). A study in Hong Kong showed that about 6% of children in primary class 3 and about 19% of those in class 6 had ever smoked (Hedley *et al.*, 1993). These results clearly demonstrate that the problem of smoking among youth begins before primary school and increases during primary schooling. The study also showed that 95% of the children in primary classes 3 and 4 recognized the Marlboro name and the Salem logo as belonging to tobacco products, from a choice of various consumer products including food, cigarettes and drinks (Peter *et al.*, 1995). The results show that primary school students in Hong Kong are aware of the smoking issue.

It had been suggested that the topic of tobacco use be addressed at primary schools in Hong Kong (Sanagan, 1996), and a smoking intervention programme was tested on children in primary class 4 (Betson *et al.*, 1995). While school can help to increase children's understanding of the harmful effects of smoking and the real objectives of the images of smoking in smoking advertisements, the knowledge may not be sufficient for children to resist invitations from close persons to try smoking. In an earlier paper on the smoking experience of the same children, 11% of those who had ever smoked said that they had started when asked to try smoking by a family member, and 12% attributed their initiation to their friends (Chung *et al.*, 1996). Children may therefore need strong support from their family and friends to consolidate their anti-smoking attitude and resist the invitation to try smoking. A study in nursery schools in the United Kingdom showed that parental influence was the most important factor affecting whether very young children smoked when they had grown up (Fiddler & Durrant, 1995). In this paper, we studied parents' concern and attitude towards children's smoking in Hong Kong.

Study design and subjects

Invitations to participate in the survey were sent to 25 randomly chosen Chinese-speaking primary schools; 17 participated, for a response rate of 68%. In each school, one class from each grade was selected randomly. Between May and July 1995, 3420 students in 102 primary classes 1 to 6 participated in the survey.

Two standardized, self-administered, anonymous questionnaires were used, both in Chinese, modified from those developed earlier by the Department of Community Medicine of the University of Hong Kong (Hedley *et al.*, 1993). One questionnaire, designed for the students, was pilot-tested and revised to ensure that the questions were simple and straightforward enough for the lower-grade schoolchildren. The students completed the questionnaires in their classrooms under the guidance of teachers or one of our trained interviewers. The questionnaires were collected immediately upon completion. Specific instructions were given to the teachers and interviewers not to influence the students; if the students had queries about the questions, the teachers and interviewers were asked to tell the students to choose the answer 'Don't know'. The students were also reminded not to discuss the questions with anyone else in the class. The second questionnaire was taken home by the students for their parents or guardians to complete, to be returned within one week of distribution, regardless of whether or not the questionnaire had been completed. The response rates for the students and parents were 100 and 93%, respectively.

Results

The smoking experience was reported as 'never' by 93.6% of the children, 'tried only' by 5.2%, 'used to but stopped' by 0.8%, 'smoke < 7 cigarettes per week' by 0.3% and 'smoke ≥ 7 per week' by 0.2%. The parents' responses indicated that 94.4% thought their children had never smoked, 0.5% thought their children were smokers and 5.1% did not know. In the children's reporting of their parents' smoking, 3.5% said their mothers were smokers, 1.9% did not know whether their mothers smoked, 38.7% said that their fathers smoked and 1.5% did not know whether their father smoked. The parents' responses showed that 2.9% of the mothers and 41.6% of the fathers were smokers. With regard to the attitude of the parents, 85% of the children thought that their parents would be against their smoking, 5.4% thought that their parents would not be against it, and 8.6% did not know. According to the parents' responses, 87.6% of the parents would be against their children's smoking, 5.6% would not be against it, and 6.8% did not know.

Discussion

Since the questionnaires were anonymous, we could not link the answers of the children with those of their parents. Nevertheless, the results showed that the parents of 5.1% of the children did not know whether they were smokers or not. These children had probably tried smoking, as the proportions of 'Never smoked' reported by the children and the parents were similar. For the questions to which the response was "Don't know", we did not enquire whether the parents had not asked the children or the children had not answered the parents' question. The result suggests that lack of parental concern may be a factor in children's experimenting with smoking.

The results also show that about 7% of paternal smoking was not recognized by the children, probably because the father did not smoke in front of the children. Parents should be encouraged not to smoke in front of their children, in order to protect the children's health even if they cannot quit smoking.

The children's perception of their parents' attitude towards their smoking was similar to the attitudes reported by the parents. In the above-mentioned study in junior secondary schools, the students were asked whether they thought their parents would interfere if they smoked: 88% thought that their mothers and 82% thought that their fathers would interfere (Lam *et al.*, 1994). These proportions are similar to that of the present study (85%), which suggests that more than 10% of parents would not be against their children smoking. Further research is needed to find out why some parents accept smoking by their children.

Acknowledgments
We would like to thank the schools, the students and the parents for their participation and the Education Department for its assistance. This survey was supported by a grant from Hsin Chong-KN Godfrey Yeh Education Fund for Joint Student Projects. It was also awarded a prize by the Hong Kong College of General Practitioners.

References

Betson, C.L., Peters, J., Hedley, A.J., Lam, T.H., Wong, C.M., Day, J. & Fielding, R. (1995) A smoking intervention program for primary four students in Hong Kong: What it can and cannot achieve. *Asia–Pacific J. Public Health*, **8**, 13–19

Chung, S.F., Wat, Z.M., Tong, S.H., Tsang, S.L., Tsang, Y.H., Wong, C.H., Wong, C.Y., Wong, H.S., Wong, H., Wong, K.C., Wong, M.K., Wong, S.T., Wong, S.H. & Wong, W.Y. (1996) Smoking and anti-smoking in family and in primary school. In: Smoking and Health 2000: Proceedings of the 1996 Conference on Smoking and Health, pp. 92–96

Fiddler, W. & Durrant, K. (1995) The influence of the adult role model of smoking on very young children. In: Slama, K., ed., *Tobacco and Health: Proceedings of the Ninth World Conference on Tobacco or Health*, pp. P613–621

Hedley, A.J., Peter, J., Lam, T.H., *et al.* (1993) *Air Pollution and Respiratory Health in Primary School Children in Hong Kong, 1989–92: Report to the Environmental Protection Department, Hong Kong Government*, Department of Community Medicine, University of Hong Kong

Lam, T.H., Chung, S.F., Wong, C.M., Hedley, A.J. & Betson, C.L. (1994) *Youth Smoking and Health Survey 1994, Report No. 1: Youth Smoking, Health and Tobacco Promotion*, Hong Kong Council on Smoking and Health

Peter, J., Betson, C.L., Hedley, A.J., Lam, T.H., Ong, S.G., Wong, C.M. & Fielding, R. (1995) Recognition of cigarette brand names and logos by young children in Hong Kong. *Tobacco Control*, 4, 150–155

Sanagan, P. (1996) Interactive programming for smoking prevention in primary schools. In: Proceedings of 1996 Conference on Smoking and Health, pp. P143–147

Five-year old urban children's perceptions, attitudes and expressed intentions regarding cigarette use (The Birth-to-ten study)

T. de Wet, K. Steyn, I. Richter & D. Yach

Chronic Diseases of Lifestyle Programme, Urbanisation and Health, Medical Research Council, Tygerberg, South Africa

Objectives: Understanding how children's perceptions of smoking change over time may explain why some children decide to experiment with cigarettes and take up smoking, while others do not. The purpose of this study was to determine the perceptions, attitudes and expressed intentions of five-year old urban children with regard to cigarette use.

Methods: The 'Birth-to-ten' study is a longitudinal birth-cohort study of health and development among children born in Soweto–Johannesburg during a seven-week period in 1990. In 1995, at the age of five, 1350 children in the study were interviewed about their knowledge of tobacco use, their perceptions of and attitudes towards smoking and their intention to experiment with cigarettes and to smoke regularly when grown-up.

Results: These five-year-old children have well-developed beliefs about tobacco use: 98% knew someone who smoked, 60% reported buying cigarettes for other people (52% for parents, 41% for other family members). Of those who bought cigarettes for other people, 81% bought loose cigarettes and 19% bought packs. Of the children, 29% knew brand names, especially Peter Stuyvesant, Rothmans and Consulate, the most heavily advertised brands; nevertheless, 77% thought smoking was bad for you (21% give health reasons), 19% thought it was anti-social, 81% thought they would not smoke when they grew up, but 19% thought they would and 7% had tried smoking.

Conclusions: These data show that the smoking behaviour of adults and cigarette advertisements have a substantial impact on the perceptions, attitudes and expressed intentions concerning cigarette use of five-year-old South African children.

Tobacco smoking and music preferences of students

J. Posluszna & R. Palusiński

Department of Educational Sociology, Poznan, Poland

Music produces strong emotions and is therefore a powerful therapeutic and diagnostic tool in contemporary psychology. As emotional factors seem to play a role in the development of cigarette addiction, the aim of the study was to compare music preferences in the group of educational sociology students with regard to their smoking habit.

One hundred students (70 women and 30 men) at the mean age of 22.2 ± 4.5 years were asked to fill in a questionnaire and listen to 35 pieces of music composed in various stylistic periods and performed on various instruments. The 19 smokers and 81 non-smokers in the study population did not differ in their level of musical education or sex; however, significant differences were found in the student's preferences in music, as shown in Table 1. We also found that the smokers went to concerts more frequently than the non-smokers (37% versus 6%, $p = 0.006$).

The smokers preferred solo music played on stringed instruments at a slow tempo, rather low-pitched and sentimental. Their reactions to music therefore seem to be more emotional than those of non-smokers. These results may be useful in music therapy for smokers.

Table 1. Types of music preferred by smokers and non-smokers

Smoking status	Type of music (% positive answers)				
	Low-pitched	Solo	String	Sentimental	Fast tempo
Non-smokers	18	24	29	34	27
Smokers	30	33	38	45	12

Youth culture and smoking: How to find out who does what and why

P. Schofield[1,2], D. Hill[1] & P. Pattison[2]

[1]Anti-cancer Council of Victoria, and [2]University of Melbourne, Melbourne, Australia

Youth culture has long been recognized as a powerful force opposing anti-smoking campaigns. Youth is made up of many 'tribes', and each of these peer groups has different norms to which their members subscribe. To gain insight into the connection between various peer groups and smoking, we conducted intensive one-to-one interviews with 29 school leavers. The findings of these interviews indicated that smoking is seen as a stereotypical attribute of certain peer groups and serves to distinguish one group from another. Groups in which smoking was the norm had very different descriptors ('alternative' and 'rebels') from non-smoking groups (e.g. 'nerds', 'study together'). This information provided concrete direction for choosing appropriate target groups. The interview material was also used to develop items for questionnaires. Quantitative findings confirmed the perceptions derived from the interview material.

The social symbolism of smoking

T. Bechmann Jensen

Psychological Laboratory, University of Copenhagen, Copenhagen, Denmark

Background

Although the Danish population is well informed about the health effects of smoking, many Danes ignore the risks: the prevalence of smoking is one of the highest in Europe (40%). A negative attitude towards smoking is increasingly common among children and young people, but large numbers are still starting to smoke during adolescence. This paper deals with research on the knowledge, attitudes and behaviour of young people aged 16–25 based on a reseach project that includes both qualitative interviews with about 60 people aged 16–25 and a quantitative study of 1200 individuals in different contextual settings, including students, unemployed people and professionals.

The reasons for smoking fall into contextual (e.g. geographical) and situational (relational) categories. In our study, smoking seemed to be related to the closeness and length of relationships: thus, the longer the contextual setting and the closer the contact between individuals, the less people smoke. The main focus of my research is how young people smoke: with whom, in what circumstances and with what perceived advantages or satisfaction in mind.

In the qualitative research, personal interviews were carried out according to the ideological deconstructive method, focusing on the situations in which smoking is done. The aim is to help the informants to develop personal ideas, so that there is consistency between theory and practice. The underlying assumption is that what seems irrational or poorly argued is often rational in the context of the actual conditions and circumstances under which the action takes place.

Results

I have chosen as an example a man in his mid-twenties, called Peter, who has been smoking on and off for the past 10 years. He smoked most frequently in high school and during his training as a public school teacher. As he is an athlete and runs in marathons, he knows about the physiological effects of smoking; he is also conscious that he is a role model for his pupils and never smokes during working hours. Peter is aware that smoking damages health and considers that it should be avoided. He explains that he smokes 10–15 cigarettes per week and divides his smoking into three categories:
• Smoking with friends: He explains that smoking strengthens bonds and relationships with friends who smoke. They discuss the brand of cigarettes they smoke and have smoking rituals. Peter never smokes more than five cigarettes in these situations, but he smoked one cigarette during our interview, identifying it as a friendly but serious discussion similar to those he has with friends.
• Smoking alone: This kind of smoking is usually done in the evening or at night when Peter wants to reflect upon something in his everyday life, or on holidays. He explains that this kind of smoking allows him to analyse himself from the 'outside'. He usually smokes one or at most two cigarettes.
• Party smoking: This is the best-known type to many young people. Peter explains that he smokes at parties for company and to relax. Party smoking is always accompanied by drinking alcohol. Smoking at parties can easily lead to smoking 10–15 cigarettes in one night.

When Peter was asked if he would smoke more cigarettes if they were not unhealthy, he replied that in that case he would not smoke at all. The fact that cigarettes are unhealthy makes smoking psychologically, socially and cognitively satisfying.

Conclusion

Peter is a type of smoker who is not included in most educational programmes. The questions to be asked are therefore: Can educational programmes on smoking be designed to include perspectives and values other than health? Should we focus educational efforts on smoking situations rather than on the individuals who smoke? Can the perceived advantages of smoking be replaced by something other then nicotine products and counselling?

Health effects

Smoking and lung function in Hong Kong Chinese schoolchildren

J. Peters[1,2], A. Hedley[1], T.-H. Lam[1] & C.-M. Wong[1]

[1]*Department of Community Medicine and Behavioural Sciences, University of Hong Kong, Hong Kong SAR, China;* [2]*Section of Public Health, School of Health and Related Research, University of Sheffield, United Kingdom*

Introduction

The association between tobacco smoking and diseases of the respiratory system, such as chronic obstructive lung disease and lung cancer, is well recognized in adults, as is its association with respiratory ill health in children who are exposed to environmental tobacco smoke (Environmental Protection Agency, 1992). The effect of exposure to tobacco smoke on lung function is less clear. Lower values for forced expiratory volume (FEV) have been reported for children living with parents who smoke (Hasselblad *et al.*, 1981; Vedal *et al.*, 1984; O'Connor *et al.*, 1987; Kauffman *et al.*, 1989), but not necessarily with parallel change in functional vital capacity (FVC) (Kauffman *et al.*, 1989). Gold *et al.* (1996) found larger values for both FVC and FEV in children who smoked than those who did not, but the rates of growth in lung function were reduced in the smokers (Lebowitz *et al.*, 1987; Gold *et al.*, 1996). This paper presents the results of a preliminary examination of lung function in Chinese primary school children according to the children's exposure to tobacco smoke.

Method

A population-based enquiry into the respiratory health of children was set up in 1989 in two districts of Hong Kong, Kwai Tsing and Southern, to examine the impact of poor air quality on respiratory health. Children and their parents were recruited from primary classes 3 and 4 in 17 schools, seven in Southern and eight in Kwai Tsing. Full details of the study design and the selection of schools and classes are reported elsewhere (Ong *et al.*, 1991).

Questionnaires developed after reference to internationally recognized standard questionnaires (Medical Research Council, 1960; Florey & Leeder, 1982) were completed by all children in a classroom under the supervision of a trained researcher; no teachers were present. The questions addressed the child's respiratory symptoms, their smoking practices and their exposure to tobacco smoke in the home. For the latter, the questions included who and how many categories of people (father, mother, siblings and other relatives or lodgers) smoked in the family home; the answers to all of these questions were aggregated and coded as exposure to none or one or more smoking categories. The children's smoking practices were recorded as 'never' or 'ever' smoker on the basis of their answers to one of six options: 'never smoked, used to but not now, tried a few times, smoke less than one cigarette a week, smoke 1–6 cigarettes a week, smoke more than 6 cigarettes a week'. Parents also completed a questionnaire, which addressed the type of housing (coded as public and all other), their educational attainment (no formal education, primary, lower, upper or post-secondary) and current occupational status (working, not working, not known).

All of the children underwent a health examination which included measurements of height and weight taken by a trained researcher using standard techniques (Cameron *et al.*, 1981). Lung function (FVC and FEV in one second, FEV_1) were measured with a Vitalograph. The session was supervised by a trained researcher, and the highest of three attempts was recorded in each case.

All data were analysed with SPSS with independent sample *t* tests and one-way analysis of variance to test for differences between lung function values according to sex, district of residence, parents' occupation and education, type of housing, exposure to smoking and child's smoking status. Linear regression was used to examine the relationship between height and age with FVC and FEV_1.

Results

For a number of reasons, 38 children were significantly older than their contemporaries and were excluded from the analyses. Lung function measurements were missing for 270 children (8%). The final data set comprised 3240 children aged 8–11 (Table 1). Any smoking was reported by 260 children (8%), with proportionately more boys than girls (Table 1). The proportion of ever-smokers increased with age and ranged from 2.3% among eight-year-old girls to 31% among 11-year-old boys. Half of the children (48%, 1526) lived in a home with one or more categories of smoker.

A relationship was seen between the children's FEV_1 and FVC and their age, height and sex (Table 2). Having a non-working mother was also found to be associated with both FVC and FEV_1, and housing was associated with FVC but not FEV_1 (Table 2). No statistically significant relationship was seen between FEV_1 and FVC and the socioeconomic factors of the father's occupation, parental education or district of residence. Both measures of lung function were significantly higher in children who had ever smoked than in those who had never smoked (Table 2), and these differences were maintained when adjusted for age and sex. The mean percentage difference was 2.0 and 2.1% for FVC and 0.9 and 2.8% for FEV_1 in girls and boys, respectively, after adjustment for age.

Discussion

Respiratory complaints associated with exposure to smoking have been demonstrated in these children (Ong et al., 1991; Peters et al., 1996). There is also evidence that exposure to smoking affects lung function, particularly among children whose mothers smoke (Hasselblad et al., 1981; Vedal et al., 1984). A similar result was not demonstrated in our study, but less than 4% of the mothers smoked (Peters et al., 1996). Although we did not use cotinine measurements to verify the smoking status reported by the children, the high level of agreement observed between some other answers in the questionnaire, such as children's versus parental reporting of the smoking practices of family members, lends credence to our assumption that the children's responses were honest.

The cross-sectional nature of these data does not enable us to show if the larger FVC and FEV_1 values seen in the smoking children are a response to their smoking practice. Gold et al. (1996) suggested that children who already have better lung function before starting to smoke experience less discomfort when they experiment and therefore persist in smoking. Either way, evidence is accumulating of differences in lung function in children as young as eight years of age at what is likely to be an early stage in their smoking history. Given that increasing numbers of young children are experimenting with smoking and that this experimentation is starting at younger and younger ages, longitudinal studies are needed to examine the early impact of smoking on lung function in young children.

Table 1. Characteristics of study population

Characteristic	Boys	Girls	Test and significance
Age (years)			
8	465	485	
9	815	663	
10	414	302	
11	62	34	
Mean	9.52	9.43	$t = -3.56$, df = 3238, $p < 0.001$
District			
Southern	774	591	$\chi^2 = 5.97$, df = 1, $p = 0.015$
Kwai Tsing	982	893	
Child smoking			
Ever	186	74	$\chi^2 = 33.92$, df = 1, $p < 0.001$
Never	1569	1404	
Child living with smokers			
None	916	771	$\chi^2 = 0$, df = 1, $p = 0.98$
≥ 1	828	698	

Table 2. Relationship between FVC and FEV$_1$ by demographic and socioeconomic factors and exposure to smoking

Factor	Mean FVC	Test and significance	Mean FEV$_1$	Test and significance
Sex				
Boys	1.904	$t = -14.89$,	1.718	$t = -11.91$,
Girls	1.734	df = 3238	1.599	df = 3238
		$p < 0.001$		$p < 0.001$
Age (years)				
8	1.670	F = 180.22	1.523	F = 195.61
9	1.828	df = 3,3236	1.664	df = 3,3236
10	1.989	$p < 0.001$	1.810	$p < 0.001$
11	1.141		1.953	
Height (cm)	a = 0.03,	F = 3172.4,	a = 0.03,	F = 3306.1,
	b = -2.77	df = 1,3238,	b = -2.38	df = 1,3238,
		$p < 0.001$		$p < 0.001$
Mother working				
Yes	1.857	$t = 2.69$,	1.700	$t = 3.74$,
		df = 2330		df = 2330
No	1.818	$p = 0.007$	1.652	$p < 0.001$
Housing				
Public	1.809	$t = -3.68$,	1.656	$t = -1.83$,
		df = 2180.7		df = 3122
All other	1.855	$p < 0.001$	1.676	$p = 0.067$
Child smoking				
Never	1.818	$t = -0.64$,	1.657	$t = -4.25$,
		df = 3231		df = 3231
Ever	1.918	$p < 0.001$	1.737	$p < 0.001$
Live with smokers				
None	1.826	$t = -0.06$,	1.663	$t = -0.08$,

References

Cameron, N., Hiernaux, J., Marshall, W.A., Tanner, J.M. & Whitehouse, R.H. (1981) In: Weiner, J.S. & Lourie, J.A., eds, *Practical Human Biology*, London: Academic Press, pp. 27–52

Environmental Protection Agency (1992) *Respiratory Health Effects of Passive Smoking: Lung Cancer and other Disorders* (EPA/600/6-90/006F), Washington DC

Florey, C.duV. & Leeder, S.R. (1982) *Methods for Cohort Studies of Chronic Airflow Limitation* (WHO Regional Publications, European Series No. 12), Copenhagen: WHO Regional Office for Europe

Gold, D.R., Wang, X., Wypij, D., Speizer, F.E., Ware, J.H. & Dockery, D.W. (1996) Effects of cigarette smoking on lung function in adolescent boys and girls. *New Engl. J. Med.*, **335**, 931–937

Hasselblad, V., Humble, C.G., Graham, M.G. & Anderson, H.S. (1981) Indoor environmental determinants of lung function in children. *Am. Rev. Respir. Dis.*, **123**, 479–485

Kauffman, F., Tager, I.B., Munoz, A. & Speizer, F.E. (1989) Familial factors related to lung function in children aged 6-10 years. *Am. J. Epidemiol.*, **129**, 1289–1299

Lebowitz, M.D., Holberg, C.J., Knudson, R.J. & Burrows, B. (1987) Longitudinal study of pulmonary function development in childhood, adolescence, and early adulthood. *Am. Rev. Respir. Dis.*, **136**, 69–75

Medical Research Council (1960) *Questionnaire on Respiratory Symptoms*, London

O'Connor, G.T., Weiss, S.T., Tager, I.B. & Speizer, F.E. (1987) The effect of passive smoking on pulmonary function and non-specific bronchial responsiveness in a population-based sample of children and young adults. *Am. Rev. Respir. Dis.*, **135**, 800–804

Ong, S.G., Liu, J., Wong, C.M., *et al.* (1991) Studies on the respiratory health of primary school children in urban communities of Hong Kong. *Sci. Total Environ.*, **106**, 121–135

Peters, J., Hedley, A.J., Wong, C.M., Lam, T.H., Ong, S.G., Liu, J. & Spiegelhalter, D.J. (1996) Effects of an ambient air pollution intervention and environmental tobacco smoke on children's respiratory health in Hong Kong. *Int. J. Epidemiol.*, **25**, 821–828

Vedal, S., Schenker, M.B., Samet, J.M. & Speizer, F.E. (1984) Risk factors for childhood respiratory disease. *Am. Rev. Respir. Dis.*, **130**, 187–192

TOBACCO AND OCCUPATIONAL HEALTH

Smoking and occupational exposure of workers in Guangzhou, China

C.Q. Jiang[1], T.H. Lam[2], S.Y. Ho[2], W.W. Liu[1], W.S. Zhang[1], J.M. He[1] & C.Q. Zhu[1]

[1]Guangzhou Occupational Diseases Prevention and Treatment Centre, Guangzhou;
[2]Department of Community Medicine, The University of Hong Kong,
Hong Kong SAR, China

Introduction

In China, occupational health professionals are mainly concerned with the control of occupational hazards, such as dust and chemical, biological and physical hazards, and with prevention and management of occupational diseases. Occupational health research is also focused on the effects of such exposure. Other lifestyle factors, such as smoking, drinking and dietary habits, which are important for workers' health, are considered to be non-occupational factors and are usually ignored. Although smoking is a major health hazard among workers, it is neglected by many occupational physicians and other occupational health professionals.

According to the 1984 Chinese National Smoking Prevalence Survey (Weng et al., 1987), male workers had a smoking prevalence of 65.7%, which was higher than that of peasants (63.7%) and cadres (59.2%). In our 1994 cross-sectional study on 8304 workers from a random sample of 47 factories in Guangzhou (Lam et al., 1996), we found that male workers who were exposed to occupational hazards had higher smoking prevalence rates than those who were not exposed. Among male workers exposed to dust, the prevalence was as high as 71.6%.

Studies in the West have shown that smoking and occupational exposure can have synergistic effect on the health of workers. A few reports that support such finding have been published in China. For example, Huang et al. (1994) found that smoking and exposure to chromium compounds had synergistic effects on the rate of lung cancer among male workers. Yang, J.M. et al. (1996) found synergistic effects on lung function of smoking and exposure to weldings fumes, and Gong et al. (1996) found synergistic effects on lung cancer of smoking and exposure to asphalt.

To study the effect of smoking and occupational exposure on mortality, we are carrying out a prospective study of about 200 000 workers aged ≥ 35 in Guangzhou. In this paper, we present the preliminary findings on smoking prevalence and occupational exposures of the 24 014 workers included in the first phase of data retrieval from occupational health surveillance records.

Methods

All 860 factories with an occupational health surveillance record system, established at the Guangzhou Occupational Diseases Prevention and Treatment Centre between 1990 and 1992, were invited to participate. All workers aged ≥ 35 with a smoking history recorded in their occupational health record were included. A standard data retrieval form with 'intelligent character recognition' was designed. Factory doctors were invited to attend a training workshop to learn to transfer information from the workers' records onto the data forms. The data forms were scanned and entered into a computer. These procedures are still in progress. The first batch of completed data forms was then checked and analysed by SPSS for Windows.

Results

Of the 24 014 workers, 15 345 (64%) were men and 8669 (36%) were women, and 47% of the men and 33% of the women were exposed to occupational hazards. The smoking prevalence was 66.8% among men and 1.1% among women. Table 1 shows that the smoking prevalence decreased with age among men, with the highest prevalence

Table 1. Smoking prevalence by age, education, occupation and exposure among men and women

Characteristic	Men (%)	Women (%)
Age (years)		
35–	72	0.5
40–	67	1.3
45–	66	2.1
50–	64	3.3
55–	63	5.3
60	56	–
Education (years)		
≤ 6	73	2.0
7–12	67	0.7
≥ 12	45	0.9
Marital status		
Single	65	0.8
Married	67	1.1
Occupation		
Management	58	0.8
Worker	70	1.1
Exposure to occupational hazards		
No exposure	64	1.0
Dust	70	1.7
Chemicals	65	0.6
Physical factors	71	1.3
Other factors	56	2.8
Multiple exposure	74	1.4

for those aged 35–39 (72%) and the lowest for those aged ≥ 60 (56%). Among women, the smoking prevalence was highest for those aged 55–59 years (5.3%), but, in general, younger women had a lower prevalence. Both men and women with a lower educational level had a higher prevalence than those with longer education. No differences were found by marital status.

Workers had a higher smoking prevalence than management personnel, and those with no exposure to occupational hazards had a lower prevalence than those who were exposed (64% versus 70% among men and 1.0% versus 1.2% among women). The highest smoking prevalence was that of men exposed to more than one type of occupational hazard.

Discussion

This preliminary analysis of data from the first phase of the prospective study showed that male workers had the highest smoking prevalence, and exposed male workers had a higher smoking prevalence than unexposed workers. The smoking prevalence of female workers was low, but those who were exposed also had a higher prevalence. These results are consistent with those of our earlier report, which was based on a smaller sample (Lam et al., 1996). It is clear that in China most workers who are exposed to occupational hazards are also smokers, and the high smoking prevalence among exposed men indicates that their health is seriously at risk from simultaneous exposure to at least two health hazards.

Furthermore, the high smoking prevalence among workers is an important source of passive smoking both at work and at home. The 1996 Chinese National Prevalence Study (Yang, G.H. et al., 1998) showed that 41.5% of male and 19.3% of female non-smokers were exposed passively to smoking at work. There is also evidence in China to show that passive smoking at work is a risk factor for coronary heart disease in women who have never smoked (He et al., 1994). Passive smoking at work is therefore an important occupational health hazard. Further studies are needed to examine whether there is a synergistic effect of passive smoking and occupational exposure in non-smoking men and women.

The growing tobacco epidemic in China and other developing countries is likely to be greater and faster in the working population. They have increasing occupational exposures due to rapid industrialization and increasing tobacco consumption due to the improved economy and aggressive promotion by multinational tobacco companies. Occupational health professionals should be aware of the important health hazards of smoking and passive smoking in the workplace and should control them. The narrow focus and traditional perspective of occupational health, confined to occupational hazards, which ignores smoking and other lifestyle risk factors of workers, cannot help to control this epidemic and might contribute to its spread by passively permitting or encouraging smoking. It should also be noted that when there is syngerism between smoking and an occupational hazard, prevention of smoking will eliminate both its adverse health effects and the synergistic effects of smoking and the hazard. The health gains of tobacco control in the workplace are potentially substantial and could be more substantial than control of the occupational hazard, if the latter is less harmful than smoking. As the goal of occupational health is to promote the health of the working population, occupational health professionals should control smoking as well as occupational hazards.

Acknowledgements
We wish to thank the Health Services Research Committee and the Research Grants Council of Hong Kong for funding this project and the Dr Sun-Yat-Sen Foundation Fund for Academic Exchanges with China in the Faculty of Medicine, The University of Hong Kong for the visitorship of Dr C.Q. Jiang to Hong Kong and Ms Marie Chi for clerical assistance.

References

Gong, D.T., *et al.* (1996) [Study on relationship between smoking and lung cancer in asphalt felt-making workers.] *Tumour*, **16**, 83–86 (in Chinese)

He, Y., Lam, T.H., *et al.* (1994) Passive smoking at work as a risk factor for coronary heart disease in Chinese women who have never smoked. *Br. Med. J.*, **308**, 380–384

Huang, M.Y., *et al.* (1994) [A study on smoking and lung cancer in chromic salt production workers.] *Ind. Hyg. Occup. Dis.*, **20**, 323–325 (in Chinese)

Lam, T.H., Jiang, C.Q., *et al.* (1996) Smoking and exposure to occupational hazards in 8304 workers in Guangzhou, China. *Occup. Med.*, **46**, 351–355

Weng, X.Z., *et al.* (1987) [*A Collection of Data of the 1984 National Smoking Sample Survey*], Beijing: People's Health Publishers (in Chinese)

Yang, J.M., *et al.* (1996) [Study on effect of welding fumes on worker's lung function.] *Ind. Hyg. Occup. Dis.*, **22**, 202–204 (in Chinese)

Yang, G.H., *et al.* (1996) *National Prevalence Survey of Smoking Pattern*, Beijing: China Science and Technology Press

Smoking cessation at the worksite: Taking the viewpoint of employers into account

M.C. Willemsen

Department of Health Education and Promotion, Maastricht University, Netherlands

Many company managers feel that smoking by employees is not their responsibility, as long as the company's interests are not threatened by it. This attitude makes it difficult for anti-smoking advocates to reach smokers at the workplace. This paper presents one strategy for motivating companies to offer their employees smoking cessation programmes. This strategy has been developed and tested in The Netherlands.

Differences in perspective

It is often not realized that the smoking problem is perceived fundamentally differently by companies and public health professionals. For public health professionals, smoking deserves to be singled out as a target for public health campaigns, because it is an important cause of illness and premature death, which can be prevented by motivating smokers to quit smoking. In terms of public health risks, passive smoking is not a high priority, whereas in contrast, the main motive for (Dutch) companies to do something about smoking is that they have a problem with environmental tobacco smoke. In The Netherlands, non-smokers are becoming more and more assertive about their right to work in a smoke-free workplace. In many companies, there is a long history of friction between smokers and non-smokers about the issue of smoking.

In The Netherlands and in many other countries, national legislation can motivate managers to do something about environmental tobacco smoke. The Dutch Tobacco Law prohibits smoking in public areas of organizations that are run by the State. Furthermore, national legislation on working conditions can be interpreted to include exposure to environmental tobacco smoke as well. Accordingly, Dutch companies define the smoking problem primarily in terms of a social and legal, not a health problem. This may, of course, be different elsewhere: in countries such as the United States, the idea that smoking cessation can reduce the medical costs of companies seems to be an important motive for offering smoking cessation programmes. This is of only marginal importance in The Netherlands, because Dutch employees do not have health insurance through their worksite. Absenteeism for illness is a very important topic in most Dutch companies; however, managers know very well that such absenteeism is primarily related to physical and psychological strains such as bad working conditions and a high workload, and less to smoking. The wish to reduce absenteeism is therefore at best an additional motive for Dutch employers to start a smoking control programme and hardly ever an important one.

Our solution of the problem of differences in perspective was to study how companies perceive the problem (i.e. social and legal) and then try to motivate companies to start thinking, not only about smoking policies, but also about smoking cessation programmes. To accomplish this aim, we developed a protocol in collaboration with the Dutch Coordinating Cancer Centers and the Dutch Foundation for Smoking and Health, which is now widely used in The Netherlands, especially at larger worksites, such as the Shell Oil Company, Fuji Photo & Film, PTT-Telecom and many governmental organizations. The protocol consists of four steps: orientation, planning, implementation and integration. The first two steps are relevant to the present paper and are described below.

Orientation

This first step starts when a company invites an expert from the organizations that developed the programme to give advice about improving smoking policies. One of the expert's first tasks is to interview company representatives in order to learn whether and how they perceive smoking as a problem at their worksite. This will also show which important people in the organization support the idea of doing something structural about smoking. This step ends with gaining approval from top management to improve the current smoking policy.

Planning

In the second step, a working committee is organized with company representatives. The importance of sufficient support from the employees is made clear, and the committee is advised to organize a company-wide survey. To help them do this, we have developed a standard inventory, on the basis of which the appropriate intervention strategies are chosen to solve the smoking problem. In a study involving eight large Dutch companies (Willemsen et al., 1996), we found that 66% of non-smokers reported that they were bothered by environmental tobacco smoke at their workplace.

It is important to design a health education campaign to inform employees about the changes in smoking policy and to motivate them to comply with the smoking restrictions (Greenberg, 1994); this increases the impact of the restrictions. The campaign may consist of general information about smoking, environmental tobacco smoke and smoking policy, for example in displays and company newsletters. Furthermore, a health educational campaign is needed to attract smokers to the smoking cessation programme (Dawley et al., 1993).

The third strategy is a smoking cessation programme. The information collected in the inventory proves to the company management that there is sufficient interest among smokers to justify such a programme. They can be told that they should offer their employees an effective smoking cessation programme before the smoking policy is changed, since many smokers will take the opportunity of the policy change to think about quitting smoking. It might then even become a moral obligation for employers to offer smokers an effective cessation programme before they adopt a strict smoking policy.

The Dutch worksite smoking cessation programme consists of group courses, self-help manuals and nicotine replacement therapy. Its effectiveness has been demonstrated in another study (Willemsen et al., 1998). Smoking cessation programmes help reduce the numbers of smokers: in one study, a 4% net reduction in smoking prevalence was seen throughout a worksite over two years (Jeffery et al., 1993). This in turn helps to reduce exposure to environmental tobacco smoke.

Conclusion

This strategy makes good sense for both employers and employees. The main objective of employees remains the elimination of exposure to environmental tobacco smoke, but they come to realize that smoking cessation and health education programmes are also important. Most of the companies we have dealt with have implemented not only a smoking policy but also a health educational campaign and a smoking cessation programme. With this approach, both public health interests and the interests of employers and employees can be satisfied.

References

Dawley, L.T., Dawley, H.H., Glasgow, R.E., Rice, J. & Correa, P. (1993) Worksite smoking control, discouragement, and cessation. Int. J. Addict., 28, 719–733

Greenberg, J. (1994) Using socially fair treatment to promote acceptance of a worksite smoking ban. J. Appl. Psychol., 79, 288–297

Jeffery, R.W., Forster, J.L., French, S.A., Kelder, S.H., Lando, H.A., McGovern, P.G., Jacobs, D.R. & Baxter, J.E. (1993) The Healthy Worker Project: A worksite intervention for weight control and smoking cessation. Am. J. Public Health, 83, 395–401

Willemsen, M.C., De Vries, H. & Genders, R. (1996) Annoyance from environmental tobacco smoke and support for no-smoking policies at eight large Dutch workplaces. Tobacco Control, 5, 132–138

Willemsen, M.C., De Vries, H. & Genders, R. (1998) Long-term effectiveness of two Dutch worksite smoking cessation programs. Health Educ. Behav.

Structure and effectiveness of an in-company no-smoking programme

G. Zeeman

Dutch Foundation on Smoking and Health (Stivoro), The Hague, The Netherlands

In 1992, the Dutch Foundation on Smoking and Health developed a non-smoking programme for implementation within companies. The programme consists of two main activities: regulation of smoking inside company buildings in order to reduce exposure to environmental tobacco smoke and smoking cessation activities to stimulate and support quitting.

Companies differ in their main objective: reducing exposure to environmental tobacco smoke and the concomitant disturbance of working conditions or improving the health of workers by cessation activities. Depending on their priority, one or other aspect of the programme is emphasized. Both activities must be implemented, however. When the main objective is regulation, it might be assumed that prohibition is the main motivation of the smokers to quit. An offer to support cessation facilitates the implementation of prohibitions. When improving the health of workers is the main goal, the process of regulation should also be initiated to prevent frequent confrontations between workers who have quit and their colleagues who are still smokers, which also represents a potential relapse situation. Cessation activities also add credibility to the employers' concern to reduce damage to health.

The non-smoking programme is shown in the scheme below. Throughout the programme, there is communication about the process and the programme. This continuous communication creates a basis of support for the programme and commitment and is essential in the Dutch culture.

The programme has been conducted in 30 large companies in The Netherlands. In four companies, with a total of 3000 employees, the reduction in smoking prevalence was 10–20% after one year.

Phase	Activities	Cessation, regulation or both
Orientation	Establish commitment of management	Both
	Set up working group	Both
Information	Conduct in-company survey	Both
	Interview key persons	Both
Planning	Develop policy: regulation and/or cessation	Both
	Plan interventions	Both
Action	*Preparation (five weeks)*	
	Train company medical officers in cessation counselling skills	Cessation
	Arrange meetings to inform workers about cessation programme and regulations	Both
	Issue personal invitations to join cessation programme	Cessation
	Give talk with interactive elements, giving information about 'why to quit' and 'how to quit'	Cessation
	Arrange meeting to inform heads of departments about new regulations	Regulation
	Prepare buildings for change (smoking rooms, signs)	Regulation
	Action week	
	Organize local publicity	Both
	Organize in-company activities to create a positive, enthusiastic atmosphere	Both
	Start smoking cessation with groups, self-help manuals and individual counselling by company medical officers	Cessation
	Give talk on 'How to stop smoking'	Cessation
	New regulations come into force	Regulation
	Maintenance (five weeks or more)	
	Model experiences of participants	Cessation
	Give talk on how to sustain non-smoking	Cessation
	Continue smoking cessation assistance	Cessation
	Maintain compliance with nexw regulations	Regulation
Evaluation	Effect of programme and need for continuation	Cessation
	Compliance with the regulations	Both

Tobacco use among police personnel in Indore, India

B.M. Shrivastava

*Department of Oral and Maxillofacial Surgery, College of Dentistry, Indore,
Madhya Pradesh, India*

Policemen, factory workers and public-transport workers are expected to work for long hours, often out of normal working hours, in bad weather and without proper rest intervals. Such workers often take up tobacco consumption under the widespread misconception that this habit helps them to discharge their duties with the necessary alertness. The study described here was designed to study why police personnel consume tobacco in various ways; we also studied whether their environment (urban, rural or tribal) affects the way they use tobacco or their awareness of its ill effects.

A questionnaire was designed to elicit the names, age, sex, rank and place of duty of 1372 policemen in Indore, which has urban, rural and tribal areas on its territory. Questions on mode, frequency and duration of the habit and knowledge about ill effects were also included.

The prevalence of tobacco use was 73%. Use of refined tobacco and cigarette smoking were more common in urban areas, whereas chewing tobacco was equally popular in all three areas. Chewing of *pan masala*, areca nut with tobacco, was prevalent in urban areas. Smoking of *bidis* was identified as a habit of the poor. The commonest cause of initiation appeared to be the belief that tobacco makes one alert. The main reasons given for using tobacco were to allay digestive problems and to improve concentration; copying older people, relieving mental upset, fashion and fatigue was each given as the reason by about 12% of the users. Of this group, 31% were aware that tobacco is harmful to health, and 37% knew that smoking can cause lung cancer.

The study showed that there are misconceptions about the medicinal virtues of tobacco. People with strenuous jobs should therefore be offered something to replace tobacco to break the cycle of monotony, boredom, lethargy and inefficiency. Campaigns should be conducted to debunk misconceptions about tobacco.

Five-year study of the smoking habits of taxi drivers

*H.C.O. Ogbolu[1], R.C. Azinge[2], P. Owen[3], D.E. Sawyer[4], A.E. Van-Santos[5]
& V.I. Omeruwa[6]*

*[1]Department of Histopathology, University of Maiduguri Teaching Hospital,
Maiduguri, Nigeria; [2]New York, City, New York, United States; [3]Department of
Physiology, University of Zimbabwe, Harare, Zimbabwe; [4]Institute of Orthopaedics,
Royal National Orthopaedics Hospital, Stanmore, United Kingdom; [5]Amsterdam,
The Netherlands; [6]Toronto, Ontario, Canada*

We carried out an informal survey of the smoking habits of taxi drivers in various areas of the world by means of a questionnaire. This group was chosen because they spend a lot of time waiting for passengers and because they represent a cross-section of people in many countries. More than 2500 questionnaires were distributed by friends and relatives in Africa, Europe and North America. The questionnaires were very simple, eliciting name, age, duration of smoking, the reason for starting to smoke, whether any attempt had been made to stop smoking and, if so, whether they had begun smoking again and for what reason.

Most of taxi drivers who smoked did so to pass the time; they smoked more at night and during colder weather in Europe and North America and during the rainy season in

Africa. Most of the taxis, however, had no-smoking signs and a warning about the danger of smoking, and most of these drivers did not smoke. Fewer drivers smoked at the end of the study than when it was begun five years previously.

Anti-smoking sessions, with films and lectures, could be held for taxi drivers at taxi stands or in cafés where the drivers congregate while waiting for a fare.

Acknowledgements
We wish to thank all of the taxi drivers who took part in the study and M.U. Abubakar, J. Orjigwe and S. Ibrahim for secretarial assistance.

Toxicological data sheet for tobacco smoke: A proposal for smoke-free workplaces

J. Tostain

Comite National Contre le Tabagisme, Versailles, France

The European Union of Nonsmokers and the French Confederation of Christian Workers note with regret and a sense of outrage that clean air is not yet mandatory in enclosed or covered areas for social and community use. To smoke in the presence of others is an act of aggression. It is anti-social. It is offensive. The European Union of Nonsmokers also notes that most of the highest international and national authorities refuse to prescribe and carry out the measures necessary for the protection of nonsmokers. 'The human right' to breathe clean air is obviously fundamental; it is noted in many declarations, charters and laws, national and international, and in particular in those that concern industrial hygiene and working conditions.

Tobacco smoke is toxic, irritating, polluting and carcinogenic and is the principal agent of pollution in enclosed and covered workplaces. One worker in four is more vulnerable than others to the health hazards associated with tobacco smoke. Thus, environmental tobacco smoke is the foremost avoidable risk factor for workers in enclosed or covered workplaces. Tobacco smoke is responsible for one death out of three among people aged 25–65 and therefore kills more workers than industrial diseases and fatal workplace accidents combined. Workers who are non-smokers should not be exposed against their will to tobacco smoke at their workplaces.

Regulations and bans on smoking already exist in some workplaces and in certain public places. They are generally uncontested and complied with, and it is therefore high time that institutions with responsibility for public health and working conditions enact regulations to protect those who do not want and cannot tolerate tobacco smoke. For these reasons, the European Union of Nonsmokers and the French Confederation of Christian Workers have proposed the adoption of a 'toxicological data sheet for tobacco smoke'. This data sheet would ensure total protection against tobacco smoke for non-smokers. It would stipulate a total ban on smoking in workplaces, whether they be enclosed or under cover, private or state-owned, and in workplaces open to the public. By extension, the ban would apply to all enclosed or covered spaces used for social or group activities.

The European Union of Nonsmokers and the French Confederation of Christian Workers do not seek to deny smokers the freedom to smoke. Smokers will be allocated areas outside buildings or in specially designated areas inside buildings in isolated 'smoking rooms' equipped with airlocks. The procedures for enforcement of these measures would be subject to internal regulations, and health and safety inspectors are qualified to verify its implementation. This new regulation would guarantee the right to breathe clean air in the workplace, a basic need. Moreover, it would give 'enforced' or 'involuntary' smokers legal grounds for redress in cases of non-compliance. Neglect or inadequacy in the enforcement of the rules would be regarded as an infringement of human rights at the workplace and would be deemed to be a deliberate and intentional offence.

On the eve of the twenty-first century, society and its decision-makers should invoke this fundamental act in the 'European Social Charter' which we wish to see enacted. It would be a new social breakthrough. In August 1997, the data sheet was included in the database of the International Occupational Safety and Health Information Centre of the International Labour Office, Geneva, Switzerland.

TOBACCO PROMOTION

Impact of cigarette marketing on female smoking

Y. Mochizuki-Kobayashi

Community Health, Health Promotion and Nutrition Division, Health Service
Bureau, Ministry of Health and Welfare, Tokyo, Japan

Global situation of female smoking

The issue of female smoking is our common interest, but there is a wide diversity in
smoking prevalence among countries (Figure 1). The problem therefore differs in
intensity, from countries where the rates are high, like Sweden and Norway, to those in
which they are still low, like Sri Lanka. The differences have been explained by regional,
cultural, historical, developmental and even political factors. Smoking prevalence should
be compared not only cross-sectionally but also over time. The World Health
Organziation model of the cigarette epidemic shows that the prevalence first rises sharply
among men, the number of deaths from smoking-related diseases among men begins to
rise two to three decades later, and then the same pattern is seen among women. When
deaths from smoking exceed 10% of all deaths, most countries begin national tobacco
control efforts. As such activities are aimed first at the predominant victims, namely
men, the female smoking prevalence continues to rise while that of males declines.

Cigarette marketing and female smoking

The epidemic can be traced as a result of the marketing of the tobacco industry
(Table 1), which went through several 'revolutions' in product development. The first
involved the American Blend, represented by Camel. After its introduction, massive
advertising and promotional activities began to increase cigarette consumption in the
United States. At the beginning of the 1900s, female social leaders started to smoke in
defiance of social taboos; young urban women followed them. When cigarette companies
realized that the female sector of their market was increasing, they began direct
persuasion of women in social, pharmacological and physiological approaches. Social
factors such as fashion, self-esteem, sexual attractiveness and peer pressure were used
in these advertisements. Pharmacological factors such as stimulation, tranquillization
and even craving were expressed. Taste and refreshment were added as physiological
factors. By 1925, almost all of the reasons why women smoke were firmly combined
with catchy slogans in advertisements for Camel. Lucky Strike reached the ultimate
desire of women, weight control, in its highly successful campaign.

Figure 1. Female smoking prevalence in 25 countries

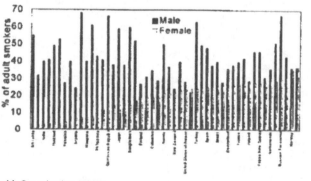

From World Health Organization (1997)

Table 1. Product development and female smoking

Revolution	Significant features	Female smoking
First: American Blend (1913: Camel)	Massive advertising and promotion Attacks on women by social, pharmacological and physiological approaches	Reasons why women smoke: • fashion, self-esteem, sexual attractiveness, peer pressure • stimulation, tranquilization, craving • taste, refreshment, weight control
Second: Filter-tipped (1952: Viceroy)	Allaying of public fear but not risks Cost saving to industry Easy to flavour	Filter-tipped menthol Salem (1956) Advantages to female smoking: • long and stylish • health consciousness
Third: Low-tar, low-nicotine (1964: Carlton)	Brand-switching to 'safer' cigarettes, instead of quitting	Women's brands: Virginia Slims (1968) Additional advantages to female smoking: • slim, graceful, beautiful • independent social status
Fourth: Low-tar, low-nicotine (1965: ?)	pH adjustment and nicotine manipulation - high absorption of nicotine - develop addiction more effectively	Reduced sidestream smoke: Premier (1988), Premier Pianissimo, Salem Pianissimo (1996) • Less sidestream smoke • environmental consciousness • reduced odour on hair and clothing

This is indirect evidence that the industry already knew about the pharmacological and physiological effects of nicotine that meet the criteria of the United States Food and Drug Administration of a 'drug'. Thus, nicotine in cigarettes 'affects the structure or any function of the body', because it causes and sustains addiction, causes other psychoactive (mood-altering) effects, including tranquillization and stimulation, and controls weight. Cigarettes were even given to American soldiers and sailors during the First and Second World Wars as part of their daily rations because the mind-altering effects of nicotine helped to combat both boredom and stress. The reasons that some women who are now combating social pressures give for smoking are similar to those of soldiers in wartime, rather than weight control. During the period when women began to smoke, the public was unaware of the health consequences of smoking, and the industry therefore did not feel the need to create imaginary 'healthy' images for cigarettes. This is partly because the life span in many countries was so short that people died before they developed lung cancer, even after several decades of smoking.

When the medical findings about smoking and lung cancer became known to the public, around 1950, the second revolution broke out. Filter-tipped cigarettes first appeared in the 1930s, but they were not popular until the early 1950s when the industry tried to remove the public fear about lung cancer by promoting these new cigarettes. The presence of filters did relieve the public's fear but did not change the risks for cancer remarkably. Filter-tipped cigarettes had many advantages for the industry; they were cost-saving, because of cheaper materials, they were long and stylish and easy to flavour on the filter. The first filter-tipped menthol, Salem, was successfully marketed in 1956 and became very popular with women. The green pack and the menthol smell gave a fresh, healthy, even medicine-like image to the public and especially to health-conscious women. This is a good example of how thoroughly cigarette marketing was conducted, by considering the existing factors and even using a potential obstacle. Medical journals, nurses and doctors were used to promote filter-tipped cigarettes, and they successfully delivered a 'healthy' or 'safer' image to the general public.

When the first report of the Surgeon General was published in 1964, deaths from smoking in the United States represented almost 10% of all deaths. As the industry began to lose more smokers from deaths and quitting, it decided to recruit new smokers from new markets, namely women and children. According to industry documents disclosed in 1963, their marketing objectives were precisely to appeal more to youth and young adult women. The low-tar and -nicotine Carlton cigarette was the fruit of new techniques for diluting smoke without reducing satisfaction. As it was launched just before publication of the Surgeon General's report, low-yield brands were considered to be 'safer' and gained brand-switchers instead of losing smokers. Carlton thus started a 'tar derby'. The leading women's brand, Virginia Slims, was brought onto the market on this tidal wave in 1968. The success of this brand was due to the implication of additional advantages of female smoking: its name gave an image of a slim, graceful, beautiful body, and the advertising copy suggested the newly independent social status of women.

New era of product development and female smoking

The second and third revolutions in product development are both characterized by efforts to counter concern about the dangers of smoking among the general public. The marketing objectives were to promote 'safe' or 'safer' cigarettes, but the hidden aims were to maintain the market by supplying nicotine more effectively and more efficiently. The industry conducted intensive research on the delivery and absorption of nicotine to develop a high-performance nicotine delivery system with pH adjustment and nicotine manipulation.

The fourth revolution is still going on, side by side with the other revolutions. When the health hazards of environmental tobacco smoke were recognized in the 1980s, efforts in product development were concentrated on reducing sidestream smoke. Premier was introduced as the ultimate smokeless cigarette, with almost no sidestream smoke but a sufficient amount of nicotine. It failed because smokers at that time needed to see smoke to satisfy themselves and were not yet environmentally conscious. In response to growing concern about passive smoking and social pressure, the Premier Pianissimo was introduced on the Japanese market in 1996 for men and the Salem Pianissimo for women, with visible sham side-stream smoke. These new species of low-sidestream cigarettes were produced mainly by modifications of the techniques associated with low yields of tar and nicotine during the third revolution. Low-tar and low-sidestream cigarettes are welcomed on the market as 'safer' cigarettes, but in reality they are high-performance nicotine delivery systems. The most advanced product concepts in this fourth revolution attract more smokers, especially female smokers, both maintaining smoking and hooking more people to start smoking. The industry began its 'low tar, low smoke' campaign in 1997.

Female smokers have thus been exposed at each period to more sophisticated tactics of the industry than male smokers. Not only because of biological reasons but also because they are smoking technologically advanced cigarettes under more effectively developed promotional efforts, female smokers find it difficult to quit and more young girls are becoming addicted. To control this epidemic, we must attack the other side of the cigarette epidemic, advertising and promotion, unless the product itself can be regulated.

Impact on the female market

The impact of such cigarette marketing on female smoking first became evident from the younger age of onset of regular smoking among women. This effect resulted in an increase in female teenage smokers and also in an increasing number of years of exposure to cigarette smoke among women. As earlier onset of smoking increases the risk for tobacco-related disease, female smokers have a higher risk than ever. This earlier onset of smoking is also seen in Japan, where the smoking prevalence among girls has increased more rapidly than that among boys during the past six years. About 20% of high-school girls are already regular smokers, and they could easily become daily smokers soon. The rapid increase in female smoking was confirmed in the two nationwide surveys in Japan (Figure 2), one conducted by the tobacco industry since 1965 and the other by the Ministry of Health and Welfare since 1986. Both surveys

Figure 2. Smoking prevalence among females in Japan and the United States

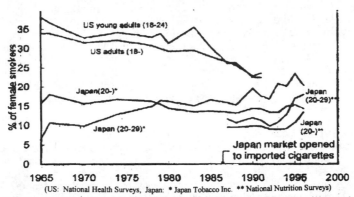

(US: National Health Surveys, Japan: * Japan Tobacco Inc. ** National Nutrition Surveys)

suggest that the smoking prevalence among women aged 20–30 will reach 30% by 2000. In the United States, female smoking rates are already declining after the peak in the early 1980s. It is obvious that the market is shifting outside the United States. As reported by R. Peto, there is a lag of several decades before smoking-related deaths are seen. Although smoking among women in the United States is now declining, deaths from smoking among females are increasing at a higher rate than for males. In Japan, as the smoking prevalence among females was low in the past, deaths from smoking represent only one-fifth of all deaths, but the rate will increase several decades later if the present smoking prevalence continues.

To consider the scale of the tobacco epidemic, we can also estimate the social cost of smoking. Medical expenditure due to smoking in Japan is 1200 thousand million yen (US$ 10 thousand million), and the social cost of smoking is nearly 4000 thousand million yen (US$ 33 thousand million), exactly equal to the gross sales of cigarettes that year. Roughly one-fifth, 8000 thousand million yen (US$ 7 thousand million), is due to female smoking.

Conclusions

Cigarette marketing directed towards females consists of four steps. First, advertisements and promotion change the social norm, making female smoking more acceptable to society. Then, the smoking prevalence among women increases rapidly, and the onset occurs earlier. After several decades of promotion of female smoking, the numbers of deaths and diseases related to smoking increase and have economic consequences on society. Female smoking also affects future generations, however: mothers' smoking results not only in premature babies and other health effects in children due to passive smoking, but also in influencing their children's attitude and behaviour with regard to smoking.

If we superimpose the time lines of risk identification and control and the marketing targets of the industry, risk control efforts are focused mainly on the major victims at a particular time. Approaches to women and children have therefore been delayed in most countries, but the tobacco industry always acts quickly to shift marketing targets from those that are already developed or shrinking to developing markets. We can reverse the direction by focusing on the most vulnerable targets, children and women. Countries that have not yet established comprehensive tobacco control efforts, like Japan, should start to take action focusing on women and children. Tobacco or health problems differ by country, but our common goal is a tobacco-free society for the next generation.

Reference
World Health Organization (1997) *Tobacco or Health: A Global Status Report*, Geneva

Policies of the editors of magazines for young women with regard to tobacco

N. Nakano

Women's Action on Smoking, Tokyo, Japan

The sight of young women smoking on the street was rare in Japan a few years ago, although many smoked privately. Now, we often see both girls and boys walking with lit cigarettes in their hands. The fact that they smoke openly means that more and more women will begin to smoke, and the smoking rate among young girls has been rising, especially among those in their 20s and 30s. Many say they know that tobacco is harmful for unborn babies and that they will stop smoking when they become pregnant. In reality, many pregnant women smoke after they have conceived, with rates of 22% for those aged < 19, 15% for those aged 20–24, 7.2% at age 25–29, 7.1% at age 30–34 and 4.2% for pregnant women ≥ 35. Some mothers start smoking again as soon as they have had their babies.

There are many factors that influence them to start smoking, including peers, the media, the family, school and the workplace. Health education at school is vital but is not widespread enough yet in our country. As smoking also has a lot to do with self image and fashion, we decided to study magazines for young women. We sent questionnaires to the editors of 45 major magazines for women aged 16–35, each of which has a monthly circulation of 300 000 to 1.5 million, to find out what interests young women and how much the editors are concerned with women's health and tobacco. As we received only six responses, we checked the contents of major magazines for young girls ourselves.

Surveys have shown that young women obtain information from television, radio, newspapers, magazines and talking to friends but seldom get health information on television or radio because the tobacco industry is one of the biggest sponsors, and newscasters, who often smoke, tend to avoid the topic of smoking and health. Many tobacco commercials appear on television at the same time as programmes that young people watch. Some of the most popular characters in serials often smoke on screen. Although information about tobacco and health is sometimes found in newspapers, 53% of young girls aged 16–24 hardly ever read newspapers, and 21% read them for < 20 min per day. Women's magazines—which sell over 400 million copies a year—therefore seem to be their main source.

There are no tobacco advertisements in Japanese women's magazines because the tobacco industries accepted a voluntary code 30 years ago to avoid conflict with traditional morals. Until 10 years ago, the code stated that the companies must not promote tobacco use by women. In fact, their sales promotion has been escalating since foreign tobacco arrived, and now they use any platform except women's magazines. To show their 'good sense', they refrain only from showing women smoking in their advertisements. For 100 years, Japan has had a law that prohibits minors under 20 from smoking, but aggressive promotion has made that law ineffective. Although the voluntary code states that the tobacco companies must not promote tobacco to minors, most magazines for young people have tobacco advertisements and are read by both boys and girls. They also offer attractive gifts. The violation is overlooked by the competent authority, the Ministry of Finance.

The six out of 45 questionnaires that were returned told us that editors pay little attention to tobacco and health. Four were from magazines that offer general information on women's life, and two were from magazines on child care; all of them were for women aged over 24. The editors of both magazines on child care said that they had run an article on health, including passive smoking by children, during the previous 12 months. All four said that information on tobacco was necessary for young women, and half said that schools, mass media and national and local governments should give them more information on tobacco and health. They said that the issue of tobacco is difficult to handle, but that they would take it up from the point of view of women's health once in a while. All six have articles on health every month; the editors said that fatigue, stress, diet, sensitivity to cold and constipation were the topics that interested readers most.

We checked the contents of magazines for girls aged 16–24, none of which had returned the questionnaire, and listed all the topics in 12 months of issues of the four major magazines, each of which has a circulation of about 1 million every two weeks: 30% of the topics were fashion, 20% were beauty and cosmetics, 10% about love and sex, and others about diet and fortune-telling. Not a single article on health was found in these magazines; they were more like catalogues of clothes, cosmetics and other goods that allure young girls by direct and indirect advertising. Nothing was mentioned about tobacco and health, but in one article, 'How to win his love', we found the sentence 'You might bring his favourite cigarette on a date'. Although various cosmetics were recommended for skin care in teenage girls' magazines, they never mentioned that cigarette smoking is harmful to the skin and accelerates ageing.

Although we cannot support the stance of these magazines, many young girls seem to rely on them to learn how to identify, love and express themselves. If these magazines also told them how to cope with the temptation to smoke, it would help them to be physically and spiritually healthy. The smoking rate among editors and writers of women's magazines is, however, very high, and many of their favourite young talents who appear in their pages are known to be heavy smokers. We cannot ignore the fact that over 5 million girls prefer these magazines to other sources of information, and, fortunately, the tobacco industry does not sponsor them. We should therefore send information to these magazines and develop information acceptable for both boys and girls. In Japan, where boys can smoke freely, it is not useful to tell only the girls to quit.

Women's magazines and tobacco in Europe: Preliminary findings

A. Amos, Y. Bostock & C. Bostock

Department of Public Health Sciences, Edinburgh University, Edinburgh, Scotland

Smoking kills over 106 000 women in the European Union each year and at least double that number in Europe as a whole. The prevalence of smoking among young women continues to increase in many countries, and in some of them the rates are higher among young women than young men. Women's magazines, with their large readership, have become one of the main ways in which the tobacco industry tries to target its advertising at women. A previous study of the policies of the largest women's magazines with respect to tobacco in 1990 showed that, while many magazines refused certain types of advertising, most accepted tobacco advertisements, unless prohibited from doing so; 40% of the magazines surveyed had no restrictions on using pictures of people smoking on editorial pages. Only one in five had given any major coverage to smoking and health in the previous year. We have repeated that study to find out what changes, if any, have taken place and to promote appropriate action on women and smoking by relevant organizations and groups in each country.

The study had two aims. The first was to determine the policies of the most widely read women's and young women's magazines in 17 European countries with regard to tobacco advertising and their dependence on it, coverage of smoking and health, use of images of smoking on pages such as fashion pages and to assess changes since 1990. The second aim was to publicise widely and disseminate information about the role of women's magazines in promoting and discouraging smoking in these 17 countries and thereby to increase public awareness about women and smoking and promote appropriate action on this issue.

The sample in each of the 17 countries consisted of the two most widely read weekly and monthly magazines aimed at women under 25 and the two most widely read weekly and monthly magazines aimed at older women.

Methods

We conducted a postal and/or telephone survey of magazine editors, with at least two follow-up letters or calls to non-respondents. The survey was carried out in winter 1996 to spring 1997 by collaborators in 17 countries (the list is given at the end of this paper). The editors were asked about:
- the magazine's circulation, female readership and the age range of its target audience;
- the magazine's advertising policy;
- the magazine's policy on accepting tobacco advertising and the proportion of its advertising revenue that represented;
- their views on the influence of tobacco advertising on women;
- the magazine's policy on use of pictures of people smoking on, for example, fashion pages and
- whether they had published articles on smoking and health in the past 12 months and whether any were one page or longer and to send copies of any articles.

Preliminary findings

The preliminary findings of this study are summarized in Table 1.

Tobacco advertising: Although 80% of the magazines refused certain types of advertisement, most accepted tobacco advertising if they were permitted to do so. Only seven magazines that were allowed to take tobacco advertisements voluntarily refused them. Many cigarette advertisements were designed to appeal to women. While many editors said they felt that tobacco advertising did not influence young women to smoke, some had strong views on their targeting and effect.

Editorial pictures of smokers: Although the majority of the editors said that they did not publish pictures of people smoking, 42% had no or only minor restrictions on doing so. Such pictures were common in magazines in Germany, Greece and Spain. They included female models and celebrities smoking in a variety of settings.

Smoking and health coverage: Coverage of the dangers of smoking and how to quit was highly variable: most magazines in France, Portugal and Sweden had given major

Table 1. Findings on women's magazines in 15 European countries

Country	Sample size	No. of responses	General advertising policy (n = 75)	Accept cigarette advertising (n = 75)	Allow photos of smoking (n = 75)	Major coverage of smoking in last 12 months (n = 75)
Belgium	11	2	2	2	1	0
Denmark	6	4	3	4	3	2
Finland[a]	5	5	5	0	4	2
France[a]	8	8	0	2[b]	2	5
Germany	8	8	8	8	5	0
Greece	5	3	2	3	3	1
Ireland	4	3	2	3	0	2
Lithuania	6	6	4	4	3	2
Luxembourg	1	1	1	0	0	0
Poland	7	4	4	3	2	1
Portugal[a]	5	3	3	0	1	2
Spain	8	8	5	8	5	1
Sweden[a]	5	5	5	0	0	3
Switzerland	8	8	8	4	3	0
United Kingdom	8	8	8	2	0	3
All	95	76 (80%)	60 (80%)	43 (57%)	32 (42%)	24 (32%)

[a] Countries in which cigarette advertising in magazines was banned at the time of the study
[b] Examples of illegal advertising were found in these magazines.

coverage, while only one magazine each in Germany, Spain and Switzerland had given any coverage. The editors expressed a wide range of views, ranging from those who saw the importance of giving regular coverage to those who were against it. Particularly worrying was the evidence that in at least one country accepting tobacco advertising might lead to self-censorship.

Changes since 1990: There has been little improvement in the countries that were surveyed in 1990–91, apart from France and Sweden, where tobacco advertisements are now banned and the coverage given to smoking and health appears to have increased. Despite increased awareness about smoking among women, many magazines do not appear to regard this as an important issue.

Conclusions

Women's magazines have a potentially important role to play in helping young women not to start smoking and helping smokers to quit. This is perhaps best seen in Sweden, where magazines do not take tobacco advertisements, regularly cover the health issues and do not show people smoking. Indeed, in 1996, several magazines published separate booklets on women and smoking, and one sponsored the participation of an ex-Miss Sweden in a workshop at the World Conference on Tobacco or Health. At the other extreme, women's magazines in Germany show little concern for this issue, even though tobacco advertisements directly target women. Magazines in former Communist countries such as Lithuania are being compelled to take tobacco advertising from financial necessity.

These preliminary findings pose challenges for tobacco control advocates in Europe to develop new ways of working with women's magazines while at the same time lobbying for a Europe-wide ban on tobacco promotion.

Acknowledgements
    Study collaborators: *Belgium*, C. Rasson, M. Wanlin, Centre des Infections Respiratoires et pour l'Éducation et la Santé; M. Lambert, L. Joossens, Koordinatiekomitee Algemene Tabakspreventie Vlaamse Gemeenschap; *Denmark*: U. Skovgaard Danielson, Danish Council on Smoking and Health; *Finland*: M. Hara, ASH; *France*: E. Beguinol, Comité National contre le Tabagisme; *Germany*: U. Maschewsky-Schneider, M. Blessing, Institut für Gesundheitswissenschaften, Technische Universität, Berlin; *Greece*: G.-M. Prepoutsidou, Aristotelian University of Thessaloniki; *Ireland*: F. Howell, North Eastern Health Board; *Italy*: M. Garcia Naldi, Bologna Healthy City Project; *Lithuania*: I. Pilkauskiene, Institute of Cardiology, Kaunas Academy; *Luxembourg*: G. Mondloch, Direction de la Santé; *Netherlands*: B. de Blij, M. Wiebing, Stivoro; *Poland*: D. Gorecka, Institute of Tuberculosis and Lung Diseases, Warsaw; *Portugal*: M. Santos Pardal, Council for Smoking Prevention; *Spain*: B. Gil Barcenilla, Distrito Sanitario Aljarafe; R. Mendoza, University of Huelva; *Sweden*: M. Haglund, National Institute of Public Health; *Switzerland*: B. Caretti, Swiss Federal Office of Public Health; C. Gafner, TAG.

Tobacco advertisements were associated with positive attitudes to smoking among children who had never smoked

T.H. Lam, S.F. Chung, C.L. Betson, C.M. Wong & A.J. Hedley

*Department of Community Medicine, The University of Hong Kong,
Hong Kong SAR, China*

Introduction

Many studies have shown that tobacco advertisements and positive attitudes to smoking, as well as other factors such as family smoking and peer influence, are associated with the smoking behaviour of children. In our cross-sectional study on 6304 junior secondary-school students (forms 1–3, aged mainly 12–15 years), we found that the students' perception of cigarette advertisements as attractive was strongly associated with smoking experience (Lam *et al.*, 1994). Other factors associated with any smoking were knowledge about the hazards of smoking, positive attitudes to smoking and smoking by the family, schoolteachers and peers (Lam *et al.*, 1995). The association was examined in this and other studies by comparing children who smoked with children who did not. All the risk factors, such as attitudes to smoking, were treated as independent variables, whereas smoking (yes versus no) was the dependent variable. Few studies have addressed children who have never smoked and the factors associated with positive attitudes (as the dependent variables). The aim of this study was to examine factors associated with positive attitudes to smoking among children who had never smoked from the above-mentioned data on 6304 students.

Methods

Details of the methods used have been reported (Lam et al., 1994, 1995, 1997). Briefly, 6304 students in forms 1–3 from a probability cluster sample of 172 classes in 61 secondary schools completed a self-administered questionnaire anonymously in the classroom under the supervision of a researcher during May–July 1994. No teacher was present. The students cooperated well, and there was no collusion. The response rate of the schools was 92% and the response rate of the students was 96%. Only the 4482 students who reported never having smoked were included in the analysis.

The dependent variables were attitudes to smoking, which were measured by the students' agreement or disagreement with each of six statements: (i) 'Smoking is fun', (ii) 'Smoking gives you confidence', (iii) 'Smoking makes you feel grown up', (iv) 'Smoking makes you look tough', (v) 'Young people smoke to "show off"', and (vi) 'Smoking calms your nerves'. Logistic regression modelling was carried out for each of the six items, with the following independent variables: sex, age, knowledge of hazards of smoking, family smoking, seeing teachers smoking, seeing classmates smoking and perception of tobacco advertisements as attractive.

Results

Table 1 shows that there were more girls than boys who had never smoked. Most of the students were aged 13–15 years. Most had seen their teachers and classmates smoking, and about half of them had at least one smoking family member. About one quarter considered that tobacco advertisements were attractive. The proportion of students who agreed with the positive attitude statements ranged from 2.5% for 'Smoking gives you confidence' to 9.5% for 'Young people smoke to show off'.

Table 2 shows the adjusted odds ratios for four factors of each of the six attitude statements, derived by logistic modelling with each statement as the dependent variable and the four factors, as well as sex, age and knowledge of hazards of smoking, as the independent variables. Perception of tobacco advertisements as attractive had larger odds ratios than the other three factors (and factors not presented here, such as knowledge), followed by seeing classmates and teachers smoking. Some of the adjusted odds ratios for the latter two factors were not significant. Family smoking was not associated with any items of positive attitude.

Discussion

Since previous studies have shown that positive attitudes to smoking are associated with smoking, children with positive attitudes who have never smoked are at risk of taking up smoking in the future. In this study, we found that perception of tobacco advertisements was strongly associated with each of the six items of positive attitudes, after adjustment for other factors, with odds ratios of 2.2 to 3.7. The greatest adjusted odds ratio, for 'Smoking is fun', of 3.68 suggests that this is likely to be the major effect of tobacco advertisements.

Smoking by classmates and teachers was also associated with positive attitudes, but the odds ratios were smaller. It is interesting to note that family smoking, although found in our previous analysis to be associated with smoking (Lam *et al.*, 1994, 1995),

Table 1. Characteristics and distribution of factors for 4482 students who had never smoked

Factor	No.	%
Sex		
Girls	2352	52.5
Boys	2125	47.4
Missing	5	0.1
Age (years)		
≤ 12	632	14.0
13	1479	33.0
14	1379	30.8
15	823	18.4
16	159	3.6
Missing	10	0.2
Had seen teachers smoking		
No	3283	73.2
Yes	1173	26.2
Missing	26	0.6
Had seen classmates smoking		
No	2746	61.3
Yes	1708	38.1
Missing	28	0.6
Smoking by family members		
None	2363	52.7
≥ 1	2119	47.3
Perception of cigarette advertisements		
None of 8 advertisements attractive	3374	75.3
≥ 1 of 8 advertisements attractive	1108	24.7
Young people smoke to 'show off'		
True	425	9.5
Not true or 'don't know'	4057	90.5
Smoking calms your nerves		
True	367	8.2
Not true or 'don't know'	4115	91.8
Smoking makes you look tough		
True	347	7.7
Not true or 'don't know'	4135	92.3
Smoking makes you feel grown up		
True	210	4.7
Not true or 'don't know'	4272	95.3
Smoking is fun		
True	162	3.6
Not true or 'don't know'	4320	96.4
Smoking gives you confidence		
True	111	2.5
Not true or 'don't know'	4371	97.5

was not associated with positive attitudes in students who had never smoked. These results suggest that although children with smoking parents may be at risk of smoking, they do not derive their positive attitudes from their parents. In many Hong Kong Chinese families, even parents who smoke often forbid their children to smoke and tell their children that smoking is a harmful and a bad habit.

Although this is a cross-sectional survey, the strongest association observed between tobacco advertisements and positive attitudes suggests that tobacco advertisements are likely to be the main source of the children's positive attitudes. Our findings should provide further evidence to support the banning of tobacco advertisement in order to create an environment that does not encourage positive attitudes to smoking in children.

Acknowledgements
We wish to thank the Hong Kong Council on Smoking and Health for funding this project, the Education Department of the Hong Kong Government for assistance, the schools and students for their participation and Ms Marie Chi for clerical assistance.

Table 2. Factors associated with positive attitudes

Positive attitude (dependent variables)	Adjusted[a] odds ratio	95% CI
Smoking is fun		
Perception of tobacco advertisement as attractive	3.68	2.63–5.15
Seeing classmates smoking	2.18	1.54–3.07
Seeing teachers smoking	1.62	1.15–2.28
Family members smoking	1.04	0.75–1.44
Smoking gives you confidence		
Perception of tobacco advertisement as attractive	2.81	1.88–4.19
Seeing classmates smoking	1.95	1.29–2.94
Seeing teachers smoking	1.65	1.10–2.46
Family members smoking	1.17	0.79–1.73
Smoking makes you feel grown up		
Perception of tobacco advertisement as attractive	2.62	1.96–3.50
Seeing classmates smoking	2.28	1.69–3.07
Seeing teachers smoking	1.21	0.89–1.64
Family members smoking	1.04	0.78–1.38
Young people smoke to 'show off'		
Perception of tobacco advertisement as attractive	2.30	1.85–2.84
Seeing classmates smoking	1.65	1.33–2.04
Seeing teachers smoking	1.15	0.92–1.45
Family members smoking	1.03	0.84–1.26
Smoking calms your nerves		
Perception of tobacco advertisement as attractive	2.19	1.75–2.75
Seeing classmates smoking	1.64	1.31–2.06
Seeing teachers smoking	1.35	1.07–1.71
Family members smoking	1.13	0.91–1.41
Smoking makes you look tough		
Perception of tobacco advertisement as attractive	1.61	1.26–2.06
Seeing classmates smoking	1.27	1.00–1.61
Seeing teachers smoking	1.12	0.87–1.45
Family members smoking	0.96	0.76–1.21

[a]Adjusted for sex, age and knowledge of hazards of smoking

References

Lam, T.H., Chung, S.F., Wong, C.M., Hedley, A.J. & Betson, C.L. (1994) *Youth Smoking, Health and Tobacco Promotion: The Youth Smoking and Health Survey 1994 Report No. 1*, Hong Kong: Hong Kong Council on Smoking and Health

Lam, T.H., Chung, S.F., Wong, C.M., Hedley, A.J. & Betson, C.L. (1885) *Youth Smoking: Knowledge, Attitudes, Smoking in Schools and Families, and Symptoms Due to Passive Smoking: Youth Smoking and Health Survey 1994 Report No. 2*, Hong Kong. Hong Kong Council on Smoking and Health, 1995.

Lam, T.H., Chung, S.F., Betson, C.L., Wong, C.M. & Hedley, A.J. (1997) Respiratory symptoms due to active and passive smoking in junior secondary school students in Hong Kong. *Int. J. Epidemiol.* (in press)

Effects of targeted advertising by the tobacco industry

J.P. Pierce

University of California, San Diego, California, United States

There is now considerable evidence that the advertising and promotional practices of the tobacco industry influence adolescents to start smoking. I review here the trends in the size and nature of tobacco advertising and promotion in the United States and some key evidence to support the conclusion that there is a causal link between tobacco advertising and promotion and uptake of smoking by adolescents.

Trends in tobacco advertising and promotion in the United States

Table 1 shows the estimated expenditure of the tobacco industry on advertising and promotion in California during the same period for each calendar year between 1989 and 1995. The estimates are based on data from a report of the Federal Trade Commission (1997). The tobacco industry is required to supply that Commission with an accounting of monies spent on advertising and promotion of manufactured cigarettes, but these figures do not include expenditure on promoting other tobacco products, such as cigars. Furthermore, these reports do not include industry spending for lobbying and political campaigns, which has been documented elsewhere by S. Glantz.

The first comment on the table is the size of the overall budget for promotion. In 1995, the tobacco industry spent about US$ 20 per person in the United States. If this money is targeted only at young people, the per capita expenditure increases by about five times, to US$ 100 per young person. To put this into perspective, the much-touted tobacco control programme in California has a budget which is about one tenth that of the industry.

It is interesting to note how the emphasis in industry promotion changed during the 1990s. In 1989, traditional advertising approaches, such as print media and billboards, comprised approximately 30% of the total promotional expenditure of the industry, whereas by 1995 this proportion was reduced to 17%. Furthermore, by 1995 expenditure on traditional advertising amounted to only 41% of the amount the industry devoted to the category of promotional items. Promotional items, which are a combination of the Federal Trade Commission categories for coupons, retail value-added and distribution of special items, comprised the largest proportion of the industry's advertising and promotional expenditure in each year. The percentage for promotional items increased from a low of 33% of total expenditures in 1989 to a high of 55% in 1993.

The other major Federal Trade Commission category that the industry designates as promotional allowances covers expenditures to encourage wholesalers and retailers to stock and promote cigarettes ('Incentives to merchants' in Table 1). Over the seven-year period, expenditure in this category rose steadily, from 27 to 38% of the total budget. No wonder it is hard to enforce laws against sales of cigarettes to minors!

Evidence of effectiveness of advertising from analyses of time series

Analyses of time series have shown a correlation between major increases in adolescent smoking with the innovative advertising campaigns of which they are the targets. The most dramatic example occurred with the introduction of the Virginia Slims campaign in the late 1960s. This was the first effort of the tobacco industry to market a cigarette specifically targeted to women. The campaign was launched in the middle of the first effective anti-smoking campaign on television, a campaign supported by the Fairness Doctrine. It is important to note that the anti-smoking campaign launched after the first report of the Surgeon General was targeted specifically at males, as the

Table 1. Tobacco industry expenditure on promoting cigarettes in the United States (million US$)

Item	Year							
	1989	1990	1991	1992	1993	1994	1995	Total
Advertising	1100	1140	1120	990	940	890	820	7 950
Incentives to merchants	1000	1020	1160	1510	1560	1680	1870	9 800
Promotional items	1220	1490	2070	2520	3320	2100	2010	14 730
Other	280	340	310	220	220	170	190	1 730
Total	3620	3990	4650	5230	6030	4830	4890	33 240

From Federal Trade Commission (1997)

evidence linking smoking with lung cancer was derived solely from studies of men. Throughout the 1950s and 1960s, the rates of uptake of smoking by adults declined consistently, while the rates among adolescents remained fairly constant. With the start of the Virginia Slims campaign, however, there was a major increase in the uptake rate only among 14–17-year-old girls and particularly among girls who did not go on to complete high school. The uptake rate of women aged 18–21 continued to decline, and no increase was identified among 14–17-year-old boys at that time.

Longitudinal follow-up of adolescents at very low risk of starting to smoke

While many studies have been undertaken to correlate adolescents' response to tobacco advertising and promotion, there has been an urgent need for longitudinal data to test the association between advertising and uptake behaviour. We were given the opportunity to follow-up adolescents in California who in 1993 (baseline) were non-smokers and considered not to be susceptible. The classification of adolescents according to the probability that they would smoke in the future was undertaken on a national longitudinal sample and validated on our California sample: a 'committed never-smoker' is defined as a person who has never puffed on a cigarette and is adamant that he or she would not smoke in a series of possible smoking situations. A 'susceptible never smoker' is someone who is not prepared to rule out the possibility of smoking in one of those situations.

About one half of our population of adolescents had progressed towards smoking by 1996, and over one third was actually experimenting with cigarettes. We found that the major predictor for progression was the degree of receptivity to tobacco advertising and promotion at baseline. We had defined this receptivity level in 1993 on the basis of a popular theory of communication and persuasion. Receptivity was a far stronger predictor than having friends or family members who smoked. Adolescents were considered to have a moderate to high degree of receptivity to tobacco advertising and promotion if they named a favourite cigarette advertisement. Some 60% of all the Californian adolescents were prepared to name an advertisement. The highest degree of receptivity was defined as owning a tobacco industry promotional item, such as a piece of clothing, or indicating willingness to use such a promotional item. Some 13% of the adolescents owned an industry promotional item, and twice that proportion were willing to use such an item. Adolescents classified in these two highest categories of receptivity were significantly more likely to progress towards smoking than adolescents with a low degree of receptivity, after control for other known predictors of smoking initiation.

Conclusion

The tobacco industry spends exorbitant amounts of money on cigarette advertising and promotion. These sums appear to be carefully tailored each year to maximize their effectiveness. Our evidence indicates that they are very effective in encouraging adolescents to begin to smoke.

Children's perceptions of cigarette advertisements in Malaysia

J. Rogayah[1], A. Zulkifli[2], M. Razlan[2] & N.N. Naing[2]

[1]*Department of Medical Education, and* [2]*Department of Community Medicine, School of Medical Sciences, Universiti Sains Malaysia, Kota Bharu, Kelantan, Malaysia*

Introduction

Cigarette advertising is an organized, planned, deliberate and often highly researched attempt to promote smoking (A Study Group of the Public Health Department, 1959;

O'Connel *et al.*, 1981). The aim of advertising is to create and reinforce associations with smoking that will increase the sales of cigarettes. All propoganda about smoking, such as its association with luxury, international travel, excitement, sexuality, companionship, uniqueness, relaxation and sports, are associations that have nothing intrinsically to do with tobacco or smoking (Salber *et al.*, 1961). They are all associations which arise because advertising has constantly attached such meaning to cigarettes in the effort to appeal to very ordinary human emotions, hopes and yearnings.

In Malaysia, cigarette advertising in the media is subject to the *Control of Tobacco Products Regulations 1993*. Direct cigarette advertisements on television and in newspapers and magazines is banned, although indirect advertising continues to be allowed. This entails the use of the already established logos, symbols and labels of well-known cigarettes in advertisements for designer clothings and accessories, travels and tours, concerts and the sponsorship of sports events. Critics have claimed that there should be a complete ban on cigarette advertisements, as it is contended that consumer interest in smoking is fanned through association with the brand name and the related attractive or glamourous lifestyle it advocates (*Medical Tribune*, 1996; Utusan Konsumer Tobacco Companies, 1996). The concern is that viewers, particularly schoolchildren, may be influenced to take up smoking.

There is little empirical evidence that advertisements for cigarettes employ images that are attractive to the young. Most claims that cigarette advertisements link smoking with success, glamour, fun and masculinity assume that there is a single interpretation of an advertisement. Although several of these advertisements are very convincing— for example, few would deny that cowboys portrayed in a cigarette advertisement promote masculinity—this interpretation would be more cogent if it had been subjected to some kind of empirical testing.

The study described here examined the perceptions of schoolchildren in primary class 6 about advertisements and particularly the indirect cigarette advertisements currently found in popular magazines in Malaysia.

Method

The study covered 159 schoolchildren (86 boys and 73 girls) in two primary schools conveniently sited in areas close to the University medical campus in Kota Bharu. Most were about 12 years old. After discussions with teachers, it was decided that children in the top two primary 6 classes would be able to read and understand the questionnaire and provide reliable responses. Twelve full-page colour advertisements taken from magazines were fixed to black cardboard mounts and prepared as slides. Eight of the advertisements were indirect cigarette advertisements, while four were non-cigarette advertisements. They were shown at random to the children in order to disguise the purpose of the study. The children were also given a questionnaire consisting of two parts. The first, 'warm-up' part had questions on the purpose of advertisements, the common sources of advertisement and what they considered to be popular and unpopular advertisements. In the second part, questions related to the impression created by and the interpretation of each of the advertisements shown and to the identity of their targets. The children were given ample time to answer the questions. Answers to the second part of the questionnaire were analysed only with regard to the eight indirect cigarette advertisements shown.

Results

The most frequent sources of advertising that the children were exposed to are shown in Table 1. The three most frequent sources were television, radio and newspapers; magazines as used in this study were the fourth most frequent source. There was no significant difference between boys and girls in these respects. The children were asked to list three of their favourite advertisements and three of their least favourite advertisements, to see if any indirect cigarette advertisements were included. Seven boys and 12 girls listed at least one indirect cigarette advertisement among their favourites, but 17 boys and 20 girls selected at least one direct cigarette advertisement

Table 1. Most frequent sources of advertisement for children in primary 6

Sex	Source					
	Television	Newspapers	Radio	Magazines	Signboards	Others
Boys	74	62	50	22	5	22
Girls	63	48	44	23	2	7
Total	137	110	94	45	7	29

Multiple responses were allowed

as their least favourite. Fifteen children (two boys and 13 girls) listed 'cigarette advertisements' as their least favourite advertisements, without naming any brand of cigarette. Sixty boys and 28 girls listed only non-cigarette-related advertisements.

The children were probed further on their perception of the indirect cigarette advertisements shown, and their responses were assessed to see whether they were able to understand and interpret them as advertising cigarettes, advertising non-cigarette products or advertising other products not shown on the advertisement or whether they did not understand the advertisement (Table 2). A·total of 404 children (42%) thought that the indirect cigarette advertisements were promoting non-cigarette products, while 274 (29%) thought that they were promoting cigarettes and the remainder (29%) did not understand the advertisement. Of the total of 1241 responses, 624 (50%) liked the indirect cigarette advertisements shown, while 617 (50%) did not like them. The reason given for disliking the advertisements was that 'it is bad for health' in only 20% of the responses; most of the children gave non-health reasons, which included 'the portrayal is contrary to religious and social norms'. Only 11 children (1.7%) liked the advertisement because the activities shown were 'fun'.

Most of children felt that the target group for these indirect cigarette advertisements was working adult males, whose common hobbies they considered to be travelling, sports, bicycling and horseriding, all of which correspond to the associations with smoking created by the advertisements.

Discussion

Television was the most powerful source of advertisements for both boys and girls in this study. Most families in Malaysia have access to a television set, and its impact will be even greater when more television channels and 24-hour satellite television become widely accessible. Given that television is the most important source of advertisements for this group, its utility and effectiveness as a source of cigarette campaigns should be studied in greater depth. Magazines were rated after television, radio and newspapers, since, at 12 years of age, reading magazines is less common than the other sources. Most of the children did not list cigarette advertisements among their favourite or least favourite advertisements; very few children listed indirect cigarette advertisements among their favourite advertisements, and many said they were their least favourite. The low level of dislike for cigarette advertisement found in this study may suggest that these children were unaware of the nature and purpose of the advertisements. Teaching schoolchildren to dislike smoking and any methods used to promote smoking, including advertising, will help reduce the prevalence of smoking among schoolchildren in the country.

Table 2. Children's understanding of indirect cigarette advertisements

Sex	Advertising cigarettes		Advertising non-cigarette products		Advertising other products		Do not understand advertisement		Total no.
	No.	%	No.	%	No.	%	No.	%	
Boys	145	28.4	159	31.2	69	13.5	137	26.9	510
Girls	129	29.3	91	20.6	85	19.3	136	30.8	441
Total	274	28.8	250	26.3	154	16.2	273	28.7	951

Even though the advertisements were advertising products other than cigarettes, one quarter of the children identified them as 'cigarette advertisements'. This is quite a high rate, since these children were still in primary school and most probably had not been exposed to smoking or brands of cigarettes. Aitken *et al.* (1985) found that 22% of 6–10-year-old children identified indirect cigarette advertisements as advertising cigarettes, and this proportion increased to 91% among the secondary schoolchildren. Although boys are usually more aware of cigarettes brands and advertising, we found that the level of awareness was slightly higher among girls (29%) than boys (28%). Most of the children considered that these advertisements were meant for adult working men, perhaps because more men are shown in these advertisements in rugged scenery. Only 5.2% felt that the advertisements were also meant for adolescents.

Conclusion

In the face of worldwide tobacco advertising campaigns, the decision to smoke becomes an easy and tempting option. Public health authorities have comparatively few resources with which to 'deglamourize' smoking and to present information about its consequences for health. The World Health Organization Expert Committee on Smoking Control (1979) bluntly stated that 'the international tobacco industry's irresponsible behaviour and its massive advertising and promotional campaigns are ... direct causes of a substantial number of unnecessary deaths'. Although educating young schoolchildren to deter them from starting smoking is still be the most feasible way of controlling smoking in the population (Yaacob & Hishamuddin, 1994), it is difficult to motivate the young to avoid a risk that they will suffer from only many years later (Chapman, 1995). A combination of strategies is called for, and banning all forms of cigarette advertising is essential. For this reason, 27 countries throughout the world have a total ban on tobacco advertising and a further 77 have some form of restriction (Roemer, 1993).

Acknowledgements

This study was supported by funds from the Ministry of Science, Technology and Environment Malaysia (Grant No:06-02-05-6074) under the IRPA scheme.

References

Aitken, P.P., Leather, D.S. & O'Hagan, F.J. (1985) Children's perceptions of advertisements for cigarettes. *Soc. Sci. Med.*, 21, 785–797

A Study Group of the Public Health Department (1959) The smoking habits of school children. *Br. J. Prev. Soc. Med.*, 13, 14

Chapman, S. (1995) Smokers: Why do they start and continue? *World Health Forum*, 161–169

Medical Tribune (1996) Tobacco advertising questioned. 11/96 1 June

O'Connel, D.L., Alexander, H.M., Dobson, A.J., *et al.* (1981) Cigarette smoking and drug use in school children. III. Factors associated with smoking. *Int. J. Epidemiol.*, 110, 221–231

Roemer, R. (1993) *Legislative Action to Combat the World Smoking Epidemic*, 2nd Ed., Geneva, WHO

Salber, E.J., Goldman, E., Buka, M. & Welsh, B. (1961) Smoking habits of high school children in Newton, Massachusetts. *New Engl. J. Med.*, 265, 969–974

Utusan Konsumer Tobacco Companies (1996) Breakaway to exploit legal loopholes, Consumer Association of Penang, May

World Health Organization (1979) Controlling the smoking epidemic: Report of the WHO Expert Committee on Smoking Control (WHO Technical Report Series No. 636), Geneva

World Health Organization (1983) Smoking control strategies in developing countries: Report of a WHO Expert Committee (WHO Technical Report Series No. 695), Geneva

Yaacob, I.B. & Hishamuddin, M.H. (1994) Smoking habits and attitudes among secondary schoolteachers. *Southeast Asian J. Trop. Med. Public Health*, 25, 74–79

Strategies used by the tobacco industry to target young consumers: The Canary Islands experience

J.R. Calvo, J. Calvo-Rosales, A. Lopez-Cabañas, M. Lopez, M. Torres, M.C. Navarro, J.M. Segura, M. Marrero & J.C. Orengo

University of Las Palmas, Unit of Health Education, Las Palmas, Gran Canaria, Spain

Tobacco companies are some of the most powerful advertising machines in the world. It is well know that the advertising budget of the largest companies is greater than the total budget of the World Health Organization. In the Canary Islands, one tobacco company spent US$ 10 million in one year to advertise three products, and US$ 3 million was spent in 1997 to promote one new brand of tobacco. When the tobacco companies say that advertising is a legal right because cigarettes are a legal product, they are saying that they need to recruit 1500 new smokers every day, only in western Europe, because 1500 old smokers are dying every day.

Tobacco companies need to addict young people because people usually begin to smoke during childhood. The companies know that the majority of new consumers are aged 11–18. They have therefore stepped up their strategies to recruit a new generation of young smokers. They have also created general confusion among the young about the relationship between tobacco and health. The population they have chosen is especially vulnerable because young people are easily influenced by the role models used by the tobacco companies: a man, alone, self confident, living in the open air and taking his own decisions about his life. It is very easy to recognize the Malboro men, the cowboy who was chosen because he was an impressive figure to adolescents who want to escape the control of their parents, take care of themselves and solve their own problems. Malboro is still the most popular brand on the adolescent market.

The Canary Islands are a region of Spain, with a stable population of 1.7 million people and more than 8 million visitors from abroad each year. We also have the 'honour' of being the one territory of the European Union with four of the biggest tobacco companies in the world; 37% of the adult population and more than 25% of adolescents between 14 and 16 years of age smoke daily. Furthermore, our adolescents start smoking very early, around 12 years. It is very easy for them to obtain tobacco because the law forbidding the sale of tobacco to minors it is not enforced. These figures show that this is a very fertile field for the tobacco companies to promote their business of addiction.

They used a broad spectrum of strategies. The most successful are those involving activities that attract young people, such as rock concerts, sports and trips. The commonest strategy is to promote an activity and give it the name of a brand, such as 'Winston fun time', 'Winston Volley Beach Cup', 'Camel Trophy' and 'Duca 2 motor race' (Ducados is a well-known brand of tobacco). The tobacco companies also offer free trips to learn the 'American way of life', to Las Vegas, Montana or Colorado. They promote activities related to the open air, such as the Camel Trophy, which guarantees the presence of that brand on television and the mass media every day, for more that a month. Another more sophisticated strategy is to give the name of a well-known brand of cigarettes to another product, such as coffee, and to design the coffee package exactly like the cigarette pack; that brand of coffee is then used to promote the music programme on the radio that is most popular among young people, 'The 40's principals' which is 'casually' sponsored by 'Coffee Coronas'.

Since 1982, Spanish law has banned the advertisement of tobacco products on television, yet companies violate the spirit of the law, for example by paying for a rock concert and its transmission on television or using 2–3 min of that time during which. the word 'Winston' is used 21 times or the most popular slogan of Winston in Spain, 'You are the genuine' is overprinted in less than 1 s. A new way has been developed of reducing the effect of the health warnings that appear on tobacco advertisements: a girl of about 18 says ' Don't let them tell you tales...', just before the warning appears.

Throughout the world, we have similar problems in controlling the tobacco epidemic. As stated by Dr Kessler, the former commissioner of the United States Food and Drug Administration, this is a paediatric epidemic, because the advertising strategies used by the tobacco companies still focus on the preferences of adolescents, despite their denials.

Tobacco promotion in Ghana

S. Koranteng

Ghana Committee on Tobacco Control, Police Hospital, Accra, Ghana

The transnational tobacco companies, sensing that their economic interests are being threatened by the worldwide anti-smoking campaign, have embarked on a counter-campaign to deny that smoking is a health hazard. At the same time, they have been reaching out for new markets in Africa and Asia. In 1996, a number of journalists from Ghana, Kenya, Mauritius, South Africa, Uganda and the former Zaire were invited to a seminar on tobacco issues in Mauritius, organized by the transnational tobacco companies. The companies brought with them their foreign mercenaries, or experts, who obediently put across their usual, highly misleading arguments on tobacco issues, denying that tobacco products are harmful; they further asserted conclusively that passive smoking is not a health hazard. The seminar raised a number of questions. Why was the meeting held in Africa? Do the companies think that African journalists can be more easily convinced? Do they think that we are unable to decide for ourselves on the basis of the evidence from the West?

Young people comprise the largest part of the world's population, are one of the main targets of sports sponsorship and are the most susceptible to deceitful tobacco-related advertisments. Second thoughts should be given to the annual launching of the 'World No Tobacco Day'. Although these have been effective, we consider that the money could be better spent on programmes with long-term effects. For instance, the money earmarked for this event could be used in selected areas within a region each year for other, longer-lasting anti-tobacco messages, such as billboards and sports sponsorship. Tobacco companies do not advertise their wares one or two days a year, but all the year round, even where they are forbidden to do so. They are quick to show their respect for the law by not advertising on local television or in the press or electronic media, but they are equally quick to sponsor 'Miss Ghana' or 'Miss Kenya' or 'Miss Nigeria' competitions and sports activities. Young people identify themselves with events such as these and not with annual 'launch and forget' affairs. Even if we cannot withstand the economic might of the transnational tobacco companies, we can use their effective methods of reaching young people in our own modest way.

I end with a question: What would your reaction be if you saw two teams on a football pitch, with the inscription on the jersey of one team reading 'Rothmans' and that on the jerseys of other reading 'Tobacco kills'?

Tobacco promotion in Nepal

M.R. Pandey

Mrigendra Samjhana Medical Trust, Thapathali, Kathmandu, Nepal

As tobacco companies face increasing resistance to promotion in the developed world, they are concentrating their full force on the developing countries, stepping up advertising and other promotional activities via most of the available media. Sponsorship of sports and cultural events is becoming common and aggressive. Tobacco promoters are focusing on populations with great potential for growth and are thus targeting children and women in these countries. There is relatively little awareness of the dangers of tobacco smoking among the general public in developing countries. The governments are faced with the dilemma of promoting awareness of the hazards associated with tobacco on the one hand and the temptation to receive a politically comfortable source of revenue from tobacco taxes on the other.

Nepal is a land-locked country bordering China in the north and India on the other three sides. The total area of the country is 1472 km^2, and the population is about 20 million. Nepal has a 40% literacy rate and a 2.1% population growth rate. It is one of the least developed countries in the world, with a per caqpita income of US$ 210. The health indicators are far from satisfactory, with an infant mortality rate of 100 per 1 000, a maternal mortality rate of 850 per 100 000, a life expectancy of 55 years and a malnutrition rate of 40%.

Nepal also has some of the highest prevalences of tobacco smoking in the world: 85% among males and 72% among females in the mountainous region and 64% among males and 14% among females in Kathmandu (Pandey et al., 1988a). Unlike most other developing countries, the rate of tobacco smoking among females is very high— one of the highest recorded anywhere in the world. During the last two decades, awareness campaigns have been launched by a number of social organizations, such as the Mrigendra Samjhana Medical Trust, the Nepal Heart Foundation and the Nepal Cancer Relief Society, and by the Government of Nepal. These have brought about some changes in attitudes and behaviour, especially in urban and other accessible areas (Pandey et al., 1988b).

Unfortunately, the tobacco industry is arriving in Nepal with its promotional effort, and there has been rapid growth of direct advertising campaigns on television, radio, the print media and billboards. Furthermore, there are two large cigarette manufacturing companies in the country, one in the Government sector and the other in the private sector. Their total sales amount to Rs 3000 million (US$ 52 million) per year. Although this figure may appear small in comparison with other countries, it is considerable in relation to the total national budget of only Rs. 62 000 million (US$ 1082 million). A substantial proportion of the revenue of Government-owned media comes from cigarette advertisements, and most of the Government's budget comes from tobacco taxes. Under these circumstances, there is great resistance to the anti-tobacco movement. There is as yet no ban on either direct or indirect advertising or promotion of sports, culural and other activities by the tobacco industry. Most advertisements seem to be targeted at the younger generation, using subjects such as glamour, social success, sexual success and nationalism.

Sponsorship by tobacco companies in Nepal

Some of the events sponsored by tobacco companies in Nepal are as follows: *Cultural and social events*: arts exhibitions, musical nights in major cities, annual eye camps, literacy classes, fertilizer distribution, festivals, road-building and i;provement of seeds. *Sporting events*: international karate championship, all-Nepal boxing championship, cricket games between Nepal and India, golf tournaments with the Royal Nepal Golf Club, football tournaments, triathlons and away games of the Nepalese football team in India. *Television and radio*: Olympic Games 1994, World Cup Football 1994, national football tournament and various popular programmes.

The large percent of the marketing budget spent on sponsoring such events in Nepal shows that the tobacco industry is fully aware of the importance for promoting their products. Studies in the United Kingdom have shown the persuasive nature of tobacco sponsoring of sports and games (Aitken et al., 1986). Both children and adults have increased brans awareness and connect the brand with the sponsored sport (Ledwith, 1984). As there is little awareness of the danger of such sponsorship in Nepal, there is negligible resistance to it. In only one or two cases have sports and cultural organizations refused tobacco money. For its part, the tobacco industry feels noble in helping so many causes.

Use of smokeless tobacco, usually chewing tobacco, is increasing rapidly in Nepal, especially in the Terai region. Last year, the market for smokeless tobacco increased by about 30%, and it is being promoted on the radio, in newspapers and on billboards.

Concerted efforts of the anti-tobacco lobby have resulted in a few positive steps. Tobacco smoking in public places, transport and Government offices has been banned, and a number of steps have been taken against promotion: a statutory health warning in mandatory on all tobacco advertisements; gifts to sellers and consumers of cigarettes have been banned; the media rate for tobacco advertising is double that for other advertisements; there are occasional radio and television advertisements against tobacco smoking paid for by the Government, social organizations and the media themselves; and there is a 'health tax' on cigarettes.

Alternatives to sponsorship

In Nepal, both sports and cultural organizations and the media are so short of funds that they are constantly seeking sponsorship. Tobacco companies are the most readily available partners in deals where their mutual interests merge. If the tobacco companies are to be denied this avenue for sales promotion, alternatives must be sought.

The total annual income from the health tax on cigarettes is Rs. 200 million (US$ 3.5 million). Some of that money should be spent on anti-Tobacco promotion activities. For this purpose, it is suggested that a health promotion foundation be created in Nepal, on the model of the Victorian Health Foundation in Australia. The Foundation could then offer its own sponsorship of sporting and cultural events. The main aim of such sponsorship is to induce behavioural changes and create a supportive environment for the Nepalese population to quit smoking and adopt a healthy lifestyle. Sportsmen and artists are 'cultural ambassadors' who could carry these ideas across the nation. We are lobbying stongly for this objective.

Until recently, the tobacco industries provided free gifts and samples to wholesalers, retailers and customers. This was banned in 1997. The tobaco industries paid about Rs. 1700 million (US$ 30 million) in excise duty and sales tax to the Government in 1996, which represented nearly half of the total health budget. The Government has owned a cigarette factory for the past 15 years, but with the advent of the multinationals, its share of the revenues is falling rapidly. The one private tobacco industry, established in collaboration with British–American Tobacco Co., is the second highest taxpayer in the country. Nepal has allowed the direct import of cigarettes into the country, and customs duty was decreased in 1997. As a result, Marlboros are being imported, and the company has launched a campaign targeting young people. Another multinational company, R.J. Reynolds, has recently signed a contract with one of the largest business houses in Nepal to enter this poor country.

Conclusion

There should be a strong, global coalition of anti-tobacco forces in the developing countries, and APACT has done a lot in this direction in the Asia–Pacific region. The resources available for anti-tobacco activities is insignificant in comparison with that of the tobacco industries, but, as we are fighting for the right cause, we stand on firm moral ground. If we act together, we will have the successes seen in developed countries. Our earnest plea is that in planning such a regional campaigns people do not forget small countries like Nepal, which are already overburdened with health problems and where the authorities have few resources or energy to give to anti-tobacco measures.

References
Aitken, P.P., Leathar, D.S. & Squair, S.I. (1986) Children's awareness of cigarette brand sponsorship of sports and games in the UK. *Health Educ. Res.*, 1, 2203–2221
Ledwith, F. (1984) Does tobacco sport sponsorship on television act as advertising for children? *Health Educ. J.*, 43, 85–88
Pandey, M.R., Basnet, B. & Neupane, R.P. (1988a) Chronic bronchitis and cor pulmonale in Nepal. *MMT*
Pandey, M.R., Neupane, R.P. & Gautam, A. (1988b) Epidemiological study of tobacco smoking behavior among adults in a rural community of the hill region of Nepal with special reference to attitude and beliefs. *Int. J. Epidemiol.*, 17, 535–541

Effect of tobacco loyalty programmes on low-income smokers

D.R. Eadie, A.M. MacKintosh & G.B. Hastings

Centre for Social Marketing, University of Strathclyde, Glasgow, Scotland

The tobacco industry sustains itself in two ways: by maximizing the number of people who start smoking and by minimizing the number who stop. The health lobby has placed much emphasis upon understanding how the industry uses marketing techniques to recruit new smokers, particularly underage smokers; yet, given that it costs the industry less to keep existing customers than it does to find new ones, there is a strong case for expanding the scope of current investigations to establish the marketing techniques used to maintain the existing customer base. This study focuses on one such technique, the tobacco loyalty programme. It examines the impact of loyalty programmes on low-income smokers, since the evidence indicates that the cessation rates in this group are particularly low.

What are tobacco loyalty programmes?

Loyalty programmes can be found in many commercial fields. For example, many airlines offer air mileage schemes which entitle customers to collect 'free' air miles for each journey made. These air miles can be cashed in at some future time in exchange for 'free' travel with the same airline. Loyalty programmes such as these have a number of commercial objectives. Most significantly, they have been described as techniques designed to maintain customer loyalty and company profitability by deflecting attention from price to value-added product benefits. Their relevance to tobacco marketing, where price increases frequently exceed inflation rates, is therefore obvious.

In the United Kingdom, Gallaghers Ltd and Imperial Tobacco Ltd operate the Benson and Hedges Gratis Points scheme, the Embassy Regal Focus Points scheme and the Kensitas Club Gift Certificate scheme. These tobacco loyalty programmes are based on fairly rudimentary techniques to enable customers to collect loyalty points, typically in the form of paper coupons or gift certificates. The coupons or certificates can be collected from packs of participating brands and then exchanged for household products selected from a gift catalogue. These products include brand-name audiovisual equipment, baby wear, child-care products, sports equipment, jewellery and fashion clothing. They are also used to promote sports events sponsored by the participating brand by offering access to 'free' tickets.

The products offered are often described as 'free gifts', so that the actual cost to the smoker is extremely difficult to calculate. Table 1 shows some estimated costs for a range of products selected from the 1994 Kensitas Club loyalty programme. A pair of children's novelty scissors worth around UK£ 1 would take the smoker of an average of 20 cigarettes per day about a month to save the required number of coupons. This is equivalent to an expenditure of UK£ 83 on cigarettes or about 33 standard packs of cigarettes. It would take the same smoker wishing to purchase an 8-mm Samsung camcorder worth around UK£ 500 38 years, with an expenditure at 1994 prices of

Table 1. Kensitas Club: 1993–94 catalogue

Item	No. of 'certificates'	Approximate collection period[a]	Approximate outlay on cigarettes (UK£)[b]	Approximate retail value (UK£)	Estimated contribution (%)
Children's novelty scissors	330	1 month	83	1	1.2
Set of kitchen utensils	3 110	10 months	778	14	1.8
Black & Decker jigsaw	10 000	2.75 years	2 500	29	1.2
Child car safety seat	16 500	4.5 years	4 125	37	0.9
Samsung 8-mm camcorder	140 000	38 years	35 000	500	1.4

around UK£ 35 000. Using these figures, it is possible to estimate that in this scheme approximately 1.3% of the cost price for those collecting certificates goes towards financing the scheme. In sterling, that is approximately 3.25 p for every pack of 20 cigarettes purchased.

Smokers who collect these coupons can usually purchase their 'gifts' in one of two ways, either by post or, more typically, by visiting a high-street retail outlet. The Kensitas Club brand operates what is referred to as a 'gift centre'. Benson and Hedges have an exclusive arrangement with one of the largest catalogue shops in the United Kingdom, Index. Index shops are located in the Littlewoods chain of stores and have over 130 outlets in the country. They have an established reputation for selling quality brand-name products.

The appeal of tobacco loyalty programmes to low-income smokers

Data from two recent surveys undertaken in the United Kingdom as part of the study indicate that tobacco loyalty programmes are more popular amongst lower-income smokers. Exploratory research with focus groups of coupon collectors provides some insight into why this is so: all coupon collectors, irrespective of income, attribute the same high material value to the programmes. They are seen to provide product lines that are comparable in terms of range, choice and quality with those available in some high-street retail chains. Significantly, as the programmes are designed in a way that does not provoke consideration of the cost to the consumer, they tend to look upon these products as free of cost. The use of terms such as 'gift', 'gratis' and 'free' to promote the programmes would appear to reinforce this perception. This combination of high quality and low perceived cost has the effect of adding value to the participating brands.

These effects offer the smoker certain psychological benefits. First, they provide a mechanism through which smokers can justify their expenditure on what is commonly considered a 'wasteful' product. This, in turn, helps to displace anxieties associated with the financial cost of smoking and provides a means of rationalizing the decision to continue smoking: "I think subconsciously it eases your conscience a wee bit. You're thinking, 'Oh, I'm going to get something back'." (low-income smoker). Significantly, given the tighter financial restrictions placed on disadvantaged groups, these psychological benefits are of greater salience to the low-income smoker. This salience is reflected in the social and cultural significance attached to tobacco loyalty programmes in low-income communities. For example, in such communities there is greater competition for coupons, and coupons are often saved as a resource to fall back on in times of financial need: "If something comes up and I know that I've not got the money, I'll check the catalogue to see if I can get it there."

In some low-income communities, loyalty programmes also provide an alternative currency, local shops offering exchange rates for coupons in pounds sterling and accepting coupons as payment for goods. In one instance, a local community centre sought to purchase audiovisual equipment by accepting charitable donations in the form of Kensitas Club Gift Certificates.

As well as having a greater social significance and offering more psychological benefits to smokers in low-income communities, it was also evident that loyalty programmes have a greater impact on some aspects of smoking behaviour in these areas. There was little evidence that loyalty programmes encourage smokers to increase the amounts consumed or that they have a role to play in recruiting new recruits to smoking; however, such programmes were clearly instrumental in discouraging existing smokers from stopping and in disrupting attempts to give up: "I was trying to cut down, and the coupons were encouraging me to smoke. So when I got the gifts I wanted, I stopped smoking that brand." "I suppose it's easier just to save the coupons than not to smoke. After all it's a drug—that's all it is at the end of the day." These behavioural effects were more often observed in smokers living in low-income communities.

Conclusions

The research indicates that tobacco loyalty programmes appeal more to low-income smokers and that rewards based on material incentive help to explain this popularity. More specifically, tobacco loyalty programmes give the appearance of improving access to material wealth, while in reality deny access by obviating any need for smokers to consider the economic consequences of maintaining their smoking habit. It is therefore argued that the ethics of this practice should be placed under greater scrutiny by authorities responsible for regulating the tobacco industries' promotional activities.

Acknowledgements
This research was supported by the Health Education Authority, London.

Influence of cigarette promotion on mediators of smoking

H. Lee[1], D. Buller[2], L. Chassin[3], J. Kronenfeld[3] & D. MacKinnon[3]

*[1]Arizona Cancer Center, The University of Arizona, Tucson, Arizona;
[2]AMC Cancer Research Center, and [3]Arizona State University, United States*

Despite various efforts to reduce tobacco use among youth, the prevalence is on the rise (Johnston, 1996). In the meantime, the expenditures of the tobacco industry for advertising and promoting cigarettes are also on the rise. It is estimated that the tobacco industry spends over US$ 6 thousand million to advertise and promote cigarette consumption. According to data from the Federal Trade Commission, the industry has been spending more money on promotion than on advertising since 1983. Although studies of advertising patterns and young people's tobacco use demonstrate a positive association between advertising and adolescent smoking (Evans *et al.*, 1995; Pierce & Gilpin, 1995; Altman *et al.*, 1996; Schooler *et al.*, 1996), there has been some concern about the direction of causality. First, the direction may be reversed: adolescents who smoke are more likely to be exposed to and to recognize tobacco marketing than those who do not smoke. Secondly, exposure to tobacco marketing may be associated with general problematic behaviour such as rebelliousness and risk-taking. Hence, it may be argued that it is not the marketing *per se*, but personal characteristics that account for differential exposure to marketing as well as smoking. To establish a causal link between tobacco marketing and smoking, we used data from a large student survey conducted in Tucson, Arizona, to explore the relative impacts of tobacco marketing and other key risk factors associated with uptake in a single analysis.

The analysis was conducted on data for students who were not current smokers in order to avoid concern about a reversed causal direction, using susceptibility to smoking as the dependent variable. To address the second concern, we investigated the relative importance of exposure and participation in tobacco marketing and other important predictors of smoking, including demographic factors and personal characteristics such as rebelliousness, social influence factors (i.e. parental, peer and reference group norms) and social image.

Method

The data were collected from self-administered questionnaires distributed to 7521 students in the seventh, eighth, eleventh and twelfth grades at 52 schools in Tucson, Arizona, as part of the Full Court Press project. The participation rate was 93%, and the average response rate was 86%. The dependent measure for this study, susceptibility to smoking, reflects whether the adolescents have consciously decided not to smoke or whether they are open to smoking. Pierce and Gilpin (1995) established that a lack of resolve not to smoke is a good predictor for smoking in the future. As shown in Table 1, the susceptibility index was created by adding three Likert-type items. The main independent measures, exposure to tobacco promotion and participation in promotion, were measured from the answers to five questions. The actual wordings and descriptive statistics for other variables are shown in Table 1.

'Rebelliousness' was measured by an index of 11 Likert scale-type items (Table 2). Personal attitudes and beliefs about smoking were measured by asking 11 questions that dealt with the potential benefits of smoking. Two indices were created from the

Table 1. Key measures for measuring susceptibility to smoking

Index or item	No.	Mean score	SD
Susceptibility[a] (Cronbach's alpha = 0.86)			
If one of your best friends offered you a cigarette, do you think you might smoke it?	5565	1.40	0.68
At any time during the next year do you think you might smoke a cigarette?	5537	1.50	0.75
Do you think you might try a cigarette soon?	5565	1.36	0.65
Family conflict[b] (correlation coefficient $r = 0.50$)			
I have a lot of arguments with my family.	5564	2.13	0.88
My family looks for things to nag me about.	5547	2.11	0.92
Parental norm[c] (correlation coefficient $r = 0.53$)			
How important does your mother (or stepmother) think staying off cigarettes is?	5201	1.42	0.81
How important does your father (or stepfather) think staying off cigarettes is?	4977	1.61	0.94
Peer norm[c]			
How important do your best friends think staying off cigarettes is?	5012	1.82	0.99
Reference group norm[c]			
How important do most people of your own age think staying off cigarettes is?	5263	2.51	0.94
Exposure to promotion (Cronbach's alpha = 0.41)			
Have you received mail from tobacco companies addressed to you personally (such as surveys coupons, free gifts, or catalogue)?	5547	14.6%	
Have you ever bought or received for free any product which was given out by a tobacco company (such as clothing, hats, bags, posters or lighters)?	5538	19.8%	
Do you have any friends or relatives who own tobacco promotional items?	5497	67.7%	
Participation in promotion (correlation coefficient $r = 0.37$)			
Have you ever saved coupons, proof-of-purchase seals, or bar codes from cigarette packs to get gifts or promotional items?	5538	10.9%	
Would you ever use tobacco promotional items?	5506	5.0% using now 27.2% yes	

[a]Scores range between 1 and 4, where 1 means 'definitely not' and 4 means 'definitely yes'
[b]Scores range between 1 and 4, where 1 means 'strongly disagree' and 4 means 'strongly agree'
[c]Scores range between 1 and 4, where 1 means 'very important' and 4 means 'not important at all'

Table 2. Items for scale of rebelliousness : Means and standard deviations ($n = 5603$)

Item	Mean score	SD
I feel guilty when I break a rule.[a]	2.05	0.74
When rules and regulations get in the way, I sometimes ignore them.	2.50	0.74
If I don't like an order I have been given, I may not obey it, or may obey it only partly	2.35	0.81
.If I don't like something I'm told to do, I often put it off or just don't do it at all.	2.27	0.81
Sometimes I enjoy seeing how much I can get away with.	2.19	0.89
When I make a decision, I usually go by what my parents taught me. [a]	1.98	0.78
I sometimes get myself into trouble at school.	2.03	0.90
When I'm told to do something by a teacher, I do it. [a]	1.80	0.66
I get a kick out of doing things every now and then that are a little risky or dangerous.	2.59	0.89
If anyone upsets me I usually try to get revenge.	2.14	0.84
I don't mind lying to keep my friends out of trouble with the authorities.	2.37	0.90

Scores range between 1 and 4, where 1 means 'strongly disagree' and 4 means 'strongly agree' with the statement. Items marked with [a] are coded reversely.
Cronbach's alpha = 0.80

results of the factor analysis: one for the 'perceived benefits of smoking' and one for
'positive social image of smoking' (Table 3).

Results

Fifty-one percent of the survey respondents were girls. Overall, 26% of the girls
and 26% of the boys were current smokers, as defined by smoking at least once within
the 30 days prior to the survey; 20% of middle schoolers and 29% of high schoolers
were current smokers.

Tobacco promotion had reached the adolescents quite widely. Nearly 20% reported
buying items or receiving free products given out by a tobacco company, and 68% had
friends or relatives who owned tobacco promotional items (Table 1). About 11% of the
students had attempted to participate in promotional activities, and 5% used tobacco
promotional items. Another 27% reported that they would be willing to use promotional
items if they had the opportunity.

To explore the influence of exposure to tobacco promotion on perceptions about
the benefits of smoking and positive social images, a stepwise regression analysis was
conducted by the forward entry method. (An analysis with backward removal produced
largely similar results.) As expected, exposure to tobacco promotion was related to
students' perceptions about the benefits and social image of smoking (Tables 4 and 5).

Since it is established that exposure to promotion is related to variables that influence
smoking among adolescents, the question is whether exposure to promotion can account
for any further variance beyond that explained by other predictors of uptake. We
conducted a hierarchical regression analysis in which the key variables known to
influence smoking uptake by adolescents (demographic and personal characteristics

Table 3. Factor analysis of perceived benefits of smoking ($n = 5603$)

Factor	Benefits	Positive social image
Helps people relax	0.84	
Helps reduce stress	0.84	
Helps people feel more comfortable in social situations	0.80	
Helps people keep their weight down	0.58	
Helps people forget their worries	0.74	
Cheers people up when in a bad mood	0.75	
Makes people feel more self-confident and sure of themselves	0.68	
Makes people look more grown up		0.84
Makes people look tough		0.85
Makes people look sexy		0.82
Enjoyable		0.55
Variance (%)	53.9	11.9
Eigen value	5.93	1.31
Cronbach's alpha	0.90	0.84

Entries are factor scores from Varimax rotation.

Table 4. Predictors for perceived benefits of smoking among nonsmokers ($n = 5603$)

Predictor	Correlation coefficient	Unstandardized coefficient	Standardized coefficient
Level of education	0.05	0.372* (0.131)	0.039*
Rebelliousness	0.32	0.233* (0.013)	0.258*
Peer norm	0.21	0.546* (0.074)	0.114*
Reference group norm	0.14	0.178* (0.077)	0.036*
Participation in promotion	0.21	0.774* (0.090)	0.123*
Standard r^2	0.141		
Adjusted r^2	0.140		

* $p < 0.05$

Table 5. Predictors for positive social image of smoking among non-smokers ($n = 5603$)

Predictor	Correlation coefficient	Unstandardized coefficient	Standardized coefficient
Level of education	−0.08	−0.376* (0.061)	−0.085*
Rebelliousness	0.30	0.094* (0.007)	0.224*
Family conflict	0.16	0.060* (0.021)	0.043*
Peer norm	0.20	0.283* (0.032)	0.127*
Exposure to promotion	0.07	0.086* (0.041)	0.033*
Participation in promotion	0.18	0.325* (0.046)	0.111*
Standard r^2	0.123		
Adjusted r^2	0.122		

* $p < 0.05$

and social and environmental variables) were entered into the equation before the promotion-related variables. This is a conservative test to investigate whether the exposure to promotion accounts for variance in susceptibility, while simultaneously controlling for all other variables. As shown in Table 6, exposure to and participation in tobacco promotion emerged as significant predictors of susceptibility to smoking. Over and above the variance explained by the other factors shown to be related to smoking uptake, the two variables explain the additional 2% variance in susceptibility to smoking among non-smokers.

Conclusions

The preceding analysis shows that exposure to promotion is a significant predictor for susceptibility to smoking among non-smokers, even after removal of variance explained by school level, rebelliousness, parental, peer and reference group norms, perceived benefits and positive social images of smoking. The analysis suggests that while exposure to tobacco promotion is correlated to other risk factors for smoking uptake, tobacco promotion has an independent influence on susceptibility to smoking. The findings support concerns about the effect of tobacco promotion on youth. Regardless of whether the promotions are intended for adults or minors, they reach youth and clearly serve as additional risk factors for smoking uptake.

Table 6. Predictors for susceptibility to smoking among non-smokers: Hierarchical regression ($n = 5603$)

Predictors	Correlation coefficient	Beta	r^2 change
Sex (female)	0.04	0.035*	
Level of education	−0.17	−0.170*	
			0.030*
Rebelliousness	0.33	0.327*	
Family conflict	0.17	0.034*	
			0.114*
Parental norm	0.06	−0.032*	
Peer norm	0.24	0.167*	
Reference group norm	0.14	0.051*	
			0.033*
Perceived benefit	0.34	0.076*	
Positive social image	0.44	0.299*	
			0.108*
Exposure to promotion	0.14	0.038*	
Participation in promotion	0.24	0.116*	0.016*
Standard r^2			0.302
Adjusted r^2			0.301

* $p < 0.05$

Acknowledgement
Funding for the study was provided by a grant from the Robert Wood Johnson Foundation.

References
Altman, D.G., Levine, D.W., Coeytaux, R., Slade, J. & Jaffe, R. (1996) Tobacco promotion and susceptibility to tobacco use among adolescent aged 12 through 17 years in a nationally representative sample. *Am. J. Public Health*, **86**, 1590–1593
Evans, N., Farkas, A., Gilpin, E., Berry, C. & Pierce, J.P. (1995) Influence of tobacco marketing and exposure to smokers on adolescent susceptibility to smoking. *J. Natl Cancer Inst.*, **87**, 1538–1545
Johnston, L. (1996) Smoking rates climb among American teenagers, who find smoking increasingly acceptable and seriously underestimate the risks. Ann Arbor: The University of Michigan News and Information Service
Pierce, J.P. & Gilpin, E.A. (1995) A historical analysis of tobacco marketing and the uptake of smoking by youth in the United States: 1890–1977. *Health Psychol.*, **14**, 500–508
Schooler, C., Feighery, E. & Flora, J.A. (1996) Seventh graders' self-reported exposure to cigarette marketing and its relationship to their smoking behavior. *Am. J. Public Health*, **86**, 1216–1221

Health sponsorship of sport: What are the rules of the game?

S.K. Frizzell & M. Carroll

Healthway, Perth, Western Australia, Australia

Background

Sponsorship of sport is not a new phenomenon. What is relatively new is the use of this medium as a health promotion strategy. The advent of tobacco tax-funded health promotion foundations in Australia in 1987, which had as a priority the replacement of tobacco sponsorship of sport, the arts and racing activities, has given a huge impetus to the use of health sponsorship of sport as a health promotion strategy. This in turn has led to a range of evaluation studies which have added new theory to our understanding of sponsorship as a health promotion strategy.

Healthway (the West Australian Health Promotion Foundation) was established in February 1991 after the passage of the Western Australian *Tobacco Control Act 1990*. The purposes of the *Act* were active discouragement of the smoking of tobacco and promotion of good health in the prevention of illness. The *Act* had the effect of phasing out tobacco advertising and sponsorship in this State, while at the same time allocating a small percentage of State tobacco tax for use by Healthway to sponsor sport, arts and racing events and to fund health promotion research and intervention projects. The Act established Healthway as an independent statutory body governed by a Board representing sport, arts, health, youth and country interests.

The *Act* allows use of 7% of the tobacco tax or AUS$ 12.9 million, whichever is the lesser, by Healthway for its range of programmes. The system of providing sponsorship grants to sports, arts or racing organizations, and the associated support grants to promote health messages at those events, is one of the most complex areas of Healthway's operations. When Healthway provides sponsorship for a sports, arts or racing organization, it also provides a support sponsorship grant to an independent health agency or a Healthway kit to promote a health message at that event. The health messages used most commonly in the sponsorship of sport by Healthway are concerned with smoking control, safe use of alcohol, good nutrition, promoting physical activity, protection against the sun and sports injury prevention. Since Healthway's inception, it has been involved in over 2000 separate sponsorships to sports (including 24 tobacco replacement sponsorships), worth a total of over AUS$ 27.7 million.

Health sponsorship

Health promotion sponsorships differ from grants to sports organizations in that a return is expected. With sponsorship, dollars are exchanged for a range of sponsor 'benefits' designed to promote the sponsors image and/or products. The major benefits sought through health sponsorship include promotional opportunities (e.g. signs, personal endorsement by players, logos on uniforms), educational opportunities (e.g. distribution of literature or sessions with young players on sports injury prevention, information about not smoking) and the introduction of structural changes to create healthier environments (e.g. smoke-free policies and areas, protection against the sun, healthy food choices and safe serving of alcohol). The potential for permanent healthy change in sports settings is increased greatly with attention to supportive environments. These also require the least amount of resources in terms of sponsorship dollars to bring about change.

Why use sports settings for health sponsorship?

Sports provide a setting for health promotion with existing strong networks and infrastructures, as well as access to large numbers of people. Approximately one third of Australians participate in sporting activities in any one year, in addition to nearly 4 million people involved in sport as spectators. Sports participation and attendance covers variations in age, sex, socioeconomic status and race. This has a number of implications for use of these settings for targeted health promotion messages. For example, it was estimated in one study that 69% of 12–16-year olds in Western Australia played structured sport, while another found that sports participation was invariably related to family income. Sports sponsorship therefore provides access to large numbers of people and specific target groups.

Community surveys conducted by the Health Promotion Evaluation Unit in its evaluation of Healthway found that people involved in sport had increased risk behaviour in nearly all areas except physical activity. While participation in recreational activities produces a range of physical, social and mental health benefits and assists in building social capital in communities, many people in these settings have increased alcohol consumption and smoking (spectators in sports settings) and less protection against the sun, whereas the venues provide opportunities to create supportive and healthy environments.

Finally, health sponsorship of sports is a lower-cost way of reaching large groups of people than the mass media. The involvement of existing media in high-profile sporting events provides opportunities for exposure of health messages to a wider population and to extend health promotion messages into rural areas. The use of high-profile role models to reinforce and extend the health message is also a vital strategy.

What are the rules of the game?

(i) Begin with small wins and move to a 'win–win' situation.

Health sponsors should start with small wins like smoke-free areas, to allow the sporting groups to appreciate and understand what is required in providing health promoting environments. Gradually move towards stronger expectations from the sponsorship, but always aim for a 'win–win' situation for both the sports and health groups. It is essential to build a co-operative working relationship with the sponsored groups.

(ii) Select compatible messages

Ensure that the health messages being promoted are compatible with the sporting group, for instance 'Be smoke-free, be active every day'. The group must feel 'comfortable' with the message, and it must be relevant to the target groups involved. Communicating the health risk factors on which the message was selected for the sponsored group will assist understanding of the goals of the health organization in sponsorship.

(iii) Make sponsorship part of a comprehensive programme

Sponsorship is only one strategy in a comprehensive approach to health promotion, which may also include mass media, community education programmes, legislation and policy implementation. Health sponsors should also seek a comprehensive mix of sponsored groups, ranging from high-profile to community groups. There is evidence that health promotion value for money can be gained by smaller value sponsorships at a grass-roots level.

(iv) Seek environmental change

The introduction of structural changes that lead to healthy environments is potentially the most powerful tool of health promotion. It not only leads to permanent changes but also assists in changing norms associated with health behaviour and makes choosing a healthier behaviour easier. Examples of structural changes that may lead to healthier environments include smoke-free areas, safe serving of alcohol, healthy food choices, protection against the sun and injury prevention through safer environments. In the 18 months after Healthway's inception, there was a significant increase in the prevalence of structural reforms. While the prevalence of smoke-free areas has increased the most (27%), there was also an increase in the prevalence of healthy food choice reforms (21.1%).

(v) Evaluate and communicate

Undertake evaluation of the sponsorship and communicate the results back to the sports organization. For example, the Health Promotion Evaluation Unit undertook evaluation of the 'Smoke Free WA' message which replaced the Benson & Hedges message as a major sponsorship at the Western Australian Cricket Association ground (Table 1). The high level of acceptance of the message and the attitude towards the smoke-free policy (even among smokers) was communicated to the organization. This enabled the sponsored organization to respond positively to an often vocal minority.

(vi) Use role models

Select appropriate role models, especially those relevant to young children, to convey health messages. Evaluation indicates that endorsement of health messages by role models, either verbally or by wearing promotional clothing, is an effective means of promoting health messages to children. With well-established sporting teams, the role models can serve to promote the sponsors' message by association, even when they do not mention or actively promote the message itself.

(vii) Develop clear contracts

Clearly defined sponsorship plans developed by health and sporting organizations serve to spell out the benefits of the sponsorship and clearly outline each organization's role in the arrangement. These help to prevent any misunderstanding or discord in the sponsored event.

Conclusion

There is considerable evidence that use of sporting organizations and events is effective for the promotion of health messages. The current focus on use of particular settings for health promotion, access to important target groups and evidence of considerable success add weight to the use of this approach. Moreover, the ability to negotiate health promoting policies which have the potential to make lasting environmental changes makes sponsorship an important health promotion strategy for use by health organizations.

Table 1. Attitude towards the smoke-free policy by smoking status at the cricket

Attitude	Smokers	Non-smokers	Total
Agree	51.0	80.9	60.7
Disagree	34.7	4.3	24.8
No feelings/don't know	14.3	14.9	13.8

Acknowledgements

The Health Promotion Evaluation Unit at the University of Western Australia (formerly the Health Promotion Development and Evaluation Programme) is acknowledged for its contribution to this paper.

Influence of sports sponsorship by cigarette companies on the adolescent mind: A national survey in India

S.G. Vaidya[1], U.D. Naik[1] & J.S. Vaidya[2]

[1]*Goa Cancer Society & National Organisation of Tobacco Eradication (India), Panaji, Goa, India;* [2]*Department of Surgery, Institute of Surgical Studies, University College, London, United Kingdom*

Introduction

The tobacco industry is looking towards Asia for a virgin market. We wish to stop the industry spreading its deadly tentacles in this region, particularly through our children and youth. We showed in a previous study in Goa (a small state in India) that sports sponsorship by the tobacco industry significantly increases children's experimentation with tobacco (Vaidya *et al.*, 1996). The Indian Tobacco Company, a subsidiary of British–American Tobacco, sponsored the Wills (a cigarette brand) World Cup Cricket series in 1996. In this popular series, 12 nations participated in 36 matches played over a period of one month. The series was broadcast live to 2 million million viewers. We studied the effect of such sponsorship on the adolescent mind.

Methods

About six months after the matches, an anonymous structured questionnaire was administered by teachers to 9004 students (66% boys and 34% girls) in grade 10 (aged 13–17) in 130 schools in 10 cities in India. Four knowledge questions and questions related to four myths possibly created by the sponsorship were analysed in relation to smoking in general and to the Wills brand in particular.

Results

After the Wills World Cup series, 13% of students felt like smoking, 5.9% smoked Wills, while 16% did not smoke. The percentages of students who answered 'Yes' to the four knowledge questions were (1) Do cigarettes cause addiction? 81%; (2) Does smoking cause serious diseases like cancer and heart attacks? 69%; (3) Does smoking lower the lifespan? 67%; and (4) Is smoking very dangerous? 79%. All four questions were answered correctly by 41% of the students, and among these only 5.4% smoked. One, two, three and four wrong answers were given by 28, 19, 8.8 and 2.7%, respectively, and their smoking rates increased accordingly by 14, 27, 38 and 42% (relative risk, 2.7, 5.0, 7.1, 7.8; $p < 0.001$).

An analysis of the influence of the environment and the slogans created by the sponsorship on children's perceptions showed that 26% of the students believed that the slogan 'Share the magic' meant sharing a cigarette or a cigarette packet; 30% believed that 'Wills is smoked all over the world'; 13% believed that 'Team with more Wills smokers will fare better' and 16% believed that 'One becomes a better cricketer if one smokes Wills'. The percentages of smokers among the believers and non-believers of these four perceptions were 22 vs 15, 21 vs 16, 34 vs 13 and 40 vs 16, respectively ($p < 0.001$ for all). Believers of the last perception had the highest smoking rate. Analysis of the percentages of smokers among those who gave correct answers to all four knowledge questions for believers and non-believers of the perceptions showed that whether the students believed in the perceptions or not, knowledge significantly reduced the risk for smoking; yet even among those with full knowledge, belief in the last two perceptions significantly increased the risk of smoking by 2.5 (12 vs. 5) and 5 (20 vs. 4) times, respectively.

In another phase, 5822 students in six cities were asked whether they had used tobacco before the Wills World Cup series: 5165 had not used tobacco, 286 had used it, and 371 did not answer the question. We analysed the group of students who had not used tobacco before the matches. The percentages of new smokers among the believers vs non-believers of the four perceptions were 13.0 vs 8.5, 10.8 vs 8.5, 16.7 vs 9.1 and 25.5 vs 7.5, respectively ($p < 0.001$ for all except the second perception). Knowledge significantly ($p < 0.001$) reduced the risk for initiating tobacco use among both the believers and the non-believers of the sponsorship-created perceptions, but even among those with full knowledge, belief in the last two perceptions significantly increased the risk for smoking by 2.1 (9 vs 4) and 4.7 (17 vs 4) times, respectively.

Conclusions

Sports sponsorship by the tobacco industry created wrong perceptions in the minds of the students, and these induced some of them to start smoking. We found that the sponsorship promoted not just the advertised brand but smoking in general, which corroborates the findings of White *et al.* (1996). Knowledge had a significant effect in lowering the smoking rates and on the initiation rates; nevertheless, even children with full knowledge were prompted to smoke after the Wills World Cup because of false, personalized perceptions such as 'Smoking improves ones performance in cricket'. This study provides strong evidence for banning sports sponsorship by the tobacco industry.

Acknowledgements

Consultant: Dr Prakash C. Gupta; collaborating investigators: Dr B.S. Srinath, Dr B. Sanyal, Dr B.L. Ray, Ms Shailja Singh, Dr S.S. Nayyar, Dr Ramakant, Dr Shyamkant Joshi, Dr Mahabir Das, Dr M. Ghate. We acknowledge Ms Luiza Pires for secretarial assistance.

References

Vaidya, S.G., Naik, U.D. & Vaidya, J.S. (1996) Effect of sports sponsorship by tobacco companies on children's experimentation with tobacco. *Br. Med. J.*, **313**, 400
White, D., Kelly, S., Huang, W. & Charlton, A. (1996) Cigarette advertising and onset of smoking in children: Questionnaire survey. *Br. Med. J.*, **313**, 398–399

TOBACCO ECONOMICS

Economics of tobacco consumption

K.E. Warner

*School of Public Health, University of Michigan, Ann Arbor,
Michigan, United States*

Consumption of tobacco products underlies one of history's largest and most profitable economic activities. As a consequence, debates about tobacco policy frequently focus on the economic implications of tobacco consumption. To defend its sale of tobacco products, the tobacco industry regularly publicizes its contributions to a country's economy. The industry's purpose is to convince governmental authorities that adopting policies designed to reduce tobacco product consumption will result in potentially disastrous economic dislocation. The health community responds by emphasizing the massive costs of medical treatment of tobacco-produced diseases and productivity losses associated with tobacco-related disease and death. Each side's argument sounds compelling, yet each is, in effect, only a half-truth. In this paper, I examine the basis of each argument and considers its limitations. I also discuss how differences in the economic status and history of tobacco consumption in a country influence each argument.

The industry's economic argument

As in the case for all major consumer goods, large numbers of people are employed in the production of the raw ingredients of tobacco products, manufacture of the finished product and distribution. Often, many of these people are concentrated in specific geographic regions (e.g. six south-eastern states in the United States) or, at least, in specific economic activities (e.g. farming). Those dependent on tobacco for their livelihood therefore constitute a noticeable, often significant political constituency. Anything that threatens their livelihood, such as a policy measure that would discourage tobacco consumption, becomes an important issue for their political representatives.

Protecting the economic interests of the tobacco industry may be financially profitable for officials, as well as politically astute. The industry has plenty of money to spread around to officials who support its economic positions, and it thus gains access to new markets and maintains existing markets that would not be available to firms in a less concentrated and profitable industry.

The basis of the industry's claim that it is essential to an economy is straightforward: because large quantities of tobacco products are consumed, substantial numbers of people are employed in the underlying farming and the manufacture and distribution of finished products. The numbers vary from one country to another, but in all cases they sound impressive. For the world as a whole, in 1983, tobacco was estimated to be responsible for part-time or full-time employment for over 47 million people, 30 million of whom grew tobacco; half of these were in China (Agro-economics Services Ltd and Tabacosmos Ltd, 1987).

In addition to emphasizing its contribution to employment, the industry identifies other economic benefits: total compensation paid to tobacco workers; tax revenues generated as a result of the sale of tobacco products; and, where appropriate, contribution to a country's international trade balance. Not only do the absolute numbers vary from one country to another, but their relative values vary as well.

- In a country that places a large excise tax on tobacco products, the revenue generated appears relatively large. Particularly if other revenue sources are modest, the importance of the tobacco tax as a revenue source may be emphasized.
- In a country that grows its own tobacco, rather than importing it, the number of farm sector jobs will appear relatively large. In a developing country in which agriculture plays an especially important role in the economy, this aspect of tobacco economics is likely to be emphasized.

- In a country that produces a great deal of tobacco or finished products for export, the positive contribution to the nation's trade balance will be among the numbers featured.

Use of the industry's economic argument varies. In all countries, the gross estimates of these benefits are disseminated, typically to both the press and legislators. In many instances, the message is implicit: "Here are your constituents who depend on tobacco for their incomes; here is the tax revenue you would have to replace were it not for tobacco sales; here is the increase in the trade deficit the country would experience in the absence of tobacco production. These are the benefits that stand at risk, should the nation's legislators decide to get tough on tobacco."

Occasionally, the industry estimates the numbers of jobs that would be lost if a specific tobacco control policy were adopted. In June 1996, for example, the Association of Accredited Advertising Agencies in Hong Kong publicized an estimate that about 1500 jobs would be lost in Hong Kong if a proposed ban on cigarette advertising were adopted (Coopers & Lybrand, 1996). No legislator wants to see his or her constituents lose their jobs. As a consequence, the industry's economic argument has a compelling ring to it.

The industry's argument is plagued by one fatal flaw, however: it says that the resources devoted to tobacco production and consumption would disappear if the sales of tobacco products declined. Declining sales will translate into declining employment within the industry, but the money previously spent on tobacco products will not evaporate; rather, it will be reallocated to spending on other goods and services. This new spending will generate new employment in other sectors of the economy and, along with it, new tax revenues.

On average, the new employment resulting from the alternative spending pattern will offset the losses experienced within the tobacco industry. In some countries, the alternative spending pattern will actually improve the nation's economy; in others, it may harm the economy but not nearly to the extent implied by the industry's estimates. Jobs may be lost within the tobacco and related sectors, but job gains in other sectors will at least partially offset the job losses (Warner & Fulton, 1995).

Whether a nation ends up a net winner or loser will depend on its specific economic situation. If a country is, on balance, an importer of tobacco or tobacco products, declining tobacco consumption will improve the country's economy. This results because a large proportion of expenditure on tobacco products is exported to the countries from which tobacco or products are bought. As consumption of tobacco products declines, consumers will spend a larger proportion of their money on goods and services produced within their own countries. This means that more money will remain within the nation's economy, recycling within the country in a process that will create a larger number of jobs.

In contrast, if a country is a net exporter of tobacco or tobacco products, a policy that reduces production may result in net job losses. Even in such a country, however, the extent of the job losses will be much smaller than that estimated by the tobacco industry, which never considers the offsetting job gains in other industries. As an example of both sides of this phenomenon, some colleagues and I recently estimated the net employment implications of declining tobacco product sales for nine regions of the United States (Warner et al., 1996). One of the regions, consisting of the six south-eastern tobacco-producing states, is an exporter of tobacco products to the other eight regions. For the six south-eastern states, using the industry's approach to measuring jobs, we estimated that, in 1993, there were 550 000 jobs dependent on tobacco; for the rest of the nation (the eight non-tobacco regions), there were 1.24 million tobacco-reliant jobs. We simulated what would happen if all spending on tobacco products were to cease instantaneously and consumers reallocated all former tobacco spending to other goods and services. In the eight non-tobacco regions combined, employment in the year 2000 would increase by 355 000 jobs. In the six-state tobacco region, employment would decline by 220 000 jobs, not the 550 000 jobs that the tobacco industry would have you believe. On balance, the United States would gain about 135 000 jobs in the short term by eliminating domestic tobacco consumption.

Related studies in other developed countries have arrived at qualitatively similar findings (Allen, 1993; Buck et al., 1995). There is a clear need for similar studies to be undertaken in developing countries, including both importers of tobacco and tobacco products and exporters (see van der Merwe &Abedian, this volume).

In most instances, declining tobacco consumption will mean a loss of some government revenue, simply because most countries impose product-specific excise taxes on tobacco products. This may necessitate raising other taxes or increasing other sources of revenue; but this will merely constitute substituting one tax for another. The offsetting benefits of reallocated resources are never acknowledged by the tobacco industry. Unfortunately, the public and its elected representatives are essentially ignorant about the industry's deceptive use of its economic data.

Costs of the health damage produced by tobacco

In typical studies, these include the costs of medical care devoted to treating tobacco-related disease and lost productivity resulting from tobacco-related illness, disability and premature mortality. The objective of disseminating these cost estimates is to emphasize that the horror of tobacco is not only human; tobacco exacts a financial toll as well. In part, this argument is intended to counteract the industry's economic argument: the tobacco control community sees an economic burden where the industry claims an economic benefit.

In estimating medical costs, the challenge is, first, to estimate the amount of illness attributable to tobacco and secondly, to evaluate the medical treatment that would be given to victims of such disease (Hodgson & Meiners, 1982). In the United States, for which most such estimations have been made, analysts have concluded that tobacco consumption is responsible for at least 6% of total health expenditure (Warner et al., in press). Estimates of the medical costs of tobacco use, sometimes accompanied by productivity loss estimates, have been produced primarily for developed nations, but recent work included an estimation of the costs of smoking in China (Chen et al., 1995; Jin et al., 1995). There is a clear need to extend this work to other countries, particularly developing nations.

The cost estimates vary widely from one country to another, reflecting in part differences in the amount of tobacco-related disease, which is the result of widely different histories of tobacco consumption; for example, in poor countries, heavy use of tobacco over many years may be a relatively rare phenomenon. The estimates also vary with differences in how and how aggressively various disease conditions are treated and differences in the costs of such treatments and in their effectiveness. Estimates of productivity losses differ because of differences in wage rates and in life expectancies and normal retirement ages.

The costs of tobacco use will increase, in many instances dramatically, in most developing countries as regular tobacco use expands, as health care becomes both more effective and more expensive and as workers become more productive (and hence work losses become more costly). The main result of all of the studies is identical: in addition to causing alarming amounts of illness and death, tobacco use imposes a distinct financial burden on a country's health-care system.

Just as there are offsets to the industry's estimated economic benefits of tobacco, however, there are offsets to the costs of tobacco use. Precisely because tobacco claims the lives of so many of its consumers, tobacco use reduces the number of years during which people use medical care. The implication is that the net medical cost of tobacco use is almost certainly less than its gross cost; yet the latter is what most analysts estimate. How much the longer lives of non-smokers offset the higher cost per year of smokers is a matter of some debate. The best study to date concluded that current and former smokers cost more in terms of lifetime medical expenditure than people who have never smoked (Hodgson, 1992).

Further analysis is needed, both to refine the estimates and to put them into context. Previously merely a debating tool, the cost estimates are becoming increasingly important in policy and legal matters. In the United States, for example, 40 states sued the tobacco industry to recover publicly funded expenditure for the care of poor people made ill by cigarette smoking. The states based their requests for damages on estimates of the gross medical costs of smoking.

Economists working for the tobacco industry counter that if smoking causes disease, one must incorporate the off-setting economic 'benefit' of earlier deaths due to smoking to determine the true cost to the states. If people systematically thought this way, there would be no point in ever trying to solve any health problem that primarily afflicts the elderly. The concept places no value at all on life *per se*. At the same time, the argument for the cost of tobacco use rests on the premise that, quite independent of its health consequences or of the inherent value of life, tobacco imposes an economic burden on society. If the objective is to understand the true burdens associated with tobacco, one must distinguish the human and economic costs and recognize that the latter must be assessed fairly for the purpose at hand. If the issue is how much of a financial burden tobacco imposes on society, then one should examine the net costs and not only the gross costs.

Conclusion

The conventional estimates of the cost of tobacco use are no more wrong than the tobacco industry's estimates of its economic contributions. The issue is the use of these estimates. The clear intent of the industry's use of its economic data is to persuade policy decision-makers that tobacco control measures good for the physical health of their constituents may be bad for their fiscal health. This claim is intentionally misleading.

The same may be said of some tobacco-control advocates who bend the truth in portraying the economic burden of tobacco. The gross cost of tobacco consumption is a meaningful number, worthy of dissemination, but some activists knowingly misuse this number. In their minds, the end justifies the means. I for one believe that we do not need to resort to distortions to battle an enemy famous for them.

A thorough evaluation of the economic issues in the public debate on the future of tobacco leads to the conclusion that, however large some of the numbers may be, the true net economic implications of tobacco pale in comparison with the impact on health. That is the true burden, the one we ought to be emphasizing. Arguments about the economics of tobacco create a lot of heat, but they rarely shed much light.

References

Agro-economic Services Ltd and Tabacosmos Ltd (1987) The employment, tax revenue and wealth that the tobacco industry creates.

Allen, R.C. (1993) *The False Dilemma: The Impact of Tobacco Control Policy on Employment in Canada*, Ottawa: National Campaign for Action on Tobacco

Buck, D., Godfrey, C., Raw, M. & Sutton, M. (1995) *Tobacco and Jobs*, York: Society for the Study of Addiction and the Centre for Health Economics, University of York

Chen, J., Cao, J.W., Chen, Y. & Shao, D.Y. (1995) Evaluation of medical cost lost due to smoking in Chinese cities. *Biomed. Environ. Sci.*, 8, 335–341

Coopers & Lybrand (1996) A study of the economic impact of a ban on cigarette advertising in Hong Kong

Hodgson, T.A. (1992) Cigarette smoking and lifetime medical expenditure. *Milbank Memorial Fund Q.*, 70, 81–125

Hodgson, T.A. & Meiners, M.R. (1982) Cost-of-illness methodology: A guide to current practices and procedures. *Milbank Memorial Fund Q.*, 60, 429–462

Jin, S.G., Lu, B.Y., Yan, D.Y., Fu, Z.Y., Jiang, Y. & Li, W. (1995) An evaluation of smoking-induced health costs in China (1988–1989). *Biomed. Environ. Sci.*, 8, 342–349

Warner, K.E. & Fulton, G.A. (1995) Importance of tobacco to a country's economy: An appraisal of the tobacco industry's economic argument. *Tobacco Control*, 4, 180–183

Warner, K.E., Fulton, G.A., Nicolas, P. & Grimes, D.R. (1996) Employment implications of declining tobacco product sales for the regional economies of the United States. *J. Am. Med. Assoc.*, 275, 1241–1246

Warner, K.E., Hodgson, T.A. & Carroll, C.E. (in press) The medical costs of smoking in the United States: Estimates, their validity, and their implications. *Tob. Control* (in press)

Estimation of direct smoking-related costs in China

S. Jin & Y. Jiang

Chinese Academy of Preventive Medicine, Beijing, China

China is the world's largest producer and consumer of cigarettes, and more than 300 million people are current smokers. The tobacco industry has been the major source of tax revenue among all of the industries in China since 1987. The revenue provided by the tobacco industry increased from 14.5 million million yuan in 1986 to 83 million million yuan in 1996.

Smoking-attributable costs include direct medical costs and indirect costs, which include indirect costs of morbidity and mortality. We estimate that the direct medical costs in China were 6.9 million million yuan in 1989 and increased to 15.4 million million yuan in 1993, accounting for 12–13% of the total health budget in the same year.

In order to estimate the impact of cigarette smoking on the economy in China, a new regression model is introduced, which is based on the following findings and assumptions:

* Direct smoking-attributable medical costs are part of the total medical income in health facilities.
* The ratio of direct smoking-attributable medical costs to the total medical income in 1989 and 1993 was identical.
* Analysis of time series data from 1989 through 1995 shows a strong correlation between total medical income (on a logarithmic scale) and year ($r^2 = 0.9896$).

Economy and diseconomy of tobacco use

S. Watanabe[1], K. Goto[2] & N. Yamaguchi[2]

[1]Department of Nutritional Science and Epidemiology, Tokyo University of Agriculture, and [2]Cancer Information Research and Epidemiology Division, National Cancer Center Research Institute, Tokyo, Japan

Introduction

The tobacco industry of Japan is of some positive economic value for the nation. It employs 20 000 persons and pays high wages; it also pays high taxes, which contribute to the national budget. It purchases raw materials such as leaf tobacco, filters and papers, it pays for advertisements and transportation. All of these increase national savings and consumption. The average smoker in Japan obtains temporary pleasure through smoking at a personal cost of about US$ 1000 per year, creating, in one sense, an economic balance.

Tobacco also creates a negative economic cost to society and to the nation. The Japanese people and the Government pay for smokers'' expenses caused by increased morbidity and mortality, as well as fire, waste disposal and other costs. In addition, there is an opportunity cost of smoking, 'lost national income', which is the present value of lost future national income, which people who have died from smoking would have produced, an economic cost to which smokers do not contribute. We discuss the debit and credit of tobacco to the national economy.

Economy

We used an established method of econometrics called 'input–output analysis' to assess the economic benefit of the tobacco industry. We used the 1990 'input–output table' published by the Government, with a foreign currency exchange rate of Y100 to US$ 1. We defined 'value added' by an industry as the direct contribution of an industry to a nation, consisting of wages, business profits, depreciation and taxes. We also considered other repercussions on the economy; for example, the tobacco industry in Japan pays about US$ 500 million a year to other industries. The rayon, acetate and paper industries receive US$ 600 million, which they use to purchase raw materials from other industries, which in turn spend money purchasing raw materials. The tobacco industry uses actors and actresses for advertisements, who in turn pay their drivers and hairdressers. Estimates of total benefits must include these repercussive costs.

In 1990, the total 'value added' was US$ 28 thousand million, which consists of US$ 19 thousand million of taxes, $2 thousand million of wages, US$ 2 thousand million of reserves (i.e. business profit plus depreciation), US$2 thousand million of repercussion wages and US$ 3 thousand million of repercussion reserves. As the total consumption tax from all commodities in Japan amounts to US$ 60 thousand million a year, it is surprising that just one commodity, tobacco, accounts for US$ 19 thousand million of this tax. High-repercussion wages represent wages paid to 20 000 workers hired directly by the tobacco industry, although figures for total employment are necessary to assess the complete picture.

Diseconomy

'External diseconomy' is an important concept of environmental economics and is explained as follows: a property produces a negative value, and elimination of this negative value is an expense or 'social cost' to a society. Tobacco produces external diseconomy by causing fires, litter and, most seriously, morbidity and mortality. We used the results of research by Goto and Watanabe (1995) to assess the diseconomy of the tobacco industry: 115 000 people died from smoking in 1990, which represented 14% of all deaths in Japan. The breakdown of smoking deaths is as follows: lung cancer, 29 000; other cancers, 36 000; cardiovascular diseases, 33 000; and chronic obstructive respiratory diseases, 17 000.

In order to assess the diseconomy of tobacco quantitively, we introduced the concept of the 'national morbidity function' of smoking. The main harmfulness of tobacco appears approximately 20 years or more after smoking began, necessitating formulation of the accumulative effect of smoking on human health. The smoking morbidity function represents the accumulated effect of tobacco, or aggregate morbidity, as tobacco already consumed years ago will still have an effect on morbidity. In 1975, morbidity due to smoking was still 12%, with 64 000 deaths from smoking. In 1990, the rate increased to 23%, with 115 000 deaths. Thus ,we can explain why deaths due to smoking are rising in spite of the fact that tobacco consumption is not increasing: It is because of the accumulated effect of smoking. With this 'smoking morbidity function', we can forecast the number of deaths from smoking and their social cost. Furthermore, we can use this function to assess the effect of a reduction in the consumption of tobacco on deaths and the social cost.

The total social cost in 1990 was US$ 56 thousand million, composed of US$ 32 thousand million of medical expense, US$ 20 thousand million of income loss, US$ 2 thousand million of indirect morbidity and US$ 2 thousand million of fire and cleaning expenses. Indirect morbidity includes employees' absence because of sickness caused by smoking. Income loss or 'lost national income' is defined as the present value of the loss of future national income caused by smoking. Without tobacco, the 115 000 dead people would have contributed to producing a national income of, for example, US$ 4.5 thousand million in the succeeding two years, the value of which in 1990 amounted to US$ 4.1 thousand million. The lost national income of US$ 20 thousand million is an aggregate amount of the present value for eight years after death. For example, if an executive who smokes dies, his or her successor may take eight years to build up similar ability, so that the executive's influence will diminish year by year. We assume that such influence becomes negligible nine years after death.

Conclusion

The economic benefit of tobacco in Japan was US$ 28 thousand million in 1990, whereas the diseconomy was US$ 56 thousand million, so that the tobacco industry produced a net negative value of US$ 28 thousand million. This means that every person in Japan bore the burden of US$ 2 per carton of social cost. Thus, US$ 6 per carton, three times the current price, should be the proper carton price, taking into account the expected decrease in demand due to a price increase.

Increased morbidity from smoking is expected to result in 174 000–226 000 deaths from smoking, with a probability of 68% in 2010. This would place Japan 20 years behind the United States, which is forecast to have a national rate of deaths from smoking of 20% in that year. The social cost would reach 2.6 times, with a 68% confidence interval of 2.5–2.78.

Without any action, the expected value of the social cost will grow from 1 in 1990 to 2 in 2010, 2.6 in 2020 and 3.3 in 2030. If tobacco consumption were to be reduced by half, there would be considerable improvement in the social cost, from 2.6 to 1.6 in 2020, although the social cost would not peak then but would continue to rise moderately. Determined efforts are needed to reduce the social cost and improve public health status.

The results of this study are very conservative; for example, brain vessel diseases caused by smoking were excluded, as were the effects of passive smoking. The true diseconomy is greater than that estimated here.

Reference

Goto, K. & Watanabe, S. (1995) Social cost of smoking for the 21st century. *J. Epidemiol.*, 5, 113–116

Estimated social costs of active and passive smoking in Japan

T. Nakahara[1] & Y.M. Kobayashi[2]

[1]*Kyoto University, Kyoto, and* [2]*National Institute of Public Health, Tokyo, Japan*

Introduction

The slogan for the 1995 World No Tobacco Day was 'Tobacco costs more than you think'. In this study, we estimated the social costs of smoking in Japan and assessed the economic burden due to smoking for use in anti-smoking activities.

Assumptions

We first defined the content of social costs and then calculated the economic cost of each item; items for which statistical data were not available were excluded. For the effects of exposure to environmental tobacco smoke, we used the method of the United States Environmental Protection Agency (1992), as epidemiological data are not available on this issue in Japan. Since these figures relate only to lung cancer, this study should be regarded as an attempt to estimate the minimum social costs of smoking; the real magnitude is much higher.

The calculation was made for 1993. Costs due to tobacco-related disease were calculated by assuming that the lag between beginning to smoke and the onset of disease is 25 years. The assumption was therefore that smoking was begun in 1968 by people aged 20 or more, and the morbidity and mortality of smokers were evaluated for people aged 45 years or more in 1993. The prevalence of smoking in 1968 was about 50% for men and women combined, on the basis of data from Japan Tobacco Inc.

Social costs

The social costs of smoking include increased medical expenditure on tobacco-related diseases, economic losses due to hospitalization, visits to hospitals, unemployment, care by the family, excess deaths, purchase of drugs, screening and examination and research and education on tobacco-related diseases. The environmental costs include loss of property, deaths and injuries due to fires caused by smoking and cleaning costs.

Increased medical expenditure for tobacco-related disease. We used the results of T. Hirayama's population-based cohort study on lifestyle and cancer between 1966 and 1982 as a basis. We regarded a disease as being related to tobacco use when the lower bound of the 90% confidence interval in Dr Hirayama's study of the sex- and age-adjusted relative risk of death due to the disease in relation to smoking was 1 or greater. Tobacco-related diseases were classified as malignant neoplasms, hypertensive disease, ischaemic heart disease, cerebrovascular disease, respiratory disease, gastric and duodenal ulcers and liver disease, according to the classification of vital statistics in japan. In the case of exposure to environmental tobacco smoke, only lung cancer was considered.

Since data on medical expenditure in Japan are available from the Ministry of Health and Welfare, the increase in medical expenditure was calculated by multiplying the medical expenditure for each tobacco-related disease by the contributory risk. We used contributory risks of death calculated by Dr Hirayama instead of the excess morbidity rate of each tobacco-related disease since those figures were not available.

The social cost of active smoking was found to be 1150 thousand million yen, and that of exposure to environmental tobacco smoke was 11 thousand million yen.

Costs due to hospitalization for tobacco-related diseases. Since our objective was to estimate social costs, the costs due to hospitalization of patients with tobacco-related diseases were calculated by multiplying the per capita national income per day by the number of days of hospitalization due to each tobacco-related disease, which was calculated by multiplying the mean number of days of hospitalization in a survey of patients conducted by the Ministry of Health and Welfare by the contributory risk. The cost of hospitalization due to active smoking was 27 thousand million yen , and the cost of hospitalization due to exposure to environmental tobacco smoke was 0.3 thousand million yen.

Costs due to excess deaths from tobacco-related diseases. The excess number of deaths due to smoking can be calculated by multiplying the number of deaths due to each tobacco-related disease by the contributory risk for each disease. Various methods are used to calculate the economic costs of such deaths; we chose national income. The economic value of the social loss of excess deaths due to tobacco-related diseases per person was calculated as the per capita national income multiplied by the mean number of years of life lost. That figure has been calculated for various developed countries by Richard Peto; it is 12 years for Japan. The cost due to excess deaths is 2590 thousand million yen for active smoking and 60 thousand million yen for exposure to environmental tobacco smoke.

Costs due to fires caused by smoking. The costs due to fires caused by smoking, the number of deaths and the number of people injured by fires due to smoking were calculated on the basis of data in the 'White paper of fire fighting'. The cost was 23 thousand million yen.

Total social costs. The estimated social cost of active smoking is about 3800 thousand million yen, and that for exposure to environmental tobacco smoke is about 71 thousand million yen. The national medical expenditure in 1993 was about 24 thousand thousand million yean, and the social cost of smoking represented about 5% of that total, although it includes costs other than those for medical services.

Comments

Active measures against smoking are being taken throughout the world. In Japan, the Ministry of Health has been very active in this area. In 1996, it proposed the concept of 'lifestyle-related diseases' and announced that one of the most important was smoking. It is now urging countermeasures against smoking and introduction of ant-smoking into health education at public health centres and municipalities throughout the country. The Ministry of Health and Welfare established an 'Action plan against smoking' in

1995, and further measures have been taken by the ministries of Labour and Education and by the National Personnel Agency. The main measure taken has been to separate smoking and smoke-free areas, and this is being implemented in both the public and private sectors.

In 1997, for the first time, the Ministry of Health and Welfare included a description of smoking and anti-smoking measures in a 'white paper' with the collaboration of the Ministry of Finance. We consider that the social cost of smoking is so high that the Government should take effective tobacco control measures. As there is a lag between smoking and the onset of tobacco-related diseases, the effects of anti-smoking measures, even if they are implemented immediately, will not become apparent for more than 20 years. Anti-smoking measures must nevertheless be taken quickly and evaluated continuously.

Impact of the tobacco farm policy on cigarette consumption in the United States

P. Zhang[1], C. Husten[2], G. Giovino[2] & T. Pechacek[2]

[1]Division of Adult and Community Health, and [2]Office on Smoking and Health, Centers for Disease Control and Prevention, Atlanta, Goergia, United States

As in many countries, the United States Government intervenes in tobacco production. It has been controlling tobacco production with a complex tobacco price support programmeme since the early 1930s. This Government intervention affects both production and imports and exports of tobacco and cigarettes. Because this intervention leads to a change in the price of tobacco and cigarettes on the domestic market, it affects tobacco and cigarette consumption (Grise, 1995).

The purpose of this study was to estimate the effect of the tobacco price support programme on cigarette consumption in the United States. Specifically, we estimated changes in tobacco prices due to the programme, changes in cigarette prices due to the change in tobacco prices and changes in cigarette consumption due to the change in cigarette prices. Using economic models and data for 1990–94, we estimated that the price of tobacco leaf was increased by 32–40 cents per pound as a result of the tobacco price support programme. Using the upper bound of the increase in tobacco price (40 cents per pound) and the estimate that 1.7 pounds of tobacco yield 1000 cigarettes, we estimated that in 1994 the tobacco price support programme increased the price of 1000 cigarettes by 51 cents—just 1 cent per pack or a 0.58% increase. This 0.58% increase in the price of cigarettes would lead to a reduction of 0.29% in cigarette consumption on the basis of a price elasticity of –0.5 (Lewit *et al.*, 1981; Batagi & Levin, 1986; Chaloupka, 1991; Becker *et al.*, 1994; Coats & Lewit, 1994; Harris, 1994; Hu *et al.*, 1995). This reduction is equivalent to a decrease of 71 million packs or about 2.4 million pounds of tobacco leaf.

We estimated that the elasticity of price transmission between the prices of cigarettes and domestic tobacco was 0.34. This means that a 10% increase in the price of domestic tobacco would increase the retail price of cigarettes by only 0.34%. The small impact of changes in the price of domestic tobacco on the price of cigarettes suggests that the two prices are very weakly related, and changes in the price of domestic tobacco have little influence on the retail price of cigarettes.

The reduction in cigarette consumption that results from the tobacco price support programme could be due to decreases in both smoking prevalence and the number of cigarettes a smoker consumes. Assuming that 50% of the reduction in cigarette consumption is due to the reduced number of cigarettes smoked (Lewit & Coats, 1982; Wasserman *et al.*, 1991; Hu *et al.*, 1995), a reduction of 71 million packs would result in a decrease of 15 cigarettes per year per smoker. If 50% of the reduction in cigarette consumption is due to a decrease in smoking prevalence, there would be 83 881 fewer smokers in 1994 as a result of the tobacco price support programme. Although such a reduction in the number of smokers may seem substantial, it is only 0.18% of the total number of smokers in the United States in 1994 (Centers for Disease Control and Prevention, 1996). This effect of the tobacco price support programme on reducing smoking is minimal compared with that of virtually all other tobacco policy measures under consideration (Warner, 1988). Thus, any health benefit that might occur as a result of the programme is likely to be small.

References

Batagi, B.H. & Levin, D. (1986) Estimating dynamic demand for cigarettes using panel data: The effect of bootlegging, taxation, and advertising reconsidered. *Rev. Econ. Stat.*, **68**, 148–155

Becker, G.S., Grossman, M. & Murphy, K.M. (1994) An empirical analysis of cigarette addiction. *Am. Econ. Rev.*, **84**, 396–418

Centers for Disease Control and Prevention (1996) Cigarette smoking among adults—United States, 1994. *Morbid. Mortal. Wkly Rep.*, **45**, 588–590

Chaloupka, F. (1991) Rational addictive behaviors and cigarette smoking. *J. Polit. Econ.*, **99**, 722–742

Coats, D. & Lewit, E.M. (1994) The potential for using excise taxes to reduce smoking (Working Paper Series No. 764), Cambridge, Massachusetts: National Bureau of Economic Research

Grise, V.N. (199) Tobacco: Background for 1995 farm legislation (Agricultural Economic Report No.709), Washington DC: United States Department of Agriculture

Harris, J.E. (1994) A working model for predicting the consumption and revenue impact of large tax increases in the US federal cigarette excise tax (Working Paper Series No. 4803), Cambridge, Massachusetts: National Bureau of Economic Research

Hu, T.-W., Ren, Q.-F., Keeler, T.E. & Bartlett, J. (1995) The demand for cigarettes in California and behavioral factors. *Health Econ.*, **4**, 7–14

Lewit, E.M. & Coats, D. (1982) The potential for using excise taxes to reduce smoking. *J. Health Econ.*, **1**, 121–145

Lewit, E.M., Coats, D. & Grossman, M. (1981) The effects of government regulations on teenage smoking. *J. Law Econ.*, **24**, 545–570

Warner, K.E. (1988) Tobacco subsidy: Does it matter? *J. Natl Cancer Inst.*, **80**, 81–83

Wasserman, J., Manning, W.G., Newhouse, J.P. & Winkler, J.D. (1991) The effect of excise taxes and regulation on cigarette smoking. *J. Health Econ.*, **10**, 43–64

United States farm policy on tobacco and tobacco control: Consistent or conflicting?

P. Zhang[1], C. Husten[2] & T. Pechacek[2]

[1]*Division of Adult and Community Health and* [2]*Office on Smoking and Health, Centers for Disease Control and Prevention, Atlanta, Georgia, United States*

Introduction

The United States Government plays a dual role in the formulation and implementation of policies related to tobacco. It supports tobacco farmers through the tobacco price support programme and agricultural research; conversely, because of the adverse effect of smoking on health, the Government promotes efforts to reduce tobacco use. This study is concerned with the degree of consistency between United States agricultural policy and health policy as they relate to tobacco production and tobacco use. We reviewed studies published during the period 1980–96 to evaluate the impact of the tobacco price support programme on tobacco control in two areas: its effect on domestic cigarette consumption and its potentially adverse political consequences on efforts to reduce smoking.

Domestic cigarette consumption

The tobacco price support programme increases the price of tobacco leaf by controlling the tobacco supply. The higher price of tobacco leaf then passes through the market channel and leads to a higher cigarette price. As the price of cigarette rises, cigarette consumption will fall. Sumner and Alston (1984) estimated that eliminating tobacco price support would reduce the price of United States tobacco by 17–30%. Using a maximum reduction of 30%, they estimated that the price of cigarettes would increase by 3% or about US$ 0.02 in 1983 dollars as a result of the tobacco price support programme. Applying a price elasticity of –0.3 for cigarettes, they estimated that the higher cigarette price would reduce cigarette consumption by about 1%.

Political impact of the tobacco price support programme on reduction of smoking
　The adverse impact of the programme on efforts to reduce smoking is indirect and must be evaluated in the political context of policy formulation and implementation. Perhaps the most important political effect of the programme on tobacco control is that it has created a new political entity, the quota owner, with a strong financial interest against efforts to reduce smoking. In 1993, there were 375 073 tobacco quota owners, about 3.3 times the number of tobacco farmers (Brown, 1995). Quota owners are the major beneficiaries of the tobacco price support programme. The annual revenue generated from leasing quota was estimated to be US$ 645–806 million, and the market value of tobacco quota was estimated at US$ 2.9 thousand million (Womach, 1994).
　Measures to reduce smoking are expected to reduce the demand for tobacco and to change the level of quota revenues. Whether those revenues will become larger or smaller depends on the response of tobacco production, which in turn relies on changes in the tobacco price support programme. In 1985, Sumner and Wohlgenant described three possible scenarios for the responses of the Federal Government to a decreased demand for cigarettes and also estimated the effect of those policy responses on the revenue of quota owners. Updating Sumner and Wohlgenant's study, Brown (1995), who assumed a 75-cent increase in cigarette tax per pack and an increase in the smoking restriction index of 0.5 (a measure of smoking restriction in public places), predicted that quota revenues would be reduced by US$ 116 million if the Government chose a policy to fix the tobacco quota and reduce the level of price support. According to Brown, choosing a policy to maintain the level of price support and reduce the amount of the tobacco quota would mean that quota revenues would increase by US$ 22 million; a policy that simultaneously reduced both the level of price support and the amount of the tobacco quota would yield an outcome somewhere between the first two results.
　The attitudes of quota owners to tobacco control should depend on their perception of the Government's response to a decline in demand for tobacco. The reduction in the level of price supports in 1986 and the negative public attitude toward quota owners (Bray & Mayo, 1992) have led the quota owners to believe that the Federal Government is unlikely to adopt a policy that is in their best financial interests. Thus, it is expected that quota owners would oppose any tobacco control efforts.
　A second indirect effect of the tobacco price support programme on tobacco control results from the political impact of tobacco farmers. Measures to reduce smoking will never increase farmers' revenues, but the magnitude of the reduction depends on the response of the Federal tobacco policy. Brown (1995), again assuming a 75-cent increase in cigarette tax per pack and an increase in the smoking restriction index of 0.5, found that tobacco farmers' revenues at best would not change but could decline by up to US$ 264 million, depending on the tobacco policy that the Federal Government chose. Given the possibility of incurring substantial losses resulting from changes in the Federal tobacco policy after implementation of measures to reduce smoking, farmers are not likely to be sympathetic to tobacco control efforts.
　Exactly how much of the political impact of tobacco farmers on tobacco control efforts should be attributed to the tobacco price support programme is impossible to estimate, since one cannot know how the tobacco production sector would change without the programme. The tobacco price support programme affects the number of tobacco farmers and the size of tobacco farms. Without the programme, the number of tobacco farmers would be smaller and the size of tobacco farms larger, but how these fewer farmers would organize themselves and how effective they would be in influencing tobacco control legislation is difficult to predict.

Conclusions

We have shown that the tobacco price support programme has only a small impact on reducing cigarette consumption (only 1%). For proponents of tobacco control, the small beneficial effect of the tobacco price support programme on cigarette consumption must be weighed against the impact of the influential group it created (i.e. the quota owners), who are likely to oppose efforts to reduce smoking. With the tobacco price support programme, both quota owners and tobacco farmers are aligned against tobacco control measures.

The decrease in cigarette consumption resulting from the tobacco price support programme is less than the effect of a 2-cent increase per pack in the Federal excise tax. Thus, the effect of the programme on reducing smoking is minimal in comparison with the expected effect of other tobacco policy measures. If the weight of the political force against tobacco control efforts attributable to the programme leads to success in blocking policies such as a cigarette tax increase or other tobacco control initiatives, then the net impact of the programme on tobacco control would be negative.

References

Bray, E. & Mayo, E. (1992) The economic welfare effect of the US peanut program. Paper presented at the Annual Meeting of American Agricultural Economics Association, Baltimore, Maryland, August 1992
Brown, B. (1995) Cigarette taxes and smoking restrictions: Impacts and policy implication. *Am. J. Agric. Econ.*, **77**, 946–951
Sumner, D.A. & Alston, J.M. (1984) *Consequence of Elimination of the Tobacco Program* (Agricultural Research Service Bulletin No. 469), Raleigh, North Carolina: North Carolina State University
Sumner, D.A. & Wohlgenant, M. (1985) Effect of an increase in the federal excise tax on cigarettes. *Am. J. Agric. Econ.*, **67**, 235–242
Womach, J. (1994) *Increase Cigarette Excise Taxes: Implication for Tobacco Farming* (CRS Report for Congress, 94-334ENR)

Tobacco or health: The grower's perspective

T.J. Stamps

Ministry of Health and Child Welfare, Harare, Zimbabwe

Zimbabwe is the world's third largest exporter of tobacco, contributing about 26% of all the world's flue-cured tobacco exports, although it grows only 4.2% of the world's total production. Tobacco growing was the basis of the development of commercial agriculture in Zimbabwe and is the only primary product produced in Africa which has relatively well maintained its real value in economic terms in the last half century.

Farmers are aware of the moral dilemma of producing a commodity that poses significant challenges to world health, while at the same time recognizing that cessation of production would be economic suicide and that other producing countries, such as the United States, Brazil and China, would rapidly make up the global deficit within one season. Nevertheless, diversification has become a widespread phenomenon in the past seven years in Zimbabwe.

Governments throughout the world profit extensively from the sale of tobacco products and from the generation of employment opportunities in many sectors and are neverthelss applauded rather than condemned for making huge tax profits from their citizens' addiction.

The relative blameworthiness of all stakeholders in tobacco must be addressed squarely and strategies must be worked out to reduce the burden of disease due to the tobacco habit effectively .

WORLD TRADE AND SMUGGLING

Success in the West—Disaster in the East

G.N. Connolly

Massachusetts Tobacco Control Program, Massachusetts Department of Public Health, Boston, Massachusetts, United States

It has been more than 10 years since the last Word Conference on Smoking or Health was held in Asia, and major progress has been made since that time in the United States to curb tobacco use. Nevertheless, the British and United States tobacco manufacturers have only shifted the focus of their marketing activities from home to abroad, with particular attention to Asian nations. I review here the progress made in the United States, with a focus on the State of Massachusetts and discuss how the tobacco industries have responded to the decline in American consumption by forcing entry into Asian tobacco markets and transforming how cigarettes are manufactured, advertised, priced and sold in Asia. Finally, I discuss how the pending settlement with the tobacco industry in the United States could further effect the promotion of cigarettes by western manufacturers in the region.

Over the past 10 years or so, the tobacco issue has received considerable attention from the media. This has been driven by the defence. The most recent media coverage focused on issues of nicotine manipulation, the seed of the tobacco industry, and litigation and settlement talks in Washington DC. This recent history began with a report on an ABC News feature called *Day One* that dealt with how tobacco manufacturers control nicotine levels in their cigarettes to cause and maintain addiction among smokers After the story was aired, Philip Morris sued ABC for US$ 10 thousand million for defamation, and the news network settled out of court. The story triggered major congressional hearings in 1994, in which tobacco industry executives testified that smoking is not addictive and does not cause lung cancer. These hearings riveted national attention to the issue of tobacco and health, resulting in a major change in the public attitude to the tobacco industry and the smoking issue.

During the hearings, internal documents from the Brown & Williamson Tobacco Company were leaked to the news media. These documents affirmed that the tobacco industry knew that nicotine was addictive but had covered up this evidence and created front groups to deceive the public about the actual dangers of smoking. Over the next few years, former industry scientists and other officials further exposed the behaviour of the tobacco industry. An internal document entitled 'Media Coverage' fuelled interest in the litigation by the State's Attorney General, who has forced the tobacco industry to talk about a settlement.

Over the last 10 years, litigation has been proved to be an effective tool for altering the behaviour of the tobacco industry. Beginning with the State of Mississippi, 42 Attorneys General have sued the tobacco industry for an estimated US$ 40 thousand million for health-care costs associated with state Medicaid programmes. The interest of the Attorneys General sparked additional class action suits by 15 union funds for health and welfare funds and suits filed on behalf of smokers for treatment of addiction. Other class actions include those for the direct health effects of smoking and a case filed in Florida on behalf of flight attendants whose health was adversely affected by exposure to second-hand smoke while working on airlines. Additionally, there are more than 500 cases filed by individuals against the tobacco industry, and analysts report that the annual legal fees for United States tobacco manufacturers are exceeding US$ 750 million. A recent quarterly report of the R.J. Reynolds Company noted that 60 suits had been filed against it in 1994, 100 in 1996 and 460 in 1997. Clearly, major progress has been made in the United States by use of the court system against the tobacco industry.

Although the effect of litigation has resulted in the awarding of damages to only a few plaintiffs, the threat of litigation has had a major impact on the value of the tobacco industry stock, that is, investors are reluctant to purchase stock from an industry that is faced with so many legal plaints. If just one state Medicaid case is successful, the value of the stock might be frozen until appeals wind their way through the courts, which could take up to a decade. The effect of litigation on the value of the stock is perhaps one of the major reasons why the industry is seeking a settlement in the United States.

Over the past 10 years, improvements have been made in the treatment of nicotine addiction. Two years ago, nicotine chewing-gum and patches became available over the counter and are now available directly to consumers, backed by major advertising campaigns. The Food and Drug Administration has approved use of nicotine inhalers and of the drug Welbutrin to treat depression. In addition, the Health Center for Policy Research has established guidelines for the treatment of nicotine dependence, which should result in the provision of care for dependent smokers by major health insurers and health plans. Finally, 15 class action suits have been filed against the tobacco industry for treatment of nicotine addiction.

At the Federal level, some progress has been made to curb tobacco use, but nowhere near the progress that has been made at the state and local level. As Congress is still influenced by the tobacco lobby, limited Federal funds are allocated to tobacco control. In 1987, however, the National Cancer Institute established the ASSIST project, which provides approximately US\$ 25 million annually to 17 states to implement social change in tobacco use. The Federal Centers for Disease Control spent US\$ 10–14 million in 1998 in 33 states to implement tobacco control, and the Robert Wood Johnson Foundation provides about US\$ 6 million annually for coalitions in 30 states to curb tobacco use. The average excise tax at state level doubled from 16 to 35 cents within the past few years, and many states are considering raising cigarette taxes substantially in the future. Forty-two state Attorneys General are suing the tobacco industry for the smoking-related costs of their Medicaid programmes, five states virtually ban smoking in all public places, and there has been a proliferation of local smoking bans in thousands of communities across America. Seven states allocate over US\$ 180 million of state tobacco taxes to curb tobacco use; most comes from the State of California, which spent US\$ 100 million in 1998 for their programmes. In addition, 50 states receive approximately US\$ 50 million from other sources. As an example of state tobacco control, I shall highlight programmes and progress made in my own State of Massachusetts.

We spend about US\$ 32 million annually to make smoking part of the history of Massachusetts. Of this, US\$ 13 million are committed to a major media counter-advertising campaign on a par with those of other major products such as Pepsi and McDonald's. We fund local boards of health to pass ordinances to curb tobacco use and prevent the illegal sale of tobacco products to minors. We commit over US\$ 4 million to smoking cessation programmes; we provide a Quitline to help adult smokers quit and funding to programmes for high-risk populations and youth. We also commit a substantial amount of money, approximately US\$ 25 million, to school-based programmes. The results of this campaign have been impressive. Since it began, the State has experienced a 25% decline in per capita consumption; the smoking prevalence among adults has fallen from 23 to 20%; the prevalence remains level among high-school students, although it has risen almost 20% nationally; and we have seen a decline in the smoking prevalence among our junior high-school students. The proportion of worksites with a total ban on smoking has risen from 50 to 65%, and the average worker's reported exposure to environmental tobacco smoke has fallen from 4.5 to about 2 h per week. The number of cigarettes smoked per day by all smokers fell from 20 to about 14 cigarettes in 1996. In over 20 000 compliance checks conducted by the State in 1996, the rate of illegal sales to minors was found to have fallen from 70% in 1992 to about 20% in 1997. The increase in the proportion of cities and towns with clean indoor air ordinances has affected 3.5 million persons. The Massachusetts experience clearly shows that dedicated tobacco tax money used by public agencies can have a significant impact on tobacco consumption.

While progress has been made throughout the United States, domestic tobacco manufacturers have greatly expanded their markets overseas. An analysis of Philip Morris and R.J. Reynolds cigarette sales between 1984 and 1986 shows that the domestic market grew from 10 to 17 thousand million units per year, indicating that domestic consumption remained constant at approximately 350 thousand million cigarettes. During that period, the number of cigarettes sold by these two companies internationally doubled, from 400 to 857 thousand million units, resulting in a major increase in revenue for the two companies. In 1984, their international sales were US$ 4.8 thousand million, but by 1996 the figure had jumped to US$ 28 thousand million. The profits made by these two companies internationally rose almost tenfold, from US$ 500 million in 1984 to US$ 5 thousand million by 1996.

In conclusion, the great success in the west has been a disaster for the east. As the United States curbs tobacco use, the companies have gone to foreign markets to increase their sales. The settlement between the Attorneys General and the tobacco industry is silent on the tobacco issue. This is unconscionable for a nation that awards hungry children and immunizes them against disease. If a final settlement is struck in the United States, it clearly should have strong measures to curb the promotion of smoking by American companies internationally. These measures should include prohibition of the use of trade threats by the United States Government to compel foreign countries to open their markets to their cigarette firms; a crackdown on smuggling of American cigarettes internationally; a substantial increase in funding to the World Health Organization and non-governmental organizations; and both policy and financial support for the World Tobacco Convention which was established at the last World Health Assembly.

Cigarette trade and smuggling in Europe

L. Joossens

International Union Against Cancer, European Liaison Office, Brussels, Belgium

The laws of supply and demand dictate that the more expensive a product is the less people will be inclined to buy it. Despite the fact that tobacco is an addictive product, price has, nevertheless, been shown to have a strong influence on consumption. Taxation is often considered one of the most effective measures for reducing consumption. The tobacco industry opposes tax increases and has used the threat of smuggling in order to convince ministers of finance not to raise taxes on tobacco products. Governments in many countries have become concerned about smuggling over the past few years, as it can lead to loss of revenue. According to the tobacco industry, the smuggling problem can be explained as follows:

- Smuggling is increasing and is a real problem in many countries (with a slight tendency to overestimate the number of smuggled cigarettes).
- Smuggling is organized with cheap cigarettes from countries with lower taxes to countries with high taxes.
- The only solution for the problem of smuggling is to lower taxes, as Canada did in 1994.
- Any increase in taxes will lead to an increase in smuggling and loss of revenue for governments.
- Smuggling is damaging the image of the industry, but it is not the tobacco industry but organized crime that is responsible for smuggling.

While it is true that the incentive for smuggling is the avoidance of taxes, it is not true that smuggling is linked to the level of taxes. In countries with the highest taxes in

Europe, such as the Scandinavian countries, there is little evidence of smuggling, while in Spain, Italy and many central and eastern European countries, where taxes and prices are much lower, the illegal sale of international cigarette brands is widespread.

The smuggling market in Europe is not the movement of cigarettes from the cheaper south to the more expensive north, but the illegal movement of duty-free imported international brands from northern ports to the south and the east. The truth about smuggling is that the tobacco companies are the chief beneficiaries of this illegal trade. The tobacco industry trade from smuggling takes various forms. First, they gain their normal profit by selling the cigarettes (legally) to distributors. The cigarettes then find their way onto the black market to be sold at greatly reduced prices, stimulating demand. This puts pressure on governments not to increase taxes because of the loss of revenue, which may also result in lower prices and higher consumption. Then, the industry uses this to urge governments to reduce, or not to increase, taxes. Finally, contraband cigarettes that are intercepted by customs have to be replaced, leading to yet more sales (Joossens & Raw, 1995).

Transnational tobacco companies lay the groundwork for smuggling by introducing top brands at reduced prices to encourage low-income consumers in developing countries to buy the much-desired western brands and to penetrate closed markets. According to an analysis in *The New York Times* of 25 August 1997, the transnational companies may themselves be involved in smuggling and have therefore avoided taking significant measures to reduce it (Bonner & Drew, 1997). Some examples:

Argentina: In the early 1960s, the entry of transnational companies into the Latin American market had a strong temporal relationship with contraband trafficking in cigarettes. Contraband was used to open the closed domestic markets to the transnational companies. Contraband rose from 2 to 12% of total consumption. Only when all the national firms had been acquired by the transnational companies did contraband finally decline in the early 1970s (Department of Health and Human Services, 1992).

Italy: This country has the longest history of smuggling in Europe. The production of cigarettes is controlled by a state monopoly. Despite a ban on advertising since 1963, Philip Morris was able to conquer the market and now dominates it, with a market share of more than 50% in 1996. Marlboro is by far the most frequently smuggled brand in Italy, and smuggled Marlboros are sold more cheaply than the leading national brand, MS. The Italian state monopoly lost its battle against Philip Morris, mainly because of smuggling.

Bulgaria: This is one of the few countries in eastern Europe which still has a state-controlled tobacco industry. Bulgaria is also one of the poorest countries in Europe, with an average income of US$ 90 a month in 1996. In 1995, the consumption of domestic cigarettes was estimated at 13 thousand million. Illegal imports were estimated at about 5 thousand million cigarettes or 38% of the legal sales. American cigarettes are popular among young people, but most are unable to buy them at the official price. The official price of a pack of Marlboros in 1997 was US$ 3, while that of smuggled or counterfeit Marlboros was only US$ 1. At the official price, the market for American cigarettes would have been extremely limited.

China: This country is the largest cigarette market in the world. Smuggling of cigarettes has already started, and it has been estimated that some 40 thousand million cigarettes are smuggled into China (Anon., 1997). In the coming years, smuggling will be used by transnational companies to open up the Chinese market even further for western brands.

The advantages of smuggling for transitional companies are even described in tobacco trade documents. The trade journal *World Tobacco* admitted in its 1996 report that 'Although sales of contraband cigarettes have affected the level of income that governments world-wide derive from tobacco sales, smuggling has also helped to promote some of the world's leading brands in markets which had remained closed to foreign imports and where demand for Western cigarettes has continued to grow.'(Anon., 1996). The benefits of smuggling go not to the local industry but to the big multinationals. Michael Barford commented in *Tobacco Journal International*, 'Whose brands sell best in contraband trade? Traditional smuggling has focused on well-known international brands, since instant recognition and confidence in the merchandise are essential to these quick, furtive transactions. Smugglers are impatient of little-known brands. They focus on what the multinationals make.' (Barford, 1993).

How big is the problem?

The magnitude of the smuggling problem can be estimated by looking at the difference between global exports and imports; most of the 'missing' cigarettes are smuggled. World cigarette production is known fairly accurately, and since cigarettes do not keep for very long, world production is very close to world consumption. There are no large quantities of cigarettes in storage. Global imports should thus be close to exports, after allowing for legitimate trade that is usually excluded from national statistics: principally imports for duty-free sales to travellers, to the diplomatic community and to military establishments. But for many years imports have been lower than exports, to a degree that cannot be adequately explained by legitimate duty-free sales. Although the volume of duty-free trade is not on public record, it has been estimated with some confidence by the tobacco trade at about 45 000 million cigarettes a year. Even the time lag of three to six months between recording export and import statistics cannot explain the export–import differences, which have remained high for years (Joossens & Raw, 1995). Table 1 shows annual global exports and imports from 1975 to 1996: there has been a steady increase in the number of missing cigarettes. In 1996, 1 107 000 million cigarettes were exported, but only 707 000 million were imported—a difference of 400 000 million. After deducting 45 000 million for legitimate duty-free sales, there are still almost 355 000 million cigarettes missing. The only plausible explanation for these missing cigarettes is smuggling.

Smuggling in Europe

In 1997, a Committee of the European Parliament published a report of more than 1000 pages on the transit trade in the European Union (European Parliament, 1997). Transit is a concession system aimed at facilitating trade. Its essence is to allow the temporary suspension of custom duties, excise and value-added tax payable on goods originating from and/or destined for a third country while under transport across the territory of a defined customs area. For instance, cigarettes from the United States enter Antwerp for onward transport to North Africa. In this case, the goods would be placed under a transit regime for transport by road from Antwerp to Spain, from where they would be shipped to North Africa. Provided the re-export of the goods is confirmed, no taxes would be due in the European Union.

Fraud occurs when these duty-free goods, destined for outside the European Union, are sold on the black market within the Union. Transit fraud and related criminal activities cover a wide range of products but tend to be focused on so-called 'sensitive' goods. According to the Committee, the product most often targeted by the transit fraudster

Table 1. World cigarette imports and exports (thousand million pieces)

Year	Imports	Exports	Difference
1975	171	223	42
1980	254	323	69
1985	313	356	43
1990	418	543	125
1991	526	712	186
1992	568	804	236
1993	600	780	179
1994	886	1156	270
1995	668	987	319
1996	707	1107	400

From US Department of Agriculture

has consistently been cigarettes. The market of contraband cigarettes in the European Union would appear to be in the region of 60 thousand million cigarettes, with a loss of revenue of US$ 6 thousand million a year.

The attraction of cigarettes to the fraudster lies in the size of the difference between the duty-free and .he duty-paid price of a cigarette, giving scope for substantial profits even at the relatively low street prices needed to attract the consumer. The attraction of cigarettes to the fraudster is further enhanced by the relative ease with which they can be handled. Other high-tax products, such as petroleum products or even alcohol, although frequently the subject of fraud, cannot compete on a tax-value per weight basis, or in terms of the conditions required for their transport. One so-called 'master pack' of 10 000 cigarettes is the size of the sort of cardboard box common in supermarkets. A container-load of cigarettes has a potential fiscal value of about US$ 1.2 million. Almost all of this is potential profit for the smuggler (Table 2).

Large-scale smuggling also requires a willing market and a good local distribution network. Such markets and networks have existed for many years, especially in Italy and Spain, where tobacco smuggling is a long-standing problem. The recent expansion in cigarette smuggling has therefore to some degree exploited these countries as a base for infiltration of markets in the rest of the European Union, most spectacularly in the case of Germany, where the activities of Vietnamese gangs made headlines in the spring of 1996 (European Parliament, 1997).

I have classified the 15 countries of the European Union into three categories on the basis of information from the European Confederation of Cigarette Retailers (European Parliament, 1997) and some other sources (Her Majesty's Treasury, 1997; Persson & Andersson, 1997): high, with a contraband market share of ≥ 10% (Austria [15%], Spain [15%], Italy [11.5%] and Germany [10%]); medium, with a contraband market share of 5–10% (Greece [8%], Belgium [7%], the Netherlands [5–10%] and probably Luxembourg and Portugal [no studies available]); and low, with a contraband market share of < 5% (Ireland [4%], France [2%], Sweden [2%] and the United Kingdom [1.5%] and probably Denmark and Finland [no studies available]). If we compare the level of smuggling with the prices in the countries of the European Union (Table 3), it becomes evident that smuggling is not linked to high prices. 'Low' smuggling countries are all high-price countries, while 'high' smuggling countries are mainly low-price countries. It is not prices, but smuggling routes which provide us with a better understanding of the smuggling problem.

The smuggling routes

One of the more absorbing aspects of the European Parliament Committee's work was to show the complexity of the routes by which contraband cigarettes now enter free circulation in the Union. The port of Antwerp in Belgium provides cigarette warehousing facilities unparalleled anywhere in Europe. In 1988, 27 thousand million cigarettes were imported from the United States, but in 1996 around 100 thousand million cigarettes passed through the port: 62 thousand million from the United States (mainly from Philip Morris and Reynolds) and 38 thousand million from Brazil (from Philip Morris and British–American Tobacco factories) into Belgium.

Table 2. Fiscal revenue at risk for one lorry load in US$

Product	Revenue
Live animals	24 000
Milk powder	36 000
Meat or butter	54 000
Alcohol	480 000
Cigarettes	1 200 000

From European Parliament (1997)

Table 3. Prices of cigarettes and level of smuggling in countries of the European Union

Country	Price of 20 cigarettes of most popular price category (US$; 1 June 1997)	Level of smuggling[a]
Spain	1.20	High
Portugal	1.75	Probably medium
Greece	2.06	Medium
Italy	2.07	High
Luxembourg	2.12	Probably medium
Netherlands	2.43	Medium
Austria	2.69	High
Belgium	2.95	Medium
Germany	3.02	High
France	3.38	Low
Finland	4.26	Probably low
Ireland	4.27	Low
United Kingdom	4.35	Low
Denmark	4.55	Probably low
Sweden	4.97	Low

Prices from Commission of the European Communities
[a] See text for explanation of levels

Aside from the relatively small proportion intended for duty-free sales, none of these cigarettes were destined for the European market but were meant for export to third countries. As the large American producers supply their legitimate European markets entirely out of European Union production facilities, any person wishing to purchase American duty-free cigarettes for European black markets—including clandestine markets—is likely to purchase products warehoused in Antwerp, simply because that is where the cigarettes are.

The value of 100 thousand million transit tax-free cigarettes arriving in Antwerp can be estimated at US$ 14 thousand million on the legal market (taxes included). The key issue of the smuggling problem in Europe is that of these transit cigarettes, most of which will end up on the contraband market in several European countries.

From Antwerp, the first two major trade routes are into eastern Europe and the countries of the former Soviet Union. A first transit operation is used to transfer cigarettes by road from Belgium to a free zone in Switzerland, where the operation is concluded quite regularly. The cigarettes leave Switzerland under a new transit procedure for a destination in central or eastern Europe or one of the former Soviet republics. This operation is also routine.

A transit operation is also used to transfer cigarettes from port warehouses to regional airports in Belgium and the Netherlands. Cargo aircraft fly the cigarettes (up to five container loads per aircraft) to destinations in the east.

From their destinations in eastern Europe, cigarettes return to the European Union in a number of ways. The two countries most affected are Germany and Italy. In Germany, the problem has been described as 'ant-smuggling' (Ameisenschmuggel): the clandestine transport of cigarettes across the eastern border in a vast number of small consignments, carried in private cars and small vans. In Italy, the route is slightly more conventional. Cigarettes are transported in vast quantities from the republics of the former Yugoslavia and Albania across the Adriatic in fast boats and landed along the long coastline. From there, they supply both the Italian and other European markets.

The third route, which has to some extent replaced traditional routes through Gibraltar and Andorra, involves sea transport from northern European ports. Documents are prepared indicating the delivery of cigarettes to destinations in North Africa. The route involves passing close to Spanish territorial waters, across which a short trip in a fast boat suffices to land the cigarettes on the Spanish coast (European Parliament, 1997)

The complexity of the routes and the structure of the transactions are remarkable. The key point for the fraudster is not be discovered. One mechanism employed to render investigation as difficult as possible is to arrange for a consignment of cigarettes to pass through a bewildering range of owners in a short space of time. The object is to make the final owner untraceable and to make the links between successive owners as obscure as possible.

The main characteristics of smuggled cigarettes are :
• international brands,
• duty-free cigarettes,
• transported in transit,
• passed through many persons,
• distributed in unofficial outlets,
• sold at lower prices than the official ones,
• mostly with inadequate health warnings.

Solutions

Ensure that all tobacco products prominently display an indication that the applicable taxes have been paid. This has been done in various ways in different countries. The key is to distinguish clearly between legal and illegal goods, making the contraband products easier to detect and the laws therefore easier to enforce. Many European countries require 'tax-paid' stamps to be affixed to each cigarette pack, under the cellophane wrapping.

Revise the penalties for tobacco smuggling. Many of the penalties for tobacco smuggling are long out of date, and the applicable reporting requirements for revenue purposes may be full of loopholes. The penalties and reporting requirements can be improved as part of a revision of the applicable law on tobacco taxation. The key to such revisions is to ensure that the penalties for smuggling, when combined with the probability of getting caught, render tobacco smuggling unappealing.

Restrict sales. Clamping down on the outlets for smuggled cigarettes, which in some countries are almost part of the culture, would require not only law enforcement but a considerable change in smokers' attitude towards authority. Restricting sales to licensed premises and charging heavy fines to unlicensed premises and unlicensed vendors would clearly help. In the Czech Republic, both policies had a measurable impact in 1994.

Reduce the supply and adopt an international convention on tobacco smuggling. Finally and probably most important is the reduction of supply. This will require greater cooperation between customs officials. As for illegal drugs (which nicotine increasingly resembles from the control point of view), it is time for an international convention to control all means of transport of cigarettes. In view of the involvement of organized crime, this convention would need the support of governments throughout the world and of some central organization (Joossens & Raw, 1997). The World Health OrganIZation is seeking to address these international issues through an international framework for tobacco control. The disappearance of about one-third of global cigarette exports from legal import figures is unacceptable. The convention should allow the transport of cigarettes only if there is agreement on the final destination, the cigarettes have adequate health warnings and tax stamps and there is adequate control that the cigarettes arrive at their final destination. The American tobacco settlement under discussion in the United States should contain clear restrictions on the international transport of cigarettes in order to combat smuggling worldwide. So far, the main winners of smuggling have been the transnational companies.

References
Anon. (1996) *World Tobacco File 1996,* London, World Tobacco
Anon. (1997) Cigarette production down; contraband & counterfeits flourish. *Tobacco Reporter,* 4, 32
Barford, M.F. (1993) New dimensions boost cigarette smuggling. *Tobacco J. Int.,* 3, 16–18
Bonner, R. & Drew, C. (1997) Cigarette makers are seen as aiding rise in smuggling. *The New York Times,* 25 August
Department of Health and Human Services (1992) S*moking and Health in the Americas,* Atlanta, Georgia
European Parliament (1997) *Committee of Inquiry into the Community Transit System,* Brussels, 4 volumes
Joossens, L. & Raw, M. (1995) Smuggling and cross border shopping of tobacco in Europe. *Br. Med. J.,* **310,** 1393–1397

Do trade pressures lead to market expansion?

F. J. Chaloupka[1] & A. Laixuthai[2]

[1]*Department of Economics, University of Illinois at Chicago, Chicago, Illinois, United States, and Health Economics Program, National Bureau of Economic Research;* [2]*Money and Banking Department, The Thai Farmers Research Center and The College of Public Health, Chulalongkorn University, Bangkok, Thailand*

Over the past few decades, the prevalence of cigarette smoking in the United States and other developed countries has fallen steadily. These declines are due to numerous factors, including more information on the health consequences of smoking, higher cigarette taxes and prices, limits on cigarette advertising and restrictions on cigarette smoking. In the United States, for example, overall cigarette consumption declined by over 20% between 1975 and 1994, from 607.2 to 485.0 thousand million cigarettes. At the same time, however, United States cigarette production rose by more than 11%. This increase in production at a time when consumption was declining resulted from a sharp increase in international trade in cigarettes. Between 1975 and 1994, total cigarette exports from the United States to the rest of the world rose from 50.2 to 220.23 thousand million, an increase of almost 340%. Currently, approximately 30% of all cigarettes produced in the United States are exported to other countries, overseas sales resulting in about US$ 6.6 thousand million in profits to United States-based multinational tobacco companies. Virtually all of these exports are accounted for by the three largest firms: Philip Morris, R.J. Reynolds and Brown and Williamson.

In recent years, Asian markets have become the leading destination for these cigarettes, with 38% of United States exports ending up in Asian countries. Another 37% end up in various European countries, while the remaining 25% find their way to the Middle East, Central and South America and Africa. The surge in exports, particularly to Asia was in part the result of the help of the Reagan and Bush administrations in aggressively using national trade policy to open foreign markets that had been closed to United States cigarette producers. The effect of these policies on cigarette smoking in the affected countries has since been debated. The industry makes essentially the same argument with respect to their presence in new markets as that with respect to their use of advertising. To quote a Philip Morris spokeswoman, "The same number of cigarettes is consumed whether American cigarettes are present or not. Whatever one may feel about the smoking and health controversy, the presence or absence of American cigarettes is not a cigarette consumption factor." Critics of the industry, however, argue that cigarette smoking in the affected countries increased as a result of the United States presence, particularly among women and children, who, they aver, are targeted by multimillion dollar promotional campaigns.

Before our research (Chaloupka & Laixuthai, 1996), there was no empirical evaluation of the impact of United States trade pressures on smoking in other countries. Before reviewing this empirical research, some historical context is useful (see Chaloupka & Laixuthai, 1996, for more details and relevant references). The key tool for the United States trade actions related to tobacco was contained in Section 301 of the 1974 Trade Act, which gave the President the power to investigate other countries' trade practices that could be considered unjustifiable, unreasonable or discriminatory. If these trade practices were found to be unfair, the Act called for negotiations to eliminate them. If the negotiations failed, then the President had the authority to impose retaliatory trade sanctions at his discretion. Subsequent amendments to the Trade Act in 1984 and again in 1988 significantly strengthened Section 301, more recently known as 'Super 301'. These amendments formalized the process, so that the United States Trade Representative is now required annually to identify countries and their trading practices which limit the access of United States firms to their markets. Once the practices have been identified, the Trade Representative is supposed to negotiate their elimination. If the negotiations do not succeed, retaliatory trade sanctions must be imposed.

With respect to tobacco, several actions have been taken under Section 301 since 1979, all involving Asian countries. The first two were relatively minor cases against Japan related to its trade barriers for cigars and pipe tobacco. The two cases were eventually combined and led to an agreement enabling United States cigar and pipe tobacco producers to compete in Japanese markets. The more significant cases dealt with cigarettes, and most were prompted by the United States Cigarette Export Association, which is a cartel created by Philip Morris, R.J. Reynolds and Brown and Williamson to increase United States cigarette exports to foreign markets. While our antitrust laws prohibit this type of cartel activity in United States markets, they allow it in foreign markets. Asian countries were the first targets of the cartel. For years, United States cigarette producers had tried to create a significant presence in many Asian markets, but were unable to do so because of a variety of trade barriers, including high tariffs on imported cigarettes, quotas and total bans on imports and limits on advertising and distribution. In most cases, domestic production was controlled by a government-run monopoly that generated a significant share of total government revenues.

Four regions were targeted by the United States Cigarette Export Association in the mid and late 1980s: Japan, the Republic of Korea, Taiwan and Thailand. The first of the Section 301 cases was brought against Japan. Historically, the Japan Tobacco Company monopolized the Japanese tobacco industry, protected by a 90% tariff on imports and by other non-tariff trade barriers. The Reagan administration initiated an investigation of these trade barriers in late 1985, threatening retaliatory measures if they were not eliminated. A formal agreement was reached in October 1986, eliminating the trade barriers and opening the Japanese cigarette market to United States producers. After the markets were opened, cigarette advertising by both United States firms and the Japan Tobacco Company increased. At the same time, Japanese cigarette consumption began to increase, reversing the downward trend observed before the agreement. The most notable increases were in the prevalence of smoking among women and young people.

Shortly after the agreement with Japan, a similar pact was reached with Taiwan. Taiwan's tobacco markets were monopolized by the Government-run Taiwan Tobacco and Wine Monopoly Bureau. Tariffs on imported cigarettes that made them three times more expensive than domestic brands and non-tariff barriers limited the market share of foreign brands in Taiwan to less than 1%. While the agreement opened Taiwan's cigarette markets, it contained restrictions related to advertising targeted at youth and required that United States cigarette packs bear a health warning label. Even with these restrictions, there was a sharp increase in advertising and promotion. In order to better compete with United States brands, the Taiwanese monopoly increased its use of United State-grown tobacco in cigarettes. A sharp rise in per capita cigarette consumption was seen: within two years, smoking by high-school students rose by 50%. Although a number of public health policies were adopted to discourage smoking, the rates have changed little.

The United States Cigarette Export Association next targeted the Republic of Korea, where the tobacco market was controlled by the Government Office of Monopoly. High tariffs had protected the monopoly, and legislation in 1982 made it illegal to sell, buy or possess foreign cigarettes. After a short investigation, an agreement was reached in May 1988 allowing United States cigarette companies to enter the market and advertise their products. The agreement also called for warning labels on packaging and advertisements and prohibited advertisements directed at women and children. Cigarette advertising rose sharply after the agreement, as the Government argued that United States producers were violating some of the advertising provisions in the agreement. More importantly, the rate of growth of cigarette smoking more than tripled after the agreement, mostly among the young.

The last of the cases related to tobacco was brought against Thailand in 1989, at the request of the Cigarette Export Association. The Thai cigarette market was controlled by a Government-run monopoly protected by a virtual ban on cigarette imports. In addition, a ban on cigarette advertising and promotion was adopted just before the Section 301 investigation. Unlike other countries, Thailand did not immediately give in to United States demands. Instead, the dispute between the two countries was taken before the General Agreement on Tariffs and Trade (GATT). The GATT Council concluded that the Thai ban on cigarette imports was a violation of the international treaty and that the markets should be opened to foreign producers. The Thai Government won part of its case, however, since its right to ban advertising was upheld by the GATT Council. The Council's general statement allows countries to use policies to restrict the overall supply of cigarettes as long as they are applied evenly to domestic and foreign producers. This was true even if these policies made it more difficult for the new foreign firms to compete with established domestic firms. A formal agreement between the United States and Thailand was signed in late 1990, and, as expected, United States exports to Thailand rose rapidly. Surveys suggest that the prevalence of smoking among youth and women has risen since the Thai markets were opened.

We examined the impact of the four Section 301 agreements on cigarette smoking in these countries. To do this, we developed a database of annual information for 10 Asian countries—the four affected countries and six control countries—for the period 1970–91. The key variables in the database are per capita cigarette consumption, the market share of United States cigarettes, an indicator for the years in which the Section 301 agreement applies and a measure of income. We use an econometric approach known as 'fixed effects modelling' to control for other, unmeasured, country- and time-specific influences on cigarette smoking.

We found a sharp rise in United States market shares in countries affected by the trade pressures. Our estimates imply that the market shares were 600% higher in 1991 than they would have been in the absence of these agreements. More importantly, we estimate that overall cigarette smoking rose as a result of the Section 301 cases: we estimate that per capita cigarette consumption in 1991 in the four countries was 10% higher, on average, than it would have been if their markets had remained closed to United States firms. Similarly, these estimates imply that opening other closed markets to these producers would result in higher cigarette consumption in those countries as well. Our estimates suggest that per capita cigarette consumption would rise by 7.5% in China and other countries if their markets were opened to United States cigarette companies.

These estimates are consistent with industry arguments that brand switching will occur in response to United States presence in formerly closed markets but are inconsistent with the argument that overall cigarette smoking is unaffected. We offer two explanations for why the amount of smoking rose after the markets were opened to United States firms. The first is based on the anecdotal evidence described earlier about advertising. Cigarette advertising increased sharply in most of the countries affected by the United States trade policies, not only for United States brands but also by the domestic monopoly. If advertising affects smoking initiation and consumption, then the rise in overall smoking is consistent with the increase in advertising.

A second explanation comes from the economic theory that predicts that prices will be highest in monopolized markets. Thus, the increased competition resulting from United States entry into previously monopolized markets should lower prices. A recent study from Taiwan (Hsieh & Hu, 1997) supports this theory, as inflation-adjusted prices for both domestic and imported cigarettes fell after the Taiwanese markets were opened to United States producers. Given the extensive literature concluding that cigarette smoking is affected by price, the price reductions resulting from greater competition are likely to account for part of the increase in smoking we estimated.

With respect to the current use of trade policy by the United States, the Clinton administration, unlike the previous two, has taken a 'hands-off' approach. They do not actively use trade policy to open foreign markets to United States cigarette companies, but they have done little to discourage the activities of those companies abroad, even though they have targeted smoking in the United States. Similarly, the 'global settlement' between state Attorneys General and the tobacco companies does not mention international issues. This led several United States Senators to introduce the Worldwide Tobacco Disclosure Act, which would prevent United States trade officials from helping cigarette companies to increase foreign sales. If adopted, this bill would prevent the events that have taken place in Asia from happening elsewhere.

References
Chaloupka, F.J. & Laixuthai, A. (1996) *United States Trade Policy and Cigarette Smoking in Asia* (National Bureau of Economic Research Working Paper No. 5543)
Hsieh, C.-R. & Hu, T.-W. (1997) *The Demand for Cigarettes in Taiwan: Domestic versus Imported Cigarettes* (Academia Sinica Discussion Paper No. 9701), The Institute of Economics

Investigation and prosecution of smuggling

A.A. Godfrey

Independent Commission against Corruption, Hong Kong SAR, China

The focus of this communication is law enforcement but with emphasis on corruption, which is the purview of our Commission in Hong Kong. In the 1960s and early 1970s, Hong Kong experienced massive economic and population growth coupled with rapid urbanization. At the same time, bribery and extortion became a way of life: paying bribes to public officials and secret commissions in the private sector were customary, and the collection and distribution of bribes by the police had become institutionalized. An important event in 1973 sparked community demands for action from the Government: a police superintendent under investigation for corruption fled to the United Kingdom. The community was enraged. A commission of inquiry was set up under a High Court judge to examine corruption in Hong Kong; one of its principal recommendations was to establish an independent, powerful agency to deal with the widespread corruption. As a result, the Independent Commission against Corruption was established, in February 1974. It is independent of the police and the rest of the civil service, and its Commissioner is directly responsible to the Chief Executive.

Three-pronged attack
When considering the establishment of the Commission, the Hong Kong Government realized that it could not win the battle against corruption solely by punishing the corrupt. It had to bring about fundamental changes in public attitudes towards corruption. Thus, the law that established the Commission required an integrated fight against corruption on three fronts: investigation, prevention and education. The Operations Department investigates corruption after receiving complaints. The Corruption Prevention department examines systems in Government departments and public bodies to reduce the opportunities for corruption. The Community Relations Department educates the public about the evils of corruption. This three-pronged attack has proved to be remarkably effective.

Smuggling very often leads to corruption or is facilitated by corruption.

Investigation and prosecution of smuggling
The smuggling trade dates back many centuries. It was and remains controlled by organized crime. The Commission has been involved on many occasions in investigating smuggling cases when corruption and organized crime were involved. We have, for example, investigated narcotics smuggling through the airport when customs officials were involved and also vehicle smuggling across our border with the mainland.

One investigation that involved cigarette smuggling and organized crime was known as 'the Giant Island matter'. It started in August 1993, when the Commission commenced an investigation of an international smuggling syndicate the activities of which were facilitated by corruption within the Department of Commerce and Exports and within private tobacco companies in Hong Kong (predominantly the British–American Tobacco Co.). A surveillance operation by the Commission identified premises at the Hip Hing timber yard at Fung Kat Heung to which contraband cigarettes were delivered and stored before being disguised for export, mainly to Taiwan. At the time, the availability of Japanese cigarettes was severely restricted in Taiwan.

On 13 March 1994, the Commission raided the timber yard, arrested six people and seized 4 296 600 cigarettes. Other seizures were made in Hong Kong and Taiwan which were directly linked to this operation. The syndicate leaders were arrested the next day. After the initial arrests, evidence emerged that substantial bribes had been paid by personnel of Giant Island Ltd to former employees of British–American Tobacco Co. and allegedly to Japan Tobacco Inc. in order to obtain preferential treatment for particular cigarette brands and to ensure continued distribution rights. It also became apparent that much of the smuggling of foreign brand cigarettes into mainland China was done by means of small boats. Large ships were loaded with cigarettes in Hong Kong, the permit showing another destination in South-east Asia. When in international waters, the ships were engaged by small boats from sites on the mainland where the cigarettes would be off-loaded.

Chui To-yan had been a shareholder of Giant Island Ltd from its inception until April 1993, when he left the company and Hong Kong and took up residence in Singapore. Chui provided statements to the Commission, outlining the bribery activities of Giant Island Ltd, including payment of bribes exceeding HK$ 100 million to executives of British–American Tobacco Co. Chui was to give evidence in Hong Kong in April 1995 at a preliminary hearing against members of the syndicate, including a former director of Giant Island Ltd, Chong Tsoi-jun. In March 1995, Chui was abducted in the car park of his office block in Singapore, and his body was found in Singapore Harbour three days later. He had been badly beaten, gagged with masking tape and placed in laundry bags attached around his neck by padlocks. The murder bore all the hallmarks of a triad killing. As a result of much research by the Commission, the Criminal Investigation Department of Singapore and the Hong Kong Police, five Hong Kong men were identified as having travelled frequently to Singapore, often together, over the previous five months; four were linked to a triad society. Two of the alleged murderers were subsequently arrested in China and handed over to Hong Kong. They are currently in custody pending trial. The other three are still at large.

One of the members of the syndicate was convicted of conspiring with triad members to pervert the course of justice by preventing Chui from giving evidence. He is serving a six-and-a-half-year sentence. Chong Tsoi-jun, who was arrested and committed to the High Court for trial on charges of corruption and tax evasion, committed suicide weeks before the beginning of the trial. A former director of British–American Tobacco Co. was arrested in the United States on charges of corruption and extradited to Hong Kong, where he is in custody awaiting trial. Arrest warrants have been issued for others who are outside our jurisdiction.

Conclusions

Why do criminals resort to smuggling?

- protective policies of governments on behalf of industry to prohibit import of foreign commodities;
- to avoid paying high import duties;
- high demand at the destination, making smuggling extremely profitable;
- the ease with which smugglers, particularly in developing countries, can suborn law enforcement;
- the fairly light sentences for smuggling goods other than narcotics.

What are the dangers of smuggling?

- suborning of state policy on revenue and the economy;
- corruption of societies by dangerous goods, like drugs, to which they would not otherwise have access;

- intermixing of criminals in legitimate business and sharing of profits;
- funding criminals for further criminality;
- attracting businessmen by huge profits to fund direct crime by smugglers;
- corruption of state officials to provide protection;
- corruption of law enforcement officers, particularly at border points, to provide free passage.

  What measures can be taken to prevent smuggling?
- promote free trade or abolish restrictive trade practices, increase quotas and increase the legitimate supply;
- lower import duties or raise duty on local goods so that the price differential is no longer significant;
- streamline procedures for importers and remove the bureaucracy involved;
- increase penalties for smuggling offences on all goods;
- ensure that law enforcement officers are paid enough to ensure that they do not succumb to corruption;
- increase penalties for corruption;
- make it an approved practice for customs officers to retain a percentage of the value of seized goods;
- improve international law enforcement liaison and cooperation.

Smuggling is not an innocuous illegal activity that only affects revenue for the receiving country. The lucrative gains that can be made invariably attract organized crime, which protects and enhances its activities by corruption and is willing to commit more serious offences to achieve its objectives.

A comprehensive strategy to reduce and prevent tobacco smuggling

R. Cunningham

Canadian Cancer Society, Ottawa, Ontario, Canada

Introduction

Tobacco smuggling has been a documented problem (Joossens & Raw, 1995) in all regions of the world. Contraband reduces government revenue, impairs health objectives by lowering the average price paid by consumers, discourages governments from further increasing tobacco taxes and pressures governments to lower taxes, as was the case in Canada (Cunningham, 1996). Lower tobacco taxes and prices lead to increased tobacco use (Lewit & Coate, 1982; Department of Health and Human Services, 1992). Indeed, higher tobacco taxes leading to higher retail prices are the most effective component of a tobacco control strategy.

The presence of contraband in a domestic market can also put pressure on a government to open the market to foreign companies. To reduce smuggling or to prevent smuggling from even becoming a significant problem, a comprehensive anti-smuggling strategy should be implemented (Canadian Cancer Society, 1994). This paper outlines 19 components of such a strategy:

Components of an anti-smuggling strategy

1. Imposing taxes at the point of production/importation instead of at the point of sale. Administratively, it is much easier to ensure compliance with a small number of manufacturers or importers than with tens of thousands of retailers.

2. Emphasizing the imposition of taxes at the national level instead of in subnational jurisdictions. If there is a choice, it is better to have the bulk of tobacco taxes at the national rather than the state or provincial level. Significant price differentials between jurisdictions can facilitate smuggling. Nevertheless, subnational jurisdictions should increase tobacco taxes. They can provide a positive example for reluctant governments at the national level and can contribute immediately to tobacco control from the benefits of higher taxes.

3. Requiring prominent tax-paid markings, including distinctive package and product markings, for each subnational jurisdiction imposing its own taxes. Tax-paid markings help to distinguish between legitimate and illegitimate products. In Canada, tax-paid markings are found on the cellophane tear-strip and vary in colour and text for almost every province. Although this is a good start, it would be better for tax-paid markings to appear on packages themselves. Smugglers can re-wrap contraband products with illegitimately obtained 'marked' cellophane tear strips. If tax-paid stamps are used, they should be difficult to counterfeit. Tax-paid markings should also appear on individual cigarettes, such as a coloured band or other mark on the filter overwrap. The Canadian Government announced this measure in 1994 but has not implemented it. Prominent package health warnings for national and subnational jurisdictions are one way to help distinguish products, in addition to markings specific to tax-paid status.

4. Banning duty-free sales to travellers. Apart from giving consumers access to low-priced cigarettes, duty-free sales create an avenue for tax-exempt tobacco to flow. This window can lead to abuse when tax-exempt products ostensibly intended for duty-free sales end up in the hands of smugglers. The European Union has taken steps to eliminate duty-free tobacco sales for individuals travelling between Member States. One way to ban duty-free sales at border crossings is for neighbouring countries to implement a treaty to ensure reciprocity.

5. Banning or limiting the quantity of duty-free imports. In addition to banning duty-free sales to travellers leaving a country, there should be controls on how much tax-exempt tobacco individuals can bring into a country or subnational jurisdiction. The lower the limit, the better. Until recently, Canada had a limit of 200 cigarettes plus 400 g of roll-your-own plus 400 tobacco sticks plus 50 cigars, equivalent to more than a six-week supply. The limit for roll-your-own has been reduced to 200 g, and the tobacco stick limit is now 200 units, but the total allowable is still far too high.

6. Controlling the circumstances in which tobacco may be sold at duty-free or duty-reduced prices, such as on aboriginal reserves, to military personnel and to diplomats. Every window for tax-exempt tobacco creates a potential opening for the flow of contraband. There should be a quota on the quantity of tax-exempt tobacco entering aboriginal reserves. Better yet, tobacco products should be sold at full tax-included prices, the incremental revenue possibly going to the band council for local objectives. For military personnel, including those working on ships and in overseas postings, there should be an end to tobacco sales that are not fully taxed. For diplomats, there should be a single government-licensed supplier for the entire diplomatic community as a means of controlling the quantity of tax-exempt tobacco supplied.

7. Requiring special package and product markings to indicate duty-exempt status. To the extent that tax-exempt sales are permitted, in duty-free stores or elsewhere, these packages should be clearly marked as such. It should be easy for retailers, consumers and law enforcement personnel to identify what is tax-exempt and what is not.

8. Banning mail-order sales. Allowing sales by mail order permits transfer of tobacco from low-tax jurisdictions to consumers in higher-tax jurisdictions. This happened in parts of Canada in recent years, cigarettes being shipped from low-tax provinces and from the United States. Consumers could order by Internet or by a toll-free telephone number. Banning mail-order sales also helps to reduce access by young people.

9. Imposing export taxes. In Canada in 1991–93, there were vast quantities of Canadian-made cigarettes which were exported to the other side of the border, only to return to

Canada as contraband. To address this problem the Canadian Government in 1992 imposed an export tax of CAN$ 8 per carton of 200 cigarettes as a means of reducing the price differential between legal and illegal cigarettes, and thus reducing the supply of contraband. Immediately, the quantity of exports dropped dramatically. Although this export tax was repealed under lobbying pressure from tobacco companies, an export tax remains a valuable anti-smuggling tool.

10. Ensuring that the tobacco industry has a financial incentive to reduce smuggling. Tobacco companies benefit by contraband. Consumer access to lower-cost products increases smoking. Higher rates of smuggling prevent yet higher taxes which would depress consumption. When contraband is seized, the tobacco companies have already made their profit. Governments must ensure that the industry has a financial motivation to reduce smuggling, not to increase it.

11. Holding transnational tobacco companies responsible for supplying products that end up as contraband, such as suspending their ability to supply the legal market. In Italy, the Government suspended the right of Philip Morris to sell products on the legal market when excessive quantities of Philip Morris cigarettes, manufactured outside the country, were appearing on the contraband market. This type of penalty lays blame at the source of the problem, the tobacco company. The penalty provides an incentive for the company to ensure that its products do not end up in the hands of smugglers. A company such as Philip Morris has far more profit to lose in the legitimate market than in the much smaller contraband market.

12. Requiring monthly shipment reports by brand from manufacturers, importers and exporters and requiring public disclosure of the reports. Government officials and tobacco control organizations need to know what is happening in the marketplace. A sudden change in shipment patterns may be a warning that intervention is required. Without sufficient information, opportunities to curb smuggling will be missed.

13. Requiring manufacturers, importers, wholesalers, transporters and retailers to have tobacco-specific licences. Licences assist in identifying and monitoring the various actors in the tobacco industry and facilitate anti-smuggling enforcement. Conditions can be attached to licences: they can be suspended for breach of the conditions or tobacco laws. Licence fees can help to pay for enforcement.

14. Ensuring that there are significant penalties, including fines of 3–10 times the tax evaded, prison terms and the right to confiscate the proceeds of crime. Significant penalties deter illegal behaviour.

15. Ensuring that there are meaningful search and seizure provisions. Law enforcement officials should have the same authority as those officials who fight illicit drug sales and other criminal activity. Any vehicles used to transport contraband should be forfeited.

16. Ensuring that meaningful resources are devoted to enforcement. Governments must make a commitment to fight smuggling. Whatever money is spent on hiring new officials is minimal in comparison with the revenue lost through smuggling or reduced taxation rates.

17. Ensuring there is cooperation between enforcement officials across enforcement agencies and across subnational and national boundaries. Smuggling is not a local problem, and inter-jurisdictional efforts are needed to solve it.

18. Lobbying of neighbouring jurisdictions to increase their taxes. The best solution of the smuggling problem is often to ask lower-tax jurisdictions to increase their taxes, rather than to ask high-tax jurisdictions to lower theirs.

19. Advocating an international treaty on the control of international shipments of tobacco products. The international nature of smuggling requires a concerted effort by nations to address the problem and to control the actions of transnational tobacco companies. Failure by one country to adopt strong anti-smuggling measures can result in significant adverse impacts for many other countries.

Conclusion

The time to implement a comprehensive anti-smuggling strategy is now, regardless of country. If smuggling is not currently a problem, implementing a strategy will ensure that it never becomes one and that governments do not feel constrained in their ability to further increase taxes. If smuggling is a problem already, then implementation of a strategy will reduce it and produce tangible tobacco control.

References

Canadian Cancer Society (1994) *Protecting Health and Revenue: An Action Plan to Control Contraband and Tax-exempt Tobacco,* Ottawa

Cunningham, R. (1996) *Smoke & Mirrors: The Canadian Tobacco War,* Ottawa: International Development Research Centre, Chapter 11

Department of Health and Human Services (1992) Smoking and Health in the Americas. A 1992 Report of the Surgeon General (DHHS Publication No. (CDC) 92-8419), Atlanta, Georgia: Pan American Health Organization, US Department of Health and Human Services, Public Health Service, Centers for Disease Control, National Center for Chronic Disease Prevention and Health Promotion, Office on Smoking and Health

Joosens, L. & Raw, M. (1995) Smuggling and cross border shopping of tobacco in Europe. *Br. Med. J.,* **310**, 1393–1397

Lewit, E.M. & Coate, D. (1982) The potential for using excise taxes to reduce smoking. *J. Health Econ.,* **1**, 121–145

PART II.
STEMMING THE EPIDEMIC

INTERNATIONAL AND GOVERNMENT OPTIONS

Global tobacco policy

N. Gray

International Union against Cancer, Geneva, Switzerland

In order to discuss global policy for tobacco, I am going to use the military idiom, because we are at war. I will take an activist's point of view towards tobacco policy. Finally, I will discuss new issues in relation to policy. In particular, I want to talk about regulation of the content of the cigarette, which is a topic we have kept away from for many years but is now very relevant in the light of the activities of the United States Food and Drug Administration and also in the light of the powers that exist in Europe.

Global policy
- Kill the enemy.
- Capture his weapons.
- Use them against him.
- Use them to recapture his prisoners.
- Protect the children.
- Cessation for addicts.

Now, I do not mean 'assassinate the enemy', I mean to destroy him as an effective force. It is necessary to define the enemy. It is not the smoker, it is not actually even the cigarette, it is the international tobacco industry, which consists of only a dozen or so companies. It is not necessarily even the monopolies, which are often controlled by governments. The enemy is the international tobacco industry. We have to beat it politically, to make it an unacceptable and ineffective political force. That means also capturing its weapons and then using its weapons against it. We have to have the same resources that it has, and we have to use them.

Then we have to recapture its prisoners, because, as Richard Peto pointed out, the existing long-term smoker is the person who makes up the mortality rate now and will continue to make up the mortality rate for the next two decades. We need to protect the children for the future and to put more effort into helping the addicts.

Kill the enemy
- Abolish all promotion
- Taxes
- Control cigarette content
- Generic packaging
- Strong health warnings
- Smoke-free environment
- Forbid sales to children

This is what I mean by 'kill the enemy'. We have to abolish all forms of tobacco promotion. We must tax cigarettes severely. Controlling the content of cigarettes is the subject of the second half of my talk: we must control what is in the cigarette and what comes out of the end of it in the same way as we control what comes out of the exhaust pipe of cars. We must stop their marketing in elegant, targeted packaging and eventually have generic packaging. We need good, strong health warnings, like those in Canada and Australia.

We need a smoke-free environment (and that is happening in many parts of the world), and we need really to reduce access by children.

Eradicate promotion
- Television, radio, print, billboards, competitions, giveaways, look-alikes, points of sale

- Sport, film
- Anything else new

Every form of promotion must be abolished. The United States settlement does not do this satisfactorily, but it goes a long way. We must especially cover sport and film and all the new ideas that will be created by the industry.

Capture his weapons

- Mass media
- Sponsorship.
- Film industry
- Role models
- Use his money

His weapons include the mass media. We have captured a little mass media in a few places—in Massachusetts and some in California. But we have not captured mass media of any consequence, for instance on the scale of Coca Cola We must replace the industry as sponsors of the sports and the arts. We need to put pressure on the film industry—the role models—and particularly for these purposes, we need to use his money. To be crystal clear, we need to take the tobacco industry's money to do our job.

That can be done. A settlement in the United States is one way his money can be used: he can be persuaded or forced to pay. The second way, which is more usual and efficient, is to tax him; and the third way, which is the case in Australia and in California and Massachusetts, is to have a hypothecated (or earmarked) tax which takes the money directly from him and gives it to us.

Packaging

- Generic: precedent needed
- Warnings: large
- Visible
- Multiple
- Explained
- Phone number

Packaging must be controlled. In Australia, we have the telephone number of the Quit Line actually on the packet. We have not used that effectively yet, because the industry has managed to obstruct our use of it.

Smoke-free environment

- Workplace
- Schools
- Public places
- Restaurants
- Note the role of litigation in bringing this about

A smoke-free environment is a very effective way of reducing the consumption of cigarettes. A workplace that is smoke-free reduces consumption by three to five cigarettes per day, which actually reduces sales of cigarettes as well as reducing the risk to the smokers. Many smoke-free environments around the world arose from the enforcement of government regulation, but many arose from litigation brought by victims of smoky environment s. We should remember that this is a serious area for litigation in countries other than the United States.

Taxation

- Regular increases
- Percentage for health
- Per stick, not per gram
- Remove from consumer price indices

We need regular increases in taxes on tobacco, and a percentage of that allocated to health, The tax should be applied per cigarette, not per gram, because the companies are reducing the amount of tobacco in their cigarettes as time goes on and maintaining the amount of nicotine, so taxing them by gram of tobacco, which is what most countries do, is actually allowing them to avoid tax. And we must remove cigarettes from the consumer price index, on which inflation is measured in every country.

Now, coming to new policy areas, I shall talk about regulation of the content of cigarettes.

Cigarette content
- Nicotine to 0.5 mg, with updating of the testing system
- Tar to 12 mg maximum
- Only tested additives

I think the 'global cigarette', which I promoted in an editorial in *The British Medical Journal* in 1996, is a concept whose time has come. It should have an upper limit of 12 g of tar and 0.5 mg of nicotine (or 1 mg at the most), and the additives used must have been tested. The system of measurement that gives us these levels is out of date and is misleading. The only people who like it are the tobacco industry. So, we need to put some work into ways of measuring the content of cigarettes and of their smoke, which is more relevant to what actually goes into smokers' lungs.

Items for regulation
- Nicotine
- Carcinogens
- Other toxins
- Needs to be flexible
- Needs to be ongoing

How should cigarettes be regulated? Given that it is rather like a minestrone soup, with 4000 items in it, we must look at nicotine, the carcinogens and the other toxins. When we look at it, we must be flexible, because when we change a cigarette we must measure the effects of that change in many ways. We must regulate in an ongoing way, and it may well be that new regulations will be needed each year; to be efficient, such regulations must be global.

Nicotine addiction
- It might not matter if cigarettes did not exist, but cigarettes do exist!

The first substance to regulate is nicotine. We must ask ourselves whether nicotine addiction is important, because nicotine on its own, as a chewing gum, does not seem to be very harmful. But nicotine addiction is harmful if cigarettes are on the market: addicts turns to cigarettes because they are the most efficient nicotine delivery devices we know. So nicotine addiction does matter. We must try to reduce global nicotine addiction. Whether that is possible will be decided only by a global series of experiments. The alternative—allowing a lot of nicotine in cigarettes—is no long-term solution and is viable only if we could remove the other harmful substances, which, I will dogmatically assert, we cannot.

Regulation of nicotine
- By weight per cigarette
- A mass weaning experiment
- By one agency
- In relation to substitutes
- No nicotine lollipops

This is a long-term human experiment justified simply because the *status quo* is too dangerous. These proposals for regulating nicotine owe a lot to Neil Benowitz and Jack Henningfield, who published some of these ideas in *The New England Journal of Medicine* in 1994. They suggested that the best way to do it was not to let the 'FTC' measurement rule the system but to control the weight of nicotine in the actual cigarette (and to relate that to blood levels by experiment). In essence, they suggested that nicotine be reduced over time, which represents a mass weaning experiment.

Nicotine must be regulated by one agency. For example, in the United Kingdom, nicotine substitutes are controlled by the office that controls drugs while nicotine in cigarettes is controlled by the Health Department. This is not suitable. We have to think about nicotine in relation to both cigarettes and substitutes, because it is absurd that nicotine should be tightly controlled when it comes in chewing-gum (which does not damage health) and uncontrolled when it comes to the cigarette, which is lethal. We should also be aware that we do not yet have nicotine lollipops, produced by a drug company, on the market, to act as a gateway drug for a cigarette. So I am proposing a long-term human experiment. If you think a human experiment is a rather frightening idea, let me tell you that nothing is more dangerous than doing nothing. The *status quo* is dangerous, and we must improve it.

Compensation for nicotine
- A mass weaning experiment
- Gradually reduce weight per cigarette
- Reduce by 10%? per year
- Research on inhalation behaviour over time
- Follow up with a scientific review panel

In reducing nicotine, we have to think of nicotine compensation, which means that if we reduce the amount of nicotine in the cigarette, the smoker sucks harder. We have known about nicotine compensation for nearly two decades and should be grateful to Michael Russell for putting us in the picture about this. These are the reasons behind a mass weaning experimentt: gradually, by regulation, reducing the weight of nicotine in the cigarette, and having done that, to do research on the behaviour of smokers. We would probably have to reduce the weight of nicotine in the cigarette by about 10% per year and then decide in five years' time whether the experiment was successful and adapt our strategy. To do that we need one good scientific review panel, a global one.

No-one has considered or attempted regulating the carcinogens in the cigarette. The United States Food and Drug Administration is thinking about it, but it has not yet been done in any country. In the graph shown in Figure 1, the lower curve is benzo[a]pyrene, which between the beginning of the 1960s and 1978 was reduced by 50% in a popular, non-filter brand of American cigarettes. The upper curve shows NNK, which is one of the nicotine-specific nitrosamines, a well-established carcinogen, which produces adenocarcinoma in experimental animals. Between the late 1970s and the early 1990s, the NNK content of cigarettes went up by 50%. So, over two or three decades of self-regulation by the industry, they have reduced benzopyrene, one carcinogen, by 50%, and have increased another, NNK, by 50%. It is difficult to believe

Figure 1. Benzo[a]pyrene (BaP) and NNK in mainstream smoke of a leading United States non-fliter cigarette, 1969–92

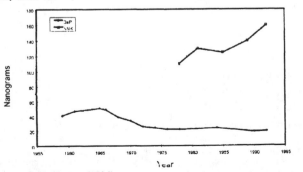

From Hoffmann & Hoffmann (1994)

that in a modern society people can increase the dose of a carcinogen by 50% and no one is doing anything about it. We really do have to control this industry and this product.

Regulate carcinogens and toxins
- Top 20 brands
- Select top 10 or 20 toxins and carcinogens
- Measure upper and lower limits
- Establish median
- Down-regulate from that
- Set targets, then standards
- Use car exhausts as a precedent

Controlling carcinogens is not as difficult as we might think, because there is a precedent: the motor car. Working with the car industry, governments have set targets and then set standards. What comes out of the exhaust of the modern motor car is much less toxic than it used to be. We can do this with a cigarette. Take the top 20 brands; look at the top 10, or perhaps the top 20 toxins and carcinogens; measure the upper and lower limits of those carcinogens in the top 20 brands; the upper limit tells us where we are today, and the bottom limit tells us what can be done. So we establish the median for the carcinogen yield and then tell the industry that they must start reducing from that median. All those with cigarettes above the median would have to come down quickly to the lowest level, because if a lower limit exists on the market, it is possible. We do this by setting a target which the industry tries to meet and then we set a legal standard and apply it. It has worked for motor car exhausts, and it can work for the cigarette. We just have to decide to try it.

Surveillance
- Basic research needed: industry and government
- All research in public arena
- Cross-licensing as needed
- Flexible testing systems as knowledge evolves
- Monitor usage by brand
- Industry to report the levels in its products, subject to spot testing

We must survey the the industry, because the it has proved it is not to be trusted. We need basic research in the public arena, and the United States settlement provides for that. Industry research has never been made public before. The United States settlement also provides for cross-licensing of results that reduce carcinogens. We need a flexible, up-to-date testing system. We need to monitor usage by brand so that we know what is happening on the market, and we need to make the industry report. All that is in the settlement; we do not have it now, but it is not impossible.

Global issues
- The United States settlement should now be the minimum global standard, but
- It docs not invoke global standards of behaviour
- We must control the industry in its homes: try the United Kingdom and the United States for a start
- We must control satellite transmission of advertising: China and India could insist on this and probably succeed

There is much argument about the United States settlement, but I think that, although it is not perfect, it is at least a minimum and contains acknowledgments of the health risks. We need a global standard of behaviour, which means that we need to control the industry in its home countries. The two big home countries are the United Kingdom and the United States. The way to do this is by a global system of regulation. I think this must be done by governments, which means it should be brokered by the World Health Organization (WHO). The framework convention is a mechanism for doing this; WHO is working on it, and we should all support it. The job of the non-governmental organizations is to lobby to support it, and I believe WHO will set this standard of behaviour. It is then up to all of us to work to make sure that this standard of behaviour is met; in particular, we want to see this standard introduced into the United States settlement, if that can be done. It will be difficult.

1997 was a good year
- United States settlement negotiations
- United Kingdom Government decision to vote for a ban on advertising in Europe
- Probability of a ban in the European Community
but
- Nothing done for developing countries

1997 was really a good year. Whether the United States settlement happens or not, whether it is perfect or not, the fact that the industry wants it and is coming to bargain with people they hate is an indication that the industry is severely wounded. The settlement has damaged it seriously, and we should make sure we continue that damage.

The United Kingdom Government decision to vote for a complete ban on advertising in Europe is another bad blow to the industry. As a result, the European Community is likely to agree to a complete advertising ban,; it also has the power to regulate the content of cigarettes.

Although nothing has been done for developing countries, if we beat the industry in Europe and the United States, much is possible in central and eastern Europe and in Asia.

Conundrums
- Slow declines in the prevalence of smoking among adolescents in some countries
- The FTC measurement system for tar content must be replaced
- The nicotine policy proposed here is speculative and experimental
- Political corruption persists in high places

I want to finish with some of the problems, because it is not clever to conceal the problems from ourselves. This first one troubles me more than anything. I am from Australia. We have had an advertising-free society for some time; we have had money, although we have not used it as effectively as we could have. We have a health promotion foundation funded by tobacco tax, although we have not had a Coca Cola-style mass media campaign as is now occurring in Massachusetts. We have a very good environment for anti-smoking work. The prevalence among children went down for quite a long time, but it has recently crept up, despite continued success with adults. Why did that happen, when we have a comprehensive policy in place? It has also happened in California and in other parts of the United States, in the United Kingdom and in Norway. So in some ways we are not getting the results that I have expected all my life, and we must think very carefully about why our policy has not given us the decreases in prevalence that we want.

We need better systems for measuring what is in the cigarette and for the behaviour of the population. We (or I) must admit that the nicotine policy I have presented to you is speculative, that it is an experiment, despite my view that we should do it.

We haven't got rid of political corruption. The United States settlement goes to Congress, and we must be aware that many people in Congress receive money from the tobacco industry. If you think that is unique to America, you are wrong. Political corruption is rampant. The receipt of money by politicians in the United Kingdom and by political parties even in Australia, where I think we have beaten the industry, is still an issue. We must not forget that corruption still exists.

Our global policy must be updated. We must make sure that we don't ease up on the industry. We must make sure that we support the fights that are going on in Europe, the United Kingdom and the United States. We must win those fights within the next 12 months, and we must then work very hard on what is happening in central and eastern Europe and in the other parts of the world, especially Asia.

International action for tobacco control

R. Roemer

School of Public Health, University of California, Los Angeles, California, United States

Electrifying events in the United States concerning tobacco in 1996–97 have sparked new energy and new efforts to combat the tobacco epidemic. The United States Food and Drug Administration has declared cigarettes and smokeless tobacco a drug and drug delivery device subject to regulation, a decision upheld by a Federal court in North Carolina, a tobacco-growing state. Numerous state class action and individual suits have been brought against the tobacco companies in products liability cases. In a brilliant legal strategy, 40 jurisdictions—states, counties and cities—have brought suits against the tobacco companies to recover their expenditures for medical care of persons suffering from smoking-related diseases. This enormous threat of potential liability led the tobacco industry to enter into negotiations with state attorneys general to reach a settlement of these suits. On 20 June 1997, a pact was reached in which the tobacco companies agreed to pay US$ 368.5 thousand million over the next 25 years to compensate states for the costs of treating tobacco-related illness, to finance nationwide anti-smoking programmes, to underwrite health care for millions of uninsured children in lieu of punitive damages and to pay penalties if smoking among young people is not reduced. The proposed settlement must be approved by the President and Congress. The public health community almost unanimously opposes the settlement because of grave shortcomings which limit the authority of the Food and Drug Administration to regulate nicotine, restrict the right to sue the tobacco companies, require inadequate penalties for continued smoking among the young and, most importantly, fail to control the assault of the multinational tobacco companies on the developing countries (*New York Times*, 1997a).

Clearly, the tobacco industry is on the defensive, and tobacco control forces are on the offensive. The industry, under relentless pressure, is being driven on the domestic front in the United States to concessions that may have significant international implications. In other countries, similarly powerful legal suits may be brought. The exposure of the nefarious and duplicitous conduct of the tobacco companies may well lead to effective international regulation of the industry.

Among the stunning tobacco control events of 1996–97 is the little-noticed but enormously important action of the World Health Organization (WHO), discussed by Neil Collishaw. In 1996, the World Health Assembly adopted a powerful new strategy by passing a resolution calling on the Director-General of WHO:

(i)   to initiate the development of a framework convention in accordance with Article 19 of the WHO Constitution;

(ii) to include as part this framework convention a strategy to encourage member nations to move progressively towards the adoption of comprehensive tobacco control policies, and also to deal with aspects of tobacco control that transcend national boundaries....(World Health Organization, 1996)

Why has the World Health Organization decided to develop a legally binding international instrument for comprehensive tobacco control policies?

For three reasons. First, WHO recognizes the power of the multinational tobacco industry which, faced with a decline in smoking in industrialized countries, is pushing tobacco sales in developing countries with increasing aggressiveness and ingenuity. Between 1990 and 1995, the sales of cigarettes declined by 4.5% in Canada and the United States and by 1.7% in western Europe, but sales increased by 5.6% in eastern Europe, by 17.7% in the Middle East and by 8% in the Asia and Pacific Region (*New*

York Times, 1997b). In the early 1990s, about 1.2 million smoking-related deaths occurred annually in the developing countries and 1.9 million in developed countries—roughly an equal number. Within the next 30–40 years, however, the number of deaths caused by smoking in developing countries will rise substantially because of the massive increase in cigarette consumption (Collishaw & Lopez, 1996).

The second reason for WHO's support of an international instrument is that, in its 35-year campaign to combat the tobacco epidemic, legislative action has proved to be an essential tool in reducing the prevalence of smoking. Norway presents an early example of the effectiveness of legislation. Its tobacco control law was passed in 1973, and regulations on labelling and prohibition of advertising in 1974 (Norway, 1975). Declines in the prevalence of smoking occurred with each step in the legislative process. Finland's law of 1976 was similarly powerful in reducing smoking (Finland, 1977). In 1994, Finland passed a new tobacco law to increase restrictions on smoking in public places and prevent young people from taking up smoking (Finland, 1995a,b), which resulted in a sharp decline in the prevalence of smoking, with a sharper decline for men than for women.

No claim is made that legislation alone is sufficient to reduce the prevalence of smoking, but legislation expresses the political will of Government to combat the epidemic. It restricts some of the most harmful and insidious actions of the industry. It lays the basis for adequate resources to spread the health message to the people. Strong legislation, combined with effective health education, constitutes a powerful weapon. Significant advances have been made in legislation, but enormous challenges remain. About 95 countries have now enacted tobacco control legislation, and laws have been passed at the sub-national level, but many countries have weak legislation. In some places, laws are not enforced, and legislation is totally lacking in a number of countries. A binding international instrument is a global necessity for providing an impetus for strong national action and to counter the aggressive marketing of the multinational tobacco industry.

A third reason for an international instrument is that it has the capacity to mobilize policy-makers in various ministries—not only the health ministry—to support tobacco control. Because the framework convention and succeeding specific protocols call for the commitment of parliamentarians and national policy-makers, ministries of agriculture, commerce and finance will be impelled to join with health ministries to create a countervailing force to the power of the tobacco industry. A framework convention with protocols provides a weapon to combat the effects of the global tobacco trade, international tobacco investment and export–import policies that increase the supply of cigarettes and lower their price.

What is a framework convention?

A framework convention is a legally binding treaty that calls for the cooperation of nations in achieving broadly stated goals. It is a statement in general terms of the goals designed to achieve the widest consensus of the nations of the world. Although technically binding, a framework convention imposes no explicit obligations. Nevertheless, it creates an institutionalized forum for cooperation and negotiation as a prelude to adopting protocols that contain specific, detailed obligations, when such action is possible and appropriate.

A framework convention has the advantage of creating legally binding international standards governed by international law. Moreover, nations may adopt domestic legislation in accord with the framework convention that can be enforced by domestic courts. The treaty-making process enables nations to overcome powerful, organized industry resistance to regulation. At the same time, a framework convention, being couched in general terms, does not require nations at the outset to commit themselves to more than they can deliver. Thus, a framework convention is likely to be more politically acceptable than any other binding approach to tobacco control.

How will the framework convention–protocol approach work?

Once an international convention is adopted, specific protocols can be proposed, debated and adopted as nations become ready for such action. Initially, such protocols may address widely accepted measures for control of tobacco use, such as bans on smoking in public places and preventing smoking by children and adolescents. Then, as momentum is gained in the process, more difficult issues may be tackled, such as alternatives to tobacco production and matters related to tobacco trade, investment and taxes.

Although this double-track approach requires multiple international negotiations and national ratifications—one for the framework convention and others for each of the implementing protocols—it has the advantage of being a dynamic law-making process that can respond to changing conditions, needs and knowledge (Taylor & Roemer, 1996).

What should be the scope of a framework convention?

Since it is proposed that the framework convention be a WHO instrument, rather than an instrument of the United Nations General Assembly, it would be reasonable for WHO to look to its own 1986 resolution which was adopted unanimously by the World Health Assembly (World Health Organization, 1986). This resolution urges Member States to consider a comprehensive national tobacco control strategy containing measures of the following types:

- controlling involuntary exposure to tobacco smoke;
- protecting children and young people from addiction to tobacco;
- promoting the example of non-smoking health personnel and smoke-free health facilities;
- progressively eliminating socioeconomic, behavioural and other incentives for tobacco use;
- adopting strong health warnings, including the statement that tobacco is addictive;
- mandating effective health education and information programmes, including cessation programmes;
- monitoring trends in tobacco use, tobacco-related diseases and the effectiveness of tobacco control actions;
- promoting alternatives to tobacco production, trade and taxation and
- establishing a national focal point to stimulate tobacco control activities.

This resolution could well serve as a starting point for consultation with public health and legal experts to consider the broad goals of comprehensive tobacco control policies that should be incorporated into a framework convention. In the time since this resolution was adopted, other measures might be considered, such as the full use of legislative, administrative and judicial strategies to promote smoke-free societies.

What steps should tobacco control advocates take to advance international action?

The public debate engendered in the United States by the suits of the attorneys general against the tobacco companies shows how prominent the issue of tobacco control can become on the national scene when national and state governments, public health professionals, voluntary health organizations and the media focus their concerns on a public health issue of monumental proportions.

Our strategy as public health advocates should be to move consideration of WHO's landmark action for an international framework convention into the public domain. International action should become a high priority of every ministry, of every government, every official health agency, every voluntary health organization, every public health professional and every citizen and consumer group to stop the global epidemic that now kills 3 million people a year and is predicted to cause 10 million deaths annually by the 2020s or 2030s, of which 7 million will occur in the developing countries.

References

Collishaw, N.E. & Lopez, A.D. (1996) The tobacco epidemic—A public health emergency. *Tobacco Alert*, Special Issue, Geneva: World Health Organization, pp. 18-19

Finland (1977) Law No. 693 of 13 August 1976 on measures to restrict smoking. *Int. Dig. Health Legis.*, **28**, 486–489

Finland (1995a) Law No. 765 of 19 August 1994 amending the Law on measures to reduce smoking. *Int. Dig. Health Legis.*, **46**, 62

Finland (1995b) Law No. 1148 of 8 December 1994 amending the Law on measures to reduce smoking. *Int. Dig. Health Legis.*, **46**, 189–190

New York Times(1997a) 10 July, p. A15

New York Times (1997b) 24 June 24, pp. A1, 9

Norway (1975) Law No. 14 of 9 March 1973 on restrictive measures in trade in tobacco products, etc. *Int. Dig. Health Legis.*, **26**, 571–572

Taylor, A.L. & Roemer, R. (1996) *International Strategy for Tobacco Control* (WHO/PSA/96.6), Geneva: World Health Organization, Programme on Substance Abuse, pp. 16–17

World Health Organization (1986) Tobacco or Health, Resolution WHA39.41, Geneva World Health Organization (1996) International Framework Convention for Tobacco Control, Resolution WHA49.17, Geneva

An international framework convention for tobacco control

N.E. Collishaw

Tobacco or Health, World Health Organization, Geneva, Switzerland

Summary

Since 1970, the World Health Assembly has adopted 16 resolutions on tobacco or health issues, several of them calling for the implementation of comprehensive tobacco control policies and programmes. There has been a good deal of progress towards this goal, but only a few countries have fully implemented the comprehensive tobacco control called for by the World Health Assembly. There is clear evidence that the implementation of such policies can contribute to slowing, stabilizing or reducing tobacco consumption. In addition to progress in tobacco control at the national level, there are encouraging indications of greater international collaboration and coordination of international and global tobacco control efforts.

In May 1996, the 49th World Health Assembly adopted resolution WHA49.17 calling on the Director- General of the World Health Organization (WHO) to initiate the development of an international framework convention for tobacco control in accordance with Article 19 of the WHO Constitution. Should such an international convention eventually be adopted, it would be the first international treaty to be administered by WHO under Article 19. Progress to date in the preparatory work for this convention is reviewed. In addition, the following questions are addressed:

What is the significance of this resolution for global tobacco control?

What is an international framework convention?

How does a framework convention work?

What would be the content of a framework convention for tobacco control?

What are the uniquely internatiional dimensions of tobacco control that can be effectively addressed only through treaties or other international agreements?

How will this preparatory work be coordinated within the United Nations system?

Member States, non-governmental organizations and others are urged to support WHO in this new initiative to strengthen global tobacco control through the creation of a framework convention for international tobacco control.

Resolutions adopted by the World Health Assembly

The World Health Assembly is the governing body of WHO and is made up of representatives of every Member State. Since 1970, the Health Assembly has adopted 16 resolutions in favour of tobacco control measures, all without dissent, indicating that there is a most remarkable global consensus in favour of comprehensive tobacco control measures: they are favoured by the representatives of 191 WHO Member States. Several of the resolutions called for comprehensive tobacco control programmes and policies. The following 10-point programme is a summary of the comprehensive measures called for by the World Health Assembly and other international public health agencies (World Health Organization, 1996a):

- protection of children from becoming addicted to tobacco;
- use of fiscal policies to discourage the use of tobacco, such as tobacco taxes that increase faster than the growth in prices and income;
- use a portion of the money raised from tobacco taxes to finance other tobacco control and health promotion measures;
- health promotion, health education and smoking cessation programmes; health workers and institutions to set an example by being smoke-free;
- protection from involuntary exposure to environmental tobacco smoke;
- elimination of socioeconomic, behavioural and other incentives which maintain and promote use of tobacco;
- elimination of direct and indirect tobacco advertising, promotion and sponsorship;
- controls on tobacco products, including prominent health warnings on the products and any remaining advertisements; limits on and mandatory reporting of toxic constituents in tobacco products and tobacco smoke;
- promotion of economic alternatives to tobacco growing and manufacturing and
- effective management, monitoring and evaluation of tobacco issues.

Analysis of tobacco control measures in countries of the Organisation for Economic Co-operation and Development

Most of the programmes and policies that are required to control tobacco use can be effectively carried out at national or sub-national level. A very wide range of actions in the areas of legislation, taxation, agricultural policy, health education and promotion and smoking cessation programmes can be imagined. Typically, these measures are rarely subject to rigorous evaluation, and when various measures are undertaken simultaneously, evaluation of their independent and joint effects is difficult.

One study, notable for its scope, involved use of multiple regression techniques to evaluate the effect of advertising restrictions, price and income on tobacco consumption in 22 countries of the Organisation for Economic Co-operation and Development (OECD) between 1960 and 1986 (Laugesen & Meads, 1991). At above-threshold levels, both price relative to income and advertising restrictions were found to be significant in decreasing tobacco consumption. Moreover, the most comprehensive tobacco control programmes that included both high prices for tobacco products and comprehensive bans on tobacco advertising, together with stringent cigarette pack health warning labelling requirements, had the strongest effect. The authors estimated that a ban on tobacco advertising, strong and varied health warnings on packs and a 36% increase in real price would have reduced tobacco consumption by 13.5% in 1986, had any of the OECD countries under study taken such measures in that year. This analysis, both by its scientific rigour and its comprehensive inclusion of virtually all available international data on the question, lends scientific weight to the assertion that national tobacco control programmes that include at least progressively increasing tobacco prices through taxation, strict controls on tobacco advertising and strong warnings on packs of tobacco products are effective at preventing and discouraging tobacco use.

Why have only a few countries been successful in implementing comprehensive tobacco control policies and programmes?

The available scientific evidence therefore provides some support for the resolutions of the World Health Assembly in favour of comprehensive tobacco control measures. Despite this congruence of policy recommendations and evidence in favour of the effectiveness of such recommendations, most countries have experienced difficulty in fully implementing tobacco control policies and programmes recommended by the World Health Assembly. Failure to recognize the seriousness of the tobacco epidemic, failure to recognize tobacco control as a top public policy priority, strong opposition from those with an economic interest in continued unrestricted access to tobacco products and unrestricted smoking at work and in public places and lack of specific knowledge of how to implement multisectoral tobacco control policies have all been cited as reasons why only a handful of countries have been successful in fully implementing resolutions calling for comprehensive tobacco control policies.

Recent actions to control tobacco use in selected countries

Most of the countries that have banned tobacco advertising and progressively increased tobacco taxes fast enough to discourage consumption have also undertaken many of the other measures recommended by the World Health Assembly for comprehensive tobacco control. Other countries have recently taken measures that probably improve the level of tobacco control but fall short of the comprehensive programmes called for by the Health Assembly. Highlights of recent progress in tobacco control are discussed briefly, with special attention to those countries that have recently implemented comprehensive tobacco control policies.

Initial steps towards comprehensive tobacco control

Between the mid-1980s and the mid-1990s, many countries implemented some tobacco control measures where few or none at all had existed previously. These include Brazil, Cyprus, Côte d'Ivoire and Nepal. In Nepal, the recent measures include smoking bans or restrictions on passenger airplanes, trains and buses., and restrictions have also been introduced on smoking in public places and workplaces. Nepal now has a special surtax on tobacco products, the proceeds of which are used to finance much-needed public health improvements. Further measures will be necessary, however, before Nepal and the many other countries in this category achieve truly comprehensive tobacco control, as recommended by the Health Assembly.

Adding to existing tobacco control measures

Another group of countries added further tobacco control measures to a number that already existed but still left room to achieve truly comprehensive tobacco control at a later date. Particularly noteworthy in this regard was the action of the European Union, which issued Directives applying to all 15 member states, requiring that national laws be passed to require health warnings on packs of cigarettes, labelling of yields of tar and nicotine, an upper limit on tar yields and a ban on new oral tobacco snuff products. In the late 1980s and early 1990s, tobacco control measures were also improved in China, Costa Rica, Cuba, India, Mongolia, Poland, Turkey, Slovenia, Lithuania, South Africa and the United States, to mention only a few. Many of these countries have recently adopted strong legislative measures including bans or severe restrictions on advertising. In the main, however, even when the measures are strong and comprehensive, they are so recent that it not yet possible to say that they are being effectively implemented. Among the stronger measures introduced in these and other countries, it is notable that Poland and South Africa now require very strong warnings on tobacco advertisements and tobacco packaging, occupying 20% or more of the face of the advertisement or pack. Yet, while making progress in tobacco control, this group of countries still falls short of achieving truly demonstrable, comprehensive national tobacco control programmes.

Mixed records of implementing comprehensive tobacco control measures

In a third group of countries, the record is mixed, with both advances and setbacks in continuing efforts to strengthen comprehensive tobacco control policies. In the period of reconstruction after its invasion and subsequent liberation, Kuwait had temporarily suspended import regulations, including stringent requirements for health warnings and high import duties on cigarettes. As a result, for a short period in the early 1990s, cigarettes bearing no health warnings were widely available in the country at low prices. The prevalence of smoking among men increased from 34% in 1989 to 52% in 1992, while that among women increased from 6% to 12% in the same period. Subsequently, however, significant policy advances were made. In 1995, Kuwait adopted new tobacco control legislation, authorizing regulation of smoking in public places and banning tobacco advertising.

Under the threat of trade sanctions from the United States, Japan and the Republic of Korea lifted restrictions on cigarette imports. Imports and advertising of foreign cigarettes, mainly American, have subsequently increased in these countries, and the prevalence of smoking among Japanese women has also increased in recent years.

Countries of central and eastern Europe are undergoing rapid change to market economies. Unhappily, this change has also been accompanied by the introduction of western-style cigarettes and modern tobacco advertising and merchandising. These countries, where tobacco use was already widespread, are now experiencing even further increases in tobacco consumption, particularly among young people, who are especially vulnerable to the lure of seductive cigarette advertisements. Encouragingly, attempts to implement strong national tobacco control measures are also under way in many central and east European countries, but few have yet come to complete fruition. Proposals for greater legislative restrictions on tobacco advertising and marketing and greater restrictions on smoking in public places and workplaces are under active consideration or recently implemented in a number of countries including Poland, Lithuania, Slovakia and Slovenia.

In 1989, Canada adopted the *Non-smokers' Health Act*. Under this law, smoking is banned in buses, airplanes and all Federal Government offices and banned or limited to just a few smoking areas in other forms of public transport, other public places and private sector workplaces that come under Federal jurisdiction for health and safety matters. The *Tobacco Products Control Act*, also adopted in 1989, banned most forms of tobacco advertising and promotion and required strong, varied health warnings on packs of tobacco products, as well as mandatory labelling of tar, nicotine and carbon monoxide on packs of cigarettes and cigarette tobacco. In 1995, however, the Canadian Supreme Court ruled most of the *Tobacco Products Control Act* invalid under the Canadian Constitution. A new *Tobacco Act* was adopted in 1997, but key provisions to restrict tobacco sponsorship were delayed by one year in the face of intense tobacco industry lobbying. Another important component of the Canadian tobacco control policy in the 1980s was a system of payments to tobacco farmers who agreed to leave the tobacco-growing business permanently, in order to help them to adjust to alternative forms of economic activity. Other measures include intensified support for smoking cessation, education and prevention programmes. There were also large increases in tobacco taxes in the 1980s and early 1990s, with the stated purpose of discouraging tobacco use, particularly among young people; however, the development of widespread smuggling prompted the Government to reduce tobacco taxes in 1994.

Countries with recently implemented comprehensive tobacco control policies
A fourth group of five countries, Australia (most states), France, New Zealand, Sweden and Thailand, have recently implemented truly comprehensive tobacco control programmes embracing most or all of the WHO recommendations for comprehensive tobacco control. These countries join five others, Finland, Iceland, Norway, Portugal and Singapore, which had previously implemented comprehensive tobacco control programmes.

Australia: As a consequence of Australia's federal system of government, responsibility for tobacco control is split between the Federal and state governments, states bearing a large part of the responsibility. Accordingly, tobacco control measures are uneven in the country. With some variations, they have been implemented in the most populous states, which contain about 80% of the population, but have yet to be implemented in some of the more sparsely populated states. Victoria, South Australia and West Australia were the first to adopt comprehensive tobacco control policies. Together with measures adopted by the Federal Government, smoking control measures in Australia generally limit smoking in transport, public places, health-care facilities and Government buildings to a few smoking areas or ban it altogether. Strong health messages and mandatory tar and nicotine labelling are required on packs of cigarettes. Most forms of tobacco advertising, except at the point of purchase, are banned.

A notable feature of tobacco control in Australia is the creation of health promotion foundations, with the objective of replacing tobacco sponsorship of sports and cultural events by health promotion sponsorships. The foundations are well funded by special State-dedicated surtaxes on tobacco products. The idea was pioneered in the State of Victoria and emulated in other states. Education and promotional activates to encourage a smoke-free life have been considerably enhanced through various activities financed by these funds.

France: Information and education programmes about smoking have been intensified in France, as have smoking cessation programmes. Tobacco taxes were also recently increased. Importantly, France adopted a comprehensive tobacco control law in 1991. This law, which is being phased in and came fully into force in 1993, bans tobacco advertising, requires labelling of the composition of tobacco products and tar and nicotine yields, fixes maximum tar yields and requires strong health warnings on both the front and the back of the pack. Moreover, the law controls smoking in transport, public places and workplaces by either banning it altogether or limiting it to a few smoking areas. Tobacco consumption in France declined by 9% between 1991 and 1996.

New Zealand: Late in 1990, the New Zealand *Smoke-free Environments Act* came into force. This comprehensive tobacco control law bans most forms of tobacco advertising and requires varied health warnings and tar and nicotine labelling on cigarette packs. While existing tobacco sponsorships were permitted to run until 1993, the law also created the Health Sponsorship Council, funded from general revenues, to offer health promotion sponsorships to sports and cultural events in place of tobacco sponsorships. The law also requires all workplaces to adopt policies on smoking. While the law allows considerable latitude in the content of workplace smoking policies, a great many have now chosen to ban smoking entirely. The law also bans smoking in domestic flights and flights to Australia. Smoking is banned on intercity buses and restricted to a few smoking areas on trains. Similarly, smoking in many public places and health-care institutions is either banned or restricted to a few smoking areas. The law has been complemented by intense health promotion and health education campaigns in favour of a smoke-free life and several tax increases that have raised the price of cigarettes faster than the rate of inflation. New measures were adopted in 1997 further to restrict tobacco advertising and display of tobacco products at the point of sale.

Sweden Sweden began funding health education and health information campaigns on tobacco use as early as 1964. It was also one of the first countries to require rotating health warnings on cigarette packs, beginning in 1977. Regrettably, these were weakened when Sweden entered the European Union. A new *Tobacco Control Act* was adopted in 1994 restricting smoking in public places and workplaces, requiring health warnings on packs, setting maximum limits for tar and banning most forms of direct tobacco advertising; however, indirect advertising by the use of tobacco trade marks on non-tobacco goods and services is still permitted.

Thailand: It is especially noteworthy that Thailand has adopted a comprehensive tobacco control programme, because it has done so in the face of a large number of adverse factors. Thailand is a developing country with many other serious health problems that compete for priority. It both grows tobacco and manufactures tobacco products, and tobacco use is widespread. Moreover, Thailand, like its South-East Asian neighbours, was threatened with trade sanctions from the United States if the domestic market was not opened up to the import of American cigarettes. Unlike the Republic of

Korea and Japan, Thailand resisted this threat. Eventually the matter was resolved by a GATT panel which ruled that the ban on imports was not justified but that, in the interests of protecting public health, a panoply of other tobacco control measures could be undertaken. In accordance with the GATT ruling, the ban on imports of foreign cigarettes has been lifted, but public information campaigns against smoking have been intensified, and other smoking control measures have been consolidated into two new laws that are the keystones of a new comprehensive national tobacco control policy, including two new tobacco control laws.

The *Nonsmokers' Health Protection Act*, passed on 13 March 1992, came into force on 7 April 1992. It authorizes the Ministry of Public Health to designate certain public places as non-smoking areas. Owners of establishments that fail to designate such areas are liable to a fine, as are individuals who smoke in non-smoking areas. Regulations to designate non-smoking areas are under development in the Ministry of Public Health.

The *Tobacco Products Control Act*, also enacted on 13 March 1992 and brought into force on 6 August 1992, prohibits all forms of cigarette advertising and sales promotion, including free samples, price reductions and gift and coupon schemes. Tobacco product facsimiles are banned, as is the display of tobacco brand names on other products and in advertisements for other goods and services. Only telecasts from outside the country and foreign magazines are exempted from the ban. The *Act* and related regulations require very prominent rotating health warnings on cigarette packs. Manufacturers and importers are required to disclose the ingredients of tobacco products to the Ministry of Public Health. Sales through vending machines are prohibited, as are sales to persons under 18 years of age.

Government officials will nevertheless have to be especially vigilant to see that the new laws are respected. Five major importers are jostling for a share of Thailand's lucrative tobacco market. So far, legitimate imports are claiming 1–3% of the market, the Thai Tobacco Monopoly claims 90%, but imported contraband cigarettes continue to claim 7–9% of the market, despite increased enforcement efforts by the Excise Department. Smuggling continues because of differences in taxation between domestic and imported cigarettes. An excise tax of 55% of the retail price is applied to both, but an additional 30% of the retail price is due on imported cigarettes. For a time, in an effort to improve compliance, smugglers were fined 15 times the duty owing, even for a first offence. Enforcement officers were directly rewarded from the fines collected: once the fine was paid, 40% was returned to the Government, and 60% was awarded to informers and arresting officers. Now, enforcement officials in other departments will also have to ensure that the new restrictions on tobacco advertising and marketing and smoking in public places are respected. To the extent they are successful, Thailand may soon begin to enjoy the public health benefits that flow from declining tobacco consumption.

Countries with long-standing comprehensive tobacco control policies

Finland, Iceland, Norway, Portugal and Singapore all have comprehensive tobacco control policies that have been built up gradually since the 1970s by progressively adding or improving tobacco control measures. In the 1990s, measures to further improve protection from involuntary exposure to tobacco smoke were introduced in Finland, Norway and Singapore. Finland and Norway adopted new legislative provisions to clarify that existing bans on tobacco advertising also applied to indirect advertising.

Detailed examination of effectiveness of comprehensive tobacco control policies

By and large, the rates of tobacco consumption in countries with comprehensive tobacco control policies have been low and stable or are declining still further. In a detailed analysis of the effectiveness of advertising bans in four countries (Canada, Finland, New Zealand and Norway) (Department of Health, 1992), it was concluded that: "Though there are qualifications (for example, the bans in Canada and New Zealand are relatively recent and so may not yet have had their full impact), the current evidence available on these four countries indicates a significant effect. In each case the banning of advertising was followed by a fall in consumption which cannot reasonably be attributed to other factors." The same report also described year-to-year variations in tobacco advertising expenditures within countries and concluded, "The balance of evidence thus supports the conclusion that advertising does have a positive effect on consumption."

Country-by-country studies of tobacco control policies are encouraging but do not provide definitive evidence of the importance of comprehensive programmes in discouraging tobacco consumption. Trends in these countries illustrate the findings of Laugesen and Meads (1991) concerning the determinants of tobacco consumption in OECD countries.

Australia: Continuing declines in smoking prevalence have been noted in the three Australian states with the longest experience of comprehensive tobacco control programmes—Victoria, South Australia and West Australia, demonstrating the regression relationship observed by Laugesen and Meads. Proposals for new health warnings have been subjected to rigorous examination for effectiveness in Australia in a study partly financed by money from tobacco taxes through a state health promotion foundation (Centre for Behavioural Research in Cancer, 1992). The study showed that warnings could be effective at discouraging consumption if they were strong and varied, were prominently displayed at the top on the front of the pack and were accompanied by a more detailed, varied explanation of some of the health hazards of tobacco use on the back of the pack. The Australian Council of Health Ministers endorsed this report and recommended that states adopt laws or regulations in line with it. This has been done, and now Australia has some of the world's strongest and most effective health warnings on packs of cigarettes.

Canada: All indicators of tobacco consumption in Canada showed continuous declines throughout the 1980s and early 1990s. The strongest single-year declines in adult per capita consumption of cigarettes occurred in 1989 and 1990, the two years immediately following full implementation of Canada's comprehensive tobacco control policy. This indicator fell by about 6% in each of those two years. There were also declines in the prevalence of smoking, particularly among adolescents. While the overall smoking prevalence declined in Canada until 1993, the prevalence among adolescents fell faster. The prevalence of daily smoking by boys aged 15–19 declined from 43% in 1979 to 12% in 1991. Among girls it declined from 41% in 1979 to 20% in 1991. In 1994, when the tobacco taxes were reduced and cigarettes became cheaper, the prevalence increased again, especially among adolescents (Ontario Tobacco Research Unit, 1995).

New Zealand: New Zealand's new comprehensive tobacco control policies have been subject to careful evaluation by multiple regression techniques. The investigators concluded that one component of the comprehensive policy, the ban on tobacco advertising, caused a one-time, permanent 8% reduction in tobacco use (Laugesen *et al.*, 1992). In 1991, the year following passage of the *Smoke-Free Environments Act*, cigarette consumption per adult fell by 8.4% to 1791 cigarettes, a 71-year low and the second-lowest level among OECD countries. In the same year, the prevalence of smoking fell by 10%. There has been a strong cumulative effect of gradual improvement in New Zealand's comprehensive tobacco control policies as well. Adult per capita tobacco consumption declined by 36% between 1984 and 1991.

Summary

At least 10 countries now have comprehensive tobacco control policies of the sort recommended by the World Health Assembly (Laugesen & Meads, 1991; Department of Health, 1992). Through the use of econometric evaluation techniques, the effectiveness of such policies has been demonstrated for all OECD countries and for several individual countries that have implemented such policies. The positive experience of these countries with comprehensive tobacco control programmes and the repeated quantitative demonstrations of their effectiveness should be further encouragement to those countries that are currently contemplating their implementation.

Recent developments in international tobacco control

While most tobacco control measures are undertaken at the national level, there is also a need for action at the international level, if only to counterbalance the international activities of the few transnational tobacco companies that control most of the international trade in tobacco (United States Department of Health and Human Services, 1992). Three areas of activity that require attention have been identified—those of international non-governmental organizations, the United Nations and related organizations and international coordination with respect to tobacco advertising, pricing, taxation, trade and smuggling. No evaluations of activities in these areas have been undertaken. In fact, in most cases, only nascent activities have been identified. While international tobacco control activity has increased in recent years, there are still significant lacunae, notably in the area of international coordination of tobacco trade and taxation policies. The most promising new development is the call by the World Health Assembly for the WHO secretariat to undertake preparatory work leading to the creation of a international framework convention for tobacco control. The sections that follow are therefore necessarily confined to descriptive reports of activities under way, supplemented by some suggestions for possible strengthening of international tobacco control strategies in the future.

Activities of international non-governmental organizations

Between 1967 and 1994, nine world conferences on tobacco or health have been held under the auspices of coalitions of national and international non-governmental health organizations concerned about the serious health effects of tobacco use. These conferences have contributed a great deal to international understanding and international action for discouraging tobacco use. The Ninth World Conference on Tobacco or Health adopted a resolution calling on WHO to begin preparation of an international convention on tobacco control.

A small number of international non-governmental health organizations, such as the International Union against Tuberculosis and Lung Diseases and the International Union Against Cancer, have carried out anti-tobacco activities for years. The latter has been particularly active in this regard, with programmes spanning several decades of publications, regional seminars and major international meetings. Now, these two and many other organizations concerned with tobacco control have banded together to form the International Non-governmental Coalition against Tobacco, based in Paris, which has the potential to speak with a strong, united voice on behalf of all its member organizations in favour of international tobacco control.

Several regional coalitions of national health agencies concerned with tobacco or health issues have emerged, such as the Latin American Coordinating Committee on Smoking Control, the Asia–Pacific Association to Control Tobacco, the European Medical Action on Smoking and Health and the Arab Council on Anti-smoking. Many of them are effectively advocating increased tobacco control activities within their regions.

International tobacco control has also joined the computer age, with the establishment of an international computer network called Globalink that permits rapid worldwide communication among people who work in health agencies concerned with tobacco or health and who have access to computer communication facilities. Globalink operates from a World Wide Web site (URL: http://www-uicc.who.ch/; e-mail: israel@uicc.ch) and is an undertaking of the International Union against Cancer. This network has facilitated international tobacco control work. For example, a loose coalition of national health agencies united under the name 'Campaign for Smoke-free Skies Worldwide' made extensive use of Globalink to build up support in many countries for a ban on smoking on international passenger flights. Their work may well have contributed to the eventual adoption of a resolution by the International Civil Aviation Organization (ICAO, 1992) to ban smoking on international flights by 1996.

Activities of the United Nations and related organizations

The World Health Assembly first passed a resolution expressing concern about the serious health consequences of smoking in 1970 and has employed staff to encourage greater efforts to control the growth in tobacco use since that time. Successive resolutions of the Health Assembly have expressed increasing levels of concern about this problem and have culminated in calls for comprehensive national tobacco control policies and programmes. Over the years, WHO has sought to involve its sister United Nations organizations in an effort to discourage tobacco use. This has included calls for other organizations to join in the celebration of World No-Tobacco Day, and to follow the example of WHO by banning smoking in the workplace. There has been widespread support for the former request and more limited support for the latter. Many United Nations organizations have restricted smoking in the workplace to some extent, but more and more are moving towards greater restrictions. The former Secretary-General, Mr Kofi Annan, called for a smoke-free United Nations by the end of 1997.

During the 1970s, the Food and Agricultural Organization (FAO) and the World Bank encouraged the development of tobacco cultivation and manufacture in developing countries as a worthwhile economic development strategy. These policies were at cross-purposes with those of WHO, however, and increased collaboration between those agencies and WHO over the years has led them to recognize that any short-term economic benefit to be gained from increased tobacco production will be more than outweighed by serious long-term public health damage and the consequent long-term economic disadvantage. As a result, neither FAO nor the World Bank pursues tobacco agricultural development strategies any longer. In fact, the World Bank has issued an explicit policy statement to that effect (World Bank, 1991).

In 1992, the World Health Assembly requested that the Economic and Social Council (ECOSOC) of the United Nations discuss the subject of tobacco or health and call for appropriate follow-up within the United Nations General Assembly and organizations of the United Nations (World Health Organization, 1992). A 1993 ECOSOC resolution created the United Nations Focal Point on Tobacco, housed in the United Nations Conference on Trade and Development (UNCTAD), which has been instrumental in encouraging greater coordination of tobacco and health policies among offices and agencies of the United Nations and movement towards adoption of smoke-free workplace policies throughout the United Nations system. UNCTAD (1995) has examined the prospects of substitution of tobacco by other crops in a number of countries where tobacco is grown. Another example of highly successful collaboration is that between WHO and ICAO, which resulted in the ban on smoking on all international passenger flights by 1 July 1996. Even if the resolution has not been completely implemented, smoke-free international flights are now offered by a growing number of airlines, many more than if the resolution had not been adopted.

International coordination of tobacco control activities with respect to tobacco advertising, pricing, taxation, trade and smuggling

In a shrinking world, where international communication, travel and the distribution of culture, ideas, services and goods becomes easier and more frequent, tobacco products and tobacco use are spreading much faster than the measures needed to curb their use. This international development is aided in no small measure by the efficient, businesslike approach of the transnational tobacco companies. When States do propose action to control tobacco advertising or the use of tobacco in public places and workplaces, the tobacco industry is able to respond quickly through its well-developed international structures, such as the Tobacco Documentation Centre in London, to provide effective opposition to such measures. Through such international coordination, the same or similar opposition tactics, arguments, documents and even hired consultants have appeared in places as diverse and far-flung as Canada, Hong Kong, Indonesia, Mauritius,

New Zealand, Sri Lanka and Switzerland. Public health agencies cannot match the industry with international structures, coordination or strategies in favour of tobacco control measures. Despite well-orchestrated opposition from the international tobacco industry, many States have succeeded in adopting comprehensive tobacco control measures, but many more might well do so if there were a more effective counterweight to the international lobbying of the tobacco companies.

There is now a possibility that such a truly effective counterweight can be created in the not-too-distant future. In January 1996, the WHO Executive Board recommended that the Health Assembly adopt a resolution calling on the Director-General to initiate the development of an international framework convention for tobacco control in accordance with Article 19 of the WHO Constitution (World Health Organization, 1996b). Should the World Health Assembly adopt such a resolution, it would mark the first use of that Article, which authorizes the adoption of conventions, and it would be the first international convention adopted by WHO. Before making its recommendation to the World Health Assembly, the Executive Board carefully considered a feasibility study on the subject that had been requested by the Health Assembly, with an antecedent in a resolution adopted by the Ninth World Conference on Tobacco and Health.

As most public health workers are unlikely to be familiar with the concept of an international framework convention, the following questions and answers have been designed to increase understanding of how such a document could contribute to strengthening global tobacco control.

What is an international framework convention?

It is a legal instrument in the form of an international treaty in which the signatory States agree to pursue broadly stated goals, in this case on international tobacco control.

How does a framework convention work?

A framework convention, unlike other more detailed treaties, does not try to resolve all the substantive issues in a single document; rather, it breaks the problem down into more manageable segments. States first adopt a framework convention that calls for cooperation in achieving broadly stated goals, allowing for the possibility that the parties to the convention will conclude separate protocols containing specific measures concerning each of the goals stated in the framework protocol.

What could be the content of a framework convention for tobacco control?

The final answer to this question will depend on what the States which sign the convention choose to include. Nevertheless, one broadly stated goal could be to move progressively towards implementation of comprehensive tobacco control strategies that include the measures referred to in previous Health Assembly resolutions and other appropriate measures. Separate protocols (more detailed forms of international sub agreements) could break down the lists of elements in comprehensive tobacco control programmes into more manageable segments and develop separate plans and timetables for moving progressively towards the implementation of each segment. The protocols could probably be most usefully organized by degree of comprehensiveness, ranging from mild to sweeping and complete. States need only sign the protocols that can feasibly be implemented in their country.

Why is an international framework convention needed?

In theory, States can implement comprehensive tobacco control on their own. In practice, only a few have done so. The planning, scheduling and international information-sharing that accompany the development of an international convention will all help and encourage States to strengthen their national tobacco control policies. In addition, a framework convention is a useful tool for promoting international cooperation and coordination of supra-national aspects of tobacco control that can be addressed only through international cooperation. Because many elements of national tobacco control programmes can be affected by what is going on in other countries, international instruments can be used to move towards better international control— and greater public health effectiveness—with respect to at least the following issues:

Tobacco smuggling: Recorded world cigarette exports currently exceed imports by about 300 million cigarettes, implying that up to 6% of world cigarette production is smuggled from one country to another to avoid cigarette taxes. It has been estimated that cigarette smuggling results in global losses of tax revenue totalling US$ 16 thousand million annually (Joossens & Raw, 1995). There is ample evidence that tobacco smuggling is a growing problem. Recorded world exports of cigarettes exceeded recorded imports by 175 thousand million cigarettes in 1990 (Kaiserman & Ducharme-Danielson, 1992). By 1994, this excess had grown to 280 thousand million cigarettes, and was still growing (United States Department of Agriculture, 1995). In the Americas, tobacco smuggling 'hot spots' that have been identified include smuggling from the United States into Canada in a triangular arrangement among Paraguay, Uruguay and Argentina, from various sources into Colombia and from Surinam into Guyana (Pan American Health Organization, 1992). Many others exist around the world.

Tobacco advertising: Bans or restrictions on tobacco advertising in one country can be undermined by advertising spillover from other countries. Formula One race cars have become the world's première vehicle for international tobacco advertising. Via television, the tobacco advertisements they display race around the world at far higher speeds than the cars race around the tracks. They race right into people's homes, even in countries that have national bans on tobacco advertising. National law is no match for tobacco advertising as it moves at warp speed through international channels of telecommunication.

Duty-free sales of tobacco: Current international agreements on duty-free sales should be reconsidered in the light of the serious health consequences of tobacco use. Cigarette taxes can be legitimately avoided by travellers who purchase cigarettes in duty-free locations in international transit. In addition, duty-free outlets are a potential source of contraband cigarettes. They may be purchased legitimately and later smuggled by unscrupulous operators. In these circumstances, some international collaboration and coordination would be beneficial in providing public health surveillance and monitoring of cigarette duty-free sales and in taking coordinated international action as needed to control this problem; however, no such action is currently under way.

Tobacco pricing and taxation: International harmonization of tobacco prices and taxes at high levels would do much to discourage tobacco use and to ensure that high-price policies for tobacco products would not be undermined by smuggling from nearby low-price jurisdictions. Tighter controls are needed to ensure that taxes due are actually collected.

Reporting of production, sales, imports and exports of tobacco products: Improved standards of international reporting on the production and sales of tobacco products would facilitate international monitoring of this epidemic.

Testing and reporting of toxic constituents: Improved, more effective international standards for the testing and reporting of toxic constituents of tobacco products and tobacco smoke would facilitate monitoring of the hazards of tobacco products.

Policy and programme information sharing: More effective sharing of information among nations about the state of their national tobacco control legislation and programmes would help improve both national and international tobacco control.

What would be the role of the United Nations Focal Point on Tobacco?
Tobacco use is a major public health problem, but most of the solutions are to be found outside the health sector, by addressing issues of agriculture, trade, taxation, advertising, pack labelling, personnel management and many others. The Focal Point could play a key role in seeking the cooperation of other parts of the United Nations system in the development and operation of a framework convention.

Future directions

In theory, as more nations gain experience with strengthening their tobacco control programmes, thereby providing more successful examples of policy implementation strategies to other nations that are still considering such policy initiatives, examples of comprehensive tobacco control programmes and policies should increase in both number and effectiveness. Better coordination at the international level should also enhance policy development.

Tobacco control efforts are often slowed or blocked by tobacco interests that view such policies as a threat to continued growth of the tobacco industry. The development of effective tobacco control policies are met by increased efforts to retard their implementation. Greater effort will therefore be required to maintain steady progress towards improvements in global tobacco control.

The creation of an international framework convention on tobacco control is exactly the kind of greater effort that will be required. WHO plans to present a draft convention to the World Health Assembly for consideration early in the next decade. Background papers have been written, and more are planned. One organizational meeting has been held, and meetings of experts and representatives of Member States are planned. WHO has received some technical and financial support for this work from a few Member States, but more resources will be needed if the objectives of preparing a framework convention and related protocols that will be effective and widely supported are to be realized.

Multinational tobacco companies are strong; they have money and power, and they are a threat to global public health. But the forces of public health are strong too; we also have our own multinational corporation—the World Health Organization—and WHO has a card that the tobacco industry does not have. With considerable help from its Member States, from non-governmental orgnizations and from other institutions, groups and individuals, WHO can now draft an international public health law that will help slow the progress of the tobacco epidemic.

References

Centre for Behavioural Research in Cancer (1992) *Health Warnings and Contents Labelling on Tobacco Products*, Carlton South, Victoria

Department of Health (1992) *Effect of Tobacco Advertising on Tobacco Consumption: A Discussion Document Reviewing the Evidence*, Economics and Operational Research Division,, London

International Civil Aviation Organization (1992) *Smoking Restrictions on International Passenger Flights*. Resolution adopted 8 October 1992, Montreal:

Joossens, L. & Raw, M. (1995) Smuggling and cross border shopping of tobacco in Europe. *Br. Med. J.*, **310**, 1393–1397

Kaiserman, M.J. & Ducharme-Danielson, C. (1992) Global per capita consumption of manufactured cigarettes, 1990. *Chronic Dis. Canada*, **13**, 72–74

Laugesen, M. & Meads, C. (1991) Tobacco advertising restrictions, price, income and tobacco consumption in OECD countries, 1960-86. *Br. J. Addict.*, **86**, 1343–1354

Laugesen, M., Meads, C. & Scott, G. (1992) Why New Zealanders smoke less: Econometric and policy analysis of the effects of advertising ban legislation and taxation. Paper presented at the Eighth World Conference on Tobacco or Health, Buenos Aires, Argentina

Ontario Tobacco Research Unit (1995) Tax cuts undermine OTS. *Tobacco Res. News*, **2**, 1

Pan American Health Organization (1992) *Tobacco or Health: Status in the Americas* (Scientific Publication No. 536), Washington DC

United Nations Conference on Trade and Development (1995) *Economic role of tobacco production and exports in countries depending on tobacco as a major source of income* (UNCTAD Technical Report)

United States Department of Agriculture (1995) *Tobacco: World Markets and Trade* (No. FT 8-95), Washington DC

United States Department of Health and Human Services (1992) *Smoking and Health in the Americas* (DHHS Publication No. (CDC) 92-8419), Atlanta, Georgia: Public Health Service, Centers for Disease Control, National Centre for Chronic Disease Prevention and Health Promotion, Office on Smoking and Health
World Health Organization (1996a) Advisory kit for World No-Tobacco Day, 31 May 1997: United for a tobacco- free world. *Tobacco Alert*, 4,
World Health Organization (1996b) EB97.R8: An international framework convention for tobacco control, Resolution of the Executive Board of WHO, 97th Session
World Bank (1991) *Policy on Tobacco*. Washington DC

The World Health Organization and a framework convention–protocol approach to global tobacco control

A.L. Taylor

Columbia University School of Law, New York City, New York, United States

In 1996 the World Health Assembly authorized the development of a powerful new international regulatory strategy for global tobacco control (Taylor & Roemer, 1996). In particular, the Health Assembly adopted a historic resolution calling upon the Director-General of the World Health Organization (WHO):

(i)   to initiate the development of a framework convention in accordance with Article 19 of the WHO Constitution;

(ii) to include as part of the framework convention a strategy to encourage member nations to move progressively towards the adoption of comprehensive tobacco control policies, and also to deal with aspects of tobacco control that transcend national boundaries.... (World Health Organization, 1996).

As Professor Roemer described in her presentation, the framework convention–protocol approach prescribed by WHO in 1996 could have an important impact on global tobacco control efforts. Professor Roemer and I first presented the idea that WHO should adopt the framework convention–protocol approach to tobacco control in a background document prepared for WHO's Executive Board in 1995 (Taylor, 1994; Taylor & Roemer, 1996). I shall briefly describe international precedents for global tobacco control efforts and mechanisms that could be used by WHO and Member States to initiate support and action on international tobacco control instruments.

International precedents for a framework convention–protocol approach to global tobacco control

The framework convention–protocol approach is a dynamic, continuous model of international standard-setting that has been used frequently and, at times, successfully by other international organizations to secure international agreement and action, particularly in the environmental field. An early instance was the 1979 Convention on the Conservation of Migratory Species of Wild Animals (1979). In the most celebrated use of this method, the United Nations Environment Programme (UNEP) fostered broad political consensus among nations for measures to reduce the depletion of the ozone layer, resulting in the Vienna Convention for the Protection of the Ozone Layer (1985), the Montreal Protocol (1987) and the London Amendments to the Montreal Protocol (1990). A number of other international and regional agreements are patterned on this convention–protocol format, including the 1992 Framework Convention on Climate Change (Intergovernmental Negotiating Committee for a Framework Convention on Climate Change, 1992) and the 1979 Convention on Long-range Transboundary Air Pollution Economic Commission for Europe, 1979).

The ability of multilateral environmental institutions to encourage and assist nations in overcoming powerful, organized industry resistance to regulation through this dynamic international regulatory strategy shows the important role that international standard-setting can play in efforts to regulate the activities of the transnational tobacco conglomerates. For example, the International Maritime Organization, through the formation of a powerful coalition of States, has assisted nations to overcome the resistance of influential oil and shipping interests and to foster international agreement and action on measures to overcome marine pollution through a number of international conventions (International Convention for the Prevention of Oil Pollution from Ships, 1973; International Convention on Oil Pollution, Preparedness, Response and Cooperation, 1990). Overall experience in the United Nations system demonstrates that the dynamics of international negotiation and coalition pressures can encourage and assist nations in overriding powerful and organized industry resistance to costly and restrictive regulation (e.g. Kildow, 1994).

The successful international lawmaking efforts of other international organizations can serve as a precedent, a model and a guide in WHO's efforts to achieve international agreement and action on tobacco control. Although WHO may not be able to mirror the success achieved in a number of international environmental conventions, it can still play an important role in assisting States to contain the tobacco pandemic by stimulating national policy change through the international law-making process. The process of seeking international agreement on tobacco control standards can encourage nations to adopt and implement effective national measures to contain the tobacco epidemic by educating and informing national leaders, by expanding global concern and by increasing the political, technical and financial capacity of States to adjust their domestic policy. Although this legislative prescription may not lead to a smoke-free world, the development of an international framework convention–protocol regulatory strategy may be a reasonable and politically achievable approach to progressive implementation of standards to prevent the further spread of the pandemic.

Implementation of framework convention and protocols on global tobacco control

To ensure that the proposed framework convention and protocols are not purely symbolic, WHO and Member States must establish effective mechanisms to overcome some nations' incapacity or apathy and other governments' resistance to regulation. Although WHO must ultimately look to States to adopt and implement international commitments, it can generate means and incentives that change the balancing of national interests and encourage compliance with the international instruments. Using the experience of other international organizations, this paper outlines some of the specific strategies that could be used by WHO to encourage national implementation of international instruments.

Establishment of an international tobacco control trust fund: International financial arrangements are essential for implementing an international tobacco control instrument. Appropriate funding is crucial for the least developed nations, for training personnel in tobacco control strategies, for funding urgently needed crop-substitution programmes and for supporting monitoring. Existing international financial models provide a starting point for designing a new global financial regime to support international instruments on tobacco control. One paradigm is provided by the London Amendments to the Montreal Protocol which established a US\$ 240 million multilateral trust fund to assist developing nations to meet their obligations under the Protocol. As a further example, the World Bank established the Global Environmental Facility as a general fund to aid developing nations to address environmental problems.

International monitoring and supervisory systems: Multilateral surveillance of the implementation of State obligations is a powerful mechanism for ensuring that nations give appropriate and adequate attention to their international commitments. Disclosure and discussion of sub-standard national efforts in an international arena can put pressure on governments to increase their efforts to comply with their obligations. In addition, a reporting process can help identify problems that nations have in meeting their tobacco control obligations and trigger international technical and financial assistance.

International human rights law and international environmental law provide numerous examples of effective supervisory institutions. Various approaches are used to international surveillance of multilateral commitments. One common approach in treaties is a system of periodic national reporting. This strategy requires participating States to submit reports to independent committees on measures that have been taken and progress that has been made in implementing international commitments. Experience with reporting systems in the human rights committees of the United Nations indicates that the reports submitted by State parties can help to promote national compliance with international obligations if the reports are subject to critical evaluation by independent committees that have access to input from non-governmental sources ((e.g. Taylor, 1997). On the basis of favourable experience with auditing and reporting systems, an institutionalized monitoring system can be incorporated in the context of the framework convention or succeeding protocols to encourage national implementation of tobacco control obligations.

Role of other international organizations and non-governmental organizations in an international regulatory strategy for global tobacco control: Collaboration among a wide range of international organizations will be required for the effective implementation of international instruments on tobacco control. Other international agencies can assist WHO's efforts by promoting the support of their constituencies for appropriate tobacco control policies, national legislation, economic and agricultural policies and specific protocols on tobacco control as they develop. Effective collaboration with non-governmental organizations will also be critical for the success of this strategy, in encouraging nations to adopt and implement tobacco control instruments. Such organizations can highlight the importance of global tobacco control measures and influence nations to adopt and implement international instruments. Their participation will also be central for effective monitoring of national compliance.

Establishment of an international communications strategy: In order to transform the international regulatory approach into an effective strategy that can influence national behaviour, it is essential to generate and magnify public and media attention about the importance of international cooperation and action on tobacco control. Cultivating public support for national and multilateral action and publicizing nations' compliance and non-compliance with the rule of law have been key ingredients in the successful law-making activities of other international organizations. For example, UNEP's achievements in securing multilateral agreement on environmental matters can be attributed largely to its vigorous efforts to rouse public awareness and support for global agreement. UNEP's success in persuading nations to develop and comply with international standards is based, in part, on wide dissemination of scientific information that affirms the need for global action and extensive publicity on national compliance with UNEP-sponsored treaties (e.g. Haas, 1991; Taylor, 1992).

The tobacco industry has a massive war chest for funding advertising and promotion, the most powerful weapons in its campaign to increase global tobacco consumption. Tobacco is the most heavily advertised product in the world, and the tobacco conglomerates are among the most sophisticated of all corporate marketers, widely recognized for using deceptive marketing practices. In order to encourage nations to adopt and implement effective international tobacco control instruments, policy-makers must take measures to counteract the marketing prowess of the tobacco industry by developing an effective communications strategy to educate and inform the world community about the importance of global tobacco control and the contribution that international instruments can make to it. Multiple communications strategies involving myriad channels, including non-governmental organizations and other international organizations, must be developed in order to build global public support for coordinated, multilateral approaches to tobacco control. The pivotal role of an international communications strategy is highlighted by the fact that the World Health Assembly's call for an international legislative framework for tobacco control has thus far received limited public or media attention.

References

Amendment to the Montreal Protocol on Substances that Deplete the Ozone Layer, 29 June 1990. *Int. Law M.*, **30**, 537, 541

Convention on the Conservation of Migratory Species of Wild Animals, 23 June 1979. *Int. Law M.*, **19**, 11

Economic Commission for Europe (1979) Convention on Long-range Transboundary Air Pollution. *Int. Law M.*, **18**, 1446

Haas, P.M. (1991) *Int. Environ. Issues*, **39**

Intergovernmental Negotiating Committee for a Framework Convention on Climate Change (1992) United Nations Doc. A/AC.237/18 (Part II)/Add.1, New York: United Nations

International Convention on Oil Pollution, Preparedness, Response and Cooperation, 20 November 1990. *Int. Law M.*, **30**, 735

International Convention for the Prevention of Oil Pollution from Ships, 2 November 1973. *Int. Law M.*, **12**, 1319

Kildow, J.T. (1994) The impact of international environmental treaties and agreements on corporate strategy. In: Urbani, E., *et al.*, eds, *Transnational Environmental Law and its Impact on Corporate Behavior*, pp. 281, 295

Montreal Protocol on Substances that Deplete the Ozone Layer, 16 September 1987. *Int. Law M.*, **26**, 1550

Taylor, A.L. (1992) Making the World Health Organization work: A legal framework for universal to the conditions for health. *Am. J. Law Med.*, **18**, 301, 335–338

Taylor, A.L. (1994) International legislation to control the tobacco pandemic, paper presented at the Ninth World Conference on Tobacco or Health, Paris

Taylor, A.L. (1996) An international strategy for global tobacco control. *Yale J. Int. Law*, **21**, 257

Taylor, A.L. (1997) Controlling the global spread of infectious disease: Toward a reinforced role for the international health regulations. *Houston Law Rev.*, **33**, 1327, 1352–1362

Taylor, A.L. & Roemer, R. (1996) *An International Strategy for Global Tobacco Control* (WHO Doc. PSA/96.6), Geneva: World Health Organization

Vienna Convention for the Protection of the Ozone Layer, 22 March 1985. *Int. Law M.*, **26**, 1516

World Health Organization (1996) *International Framework Convention for Tobacco Control*, WHA. Res. 49.17, Geneva

Understanding the role of governments in global tobacco control

P. Jha, T.E. Novotny & R.G.A. Feachem

Human Development Network, The World Bank, Washington DC, United States

Abstract

Relatively little has been written about the appropriate roles of governments in tobacco control. Using economics and public policy and public health theories, we examine why governments should intervene in tobacco control, and what they should do. We then review key government roles that: (i) increase information for individuals on tobacco by banning tobacco advertising and promotion on tobacco goods, trademarks and logos; by increasing research on the causes, consequences and costs of tobacco products and by promoting public information and media campaigns, including serious warning labels on tobacco products; (ii) raise the cost of smoking through taxation and regulation; (iii) spend limited public funds on the most effective and cost-effective tobacco control interventions; (iv) develop global and regional taxation and regulatory approaches, including control of smuggling.

Why should governments intervene to reduce tobacco consumption?

Governments have several responsibilities, including providing information, taking actions that others (individuals or the voluntary and private sectors) cannot or will not take, and protecting the poor. In addition, governments have the responsibility to promote good health—both because it is important in itself and because it contributes to economic development (World Bank, 1993). Tobacco use is incompatible with good health.

There is little doubt that tobacco will become the leading cause of death in the world within two or three decades. The numbers of deaths expected on the basis of current smoking patterns are staggering. Peto and others estimate that about 500 million people who were alive in 1990 will die from from causes such as heart attacks, strokes, lung cancer, chronic respiratory disease and other cancers, due to tobacco (Peto *et al.*, 1994). Of these, 200–300 million will be today's children and adolescents. Of great relevance to developing countries is the fact that at least one half of these deaths occur in middle age (35–69), a time of great productivity and social importance in all societies.

Economics of tobacco use

Most smokers start early in life—as adolescents or children—when they have imperfect information on the risks. As they grow older, they lose some (but not all) of their ability to quit, because of addiction. Most adult smokers say that they wish they had never started (Department of Health and Human Services, 1989). For several reasons, people and governments seriously underestimate the risks of tobacco use (Table 1; Department of Health and Human Services, 1989; Zatonski, 1996). In addition, tobacco use may impose social costs on others, although this not fully clear (Warner *et al.*, 1995).

Issues of equity

The burden of tobacco-related disease is highest among the poor in most countries. In established market economies, the disparities between rich and poor in the prevalence of smoking have widened. In Norway, the prevalence was 75% among high-income males and 60% among low-income males in 1955 and had fallen to 28 and 40%, respectively, by 1990 (Lund *et al.*, 1995). In Brazil, China and India, the prevalence of tobacco use is already higher among the poor (World Bank). The poor have higher death rates from tobacco-attributable diseases, lower access to and use of preventive information and fewer curative health services. Tobacco-attributable deaths among adults cause adverse outcomes in children, especially those in poor households, by increasing poverty (World Bank, 1993).

What should governments do to reduce tobacco consumption?

The aim of government actions should be to create an environment in which tobacco users fully understand the risks and pay a sufficiently high price for tobacco use and in which the poor are protected. The principal tools are information, price and regulation.

Table 1. Low valuation of risks of tobacco use in the United States and Poland

Rank	Habit (United States)	Percentage	Habit (Poland)
1	Never drive after drinking	62	Environment
2	Air quality	55	Dietary habits
3	Water quality	45	Stress, hectic lifestyle
4	Domestic fire detectors	27	**Tobacco smoking**
5	Body weight	25	Genetics
6	Annual blood pressure measurement	24	Sports, physical activity
7	Control stress		
8	Vitamins and minerals		
9	Exercise		
10	**Not smoking**		
11	Have friends		
12	Good genes		

United States (Department of Health and Human Services, 1989): A 1993 Harris poll of 1254 adults asked what 'helps people in general to live a long and healthy life' (1 = most, 12 = less perceived importance).
Poland (Zatonski, 1996): A 1995 representative poll of 1391 Poles aged ≥ 15 asked what were 'the most important factors influencing human health'

Increase information on tobacco use: Information should be provided in three forms: complete bans on advertising and promotion of tobacco products, trademarks, logos and associated symbols; research on causes, consequences and costs of tobacco use; and public information campaigns, including serious health warnings on tobacco products (Department of Health and Human Services, 1989). In regions where the tobacco-attributable mortality rate will be highest in absolute numbers within the next few decades, there is no direct evidence for the absolute and relative risks due to tobacco (Department of Health and Human Services, 1989; World Health Organization, 1996a; Table 2). Priorities for research include studies on the determinants of tobacco use and reduction (information, income and price, including taxation) and the impact on consumption of advertising and promotion, smuggling, trade and tobacco industry lobbying. Over the past few years, investment in research and development on tobacco control amounted to US$ 50 per death in 1990 (a total of US$ 148–164 million). In contrast, research and development on HIV received about US$ 3000 per death in 1990 (a total of US$ 919–985 million). Spending on both diseases is highest in developed countries (World Health Organization, 1996a).

Raise the costs of smoking: Taxation is arguably the most effective tool of any type for controlling tobacco use. A 10% increase in tobacco prices will reduce consumption by 4–6% and by even larger amounts among children and lower-income groups. Townsend (1996) suggests that a 63% increase in cigarette prices by the year 2000 in the United Kingdom would decrease the number of cigarettes smoked per adult by about 34%. Many countries, including South Africa and the United States, have allowed tax rates to erode with inflation, thus reducing their effect on health outcomes. Governments should use a combination of specific taxes and ad-valorum taxes to discourage consumption of various types of tobacco products, and not simply encourage switching to lower-priced brands (Townsend, 1996). Increasing tax rates reduces consumption and, in the short to medium term, increases government revenue. A recent World Bank report on financing health services in China suggested that a 10% additional tax on tobacco could reduce consumption by 5% while generating an additional 4.5% increase in revenue. This extra revenue would cover more than a third of the incremental funds needed for provision of basic health services for China's poorest 100 million inhabitants (World Bank, 1996).

Spend public funds on the most effective and cost-effective tobacco control interventions: Policy-based control efforts such as price increases, advertising and promotion bans and mass media counter-advertising are as cost-effective as childhood

Table 2. Gaps in data sources for estimated tobacco-attributable mortality

Region	Tobacco-attributable mortality rate in 2020 (percent of world total)	Vital registration in 1990 (percent coverage)	Representative epidemiological evidence on tobacco in 1997
China	27	Limited[a]	Limited retrospective and prospective
India	18	Limited[b] going prospective	Limited and on-
Established market economies	15	99	Retrospective and prospective
Former socialist economies	13	99	Indirect, ongoing retrospective
Middle East	10	22	None
Other Asia and Islands	8	10	None
Latin America	5	43	None
Sub-Saharan Africa	4	1	None

From Peto *et al.* (1994); World Health Organization (1996a) and Richard Peto, personal communication)
[a] Data based on a sample registration system covering 10 million people
[b] Data based on an urban registration system and a survey of rural causes of death

immunization. Policy-based programmes cost about US$ 20–80 per discounted year of life saved (World Bank). The World Bank's *World Development Report* for 1993, *Investing in Health*, suggested that tobacco control policies be included in a minimum package of publicly-financed health services. In contrast, individual smoking cessation programmes are less cost-effective.

Develop global and regional taxation and regulatory approaches: Taxation should be directed to minimizing price differentials in order to discourage smuggling between countries. Smuggling is a major problem, constituting 5% of global cigarette production and 30% of global cigarette trade. The tobacco industry has effectively argued for reduced tax rates to decrease smuggling (World Health Organization, 1996b). Smuggling also exerts pressure on governments to lower tax rates, which will increase consumption. The proper response to smuggling should be to harmonize prices and to improve enforcement by customs and tax officials, including use of tax stamps and warnings in local languages.

Symmetrical regulation mandates policies that apply to all types of tobacco products without prejudice to the source of production. China, Germany, Japan and the United States account for one-half of global cigarette production. Limiting one country's supply abroad may not reduce demand, as smokers may switch to other brands. For example, Brazil and China have sharply increased cigarette exports in recent years. In some countries, such as China and France, state-owned tobacco companies generate substantial revenues (World Health Organization, 1996b).

Finally, it is imperative to target tobacco control efforts where the problem is largest. This involves government investments in low- and middle-income countries to study and monitor the epidemic of tobacco and to promote effective control. The governments of established market economies should identify ways of providing financial and technical resources to such research. 'Tobacco or health' units are needed in every country, and these should have expertise in fiscal, trade and regulatory polices and a strong analytical and policy-oriented public health capacity.

References

Department of Health and Human Services (1989) *Reducing the Health Consequences of Smoking: 25 Years of Progress. A Report of the Surgeon General* (DHHS Publication No. (CDC) 89-8411), Public Health Service, Centers for Disease Control, Center for Chronic Disease Prevention and Health Promotion, Office on Smoking and Health

Lund, K.E., Roenneberg, A. & Hafstad, A. (1995) The social and demographic diffusion of the tobacco epidemic in Norway. In: Slama, K., ed., *Tobacco and Health*, New York: Plenum Press, pp. 565–571

Peto, R., Lopez, A.D., Boreham, J., Thun, M. & Heath, C. Jr (1994) *Mortality from Smoking in Developed Countries 1950–2000*, New York: Oxford University Press

Townsend. J. (1996) Price and consumption of tobacco. *Br. Med. Bull.*, **52**, 132–142

Warner, K., Chaloupka, F.J., Cook, P.J., *et al.* (1995) Criteria for determining an optimal cigarette tax: The economist perspective. *Tob. Control*, **4**, 380–386

World Bank (1993) *The World Development Report 1993: Investing in Health*, New York: Oxford University Press

World Bank (1996) *China: Issues and Options in Health Financing* (World Bank Report No. 15278-CHA), Washington DC

World Health Organization (1996a) *Investing in Health Research and Development. Report of the Ad Hoc Committee on Health Research Relating to Future Intervention Options* (Document TDR/Gen/96.1), Geneva: World Health Organization

World Health Organization (1996b) Tobacco industry. *Tob. Alert*, Special Issue, pp. 12–16

Zatonski, W. (1996) *Evolution of Health in Poland since 1988*, Warsaw: Marie Skeodowska-Curie Cancer Center and Institute of Oncology, Department of Epidemiology and Cancer Prevention

Stages of change: Moving countries towards comprehensive tobacco policies and programmes

B. Zolty

World Health Organization, Geneva, Switzerland

Today, about 9000 people around the world will die because of tobacco use. This will happen tomorrow and each day thereafter. Unless the situation changes dramatically, in another two or three decades, tobacco products will kill around 10 million people each year, with 70% of those deaths occurring in developing countries. The World Health Organization (WHO) has been involved in a series of activities to help countries move towards comprehensive tobacco control policies and programmes. One project focuses on strengthening tobacco control in countries of central and eastern Europe, largely because of the remarkably high rates of mortality that tobacco causes in this region: In 1995, 700 000 deaths in the former socialist economies were caused by tobacco, or about 25% of the world total.

WHO teams visited a number of central and eastern European countries in an attempt to help them move towards comprehensive tobacco control polices and programmes. A number of common themes and issues emerged from these consultations, and we hope that the lessons learnt and the strategies initiated will be applicable in other regions. In the vast majority of countries, various departments, organizations and individuals were knowledgeable and keenly interested in tobacco control, although there was often a lack of coordination and communication. When facing the strength of the tobacco industry, such coordination is essential.

Coordination and communication can be improved by appointing a tobacco control focal person who has the full support of the Ministry of Health and establishing an intersectoral coordinating committee, composed of key players from both governmental and non-governmental organizations This committee has the responsibility for developing and implementing country-based action plans on tobacco, with specific targets and timetables for implementation.

Multi-sector support: Finding allies

While there is often little communication between ministries of health and other sectors, there are key departments outside health ministries that can provide essential support if real change is to occur. Ministries or departments of finance, taxation, industry and customs all play crucial roles in tobacco control. For example, the Ministry of Health may need to convince other departments of the long-term dangers of accepting highly attractive investment from multinational tobacco companies.

In order to counter the influence of the tobacco industry on governments, it is important to be aware of it and expose it where possible. Working with the media to bring these issues to public attention is also important. It is useful to learn how the tobacco industry works, particularly with regard to foreign investment. Competing priorities often relegate health promotion and prevention to the bottom of the list. The best way to counteract this is to show the cost-effectiveness of tobacco control. Although data are available from the World Bank, local data are even more powerful.

Stages of change

One of the most important themes that emerged from our missions was that countries are at different stages of action for tobacco control. This must be considered by tobacco control workers both within a country and in organizations that offer support to move countries towards a tobacco-free society, no matter what stage a country is at.

The trans-theoretical model of change is a model of behavioural change presented by Prochaska and DiClemente in 1982. It is still widely used to help individuals to stop smoking. The premise is that individuals go through various stages before they finally quit smoking: pre-contemplation, contemplation, preparation, action and maintenance. This model can also be applied on a collective level. Just as the interventions offered to individual smokers differ according to the stage the smoker is at, health workers can benefit from taking stock of the stage of a country is in the continuum of behavioural change. Although there may be individuals and organizations within a country who are knowledgable and committed to tobacco control, within this model it is useful to consider the readiness of a country as a whole, particularly at the highest levels of government, the Ministry of Health and the general public.

This approach is likely to increase the cost-effectiveness of tobacco control interventions, which is particularly important when resources are scarce. For example, detailed expertise in drafting anti-tobacco legislation is crucial for countries in the action stage, but a waste of resources for those countries still at pre-contemplation, which are most in need of basic health information to motivate action. Matching interventions to the appropriate stage also enhances movement through the stages, which in the long term may shorten the time it takes to attain tobacco-free societies. Although space does not allow a discussion of all of the stages, several examples are presented from the model.

Individual smokers in the pre-contemplation stage are not seriously thinking about making changes in their smoking habit in the foreseeable future; they are likely to be under-informed about the health risks, demoralized about their inability to change or defensive and resistant to change. At the collective level in this stage, ministers of health and other government leaders do not consider tobacco control to be a priority, there is high level of smoking, especially among doctors, no or little tobacco control legislation and smoking in public places is widely accepted. Countries are not ready to discuss the problem seriously and often deny that there is a problem. The appropriate action at this stage is motivational. Just as smokers need motivation and information to quit, so do countries. Health education is important at this stage, because smoking is not considered to be a major public health problem. In countries where the epidemic is at its early stages and governments consider that other problems take priority, it is necessary to stress the future costs to the country. Economic data can be provided to show the present and future cost, and the need to take early action, before the multinationals can develop a stronghold in the country must be stressed.

Individual smokers at the action stage have set a date for stopping smoking and have tried to quit. They may have relapses, especially at the beginning. At the collective level, the issue is being taken seriously. Attempts are being made to enact tobacco control legislation and provide smoking cessation programmes and strong health education programmes. Just as smokers often need to make several attempts before they are smoke-free, national legislation often takes many years to enact. The appropriate action at this stage is a national tobacco control action plan. Legislation should be in line with the set targets. Most successes have been achieved when multiple strategies are used. The industry is at its strongest at this stage, and the goal is to avoid relapse. This is the stage at which it would be most cost-effective to bring in experts in drafting legislation. Expertise and support from other countries is beneficial. Media involvement must be ensured.

Many countries in the developed world are at the action phase of tobacco control, although some are more advanced than others. Other countries have suffered relapses but have since enacted new legislation. Although many countries are far advanced in the action stage, it would be premature to classify any country as being in the maintenance stage. It is likely, however, that the twenty-first century will see some countries move into this phase. We must work together to ensure that all countries move through the stages as fast as possible and do not remain stuck in the early stages. With increased collaboration and information sharing, it may be possible to speed up the process and ultimately bring about smoke-free societies.

TOBACCO CONTROL PROGRAMMES

Regional and national

China: Tobacco control

M. Chen

Minister of Health, China

Tobacco control in China started with the open-door policy. Although China is late in its efforts at tobacco control, it is now doing as well as many developed countries. In 1979, the Ministry of Health and three other ministries entrusted by the State Council issued a circular on the need to publicize the hazards of smoking and the need to control it, indicating the Government's determination to control tobacco use by tobacco control, persuading smokers to quit and public education. In 1990, the Chinese Association on Smoking and Health (CASH), a non-governmental tobacco control organization supported by the Government, was established, marking a new phase in tobacco control in China.

Recent results indicate that tobacco will kill one third of all young men in China if the current rate of recruitment of new smokers persists. Of the 300 million males now aged 0–29, about 200 million will become smokers . If they continue to smoke throughout their lives, 100 million will eventually be killed by tobacco, and half of these deaths will occur before the age of 70.

Researchers from China and the United Kingdom, led by Professor Liu Boqi of the Chinese Academy of Medical Sciences, investigated the smoking habits of 1 million Chinese people in 99 rural and urban areas who died between 1986 and 1988. The results from this and from studies led by Professor Niu Shiru and Dr Yang Gonghuan, both of the Chinese Academy of Preventive Medicine, show that there are already about 750 000 deaths a year in China from smoking, mostly among men.

Smoking among adolescents is a serious problem. If proper intervention is done, we will not have a new smoking generation. Since 1993, a programme for 'smoke-free schools' has been carried out nationwide. Each year, a number of schools are selected for awards. By 1997, 42 directors of schools had won an award. Beijing organized a 'One hundred smoke-free schools' campaign, and 1000 schools have become smoke-free (100 schools as 'best organizers' and 10 000 pupils as 'young tobacco control activists'). In May 1994, the Soong Ching Ling Foundation started a campaign called 'Children against smoking', which called on all students not to smoke, not to buy or sell cigarettes, to persuade one family member to quit or remain smoke-free and to stop anyone who smoked in a public place. By July 1997, 1 million children had signed their names in support of the campaign. These activities have influenced the smoking behaviour of parents and teachers.

Tobacco control research has been conducted in medical schools, research institutes and some grassroots organizations on the hazards associated with smoking, its social impact and interventions. Between 1990 and 1996, seven national symposia on smoking and health were held, each with more than 100 national and international delegates and with about 100 papers exchanged. At one of these meetings, the financial losses due to smoking-related diseases were evoked for the first time, showing that they were much larger than the income from taxes on tobacco sales. A paper on the relationship between smoking and death showed that lung cancer ranked first among all causes of death in big cities (population > 1 million) in China. Much information has been gained from a study of smoking interventions among 50 000 Chinese peasants and a study of smoking interventions among 250 000 schoolchildren. In 1996, a national smoking prevalence survey was conducted, which produced results very useful for decision-making by health authorities.

Tobacco control has now been legislated. The *Tobacco Monopoly Law*, the *Law on the Protection of Minors* and the *Advertising Law* enacted in 1991 contain articles on tobacco control. To protect the rights of non-smokers, 72 cities have passed laws or regulations about smoking in public places. Many of those cities, such as Beijing and Shanghai, have strong enforcement teams who use various tactics such as persuasion, warnings and fines.

In 1989, WHO called for a total ban on tobacco advertising and in 1994 the WHO Western Pacific Region set the goal of a ban on tobacco advertising in the Region by the year 2000. To help reach that goal, China conducted a campaign for tobacco advertising-free cities, and by February 1997, 10 cities had reached that goal (Beijing, Hangzhou, Huizhou, Jingyin, Puyang, Shantou, Shaoguan, Zhangjiagang, Zhongshan and Zhuhai). Those cities have won awards from the Ministry of Health and CASH.

There have been many grassroots tobacco control activities. Smoke-free organizations and families have received awards. In 1992, CASH gave 382 organizations nationwide awards for their efforts to control tobacco use. Many provinces followed suit and gave awards to local organizations. At the same time, 24 individuals won national tobacco control activist awards. Tobacco control in China has won praise from several other governments and from several international organizations. WHO, for example, has presented tobacco or health awards to well-known anti-smoking figures in China, such as Wu Jieping, Chen Minzhang, Weng Xinzhi and Li Wangxian. CASH and the Health Bureau in Jushan County, Shanxi Province, won the same award from WHO.

Although much progress has been made, China is still faced with an enormous problem. The smoking rates have been on the increase. According to the 1996 national survey, the overall smoking rate in China among people over 15 years of age is 38%, which is 3.7% higher that the 1984 figure. There are 320 million smokers in this country, of whom 300 million are male and 20 million female. The average starting age is now 20, while in the 1984 survey it was 23. The smoking rates of people aged 15–45 have increased; and the average number of cigarettes smoked daily is now 15, which is two more than in the 1984 survey. The death rate from lung cancer in China is increasing at an annual rate of 4.5%, and it is estimated by WHO that by the year 2025, China will have an annual rate of 2 million deaths caused by smoking-related diseases. During the next 20–30 years, we must therefore conduct a major fight against tobacco-caused diseases. We are indeed faced with a huge task, and we must mobilize the whole society in our efforts for tobacco control. Let us be united in our endeavour for the health of our people.

China: Tobacco control campaign

X. Weng

Chinese Association on Smoking and Health, Beijing, China

China, with more than 300 million smokers, is unfortunately the largest tobacco producing and consuming country in the world, partly because of its long history of tobacco use—more than 400 years—and partly because of its traditions. Offering or lighting cigarettes for others is a common way of showing respect and friendship on social occasions. Furthermore, China was very late in joining the international tobacco control community, the programmes having been started 20 years later than in developed countries. Accordingly, tobacco control in this huge country has been an enormous challenge. Tobacco control campaigns in China can be divided into two periods: before and after establishment of the Chinese Association on Smoking and Health (CASH).

First stage

The first stage ran from 1979 to 1989 and was marked by the first official circular, issued jointly by the four ministries entrusted with the task by the State Council, which were the ministries of Health, Agriculture, Finance and Light Industry. The circular stressed the need to publicize the hazards of smoking and to control it and indicated the

Government's determination to control smoking. The mass media subsequently launched a variety of programmes to disseminate information about the hazards of smoking, and many popular science booklets on the subject were published.

In March 1982, the preparatory group for the CASH was formed. Several cities, such as Beijing, Shanghai and Tianjin, and Zhejiang Province set up local anti-smoking organizations. In 1983, the First National Symposium on Smoking and Health was convened, and in 1984 the first national smoking prevalence survey was conducted, showing that the average prevalence of smoking in China was 33.9%, with rates of 61% among males and 7% among females. Those data were officially accepted as the standard prevalence rates for quite a long time.

It was during the first stage that international cooperation on tobacco control began in earnest. China began to cooperate with the World Health Organization (WHO) in 1979; the WHO Collaborating Centre for Tobacco or Health was set up in 1986. In 1984, the former United States Surgeon General, Dr E. Koop, visited China, and in 1985 and 1990 Chinese delegates were invited by the American Cancer Society to participate in an international summit of smoking control leaders, entitled 'Trade for life'. The first international symposium on tobacco control to be held in China was organized in Tianjin in 1987 and was attended by many prominent smoking control activists including Dr Masironi of WHO, Sir John Crofton of the International Union against Tuberculosis and Lung Disease, Dr K. Bjartveit and Dr Nigel Gray of the International Union against Cancer, Mr David Simpson of the Association for Smoking or Health, Dr J. Mackay from Hong Kong, Professor Richard Peto from the United Kingdom and Professor T. Hirayama from Japan. In that same year, 1987, China participated for the first time in the World Conference on Smoking or Health and in the first meeting of the working group on smoking and health of the Western Pacific Region of WHO, in Tokyo.

During the same period, some progress in legislation was made. For example, the State Education Commission drew up regulations against smoking by primary and secondary school pupils; the State Administration Bureau for Industry and Commerce notified the whole country to restrict commercial advertising of tobacco products (although unfortunately this was not effectively enforced) and the Civil Aviation Administration banned smoking on all domestic flights in 1983 and was thus the first in the world to do so.

Second stage

The second stage began in 1990 when the CASH was established to coordinate tobacco control efforts and carry out related research. Its work includes:
- organizing annual national symposia on smoking and health;
- holding regular national meetings of executives of local tobacco or health organizations;
- giving awards to winners of smoke-free schools and other institutions, to individual anti-tobacco activists, to mass media that have advocated anti-smoking values and to television stations and film-makers for excluding smoking scenes;
- publishing The Chinese Smoking and Health Bulletin, a bimonthly journal;
- increasing the number of local smoking and health organizations to 30;
- trying to help the Government include tobacco control articles in the major laws in China, such as the Tobacco Monopoly Law, the Law on Protection of Minors and the Advertising Law, the most recent being a regulation against smoking on all public transport and in all waiting rooms;
- coordinating related scientific research such as the national smoking prevalence surveys in 1991 and 1996, retrospective and prospective epidemiological studies on tobacco or health and intervention studies involving 50 000 peasants and 30 000 students;
- further strengthening international relations, by sending delegates to most international and regional conferences on tobacco or health, celebrating WHO's No-Tobacco Day every year since 1988 and becoming more active in the international tobacco control community.

These are only a few of the activities of the CASH. Some of the results are worth mentioning in more detail. A major study showed that the health-related cost of smoking exceeded the tax revenue from tobacco. In 1993, the tax revenue from tobacco in China was 41 billion yuan, while the health-related cost was 65 billion yuan. In the past 12 years, the rate of smoking among people aged ≥ 45 has declined, but the average smoking rate has increased by 3.7% and the male smoking rate by 5.9%. The annual rate of increase in cigarette production slowed down: in the 1980s, cigarette production in China increased at an annual rate of about 9%, whereas the increase between 1988 and 1990 was less than 3%, that after 1990 was < 2% and that in 1996 was −1.2%. Sales of cigarettes have shown a similar trend. Efforts have been made to improve the quality of cigarettes: the average tar content per cigarette was 30 mg in the 1980s and only 19 mg in 1996, a drastic change. Filter cigarettes accounted for only 1.3% of all cigarettes produced in China in 1979, for 40% in 1989, for 77% in 1995 and for > 90% in 1996.

More than 70 cities in China have drawn up regulations against smoking in public places, and quite a few cities have a total ban on tobacco advertising. Ten such cities, including Beijing, Hangzhou and Zhuhai, won the Tobacco Advertising-free City Award from the Ministry of Health and the CASH. There were 230 smoke-free primary and secondary schools in Beijing in 1995 and 1000 in 1996. The Soong Ching Ling Foundation organized a project involving more than 1 million children in persuading smokers to quit. The project was welcomed by the public and was extended to involve university students. Now, six of the 13 medical universities directly under the Minstry of Health claim to be smoke-free. These universities refuse to enrol smokers or to assign them jobs in the universities or in their affiliated hospitals.

China has thus made quite some progress in tobacco control and has won awards from WHO and international and national tobacco control organizations. Since 1988, seven WHO Tobacco or Health medals have gone to China: four to individuals, one to the CASH, one to Jishan Health Bureau in Shanxi Province and one to the Soong Ching Ling Foundation.

Remaining challenges

Despite its success, China still faces a number of hurdles:
- It is still too early for the effects of the many measures to be translated into a real reduction in the prevalence of smoking and in morbidity and mortality due to tobacco-related diseases.
- Funding for tobacco control is still needed.
- Public awareness of the hazards of smoking must be further increased, especially in rural areas.
- Strong action must be taken to ban indirect tobacco advertising and other promotion tricks, especially sponsorship of arts and sports events by the transnational tobacco companies.
- New policies on cigarette prices are needed to help reduce smoking rates.
- Smuggling of foreign brands must be reduced and eventually stopped.
- More sectors of society should be involved in the campaign for smoke-free institutions.

China cannot win the war against tobacco without help and support from international organizations and individuals. It needs to strengthen its global relations and to work with foreign friends towards the common goal of a tobacco-free world. If the tobacco problem in China were solved, a quarter of the tobacco control problem of the world would be eliminated. Let us work together towards that goal.

Africa: Challenges for tobacco control

W.F.T. Muna

Tobacco Control Commission for Africa, Yaoundé, Cameroon

Smoking rates and per capita consumption of cigarettes in sub-Saharan Africa remain relatively low (600 cigarettes per adult inhabitant per year versus 1200 in developed countries), and smoking is currently not considered to be an important cause of morbidity or mortality in this region. Health and environmental issues, including diseases linked to poverty (malnutrition and diarrhoeal diseases, malaria, respiratory infections, tuberculosis and measles), remain the priorities, and over half of the estimated 8 million deaths annually still occur among children aged 0–4 years. Despite the low average smoking rate in the region, middle-income countries like the Republic of South Africa have rates of about 1500 cigarettes per adult per year. Accordingly, the morbidity and mortality rates due to smoking-related diseases—lung and oesophageal cancer and ischaemic heart disease—show trends similar to those observed in developed countries.

Smoking rates are strongly dependent on economic conditions and local purchasing power, and these trends, like those seen in South Africa, reflect social and lifestyle changes that are expected to dominate the African public health environment of the twenty-first century. The increasing restrictions on cigarette marketing in developed countries have resulted in a commercial assault by the tobacco industry in a search for new markets in the developing world, Africa being a prime target. Cigarette sales in certain African countries are expected to rise by 6% between 1994 and 2000, despite the global anti-tobacco campaign. The opportunities for tobacco control as a health priority for Africa were identified almost three decades ago, but most countries in the region do not yet see the necessity or urgency of an effective tobacco control policy. Malnutrition and communicable diseases may remain health challenges for Africans for much longer than expected, but non-communicable and chronic disorders (especially those linked to tobacco use) may present an equally important challenge sooner than expected.

Asia: Research network for tobacco control policy

S.L. Hamann

Department of Medical Education, Rangsit University, Bangkok, Thailand

The Asian Tobacco Control Policy Research Network was formed after the meeting of the Asia-Pacific Association for Tobacco Control in Chiang Mai, Thailand, in November 1995. Its purpose is to promote the development, funding and implementation of research relevant to policy and to lobby for the adoption of strong tobacco control policies based on research. Emphasis is placed on obtaining key evidence that will enable policy-makers to take further action to control tobacco.

The Network has support from the Asia-Pacific Association for Tobacco Control, Action on Smoking or Health Thailand and over 125 tobacco control advocates and researchers in 25 countries. The philosophy of the Network is that regional coordination and collaboration of research resources can maximize the impact of policy-relevant research. Research can be crucial in advancing tobacco control policy if, and only if, it is appropriately conceptualized, funded and presented. Empowering tobacco control advocates, so that the most is accomplished with each research opportunity, is vital to rapid success. While the Network does not conduct research, its members do, and the coordination they bring to the enterprise benefits all of Asia.

The process of contributing to policy-relevant research includes understanding of the country and regional setting for the production of research; bringing together like-minded researchers who are willing to work together, obtaining funding for the research and making sure the research results are publicized and have an impact in changing local and regional policy. Most of the work done so far has been in South-east Asia. Environmental tobacco smoke and the economic implications of tobacco use are policy areas for research that will be emphasized in the future.

The Net News Bulletin of the Network serves to connect tobacco control researchers and advocates. It is currently produced three times a year and includes such features as: descriptions of possible research projects; information on agencies that might fund tobacco control research; methods of assessing research needs and developing research strategies; current tobacco control research reports with their possible policy implications and reported public evidence that reflects changing social perceptions of tobacco use

An Internet web site is available at http://www.ash.or.th, which will include the Asian Tobacco Control Policy Research Network Bulletin and free materials on tobacco control advocacy, funding and policy promotion.

Australia: The Western Australian smoking and health programme: Persistence pays dividends

M.G. Swanson

Health Promotion Services, Health Department of Western Australia, Perth, Australia

In 1972, a dedicated group of public health physicians established the Australian Council on Smoking and Health in Western Australia. The Council is primarily a smoking and health advocacy organization which has the prohibition of tobacco advertising and promotion as one of its most important objectives.

The first attempt to prohibit tobacco advertising and promotion was made in the Western Australian Parliament in 1982 through a private member's bill that was initiated and strongly supported by the Council. Unfortunately, this bill was defeated by a margin of two votes in the Legislative Council, the Parliament's upper house. In 1983, the newly elected Government introduced a bill to prohibit tobacco advertising, but this bill was also defeated in the Legislative Council, by the same margin. The Government did, however, increase the tax on tobacco products and allocated AUS$ 2 million per year from the additional revenue raised to a comprehensive smoking and health campaign which is led by mass media television advertising. Since 1984, the Health Department of Western Australia, in cooperation with non-government health and medical organizations, has conducted an aggressive state-wide campaign which graphically portrays the health effects of smoking, and the magnitude of the problem.

In 1990, the Western Australian Parliament did eventually pass legislation, the Tobacco Control Act 1990, which severely restricts tobacco advertising and limits the availability of tobacco products to children. The programme was further complemented by the establishment of the Western Australian Health Promotion Foundation, which provides an alter:.ative source of funding for events previously sponsored by tobacco companies and funds health promotion research and interventions.

Does a determined, long-term, comprehensive approach to tobacco control reduce the prevalence of smoking? In particular, does a combination of mass media-led public education and enforcement of appropriate tobacco legislation reduce the prevalence of smoking among adults? According to the national health surveys conducted in 1977, 1989–90 and 1995, Western Australia now has the lowest prevalence of smoking among adults of any state or territory in the nation. In Western Australia, smoking prevalence among adults declined from 38% in 1977 to 24.4% in 1995. Unfortunately, the rate of decline in the prevalence of smoking from 1988–89 to 1995 has slowed down. The most plausible explanation is that the financial resources allocated to the smoking and health programme have not increased since 1983. Indeed, if the financial allocation to this programme had kept pace with inflation and increases in population, the allocated budget would be AUS$ 5 million per annum. It is interesting to note in this regard that the revenue from tobacco tax in Western Australia grew from AUS$ 17 million in 1983 to more than AUS$ 280 million in 1997.

Australia: A firm foundation for tobacco control: The Victorian Health Promotion Foundation model

R. Galbally

Victorian Health Promotion Foundation, Victoria, Australia

The Victorian Health Promotion Foundation model

The Victorian Health Promotion Foundation, set up in Victoria, Australia, in 1987, was the first health promotion foundation to be funded from taxes on tobacco. Using funds from a tobacco levy to develop a health promotion foundation is a way of taxing the most harmful disease-creating product to promote good health. Taxing tobacco and using the funds for tobacco control and health promotion provides many benefits at the same time: a harmful product is taxed, which increases its price. This in itself is a disincentive for many people to continue smoking and particularly for young people to take up smoking. An initial small tax increase will often lead to a further increase as governments see the popularity of the dedicated levy. A percentage of the tobacco tax can be used to fund tobacco control throughout the country and also to fund other health promotion programmes such as injury prevention, improved food and nutrition, prevention of drug abuse, improved reproductive and sexual health, promoting mental health and well-being and promoting environmental health. The popularity of such activities results in a political and economic climate in which even higher taxes may be imposed on tobacco.

After several decades of ceaseless effort, we are still faced with an epidemic of smoking. As the overwhelming majority of educational interventions have failed to achieve the intended results, it has been found that, paradoxically, better results are obtained when a health promotion foundation addresses issues other than tobacco in order to achieve successful tobacco control. Various risky lifestyles have common roots in the population, the community, the environment and the culture. Among adolescents, for example, smoking, as well as suicide, binge drinking, unsafe driving, unsafe sex and drug taking, are linked to social class, depression and poor mental health. Organizations must thus link their approaches to the underlying risk factors in order to tackle smoking and create a culture of health promotion. A health promotion foundation must support single-issue programmes, such as tobacco control, for advocacy for political reform, legislation and regulation, while also supporting tobacco control as part of integrated health promotion campaigns in specific settings, such as schools, workplaces and sporting venues.

Risky behaviour clusters in risky situations. People who smoke are more likely to be poor. People who are poor and unemployed are more likely to be depressed and even suicidal. People who consider suicide tend to have low self-esteem. People who have low self-esteem are more likely to smoke. Because risky behaviour such as smoking is not the result of a single decision but arises from a person's overall situation, single-issue anti-smoking campaigns that do not address underlying tendencies may be effective only for general populations and not for disadvantaged groups with the lowest health status. Because health is dependent on matters outside the health sector, health promotion foundations should support programmes that draw in the media, education, industry, agriculture, transport, government and the community and, most importantly, which engage with people of all ages about their own concerns, wherever and however they live, work, play and love.

Health promoters dealing with tobacco control should supplement their educational programmes with new approaches and programmes for integrated strategies to deal with people at risk. Alternative social marketing strategies are needed to sponsor sports and arts groups and to persuade groups to give up tobacco sponsorship and replace the smoking messages with anti-smoking messages, promoted on the perimeters of sporting venues and picked up by television cameras, on programmes and on T-shirts. Such strategies need innovative funding methods, which in turn will make new strategies possible. Paramount among these approaches is the health promotion foundation model—a new funding method that carries with it immense possibilities for health promotion innovation. A health promotion foundation funded from tobacco taxes can lead a nation away from domination by the tobacco industry towards smoke-free safety.

Health promotion is a rapidly developing field, and new data and new concepts are providing the basis for rapid, extensive change. As a health promotion foundation is at the centre of operations in all areas of research and practice, it is in an excellent position to develop new directions and new initiatives to extend the influence of health promotion on the nation's smoking rates and to link work on smoking with strategies being tested in other areas of health promotion.

Research conducted over the past 20 years leads us to conclude that once the basic needs have been provided, the most important factor in people's health is their control over their own lives. People who have a sense of coherence in their lives, who are able to set their own directions, who are valued and who have a source of help can resist health threats that destroy people without those protections. Programmes that attack single issues, even when those issues are as vital as tobacco smoking, are not necessarily addressing the fundamental determinants of health. They may require the assistance of other sectors, an integrated relationship with the total context of risk and a willingness to incorporate community concerns.

Communities that work together have the best hope of dealing with their public and primary health problems. They can ensure that the Government considers their needs, that proper preventive measures are developed and that individuals and families will cooperate to implement them. Health promotion foundations can help to strengthen community organizations and institutions that provide a base for this work. Foundations can also support the development of programmes on the underlying determinants of people's health. While factors such as developing a sense of control over one's life may be difficult to address, they are nonetheless proving to be the most important influences on such indices as smoking rates and cannot be ignored. Health promotion initiatives that impose goals on a passive audience cannot build people's skills to deal with other life challenges and may even reduce their self-esteem. Health promotion foundations can take the risk of supporting trial programmes to treat issues such as hopelessness and lack of self-control.

Health promotion that works and is sustained begins by stimulating people to ask about their own priorities. People are then supported in achieving those goals with community and workplace organization. Health promotion foundations can support the process by building skills that will give people the collective capacity, in communities, workplaces and families, to deal effectively with issues that affect their lives as they themselves perceive them. This will improve their health and may reduce their smoking. The campaign against smoking should not be regarded simply in terms of behavioural change. Smoking is set firmly in a social, economic and environmental context, and we cannot eliminate it without understanding that context. In order to pursue new anti-smoking strategies, we must find ways of building a sense of control, fostering hope and supporting healthy child development. This is not a quick or straightforward enterprise, and we therefore require long-term funding that can support long-term structures.

Australia: Sports and arts: Tobacco-free, tobacco control and health promotion

R. Galbally, C. Borthwick & M. Blackburn

Victorian Health Promotion Foundation, Carlton South, Victoria, Australia

Sports and arts offer excellent opportunities for health promotion, especially in the area of tobacco control. Developing partnerships with sports and arts groups for health contrasts with the tobacco industry's policy of using sports and arts to sell cigarettes. Sports and arts offer the tobacco industry lucrative opportunities because of the size of the audiences exposed to the tobacco messages: immediate audiences of spectators and much larger and more significant audiences through electronic and print media. In particular, sports sponsorship links smoking strongly to an active sporting lifestyle, thereby undermining warnings of the health consequences of smoking (Woodward *et al.*, 1989). Studies in England and New Zealand have shown that both children and adults have increased brand awareness and connect the sponsored brand with the sport (Ledwith *et al.*, 1984; Aitken *et al.*, 1986).

Tobacco industry use of sports and arts sponsorships

In tobacco sponsorship of sports, a positive association is created with cigarette smoking. Consumers, especially young people, are encouraged to associate smoking with high-profile sports achievers. The tobacco industry has exploited to the limit this use of sports and arts achievers and role models to sell cigarettes. Innovative methods are used, such as marching girls, signs on the perimeters of sports grounds, in the foyers of arts and cultural halls and on cars for motor sports, international telecasts of high-profile speeches that mention tobacco sponsorship and ceremonies to present trophies branded with the tobacco company's name and logo. The methods used not only highlight the name of a company's product but also promote the product in subtle ways, associating cigarettes with strength, sexual prowess, beauty, wealth and elegance. Cigarette companies also see sponsorship as an opportunity to enlist support, by encouraging sports and arts organizations and personalities to support their cause and in making good use of corporate boxes at sports and arts events to influence senior decision-makers to support legislation and financial policy at a state and national level (Gourlay *et al.*, 1990; Warner *et al.*, 1992; Chapman, 1992).

An alternative to tobacco promotion of sports and arts: Health promotion of sports and arts

An alternative to tobacco sponsorship is provided by the model initiated in Australia by the Victorian Health Promotion Foundation (VicHealth). VicHealth uses funds from a dedicated levy on tobacco products to counter the use of sports and arts by the tobacco industry and to optimize the health benefits of exercise and leisure. VicHealth implements a model of health promotion that has since been adopted in many other states of Australia and in some form in 17 other countries. While the broad goal of VicHealth is to promote health and prevent disease, tobacco control is a primary focus.

The model is based on a small percentage of a dedicated tax or levy on tobacco products for health promotion generally but in particular to offer replacement funding to sports and arts, so that they can give up tobacco sponsorship. VicHealth therefore uses health sponsorship of sports and arts as one of its primary methods for tobacco control.

The use of a tax on tobacco for tobacco control embodies a health promotion paradox: using a tax on a disease-creating substance for health promotion, while at the same time raising the price of cigarettes, in itself one of the most effective health promotion actions. For every 1% increase in price, consumption can be expected to fall by 0.5% (Townsend, 1993). The banning of television advertising in Australia in 1976 and the gradual imposition of restrictions on other forms of tobacco advertising have made sponsorship even more important to tobacco companies. In 1987, they were spending AUS$ 114 200 000 on sports sponsorships and AUS$ 980 000 on sponsoring arts and culture (figures from the Australian Tobacco Institute). By that time, there was growing community opposition to such sponsorship of sports and arts, on the grounds that it encouraged people to smoke. This opposition was generated over a number of years by non-governmental organizations such as the Anti-Cancer Council of Victoria, the National Heart Foundation and the Australian Medical Association, and by churches and politicians. In 1987, for example, there were public demonstrations against the Benson & Hedges-sponsored Royal Philharmonic Orchestra, Benson & Hedges-sponsored cricket and Peter Jackson-sponsored windsurfing (Gourlay *et al.*, 1990). This opposition helped to develop the climate of opinion that made it possible to pass the *Victorian Tobacco Act 1987.*

This Act established VicHealth, a statutory body with the objectives of promoting health and safety and encouraging healthy lifestyles. The Act does not prohibit tobacco sponsorship of sports and arts but specifically authorizes VicHealth to offer its replacement sponsorships for sporting or cultural activities previously sponsored by tobacco companies. To fund this and all other health promotion work, VicHealth is allocated one-sixth of the income from the Victorian tobacco franchise; 30% of that income is allocated to sporting bodies, a percentage intended to double the amount that the tobacco industry is reported to spend in that area. While no fixed proportion is allocated to the arts, the Act expresses the need to remove tobacco sponsorship from that sector and to replace it with health messages.

Size of the market

VicHealth recognized from the outset that sports and arts provide significant opportunities for health promotion. These are large entertainment industries with turnovers of millions of dollars (Stewart, 1986). They have huge infrastructures of education and training facilities, and the media profile offered by sports and arts events gives them unprecedented access to millions of participants and spectators in the country and internationally.

The greatest benefits were initially expected from exposing the public to tobacco control messages such as 'Quit smoking'. Australians are still very interested in sport: 96% of Australians watched the Olympics on television, 89% of people aged 16–65 are active in some sport, and approximately 65% attend sporting events. Signs at major events have been shown to provide high exposure of product names (Martin, 1990). Significant numbers of people also attend galleries for large exhibitions and concerts.

Beyond advertisements, tobacco replacement sponsorships also provide opportunities for other media-related benefits. The 'Quit smoking' message is linked to the sponsored sport or arts activity and is thus attached to role models through celebrity endorsement. The role models, such as football and rock music stars, then visit schools and youth groups to promote 'Quit smoking' rather than tobacco products. As the cigarette companies well know, sports and arts provide convincing advocates and powerful role models—cultural ambassadors for carrying ideas across the community. VicHealth also recognized the potential of sports and arts as agents of cultural change towards a tobacco-free society.

Replacing tobacco sponsorship

In order to replace tobacco sponsorship in sports and arts, VicHealth sees its role as a sponsor not a granting organization. VicHealth's aim is to promote health and specifically non-smoking behavioural change and to create a supportive environment that enables people to not smoke or to give up smoking. Particular difficulties with replacement of tobacco sponsorship emerged for sports and arts which received large amounts of tobacco funding at the national level, and it was not feasible for VicHealth to replace this by state-level funding. In these cases, for instance with soccer, VicHealth led inter-state negotiations to remove tobacco funding from the National Soccer League, so that the Winfield Soccaroos became the Australian Quit Socceroos.

Building favourable relationships with the media maximizes promotional exposure and allows for additional media exposure both in editorials in local and daily newspapers and in community service announcements. Indeed, media representatives may sometimes be recruited as 'ambassadors for health' and work with the organizers to achieve our goals. Given the media's interest in 'Quit smoking' campaigns, especially with the array of human interest angles that is invariably present, there is usually considerable unpaid media coverage from tobacco replacement sponsorships (Hill, 1988; Raw *et al.*, 1990; Woodward, 1990).

Health promotion sponsorships of sports and arts become more valuable over time, as the 'Quit smoking' campaign and the sports or arts group become familiar with the possibilities for raising awareness and introducing structural change. VicHealth has learnt how best to maximize the value of tobacco replacement sponsorships and to integrate them into general health promotion planning.

One continuing bias in health promotion programmes has been towards promoting individual behavioural change, neglecting the development of supportive, healthy environments that allow people to make healthy choices. Leverage obtained through tobacco replacement sponsorships enables VicHealth to create the environments conducive to health called for by the WHO Ottawa Charter for Health Promotion. VicHealth thus cooperates with arts and sports groups to ensure that all indoor arts or sports venues are smoke-free, and most outdoor venues, such as those for football and horse-racing, now have some smoke-free stands.

As well as tobacco control, healthy environments can provide delicious, healthy food, occupational health and safety for sports and arts employees, low-alcohol drinks to discourage alcohol abuse, promotion of sports safety to prevent injury to participants in sport, and development of sports stands in the shade for cancer prevention. The positive views people hold about tobacco control and health promotion encourage greater awareness of risk factors, fuller appreciation of the possibilities for a change to a healthy lifestyle and eventually behaviour modification. For example, after replacement of tobacco sponsorship for the Victorian State Opera in 1989, VicHealth and the National Heart Foundation contracted with the Opera and the Victorian Arts Centre to introduce completely smoke-free foyers and menus with healthier food in both the restaurants and staff canteens. Similar arrangements have been made under sponsorship contracts with the National Gallery, the Melbourne Zoo, the Exhibition Building, all theatres and most sports venues. These moves were generally well supported by the public. For example, 95% of survey respondents supported the smoke-free foyer at the Victorian Arts Centre.

Increased participation in sports and exercise

VicHealth uses its funding of sports to expand participation by disadvantaged groups. Women's sports, for example, have traditionally been underfunded, and women's events rarely attract sponsorship, as they are not as likely to be televised or to attract other media attention. This lesser emphasis on women's sport has contributed to the generally lower level of involvement in sports and exercise by women after puberty, and lack of exercise is an important risk factor for non-communicable diseases. VicHealth sponsors women's cricket, netball, surfing, athletics and golf in order to bring more women and girls into active sport and exercise. The opportunity to promote tobacco control messages to women is then used to the fullest, as women are the target of the tobacco industry for marketing campaigns in most countries and especially developing ones.

Although individual clubs and events are sponsored, more emphasis is placed on building long-term strategic alliances with leading sports and arts organizations. The initial incentive for these alliances is the prospect of VicHealth sponsorship, but the relationships formed during these negotiations provide opportunities for community development in which local artists, educators, business people and governmental and non-governmental health organizations work together to develop healthy public policy.

Evaluation

Changes in lifestyle brought about by tobacco control are seen over decades rather than within the life of a campaign. Most evaluations are therefore concerned with intermediate objectives, such as recall of a sponsored message; attitudes and beliefs on health issues can be measured in longer-term evaluations.

VicHealth requires bodies receiving sponsorship funds to evaluate the success of the tobacco replacement project. Some of these evaluations throw light on what can be achieved from such sponsorships. In 1987, VicHealth sponsored a major Australian football club with the Quit campaign. Footballers wore the Quit logo on their clothing, carried banners with anti-smoking messages and provided perimeter signs at their home ground. In an evaluation of this sponsorship by surveyng 548 young people who attended football games and 785 controls, 96% of the football supporters could identify Quit as one of the club sponsors. Respondents among both the football enthusiasts and the controls who had noted the Quit sponsorship had a greater interest in football and were less likely to intend to smoke, suggesting that sports sponsorship by the Quit campaign was effective in discouraging the uptake of smoking in this age group (Naccarella *et al.*, 1991).

Between 1993 and 1996, more than 1.8 million Victorians were exposed to VicHealth-sponsored projects, at a mean cost per head of AUS$ 2.70. An average sponsorship had access to more than 50 000 people. Of all sponsored projects, 83% attracted publicity, most often in the print media (74%); however, the cost of media publicity was relatively high, at around AUS$ 134 per event. A publication was derived from 59% of all sponsorships, either in the form of an in-house article or newsletter (697), a report (2049) or a scientific paper (25). A total of 2771 publications was reported. About 50% of the sponsorships incorporated a community development component; of these, 24% achieved community responsibility, and only 2% reported that they were unable to achieve the planned component.

The most commonly reported reforms were promoting smoke-free areas (71%), healthy food choices (56%) and safe alcohol practices (48%). General profile benefits were reported in 95% of the projects, and a similar proportion reported using signs, bulk materials and personal acknowledgments to promote the health message. Hospitality was used in 80% of the projects and interactive forms of promotion in 75%. Greater visibility was achieved with bulk materials and signs, whereas hospitality appeared to be the least successful. More than half (52%) of all projects included educational activities, with a total of 370 educational sessions for over 150 000 people, representing 53 283 person–hours of health education. In-service training was reported in about 25% of the projects, with over 6000 staff receiving training. Over 33% of all projects produced resource materials to promote the health message and for use during educational sessions.

Tobacco control with sports and arts organizations therefore raises awareness and provides health education, information, advocacy, access to particular target groups and opportunities for changes to smoke-free environments. By sponsoring sports and arts, new supportive settings for tobacco control are created. The VicHealth sponsorship programme has established a climate of opinion favourable to promoting health and preventing illness. Tobacco replacement sponsorship of sports and arts also ensures that VicHealth is seen as reputable, caring and socially responsible. A study in 1991 showed that Victorians overwhelmingly approved of the encouragement of healthy lifestyles, and that 86% approved the VicHealth sponsorship programme. Such approval is essential for maintaining and enhancing community acceptance of the Government's tobacco levy. These high levels of approval were also significant in enabling Australia to achieve the *Tobacco Sponsorship Prohibition Act 1992*: the example set by VicHealth and other bodies in Australia was important in the achievement of that legislation.

Conclusion

A small percentage of the tax on tobacco products has allowed VicHealth to pioneer an innovative strategy to promote health . In many countries, funds for health promotion are hard to come by, yet prevention programmes are essential for a healthy future. The VicHealth mode is one way of taxing the most harmful disease-creating product in order to promote good health. The tax becomes popular because of its association with health, and governments are thus encouraged to raise the price of cigarettes, which itself acts as an effective disincentive to young people to smoke.

VicHealth sponsors sports and cultural events that the tobacco industry found attractive, the events being no longer used to recruit smokers but to promote the benefits of not smoking and adopting a healthy lifestyle. Over 1000 sports and arts organizations now receive funding to send health messages and encourage participation. Thus, sports and arts groups gain significant support form the VicHealth model and there is broad-based support for tobacco control. The biggest winners of all are the millions of people— young, middle-aged and older—whose lives have been enriched by staying healthy, not smoking or giving up smoking and participating in the sports and cultural life of their community.

References

Aitken, P., Leathar, D. & Squaire, S. (1986) Children's awareness of cigarette brands sponsorship of sports and games in the UK. *Health Educ. Res.*, 1, 2203–2221

Chapman,S. (1992) Anatomy of a campaign: The attempt to defeat the New South Wales (Australia) Tobacco Advertising Prohibition Bill 1991. *Tob. Control*, 1, 50–56

Gourlay, S., McGrory, P. & White, M. (1990) The History of MOPUP the movement opposing the promotion of unhealthy products and its activities leading up to the *Victorian Tobacco Act 1987*. In: Durtson, B. & Jamrosic, K., eds, *Tobacco and Health 1990: The Global War*, Perth: Organising Committee of the Seventh World Conference on Tobacco and Health, pp. 844–885

Hill, D. (1988) Public opinion on tobacco advertising, sports sponsorships and taxation prior to the Victorian Tobacco Act, 1987. *Community Health Stud.*, 12, 282–288

Ledwith, F. (1984) Does tobacco sport sponsorship on television act as advertising for children? *Health Educ. J.*, 43, 85–88

Martin, D. (1990) *Incidental Advertising of Beer and Cigarettes in TV Broadcasts of the Australia Grand Prix*, Media Information Australia, pp. 6–10

Naccarella, L., Berland, R. & Hill, D. (1991) Quit Sponsorship of a Victorian Football League Club (VHSP Quit Evaluation Studies No. 5), Melbourne

Raw, M., White, P. & McNeil (1990) The Victorian Tobacco Act. In: *Clearing the Air*, London: British Medical Association, pp. 59–69

Stewart, B. (1986) Sport is big business. In: Lawrence, G. & Rowe, D., eds, *Powerplay; Essays in the Sociology of Sport*, Sydney: Hale & Ironmonger

Townsend, J. (1993) The impact of price on cigarette consumption: An overview. In: *Reducing Smoking through Price and Other Measures*, London: Department of Health

Warner, K., Butler, J., Cummings, K., D'Onofrio, C., Davis, R., Flay, B., McKinney, M., Myers, M., Pertescouk, M., Robinson, R., Ryden, L., Schudson, M.,Tye, J. & Wilkenfeld, J. (1992) 1992 Report of the Tobacco Policy Research Study Group on Tobacco Marketing and Promotion. *Tob. Control*, 1, S19–S23

Woodward, S. (1990) Running a grass-roots campaign. In: Durston, B. & Jamrozic, K., eds, *Tobacco and Health 1990: The Global War*, Perth: Organising Committee of the Seventh World Conference on Tobacco and Health

Woodward, G., Roerts, L. & Reynolds, C. (1989) The nanny state strikes back. *Community Health Stud.*, 13, 403–409

Australia: Banquo's ghost: A case study of the corruption of public policy on exposure to environmental tobacco smoke

K. Jamrozik[1], S. Chapman[2] & A. Woodward[3]

[1]*Department of Public Health, University of Western Australia, and* [2]*Department of Community Medicine and Public Health, University of Sydney, Australia, and* [3]*Department of Public Health, Wellington Medical School, New Zealand*

We describe how an enquiry into exposure to environmental tobacco smoke by the National Health and Medical Research Council, Australia's highest medical advisory body, was continually delayed, frustrated and eventually compromised by the Tobacco Institute of Australia and its member companies.

Background

In the Act of the Australian Parliament that established the National Health and Medical Research Council, part of Section 3 states:

"(1) The object of this Act is to make provision for a national body to pursue activities designed:

(a) to raise the standard of individual and public health throughout Australia; and

(b) to foster the development of consistent health standards between the various States and Territories; ...." (Commonwealth of Australia, 1993).

The Council completed a first report on exposure to environmental tobacco smoke in June 1986, in which it recommended that there be restrictions or prohibition of smoking within the work environment, enclosed public places, hospitals, restaurants and transport, and that information on exposure to environmental tobacco smoke be included in health education about smoking (National Health and Medical Research Council, 1987). The concluding remarks of this report identified the need for further research to confirm the effects of exposure to environmental tobacco smoke on health but stated that sufficient evidence was already available to require prudent public health action.

On 1 July 1986, the Tobacco Institute of Australia responded to this report by placing an advertisement in 14 Australian newspapers entitled, "A message from those who do ... to those who don't", which stated, in part, that "There is little evidence and nothing which proves scientifically that cigarette smoke causes disease in non-smokers." In court action initiated by the Australian Federation of Consumer Organizations, Justice Morling found in February 1991 that this advertisement contravened Section 52 of the Trade Practices Act concerned with misleading and deceptive conduct. The Tobacco Institute of Australia lodged an appeal against this decision with the full bench of the Federal Court, but the appeal was rejected in December 1992 (Everingham & Woodward, 1991). At the very least, however, a pattern had been established in Australia for settling arguments in the courts about the scientific evidence on exposure to environmental tobacco smoke.

Second National Health and Medical Research Council report

In May 1993, the National Health and Medical Research Council appointed a working party to update its earlier report on exposure to environmental tobacco smoke and set down the following terms of reference for the new enquiry:

- to review the epidemiological evidence linking exposure to environmental tobacco smoke with disease in adults and children,
- to assess the burden of illness due to exposure to environmental tobacco smoke in Australia and
- to make recommendations to reduce the burden of illness.

Under the National Health and Medical Research Council Act proclaimed in 1993, the Council can publish both 'guidelines', which are advisory in nature, and 'regulatory recommendations', to which the state and Federal Governments are obliged to respond. Clearly, then, the brief of the new working party was not only to bring the scientific review up to date, but to provide a framework for a public policy and legislative response to the problem posed by environmental tobacco smoke

Almost immediately, the Tobacco Institute sought to influence the process of the new enquiry by seeking membership of the working party and, when this request was rejected, by asking for a formal meeting with the working party. It next sought amendments to the terms of reference of the working party, so that the scientific review would have to extend beyond epidemiological evidence about the effect of exposure to environmental tobacco smoke on health to consider other forms of evidence. When this request was also rejected, the Tobacco Institute commenced action in the Federal Court, in January 1994, to have the amendments adopted. A compromise was eventually reached, and the focus was broadened.

Over the next two years, the Council and the working party continually received correspondence from the Tobacco Institute and repeated requests under the Freedom of Information Act for copies of documents, records of meetings and so on. Proclamation of the National Health and Medical Research Council Act in 1994 obliged the Council to publish new Notices of Inquiry, since it is proposed to issue both 'regulatory recommendations' and 'guidelines' about exposure to environmental tobacco smoke. Section 12 of the Act requires that a process of public consultation be completed when such recommendations and guidelines are being prepared. Thus, in April 1994 the Tobacco Institute submitted to the working party 122 published papers, six books, several volumes of comments on the report of the United States Environmental Protection Agency (1992) on exposure to environmental tobacco smoke, and several other reports that it had commissioned from consultants. In addition, in November 1994 the Institute released its own report, entitled, 'Health aspects of environmental tobacco smoke: an evaluation of the scientific literature' (Lee et al., 1994), which is stated to have been 'prepared by an independent group convened by Dr Julian Lee' (a respiratory physician in New South Wales).

The Council released a draft report of the working party for public comment in November 1995 (National Health and Medical Research Council, 1995). This report addressed all of the terms of reference and included 22 recommendations on the need for smoke-free policies in all workplaces, all confined public places, custodial institutions, child care centres, private vehicles and the Sydney Olympics.

Revenge in the Federal Court

The Tobacco Institute and two of three tobacco companies launched a further action in the Federal Court of Australia in July 1996, claiming that, in preparing the draft report, the working party had erred in relying only on peer-reviewed papers; they said that risks related to domestic exposures to environmental tobacco smoke do not necessarily apply in other settings and that the Council had failed to consider the submissions of the Tobacco Institute properly. Having named the Council and individual members of the working party and of two committees to which it reported as respondents, the Tobacco Institute then suppressed public debate by threatening to bring an action in contempt if any of the named respondents discussed exposure to environmental tobacco smoke while the court case was in progress.

In December 1996, Mr Justice Finn found in favour of the Tobacco Institute, giving as his principal grounds that, in restricting its review of the scientific evidence to peer-reviewed publications, the working party had failed to give proper consideration to the submissions from the Institute. His Honour found no fault with the scientific conclusions reached by the working party but granted an injunction preventing the Council from proceeding with the proposed recommendations.

In June 1997, the Council decided to issue an updated 'technical report' under Section 11 of the National Health and Medical Research Council Act. Despite another request from the Tobacco Institute under the Freedom of Information Act in July 1997 and review of 87 pages of additional references received from the Institute in August 1997, the report finally appeared on 24 November 1997 (National Health and Medical Research Council, 1997). Since the final report does not include any of the recommendations or the original review of public opinion and existing laws on exposure to environmental tobacco smoke that appeared in the draft report, the objectives of the Council as set out in the National Health and Medical Research Council Act and quoted above may be seen to have been significantly compromised.

References

Commonwealth of Australia (1974) Trade Practices Act (1974)
Commonwealth of Australia (1993) National Health and Medical Research Council Act (1993)
Environmental Protection Agency (1992) Respiratory Health Effects of Passive Smoking—Lung Cancers and Other Disorders, Washington DC: Office of Research and Development
Everingham, R. & Woodward, S. (1991) Tobacco Litigation: The Case against Passive Smoking—AFCO v TIA, Sydney: Legal Books
Lee, J., et al. (1994) Health Aspects of Environmental Tobacco Smoke: An Evaluation of the Scientific Literature, Sydney: Tobacco Institute of Australia

National Health and Medical Research Council (1987) *Health Effects of Passive Smoking*, Canberra:
    Australian Government Publishing Service
National Health and Medical Research Council (1995) *The Health Effects of Passive Smoking* (draft report),
    Canberra: Australian Government Publishing Service
National Health and Medical Research Council (1997) *The Health Effects of Passive Smoking*, Canberra:
    Australian Government Publishing Service

Bangladesh: Anti-smoking education programme

S.M. Abdus Sattar

Shastha-o-Kalyan Sangstha, Goshairhat, Shariatpur, Banglasdesh

It is clearly established that tobacco smoking harms the health of both the smoker and the non-smoker, leading to respiratory and cardiac diseases and lung cancer. This should be enough for us to commit ourselves to motivate people to work towards a smoke-free planet.

Anti-smoking education can help reduce the prevalence of smoking, by showing people that smoking harms their health. Children, adolescents and new smokers are the prime targets for anti-smoking education, although new smokers give up the habit more easily. Doctors, nurses, health workers, social workers and teachers can act as educators in an anti-smoking campaign, and journalists, writers, actors and community leaders can also play an important role. The tobacco control movement has taken the lead in establishing anti-smoking education in schools, colleges, hospitals, clinics, health centres, places of worship and community centres, to provide individual and group counselling, discussions in small or large groups, innovative methods and communication techniques such as lectures, posters, stickers, leaflets, booklets, flip-charts and vidoes, as well as advertising on the radio, television and newspapers.

A successful anti-smoking education programme can embolden people to say, 'No more smoke between us.'

Bolivia: Tobacco control

J.L. Rios-Dalenz

National Commission against Tobacco, La Paz, Bolivia

Although for cultural and economic reasons smoking is not very prevalent in Bolivia, particularly among the native people, publicity for tobacco is increasing, and more youngsters and women in the cities are becoming smokers. In Bolivia, tobacco control activities began in 1983 after a national workshop on tobacco sponsored by the International Union against Cancer. As one of its main recommendations, the National Commission against Tobacco was established on a multisectoral basis recognized by the Ministry of Health. At present, sections in eight of the nine departments of the country promote local activities and coordinate programmes on tobacco control at bi-annual meetings in the various cities of Bolivia.

Anti-tobacco legislation has been enacted to ban smoking in public places and transport, including flights within the country by national airlines. A no-smoking policy in hospitals and schools is backed by our Code of Health. A label warning that 'This product is dangerous for your health' is obligatory on visual advertisements and cigarette packs. Publicity is not allowed before 21:00 hours in the media. In addition, educational and other actions, such as research on the risks of smoking in the high-altitude population, are being carried out nationwide.

Cambodia: Tobacco or health: An overview

C. Radford, K. Baldwin Radford, S. Pun & M. Spedding

Adventist Development and Relief Agency Cambodia, Phnom Penh, Cambodia

In 1997, the United Nations Development Programme's human poverty index ranked Cambodia as one of the seven most impoverished countries in the world on the basis of life expectancy, lack of basic education and lack of access to economic resources. Cambodia is primarily a rural country, with only 15% of its 10.7 million people residing in cities. The capital city of Phnom Penh has only a little over 1 million people. Plagued by decades of civil war, political upheaval, and economic insecurity, the Cambodian Government has not considered tobacco and its related illnesses a significant socioeconomic issue. Low immunization coverage, malnutrition and diarrhoeal diseases, and high infant and maternal mortality rates remain priorities for health care. Nevertheless, World Health Organization consultants estimate that 1 million of the children alive in Cambodia today will eventually die of tobacco-related causes.

One of the reasons for the apparent lack of knowledge about the dangers of tobacco use has been a shortage of national data. Until 1994, information about smoking prevalence amongst Cambodians and data on tobacco advertising have been merely anecdotal. Nevertheless, tobacco use has become well integrated into the fabric of Khmer society. Buddhist monks are frequently given cigarettes by those seeking merit, and cigarettes are given out as favours during weddings. In the countryside, little boys as young as eight years old can be seen walking down the road, a cigarette in one hand and a rope leading the family cow in the other. Within the past three years there has also been a proliferation of lovely, young, Khmer women paid to distribute free cigarettes on busy Phnom Penh street corners. They are quite willing to mislead interested volunteers by saying that the filter tip of imported brands will protect users from the harmful effects of smoking. Attractive free clothing and accessories make a job such as this appealing to poor young women.

In 1994, statistics on tobacco advertising and smoking prevalence rates were collected and analysed for the first time in over 20 years in Cambodia. Cambodian public health professionals enrolled in a Masters of Public Health course co-sponsored by the Adventist Development and Relief Agency, and the Ministry of Health conducted surveys throughout Phnom Penh. The data collected during those surveys and another conducted in 1995 have provided a baseline for comparison with the most recent statistics gathered within the Tobacco-free Kids project.

In May 1997, an updated street advertising survey was conducted in Phnom Penh, targeting all main roads. 'Street advertising' was divided into three main categories: posters/signs, umbrellas and billboards. The results indicated that 46% of the 36 000 street signs on main roads in Phnom Penh advertise cigarettes, an alarming 400% increase in less than three years. Posters and signs made up the majority (82%) of street advertising. This category included newspaper stands painted to resemble Marlboro cigarette boxes and roadside newspaper stalls emblazoned with 'Mild Seven' logos. Of the total number of posters and signs, 40% advertised tobacco products. Large umbrellas, a precious commodity in a hot, rainy country, made up 17% of all street advertising and 75% of all umbrellas carried tobacco ads. Tobacco companies clearly value this form of advertising, as every week high-pressure water carts travel around the city with logo-clad staff diligently cleaning their company's umbrellas.

Large billboards are a relatively new phenomenon in Cambodia, comprising only 1% of all street advertising. Despite the relatively small overall number of billboards, 47% advertise tobacco products. Rental of billboards in Phnom Penh can cost more than US$ 25 000 per year, making it prohibitively expensive for all but the large multinational companies. In fact, 53% of tobacco billboards advertise just four brands, all imported: 555, Dunhill, Marlboro and Gold Leaf. National brands are beginning to follow suit by developing smaller billboards that are more affordable and easy to produce locally.

Statistics released in August 1997 by the International Management and Investment Consultants echo the findings of the Adventist Development and Relief Agency. Spending on television and print advertising in the first six months of 1997 increased by 300% over the same period last year. Tobacco companies were the biggest advertisers, comprising 18% of the market, for a total of US$ 2.6 million. Although a 1995 Government declaration requires all television and radio tobacco advertising to include a health warning, this same condition has not yet been enforced for the print media. Indeed, with a national literacy rate of only 35%, many of the tobacco companies' best customers would not be able to read the warning label even if it were there. None of the billboards or signs surveyed had a warning label in either English or Khmer.

In July and August 1997, a random sample of 2378 men and 818 women in Phnom Penh was surveyed to determine urban smoking prevalence rates, smoker demographics, and public opinion about tobacco advertising. Of the total surveyed, 47% were smokers. Earlier surveys indicated that almost 65% of urban males smoke; the 1997 statistics are slightly lower, at 62%. This drop might be explained by the larger proportion of young male students surveyed in 1997, as most urban males do not become regular smokers until their early 20s. Only 5% of urban females surveyed were smokers. Consistent with the earlier survey, educational level and smoking prevalence were related inversely. Smokers had significantly fewer years of schooling than their non-smoking counterparts.

The reasons for starting to smoke were varied, some being specific to Cambodia. Of all the smokers surveyed, most said that they were influenced to begin smoking by friends (32%) or chose to begin smoking on their own (28%). Free cigarettes helped to start 14% of those surveyed, while famous people and actors influenced 9% of smokers to start smoking. The sixth commonest reason for starting to smoke is one sadly unique to Cambodia: about 50 people (3%) said that they began smoking between 1975 and 1979 during the murderous Pol Pot regime: Some started smoking because the Khmer Rouge soldiers allowed only smokers a 10-min break from hard labour each hour. Others began smoking because smoke supposedly repelled mosquitoes and reduced their chance of contracting a mosquito-borne disease such as malaria.

Of the 1509 smokers, 78% said that they would like to quit smoking. At present, however, there are no locally available resources in Khmer to assist them with behaviour modification or supervised medical intervention strategies. Of the smokers and non-smokers asked whether the Government should create a tobacco-advertising ban in Cambodia, 89% said that all tobacco advertising should be banned. Even the smokers concurred, 88% stating that tobacco advertising bans were necessary. To date, attempts to ban tobacco advertising have met with many political challenges, most of them due to the apparent profit motive and lack of understanding about the true economic, medical and societal burden of tobacco consumption. In addition, initiating a tobacco excise tax directed towards public health initiatives, such as education about tobacco or health, has not yet been possible. Continued education is needed at every level of society, particularly targeting key Government leaders.

The Tobacco-free Kids project, funded by the Australian government, is the first and only project in Cambodia in which information on tobacco or health is disseminated in the media. As the name implies, the target audience is school-age youth, primarily in Phnom Penh, although the posters, stickers, billboards, T-shirts and public service announcements developed for television and radio can affect people of all ages throughout the country. The overall goal of the project can best be summarized by one of the winning student posters from 'World No-Tobacco Day' 1997. It depicts two young Khmers ordering a life-size cigarette into the sea, banishing tobacco from Cambodia forever. While the steps that have been taken to date are relatively small, materials and resources are now being developed to counteract the tobacco advertisers' beautifully depicted lies and to help bring reality to the dream of a tobacco-free Cambodia.

Canada: Public attitudes towards tobacco control policies: Current attitudes and changes in support over time

J.E. Cohen, M.J. Ashley, L.L. Pederson, P.D. Poland, S.B. Bull & R.G. Ferrence

Ontario Tobacco Research Unit, University of Toronto, Toronto, Canada

Background: Current information about public attitudes can be valuable in garnering political support for the enactment of effective tobacco control legislation. Data on how support or opposition has changed over time, or remained stable, can also be informative for programming and developing policy.

Methods: In spring 1996, a 25-min, computer-assisted, random-digit dialling telephone survey was conducted with a representative sample of 1764 adults living in the Province of Ontario. Their levels of knowledge and support were compared with similar information collected in 1983 and in 1991.

Results: Although knowledge about some specific health effects of both active and passive smoking increased, important deficits in knowledge remained. Overall, support for restricting smoking in a wide range of public locations increased and is substantial. Support for banning cigarette advertising also increased over the 13 years. A clear majority supported the plain packaging of cigarettes and harsher penalties for shops that sell cigarettes to minors.

Discussion: General education about the health hazards of smoking should continue. Family fast-food settings, indoor public gatherings, hockey arenas and food courts in malls are priority settings for smoking bans.

Canada: Public attitudes toward tobacco control policies: How different are smokers and non-smokers?

M.J. Ashley, J. Cohen, S.B. Bull, L.L. Pederson, B. Poland & R. Ferrence

Ontario Tobacco Research Unit, University of Toronto, Toronto, Canada

Rationale: Information about differences and similarities in knowledge about the health effects of tobacco and attitudes toward tobacco control measures among smokers and non-smokers and predictions of compliance of smokers with more restrictions can assist policy and programme development.

Methods: Data from a population-based, random-digit dialling, computer-assisted survey conducted in 1996 in Ontario, Canada, involving 1340 adult non-smokers and 424 adult smokers were analysed. The response rate was 65%.

Findings: Although knowledge deficits were identified in both groups, smokers were less knowledgeable than non-smokers. Smokers were also less likely to support bans on smoking in most settings but were more likely than non-smokers to predict that most smokers would comply with more restrictions, and more than three quarters indicated that they, themselves, would comply. Sizeable proportions of both groups, but especially smokers, failed to appreciate the effectiveness of taxation in reducing smoking. Support for other control measures also differed substantially by smoking status.

Conclusions: While effective educational interventions concerning the health effects of tobacco use that are aimed at the entire population are needed, specific efforts should be directed to improving the knowledge of smokers. In view of the levels of support among both smokers and non-smokers and the high levels of predicted compliance by smokers with more restrictions, settings for consideration of complete bans on smoking or enclosed, separately ventilated smoking areas can be identified. Specific interventions to increase understanding about the effectiveness of tobacco taxes and support for tax measures are needed.

Cuba: Programme for tobacco prevention and control

N. Suarez Lugo

Carlos J. Finlay National School in Public Health, Ministry of Public Health, Havana, Cuba

The programme

In Cuba in 1984, the situation with regard to smoking was characterized by a high prevalence, high consumption, a high rate of mortality due to chronic diseases, an early age at starting to smoke, high levels of tobacco production, social acceptance related to culture, folklore and traditions, other health priorities, consumer protection and orientation to rational consumption. In 1985, the Government approved a programme for prevention and control of tobacco use, and a national effort was undertaken. The strategy of the programme was to be national and systematic, to be persuasive through social marketing and health promotion and to have a wide focus, on both the individual and society, through legislation and education. The main focus of the strategy is on young people who have not started to smoke.

The overall objective of the progamme for 1996–2000 is to reduce the prevalence of smoking by 2% annually. The specific objectives are to stop people from smoking and to reduce the number who start, especially among the young. The methods to be used are education of the population, establishment of a legal mechanism to protect people from passive exposure to smoke and to reduce the opportunities for smoking, assisting people to stop smoking and maintaining epidemiological vigilance. Advances towards these goals each year depend on conditions and resources.

The programme is directed by a multisectoral, multidisciplinary committee coordinated by the Ministry of Public Health and integrated into other Government ministries and organizations, including the ministries of Education, Higher Education, Science, Technology and the Environment, Culture, Transport, Communication and Internal Commerce and the Institute of Radio and Television, the Institute of Civil Aeronautics, the Federation of Cuban Women and the Organization of Children and Youth. Groups also work at the provincial level. A strategy and action plan is elaborated each year on the basis of the overall aims, and the responsibilities of each participant are defined. Progress is monitored at monthly meetings, an annual meeting and in a report to the Government.

The objective of the information, education and communication actions is to orientate and educate both the general population and special groups. Education is provided directly through the mass media on the basis of information from the Ministry of Public Health. The entities involved play an important role in education through their personnel and their targets, be they women, teachers, sportsmen, physicians, children or youth, through courses, workshops, training and service. Of particular importance was the introduction of anti-smoking information into the curricula of elementary schools in 1992–93 and of secondary schools in 1993–94. Although more training is needed for health promoters, the material means of doing so are lacking.

The objective of the service for assistance and clinical intervention is to offer help to persons interested in stopping smoking. In 1992, the National Reference Centre for the Study and Treatment of Nicotine Addiction was created, which undertakes research, gives advice, trains and offers service at the Hermanos Amejelras General Hospital. In 1996, 30 centres for quitting smoking were set up in all provinces, with trained specialists. Primary treatment is provided and also specialized consultations, acupuncture, acupressure, hypnosis and other methods; subjects are given self-help manuals. The intervention is performed with the consent of the family physician.

Legislation

Legal action is needed to support the programme. This is not provided by current Cuban legislation. A Smoking Act should be promulgated to reduce the prevalence, consumption and social acceptability of smoking, with legislative measures that are stronger and more rigid than the existing ones. The principal results obtained in 1996 were:

* bans on smoking on domestic flights and in public transport, health and education centres, theatres, cinemas and shops;
* regulation of tobacco advertising through the Ministry of Public Health;
* an increase in the price of cigarettes between 1995 and 1997;
* a decrease in the nicotine and tar concentrations in popular cigarettes; and
* a proposed law on tobacco control.

The proposed law was approved by the national committee of the programme and by the Ministry of Public Health and was presented to the Government for analysis, validation and approval. It will then be presented to the Cuban Parliament. The law is described in detail in another paper in this volume.

Evaluation and research

Part of the programme consists of an evaluation of its development and impact. The research is carried out by Government institutions, including those represented on the committee which have personnel with the necessary specialities and qualifications. The main objectives are to determine the prevalence of smoking, the consumption of tobacco, mortality and morbidity due to tobacco-related diseases and socioeconomic obstacles to tobacco control. These will be used as the basis of the strategy for 1996–2000.

Conclusion

The main hindrances to the programme are that it has no legal basis, its members participate irregularly and it has no central financial support. The success of the legal measures that have been taken has not been monitored. Cigarettes are still sold separately, there has been little effect on sales or advertising, the tobacco companies are still advertising indirectly by sponsoring sports and cultural events, and the public has received few pro-health, anti-tobacco messages. These failures are due to lack of resources for printing, training health promoters, preparing promotional material, testing activities and carrying out studies on the actual situation with regard to tobacco smoking.

The main results have been:

* an annual reduction in prevalence of 1% between 1984 and 1990 but no change in prevalence between 1990 and 1995; nevertheless, there was an increased number of ex-smokers in 1995;
* a decreased prevalence among men but an increased prevalence among women between 1984 and 1995;
* an annual reduction in consumption of 1% between 1985 and 1990 and 1.5% between 1991 and 1996;
* the highest rates of cessation were among light smokers;
* the age at starting to smoke was stable from 1984 to 1990 and increased by 1.3% between 1990 and 1995;
* social acceptance of smoking remains but has diminished; the population formerly knew that smoking was hazardous but did not realize the magnitude of the risk.

These results indicate that control activities must be intensified. International collaboration will be an important factor in maintaining the results obtained.

Europe: Smoking, risk behaviour and attitudes to coronary heart disease in five European countries: The HELP study

P. Schioldborg on behalf of the HELP Study Group

Institute of Psychology, University of Oslo, Norway

A survey of attitudes towards coronary heart disease and health-related behaviour was conducted in 1996 among 5013 members of the general public, 2500 people at high risk, 1256 patients with coronary heart disease and 1249 members of their families in France, Germany, Italy, Sweden and the United Kingdom. The results showed that all the groups considered advice on coronary health provided by the physician to be credible, but compliance with the advice was low, particularly in the high-risk group. Of these, 64% were daily smokers, in comparison with only 20% of the general public and 20% of patients who had had a myocardial infarct, with no significant difference among the five countries. The average daily consumption of alcohol in the three groups was 1.4, 0.6 and 1.4 units, respectively, Italy and the United Kingdom having the highest consumption. The frequency of physical exercise (one or more times per week) was 19, 52 and 62%, respectively, Germany and Sweden having the highest percentages. In the high-risk group, 52% stated that they were unwilling to make any sacrifice to achieve a healthy lifestyle, but only 4% described themselves as 'very healthy'; the corresponding figures in the general public were 7 and 21%, respectively. In view of the serious effect of smoking on the heart, a new direction in health promotion for coronary heart disease is needed; relevant information should be provided to stress the severity of the problem, the behavioural steps to be taken and the psychological gains of coping.

Europe: Creating the European Network for Smoking Prevention

S. Fleitmann

European Network for Smoking Prevention, Brussels, Belgium

The European Union is a supranational legislative body created in 1957, with the main goal of establishing an economic trade zone in Europe. The European Union comprises 15 Member States—Austria, Belgium, Denmark, Finland, France, Germany, Greece, Ireland, Italy, Luxembourg, the Netherlands, Portugal, Spain, Sweden and the United Kingdom—with a total population of 371 million inhabitants, 11 different languages and very different social and cultural backgrounds.

In 1982, more than 3 million people died of cancer in the European Union, representing more than 1% of the total population. In 1987, the 'Europe against Cancer' programme was created by the Heads of State in order to curb the rising cancer mortality rates. The first step in cooperation on tobacco control issues at the European level was taken when the European Commission, responsible for the administration of the Europe against Cancer programme, set up a working group of organizations representative of national tobacco control activities.

The aim was to foster cooperation and to overcome cultural difficulties through exchange of information and experience. For six years, biannual meetings were held to help people to get to know each other. In 1994, the Commission requested proposals for a common strategy to reinforce tobacco control. A conference was organized in Empoli, Italy, which resulted in a consensus statement known as the 'Vinci Resolution', laying down two main principles for a future action plan:
• creation of a permanent pan-European structure to promote networking in Europe;
• creation of national anti-tobacco coalitions.

The difficulties of implementing a mutually satisfying action plan under the auspices of the European Commission seemed insurmountable. Not only did the members of the working group have 15 different national objectives and priorities, but they also had to consider the political interests of the European Commission, the stakeholder.

It took three years, several unsatisfactory meetings and a threat by the European Commission to abandon the tobacco project before a multinational executive committee was elected from among the working group in April 1996, with the mission of making practical proposals to implement the 'Vinci Resolution'.

In view of the experience of the previous years, a major challenge was to develop a strategy that was politically acceptable to both parties. The Executive Committee suggested the creation of an independent, international, non-profit association. The association would be funded jointly by the European Commission and by voluntary contributions from its members. This suggestion was accepted by both tobacco control associations and the European Commission. The legal basis for the European Network for Smoking Prevention was thus agreed upon, and the first recommendation of the 'Vinci Resolution', to create a permanent European structure, was ready to be implemented.

The second recommendation, the creation of national anti-tobacco coalitions in each of the 15 Member States, still had to be launched and put into practice. A survey conducted in 1996 in France had shown that four kinds of organizations were involved in tobacco control activities in Europe: anti-tobacco associations (43%), cancer leagues (32%), hospitals and universities (14%) and public health structures (12%). The medical approach to smoking prevention predominated, and advocacy, lobbying and economic and legal aspects were usually not covered. The number of staff employed for tobacco control activities was limited in 66% of the organizations to fewer than five employees and in 22% to between 5 and 10 employees. An analysis of the budgets of these associations for tobacco control revealed large differences among them, varying from US$ 4000 to more than US$ 6 million a year.

The main obstacles to a coordinated approach to tobacco control at the national level, however, were inadequate knowledge of activities in their own countries, fear of competition and diverging political interests. It was therefore recommended that each national coalition should:

- promote tobacco control at the national level and contribute through its work to tobacco control at the European level;
- represent all players in the field of tobacco control at the national level;
- agree on a coordinated approach to lobbying in order to establish the legal framework for tobacco control;
- create synergy and promote collaboration at the national and European levels while respecting the specificity and individual identity of each of its members;
- appoint a liaison person to ensure information exchange among members and with the coordinating office and
- establish contacts with the national representatives of the Europe against Cancer programme.

In April 1997, the European Network for Smoking Prevention was registered as an independent, international, non-profit association under Belgian law. It is now governed by a general assembly consisting of two representatives of each national coalition of the 15 Member States of the European Union and one representative of each specialized tobacco control network (ENYPAT, Smokeless Cities network, Smokeless Hospitals network, Smokeless General Practitioners network). A board of five people has been elected as administrators. Associate membership is open to all associations active in tobacco control in the European Region, including the countries of central and eastern Europe, and observers from other international organizations are invited to our meetings on request.

The general objectives and the action plan of the European Network for Smoking Prevention are:

- to promote and facilitate the activities of national coalitions and specialized smoking prevention networks by helping them to define and implement a coherent national tobacco control strategy;
- to promote collaboration between its members by sharing information, experience, activities and projects through a permanent secretariat that will create a corporate identity, give personalized advice, organize conferences, publish a quarterly newsletter and create a common database.
- to collect and distribute information among the institutions of the European Union, the European Union Member States and the members of the network. For example, as of March 1998, projects introduced for funding to the European Commission have been grouped, and a large European framework project has been coordinated, contributing to the creation of more coherent, cost–effective smoking prevention projects at the European level;
- to establish links with intergovernmental and supranational organizations, international non-governmental organizations and other relevant groups to inform them about policies and projected legislation and to participate in planning international tobacco control strategies; and
- to lend support and promote the establishment of national alliances for smoking prevention in the countries of central and eastern Europe. This is especially important as the tobacco industry is specifically targeting those countries to replace market shares lost in the European Union and North America.

Much work lies ahead, as the Network is a multifaceted enterprise. We shall report on progress accomplished at the Eleventh World Conference on Tobacco or Health and shall share our experience with people faced by a similar challenge.

Smoke-free Europe: A forum for networks

P. Puska[1], L. Elovainio[2], H. Vertio[3] & S. Lipponen[3]

[1]National Public Health Institute, [2]Cancer Society of Finland and [3]Finnish Centre for Health Promotion, Helsinki, Finland

Background

A European tobacco control conference was initiated to foster pan-European networking of professionals interested in tobacco research and policy, smoke-free environments, smoking prevention and tobacco control programmes. Over 500 delegates from nearly 50 countries participated in the 'Smokefree Europe: Conference on Tobacco or Health' in Helsinki, Finland, in October 1996. The Finnish Centre for Health Promotion acted as the conference secretariat. Financial resources for the conference were received both from national sources, such as the Ministry of Social Affairs and Health, the Ministry of Education and the Finnish Slot Machine Association, and from the Europe against Cancer and Phare programmes of the European Union.

The organizers emphasized the regional aspects of tobacco control policy. Europe is a small, densely populated area with several countries that are facing similar problems. Given the enormous scale of tobacco consumption in the world, specifically European questions are not necessarily the central issues on the global agenda. In Europe, a widespread change in the political system altered the health picture and tobacco consumption. One distinctive feature was the aggressive marketing strategies of the western tobacco industry in central and eastern Europe. Finland, on the other hand, had experienced a declining trend in smoking during the previous 20 years of anti-smoking efforts. In 1996, about 27% of men and 18% of women in the age group 15–64 years were daily smokers, and this level was among the lowest in Europe.

This specific European setting provided a fruitful basis for creating a new regional process. As a result, the conference unanimously adopted a resolution on a European tobacco control strategy.

Non-governmental organizations played a very important part in the organization of the Smoke-free Europe conference, and this directly affected the scientific programme, in which various anti-smoking networks played prominent roles. Concurrently with the conference, the European Union invited its cancer experts to Helsinki to discuss guidelines for a tobacco policy within the European Union and to produce a policy document with recommendations. The results of the consensus conference were introduced and discussed in the larger forum of Smoke-free Europe. This model proved to be successful, as it combined an expert meeting within the broader framework of a tobacco control agenda.

Smoke-free Europe was a starting point for a process of discussion of vital European issues. In the post conference book (Puska *et al.*, 1997), several approaches were defined: networks, developing a European tobacco policy, successful national campaigns, the widening health gap in Europe, public discussions and the roles of the mass media, litigation and law. The conference material was also distributed on Internet in cooperation with the Globalink network of the International Union Against Cancer. The Smokefree Europe process continues, and the second European conference was held in Gran Canary, Spain in February 1999.

Reference

Puska, P., Elovainio, L. & Vertio, H. (1997) *Smokefree Europe—A Forum for Networks*, Helsinki

India: Tobacco control: A perspective

K. Chaudhry[1] & K.P. Unnikrishnan[2]

[1]Indian Council of Medical Research, Ansari Nagar, and [2]Ministry of Health and Family Welfare, Nirman Bhavan, New Delhi, India

Abstract

Tobacco is responsible for about 800 000 deaths annually in India. The health services have to manage 400 000 prevalent cases of cancer, 1.3 million cases of coronary heart disease and at least 7 million cases of chronic obstructive lung disease, due solely to tobacco use. In the recent past, the emphasis was mainly on tobacco control through community education. Legislative action for tobacco control was initiated in 1976 with promulgation of the *Cigarette Act (1975)*, wherin all packets and cartons of cigarettes were to carry a statutory health warning. Administrative action has been taken to ban tobacco advertisements in Government-controlled electronic media and to ban smoking in certain public places. In view of the limitations of the *Cigarette Act*, more comprehensive legislation is being prepared which includes a ban on advertising of all tobacco products, a ban on smoking in public places, restriction of sale of tobacco products to minors and more effective, rotating health warnings on all tobacco products. An expert committee has been constituted to study the economics of tobacco in India. In view of the diverse areas associated with tobacco, the need for a strong political will has been recognized, and sensitization of politicians and bureaucrats about the problem of tobacco has been a major activity. The Parliament's Committee on Sub-ordinate Legislation in its 22nd report (Lok Sabha Secretariat, 1995) considered the overall problem of tobacco. Its recommendations and the current initiatives of the Government of India to control of tobacco are discussed.

Introduction

The tobacco habit has gained social acceptance in many segments of society during its 400 years of existence in India. Tobacco is used in many ways in India: being smoked in the form of cigarettes, *bidis, chuttas, dhumtis,* clay pipes and hookahs (Bhonsle *et al.*, 1992). It is also commonly used in smokeless form: chewed with or without lime as an ingredient of *pan* or *pan masala* or applied in the form of *mishri*, snuff or tobacco toothpaste. Various studies in India in the 1980s showed that the prevalence of tobacco use among men over 15 years of age varied between 46 and 63% in urban areas and between 32 and 74% in rural areas (Chaudhry *et al.*, 1990). Among women, it varied between 2 and 16% in urban areas and between 20 and 50% in rural areas. On the basis of these studies, it has been estimated that in India about 194 million men and about 45 million women over 15 years of age use tobacco (Chaudhry & Prabhakar, 1996).

The annual number of deaths due to tobacco use is estimated to be 800 000, equal to 2200 deaths per day or one death every 40 s (Chaudhry & Prabhakar, 1996). The prevalence of illness due to tobacco use includes 400 000 cancers, 1.3 million cases of coronary artery disease and at least 7 million cases of chronic obstructive lung disease.

Observations in the 22nd report of the Committee on Sub-ordinate Legislation

The Committee observed that the statutory warning on cigarette packs laid down by the Cigarette Act 1975 has not proved effective. Limitations of the warning identified by the Committee included its language, being only English, the monotony of the message, small lettering and its presence on only one side of the pack, its size, being smaller than the brand name, the absence from the purview of the Act of *bidis*, the most prevalent form of tobacco smoked in India; the absence of a maximum permissible limit for tar and nicotine content and the absence of tar and nicotine concentrations on the packs.

The Committee considered that the existing provisions on tobacco advertising were ineffective and insufficient. It observed that the glamourous tobacco advertisments on video films, newspapers and magazines create an illusion that smoking is a pleasurable and sophisticated activity, helpful for achieving success in various fields. Sponsorship of sports and cultural events gives the tobacco industry a high profile of visibility. The tobacco industry's claim that advertising is for brand switching and does not increase tobacco consumption was perceived by the Committee to be wrong and grossly misleading.

The Committee considered that the risk of disease caused by inhaling tobacco smoke is not limited to smokers but also affects those who inhale the smoke passively. It observed that the ban on smoking in public places in other countries has resulted in widespread change in attitudes, leading to smoking cessation.

The Committee noted that two important factors influence young people to start smoking: parental practices at home and peer habits at school. It is therefore necessary to tackle the problem at these two levels, by parental and preceptor example and careful, well-studied and thought-provoking information at schools and colleges. A coordinated, rational educational strategy is needed to discourage young people from smoking. The Committee also observed the success of a nationwide radio programme, 'Radio Date', carried out jointly by All-India Radio and the Indian Council of Medical Research. The successful anti-tobacco community education projects of the Council were also noted.

The Committee considered that increasing the production of tobacco and at the same time framing comprehensive legislation to curb its use cannot be justified. A policy decision by the Government to encourage farmers to switch to other profitable crops is imperative. It was observed that the Indian Council of Agricultural Research has identified mustard, sunflower, soya bean and groundnut as alternative cash crops. Farmers must be shown that cultivation of other crops will bring in equal or higher income. The Committee recognized that the livelihood of millions of workers engaged in the manufacture of *bidis* and cigarettes will have to be addressed seriously.

Recommendations in the 22nd report of the Committee on Sub-ordinate Legislation

Statutory warning on tobacco products: The Committee recommended that the health warning(s) should appear on all tobacco products. The warning should be worded strongly, rotated periodically and supplemented by symbols or pictures. The warnings should be in English and regional language(s). The lettering of the warning should be as large as that of the brand name, and it should be displayed on both sides of the pack. The concentrations of tar and nicotine should be printed on packs and cartons of all tobacco products and maximum permissible limits should be fixed. Observing that loose cigarettes are sold, the Committee recommended that individual cigarettes should also bear the health warning. The health warnings should also be displayed prominently in every shop where tobacco products are sold. Imported cigarettes and other tobacco products must meet the statutory warning requirements of India.

Tobacco advertising: It was recommended that the Government should make provision in the proposed legislation for a total ban on all forms of advertisement for tobacco, with stringent penal provisions for violation of the law. There should be a total ban on the sponsorship of major sports events by cigarette companies.

Prohibition of tobacco smoking in public places: The Committee recommended a complete ban on smoking at least in all public places where large numbers of people are expected to be present for long periods, such as hospitals, dispensaries, other health-care establishments, educational institutions, conference halls, cinemas, theatres, offices, all workplaces and railway waiting rooms. There should also be a complete ban on smoking in public transport systems, domestic flights and Government vehicles.

Social awareness about tobacco: People should be educated about the effects of smoking and passive smoking. Non-smokers who object to smoking and other forms of tobacco use should have legal backing. Anti-tobacco education should be compulsory in schools and colleges. Teachers should not smoke within school premises. The sale of tobacco and tobacco products should be banned in the vicinity of schools and colleges, with provision for punishment of vendors for violation. Persons below a minimum age (say, 18 years) should not be sold cigarettes. The Committee suggested that social awareness should be created through electronic and print media. As far as possible, scenes in which characters smoke in an obtrusive manner should not be included in programmes shown on television. The Committee recommended that the Government allocate adequate resources and personnel to carry our effective anti-smoking education.

Alternative cash crops to replace tobacco: The Committee considered that initiatives should be taken by the Ministry of Agriculture to persuade farmers to switch over to alternative crops. This may be done first on an experimental basis, and the results then widely publicized to convince farmers of its viability. The Committee also recommended that farmers be given anti-tobacco education. The Government might consider giving monetary assistance to farmers to help them change to alternative crops. It was suggested that the Indian Council of Agricultural Research develop new techniques for high-yield varieties and for fertilizers for alternative cash crops. Research should also be continued to explore alternative uses for tobacco. It was considered that the Tobacco Board should not promote internal consumption of tobacco, although the Committee had no objection to production of tobaco for export. It was suggested that a gradual approach be adopted wherein effeorts were made to phase out cultivation of tobacco for human consumption over time. The Government should at once conduct a study of the resources required for rehabilitating workers in tobacco production and the areas in which they could be absorbed; they should formulate a concrete proposal in this regard.

Newer initiatives in tobacco control in India

The heightened 'political and bureaucratic will' for tobacco control has seen several actions from various ministries and departments. The Ministry of Agriculture has requested major tobacco-growing states to consider actions for reducing production of non-flue-cured varieties of tobacco, and efforts have been initiated in the states of Andhra Pradesh, Tamil Nadu, Orissa and Karnatka. The Department of Agriculture and Cooperation held a joint meeting with the Indian Council of Agricultural Research and decided to explore the potential of alternative crops such as medicinal plants, soya bean, sugar cane, waxy-type maize, oil palm and vegetables. It was considered that the schemes for assistance to tobacco production should be discontinued. Research efforts should concentrate on the development of low-tar, low-nicotine flue-cured varieties of tobacco and on alternative uses of tobacco. A scheme should be worked out for weaning farmers away from cultivation of non-flue-cured varieties of tobacco.

The Ministry of Health and Family Welfare has constituted an expert committee on the economics of tobacco in India, which is likely to help in decision-making. The Directorate-General of Health Services is examinig the health hazards of *pan masala*, especially with tobacco, through an expert committee. The comprehensive legislation is being revised to consider the possible inclusion of the recommendations of Goa.

Perspectives for tobacco control in India

The current situation suggests that the politicians are conducive to implementing tobacco control activities. The ministries of health, agriculture and education are looking positively at the issue. The mass media are also providing better coverage of the subject. State governments are taking or are willing to take legislative action for control of tobacco use. Tobacco control has been accepted as a priority for action. The current status suggests that India is poised for major steps in the control of tobacco use in the near future.

References

Bhonsle, R.B., Murti, P.R. & Gupta, P.C. (1992) Tobacco habits in India. In: Gupta, P.C., Hamner, J.E., III & Murti, P.R., eds, *Control of Tobacco-related Cancers and Other Diseases*, Bombay: Oxford University Press, pp. 25–46

Chaudhry, K. & Prabhakar, A,K, (1996) *Tobacco Plain Facts*, New Delhi: Indian Council of Medicfal Research

Chaudhry, K., Prabhakar, A,K, & Luthra, U.K. (1990) Tobacco control in India: Search for strategies. In: Durston, B. & Jamrozik, K., eds, *Tobacco and Health 1990—The Global War*, Perth: Health Department of Western Australia, pp. 363–366

Lok Sabha Secretariat (1995) *Twenty-second Report of the Committee on Sub-ordinate Legislation (Tenth Lok Sabha) on Rules/Regulations Framed under the Cigarettes (Regulation of Production, Supply and Distribution) Act, 1975*, New Delhi

Macao: Tobacco or health

A. Ho

Macao Consumer Council, Macao

Introduction

Macao is a Chinese territory which is under Portuguese administration until December 1999. It is a city located in the Pearl River Delta on the southern coast of China, composed of a peninsula (Macao) and two islands (Taipa and Coloane). Its total area is about 21 km². The population in 1996 was estimated to be 454 607, 48.1% male and 51.9% female. The population density of peninsular Macao (7.49 km²) is about 51 000/km², one of the highest in the world. The population is 95% Chinese, 3% Portuguese and 2% other racial groups. In terms of nationality, 67.6% are Chinese, 28.5% Portuguese and 3.9% other nationalities. The population under 15 years of age was 25%, those aged 15–64 represented 67.8%, and people aged ≥ 65 represented 7.2%. The crude birth rate in 1995 was 14.1/1000; the death rate was 3.2/1000. The population growth rate was 1.1% per year. Infant mortality was 6.2/1000 live births.

Tobacco production, trade and consumption

Macao has six cigarette factories, with a total of 430 employees, but the tobacco for cigarettes is imported. In 1994, 166 million packs of cigarettes were imported, and 93 million packs were exported, mainly to China. Smuggling is a widespread problem.

Almost all of the tobacco consumed in Macao is in the form of manufactured cigarettes; hand-rolled cigarettes and pipe tobacco comprise less than 1% of the market. Tobacco companies and manufacturers have been marketing their products actively and aggressively in Macao. Most brands of cigarettes are available, and the selling price is 40–60% cheaper than in Hong Kong because of a lower tax. It is estimated that the sales volume of tobacco in 1996 was 1.6 million million MOP.

In 1991, the average number of cigarettes smoked was 11 per day. According to a survey in 1994, 75% of smokers smoked one pack (20 cigarettes) or less per day, 22% smoked two packs per day and 2.8% smoked three or more packs per day. A survey in 1997 showed that the average number of cigarettes smoked had increased to 15.5/day.

A survey in 1994 showed that 429 of the 3061 persons interviwed were smokers (14%), of whom 393 were male (92%) and 36 female (8.4%). The prevalence was 25% among males and 2.5% among females. The smoking prevalence was 2.0% in the age group 10–19 years, 12% in the group 20–29 years, 15% in the age group 30–39, 21% in the group 40–49 and 21% in the age group ≥ 50 years. In a survey in 1997, 14% of men and 3.2% of women aged 15–24 smoked, whereas 36% of men and 4.2% of women aged 25 and above smoked. Men with a higher level of education smoked less, while women with more education smoked more.

Tobacco control measures

Control measures have been instituted to prevent the undesirable effects of smoking, mainly through legislation and health education.

The first law against tobacco products, passed in 1983, restricts advertising, requires advertisements to carry a health warning and prohibits smoking in public places, health-care units and premises intended for minors. Health warnings appear on the front and back of cigarette packs, covering 10% of the area, in English and Chinese, and the tar and nicotine contents are shown. There are partial advertising bans on billboards. Sales to minors and in vending machines are prohibited, but there is no ban on smokeless tobacco. Smoking-free areas exist in all health facilities, schools, kindergartens, libraries, museums, sports arenas, transport and entertainment places such as cinemas and theatres.

The law has not, however, been seriously or effectively implemented. In July 1989, the Legislative Assembly passed a law concerning the audio and visual broadcasting industry, which included a clause stating that cigarette advertisements on television were to be banned immediately. Owing to strong opposition from the television station and tobacco-related businesses, however, the clause was revised three days later to remove the term 'immediately' and make its terms milder and more flexible.

As everyone knows, advertisements are powerful weapons for marketing. Their influence, particularly on immature adolescents, is well recognized, and the growing numbers of adolescent smokers is mostly due to the impact of advertising. A ban on tobacco advertisements is therefore the crux of the battle for 'tobacco or health'. Accordingly, in July 1996 a new law on the prevention and regulation of smoking was passed by the Legislative Assembly, stipulating that all kinds of cigarette advertisements are to be banned and that there will be stronger penalties and greater power for enforcement bodies. Before it was supposed to come into effect on 1 January 1997, however, it was delayed and then modified, by insertion of a 'transition period' until December 1998. Until then, certain advertisements were still permitted. If this law is properly enforced, it is to be hoped that the number of smokers will decrease.

In a survey in 1997, it was shown that the main reason for not smoking or for quitting smoking is health consciousness. Health education to provide knowledge and information about the health hazards of smoking and about healthy lifestyle, is therefore considered to be a core approach. We have done this consistently, through television, newspapers, radio, posters and seminars. Our efforts are focused primarily on students and children. Many activities have been organized in schools, including drawing contests with the theme of anti-smoking. Anti-smoking and health campaigns have also been organized in conjunction with celebration of the 'World No-Tobacco day' and the 'Macao Anti-smoking Day' every year. Through these activities, public awareness has been raised considerably.

Having recognized that the complexities of the tobacco problem have moved far beyond the health sector and can no longer be dealt with by traditional approaches, the Macao Government has applied a multisectoral, multi-disciplinary approach.

Cooperation has been established among governmental and non-governmental organizations, especially with the Smoke Abstention and Good Health Association. A number of activities have been organized singly and jointly, with technical and financial support from the Government. For example, commerative stamps were issued jointly with the Macao Post Department.

Future plans

Although some progress has been achieved, many obstacles remain. Although laws and regulations on tobacco have been enacted which could provide a legal basis fot the control of tobacco use, resistance and pressure from the tobacco industry are still strong. We must therefore take serious action to reinforce the laws further.

Although more and more people have realized through health education that smoking is harmful to health, not everyone is ready to stop smoking for their own health or that of others. Public health education must therefore be pursued persistently and further strengthened in order to change people's attitudes towards smoking, to give up their bad habits and to cultivate a healthy lifestyle. Everyone should be prepared to look after their health and that of others to achieve a better quality of life.

It is our strong opinion that the success of 'tobacco or health' activities depends more and more on the ability to influence policy-makers, politicians and others. We shall therefore continue to unite all possible forces and work together with other governmental and non-governmental organizations for the attainment of a smoking-free city and the highest possible standard of health for the people of Macao.

New Zealand: Tobacco control, 1990–97

M. Allen

Public Health Policy and Regulation, Ministry of Health, Wellington, New Zealand

Smoking prevalence and consumption in New Zealand

Between 1984 and 1991, the tobacco consumption per adult in New Zealand declined more rapidly than in any other industrialized country: a fall of 42% in just seven years (Laugesen, 1995). Since 1991, however, the reduction has slowed down, and consumption may even have increased slightly in 1996 (OTR Spectrum Research surveys, commissioned by the Ministry of Health, New Zealand). Between 1976 and 1996, the prevalence of smoking among New Zealand men fell from 40 to 25% and that among women from 32 to 23%; nevertheless, 40% of Maori men and 47% of Maori women smoked in 1996 (figures from the New Zealand Department of Statistics, as analysed by Ministry of Health, New Zealand). Furthermore, the rate of smoking among young women, particularly among young pregnant women, is of considerable concern.

The cost to society of tobacco use

It has been estimated that one in two smokers die from smoking and die an average of 14 years early (Doll et al., 1994). Every day, another 40 young New Zealanders take up smoking, and 4500 New Zealanders die each year as a result of smoking (Ministry of Health and Cancer Society, 1996). The social costs of smoking to New Zealand have been variously estimated. The Public Health Commission (1994) estimated that the cost of use of tobacco products to New Zealand in 1988 (in 1992 dollars) was NZ$ 1.9 million million. Easton (1997) estimated the cost to New Zealand society of tobacco use at NZ$ 22.5 million million.

The situation of tobacco control up to 1990

There was little coordination of tobacco control efforts in New Zealand up to 1990. Tobacco advertising on radio and television had been banned in 1963 by the broadcasting authorities, and the tobacco industry agreed in 1973 to remove all advertising on billboards and in cinemas. The first health warnings on tobacco packets were introduced in 1974. These were strengthened by a voluntary agreement with the industry in 1987 (Thomson & Wilson, 1997). Smokeless tobacco was banned in New Zealand in 1987. In 1988, it became an offence to sell tobacco products to people under the age of 16.

Before 1990, there was limited and entirely voluntary protection from other people's smoke on the part of employers, restaurateurs and transport operators, and the 'right to smoke' was clearly ascendant over the 'right to not be exposed to smoke'. Publication of the report of the Toxic Substances Board (1989), *Health or Tobacco An End to Tobacco Advertising and Promotion* in May 1989 and of the Department of Health's (1988) *Creating Smokefree Indoor Environments* was instrumental in provoking a debate on tobacco. These two reports and a Minister of Health with strong views on the issue of smoking and the right of individuals to be protected from environmental tobacco smoke, culminated in 1990 in the passage of the Smoke-free Environments Act, which revolutionized tobacco control in New Zealand, introducing, among other matters:

- policies on smoking in all workplaces and a requirement that all shared offices be smoke-free;
- a minimum of 50% smoke-free seating in restaurants;
- the banning of tobacco advertising, including sponsorship of sporting and cultural events, and the establishment of a Health Sponsorship Council to provide replacement sponsorship funding; and
- health warnings and information on tobacco packaging, and a requirement to file annual returns on the quantity and contents of tobacco products sold in New Zealand.

As at 1 March 1990, the tobacco excise on a packet of 20 cigarettes was approximately NZ$ 2.30, about 55% of the price of a packet of cigarettes (Ministry of Health and Cancer Society, 1996). Television campaigns to discourage smoking ran in 1984, 1986 and 1988 (Thomson & Wilson, 1997); at the same time, however, industry advertising in retail outlets was permitted to remain until 1 January 1995, and tobacco sponsorship of sporting and cultural events continued until 30 June 1995. Enforcement of the ban on sales of tobacco to minors was limited, and continued to be so until 1995.

Strategies used in New Zealand to discourage the use of tobacco products, 1990–95

Public health services were funded to educate people on and to enforce legislation providing for smoke-free areas and the ban on sales of tobacco products to people under the legal minimum age. Depending on the service, other smoke-free activities were also undertaken, such as smoke-free pregnancy programmes.

No Government-sponsored media campaigns on the risks of smoking were run between 1988 and 1995, but the Cancer Society in New Zealand ran a campaign over three years (1993–95), using television advertising and radio talk shows (Thomson & Wilson, 1997). Health sponsorship— sponsorship of sporting and cultural events to promote healthy lifestyle messages—has been a key part of the New Zealand approach to health education. The target groups for these messages are young people and Maors. Approximately NZ$ 17 million was spent between 1991 and 1996 on promoting the smoke-free message or replacing tobacco sponsorship in this country (personal communication, I. Potter, Director, Health Sponsorship Council).

The curriculum of primary and secondary schools includes a health education component, but this has been implemented variously. In a survey of secondary schools in Wellington, as many as half of the students reported that they had received no information at school about not smoking over the past year (McGee, 1992). Programmes in schools have been given a boost by the Government's 1995 smoke-free strategy (see below), in which additional funding was provided to promote smoke-free schools nationwide.

The last increase in the real price of cigarettes in New Zealand was in 1991, but in 1995 the Government increased the tax on loose tobacco to equalize it with that on manufactured cigarettes. This involved an increase of 37.5% in the tax on loose tobacco.

As at 1 July 1997, the rate of excise on tobacco products amounted to NZ$ 202.87 per kg of tobacco, or approximately NZ$ 3.25 on a packet of 20 cigarettes.

National strategy for tobacco control

Over the last few years, in an attempt to formalize tobacco policy in New Zealand, the Government and health authorities have developed a national strategy on tobacco. This strategy has found form and some degree of substance in two documents, the *National Drug Policy (Part I - Tobacco and Alcohol)* (Ministry of Health, 1996) *and Tobacco Products: The Public Health Commission's Advice to the Minister of Health 1993–1994* (Public Health Commission, 1994). These documents provide a framework within which activities can be developed to discourage the use of tobacco. The Public Health Commission's advice to the Minister of Health gives the following targets for tobacco consumption and prevalence in New Zealand:

To reduce tobacco use ...	Actual in 1993 from	Target for 2000 to
Tobacco products sold, cigarette equivalents/adult	1579	1000
Adults (15 years and over), smoking any cigarette	27%	20%
Youth (15–24 years), smoking any type of cigarette	31%	20%
Pregnant women, smoking any type of cigarette (1991)	33%	20%
Māori women in pregnancy (1991)	68%	50%
Māori, smoking any type of cigarette	54%	40%
Workers exposed to environmental tobacco smoke indoors:	in 1991	for 2000
during actual working hours	19%	Near zero
during tea and lunch breaks	41%	5%

In 1995, it was recognized that in current policy settings these targets were unlikely to be met. Accordingly, the Government introduced a strategy to confront smoking, particularly smoking by young people and Maoris. It allocated an extra NZ$ 11.5 million over three years for a smoke-free strategy aimed at reducing the uptake of smoking by young people, particularly Maori women and pregnant women. The Health Sponsorship Council was allocated additional funding for three years from July 1996 to enable it to expand sponsorship of sporting and cultural events that appeal to Maoris and young people. Additional funding was also provided for a school-based programme aimed at promoting entirely smoke-free schools and encouraging a smoke-free lifestyle among the young. The Government also funded a multimedia campaign, 'Why start?', running over three years from July 1996. The aim of the campaign is to discourage young people, Maoris and women from starting to smoke and to encourage pregnant women to stop. Initial evaluations suggest that the campaign is being very well received by the target groups, with 84 and 87% of respondents thinking the campaign has adopted the right approach and 87% (dropping to 84% in the second evaluation) of young uncommitted smokers recalling advertising about not starting to smoke (Business Research Centre & Eru Pomare Maori Health Research Centre, 1996, 1997).

In 1995, the Government also provided additional funding for enforcement of the Smoke-free Environments Act. The primary focus of this increased enforcement is on the ban on sales of tobacco to minors. 'Controlled purchase operations' have been initiated nationwide, which involve sending volunteers under the age of 16 into premises to determine whether retailers are inclined to sell them tobacco. This has become perhaps the most controversial area of tobacco control in New Zealand. Between July 1996 and June 1997, over 750 premises were visited, and sales were made in 76 instances. Fifteen prosecutions have already progressed through the courts, with 13 convictions and two discharges without conviction. Although it is too early to determine whether the enhanced enforcement programme is having the desired effect of making it harder for young people to obtain cigarettes, anecdotal evidence from health workers suggests that it is. Certainly, the number and prominence of warning signs in shops, advising young people that they will not be sold tobacco products, has increased markedly. Media coverage of the controlled purchase operations has been extensive. A survey was carried out in late 1997 of the smoking behaviour and tobacco purchasing habits of 14 and 15 year olds, to determine whether the enforcement programme, and the publicity that surrounds it, is having an impact on accessibility to and use of tobacco products by, young people.

In 1995, the Government also introduced a Bill to Parliament to strengthen certain provisions of the Smoke-free Environments Act. In July 1997, the Bill was passed. It amends the Smoke-free Environments Act 1990 to (among other matters) raise the age at which people may be sold tobacco from 16 to 18 years, ban the sale of single cigarettes and packs of less than 20 cigarettes and further restrict the form of advertising permitted in retail outlets.

Into the future

A conference hosted by the Health Sponsorship Council and the Cancer Society in March 1997 developed a blueprint for future smoke-free activities. This programme has been generally agreed by health agencies . If all agencies involved in tobacco control can focus their efforts on a coordinated plan for tobacco control in New Zealand, this will bode well for the future. There appears to be some political support for new initiatives to reduce tobacco consumption in the coun try. The initiatives proposed include tax increases, new legislation for smoke-free schools and workplaces, regulation of tar and nicotine, strengthening health information on tobacco packaging and public funding of smoking cessation courses and nicotine replacement therapy treatments.

Conclusion

Tobacco consumption in New Zealand has not changed markedly since 1991 and may even have increased slightly since 1995. The decline in smoking prevalence over the past two decades has also slowed down. In 1995, it became clear that the Ministry of Health's targets for consumption and prevalence in the year 2000 were unlikely to be met with current policy directions. The Government therefore approved a smoke-free strategy aimed at reducing smoking among young people, Maoris, women and pregnant women. In addition, new legislation was passed during 1997. These initiatives have not yet run long enough for their effect to be measured or experienced; however, initial evaluations suggest that they have been well targeted.

It is important that the fight to reduce tobacco use be multi-pronged. New Zealand now has in place a comprehensive tobacco control programme and stands to benefit greatly from it in terms of improved health outcomes. This will be subject to commitment of continued funding for local smoke-free programmes.

References

Business Research Centre & Eru Pomare Maori Health Research Centre (1996) *Why Start?: Evaluation One*, Wellington

Business Research Centre & Eru Pomare Maori Health Research Centre (1997) *Why Start?: Evaluation Two*, Wellington

Department of Health (1988) *Creating Smokefree Indoor Environments: Options for Action*, Wellington

Doll, R., *et al.* (1994) Mortality in relation to smoking: 40 years' observations on male British doctors. *Br. Med. J.*, **309**, 901–911

Easton, B. (1997) *The Social Costs of Tobacco Use and Alcohol Misuse*, Wellington: Economic and Social Trust on New Zealand

Laugesen, M. (1995) New Zealand's monitoring system for tobacco control 1984–1992. In: Slama, K., ed., *Ninth World Conference on Tobacco and Health*, Paris: Plenum Press, pp. 169–172

McGee, R. (1992) *Smoking among Wellington Fourth Formers: A Report to the Cancer Society of New Zealand*, Wellington

Ministry of Health (1996) *National Drug Policy Part 1: Tobacco and Alcohol*, Wellington

Ministry of Health and the Cancer Society of New Zealand (1996) *Tobacco Statistics 1996*, Wellington

Public Health Commission (1994) *Tobacco Products: The Public Health Commission's Advice to the Minister of Health 1993–1994*, Wellington

Smoke-free Environments Amendment Act 1997 (1997, No. 32).

Thomson, G., &Wilson, N. (1997) *Resource Document: A Brief History of Tobacco Control in New Zealand*, Wellington: Australasian Faculty of Public Health Medicine (New Zealand Office), pp. 29, 30

Toxic Substances Board (1989) *Health or Tobacco: An End to Tobacco Advertising and Promotion*, Wellington: Department of Health

New Zealand: Smoking is not a disease of poverty

M. Glover

University of Auckland, Auckland, New Zealand

Introduction

Smoking is increasingly being called a disease of poverty. In 1997 in *Tobacco Control*, Flint and Novotny (1997) concluded that 'persons below the poverty threshold continue to be more likely than those at or above the threshold both to be current smokers and not to have quit.' Poverty status, they say, 'probably represents determinants that extend beyond issues of individual or household income.' In this paper I explain why smoking is neither a disease of poverty nor necessarily a response to inequality and oppression. These viewpoints are defeatist and condescending and shift focus from the real reason why oppressed and poor groups generally have higher smoking prevalence rates than their richer, more privileged neighbours.

Maori, the indigenous people of New Zealand, have the highest rates of lung cancer for women in the world. Two thirds of Maori women smoke during pregnancy, and 30% of deaths amongst Maori are tobacco-related (Waa *et al.*, 1997). Maori are also over-represented in the lower socio-economic groups of society and have greater unemployment rates and need for welfare support.

Inadequate and culturally inappropriate health-care services

Flint and Novotny (1997) do consider the possibility that public health efforts 'may not be reaching all socioeconomic groups equally', and they suggest that low-income populations need specifically targeted efforts. This is what Maori have been saying for years: 'Poor Maori health status reflects poorly on the health sector not on Maori' (Kotuku Partners, 1994); 'Disparities between Maori and non-Maori reflect inequality, iniquity, and sometimes institutionalised racism' (Review Team to Consider Hearing Impairment Among Maori People, 1989).

In education, 'equity' is the term that has come to replace the previously used term of 'equality'. The notional meaning of 'equity' is 'the quality of results or outcomes', so that educational performance can be used as a test of equality of opportunity and access. Similarly, it could be argued that health outcome can be used as a test of equality of opportunity and access to health services

New Zealand health authorities began publicizing the health risks associated with tobacco use from about 1948. The information was, however, monocultural, developed by the dominant *pakeha* (European) and aimed at reducing smoking among *pakeha* men (Glover, 1995; Waa *et al.*, 1997). The smoking prevalence among this group subsequently dropped. There was some diffusion of this effect to older white women, but uptake among younger white women is increasing. Some tobacco control efforts do work: the national average adult smoking prevalence rate is now down to 21%, despite the tobacco industry. Until 1984, no specific attempts were made to ensure that Maori had access to information and intervention programmes, and the level of financial support for these programmes remains disproportionately low compared with the need (Kotuku Partners, 1994; Waa *et al.*, 1997).

Other indigenous people appear to have similar experiences: 'Historically, tobacco education campaigns have not reached this group [American Indians] for lack of resources and leadership' (Flannery *et al.*, 1995). 'Smoking cessation programmes have been slow to address the over-representation of indigenous and 'minorities' peoples in the smoking statistics' (Stewart, undated). Historically, smoking cessation support has been provided by national non-governmental organizations like the National Heart Foundation, the Cancer Society and the Seventh Day Adventist Church, none of which provided appropriate programmes to the Maori and did not routinely involve Maori people in the delivery of the programmes.

The New Zealand Government still refuses to provide systematic treatment for nicotine dependency, i.e. smoking cessation, for anyone, let alone Maori.

Inadequate legislation

The Anglo-European process of legislation is a barrier in itself. The Maori form of government would not allow tobacco industries so much freedom. The much touted *Smokefree Environments Act* (1990) excluded legislating against smoking in blue-collar work environments occupied by lower socioeconomic groups, e.g. factories. Maori tend to be over-represented in blue-collar work (Waa *et al.*, 1997). Maori social environments, e.g. *marae* (traditional meeting venues), were excluded from the Act altogether.

Even price increases due to tobacco taxation, which is promoted as the most effective tobacco control policy in New Zealand (Laugesen, 1997), failed to influence Maori smoking prevalence rates, although consumption did drop slightly as Maori smokers switched to roll-your-owns; nevertheless, the smoking prevalence is increasing among younger Maori women.

A white, middle-class workforce

The majority of New Zealand health promotion and education workers are middle-class *pakeha* (white) women, who develop and deliver middle-class *pakeha* programmes. Similarly, the majority of New Zealand Members of Parliament and advisers to Government are middle-class and *pakeha*. For example, despite Maori arguments to the contrary, the New Zealand Government is still advised that "there are no programmes or 'magic bullets' in the tobacco control armamentarium which work specially for Maori" (Laugesen, 1997).

Maori smokers are not beyond help

It is not because they don't care that Maori smoke. As one Maori health worker recently said to me 'our people aren't dumb'. Instead, we remain hopeful and determined. We have repeatedly called for funding to develop, run and deliver our own programmes. When this has occurred, there is mounting evidence that smoking can be reduced among Maori just as effectively as it has been reduced among *pakeha* New Zealanders. Some anecdotal evidence suggests that Maori tobacco control programmes may be more effective. Anecdotal evidence of quit rates from a Maori cessation programme indicate that an average of 75% are still not smoking after one year. In one Maori community, the smoking prevalence has been reduced to below the national norm by a *marae*-based holistic health programme.

We need the same opportunity to undertake the same amount of tobacco control activities to bring about the same (if not greater) reduction in smoking prevalence. Unfortunately, 'the ability to initiate health programs is directly related to funding' (Ellis, 1995). It is lack of resources that prevents us from doing more (Glover, 1995). A shortage of tax dollars is not necessarily the problem either. 'Our Government takes over $111 million each year in tobacco taxes from Maori smokers, far exceeding the resultant hospital cost by Maori of $8.5 million per year.' Thus, some Maori conclude that 'they have a strong, incentive to keep us smoking' (Kotuku Partners, 1994).

The real enemy

The problem is not stress from multiple sources of oppression, alienation and marginalization. Maori smoke because our colonizers control the allocation of resources, the content and focus of education and public health prevention activities and the focus of personal health interventions. Maori still smoke disproportionately more because politically dominant *pakeha* New Zealanders are unwilling to reorient funding to those most in need. This reluctance exists despite the Government's supposed commitment 'to improve Maori health to at least the same standard of health as non-Maori.'

The real enemy for Maori is not the tobacco industry, as we have been led to believe, it is our colonizers, who have supplanted our own social and political systems with theirs and subsequently withheld from us the resources necessary to reduce Maori smoking. On a worldwide scale, it is the richer echelons of society that control the prevalence rates, by manipulating the availability of the drug through legislation, advertising, health education, treatment, and negotiation with the industry.

The obvious solution

Given my conclusion that inequitable smoking prevalence rates result from inequitable distribution of political power, the obvious solution is the removal of political inequality. As Greaves (1996) argues, 'a global effort to improve the circumstances of the world's girls and women may be the very best first step.' Like women, Maori have been trying to improve their circumstances for over 100 years, and we continue to seek improvement at all levels. With 650 Maori dying each year from smoking, we cannot afford to wait for some idealistic state of equality to do away with the higher smoking prevalence. Nor do I believe that the answer will be found by researching how smokers in poverty differ, as suggested by Flint and Novotny (1997), unless, the focus of such research is the inequitable distribution of power and resources. Simply, Maori (and other special population groups) need equitable access to health-care services and interventions that are culturally specific and thus more likely to be effective.

References

Ellis, R. (1995) *Ko tenei te whare auahi kore mo te oranga o nga tamariki! This is a smokefree whare for the health of our kids!* A Health Research Council student summership report

Flannery, D., Sisk-Franco, C. & Glover, P.N (1995) The conflict of tobacco education among American Indians: Traditional or health risk? In: Slama, K., ed., *Tobacco and Health.*, New York: Plenum Press, pp. 903–905

Flint, A.J. & Novotny, T.E. (1997) Poverty status and cigarette smoking prevalence and cessation in the United States, 1983–1993: the independent risk of being poor. *Tobacco Control,* 6

Glover, M. (1995) Mobilising an indigenous population: Reducing Maori smoking. In: Slama, K., ed., *Tobacco and Health.*, New York: Plenum Press, pp. 907–909

Greaves, L. (1996) *Smoke Screen: Women's smoking and social control,* Canada: Fernwood Publishing

Kotuku Partners (1994) *Hauora Wahine Maori: Recent directions for Maori women's health 1984–1994.* Wellington: Ministry of Health

Laugesen, M. (1997) *Reducing tobacco use, exposure to environmental smoke and their adverse health consequences.* A report for Midland Regional Health Authority

Review Team to Consider Hearing Impairment Among Maori People (1989) *Whakarongo Mai: Maori Hearing Impairment.* Wellington: Minister of Maori Affairs

Stewart, T.R. (undated) Kaati te kai paipa: Smoking cessation. Auckland: Health Research Council

Waa, A., Moewaka Barnes, H., Blewden, M. & Spinola, C. (1997) *Auckland Healthcare and Northland Health Tobacco Program Evaluation: Literature Review. Maori Smokefree: History of Tobacco Use; Background Facts and Figures.* Auckland: University of Auckland, Department of Community Health, Alcohol and Public Health Research Unit & Whariki

Tobacco-free Norway: A five-year action plan

S. Stenmarck[1], E. Juul Andersen[2] & T. Sanner[3]

[1]The Norwegian National Health Association, [2]The Norwegian Medical Association and [3]The Norwegian Association against Tobacco, Oslo, Norway

Introduction

A coalition called 'Tobacco-free' was established between The Norwegian Cancer Society, The Norwegian Medical Association, The Norwegian Confederation of Sport, The Norwegian Association against Tobacco, The Norwegian National Health Association, The Norwegian Asthma and Allergy Association and The Norwegian Coordinating Board of Health Education, which prepared an action plan for a tobacco-free Norway 1994–98 (Sanner *et al.*, 1993). This was presented to the Norwegian Minister of Health on 15 November 1993.

Many countries have looked to Norway as an example of a country in which work against tobacco is going well: the legislation in relation to tobacco is good, and the cigarette prices are high. Since 50% of the cigarettes smoked are hand-rolled, however, and the cost of a hand-rolled cigarette is only half that of a manufactured cigarette, the price increase on manufactured cigarettes has to a large extent resulted in a transition from manufactured to hand-rolled cigarettes instead of reduced cigarette consumption.

The smoking prevalence among men in Norway decreased considerably over the period 1970–80, but the prevalence among women has been relatively constant over the last 25 years and high: about 32% of women in Norway smoke, and the prevalence of smoking among women is higher only in Denmark, the Netherlands and Poland. The prevalence of smoking among pregnant women has also been among the highest in the world, with about one-third of pregnant women in Norway smoking daily.

During the period 1980–93, the prevalence of smoking among adult Norwegians decreased by only 2%, while the decreases in Belgium, the Netherlands, Sweden, the United Kingdom and the United States were 8–15% (Figure 1). Moreover, while 35% of the adult Norwegian population smoked daily in 1993, the prevalence of daily smoking was 25% or less in countries such as Belgium, Finland, Sweden and the United States.

In Norway as in most other countries, cigarettes were first used among young, well-educated men. Later, the smoking epidemic spread to other groups of the population. When women started to smoke a decade later, it was the high-status groups who started. The situation today is different, however. In the 25–35 age group, less than 20% of university graduates and post-graduates smoke, while the smoking prevalence is three times higher (60%) in the group with only basic education. In older age groups as well, considerable but smaller differences in smoking habits exist between groups with different educational level.

Figure 2 shows the prevalence of daily smoking among 15-year-old boys and girls in Norway in five-year periods between 1975 and 1995. As the legal age for buying tobacco in Norway in 1993 was 16 years, and about 17% of boys and girls aged 15 smoked daily, approximately half of the smokers of tomorrow started to smoke before they could buy cigarettes legally.

These findings clearly demonstrated the need for a plan for a tobacco-free Norway.

Action plan for a tobacco-free Norway 1994–98

A number of the goals in the action plan for a tobacco-free Norway have deadlines (Table 1). A sub-target of the action plan is the World Health Organization's goal that a minimum of 80% of the population should be non-smokers by the year 2000. The main goals for the five-year period covered by the action plan were to reduce the prevalence of smoking in the population to less than 25% and the prevalence of daily smoking in the age group 16–24 years to less than 20% in 1998. The goals of increasing

Figure 1. Changes in the prevalence (%) of daily smoking in certain western countries, 1980 and 1993

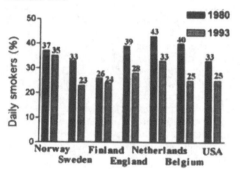

Figure 2. Prevalence of daily smoking among 15-year-old girls and boys in Norway, 1975–95

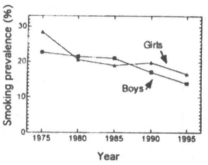

Table 1. Goals and actions, with deadlines, for a tobacco-free Norway

Goal	Year		
	1994	1996	1998
Protection of non-smokers		All kindergartens, schools and universities smoke-free	Health institutions completely smoke-free
		At least 25 communities have smoke-free schools and health institutions	At least 100 communities have smoke-free schools and health institutions
		All public offices and institutions smoke-free	All youth establishments smoke-free
		Smoke-free cafeterias and restaurants in theatres, cinemas and concert halls	
Reduced availability	Legal age for buying tobacco, 18 years. No sales from vending machines		Restrictions on sale locations and periods
Increased taxation	> 20% yearly	Tobacco removed from price index	
Restrictions on sale of snuff	Health warnings		Prohibition of sale
Smoke-free flights		The whole world	
Duty-free sales stopped			Nordic countries
Partial aim Reduction in prevalence of daily smoking to less than:		20% among pregnant women	5% among 15-year-olds 20% among 16–24-year-olds 25% in the whole population

the legal age for buying tobacco to 18 years, no sales from vending machines and a health warning on smokeless tobacco have been achieved. There have been some increases in taxation but less than the 20% yearly increase targeted in the action plan. The goal that all flights should be smoke-free in 1996 was not achieved, but all commercial flights of Nordic airlines were smoke-free by September 1997. Health institutions, kindergartens, schools and most universities are now completely smoke-free.

The resources from the Government for campaigns against the use of tobacco in Norway were very small between 1980 and 1993, representing about 10 US cents per inhabitant per year. In order to attain our goals, these resources had to be increased considerably. During the first three years of the action plan, we were able to increase the resources by a factor of about five.

In our work for a tobacco-free Norway, the most important task is to prevent adolescents from beginning to smoke by changing the attitude and behaviour of children, adolescents and trend-setters for youngsters including parents, health and educational personnel, youth and sports leaders and well-known persons. In the action plan, youngsters between 12 and 18 years have high priority, as do groups that are most vulnerable to damage to health caused by environmental tobacco smoke, i.e. children. Action to reduce smoking among parents-to-be and parent of children up to the age of 12 will not only reduce health damage in children but will also help to reduce smoking among young people. It is well known that if parents smoke, the risk that their children will start to smoke is considerably increased.

One goal of the action plan is to reduce the prevalence of smoking among 15-year-olds from 17% to less than 5%. All establishments for adolescents should be smoke-free. Restrictions on sale periods and sale location should be enforced. This has not been achieved, and it is unlikely that it will be in the remaining time covered by the action plan. Some of the action should continue throughout the period. Information on the effects of tobacco use on health and action to change attitudes must be intensified. The most resources must be put into secondary schools. Smoking cessation courses for adolescents and for employers in the health and education sector and among sports and youth leaders must be enhanced. Communities and counties must be motivated to provide smoke-free environments in the health and education sector. Businesses must prepare a smoke-free environment and organize smoke cessation groups among employees.

The prevalence of smoking among men was reduced during the period of the action plan (Figure 3), while that among Norwegian women has been constant since the 1970s. Considerable efforts were made to reduce smoking among pregnant women, and the prevalence has now been reduced to 20%. To conclude, the action plan has been a valuable tool in the fight against tobacco in Norway, but. although our legislation is good and we have high prices on tobacco products, we still have far to go to reach the goals of WHO and to achieve a smoking prevalence similar to that achieved in Finland, Sweden and the United States.

Reference

Sanner, T., Juul Andersen, E., Hauknes, A. & Stenmarck, S., eds (1993) *Action Plan for a Tobacco-free Norway, 1994–1988*, Oslo, Department of Health and Social Affairs (in Norwegian with English translation)

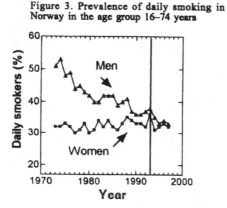

Figure 3. Prevalence of daily smoking in Norway in the age group 16–74 years

Norway: 'Tobacco-free': A coalition for reducing use of tobacco

E. Juul Andersen[1], S. Stenmarck[2], S. Jacobsen[3] & T. Sanner[4]

[1]*Norwegian Medical Association,* [2]*Norwegian Health Association,* [3]*Norwegian Coordinating Board of Health Education and* [4]*Norwegian Association against Tobacco, Oslo, Norway*

A coalition called 'Tobacco-free was established in August 1994, founded by the Norwegian Association against Tobacco, the Norwegian Asthma and Allergy Association, the Norwegian Cancer Society, the Norwegian Confederation of Sport, the Norwegian Medical Association, the Coordinating Board of Health Education and the Norwegian Health Association. The organizations represent both voluntary bodies such as the Norwegian Cancer Society, and professionals, such as the Norwegian Medical Association. These organizations had previously collaborated in preparing a five-year action plan for 1994–98 on the use of tobacco in Norway and the health effects of use of tobacco. The aim of the plan (Sanner et al., 1993) was the goal stated by the World Health Organization: that more than 80% of the population should be non-smokers by the year 2000. Concrete targets, target groups and time limits for different actions were suggested (see Stenmarck et al., this volume). The plan also involved protection of non-smokers against environmental tobacco smoke, reduced availability of tobacco, increased prices and help for smokers to quit smoking. The plan was adopted by the Norwegian Minister of Health.

When the plan was finished, the participating organizations saw the need for a coalition which could maintain the pressure on the politicians in the struggle to reduce smoking in Norwegian society. Most people think that Norway is very active in preventing people from smoking, but this is not true. Norway has 4.2 million people, and the average smoking rate is 33%. Since 1980, there have been very limited financial resources for tobacco control campaigns. The campaigns to prevent AIDS received 10 times as much (300 million Norwegian kroner) as tobacco prevention during the last 10 years.

That is why Tobacco-free was established, to develop strategies in both a long-term (three years) and a short-term perspective. With this initiative, the structure of anti-tobacco work in Norway was now that recommended by the World Health Organization, with a non-governmental pressure group.

Main targets

The main targets for Tobacco-free are:
* to get tobacco policies on the political agenda,
* to inform politicians and the press about the health and economic consequences of the use of tobacco and
* to secure funds for campaigns against the use of tobacco and to strengthen the funding for preventive medicine.

All of the member organizations are represented on our board. Three persons assume the daily running of Tobacco-free. There is no secretariat and almost no funding; the strength lies in the knowledge and competence of the coalition member organizations.

What did we do?

We informed all members of the Norwegian Parliament that Tobacco-free had been established and gave the names of the participating organizations. The letter stated that Tobacco-free is a coalition with the goal of reducing the use of tobacco in Norwegian society and that there are no commercial interests involved. This gave it the necessary legitimacy. Personal letters on legislation and the high prevalence of tobacco use were later mailed to members of Parliament on several occasions.

The following topics were considered important:
* revision of the legislation on tobacco,
* meeting with the Parliament Committee on Finance to discuss taxation,
* meeting with the Parliament Committee on Health and Social Affairs to discuss legislation and health effects of tobacco use,
* smoke-free flights in Europe,
* a financial platform for organizations involved in health promotion and
* close contact with the media.

We sent a letter to the Prime Minister, who at the time was Ms Gro Harlem Brundtland, and informed her about Tobacco-free.

Articles on the achievements of Tobacco-free have been published in the journals of the member organizations and kept the members informed.

Tobacco-free has very low costs, as the member organizations pay their own expenses. In 1997, Tobacco-free received 200 000 Norwegian krones, equivalent to US$ 23 000, from the Norwegian Coordinating Board of Health Education.

Tobacco-free has had several meetings with the Parliament Committee for Health and Social Affairs, which prepares all health issues on tobacco for Parliament, except for taxation. We presented Tobacco-free and gave them material that showed the huge increase in the number of deaths caused by smoking: More than 7500 Norwegians die every year of diseases related to use of tobacco. About 60% of people whose highest level of formal education is secondary school are smokers, and only 20% of academics smoke. We have good legislation, but despite this, the number of daily smokers is still high. The politicians understood that reduction in the use of tobacco is a matter of health politics and that it is their responsibility to do something about it. They were shown that these disappointing figures could easily be changed by making more people quit smoking and preventing young people from starting to smoke by increasing tobacco taxation.

We provided the politicians with these facts and emphasized that the rate of daily smoking in Norway has been almost the same since 1980. During the 1970s, there had been campaigns in the media, on television and on billboards that told people about the health consequences of smoking. After 1981, there were no nationwide campaigns. Many politicians thought that the campaigns had been carried out much later than they were and that there had been a 'lot of information campaigns' between 1981 and 1993. We showed that these impressions were false; one of the reasons why the number of daily smokers in Norway is so high is that there have been no mass media campaigns or other efforts.

The budget for campaigns has increased by a factor of about five since Tobacco-free started its work in 1994, and Norway now spends about 10 million Norwegian kroner on tobacco control. The World Health Organization recommends that 4% of the financial income from tobacco should be used; this would yield 220 million kroner for tobacco control and preventive medicine.

How we work

We establish contact with politicians, authorities and commercial companies (e.g. the Scandinavian Airlines System, SAS) by asking for meetings and telling them in advance what topics will be covered. As they can prepare themselves, the quality of the discussion is improved and they cannot tell us that they are not prepared to discuss an issue.

Proposals for the next national budget are presented in October each year, when we arrange meetings with the influential Parliamentary Committee for Health and Social Affairs. In 1996, we also met with the Committee for Finance to discuss tobacco taxation. We persuaded the politicians to make public statements about the importance of reducing smoking in Norway.

To strengthen our arguments, we commissioned documentation and a report on tobacco taxation and financing of health promotion from a resource institute, the HEMIL Centre in Bergen, inspired by the excellent work done in the State of Victoria, Australia. The Victoria Health Promotion Foundation is financed entirely by a dedicated levy of the tobacco tax. Our proposal for Norway is a special fund for health promotion funded by 4% of the revenue from tobacco taxation. We have also pointed out that public health will benefit from a larger increase in taxes on 'roll your own' tobacco, which unfortunately costs half the price of manufactured cigarettes and represent half of the total cigarette consumption. It gives the smoker higher doses of nicotine and tar than manufactured cigarettes.

The facts and findings in the report of HEMIL Centre were presented at a conference in Oslo in January 1996, where we targeted Parliamentarians. We decided to invite politicians who had influence in their parties and also held positions in the Committee of Finance or the Committee of Health and Social Affairs in the Parliament. We also invited opinion leaders in health organizations and the media. The politicians were invited to participate in a panel debate at the end of the meeting, in which they were asked if they would support increased activities and funding for anti-tobacco work in Norway. All of them agreed, but so far we have had no concrete results.

What have we achieved?

SAS met with Tobacco-free several times, and we had excellent cooperation from employees organizations. Since September 1997, all SAS flights have been smoke-free, and our member organization, the Norwegian Medical Association, suggested in a European forum for medical associations that all flights in Europe should be smoke-free. The forum adopted the idea, and on 29 August 1996, all European medical associations wrote letters to their national authorities and airlines and asked for smoke-free flights.

Tobacco-free has given prizes to non-smoking charter tour operators to highlight the importance of smoke-free flights.

Tobacco-free initiated a proposal, which was made by the Norwegian Medical Association in the Assembly of World Medical Associations, to ban funding from the tobacco industry for medical research.

Tobacco-free has, we hope, increased interest and knowledge among Norwegian politicians about the health consequences and cost of smoking.

Tobacco-free has pressed for stronger legislation on tobacco in Norway.

References

Sanner, T., Juul Andersen, E., Hauknes, A. & Stenmarck, S., eds (1993) *Action Plan for a Tobacco-free Norway, 1994–1988*, Oslo: Department of Health and Social Affairs (in Norwegian with English translation)

Russian Federation: Tobacco smoking control

A.N. Zubritsky

Department of Pathology, Taldom Territorial Medical Union, Taldom, Russian Federation

Introduction

In early times, smoking was controlled by severe punishment. For example, under the first Romanoff tzar, Michael Fedorovich, people caught smoking for the first time were punished with 60 lashes on the feet, and when they were caught for the second time their nose and ears were cut off (Zaikin *et al.*, 1990). In the former Soviet Union, there were no State programmes devoted to smoking control and no effective medical help for smokers. The only actions were warnings on cigarette packs by the Ministry of Public Health, a few articles in newspapers and chapters in school biology textbooks that were meant once and for all to persuade young people to hate this harmful habit.

Nowadays, physicians join their foreign colleagues in preventing smoking. One example is an international seminar on smoking control held in the Cancer Research Centre of the Russian Academy of Medical Sciences, at which the medical and sociological aspects of smoking were discussed. Dr D. Zaridze presented the project for legislation on smoking developed by specialists at the Research Institute for Cancerogenesis to reduce the maximum tar content of cigarettes to that in the European community, 15 mg, to increase prices of cigarettes and to restrict production of new forms of tobacco and other products containing nicotine on Russian territory.

Tobacco smoking has become a socioeconomic problem and requires preventive measures (Raw *et al.*, 1990; Zubritsky, 1995). The measures taken to date by national governments have been partial and gradual. Poland has proposed laws restricting the purchase of tobacco products to persons under 18 and imposing a fine for smoking in restricted places; it noted that one of the best measures against smoking is sports, especially running. Singapore is attempting to become the first no-smoking nation in the world. One large district of Manila, in the Philippines is smoke-free; a fine is imposed for carrying a cigarette in public places and 10 days' imprisonment for repeated violations.

The International Union against Cancer has suggested the following measures for tobacco control (Committee on Tobacco or Health, 1990): restrictions on all advertisements and sponsorship by the tobacco industry; government warnings on all tobacco products; reduced tar and nicotine in tobacco products; tax and price policies for tobacco products; policy of economic choice; restriction on the purchase of tobacco products by young people; protection of the rights of non-smokers by designating smoking areas; introduction of new sources of nicotine and a future trade strategy; and guaranteeing help for tobacco users who want to give up.

More and more demands are being heard throughout the world for a full ban on tobacco advertising (Amos, 1990; Crofton, 1990; Mackay, 1990). The European Community has suggested that all advertisements carry warnings, like 'Tobacco is a serious threat to your health', 'Protect children from tobacco smoke', 'Give up smoking and become rich' and 'Smoking kills'. In countries such as Norway and Finland, where advertising of tobacco products has been banned for more that 10 years and the prices are increasing, the number of smokers has decreased. The European Community has taken the following legislative measures:

- Since January 1992, all packs of cigarettes must show the tar and nicotine content and a warning in the official language of the country of final sale.
- Restrictions have been imposed on smokeless tobacco in all European countries since July 1992. Smokeless tobacco was used by less than 10% of young men in the United States 20 years ago and by 25% today; in Sweden, its consumption accounts for 30% of all tobacco use. More than 100 million persons in India and Pakistan use smokeless tobacco, and in Africa it has cultural significance.
- The tar content of cigarettes must not exceed 15 mg since 31 December 1992 and 12 mg since December 1997.
- Smoking has been restricted in all public places since July 1989.
- Since October 1991 advertising of tobacco products on television has been restricted in all European countries.
- Since 1 January 1993, the minimum level of taxation is not less than 70% of the final retail price.

The European action plan for tobacco smoking control includes: establishment of alliances of representatives of international, national and community organizations to strengthen social and political support; multisectoral policy on tobacco; no smoking in all public places, transport and workplaces; teaching youngsters to be non-smokers, by education, role models, particularly physicians; support for smokers who want to give up smoking; strong management and human and financial resources for tobacco control. This action plan is based on the recommendations of external consultants and specialists from other WHO programmes. Activity within the programme of tobacco control is based on three main principles:

- support of national programmes on tobacco prevention and control;
- campaigns and community involvement to establish refusal of tobacco consumption as a norm of public behaviour;
- collection, processing and distribution of information.

The European Charter (1989) adopted at the first European conference on tobacco policy in Madrid speaks for itself:

- Fresh air free of tobacco smoke is the most important component of the right to a healthy, unpolluted environment.
- Every person has the right to information on the unprecedented risk to health associated with tobacco consumption.
- All people have the right to air free of tobacco smoke in closed public places and transport.

Attention must be paid to public education. National No-smoking Days are observed annually; they should take new, original forms that attract young people.

Conclusions

Analysis of the world literature shows that the development and implementation of preventive measures aimed at tobacco smoking is difficult but necessary. Effective tobacco control is possible only with adequate legislative measures, national and international programmes and the support of governmental and non-governmental organizations with the participation of specialists led by physicians. The direction of the anti-tobacco campaign should be vested with the World Health Organization. Legislation will help governments to control the epidemic of tobacco smoking, defend the rights of non-smokers to breathe pure air and create a future society free from tobacco smoke.

References

Amos, A. (1990) How women get involved into the sphere of the tobacco industry's influence. *World Health Forum*, 11, 55–59 (in Russian)

Committee on Tobacco or Health (1990) *Bull. Int. Union Tuberc.*, 65

Crofton, J. (1990) WHO technical advisory group on tobaco or health. *Bull.Int.UnionTuberc.*, 65, 58–59

European Charter on Tobacco Restriction (1989) *World Health Forum*, 10, 118–119 (in Russian)

Mackay, J. (1990) First National Seminar on Smoking and Health, Hanoi, 15 March 1990. *Bull. Int. Union Tuberc.*, 65, 70

Raw, M., White, P. & McNeill, A. (1990) *Clearing the Air. A Guide for Action on Tobacco*, London: British Medical Association

Zaikin, N. & Nikitin, A. (1990) *Thanks, I Don't Smoke*, Moscow (in Russian)

Zubritsky, A. (1995) How to prevent smoking in Russia (Abstract). *Tuberc. Lung Dis.*, 76 (Suppl. 2), 100

Russian Federation: Use of computers in tobacco control

L. Dartau

Institute of Control Sciences, Academy of Sciences, Moscow, Russian Federation

'*Nobody knows where the shoe pinches, except he who wears the shoe.*' *(German proverb)*

Control theory, a part of mathematics, can be used to consider the problems of public health. I have conducted a study of heterogeneous populations and control on the basis of incomplete data, financed by the Russian Academy of Sciences (Dartau, 1995). During the past 10 years, we have been studying public health by means of a computer dialogue method known as Expert Dialogue for Investigation of FActors of Risk (EDIFAR). Population research often suffers from lack of representativity, because it is impossible to examine or to question the whole population in real time. Study samples are therefore commonly used (Noelle, 1971), but the establishment of a representative sample is no less complicated or expensive.

Samples can be drawn in two basic ways: by completely random choice, with a relatively large sample to achive representativity, or by planned non-random selection on the basis of features such as sex and age. The latter allows for significantly smaller samples but involves the problem of lack of representativity. Our method lies between the two: it is not completely random, but we do not select anyone. In our studies, nobody determines the size or the parameters of the representative sample, but individuals are included sequentially when they come for an examination. Since health deteriorates naturally and randomly with time, all local sociodemographic groups seek the services of primary health clinics. Thus, ordinary healthy people sometimes need to consult a physician about their health. There are 500–700 such visits to primary health care clinics in Moscow every day.

We placed computers in three primary health care clinics, two serving the populations of areas of Moscow and the other serving employees of the Academy institutes. We questioned our respondents once during the study period, inviting them to answer the questions on the computer. The respondents are thus ordinary patients who come to the clinic independently of our study, without their doctors' invitation. The questionnaire contains 150 questions on illnesses and lifestyle. So far, 12 500 patients have been questioned in this way.

Our experience has shown that when a certain number of respondents is reached, the population characteristics become stable and can be verified (by means of a repeat questionnaire). We therefore conclude that objective population characteristics that are stable and reproducible can be collected on the basis of information in this way. These characteristics can be used for evaluation and control of population health.

In the group of 4822 people whom we questioned between January and November 1989, the sex and age structure were similar to that of the whole population. A well-known feature of the demographic profile in many countries in Europe is the considerable deficit in the birth rate during the years of the Second World War. The demographic profile of the patients we questioned acquires this feature after the first 100 patients. Primary health care clinics can thus provide representative personal contacts between local authorities and the population, and the EDIFAR technique is a combination of technical, methodological and organizational steps for the rapid detection and monitoring of trends in population health for the purposes of adequate control and medico-social investment. It could also be used to predict emerging social issues in health.

With regard to tobacco consumption, EDIFAR could be used to study social and psychological aspects of smoking, smoking cessation and non-smoking in order to define more precisely the role of health professionals and the mass media in health promotion. The prevalence of tobacco consumption is one objective population characteristic. As it is subjective, questionnaire methods must be used to study it. The data on tobacco consumption are stable and can be reproduced like those mentioned above. Thus, the cumulative values become stable relatively quickly, and the percentages of smokers, ex-smokers and non-smokers change little from month to month. Analysis of the distribution of men in these categories in the age groups 15–17, 18–34, 35–59 and ≥ 60, representing teenagers, young men, middle-aged men and men born before the Second World War, shows that about 25% in all groups are non-smokers.

The most interesting data are combinations of complaints and other factors. At any time after the interviews, we can examine and analyse any correlations, because each datum is present on the computer record of a respondent. More respondents who smoked also abused alcohol, particularly among adolescents. The correlation between educational level and tobacco consumption is well known. We found more smokers in the public clinics than in those serving Academy staff.

The EDIFAR technique is cheap, as we have only one questionnaire for all the patients. It is not necessary to code initial data and enter it into a computer. There are few respondent errors because each respondent answers the questions that are relevant to him or her. The questions appear on the computer screen independently of sex or age and the answers to previous questions. We can therefore do without representative samples; we need only ensure that the characteristics (data) have stabilized.

References

Dartau, L. (1995) Tobacco and public health. In: *Tobacco and Health*, New York, Plenum Publishing Corp., pp. 581–584

Noelle, E. (1971) *Umfragen in der Massengesellschaft (Einführung in die Methoden der Demoscopie)*, Munich

Singapore: National smoking control programme, 1986–96

C.Y. Chng

Public Health Services, Ministry of Health, Singapore

When we talk about financing, we usually refer to providing funds for certain organizations or projects. I will stretch the definition to include not just cash funding but also providing resources in terms of expertise, time and manpower. As resources, especially monetary ones, are always limited, we need to consider ways of extending the impact of a programme. I shall first give an overview of Singapore's smoking control programme, the advantages of Government funding, the limitations and how alternative financing is used to support and extend the reach of the programme.

National smoking control programme

Efforts to promote a smoke-free lifestyle in Singapore began in the 1970s. With increasing evidence of the harmful effects and the cost of smoking, the Government recognized the importance of tobacco control. In 1986, a Government-funded national smoking control programme was launched by the Ministry of Health. This is a comprehensive, long-term programme that aims to reduce smoking rates in the population through public education, legislation, a tobacco taxation policy, intersectoral collaboration, community mobilization and smoking cessation services.

The advantages of Government funding for the programme are that it has an annual budget, long-term support and implementation, the necessary infrastructure, Government commitment and assurance that unpopular but essential programmes will be implemented. Thus, Government funding ensures that at least a minimum budget is provided annually for the organization and conduct of smoking control activities, so that staff can concentrate on devising strategies and implementing activities. It also ensures the infrastructure needed to initiate, implement and monitor the programme. This includes manpower and the structures needed to initiate and coordinate the programme with other organizations to achieve its aims.

The launch of the programme demonstrated the Government's commitment to promoting a smoke-free lifestyle. Reducing the prevalence of smoking is one of the national health targets set by the Review Committee on National Health Policies in 1991. The Government's commitment has set the political and social climate necessary for establishing a smoke-free nation. It has helped to raise the profile of the smoking issue, which has resulted in increased awareness of the programme, with more than 90% awareness recorded consistently in annual campaigns, and facilitation of intersectoral collaboration between the Health Ministry and other ministries and organizations.

Funding from the Government also ensures implementation of programmes, in particular those that are unpopular or nonprofitable but have proved to be effective, such as providing smoking cessation services, implementing legislation to discourage smoking among young people, designation of non-smoking areas and legislation to license tobacco retailers.

Achievements

With the budget and support from the Government, we have conducted public education activities throughout the year, targeting all sectors of the population but with special emphasis on preventing young people from starting to smoke and encouraging and enabling smokers to stop smoking. Public education is also used to enlist public support for legislative and other measures in smoking control. Every year, a month-long, intensive media campaign is organized to coincide with WHO's annual World No-Tobacco Day on 31 May. These activities are supplemented by programmes for specific target groups:

Smoking prevention programmes for young people are conducted within the school curricula, from primary to pre-university level, in extracurricular programmes in schools and in community settings. Peer educators are trained to spread the no-smoking message to young people and to promote sports, such as street soccer and rugby, as healthy alternatives to smoking.

Programmes to encourage and assist smokers to stop smoking are conducted in workplaces, health-care settings, communities and schools to increase awareness of the consequences of smoking and the benefits of stopping smoking. Training is also provided for facilitators, especially teachers, to help young people to stop smoking. A programme to update and encourage health-care professionals to talk to their clients about stopping smoking was started in the late 1980s in Government out-patient clinics and has since been extended to non-Government clinics and hospitals. Smoking cessation programmes are provided at certain Government clinics, the Singapore Cancer Society, the Youngberg Adventist Hospital and the Institute of Mental Health. A service called 'Quitline' provides pre-recorded messages 24 h per day and personalized telephone counselling. Self-help quit kits are available free-of-charge upon request.

With the support of the Government, many legislative and fiscal measures have been implemented since the early 1970s, including:
- prohibition of tobacco advertisment and promotion in the media or in public;
- restriction of sponsorship by tobacco companies, only with permission from the Minister of Health;
- display of health warnings on all cigarette packs;
- limits on tar (15 mg) and nicotine (1.3 mg);
- prohibition of sale or supply to persons under the age of 18 and prohibition of smoking, chewing or possession of tobacco products by persons under 18 in public places;
- prohibition of sales of tobacco products from vending machines;
- prohibition of smoking in public places: gazetted smoke-free areas include public transport, health-care settings, air-conditioned food outlets, workplaces, shopping centres, indoor and outdoor sports stadia, public queues, pedestrian underpasses, libraries, rooms used for public functions and the airport. With effect from 15 August 1997, all schools, junior colleges, polytechnics, training institutes and air-conditioned and enclosed areas in universities are smoke-free, having been voluntarily designated smoke-free since the early years of the programme. The extension also includes air-conditioned and enclosed areas in private clubs and air-conditioned shops in town centres, hotels and petrol stations. Most confined spaces in Singapore are therefore smoke-free.
- a progressive increase in tobacco taxation: the excise duty on tobacco in Singapore in 1997 was Singapore $ 115 per kg; tax payable on each pack accounted for 44–53% of the retail price, which was $ 4.70–5.00 per pack of 20 cigarettes.

These measures are reviewed and updated constantly. With effect from September 1998, a tobacco-licensing scheme controls the number of tobacco retailers in Singapore, with the aim of strengthening enforcement of the prohibition of sales to minors.

We have always tried to promote, strengthen and mobilize community participation and build alliances with a variety of organizations to ensure that the activities meet the needs of the community and create a sense of ownership. This may in turn result in more commitment of the community in taking action to change lifestyles. In the early years of the programme, the Government initiated and organized most of the smoking control activities. An interministerial committee chaired by the Minister of Health was set up in 1986 to formulate directions for the programme, and an executive committee was constituted comprising representatives of Government ministries, statutory boards, the private sector, unions, professional organizations, community self-help groups and the media. There were 34 participating organizations in 1986 and 53 in 1993.

Between 1977 and 1987, an impressive decrease in the prevalence of smoking was recorded, from 42 to 27% among men and from 4.5 to 2% among women. Subsequently, however, Singapore witnessed an increase in the prevalence of smoking, from 14% (27% in men and 2% in women) in 1987 to 17% (32% in men and 3% in women) in

1995. This increase was due mainly to an increased prevalence among people aged 18–24, which increased from 13.9% in 1991 to 17.7% in 1995.

Limitations of a Government-funded programme

The amount of funding depends on the political support and economic stability of the country. Furthermore, while strong Government support has led to many initiatives to stop smoking in Singapore, the top-down approach, especially in the early years, was perceived as paternalistic. As the population becomes more highly educated, they may become resistant to this approach. Although the majority of the population support smoking control activities, few are willing to participate actively in smoking control activities. It is hoped to overcome this limitation by mobilizing community participation. With increased interest in health among Singaporeans in recent years, organizations and individuals are more forthcoming in initiating and participating in health promotion programmes, including those for smoking control. The top-down approach has evolved, with greater contributions and leadership from the community. In 1996, a civic committee on smoking control led by community leaders was formed to review and provide overall policy direction for the national smoking control programme. The committee comprises top executives from the private sector, leaders of youth organizations and ethnic self-help groups, representatives from the media and public health specialists. It aims to increase community involvement and organizational support for the programme, so as to make the promotion of a smoke-free lifestyle a civic movement.

A further limitation of Government support is over-dependence on one source of resources. The programme thus has a limited annual budget and limited manpower to reach the entire population of 3 million Singaporeans. Special groups such as young people and specific ethnic groups who are at risk of smoking must be reached. These communities would be more at ease with their peers, so that the Government must work with the community to promote a smoke-free lifestyle.

Alternative financing

In view of the limited budget, manpower and resources, we have worked with nongovernmental and other organizations to extend the scope of our programme, and many activities have been organized jointly with facilitators in such organizations, which have also provided sponsorship, manpower, expertise and time.

Time has been provided, for instance by schools and the media. Many organizations have provided volunteers to help in organizing activities. Some well-known local sports personalities and celebrities act as role models to encourage young people to stay smoke-free. Professional groups have supported the programme by lending their expertise, such as in conducting smoking cessation programmes and speaking at public fora on smoking control issues. The Customs and Excise Department and the Ministry of the Environment have provided support by enforcing the smoking control laws within their purview. Nongovernmental organizations and private companies have provided funding, by sponsoring overseas speakers for seminars, developing material such as posters, exhibits, brochures and street banners and sponsoring events such as smoke-free street soccer and streetball. Many of the organizations helped by mobilizing community action through personal contacts and influence. For example, the support of Malay community organizations has resulted in a significant decrease in their prevalence of smoking.

Conclusion

Our experience has shown that political action, with Government support, leadership and funding, can have a significant impact on the prevalence of smoking; however, a comprehensive programme must also consider the social context and identify community resources to maximize the impact of the programme. Community participation must also be fostered to create a climate of support for a smoke-free lifestyle and environment. If we are to reverse the tobacco-induced pandemic, a comprehensive programme of strong, well-integrated, concerted community action is required.

Setting an annual budget at Government level is crucial for ensuring the continuity of the programme, although depending on Government resources alone may sometimes be limiting. To reach all the relevant segments of the population, we will need funds, resources and manpower. These can be achieved if strong coalitions are built with various partners with the power and capacity to 'finance' or support the programme by providing alternative resources, whether monetary or non-monetary.

Slovakia: Evaluation of tobacco control initiatives

Z. Honzátková

National Institute of Tuberculosis and Respiratory Diseases, Bratislava, Slovakia

Epidemiological data on health status reveal a serious problem among the population of Slovakia. In 1995, according to a subjective evaluation of health status by age, only 42% of people aged 15–19 considered themselves to be in good health.

Evaluations of measures against tobacco usually include smoking prevalence, trends in mortality, tobacco production and cigarette consumption and the economic costs of smoking. In practice, evaluation is limited to overall prevalence surveys, with several concurrent measures. Surveys carried out in 1994 on mortality and morbidity related to tobacco use, attitudinal surveys and the economic impact of tobacco were important for assessing the scope of the problem in our country and for illustrating to the Government the need for preventive measures.

Smoking prevalence

Collecting data on the use of tobacco is a priority in our activities, as they are useful for both decision-makers and the media. Resources for tobacco control are lacking in Slovakia, in contrast to the vast financial resources of the transnational tobacco companies. The tobacco industry uses sophisticated, expensive promotion, including direct and indirect advertising and sponsorship of sports, arts and the media. Three surveys were carried out in 1979, 1991 and 1995 by the Institute of Health Education in Bratislava on representative samples of the Slovak population. One survey (Bronis et al., 1993) showed smoking prevalences of 33% in 1991 and 28% in 1995. The number of smokers was greatest in the 35–44 year age group among both men and women. The incidence of smoking in the 15–19 year age group gave cause for alarm because it was relatively high: 39% for males and 16% for females. The prevalence of daily smoking among women (16%) is twice as high as in China and almost half of that in the United Kingdom. The female market currently represents a source for future expansion by the tobacco industry. In Slovakia, smoking is much more widespread among young women (25% in 25–34 year age groups, 27% in 35–44 year group) than among older ones (17% in 45–54 year age group). In 1993, an investigation by questionnaire among doctors, nurses and assistants in a hygienic service about their attitudes towards smoking, smoke-free hospitals and tobacco habits showed a high prevalence of smoking among nurses (24%), whereas 19.5% of the doctors smoked (Avdicová & Hrubá, 1994).

Mortality attributed to smoking

In 1995, 52 686 deaths (9.82/1000 inhabitants) were recorded in the Slovak Republic. Heart disease, stroke, cancer and chronic respiratory diseases were the main causes of death. There were 2.8 more deaths among men than among women in middle age (35–54 years). Cigarette smoking has been shown to be a primary risk factor for coronary heart disease, arterosclerotic peripheral vascular disease, neoplasms and respiratory diseases. These three major causes were responsible for 83% of the total deaths in 1995. Among females, the number of deaths indicates that the overall risk of death at ages 35–69 was decreasing (20% in 1985, 18% in 1995), but that the risk of death from tobacco was increasing (from 2 to 3%); the risk of death attributed to tobacco among males was 13% in both years. In 1995, tobacco dependence caused the deaths of more than 9500 people in Slovakia, that is to say 17% of all deaths that year. The leading cause of smoking-attributed death in my country remains lung cancer , with 88% of cases attributed to smoking in 1995. There are thus long delays between decreases in smoking rates and reductions in smoking-related diseases (Peto *et al.*, 1994).

Tobacco production and cigarette consumption

Slovakia is not a big producer of leaf tobacco, and production decreased from 4500 tonnes in 1965 to 2000 tonnes in 1995. In that year, only 1000 ha were devoted to tobacco growing, whereas 5000 ha were used in 1965. Average per capita cigarette consumption rose by more than 31% during the past three decades and by 4.3% during the years 1991–93. In 1994, it decreased by 8%. According to a survey in 1995, 15% of the adult population began to smoke before they were 10, 51% began to smoke before they were 15, and 92% began to smoke before they were 20.

Economic consequences of smoking

The prices of cigarettes and tobacco products were fairly stable before 1989, but the price of cigarettes rose between 1991 and 1995. Overall, the industrial producers price indices increased about fourfold, and the consumer price increased by 2–50% yearly.

In 1993, the National Centre of Health Promotion estimated that the annual cost of smoking for the community, due to hospitalization and medical treatment, was 3.2 thousand million SKK (about US$ 100 million), and total costs, including loss of production, were more than 32.5 million million SKK (over US$ 1 million million) (Kozíková *et al.*, 1994).

Evaluation of tobacco control activities

Tobacco control measures in Slovakia have not been evaluated specifically, because several measures are taken simultaneously, including a health education programme and new legislation and price policies. At present, there is an enormous difference in funding for health education and for promotion by the tobacco companies in Slovakia. None of the tobacco tax revenue is used for anti-tobacco activities or research projects.

The advertisement of tobacco products, mainly cigarettes, became a new problem in the prevention of smoking in Slovakia in 1992, when the tobacco industry distributed various kinds of cigarette advertisements and used bus stops, billboards and shop windows to advertise their products. Taxis, buses and trams were painted in the colours of tobacco firms, with their logos. In 1995, the advertising sector and the Slovak Tobacco Industry prepared a revision of the act on advertisement, launched a campaign in the Slovak health sector and organized several press conferences. The idea of this challenge was to influence members of the Government and Parliament not to ban tobacco advertising. After strong public pressure, however, Law No. 220/1996 on advertising was enforced.

Our newest success in the field of tobacco control is that in 1997 the Slovak Parliament adopted Law No. 67 on the protection of non-smokers, which bans advertising, restricts tar and nicotine content (a maximum tar yield of 15 mg by December 1998, 12 mg by January 2001; a maximum nicotine content of 1.2 mg/cigarette by January 1998), bans the sale of tobacco to young people under the age of 18, imposes labelling and bans smoking in public places. It covers many aspects of of the problem of non-smokers' rights. Violations of these measures are punishable by fines of 500 to 5 000 000 SKK (US$ 14–145 000). The law is based on the WHO recommendations in its action plan for a smoke-free Europe and on certain guidelines of the European Union. The first issue is to improve protection of non-smokers from the effects of environmental tobacco smoke, in workplaces, public places and in front of children. The law shifts the issue of smoking from the individual and private sphere to the social and public arenas. The next goal of the law is to prevent recruitment of new smokers among children and adolescents. This legislation at the State level is our most important and powerful new weapon for helping non-smokers to avoid exposure to tobacco smoke.

Other activities in smoking prevention include participation in a 'Quit and win' competition in May 1997, a national no-tobacco day and the CINDI project.

Conclusions

In the beginning of the 1990s, the tobacco companies repeated advertising trends established in other countries and used tactics to target Slovak women and children. In 1997, Slovakia introduced a tobacco policy based on legislation that included a strong ban on advertising and restrictions on smoking and the tar and nicotine content of cigarettes. The law on protection of non-smokers is an effective measure to avoid involuntary exposure to tobacco smoke in public places, workplaces and schools. Now, full implementation of the law must be ensured.

Smoking is a public health problem, and its elimination requires an intersectoral approach in control strategies and a community climate of non-smoking promotion. We hope that these legislative controls, together with smoking cessation and health education, will lead to a comprehensive national tobacco control policy which can change the climate in favour of a smoke-free lifestyle.

References

Avdicová, M. & Hrubá, F. (1994) Prevalence of risk factors. CINDI programme, NCPZ, pp. 30–42
Bronis, M., Kaleta, M. & Beniaková, J. (1993) Frequency of tabaquisme in Slovakia: General decrease during last twelve years. In: *Tobacco or Health*, Bratislava, p. 35
Kozíková, E., Bebjaková, D., Sinka, F. & Srámek, L, (1994) *Analysis of economic and social effects of smoking epidemic in Slovakia*, Bratislava: NCPZ
Peto, R., Lopez, A.D., Boreham, M.T. & Health, C. (1994) Mortality from Smoking in Developed Countries 1950–2000, Oxford: Oxford University Press

Slovenia: United in non-smoking: New thinking, model and philosophy

V. Rehar

Institute of Public Health, Celje, Slovenia

The Slovenian approach to the smoking epidemic demonstrates the need to organize and work systematically to overcome the tobacco epidemic. It is important to benefit from previous experience for better planning and implementing of national decisions for the health of the population, including knowledge of modern pedagogy, health and humanistic and other sciences.

Non-smoking is a repeated action. It has a special place in individual value systems, in health policy and in the planning of social and economic development. As a model of thought, it is used in the education of smoke-free generations, helping in smoking cessation and in building the conditions for a smoke-free society. For this purpose, we promote all kinds of individual creativite actions for attaining a healthy lifestyle in the family. Each generation of each family approaches the quality of life in an original way. Non-smoking is a conscious model that may be chosen freely by individuals, groups and society in deciding on responsible individual and social values. The non-smoking philosophy is reflected in the choice of goals, targets, topics, methods, activities and results.

Tobacco-related problems in Slovenia

The seventeenth-century Slovenian researcher Baron Janez Vajkard Valvasor wrote in his life work, *Slava Vojvodine Krajnske*, about the relationship between a long life and abstinenece from tobacco. The problem has grown since then; Table 1 shows the prevalence of regular smoking in Slovenia between 1974 and 1996. The tobacco problem after the Second World War can be divided into three periods:

1945–75: Health and social protection was organized by the centralized State planning system. Typical of this period was preventive action by doctors, nurses and workers in the Red Cross and other organizations, in the form of essential hygiene, raising the level of health awareness in the population and controlling the classic infectious diseases. They also gave warnings about the health hazards of tobacco smoke. Qualitative studies on smoking among doctors were begun in Slovenia, and interest in changing the smoking status of the population grew. The first public opinion survey that included smoking was conducted in 1974–75 and showed that society supported the development of smoking prevention through health programmes and schools. The Slovenian Red Cross developed a programme of activities to stop smoking.

1976–90: Decentralization in the form of self-management systems was introduced into the preventive health system. Programmed health care and smoking prevention were well supported, and projects to promote a healthy lifestyle were begun. A ban on the advertising of tobacco products was included in a law on protection at the workplace passed in 1977, and smoking restriction was added to the law in 1984. Article 45 prohibits smoking in public transport, in the workplace and in public institutions; its implemetation was the responsibility of workers' councils.

1991–96: After Slovenia became an independent State, the national health policy included anti-smoking as a priority. The Minister of Health appealed to all Slovenian health institutions to respect non-smoking laws. The next step was to create a law specifically for tobacco control. The Slovenian Parliament accepted the first proposed law, on the protection of non-smokers, but the State Council rejected their decision, arguing that the law must include a total ban on advertising of tobacco products to prevent youngsters from starting to smoke. After two years, the second proposal was adopted and came into force on 18 May 1996. The law was thus accepted after long, systematic preparation by the Ministry of Health, with relatively strong support from the population because of the raising of awareness by civil initiatives, and especially non-governmental organizations.

The tobacco movement within the Institute of Public Health is now actively involved. We used previous local and national experience to develop a non-smoking tobacco policy, with the help of public and international organizations. The Ministry of Health supported targeted research by the Institute of Social Sciences in Ljubljana on the attitudes of the public about health and smoking. The media supports our efforts and regularly informs the public about health policies on non-smoking. Further research on the quality of life, health status and standards of the population showed the importance of individual choice and personal responsibility for health. In the public opinion survey of 1994, the Slovenian people ranked health as the highest value. The use of an appropriate strategy and relevant targets at all levels of society can increase the number of non-smokers.

Table 1. Prevalence of regular smoking in Slovenia, 1974–96

Year	Prevalence (%)		
	Adult population	Men	Women
1974–75	39.7		
1978	35.6		
1981–82	32.4		
1988	34.1	41.7	27.3
1994	28.2	34.7	22.7
1996	26.4	33.2	20.5

Project for smoke-free Slovenia

In 1992, we prepared a project based on a new philosophy of non-smoking. Its implementation involves the World Health Organization, the State Council, Parliament, 149 communities and their delegates, mayors, the Council of Health and the Committee for Drug Abuse. The target groups are kindergartens, schools and the educational system as a whole, with multi-sectoral support from professional institutes, organizations and the public. We counted on strong mass media support and national and local cooperation between the suppliers and the consumers. We are also involving families.

Professional analysts and research institutions evaluate the programmes and projects. The final evaluation was made in 1997–98. The project's technical basis and logistic support were assured partly by the Institute of Public Health in Celje. We started by organizing special non-smoking activities, such as conferences, workshops, seminars, public presentations and regular mass media presentations, introducing and using the World Health Organization and other tobacco-or-health programmes. Our partners include kindergartens, schools, military staff, lay people, non-governmental organizations and more that 100 associations with health topics in their programmes. The Slovene National Press Agency currently provides information to the press, and the mass media promote free of charge the innovative non-smoking projects and materials aimed at various target groups.

Shops, restaurants, customs, the airline company and public transport are now smoke-free. A project to make the university smoke-free has begun with the introduction of health and non-smoking exhibitions. The staff of the Economic Chamber have also joined the project. World No-Tobacco Day is celebrated regularly, and in 1998 we organized a national round-table meeting of all our partners in the non-smoking programme. Each presented the outcomes of the planned activities and systematic work in various sectors and confirmed the need to develop a positive-thinking model of non-smoking in families. The Ministry of Health and the Ministry for Education and Sport initiated a smoke-free project with the participation of the Ministry for Family and Social Affairs, the Slovene Olympic Committee and national organizations promoting sports for the family.

In 1994, we issued a booklet entitled 'So that I won't forget', based on the non-smoking teaching package, to all pupils in the first year of secondary school, to each member of Parliament and to all mayors in Slovenia. All smoke-free environments in public, private and other institutions received an award from the Minister of Health for their contribution to non-smoking. Applications were made to non-governmental organizations to finance individual and institutional preventive activities.

Tools for a non-smoking programme

Important tools in a non-smoking philosophy are humour and health, human rights and health, communicating with individuals and the public and management of stress. Working groups provide active, strong support for responsible individual behaviour, by raising self-esteem and the quality for life without stress or behaviour that leads to health risks. Positive acceptance of the facts is achieved by lifelong education starting in early childhood.

International collaboration and exchange have been useful for introducing the concept of a healthy lifestyle, and support for the smoke-free project was provided by banks, insurance agencies, donors and foundations. The interest of the private sector is growing. The number of 'hot lines' for counselling on smoking cessation has increased.

Conclusions

Social changes have stimulated progress in achieving the goals of tobacco control. Individual requests for support in stopping smoking have increased, but we need new projects for families and the young, who will respond only to non-aggressive methods that allow free choice. Anti-tobacco laws provide only short-term motivation for people to stop smoking. The key is lifelong individual education to make appropriate choices for improving the quality of life. The priorities in a non-smoking programme are:

- a systematic approach to non-smoking projects,
- promulgation of an anti-tobacco law,
- developing the economic conditions for an agreed tobacco policy and
- the support of private initiatives by non-governmental organizations.

South Africa: Development of a comprehensive tobacco control policy

D. Swart, P. Reddy, Y. Saloojee & K. Steyn

National Health Promotion Research and Development Office, Medical Research Council, Cape Town, South Africa

The *Tobacco Products Control Act* was passed in South Africa in 1993. This Act has serious limitations. It is not a comprehensive Act, as it deals only with the regulation of smoking in public places, the prohibition of sales to minors under the age of 16 and the regulation of advertising of tobacco products in certain respects and circumstances. The strengths and weaknesses of the Act are outlined here.

We conducted a study to develop strategies to support the formulation and implementation of a comprehensive tobacco control policy in South Africa. We used Political Mapping, a form of computer-assisted political analysis, to construct maps of the political terrain around the responses to the policy and future amendments to it. Descriptions of the content of the policy, its consequences, key players (supporters, potential supporters and opponents), the objectives of the players, networks of players and transitions in organizations and political environments have been collected and organized. This information will allow for detailed planning of a comprehensive policy.

Potential strategies for successful acceptance of amendments to the present Act which are designed to achieve comprehensive tobacco control are identified and analysed in order to improve its political feasibility. It is recommended that tobacco control activities have an active focal point in the Department of Health, that an active tobacco control network be developed among all the relevant Government departments and that the network of tobacco control activists and organizations be extended and strengthened so as to facilitate the acceptance of a comprehensive tobacco control policy in South Africa. As this study contains information crucial for policy and programme development, the findings will be distributed to Government departments and to tobacco control activists and organizations.

Taiwan area: Anti-smoking activities

L. Ho & C.-L. Lin

John Tung Foundation, Taipei, Taiwan

When the topic of anti-smoking is brought up in Taiwan, the John Tung Foundation is the first thing that comes to mind. Since the Foundation was established more than 14 years ago, it has made significant efforts to promote the anti-smoking cause. We review our efforts here, in eight phases.

Phase 1: Development (1984–86)
Immediately after the Foundation was established, it focused on innate knowledge and resource building. It collected information on the harmful effects of smoking worldwide and invited people in the medical and academic fields and environmentalists to become involved in the non-smoking effort.

Phase 2: Social activities (1987–92)

In 1987, when importing foreign cigarettes was permitted in Taiwan, the United States repeatedly urged the Government to allow their cigarette advertisements and promotional activities. For three days in 1992, *The Washington Post*, *The New York Times* and *The Wall Street Journal* all published advertisements stating "We want friendship, not cigarettes" and similar messages. These papers received a tremendous positive response from United States citizens, and the United States finally stopped asking us to allow their advertising campaign in Taiwan.

Phase 3: Asia-Pacific Association for the Control of Tobacco established (1989)

In 1989, we decided that we needed help to fight the powerful international tobacco companies and invited other Asian countries to unite and establish the Asia-Pacific Association for the Control of Tobacco.

Phase 4: Campaign against adolescent smoking (1990–93)

As the prevalence of smoking among adolescents was increasing in Taiwan, we began to focus on this age group. In 1990, a well-known Taiwanese singer developed liver cancer. Before he died, this popular adolescent role model asked the John Tung Foundation to help him send an important message, and he recorded a commercial urging them to 'respect life'. This commercial was the first to be broadcast on television free of charge, and since then all our public welfare commercials have been broadcast with no charge.

We followed this with anti-smoking identification cards, with the slogan "I'm 15 (or 16) years old and I don't smoke!", which we hoped would become a new adolescent trend. Led by various celebrities and role models proudly carrying these cards, we distributed over 200 000 of these anti-smoking cards. During this phase also, a now familiar face appeared in Taiwan. When Camel began using cartoon characters to promote cigarettes, the sales of cigarettes to adolescents increased from 3 to 33% within five years. To counter Camel's efforts, we created our own cartoon character, an anti-smoking friend named Xu Zhe Lin. His name was chosen by reversing the name Lin Zhe Xu, who was a heroic general in the opium wars in China, over 150 years ago. Both life-size and miniature cut-outs of Xu Zhe Lin were made, and he quickly won popularity among adolescents.

Our efforts against adolescent smoking reached a climax when four well-known singers, Taiwan's best-known baseball pitcher and other celebrities brought over 2500 high-school students together, and all wearing anti-smoking T-shirts, enthusiastically shouted in unison "Just say no to smoking and drugs!" This event was recorded as a commercial and was a huge success.

Phase 5: Annual anti-smoking themes (after 1993)

Each year we support the anti-smoking theme announced by the World Health Organization, which changes from year to year. In 1994, the theme was 'Media against smoking'. We urged three national television stations, cable television, 155 radio stations, over 20 newspapers and 60 magazines to join in spreading the anti-smoking message that 31 May is World No Smoking Day. In 1995, the theme was 'Women and smoking', with emphasis on second-hand smoke and the harmful effects of smoking on pregnant women and their children. We targeted pregnant women with our successful 'Happy mommies' poster. A well-known child movie star recorded a commercial and posed for posters urging pregnant women not to smoke or subject themselves to second-hand smoke. We then surveyed over 5200 women to learn more about the influences that promote smoking among women. Finally, we created a poster advocating refusal of second-hand smoke, which featured an internationally known actress with Miss Xu Zhe Lin, the female anti-smoking cartoon character.

In 1996, the theme was 'Sports and the arts without tobacco'. We invited six professional basketball players and other celebrities to record commercials in which they described quitting or refusing to smoke. They served as excellent role models. In 1997, we supported the theme 'United for a tobacco-free world!', making a television commercial and distributing it free of charge to members of the Asia-Pacific Association for the Control of Tobacco, requesting them to broadcast it on 31 May. The commercial was distributed to China, Hong Kong, Japan, the Philippines, the Republic of Korea, Singapore and Thailand.

Phase 6: Eliminating smoking in public areas (1995 to present)

First, we worked together with our nine domestic and international airline companies. On 1 July 1995, the presidents of these airlines came to the John Tung Foundation to declare that smoking was prohibited on their flights. The Ministers of Health and Communications, Foundation members and the mass media served as witnesses. This announcement came exactly one year before the target of the International Civil Aviation Organization to eliminate smoking on airlines.

In 1996, the presidents of 17 city bus companies also came to the Foundation to declare that smoking was prohibited on the over 10 000 city buses. Additionally, telephone hotlines were made available for citizens to denounce violators.

In 1997, a team of specialists spent three months evaluating 284 entries to determine the 10 public locations around Taiwan which had been most successful in eliminating smoking on their premises. The 10 winners include China Airlines, McDonalds's, Motorola and Texas Instruments.

Phase 7: Anti-tobacco legislation (1996)

We have joined forces with 51 public welfare groups to submit drafts of anti-tobacco laws to our legislature. In 1996, these groups went again to the Legislative Yuan to ask the leaders of the three major parties to pass anti-tobacco legislation. We visited each of the 164 legislators to explain the law in detail. The tobacco manufacturers retaliated by publishing three half-page newspaper advertisements that contradicted our message about the harmful effects of tobacco, in an attempt to confuse the public. Local groups and Government authorities negotiated with representatives of the National Tobacco Association, however, and the Tobacco Hazards Control Act was finally passed on 4 March 1997. It was fully implemented on 19 September 1997.

Phase 8: Efforts after passage of the Tobacco Hazards Control Act.

After this important legislation was passed, we began new social programmes, such as directly mailing anti-smoking publications targeted towards youth. To encourage improved public understanding of the anti-tobacco law, we created a 'trivia contest', in which individuals submitted answers to various questions to win prizes. On 15 September 1997, the presidents of 12 convenience store companies publicly announced their support of the anti-tobacco legislation and agreed to display warning posters and signs on windows and checkout stands in over 4000 of their shops. The signs declare that the sale of tobacco products to minors is illegal, and that adults should not send their children to purchase tobacco products for them. We are also working with a well-known jeweller to design anti-smoking rings and earrings which we hope will become the newest adolescent fashion statement.

We continue to help individuals understand how the anti-tobacco law affects their daily life. We hope that our efforts will receive widespread support from the public and that we can work together to implement the anti-tobacco legislation effectively to make Taiwan and the world smoke free!

United Kingdom: Impact of No Smoking Day

L. Owen

Health Education Authority, London, United Kingdom

No Smoking Day is a nationwide event held annually on the second Wednesday of March in the United Kingdom since 1984. It is organized by a coalition of national organizations. One of its main aims is to attract the maximum amount of publicity about smoking and health at the minimum cost to the organizers by deliberately creating news stories and events that are likely to be publicized by the media. The campaign has generated over 1 million words in free publicity every year over the past few years. Another aim of No Smoking Day is to encourage and assist smokers to quit on that Day, through a network of local organizers. A new image is created each year to keep the campaign fresh and to provide local organizers with ideas for activities. I report here the findings of surveys on awareness of and participation in the Day and its impact on smoking behaviour in the longer term.

Method of annual surveys

Thirteen surveys were carried out between 1986 and 1997, with the same questionnaire and method each year to facilitate comparisons between years. Questions to determine attitudes towards the event are included in each survey. The surveys are conducted about one week after the Day and involve interviews at home with about 1800 persons aged $\geq$ 16 in Great Britain; in the last few years, the survey has been extended to Northern Ireland, where about 600 people aged $\geq$ 16 are interviewed. In 1997, 1851 people in Great Britain and 583 in Northern Ireland were interviewed as part of a random 'omnibus' survey conducted by a commercial market research company which sells questionnaire space to interested parties. Quotas were set for age, sex, region and social class.

Key findings

Prompted awareness of the campaign was very high among all adults and among smokers separately. Thus, between 1986 and 1996, at least 80% of smokers had heard of the Day. In 1997, the awareness level among smokers was 68%. The average cost of creating this level of awareness through paid television advertising would be about UK£ 2 million; instead, through a combination of coverage on national and regional television and radio and in the press, it cost about UK£ 80 000.

The decline observed in 1997 was unexpected, as the actual coverage had been consistent with that of previous years. We explored several hypotheses, such as changes in the socioeconomic and psychological profiles of smokers, but none was of much significance. A decline in media coverage also did not account for the change, since higher awareness has been achieved with less coverage than that of 1997; the amount of coverage was similar in 1995 and 1997, yet there was greater awareness in 1995. One explanation that received some support was that a general election campaign was also held in March 1997, and, after 18 years of Conservative government, there was every expectation that a Labour government would be voted in. Thus, the number of articles that mentioned the election rose from around 2000–3500 in the same month in 1993–96 to nearly 8000 in March 1997, while the number that mentioned smoking remained relatively constant, at about 500. It seems likely, therefore, that awareness of No Smoking Day is not simply a function of the absolute volume of coverage but is also related to the importance of other messages carried in the media at the same time.

The percentage of smokers who reported having participated in No Smoking Day, defined as having stopped or tried to stop smoking on the Day, fluctuated around 15% between 1986 and 1996, but declined to 10% of smokers in 1997. This apparent decline in participation between 1996 and 1997 was not, however, statistically significant.

Participation was highest among 16–24-year olds (20%) and among people smoking ≤ 10 cigarettes per day (17%). The latter finding is not surprising, as younger smokers are more likely than older smokers to smoke less. Of 41 people who stopped or tried to stop smoking, 41% claimed to have stopped for the whole Day and 47% for part of the Day; 13% said that they had been unable to stop smoking at all. When 36 participants were asked what their intentions were with regard to smoking, 49% said that they intended to stop for as long as possible and 37% claimed that they would stop only on No Smoking Day. These figures should be treated with caution as they are based on few people, but they suggest that future initiatives might be shifted from encouraging short-term quitting to helping smoking cessation.

People hear about No Smoking Day through national and regional television, radio and the press, but 57% of the smokers cited television as the source of their awareness. An important aspect of the campaign is delivery at the local level. When asked if they were aware of any event in their area that was aimed at helping smokers to quit, 3% of all adults and 4% of smokers answered positively. Although these figures appear low, they are fairly typical for a campaign of this nature. Of those who were unaware of No Smoking Day events in their area, 34% of all adults and 49% of smokers claimed to be aware of other help available for smokers.

One aim of the Day is to publicize the telephone help lines in England, Scotland, Northern Ireland and Wales. In 1997, 52% of all adults and 71% of the smokers claimed to have heard of a help line for smokers. Of those who had heard of them, 2% of all adults and 4% of smokers said that they had phoned or tried to phone a help line. These figures are slightly higher than those obtained in 1996: 1 and 2%, respectively.

Method of three-month follow-up surveys

Three-month follow-up surveys are conducted about once every three years, the latest having been carried out in 1996. The key purpose of these surveys is to assess the impact of No Smoking Day in the longer term. The latest, carried out on 13–27 June 1996, involved a sample of 5061 smokers and recent ex-smokers aged ≥ 16 in 142 constituency sampling points in the United Kingdom. The sample was weighted to reflect the demographic profile of all smokers interviewed in March 1996, and quotas were set for age, sex, social class and working status.

Key findings

In 1996, 47% of respondents recalled the exact name No Smoking Day without prompting, and when these are combined with people who remembered the name after prompting the proportion rises to 83%. Although this percentage is much higher than thr annual figure reported above for 1997, the relevant comparison is with the annual survey for 1996 in which 77% of all adults and 82% of smokers were aware of the campaign. When respondents who were aware of the Day were asked whether they had attempted to give up or cut down on the Day, 18% claimed to have done so. As in the annual survey, participation was highest among younger smokers.

When respondents were asked what they actually did, 37% claimed to have given up for the whole Day, 20% had given up for part of the Day, 36% had cut down their consumption, and 7% had tried but failed to participate to any degree. Participants who had either stopped for all or part of the Day or reduced their consumption on the Day were asked about their current smoking behaviour three months later. Table 1 shows that 25% had stopped for less than one day and a similar proportion had lasted the whole Day. The impact of the Day clearly reaches beyond the event itself, as 40% continued a positive change and 14% were still not smoking or were still smoking less three motnhs after the Day itself.

This information from this survey can be used to calculate the total proportion of the population who had stopped smoking on the Day and were still not smoking three months later. According to mid-year estimates, there were nearly 13 million smokers in the United Kingdom in 1996. Of these, 83% were aware of No Smoking Day, and

Table 1. Length of cessation or reduction in smoking after No Smoking Day in the United Kingdom, 1996

Duration of cessation or reduction	Active participants (%)
< 1 day	25
1 day	27
> 1 day ≤ 1 week	13
> 1 to ≤ 2 weeks	6
> 2 weeks ≤ 1 month	3
> 1 to ≤ 2 months	3
> 2 to ≤ 3 months	4
Still not smoking or still reduced	14
Don't know	6

Based on 712 persons who stopped or reduced smoking on No Smoking Day

15% had participated; 2% had still stopped or cut down at three months. Of these, 0.3% had stopped completely, representing 38 000 people in the United Kingdom, and 1.8% had continued to smoke at reduced levels, representing 222 000 people.

Extrapolation to China

The potential impact of a no-smoking day in China is difficult to estimate, as the population differs from that of the United Kingdom in demographic profile and other characteristics, such as previous attempts to quit, the nature of the media and the nature of local health promotion services. Nevertheless, I have estimated the potential impact of such a campaign in China by applying the percentages for the United Kingdom to figures from the 1990 census and the first national smoking prevalence survey in 1984 (Weng et al., 1987). In 1990, there were about 422 million males and nearly 400 million females over the age of 15 in China. The prevalence survey showed that 258 million males and 28 million females of those ages smoked. Assuming an impact of a no-smoking day on 0.3% of that population, such an event would result in 773 000 males and 84 000 females stopping smoking on the day and still not smoking three months later.

Awareness levels in the campaigns in the United Kingdom show that they meet their objective of bringing the event to the attention of as many people as possible and that the impact of the Day reaches beyond the event itself.

Reference

Weng, X.Z., Hong, Z.G. & Chen, D.Y. (1987) Smoking prevalence in Chinese aged 15 and above. Report of the 1984 First National Prevalence Survey. Chin. Med. J., 100, 886–892

United Kingdom: No Smoking Day

J. Buckler

No Smoking Day, London, United Kingdom

No Smoking Day is a nationwide campaign in the United Kingdom to help people who want to stop smoking. It has two main strategies: a public relations campaign, achieving over 1 million words of free publicity each year in the mass media, together with strong message delivery; and a network of organizers at local level who run events to promote the Day and help smokers who want to quit.

Delivering the campaign requires detailed advance planning to identify potential stories for use in the national and regional press and broadcast media that will deliver supportive messages, and to develop a range of theme materials and ideas for local use.

The result is a combination of wide media coverage, raising awareness of No Smoking Day, and the delivery of practical local events to support people who want to quit.

United Kingdom: The post of smoking prevention coordinator: A strategic, coordinated approach to reducing smoking prevalence

C. Owens

Smoking Prevention Co-ordinator, Development & Environmental Services Directorate, Liverpool City Council, Liverpool, United Kingdom

Introduction

In Liverpool, we are committed to reducing the high levels of ill health and premature death caused by smoking. We have therefore developed a strategic and coordinated approach to smoking prevention in the form of a City strategy on tobacco abuse, the implementation of which is overseen by a smoking prevention coordinator. The post is jointly funded by Liverpool City Council and the Roy Castle Lung Cancer Foundation. The Foundation is a United Kingdom charity dedicated to defeating lung cancer. It is unique for a local authority to have an officer wholly dedicated to smoking prevention.

The City strategy consists of strategic statements covering research, action in workplaces, smoke-free areas, young people, health promotion, work with communities, advertising and sponsorship and advocacy. A work programme to ensure that progress is made in implementing the strategy has also been produced, which involves lead officers in various organizations in the city. At six-monthly intervals, a half-day seminar is held with the lead officers to review progress and identify future action plans.

One of the objectives of the smoking prevention coordinator's post is to increase the support available for smokers wanting to quit. This is done by training primary health care teams in helping smokers to quit; training other people in contact with smokers, e.g. social workers, youth workers and advice workers; supporting self-help groups, such as Fag-Ends, Liverpool One Parent Family Trust, and supporting research to find the most successful methods of helping smokers to quit.

Fag-Ends is a stop smoking self-support group funded by the Roy Castle Lung Cancer Foundation. They provide the following free stop smoking support: a telephone helpline staffed by volunteers, weekly self-help group meetings, individual counselling and stop smoking courses at various venues across the City. The appeal of Fag-Ends to smokers is that it is run by people who have quit smoking—ordinary people, rather than health professionals, who, smokers feel, are inclined to 'preach' to them. As Fag-Ends has no paid workers, part of the work of the smoking prevention coordinator involves supporting the group and ensuring that volunteers receive the necessary training and that the service runs smoothly. The Roy Castle Lung Cancer Foundation agreed from January 1998 to fund one full-time and one part-time post for Fag-Ends.

One objective of the post is to work with breweries to help and encourage pubs and licensed premises to develop no-smoking areas. A joint working party has been established comprising representatives from the retail section of the four main breweries in Liverpool, the secretary of the North West Brewers and Licensed Retailers Association, Liverpool City Council environmental health officers and the smoking prevention coordinator. The 10 pubs involved in the pilot project have dedicated no-smoking areas in the main drinking part of the premises. Before the introduction of no-smoking areas, the customers in the pilot pubs were surveyed to gauge their reactions, as it was essential to aoid any loss of business when the areas were introduced. The first pubs introduced their no-smoking areas in May 1996. Feedback from these pubs is closely monitored to help with the introduction of smoke-free areas in other premises. Consideration is also given to effective methods of ventilating the whole premises to reduce smoke throughout the pub, with particular attention to the health and safety of the pub staff.

A third objective is to encourage employers in the city to develop clearly defined policies to prohibit smoking in the workplace. There are two main parts to this work. A pack is being developed to outline the steps to be taken by a business in developing, adopting and implementing a no-smoking policy. This will be distributed to small businesses in the city free of charge. The smoking prevention coordinator works with local businesses, advising, supporting and assisting them in policy development and implementation.

A further objective of the post is to work with organizations in the city to provide literature written with specific groups in mind. Current projects include working with the Pagoda of the Hundred Harmony Chinese Community Centre to produce appropriate and acceptable local literature in Chinese. Plans are also under way to use the local Chinese community newspaper, *The Silk Road News*, and the local Chinese radio programme, *The Orient Express*, to give information about the health risks for smokers and advice about quitting .

Research

The post of smoking prevention coordinator also involves seeking new and innovative ways of warning of the dangers of smoking and of helping people quit. I am involved in two projects. One is research to establish the effectiveness of a Canadian stop-smoking programme for low-income women, which was introduced in Liverpool in 1995. This programme focuses on increasing self-esteem and self-confidence and developing stress management models and relaxation techniques which do not require a great deal of time or expense. This programme has been used in whole or in part across the city for two years, and it is now necessary to assess any benefits provided by this as opposed to more traditional, information approaches. A project to be undertaken jointly with health promotion specialists from Manchester and Liverpool is bidding for funding from the European Commission Public Health and Safety at Work Directorate.

Conclusion

To tackle the problem of smoking, a coordinated approach is needed. No one organization can do it alone. The fact is that the whole is greater than the sum of the parts. This unique local authority post is one that all major cities should have in order to ensure a coordinated approach to smoking prevention.

United States: Achieving an effective national tobacco control policy

J.R. Seffrin

American Cancer Society, Atlanta, Georgia, United States

I appreciate the opportunity to share our thoughts on the tobacco settlement but more importantly on the broader agenda that we all share: protecting the world from tobacco. We are very concerned about international issues in tobacco control and have been very active for many years on these issues. The American Cancer Society was involved in the First World Conference on Smoking or Health in New York in the mid-1970s. We have also worked with the United States trade representative's office for many years to stop the two-faced policy of supporting health on one hand and exporting death on the other.

When the original proposal for a settlement with the tobacco industry was released, the American Cancer Society began a three-stage, comprehensive analysis which included reviews by volunteers and staff and by a specially convened panel of outside legal, economic and health policy experts. We also participated in the evaluation process conducted by the Advisory Committee on Tobacco Policy and Public Health, chaired by a former commissioner of the United States Food and Drug Administration, David Kessler, and the former Surgeon General, C. Everett Koop. I chaired the panel on regulation of tobacco products for that committee. During this process, several areas of concern were identified:

Industry payments: The amount of the required payments may be too small to result in significant reductions in smoking among the young. The present discounted value of the required US$ 368.5 thousand million payments is actually only US$ 194.5 thousand million. The payments would produce an increase per pack in the price of cigarettes of 41 cents, which would eventually grow to 62 cents per pack after five years. No other public health strategy would have the speed and cost-effectiveness of the impact of increasing the price of tobacco products.

Regulation of nicotine and other tobacco constituents by the United States Food and Drug Administration: The procedural hurdles are wholly unjustified.

Pre-emption: State and local governments have made significant efforts to control use of tobacco by minors by imposing excise taxes, restrictions on sales, labelling and disclosure requirements and policies to protect citizens from secondhand smoke. National tobacco control policy must not undermine these efforts.

Public disclosure of industry documents: It is clear that the tobacco industry did not disclose what it knew about the dangers and addictive properties of cigarettes. This situation must be rectified.

Reducing tobacco consumption by minors and 'look back' provisions: There is no economic incentive to ensure that the industry will meet the targets.

Disclosure and regulation of non-tobacco ingredients and reduced-risk products: Manufacturers must be required to provide the United States Food and Drug Administration with a list of non-tobacco ingredients.

International tobacco control: In this context, the word 'global' has been used inappropriately. The intention is not and cannot be to solve the entire problem. We need to begin in our own garden, ensuring that critical information about tobacco industry deceit is available to everyone in all countries and regulating the product as a drug. We support the use of additional funds for international tobacco control activities. We do not intend to prescribe who should control those funds or how they should be used, other than for activities that will reduce the use of tobacco products around the world. To be truly effective, any national tobacco control policy must take these and other issues into consideration.

The American Cancer Society believes that the current debate on tobacco control provides us with a historic opportunity to create an effective national tobacco control programme which could save thousands of lives from tobacco-caused disease; we must also regulate the tobacco industry's marketing practices that target our youth. While the proposal that was agreed to by the tobacco companies and state attorneys-general is an important first step, the American Cancer Society believes that carefully crafted legislation that ensures the intent of the provisions of the agreement should be the goal. To this end, we will work to enact legislation that results in a comprehensive, sustainable, effective, well-funded national tobacco control policy. Specifically, the Society is committed to working with the Administration, members of the 105th Congress and our tobacco control allies to include the following critical public health measures in comprehensive federal tobacco control legislation:

• The Federal Food and Drug Administration must be given unfettered authority to regulate nicotine and other ingredients, as well as the labelling, advertising and promotion of tobacco products. The Administration should be allowed to develop an incentive system that will help stimulate the production or availability of less hazardous products. Additionally, tobacco companies must disclose all ingredients in tobacco products to the Food and Drug Administration, with any documents and research done on the health impact of tobacco use and marketing of tobacco products to children.

- Enforceable performance standards combined with significant industry penalties must be developed for tobacco companies in order to hold them accountable for the real reductions in tobacco use among the young;
- The price of tobacco products in the United States must be dramatically increased to ensure that children do not begin to smoke. The American Cancer Society supports an immediate and dramatic increase in the tobacco excise tax on all tobacco products.
- States and localities must be empowered to adopt consistent or stronger tobacco control laws than the Federal legislation.

The American Cancer Society further believes that Federal legislation for tobacco control will provide the opportunity to address international tobacco control measures, funding for health research, prevention and treatment programmes and incentives to assist tobacco farmers and their families. The American Cancer Society will continue to work with all individuals and groups having an interest in public health to make meaningful contributions to this process. It is our hope that this dialogue will help enhance the overall quality of the outcome and ultimately save lives from tobacco-caused diseases.

United States: Money against tobacco *versus* money for tobacco

J. Cook, D.G. Bal, R. Todd, M. Morra, N. Lins & J. Seffrin

American Cancer Society, Atlanta, Georgia, United States

In order to paint the whole picture of financing tobacco control, we shall address not only how to raise money to fight 'big tobacco' but also how the tobacco industry spends its money and buys influence. First, we shall attempt to show how the tobacco industry bought influence—social, political, cultural and ethnic—by strategically and tactically funding various segments of American society without overtly appearing to do so. Thus, the tentacles of the tobacco companies' influence extend into the very fabric of society, in such an insidious fashion that when we look at the overall picture we are astounded by the heterogeneity of their spheres of influence: into politics, art in all its forms, sports, ethnic and other social organizations, small business (especially little shops in which up to 20% of sales and 50% of profits are derived from tobacco) and, most of all, Government, especially in the parts of the world where tobacco revenues are a major contributo to the public coffers.

Having dealt with the tobacco industry's point, we shall mention the American Cancer Society's 'counterpoint', how we evolved our thinking over the decades in addressing tobacco issues, from our initial focus on cessation to emphasis of prevention of tobacco use and public education, to our aggressive advocacy stance and finally our current perspective that a comprehensive social change is the only way to achieve a tobacco-free generation. We in the American Cancer Society and our partner agencies in the private and public sectors hope to achieve a 50% reduction in the rate of mortality from cancer by the year 2015; we are certainly unlikely to achieve that goal is we do not further improve the reductions in tobacco use that we have already achieved, especially in California and Massachusetts.

The tide has turned, because powerful interests, including the President of the United States, are now on our side, albeit somewhat belatedly and unfortunately sometimes intermittently and half-heartedly. The supreme irony of this enterprise is that the tobacco companies have had a great deal of money all the time, and now we are using their money—their ill-gotten gains—to oppose them in a systematic, scientific fashion. How we are doing this is simple: state by state, we are sponsoring initiatives to impose an additional tax on every pack of cigarettes and earmark those funds to set up a broad-based public and private sector programme to counter the tobacco industry's insidious influence at every level of society. These interventions include broad-based, statewide local programmes and comprehensive media and public relations campaigns.

Let me begin by describing how over US$ 6 thousand million of tobacco money goes into maintaining the carefully orchestrated status quo in the United States alone. This 'money for tobacco' in the United States takes various forms. It has been realized only recently that this is not a series of haphazard events but instead a carefully choreographed advertising, public relations, legal and political blitz aimed at increasing cigarette and tobacco sales by belittling health concerns, raising the spectre of the Government (by emphasizing people's individul rights) and, most of all, buying influence, directly or indirectly. We categorized those efforts into five somewhat arbitrary classes:

• buying influence through myriad private organizations,
• influencing the media,
• using the Government as a 'Trojan horse',
• lawsuits and legal threats and
• manipulating the political process at every level.

Manipulating society and buying influence through social, cultural, ethnic and art organizations

This issue has been well summarized for the lay public in an article by Sharon Lerner, from which I quote extensively herein, especially because it focuses on insidious influence buying in hard-pressed women's organizations. Under increasing fire in the United States, tobacco companies are only too willing to come to the rescue of cash-starved activist, cultural, professional and political groups, in the hope that visible support of good works will help improve their corporate public image. The result has been a steady flow of cash gifts to the non-profit sector and sponsorship of high-profile sports, arts and entertainment events. Such gifts have long been a part of the tobacco industry's public relations, but the current wave of anti-tobacco sentiment and legislation has been accompanied by an increase in such philanthropic activity, Philip Morris having risen to the top of the list of all corporate cash donors, from its ranking of twenty-fifth in 1984.

The increased availability of tobacco money is creating a moral conundrum for many women's organizations. If the groups refuse the largesse of tobacco companies, they may have to sacrifice valuable programmes. If they accept it, they may feel—or be perceived as—beholden to the industry.

However they are categorized, the lavish offerings reach far and wide. In addition to providing funding for sports, arts and scientific research, tobacco companies steadily funnel money to thousands of worthy community, political and professional groups every year. An internal memo leaked from Philip Morris in 1988 gives a sense of the scope and nature of these contributions. It categorized organizations that received 'corporate contributions, business expenses, samples, journal ads, promotional items, Philip Morris publications, printing, honoraria for guest speakers, and USA Corporate Affairs staff participation' as either 'Asian American, Agricultural,American Indian, Black, Business, Cultural, Hasidic, Hispanic, legislative, other, or Women', cold-bloodedly segmenting all possible potential markets!

In fact, a great number of groups do consider tobacco money worth whatever complications it may bring, including the American Association of University Women, Catalyst for Women, the League of Women Voters, the national Coalition of 100 Black Women, the NOW Legal Defense and Education Fund, the Women's Legal Defense Fund and the Women's Research znd Education Institute, to name just a few. At the same time, women in the United States have played a leading role in warning us about the very real dangers. According to the chairperson of the subcommittee on tobacco of the American Medical Women's Association, "Anyone—organizations or elected officials—who would receive tobacco industry funds runs the risk of compromising their credicibility, their work, and their ability to promote tobacco control and prevention programs." Those who do receive tobacco money often take such suggestions as harassing and intrusive.

Tobacco companies have also been a lifeline to organizations such as the National Association for the Advancement of Colored People, the Urban League and the United Negro College Fund (now known as the College Fund/UNCF). Targeting of ethnic minorities' and women's organizations has become a specific tactic of 'big tobacco'.

As most of the women's organizations that accepted funds from the tobacco industry said that they would not accept money from the National Rifle Association or from anti-choice sources, it is clear that they do discriminate among potential funders, but many women's groups do not consider tobacco to be a women's issue. The President of MANA, a national Latina organization, described her organization's acceptance of US$ 15 000 (to write a history of the group and for 'briefcases for our conferences and things like that') as a form of retaliation. "Our position is that if they're making money on our community, at least they can give some back." These frightening efforts at rationalizing influence buying by the tobacco industry must be countered without alienating these minority, ethnic and women's groups, because this tactic is regrettably the rule rather than the exception. Organizations that are not receiving direct or indirect funding (through tobacco industry subsidiaries) are rare.

One major way in which the tobacco industry has begun to buy both the influence and the legitimacy they crave is by targeted takeovers and diversification. Thus, over the past decade, several have used Wall Street's new mania for mergers and acquisitions to buy huge food and other 'legitimate' businesses with well-known names, with the twin intent of increasing their spheres of influence and prudently investing their obscene profits.

Influencing the media

The tobacco industry buys influence very cleverly in the ostensibly incorruptible American media. Professor Daynard and Professor Sweda in Boston have described the tactics in detail. The tobacco industry can influence public opinion in ways that are not readily apparent to the general public. For example, an editorial in *The New York Post*, entitled 'No-smoking's victim', described the purported negative effects inflicted on the New York restaurant business by the smoke-free ordinance: "The health fascists, as predicted, have actually injured a vital New York City industry," the editorial began. The sources of the claim that no-smoking laws are bad for the restaurant business were surveys conducted ostensibly independently, one by a tobacco-rights group and one by a front organization, the New York Tavern and Restaurant Association. Rupert Murdoch, the Editor-in-Chief of *The New York Post* and hundreds of other newspapers, has been a member of the Board of Directors of Philip Morris since 1989.

A less covert but equally influential media blitz is to buy full-page advertisements in ethnic and general newspapers, some of which appear as thinly disguised legitimate articles, to send out their messages on a wide variety of public policy issues affecting tobacco. A large number of such advertisements appeared shortly after a spate of negative publicity for the industry after Congressional hearings in the the spring of 1994. R.J. Reynolds' advertisements included headlines such as 'Today it's cigarettes. Tomorrow?', 'Smoking in a free society', 'Secondhand smoke: How much are non-smokers exposed to?' and 'Is the Government going too far?' The three directions of the tobacco industry's propaganda are thus: dismissing health concerns, emphasizing people's rights and denigrating Government (Government is always capitalized in R.J. Reynolds' advertisements, to make it bigger and more menacing). Dr Ken Warner in Michigan showed a strong statistical relationship between cigarette advertising in magazines, especially those for women, and their tendency to cover up the hazards of smoking.

Another means by which the tobacco industry influences the media is reflected by a tour of New York and Washington DC sponsored by Philip Morris for 10 Asian journalists. The special topics on the agenda of this trip were talks on the smoking ban in New York by people who opposed the ordinance.

As tobacco cannot be advertised on television or radio, the industry has obtained major television coverage of sports sponsorships; however, these openings are now being shut off due to our collective efforts.

Big Government used as a 'Trojan horse'

Using 'Big Government' as an excuse, the tobacco industry has heavily funded so-called public interest groups of 'concerned citizens'. If there is not an appropriate group or entity to ally with on a particular issue, the tobacco industry will create one. A prime example in the United States is the National Smokers Alliance. Maintaining the guise of a spontaneous uprising of millions of smokers outraged by the steady infringement of their God-given rights as Americans, the Alliance is in reality a 'Trojan horse', designed to give the appearance of a legitimate expression of genuine anger at the grass roots but created and financed by powerful outside interests, in this case seed money from Philip Morris' public relations firm, Burson-Marsteler. It quickly claimed over 1 million members, a 'member' being someone who signed his or her name to a form circulated by paid persons, who gave prospective 'members' free gifts, such as cigarette lighters.

Another example of the fabrication of allies by the tobacco industry is the United Restaurant, Hotel and Tavern Association of New York State, which placed full-page advertisements in *The New York Times* in 1994 to oppose the smoke-free ordinance proposed by the New York City Council.Joe Cherner of Smoke-free Educational Services not only discovered that the Association did not even have a telephone listing in New York City and that its supposed chapters in New York boroughs were all defunct, but also found that the Association's representative at the hearing of the City Council admitted that the advertisements were paid for by tobacco interests. Similarly, in California, a group called Restaurateurs for a Sensible Voluntary Policy was created by tobacco interests.

Law suits and legal threats and sponsoring or countering of initiatives

Professor Sweda and Professor Daynard again provided numerous instances of how the tobacco industry pushes its objectives in preempting legal initiatives. In 1994, after communities in California had implemented tough local laws requiring smoke-free public places, the tobacco industry poured more than US$ 18 million into a campaign to sponsor its preemption proposal and to put it on a ballot as a binding referendum. In this effort, Philip Morris falsely persuaded potential signatories that its goal was to achieve a law that restricted smoking in public. California's Secretary of State accused Philip Morris' front group, called 'Californians for Uniform Statewide Restrictions' of outright deception.

It is perhaps not surprising that the tobacco industry feels free to sue local governments in an effort to overturn bans on cigarette vending machines or cigarette advertising on the tops of taxis. It is now threatening governments throughout the world with the preposterous claim that labelling regulations infringe the companies' trademark rights, in violation of international conventions. A libel suit against ABC Television was settled in 1996 after ABC apologized for a technical inaccuracy, despite the truth of the story that Philip Morris adds unnecessary nicotine to American cigarettes.

Manipulating the political process at every level

The tobacco industry has mastered the art and science of manipulating the political process in the United States at the Federal, state and local levels. They heavily fund the re-election campaigns of their friends and oppose those of tobacco control advocates. The industry is bipartisan and funds Republicans and Democrats equally, on the basis of their level of influence. They manipulate the executive and legislative branches at every level of Government. As they influence large segments of the media, the legendary independence of the American judiciary is the one major recourse remaining, although even this has on occasion been compromised in small tobacco-growing states.

In Massachusetts in 1993 and 1994, one person worked as a registered lobbyist at the State House for both the Massachusetts Restaurant Association and the R.J. Reynolds Tobacco Company. Dr S.A. Glantz and Dr F.M. Monardi studied the campaign contributions of tobacco companies in 1993–94 and their effects on legislative behaviour in six states in which there has been varying activity by local tobacco-control activists:

California, Colorado, Massachusetts, Ohio, Pennsylvania and Washington. State legislatures are important sites for tobacco control, because they control policy-making on issues such as tobacco taxation, the access of young people to tobacco products, legislation of environmental tobacco smoke and funding for anti-tobacco education programmes run by state health and education departments. Glantz and Monardi found that the tobacco industry tended to be opportunistic rather than ideological in its campaign contributions, supporting whatever party was in power. They concluded that the contributions in the six states may reflect the amount of tobacco control activity in those states. Thus, the largest industry efforts were made in California and Massachusetts, where the contributions were greater than those made to Congress. Both of those states have passed legislation to increase the tax on tobacco and earmark money for tobacco education and research.

Fund-raising by the American Cancer Society, the American Lung Association and the American Heart Association

We have systematically raised money to counter the tobacco industry, by persuading states to increase taxes on cigarettes and then allocating a portion of those funds to reducing tobacco use. In California, it had been impossible to raise the cigartte tax because the vast majority of the members of the California Legislature received large amounts of tobacco funds. We therefore decided to go directly to the people of California and obtained the requisite number of signatures to qualify for introduction of the initiative on a ballot in November 1988. The tobacco industry and its front organizations mounted an attack, which included fabrication of 'anti-tobacco police' and a 'health Nazi' bureaucracy to deal with the smuggling and other criminality they said would be generated by the proposition. Despite a US$ 25 million campaign by the industry, against our US$ 1 million, we won the battle, and a large majority of Californians passed Proposition 99. Since then, we have had to fight to protect the funds for tobacco prevention and control, as the tobacco industry has persuaded the legislative, executive and even judicial branches of Government to block the appropriation, authorization and spending of these funds. Our next most significant victory was the passage of a 25-cent tax increase in Massachusetts in 1992, which was conceived, implemented and funded by the American Cancer Society alone. Advances have also been made in other states.

These efforts have resulted in dramatic decreases in tobacco consumption and the prevalence of tobacco use among adults. In California, although uptake by young people has not declined recently, the rate of use by adults has decreased dramatically, except in 1996. We have examined whether the increase in 1996 was real or due to some changes in our survey questions and method. The American Cancer Society is thus implementing an aggressive nationwide effort to support state and local tobacco-control coalitions designed to provide leadership and support for increases in taxes on tobacco and other initiatives for tobacco control. Thus, we will not only reduce the rate of mortality from cancer in the United States by 50% by the year 2015 but will also bring about a concomitant reduction in the frequency of all of the other tobacco-related diseases.

Venezuela: 'World No Tobacco Day': Ten years of experience

M. Adrianza, T. Villamizar & N. Herrera

Fundacion Antitabaquica de Venezuela, Instituto Diagnostico, Caracas, Venezuela

In 1986, we initiated celebration of a national day without tobacco smoke, promoted by the American Cancer Society, which contributed its experience with this type of event. In 1988, the World Health Organization's Tobacco or Health programme requested Member States to celebrate World No-Tobacco Day, coherent with the international character of the smoking epidemic. The objective of the World Health Organization (WHO) was to call attention to the health impairments induced by direct and indirect use of tobacco, to use up-to-date scientific knowledge in that area and to take the concern of WHO to be around each country reflected in a motto specific for each area. We consider our experience in this area important and wish to share it with other countries with anti-smoking programmes.

Objectives

Our objectives were to take knowledge on the subject chosen each year, with its corresponding motto, to all institutions specializing in that problem and to the entire community served by those institutions, thus transferring the objectives of WHO to our country. We also wish to describe the methods we used to carry out, monitor, readjust and evaluate the process within its social context. Another objective was to show the advantages of population evaluation for judging the real results of the operational strategies used. Lastly, we wanted to disseminate information on the harmful effects of tobacco smoke in order to reduce the prevalence of smoking.

Methods

We used a combination of time, space, human, other physical and information resources. Specifically, we used the space that the subject of tobacco occupies in the country as a whole and in the population, directly and indirectly. For example, for the subject 'Health sectors and smoke-free health workers', we took information on all the health institutions in the country, from highly complex hospitals, to personnel in teaching and administration and to the community of each health institution.

We use January to plan and collect the information. In February, we initiate weekly meetings with the most suitable human resources to develop information instruments. In March, we coordinate the promotional activities that appear to be the most productive, including:

- a poster with the motto, which is disseminated in May;
- creation of posters and drawings in schools;
- dissemination of a message to all of the health structures of the country, signed by the Minister of Health and Social Welfare, to stimulate the best possible World No-Tobacco Day; equal incentive is requested from the Ministry of Education;
- a message for all mass media;
- interventions for radio, television and other mass media;
- preparation of a 7-km 'march for health' to be held on the Sunday before 31 May, sponsored by the Anticancer Society and the national Directorate of Oncology, along the avenue that links three municipalities (Libertador, Chacao and Sucre) in the metroplitan area of Caracas; and
- preparation of cultural and scientific events for 31 May.

Results

We have two ways of evaluating the results. First, we analyse all the institutional reports prepared for the World Cigarette Smoke-free Day; secondly, we carry out a population survey with a coverage of all population centres ($\geq$ 5000) throughout the country, using a multiphasic randomized sampling design with an estimation error of 2.5% and a reliability index of 95%. The survey covers all the socioeconomic strata and all educational levels.

A high percentage (86–97%) of people over 15 were aware of the existence of World No-Tobacco Day each year since 1988, although the percentage for 1996 fell to 76%, perhaps because of deficiencies in the mass information system, which is today in the hands of the advertising strategies of the tobacco industry. Thus, the percentage who knew about the last World No-Tobacco Day decreased consistently between 1991 and 1996, from 92 to 57%.

In answer to the question of how the respondent learnt of World No-Tobacco Day, television occupies the highest place, with a rising trend since 1991, although it informs only half of the respondents. Newspapers and radio maintain small fluctuations around 30% in information coverage. Workplaces and other sources show growing trends of 14 and 25%, respectively, indicating that personal contact is of great value in this type of issue.

The percentages of people who stopped smoking on World No-Tobacco Day vary between 36 and 54%, but an increasing trend of people who did not stop was seen in 1995 and 1996. These percentages indicate that we must work harder to increase the number of smokers who stop or after on the Day. The percentage of people who consider that the Day is not effective decreased from 68% in 1988 to 42% in 1996.

Discussion

It is clear that there is a close relationship between knowledge of the existence of World No-Tobacco Day and celebration of the most recent one. This is logical in view of the influence of the information media. The influence of the different media is not known, but it is evident that radio and television could be used more effectively. We are satisfied by the increase in exchange of information in workplaces and elsewhere, indicating greater individual and group communication on the problem. The ideal situation will be that in which workplaces and groups surpass the mass media. Despite the fact that the percentage of smokers who follow the recommendation of WHO has not exceeded 54%, it is satisfying to see that the percentage who remain non-smokers three months after 31 May was 24% in both 1995 and 1996.

Conclusions

Celebration of World No-Tobacco Day is a useful and important strategy for disseminating information about the health impairments due to tobacco in certain specific areas well covered by scientific knowledge. On this Day, smokers are asked to give up cigarettes for one day. This has resulted in complete cessation of smoking by an appreciable percentage of smokers. Promotion of celebration of World No-Tobacco Day makes it possible to test the whole anti-smoking movement of the country, with the participation of the Government and nongovernmental organizations. It can be used to monitor several information parameters, in addition to those used in the World Day, for evaluating the impact of the tobacco or health programme.

We recommend that World No-Tobacco Day, 31 May, be maintained and that specific work units be created for its celebration, with emphasis on human resources in the mass media. At least five months should be devoted to preparing the activities. Evaluation surveys should be carried out within the three months following 31 May in order to judge the results of the activity with respect to the stated objectives.

Viet Nam: Action plan on tobacco control, 1995–99

T.T. Thuy

Viet Nam Committee on Smoking and Health, Ministry of Health, Hanoi, Viet Nam

Challenges in tobacco control in Viet Nam

Tobacco production is considered favourably in Viet Nam as it creates jobs for farmers and workers. It also represents a large proportion of the State revenue, as 3–6% of the budget comes from taxes on tobacco. Cigarette manufacture is mainly (81%) under the control of local authorities, with only 19% under State control. Three multinational corporations also manufacture cigarettes in Viet Nam. Local and multinational production has increased dramatically in recent years, from 390 million packs in 1980 to about 1950 million packs in 1996.

The prevalence of smoking has increased concomitantly, due also in part to improved living standards. Thus, the number of cigarettes moked per person per year was 144 in 1980, 365 in 1993 and 518 in 1996. A survey showed that the overall prevalence of smoking in Viet Nam is 40–50%; that among men is 73%, that among women is 4% and that among young people is 8.7%. Male adults smoke 70–80 packs of cigarettes per year.

Viet Nam Committee on Smoking and Health

The steering committee for a national tobacco control programme was set up in May 1989. The Viet Nam Committee on Smoking and Health now consists of district organizations, city and provincial organizations in various sectors and the national Committee under the aegis of the Ministry of Health. The specific objectives of the Committee's plan of action for 1995–99 were to reduce the consumption of tobacco, to reduce the number of smokers, especially among the young and in the armed forces, and to reduce morbidity and mortality from diseases due to smoking.

In order to reduce the volume of tobacco consumption, both supply and consumption must be taken into account. Several measures have proved effective for reducing the supply. The first is to reduce the land area used for growing tobacco. The total area devoted to tobacco cultivation was 45 000 ha in 1985, which was to have been reduced by nearly half by 1995. A second effective measure is to increase taxes, including those on turnover, profits, raw materials and imported facilities for manufacturing cigarettes. Tobacco is considered to be liable to a special consumption tax; the rate varies from 32 to 70%, depending on the kind of tobacco. The third measure taken to reduce the supply is a ban on tobacco advertisements.

Further activities to control the supply need to be conducted more effectively. These include strictly forbidding the import of cigarettes, but smuggling of cigarettes is very hard to control especially across the 500-km border with Cambodia to the west. Collaboration between countries is needed, with national policies that are in accord. Other hindrances to control are that the volume of raw materials and equipment to produce cigarettes has not been decreased; the warnings printed on cigarette packs are still too small; funds for anti-smoking activities and health promotion have still not been made available from tobacco taxes; both cigarette manufacturers and tobacco traders still explicitly support and sponsor arts and sports events and the quality of cigarettes is still not controlled properly, for instance by stipulating the tar and nicotine content of cigarettes. What is needed is a national policy on tobacco control, with legal backing from the Government.

Three types of measure have proved to be effective in reducing the consumption of cigarettes: enacting legislation on tobacco use, providing information and education on tobacco and conducting surveys, collecting data and running quitting trials. For the first, a law on the protection of public health promulgated in 1989 bans smoking in meeting rooms, cinemas, theatres and other selected places. Smoking is also banned in health units. Information, education and communication for tobacco control has included a wide variety of activities:

- organizing meetings in response to the annual themes of World No-Tobacco Day;
- banning smoking in public places and on all public transport;
- campaigns aimed at women and children;
- promoting sports and arts without tobacco: 'Play it free';
- socializing anti-smoking activities in collaboration with other sectors and mass organizations;
- using pictures, posters, leaflets, books, newspapers and talks;
- encouraging Government employees, especially in the health sector and the armed forces, to quit tobacco;
- holding the first 'No-tobacco wedding', which was widely publicized;
- celebrating 'No-Tobacco Week', from May 24 to 31, in 1997;
- funding a competition in The Pioneers newspaper to study the harm done by tobacco.

The data collection has involved a preliminary hospital-based study to assess the correlation between smoking and respiratory and cardiovascular diseases and cancer; trials of use of nicotine patches for quitting and surveys in 34 health institutions show that nearly 4500 health workers have registered in programmes to give up smoking and nearly 3000 have succeeded.

The main weakness of activities to control consumption is that the ban on tobacco sales to children in not properly enforced.

Action plan for tobacco control in 1998–99

With regard to legislation, the objectives were to gain recognition that tobacco control is the Government's responsibility; to ban all forms of tobacco advertising; to prohibit cigarette manufacturers from sponsoring sports and arts, explicitly or implicitly; to increase the tax on tobacco and start an anti-tobacco fund; to set acceptable levels of tar and nicotine in cigarettes; to stipulate that warnings on cigarette packs should be large, visible and on both sides of the pack; and to forbid the sale of cigarettes to children under the age of 18. The objective with regard to communication was to integrate teaching of the hazards of tobacco use into the curriculum of secondary schools and pharmaco-medical training institutions.

It was intended to conduct surveys to collect data on the prevalence of smoking, including the numbers of smokers among women and children, on the manufacture and consumption of cigarettes and on the land area used for growing tobacco. Another objective was to conduct surveys to evaluate the effectiveness of implementation of policies, measures and activities for tobacco control and to define the correlation between smoking and respiratory and cardiovascular diseases and cancer.

Conclusion

The tobacco control programme in Viet Nam has included dynamic activities to achieve comprehensive positive results. One constraint is that a national policy on tobacco control does not yet exist, since the tobacco industry is an important source of revenue for the Government. Achieving the objectives of the programme would, however, enhance and protect the health of the community.

Yugoslavia: Smoking prevention and control, with special reference to the Novi Sad MONICA project

B. Legetic[1], M. Planojevic[2] & D. Jakovljevic[2]

[1]Institute of Public Health and [2]MONICA WHO Collaborative Centre, Novi Sad, Yugoslavia

Investigations performed in Yugoslavia and routine statistical data led to the establishment of strategies within the MONICA programme to monitor trends in ischaemic heart disease. Emphasis has been placed on smoking as one of the leading risk factors, since the prevalence is high among the adult population of Novi Sad, with increasing trends among women and young people: a federal commission for control of addictive diseases estimated prevalences of 45% among males and 25–30% among females.

Tobacco growing, tobacco products and consumption in Yugoslavia

According to the Food and Agricultural Organization of the United Nations (FAO), 88 000 tonnes of raw tobacco, or 78 000 tonnes of dry tobacco, were produced in Yugoslavia in 1990. A 1.9% annual increase was predicted up to 1995 and a 1.7%

increase between 1995 and 2000. Yugoslavia is one of a few European countries in which tobacco production is increasing.

Consumption of dried tobacco is also increasing. About 50 000 tonnes were consumed in 1990, and a 1.7% annual rise is expected up to 2000. About 2.5 kg are used annually per person. Yugoslavia exports about 33 000 tonnes each year, with a 1.7% increase up to 2000. About 10 000 tonnes are imported, with no planned increase. Yugoslavia still exports more dried tobacco than tobacco products.

The measures undertaken to control smoking are limited to restrictions on advertising, prohibition of smoking in closed areas and increased prices. These measures do not seem to have affected production or distribution of these products.

Distribution of smoking habits in Novi Sad

Novi Sad is the capital of Vojvodina Province, covering 753 km², with 553 027 inhabitants in 1991 and an average population density of 378 per km². The smoking habits of a representative sample of 1600 adults in Novi Sad aged 25–64 were surveyed in 1984 and 1995, with the questionnaire on smoking from the MONICA project. The 1984 survey showed a prevalence of 42%, with 52% among men and 32% among women. Former smokers accounted for 20% of the men and 5.8% of the women. Most of the smokers were aged 25–44, and the numbers of smokers of each sex decreased with age. On average, the smokers smoked 20 cigarettes per day, with a mean of 23 for men and 14.9 for women. The number of smokers increased with the amount of education up to university level, where a 25% decrease was seen. A desire to stop smoking was expressed by 82% of women and 77% of men; 63% sought help when they were trying to stop smoking, which is important information for smoking cessation programmes.

Men were better informed than women about the risks associated with smoking, and our results showed that persons over 35 paid more attention to their health. More than half of both smokers and non-smokers were aware of the harmful effects of smoking, indicating that changes are needed in attitude and behaviour.

The study in 1995 also showed a total smoking prevalence of 42%, but a decrease was seen in the rate among men in the youngest age group: 70% in 1984 and 61% in 1995.

Smoking among children and adolescents in Novi Sad

A study of behavioural risk factors among 3141 children and adolescents aged 9–18 in 1984 showed that the number of smokers increased with age and that about 40% of those aged 18 smoked. About 28% of the youg people said that they had started smoking at the age of 12, and 57% of current smokers said they thought they would be non-smokers within five years.

In 1995, 3649 schoolchildren aged 9–18 participated in an identical study. The proportion of daily smokers (10.4%) was not significantly different from that in the previous study, but the proportion of temporary smokers had fallen significantly to 4.5%. In this study, the children had taken up smoking significantly later, at an average age of 16, and 86% of those who smoked said that they would be non-smokers within five years.

Smoking among physicians in Novi Sad

A survey was performed in 1993–94 to determine the attitudes and behaviour of physicians towards smoking. Of the 937 physicians (52% male), 43% were smokers. They agreed with socially and scientifically acknowledged issues in smoking but were not ready to take concrete measures to control the habit in the population.

Mortality due to cigarette smoking in Novi Sad

Estimates of mortality from tobacco-related causes have been published for several European countries (Masironi & Rothwell, 1988). A total of 504 935 deaths from smoking were observed in Europe in 1994, with 343 469 in males and 161 469 in females. In Yugoslavia in 1992, there were 12 835 deaths due to smoking, with 9103 in males and 3732 in females. The prevalences of smoking estimated in this study, however, account for 57% of males and 10% of females. In comparison with other countries, the proportion of smokers is very high among males and very low among females. According to this estimate, 1900 people in Vojvodina die each year from cigarette smoking, comprising 1400 males and 500 females. In Novi Sad, there were 210 deaths per year due to cigarette smoking, with 160 in males and 56 in females.

Smoking control activities

Measures taken for the control and cessation of smoking at the national level are limited to a ban on advertising of tobacco products and on smoking indoors. It is planned to extend the law to ban the sale of cigarettes to minors, sale of cigarettes only in special shops and inclusion of warnings on cigarette packs. Since 1991, TV Belgrade together with the Federal commission for control of addictive diseases has been broadcasting spots on the medical, economic, social and biochemical effects of tobacco.

At a local level in Novi Sad, a video programme entitled 'Smoke in your face' is included in a health promotion programme in pre-school institutions, which reaches about 7000 children aged 6–7. In the school health programme organized in collaboration with the Red Cross, children aged 7–11 are introduced to the harmful effects of smoking by peer leaders. In a health promotion programme, schoolchildren in higher grades discuss the undesirable features of today, such as smoking, alcoholism and drugs, and learn how to resist the social pressure to start smoking. Physicians, biology teachers and psychologists at the school are involved. In high schools, three panel discussions and an exhibition on 'Smoking or health' are organized. The 1995 exhibition was shown in 30 places and was visited by about 20 000 persons. Future health educators, medical students in their final year and students at the teachers' training college and in physical education attend a seminar on smoking and health, where they are trained for future programmes to fight against smoking.

Outside of school, drawing and writing competitions are held for children and adolescents on the topic 'Smoking or health'. Health personnel in health and other organizations are engaged in both primary and secondary prevention of smoking. The causative role of smoking is cited on radio and television and in newspapers and specialized magazines for children and adults. The mass media support the international No-Tobacco Day.

In 1978, a guidance clinic was set up in Novi Sad to help smokers give up smoking, with a five-day plan. The basic idea of the plan is to change people's behaviour using the principle of group dynamics. The clinic has been attended by 2420 people so far. The success rate was 92% after five days and 60% after three months. Men have shown more interest than women. About 80% of the attendees are middle-aged with a long-standing smoking habit. The involvement of persons with a high level of education is very high.

Conclusions

The results of the programme are encouraging, but there is still room for action, both at in legislation and in the policy of distribution of tobacco products. More precise epidemiological data are needed at the national level and a national programme for the prevention and control of smoking should be established.

References

Food and Agricultural Organization of the United Nations. *Economic and Social Development Paper No. 92*, Rome

Masironi, R. & Rothwell, K. (1988) Tendencies and effects of tobacco smoking in the world. *World Health Stat. Q.*, 4, 228–241

Tobacco control networks in Latin America, sub-Saharan Africa and communities of colour in the United States

R.G. Robinson

Associate Director for Program Development, Office on Smoking and Health, Centers for Disease Control and Prevention, Atlanta, Georgia, United States

It is an axiom of the tobacco control movement that a substantive infrastructure is critical to enable regions, nations and communities to counteract the tobacco industry and to institute credible programmes and policies to ensure public health. A review of efforts in Latin America, sub-Saharan Africa and the United States to develop strong regional or national tobacco control infrastructures can be useful, particularly because those lessons have direct relevance to developing countries and regions worldwide. Although Asia is not a focus of this paper, the contexts are similar, as these are the regions and the people of the world that the tobacco industry is targeting in their efforts to counteract the progress being made in tobacco control in developed regions. In essence, the basic contradiction between developed and developing continues on both sides of the tobacco equation: the successful efforts of the tobacco industry to gain customers, win friends and influence people in developing regions or communities and the striking inability of global and national tobacco control movements to reflect and implement similar priorities.

Critical assumptions

Why is this focus so important? It is necessary to understand the basic assumptions behind this analysis. First, the globalization of tobacco control mandates the globalization of capacity and infrastructure and the resulting ability to implement tobacco control initiatives effectively. Tobacco control can only be as strong as its weakest link. Secondly, the historical experience of developing countries parallels the inequitable development of communities of colour in the United States. Latin America and Africa have lagged behind the world in the same way that African Americans, Hispanics, Asians, Pacific Islanders and American Indians have lagged behind white communities in the United States. The reasons are similar for each and reflect the level of resource allocation to these respective movements. Finally, failure of the tobacco control movement to resolve these inequities at the global and national levels will result in victories for the tobacco industry; and victories for the industry mean disease and death for the most vulnerable, for lack of the resources needed to defend themselves. Resources reflect not only money for programmes and materials but representation at the tables where decisions about research, policy and strategies are being made.

Core problems

Communities of colour in the United States and peoples of Latin America and sub-Saharan Africa are substantially similar with respect to core problem areas (Robinson et al., 1992a,b, 1995). First, there is the lack of research capacity for tobacco control. The reasons are obviously complex, but they have to do with the limited resources targeted to these regions or communities. For example, in the United States, targeting communities of colour has been a priority only since 1985, and then it was several years before researchers representing African American, Hispanic, Asian or American Indian communities received serious support. It is always a struggle to ensure that these communities have priority. Indeed, it is almost as great a struggle as it is to combat the targeting efforts of the tobacco industry.

Other problems are lack of human resources, lack of financial resources for programmes, materials and communications, and lack of priority within the respective communities and regions because of the many other health and social and economic problems that must be confronted. It is very difficult to get tobacco control to the top of their agenda. So we have 'negative synergy'. The tobacco control movement has not traditionally given priority to these regions or communities, and these regions and communities have not given priority to tobacco control

Finally, there is the problem of the absence of coordination of research, programmes and resources. We have learnt how important it is to have a coordinated information network if tobacco control coalitions within communities are to battle the tobacco industry effectively (Robinson & Sutton, 1994; Department of Health and Human Services, 1995). The inability to coordinate remains a critical problem.

Latin America

What is the history of Latin America in developing a regional network for tobacco control? The American Cancer Society played a very important role, providing resources to Latin American representatives to found the Latin American Coordinating Committee for Tobacco Control (CLACCTA). This Committee had annual meetings, produced a bulletin and received support from the International Union against Cancer (UICC). In 1993, the Office on Smoking and Health at the Centers for Disease Control and Prevention (CDC) in the United States became involved, as the American Cancer Society was reorganizing and could no longer promise the support that it had provided. Matters were very critical and a new vision had to be created. Several strategic planning meetings were held, and new, critical partnerships emerge. The American Cancer Society, the CDC, the National Cancer Institute, and the Pan American Health Organization (PAHO) developed a plan with CLACCTA for the creation and implementation of a tobacco control secretariat for Latin America. This secretariat is managed by PAHO and is located in Caracas, Venezuela. Health Canada joined the original planning committee, and each partner provides finances each year for core support of this initiative.

The programme activities include building and strengthening national coalitions, ongoing communication and strategic planning, developing regional research initiatives such as the analysis of legislation that might receive support from the International Development Research Council (IDRC), fund-raising to expand the secretariat to other regions of Latin America and the development of a World Health Organization (WHO) Tobacco Control Collaborating Centre. Brazil has achieved Collaborating Centre status.

Sub-Saharan Africa

What is the history of sub-Saharan Africa in developing a regional network for tobacco control? The groundwork was laid during the late 1970s and early 1980s (personal communication, P. Wangai, 1997). The first tobacco control events were crystallized by the UICC in East Africa in 1977. In 1981, the largest conference on tobacco in Africa took place in Nairobi, out of which emerged the first comprehensive coalition of East African countries. Dr Paul Wangai was chosen as the first Deputy-Chairman for the UICC-led tobacco control programme for East Africa. Subsequent conferences were held in 1985 in Arusha, United Republic of Tanzania, and in 1988 in Jinja, Uganda. At the 1992 world conference on Tobacco or Health in Argentina, a small group of Africans came together to discuss regional issues at a meeting led by colleagues from Europe and Australia in collaboration with leadership from South Africa. Support was received from the CDC, in collaboration with WHO to sponsor the first all-African conference on tobacco control, which took place in Zimbabwe in 1994. Small meetings were held in Ghana and South Africa, with continued support from the CDC. At the following world conference in Paris, this initiative reached a new phase of development with the creation of the Tobacco Control Commission for Africa (TCCA). Derek Yach from the Republic of South Africa was the first President. A second major meeting was held in South Africa in 1996, at which time Dr Wali Muna from Cameroon was appointed President. The TCCA board is representative of both French- and English-speaking Africa.

Meetings and strategic planning have been ongoing. Efforts are being made to develop proposals for additional funding. The Council Against Smoking in South Africa has been proposed as a WHO Tobacco Control Collaborating Centre, which is viewed as critical because sub-Saharan Africa is the only area without a collaborating centre. If collaborating centres are to have a meaningful role in strategic planning for global tobacco control, it is critical for all regions of the world to be represented. The importance of this objective was made clear at a meeting of collaborating centres sponsored by the CDC in Atlanta in 1996. The TCCA met in Cameroon in July 1997 to develop a strategic action plan for the region. The emerging partnership of the TCCA, CDC, WHO and the IDRC was strengthened at this meeting. The meeting in China found the TCCA at an important juncture in its development.

The programme activities include development of the core infrastructure for the TCCA, developing a partnership with the African Regional Office of WHO, communication and strategic planning, approval and implementation of the strategic action plan, fund-raising with prospective core support from CDC and programme support for research initiatives from the IDRC, and development of a WHO Tobacco Control Collaborating Centre.

Communities of colour in the United States

What is the history of communities of colour in the United States in developing a national network for tobacco control? Perhaps the first community-based activity occurred in Detroit, Michigan, in a general protest against use of billboards for tobacco and alcohol advertising in the African American community. In 1985, the National Cancer Institute began the first major research effort to develop specifically targeted initiatives for communities of colour. The turning-point in developing infrastructure beyond research came in 1990 with the success of the African American community in Philadelphia in defeating the marketing of Uptown cigarettes, which had been developed by R.J. Reynolds specifically for the black community. Protest and advocacy culminated in the success of the Uptown coalition. In 1993, CDC launched a capacity-building initiative targeting African Americans, Hispanics, Asians and American Indians; youth, women and tobacco farmers were also included in this initiative, which was the first to address the absence of diversity within the United States tobacco control movement. Diversity and inclusion have remained a problem in the United States and continue during the tobacco industry settlement talks.

The programme activities include the development of targeted initiatives for each of the communities, advocacy for inclusion of people of colour in each of the national programmes supported by the National Cancer Institute, the American Cancer Society, the American Lung Association, CDC and the Robert Wood Johnson Foundation. These efforts have met with limited success. African American organizations have led the planning of World No-Tobacco Day in the United States for the past several years. Hispanic, Asian and American Indian organizations have launched research, programmes and advocacy initiatives within their respective communities. There are ongoing national meetings and strategic planning, and, of course, advocacy for inclusion is ongoing, perpetual and surprisingly difficult because of the absence of principled support from mainstream tobacco control advocates in the United States.

In the 1960s and 1970s, white Americans joined hands with their black, brown, yellow and red brothers and sisters in the struggle for freedom and social justice. Mainstream tobacco control advocates seem to be disconnected from this history or are unwilling to make the same sacrifices. It is critical that WHO understand the implication of this retreat for the world.

Lessons for tobacco control

What are the lessons learnt from the development of these regional and national tobacco control infrastructures?

- Interestingly, the issue of inclusivity and targeting is a principle, not a problem, for the tobacco industry.
- Capacity building and infrastructure must be viewed as priority areas for these regions and communities by national and global tobacco control movements.

- The global and United States-based tobacco control movements must struggle with racism, paternalism and elitism in the effort to allow these regions and communities to have their own voice and their own capacity in tobacco control.
- Globalization of tobacco control requires that all regions and all faces be represented at decision-making and planning meetings.
- The absence of inclusivity and diversity must be regarded as the absence of principle. If the tobacco control movement moves forward in an unprincipled manner, it will pave the way for the success, not of tobacco control, but of the tobacco industry.

Conclusions

What are the underlying determinants of these problems, demanding an explication of lessons? It is important to recognize that in the determinants of social movements all truths are partial. Complexity demands an appreciation of partialness and the need to avoid simplistic stereotyping. Once these limitations are recognized, it is possible to venture forward. In the United States, which has a specific relationship to communities of colour, how can the mainstream tobacco control movement exclude their meaningful participation in decision-making and resource allocation? Racism is a factor and results in the perception that communities of colour have little to contribute. Paternalism is a factor and results in the perception that communities of colour have little to contribute. Elitism is a factor and results in the perception that organizations representing communities of colour do not have enough resources or experience to warrant a seat at the table. There are so few seats that to 'give up' some of them to achieve diversity does not have social value.

There is also a paucity of theory to justify the conclusions and related actions of the scientists and leaders in mainstream tobacco control. For example, there is reliance on what I refer to as the 'epidemiological fallacy', which has three underlying components that can be illustrated by African Americans in the United States. The first component is methodological. If data on race and social status or education are factored into statistical analyses with the result that the contribution of race disappears when controlling for social status or education, the conclusion is that race is no longer important. This analysis is one-dimensional or reductionist in that race is reduced to economic status. While it is true that, because of the history and social context of African Americans, low social status or lower levels of education correlate highly with race, an analysis that concludes that race is therefore insignificant is deficient because it ignores the fact that the majority of those who are of low status or low education remain African American. They continue to reside in African American communities. The fact of their race has not disappeared and neither has the necessity to formulate policies and programmes that are sensitive to race and the African American community.

The second component is the notion that prevalence is the sole determinant of priorities for programme development and related resource allocation. Thus, communities of colour or regions of the world that have lower prevalence do not require the same degree of attention. There are ironies and contradictions in this formula especially in view of the high level of attention given to white communities in the United States, despite the fact that they have been only third in terms of smoking prevalence for decades. Nevertheless, the numbers game is a factor in justifying policies related to communities of colour, either because of where they stand in relation to prevalence or because of their absolute numbers in the population. This is not a formula that results in equity.

Finally, there is the component of the epidemiological fallacy that confuses the difference between prevention and control. If the dominant method encourages a focus on high-risk segments of the population, the tendency is to ignore the critical relationship between efforts to bring about environmental change and the consciousness of whole communities, not just those who are poor or disadvantaged. Prevention strategies require a relationship with a community and its leaders, whereas control strategies are more limited and may require, for example, only the elimination of financial barriers. It is best to consider control strategies as targeting specific high-risk strata in a community and prevention strategies as targeting the whole community. Thus, an analysis of low-income or low-education segments is relevant in the context of assessing control. The dominant method (i.e. discounting the importance of race) benefits control initiatives. It is ironic that nineteenth century race theory justified the subjugation of particular races and regions of the world on the basis of assumptions of inferiority, and that this has been replaced with epidemiological methods or 'theory' that justify their exclusion on the basis of assumptions of non-parity.

Issues related to racism, paternalism, elitism and the epidemiological fallacy are relevant to our understanding of the evolution of tobacco control infrastructures in Latin America and sub-Saharan Africa. In addition, there is an absence of theory supporting social change at the global level. For example, we have not altered the exploitation of the world's resources by the rich. We have not changed the growth of inequality or its relationship to differences in health status. We have not explained how to defeat a multinational corporation without the involvement of all nations, all regions and all peoples. These factors require a paradigm of inclusiveness and policies and resource allocation that support the inclusion of all communities and regions in the worldwide struggle to defeat exploitation by the tobacco industry.

References
Department of Health and Human Services (1995) *Community-based Interventions for Smokers: The COMMIT Field Experience* (Smoking and Tobacco Control Monograph, No. 6), Rockville, Maryland
Robinson, R.G. & Sutton, C. (1994) The coalition against Uptown cigarettes. In: Jernigan, D. & Wright, P.A., eds, *Making News, Changing Policy: Case Studies of Media Advocacy on Alcohol and Tobacco Issues*, University Research Corporation and The Marin Institute for the Prevention of Alcohol and Other Drug Problems, Center for Substance Abuse Prevention
Robinson, R.G., *et al.* (1992a) Report of the Tobacco Policy Research Group on marketing and promotions targeted at African Americans, Latinos, and women. *Tobacco Control Int. J.*, 1(Suppl.), 24–30
Robinson, R.G., Pertschuk, M. & Sutton C. (1992b) Smoking and African Americans: Spotlighting the effects of smoking and tobacco promotion in the African American community. In: Samuels, S.E. & Smith, M.D., eds, *Improving the Health of the Poor*, Menlo Park, California: The Henry J. Kaiser Family Foundation

Local

The Khush Dil Stop Smoking Initiative: A project to raise awareness and reduce smoking in a predominantly Asian community in Birmingham, England

C. Farren

Bristol, United Kingdom

The Khush Dil Stop Smoking Initiative was a pilot initiative which ran for nine months in 1996–97 within the community-based Khush Dil Happy Heart Project. The project targeted the Saltley and Small Heath areas of East Birmingham in a predominantly Asian community with high rates of heart disease.

Smoking is a risk factor associated with heart disease, and national (Rudat, 1994) and local research has shown very high rates of smoking among Asian men in the United Kingdom: almost half of Bangladeshi men and almost 40% of Pakistani men are smokers. These are the main minority groups in the Saltley and Small Heath areas. The national research indicates that many Asian smokers say they would like to give up, but very few have tried or succeeded; the numbers of ex-smokers are very low. This situation is similar to that of the general population of smokers in the United Kingdom about 15–20 years ago. It indicates that information about smoking and the damage it causes must be given to these groups and appropriate motivation and support to quit provided.

Very few women in the Bangladeshi and Pakistani communities smoke cigarettes, although some smoke hookah pipes and many Bangladeshi women chew *paan*, a chewing mixture which can and often does contain tobacco. The tobacco in *paan* can cause oral cancer and absorption of nicotine in high concentrations. As women are also in a position to protect children from passive smoking, it was decided to target both women and men with information about the damage caused by passive smoking.

The first principle used in project was the 'cycle of change' (Prochaska *et al.*, 1994), a model for helping smokers to stop smoking in which smokers are categorized by their stage in a process that all smokers must move along to stop smoking and remain non-smokers. Most Bangladeshi and Pakistani smokers are 'contented' smokers or 'contemplators'. A small minority are ready to stop, and those who do usually relapse. We needed to raise awareness about the health hazards and encourage people to want to stop, and prevention of relapse had be increased. The strategies for the project were taken from the findings of a study of the most cost-effective strategies for reducing smoking (Reid *et al.*, 1992). These include opportunistic advice from health professionals and using unpaid and paid publicity. We adapted the results for a minority ethnic community.

Many of the ideas for action came from a paper presented at a symposium on cancer in minority ethnic groups (Farren & Naidoo, 1996), which outlined smoking prevention projects targeting ethnic minority groups in thecommunity, the workplace and primary health care settings and quoted many existing examples of projects in the United Kingdom and the United States.

Aims of the Khush Dil Stop Smoking Initiative

The main aim was to raise awareness about the damage to health caused by tobacco in order to reduce and prevent smoking in the Bangladeshi community and other Asian populations of Saltley and Small Heath in East Birmingham. By the end of the project, the Khush Dil team will have achieved the following:
* increased awareness of the dangers of smoking and the benefits of quitting;
* informed the community of the harm to children and unborn babies of passive smoking;
* distributed Ramadan stop-smoking calendars to at least 1000 families;
* run a 'Stop smoking in Ramadan and stay stopped for good' campaign in the mosque;

- persuaded 10% of restaurant managers to introduce smoking sections;
- increased the amount of advice given out by members of the primary health care team in the area and achieved a 5% reduction in smoking;
- increased information about smoking and advice on giving up, particularly the use of nicotine replacement therapy from pharmacists to the community;
- promoted a 'dentists against smoking' information campaign;
- attracted at least five media stories about the Khush Dil smoking campaign;
- increased the numbers of calls to the ethnic language quitline and
- presented the findings to relevant health and community projects in the United Kingdom.

Achievements

Health professionals—general practitioners, health visitors, practice nurses, dentists and pharmacists—were approached informally and offered personalized advice and support. While waiting to see the doctor, dentist or pharmacist, we talked to practice nurses, assistants and receptionists. A pack of leaflets and charts and a resource pack were given at every visit. We visited 14 surgeries and health centres, had one-to-one meetings with eight general practitioners and four practice nurses and liaised with their reception staff. We visited and had informal talks on several occasions with eight pharmacists and their staff. We conducted a lunchtime meeting with all the nursing staff of three health centres. We visited two dental practices and gave a talk to the dental nurses. We talked to over 80 general practice registrars for the Birmingham area and conducted informal training at the advice centres for participating general practitioners, and we ran two stop-smoking advice stalls in the waiting areas of two health centres.

At our community-based stop-smoking advice centres, a range of initiatives was tried and repeated when they proved successful. Sessions were advertised on the radio and on posters displayed in shops, community centres and health centres. Invitations were sent to Bangladeshi families. Five sessions were held at the Bangladesh Welfare Association. At each session, 4–10 smokers asked for help and advice, and two reported giving up smoking, though both later relapsed. Registrars from the Birmingham area volunteered to attend the stop-smoking advice days, and many of those attending came because the attendance of a doctor was advertised.

Four stalls were run in the lobby of a community and sports centre. Stop-smoking advice, information and carbon monoxide testing were offered, and a registrar attended once to give medical advice. At each session, we saw 30–50 people, who were mainly smokers but also people wanting advice on passive smoking or smoking by students. We saw mainly young people and the staff of the centre. Some came back each week to check their carbon monoxide levels, and some admitted to trying to stop smoking, but without success.

For No-Smoking Day 1997, the Khush Dil Stop-smoking Initiative set up a caravan to run a stop-smoking advice and information stall in a car park on the corner of two main roads. We ran competitions, with prizes of pens, balloons and T-shirts, and advice stalls with the carbon monoxide monitor. We had smoke-free face-painting for small children and a puppet show 'How the Marlboro Cowboy quit smoking'. In total, about 35 adults and 50 children visited the stall. These included 10–12 smokers.

We decided to start home visits, as the numbers of Bangladeshis reached via the talks and the advice centres were small. The visits involved a general talk about health and smoking, including passive smoking and chewing tobacco. Smokers were invited to attend the centres. Leaflets in English and Bengali about smoking cessation and passive smoking were given to the families. About 15 home visits were carried out; at 12, there were smokers in the family, and all of the women used oral chewing tobacco in the form of *paan*. Two men said they would try to give up smoking, and one visited the advice stalls and attempted to quit but did not succeed in the longer term.

We raised awareness about the dangers of smoking by giving talks during training and English-language courses for adults. Talks were given to over 65 people, mainly

Asian, in five community education and employment training centres. Some were smokers, but all had smokers in the family and took leaflets home.

Posters and leaflets with information about the stop-smoking initiative and ethnic quitlines were distributed in person to local shops and businesses. Most agreed to display materials and were supportive of the project. Restaurants were offered no-smoking signs, but none accepted, saying there was no demand.

Most of the target group were Muslims, and Islam considers smoking to be harmful to the body and should therefore be discouraged. Attractive, full colour, stop-smoking Ramadan calendars were printed and distributed via religious and community outlets. The calendars gave the fasting timetable and carried a message to persuade smokers to use Ramadan to give up smoking for good. The quitline numbers were given for Bengali, English, Punjabi and Urdu speakers. A total of 2000 Ramadan calendars were distributed via shops, general practitioners' surgeries, pharmacists, Halal butchers, secondary schools and community centres. About 3000 posters were distributed at local Mosques.

A pilot stop-smoking advice stall was held in the community centre opposite the mosque on a Friday afternoon after the Juma prayers, with permission from the mosque leaders. We handed out about 220 invitations and asked that an announcement be made inside the mosque. We provided refreshments. About 25 men turned up. Some came to argue the case for smoking, but five wanted help to stop smoking; two or three ex-smokers wanted reinforcement and encouragement to remain ex smokers.

Four press releases were sent out, which attracted some publicity. A media plan was built into the original strategy document. The coverage achieved consisted of a story about the Khush Dil Stop-smoking Initiative in *Janomot* (Bengali newspaper), a 12-min radio interview about the Ramadan project (BBC Asian network), a photo story and articles about the Smoke-free Asian Cricket team, with a photo call at a cricket practice for the junior and senior team of a winning Asian cricket club (Pakistani English language newspaper, Birmingham free newspaper) and a 5-min interview on the morning news for No-Smoking Day (BBC Asian network). The stop-smoking advice stalls were mentioned three times on the BBC Asian network programme in a 'What's on' slot.

The Khush Dil Stop-smoking Initiative has been described at two presentations at the Health Education Authority's Black and Minority Ethnic Groups Smoking Prevention Forum of health workers, a national meeting of dental health educators, who asked for a presentation on reducing smoking among minority ethnic groups, and a poster presentation about the initiative presented at the Tenth World Conference on Tobacco and Health.

Why was the stop-smoking initiative successful?

The Khush Dil Stop-smoking Initiative achieved most of the objectives set; some were achieved in part, and some went beyond the expected outcomes. Long-term success in helping smokers to stop requires further research.

The skills, knowledge, language and cultural mix of the team enabled the initiative to work effectively. We had two Urdu speakers, one Bengali speaker and an experienced smoking prevention consultant, and three were Muslims. A range of ages was represented, but the only man on the team was a part-time volunteer.

It was a combined community approach and medical model. The Khush Dil project addressed heart disease in a community setting. It used community approaches as well as strategies to encourage health-care teams, pharmacists and dentists to increase and improve opportunistic stop smoking advice and information.

Most Bangladeshi and Pakistani families are practising Muslims. Smokers could thus be reached through the mosques and in the Ramadan calendars, stop-smoking sessions in mosques and support from Muslim leaders.

The initiative had messages for everyone. Help in stopping smoking was a priority, but the risks of passive smoking and chewing *paan* were also addressed.

Research on health and lifestyle provided the background and rationale for running the initiative. The 'cycle of change' provided a model for helping smokers to stop smoking. Papers on cost-effective strategies provided a range of strategies and ideas.

The Khush Dil Project had a high profile in the community, as it had been in operation there for several years and had won a Department of Health Healthy Alliances Award. We also attracted publicity in the local Birmingham media and in the national and local ethnic media including radio.

As part of the North Birmingham Community National Health Service Trust Health Promotion Service, the initiative could use their resources. These included graphic designers and other staff. It also made it easier to approach and involve the registrars in general practice and other community health workers.

The Khush Dil Project had made contact with most community networks in the two areas, including health networks, community education networks, cultural and religious networks and employment and voluntary agencies. Everyone we met and talked to referred us to other relevant contacts and groups.

The support of the smoke-free cricket team provided positive role models to promote a smoke-free message.

Some smokers were defensive about attempts to challenge their behaviour, but the Stop-smoking Initiative was supported by most of the community. It was hard to find sustained enthusiastic support for the initiative, but it was not dismissed as irrelevant. Some key individuals and organizations gave wholehearted support and this was crucial in making progress.

The initiative produced a few simple translated posters and handouts, but various resources and materials were already available, including a set of leaflets on stopping smoking and passive smoking in most Asian languages, as well as a range of smoking education leaflets in English; a resource pack from the Smoking Prevention for Minority Ethnic Groups, with six smoking-related information sheets in English and six Asian languages; flow charts based on the 'cycle of change' model and other guidance sheets for professionals; the Ramadan calendar with stop-smoking information, produced by Smoke-free Birmingham, which we overprinted with Khush Dil information and the logo; a minority ethnic language quitline in Bengali, Punjabi and Urdu, for one session a week; visual aids, such as the carbon monoxide monitor and an anatomical model for illustrating the effects of smoking on the body and a video in Bengali with advice on stopping smoking.

The initiative ran for only nine months on a part-time basis. The project had to be focused and well planned, with defined priorities. Not everything got done, but the momentum kept up the energy levels.

References
Farren, C. & Naidoo, J. (1996) Smoking cessation programmes targeting black and minority ethnic communities. *Br. J. Cancer*, **74**
Prochaska, J., Norcross, J. & DiClemente, C. (1994) *Changing for Good*, New York, William Morrow & Co.
Reid, D., Killoran, A., McNeill, A. & Chambers, J. (1992) Choosing the most effective health promotion options for reducing a nation's smoking prevalence. *Tobacco Control*, 1, 185–197
Rudat, K. (1994) *Black and Minority Ethnic Groups in England*, London, Health Education Authority

Development of an anti-smoking policy in Novosibirsk, Russian Federation

N.V. Alexeeva, A.L. Molokov, S.K. Malyutina, O.L. Alexeev & T.A. Kovalenko

Institute of Internal Medicine, Novosibirsk, Russian Federation

The prevalence of smoking in Siberia is very high. Within the World Health Organization (WHO) MONICA project, we have conducted three population surveys in Novosibirsk, one in 1984–85, the second in 1988–89 and the third in 1995–96. The prevalence of smoking was 59% in men and 3% in women in the first survey, 56% in men and 4.4% in women in the second and 59% in men and 10% in women in the third. The number of smokers among children is growing steadily, and they are starting to smoke earlier (9–10 years of age). Tobacco advertising is widespread, and cheap cigarettes of bad quality are readily available. The legislation regulating the advertising and promotion of tobacco products is imperfect, and the existing legislation is not strictly respected by the local administration. Financial support for anti-smoking activities is poor, although medical staff and social workers in Novosibirsk are trying to make anti-smoking activity more effective.

Anti-smoking activity in Novosibirsk is headed and coordinated by the Institute of Internal Medicine within the framework of the WHO programme for the prevention of non-communicable diseases. As smoking is not only a medical but also a social problem, we have concentrated our activity on anti-smoking policy development. Our priorities are for the adoption of a common anti-smoking law in our region, prohibition of tobacco advertising in the mass media and strict control over the sale of tobacco products to children. Only strict legislative measures and joint efforts will stop the expansion of American and European cigarette companies to Russia, which has increased inordinately over the last few years.

The main components of our activity are working with the local administration and with the population, involving the mass media in anti-smoking activities, conducting epidemiological studies and participating regularly in the international 'Quit and win' campaign, organized by WHO every two years. In this campaign in Novosibirsk, the total numbers of participants were 1261 in 1994 and 455 in 1996, of whom 69 and 92% stopped smoking for a month during the campaign and 38 and 60% in the two years, respectively, stopped smoking completely. A one-year follow-up in 1997 with a 60% response showed that the effectiveness of this method was 36%. In the 1998 campaign, there were three times more participants than in 1996, and the Mayor of Novosibirsk and the Governor of the region were among them. The Mayor subsequently quit smoking.

Combining political activity and practical measures, we published (with methodological and financial assistance from Health and Welfare, Canada) 25 000 copies of a leaflet giving practical guidelines for the population on how to stop smoking and distributed them through polyclinics, hospitals, shops and pharmacies; we also produced and distributed anti-smoking stickers. We try to create and support people's desire to change their lifestyle positively and try to create a supportive environment to make health changes easier, working with the regional social rehabilitation centre. Our anti-smoking activity among children has increased, with a special anti-smoking programme for schoolchildren and students, as well as a programme for kindergartens. Several seminars for teachers were conducted in schools. A children's drawing competition on fresh air was arranged on World No-smoking Day in 1997. Children also wrote a composition on 'Why I want my friend to stop smoking' on that day. Two booklets have been published: *Modern Social and Medical Problems of Smoking* and *Nicotine and Descendants*. We are now trying to include anti-smoking programmes in the obligatory educational curriculum at schools and institutes.

Conclusion

People are becoming more interested in having a healthy lifestyle. Those most active in trying to stop smoking are men aged 25–44 years of age. The population of our area is showing a good response to anti-smoking propaganda and other preventive programmes. Since people need support in their attempts to stop smoking, we hope to establish a special anti-smoking medical centre with highly skilled, specially trained staff in our city. Smoking prevention among schoolchildren and students should be more active and regular.

Lessons from nine years of a quit campaign

L. Roberts[1] & M. Wakefield[2]

[1] South Australian Smoking and Health Project and [2] South Australian Health Commission, Adelaide, South Australia

The South Australian Smoking and Health Project is an initiative of the Anti-Cancer Foundation and the National Heart Foundation, which are two non-governmental organizations in South Australia. The Project is funded by Living Health, which is a health promotion foundation set up by the Government in 1989 as part of legislation to replace tobacco sponsorship and to fund health promotion programmes, especially those designed to reduce the prevalence of smoking. With a population of 1.5 million people in South Australia, the Project's annual funding of US$ 468 000 per year equates to US$ 0.31 per head of population.

The objectives of the Project were to reduce the population prevalence of smoking by encouraging existing smokers to quit and maintain cessation, and to prevent uptake of smoking among children and adolescents. Another objective was to protect the public from exposure to environmental tobacco smoke.

We used a range of strategies to meet these objectives. The most visible part of the programme was a three-week mass media campaign in September of each year, in which television, radio and press advertising were backed up by community-based activities. Over the years, the campaign themes included cessation, prevention and protection from environmental tobacco smoke. We established a telephone 'Quitline', to enable smokers to ring for advice and gain access to resources for stopping smoking, and this service was also available to non-smokers who rang with enquiries about passive smoking. We distributed a range of resources through doctors and pharmacists. We also established a school smoking prevention programme and provided assistance in workplaces and other public places where there was a wish to be smoke-free.

From the beginning, we set up a system to monitor the prevalence of smoking and other indicators of changes in smoking-related knowledge, attitudes and practices in the adult population. To achieve this, we performed an annual survey of a representative population, which also provided us with information about campaign recall and recognition. The sample size of the survey was large enough to allow us to describe and monitor changes in population subgroups. Every three years, we also took part in a national survey of smoking among schoolchildren. In addition, we undertook dedicated evaluation of specific components of the programme, such as the Quitline and press advertising.

Over the years of the programme since 1989, our population surveys have tracked changes in a number of indicators, although we have seen no overall change in smoking prevalence. We have been able to show:
- an increase in the percentage of the target group who recall and recognise television advertising,
- increased awareness of the risks to health presented by active and passive smoking,
- increased support for bans on smoking in public places, including workplaces,
- an increased likelihood that indoor workers will report a total ban,
- an increased likelihood that people will report imposing bans in domestic environments and
- favourable shifts in stage of change and quit attempt activity.

What lessons did we learn from this experience? Hindsight is a great teacher: if we had our time again, we would have done some things very differently.

Lesson 1: Don't appear too grateful for funding that is insufficient for performing the task. The amount of funding we received in 1989 (US$ 0.4 million per year) was much more than had ever been allocated to tobacco control programmes in South Australia, but is much less than the amount allocated in places like California. We should have been aiming for something similar, which for South Australia would have meant an allocation of US$ 4.2 million per year.

Lesson 2: Don't try to do everything. Concentrate on key programme components and recycle campaign elements when possible. With the money we were allocated, we ran cessation, prevention and passive smoking campaigns,. We probably should have focused only on one of those areas and done it well. A lot of anti-smoking advertising was produced in other Australian states, and one of the things we did well was to make use of these (depending on the results of evaluation studies) and recycle them for South Australian campaigns. We therefore saved a lot of money by not making new advertisements.

Lesson 3: Don't become complacent by letting other organizations relinquish responsibility for tobacco control. When the Anti-Cancer Foundation and the National Heart Foundation received funding to run the project, many other organizations that had a role to play in tobacco control shifted their energies to other areas, because they considered that 'tobacco was covered'. In hindsight, we should not have let them off the hook and should perhaps have made them more active stake-holders in our programme.

Lesson 4: Consider an external lobby group or develop a coalition to keep up the pressure for extra funds. In 1989, US$ 0.4 million per year was the most we could expect. Although we probably would not have been allocated a greater amount at that time, we should have put some energy into lobbying for additional funding.

Lesson 5: Develop a sound plan for evaluation which includes evaluation expertise external to the programme. Recognize the importance of independence and peer review. Use a range of indicators, not just smoking prevalence. We think we did this reasonably well, and the fact that we have been able to publish much of our data in peer-reviewed journals has been important in defending the outcomes in the face of criticism from the tobacco industry and other sources. By measuring a range of indicators, we know that some important progress was made in South Australia over the period, although the key change we were looking for—a decrease in smoking prevalence—did not occur.

Lesson 6: Educate key fund-holders and politicians to adopt a longer-term view and to appreciate the difficulty and complexity of achieving a significant reduction in smoking prevalence. It is very important to make such people understand that funding for tobacco control is a long-term investment and that the desired results will not be achieved overnight. It is also important to make them understand that a complementary range of strategies is required. In this respect, an advocacy strategy aimed at all political parties is advisable, in order to achieve bipartisan support for adequate allocation and preservation of funding for tobacco control.

Prevention of smoking in the Veneto Region, Italy

E. Tamang, G. Pilati, M. Boschiero, M. Fridegotto & F. Michieletto

Centre for Health Education, Regional Documentation Service, Padua, Italy

The Veneto Region is situated in north-east Italy, with Venice as its capital. It has a territory of 18.364 km^2 and 4 380 797 inhabitants. It is divided into 21 local health units and 582 municipalities. The prevalence of smoking in the population aged 14 years and above in the Region was 20% (26% of males and 14% of females), in comparison with 25% in Italy as a whole (34 of males and 17% of females). Between 1993 and 1997, Veneto adopted a comprehensive strategy for tobacco prevention. The strategy used included:

- institution of the Centre for Health Education in Padua to programme health promotion and health education interventions for the Region and provide advice and expertise to all local health units and hospitals;
- organization of workshops and training seminars for teachers and health and social workers on tobacco control;
- setting up regional work groups to plan and implement tobacco control projects;
- preparing ad-hoc materials;
- evaluating the process and the results;
- developing health promotion settings such as tobacco-free schools, hospitals, health services and workplaces;
- producing a newsletter four times a year with contributions from all local health units and
- celebration of World No-Tobacco Day.

Regional projects for smoking prevention included smoking prevention in schools; smoking cessation courses; smoking reduction and cessation through counselling by general practitioners; smoke-free hospitals and health services; smoking prevention among young people, financed by the European Commission and smoke-free class competitions.

Smoking prevention in schools

This project involves secondary schools with students aged 11–13. In 1997, the project was carried out in 10 local health units and involved 2000 students, 250 teachers and 28 health workers. Two training seminars were held for health and social workers at the regional level, and each local health unit also gave training courses. The instruments developed for this project included a guide dealing with the complex problems related to adolescence and smoking. Teachers offered to help students to develop a more critical sense and to strengthen their ability to resist peer pressure.

An interactive multimedia tool for computers was developed which allows children to learn in an enjoyable way. The programme permits them to navigate in 'Healthy City' which has different settings: a town square, a billboard, a school, a park, a hospital, a bar, a tobacconist's and a gymnasium providing information on tobacco issues and health hazards related to tobacco consumption. It includes a quiz game that can be accessed from any setting with 10 options. A kit of transparencies and diskette contains epidemiological data on tobacco consumption and the tobacco epidemic in the countries of the European Union, Italy and Veneto Region in practical tables and graphics.

Smoking cessation courses

The courses have been given in 14 local health units and had a success rate of about 40% after one year. Two training seminars for health workers were held in 1997. Each health unit encourages its participants to create associations of ex-smokers. Instruments developed for this project include: smoking cessation course guidelines for professionals and cards for participants which contain information and tips to help them maintain their decision to become and remain a non-smoker.

Smoking reduction and cessation through counselling by general practitioners

Pilot studies carried out in three local health units showed that the rate of quitting after one year of counselling was 19%, which may be compared with the natural quitting rate of 1.4% in Italy and 2.7% in Veneto. Training seminars have been carried out, and a manual has been developed to help local health units adopt the project. It explains what resources are needed, whom to involve and how long the project takes to carry out. A manual was also prepared for doctors to help them in counselling their patients to quit smoking. Posters and handouts have been produced as well.

Smoke-free hospitals and health services

This project is part of a regional network and involves 16 local health units and the two regional hospitals, which have adopted a smoke-free policy. The tools that have been developed for this project are a manual for local health units and hospitals to develop the project, a manual for nurses to help their patients stop smoking and various posters.

Smoking prevention among young people

In a five-year project partly financed by the European Commission and developed in collaboration with the Italian League Against Cancer of Milan, the Cancer Institute of Faenza and the Department of Health of Barcelona, the aim is to prevent smoking by 11–13-year olds. We will try to improve school smoking prevention programmes and develop a new strategy for involving and training teachers and designing an interactive CDRom for young people.

Smoke-free class competition

The Veneto Region is participating in a European project with Denmark, Finland, France, Germany, Spain and the United Kingdom in another school-based project financed partly by the European Commission and conducted in collaboration with the European Network of Young People and Tobacco. The aim of the project is to prevent or delay the onset of smoking among young people and to stop or reduce cigarette consumption by pupils who have already experimented with smoking so that they do not become regular smokers.

Future actions

The Region is working to establish networks of health-promoting schools and healthy work sites that adopt a smoke-free policy.

Anti-smoking campaign in Shanghai Medical University, China

T. Yao, F.-J. Xiong, H.-F. Xia, J.-H. Huang & L. Zhou

Shanghai Medical University, Shanghai, China

Introduction

Shanghai Medical University, one of the key universities in China, is an important base for training medical and health professionals; even in such an institution, however, there was a non-negligible number of smokers among students and staff members. A survey conducted by the Department of Health Education in early 1995 revealed that 12% of the students in the university were smokers and that 3.3% of them smoked every day. The number of smokers among the university staff was even greater, accounting for 22%, with 18% daily smokers. In view of this situation, the President of the University proposed that smoking be prohibited on the campus. He said that a medical university should create a better, smoke-free environment, and the staff and students should become non-smokers. On 1 April 1996, a campaign for a 'smoke-free university' began, and thousands of staff and students signed their names to 'start with themselves for a smoke-free university'. The prevalence of smoking dropped from 12 to 6.2% among students and from 22% to 17% among staff. The main method used to promote a smoke-free university combined health education with administrative support and was proved to be highly effective.

Methods and experiences

The university administration considered that smoking control should become a 'model unit', and a supervisory group headed by the President was set up in January 1996. The university formulated a series of the rules and regulations on smoking:

- from 1 April 1996, all smoking in public areas on the campus was banned, including the library, gymnasium, classrooms, dormitories, laboratories, meeting rooms, clinics, video rooms, dining halls and paths.
- The sale of tobacco products is prohibited at shops on the campus, and people who sell tobacco products on the campus will be fined 500 yuan RMB.
- The University does not recruit new staff members who are smokers.
- The regulations on smoking and related materials are distributed to all departments and classes of the university.

The supervisory group met several times to discuss strategies for smoking control, and several groups from other schools at the university were set up.

Under the guidance of experts, smoking control is combined with medical education. The Department of Health Education plays an important role by giving courses to all university students. They also developed the smoking control programme, advised the President and supplied educational materials to the supervisory group. The Department also conducted two large-scale surveys to determine smoking status. Professor Li Wanxian of the Department of Epidemiology, a well-known specialist in smoking control, often gives lectures to students and staff on tobacco use and its effects on health, and a number of smokers were inspired to give up smoking after her lectures. A team from Finland representing a well-known Nordic smoking-control organization was invited to the University to give a series of lectures on tobacco and health to the students. Two persons from the United States, Mr Gimbel and Mr Benall, gave enthusiastic support to making Shanghai Medical University a smoke-free university; they gave lectures and exchanged experiences of smoking prohibition.

The public was involved in anti-smoking activities, to enhance the awareness of medical students and teaching staff about smoking and professional responsibility. Health education is necessary for everyone, and everyone should take part in smoking control activities. The main aim is to allow smokers to give up smoking of their own accord and to ask non-smokers to help them. We therefore encouraged public participation in every phase of the smoking control activities.

In March 1996, we started taking action on establishing a smoke-free university. The Youth League Committee distributed information about smoking and 'quit-smoking candies' to smokers to help them make determined efforts to give up smoking. The students of the School of Public Health collected cigarette butts on campus paths in a box labelled 'Part from it' and displaying it in a public place. Graduates composed poems and painted pictures to encourage the campaign against smoking.

On 1 April 1996 we launched a signature drive. On a 35-m banner with the slogan 'Start with yourself for a smoke-free university' written by the President, more than 3000 students and staff members signed their names to support the prohibition of smoking on the campus. The action met with an enthusiastic response in the press: several major news agencies in Shanghai reported the event, the Shanghai International Broadcast Service compiled a special news item in English, and the Japanese television programme 'China Report' filmed the event. the international journal *Tobacco Control* published a report.

In May 1996, we organized a Shanghai International Quit-smoking Contest in collaboration with the World Health Organization (WHO). Students and staff who had stopped smoking were encouraged to take part in the contest. The top 10 prizewinners were selected to join the Shanghai Municipality Quit-smoking Contest.

On 31 May 1996, we launched a street activity for the Seventh World No-Tobacco Day, jointly organized with the Shanghai Municipal Health Bureau. We sent students and doctors to the city centre to make voluntary diagnoses and emphasize the importance of not smoking to the public.

Between 28 March and 5 April 1997, we held a smoking prohibition culture festival. 1 April 1997 was the first anniversary of the smoke-free Shanghai Medical University. To promote the campaign further, the festival emphasized environment, health and development. A series of activities were carried out. A student Association for Tobacco Control with 920 members was set up. Photographs and pictures reflecting non-smoking achievements were displayed in an exhibition.We also published 3000 commemorative envelopes designed by students with an inscription written by the Health Minister Chen Min-zhang. A blackboard providing information on non-smoking for freshmen was judged in a competition. The 'Zihizhe Cup' is a forum conducted by the Youth League Committee to inspire students to ponder the philosophy of life. At this festival, the theme was non-smoking.

We organized lectures on non-smoking by Professor Li Wan-xian and lectures by the Department of Health Education on the harm smoking does to health. We also held special performances, including sketches, comic dialogue, song-and-dance, drama and recitation of poems. All the texts were written, directed and performed by the students themselves. The 1500-seat auditorium was filled, and those without seats stood to watch from beginning to end. Groups of students went to XuHui Square, a commercial centre near our campus to inform the public about the benefits of not smoking.

We commended people when they quit smoking. Ten of the teaching staff who had given up smoking for more than half a year and 28 units that had played active role in the non-smoking campaign won the prize. Moreover, 27 students' classes and dormitory rooms were praised for observing the regulations.

Evaluation

After one year of a smoke-free university, we can conclude that this is an effective way of integrating three activities, leadership, expert guidance and mass participation. A series of activities ensured continual progress of the non-smoking campaign.

Through their medical education, most students and teaching staff are aware of the harm and are aware that they should set a good example by not smoking. Of the students who smoked, 25% intended to become non-smokers, and 59% intended to smoke less. Of the staff who smoked, 88% knew about the harmful effects of smoking, 93% agreed that smoking should be prohibited in public, 86% agreed with a ban on advertisement of tobacco and 93% thought that it was necessary to develop a smoke-free university.

The medical students improved their knowledge and attitudes towards non-smoking and their responsibility and ability to advise patients who smoke. The percentage that considered it to be a doctor's duty to convince people to stop smoking increased from 84% to 90%; agreement with the view that medical students should set a good example by not smoking increased from 85 to 92%. Most of the students asked to be trained in counselling and other methods for helping people to quit smoking.

Community approach to tobacco control in Thailand

B. Ritthiphakdee

Action on Smoking and Health Foundation, Bangkok, Thailand

Country outline and aspects of tobacco control

Thailand is a kingdom with about 60 million people. Ten years ago, 60% of Thai men aged over 15 were smokers, while only about 4% of women smoked. At that time, cigarettes were perceived as a luxury product, and it was thought to be' cool' and superior to be seen smoking.The incidences of lung cancer and emphysema were, however, increasing dramatically, and it was obvious that something had to be done. In 1986, the Action on Smoking and Health Foundation was founded by health activists and non-governmental organizations. We saw the need to have a strong, well-organized movement and believed that we could do something both at grassroots and policy level.

During the past 10 years, many activities have been organized and an extensive network established to ensure that all sectors of society can be reached, from village residents to Members of Parliament. In 1991–92, we succeeded in persuading the Government to pass strong tobacco control laws, which ban all forms of tobacco advertising, sponsorship and promotion, smoking in public places, sales to people under 18 and prescribe prominent, strong health warnings on cigarettes packs. According to a survey by the national statistics office in 1996, the rate of smoking among men aged over 15 is 49%, and that for women is 2.7%. The rate of smoking for both sex therefore fell from 26% in 1986 to 23% in 1996.

Of all the tobacco consumed, 45% is in hand-rolled cigarettes and 55% in commercial cigarettes. The Thai Tobacco Monopoly, a Government enterprise, produces about 96% of all commercial cigarettes. Foreign cigarettes, which were introduced on to the Thai market in 1990 under United States Government coercion, have only 4% of the market, about six times less than what the transnational tobacco companies expected.

Community approach: our major strategy

The community approach is one of our major strategies. Many programmes have been conducted to educate people about tobacco and health, to lobby politicians for a stronger tobacco control policy and to encourage youth and future generations to be 'smoke-free'. We realized that we would not succeed in our campaign for a smoke-free society if we worked alone.

The growth area for the tobacco market is young people. Schools are therefore an important place for work in the community. Students must be equipped with information and trained in life skills, so that they are confident and proud to grow up without tobacco. It is important to start from the earliest age. We have a 'care for kids' programme in kindergartens which aims to minimize children's exposure to environmental tobacco smoke. We encourage kindergarten teachers to design activities that they think appropriate and effective for educating their students and to alert parents to the dangers of passive smoking. We provide songs, cartoon books and other campaign material. Children are very active and effective in motivating their parents to quit smoking. In Thailand, there is a saying, 'fathers tend to care for their children rather than their wives'. We have heard from teachers that many parents have quit smoking for their children's sake, but we have never heard that they quit for their wives.

For secondary-school children, we started a 'Smokebusters' group, based on a successful and popular model in the United Kingdom. Today, there are more that 20 000 student members of 'Smokebusters' clubs. The clubs invite schoolchildren to participate in smoke-free activities, such as slogan and painting competitions. Early in 1997, we introduced a 'Smokebusters caravan', a mobile education unit that goes from school to school, which contains games, science experiments, songs and other activities aimed at helping young people to refuse their first cigarette. Students love participating in the activities. We also have a smoke-free schools project, which includes teacher education and workshops. We are conducting a pilot project that directly involves schoolteachers as tobacco educators and counsellors. We aim to have smoking- and tobacco-related illnesses as part of the school health curriculum.

We are trying to foster a school environment where non-smoking is rewarded—a proactive rather than a reactive approach. We work closely with some schools, trying out new approaches, learning with them, supporting them with information and resources and working with them to lobby the Ministry of Education to develop a smoke-free schools policy.

For adults, we go to workplaces and advocate smoke-free areas and smoking cessation programmes provided by employers. We give them material and ideas for running smoke-free workplaces by using the report of the United States Environmental Protection Agency. We found that workplaces that have a smoke-free policy promote non-smoking norms and motivate smokers to quit.

Although many health professionals are devoted to curing or treating illness, we cannot ignore their potential and opportunity to act as advocates and educators in tobacco control. We need to establish a network or channel to motivate and support them to take action. We found that nurses actively warn their patients about smoking, run smoking cessation programmes and organize grassroots activities. Medical doctors are useful in lobbying for stronger legislation.

Religious groups are important in some countries. In Thailand, monks are very active in educating people, and some are outstanding speakers on tobacco control. They are experts in m motivating and assisting smokers to give up smoking. According to a 1989 sampling survey, however, we found that about 53% of monks smoke. When they were asked how they got cigarettes, we were surprised to learn that lay people gave them together with other gifts. So we started a smoke-free temples programme, with two main objectives: to stop people from giving monks cigarettes and to create non-smoking norms among monks. The theme of our campaign is 'It's a sin to give a monk cigarettes'. We received good media coverage, and the campaign was continued. We did another sampling survey last year and found that only about 32% of monks smoke, and many monks have become active partners in tobacco control.

When we drew a map pinpointing the organizations that support tobacco control, besides the Ministry of Health, we found many interested and supportive organizations. For example, in Thailand, the Telephone Authority helps us to run Quitline, a telephone counselling service to help smokers to quit; the Petroleum Authority gives us money to run smoke-free school programmes, and there are private companies willing to participate in building a smoke-free generation.

Film stars are another influential group, which can support non-smoking norms or promote smoking behaviour. To recruit film stars to our cause, we approach them, ask them to join our seminars, press interviews and other activities and appeal to those who are ex-smokers to speak in interviews about giving up smoking. We invited Miss Thailand and pop stars to feature in 'the non-smoking generation' posters. One of our strategies in mobilizing film stars is to make regular contact with entertainment columnists and gossip writers, because these people help us to publicize the issue and encourage more film stars to join the campaign. We pay the film stars nothing, but we give them prestige, and every year, we organize a 'Non-smoking Honorary Award'.

The media are a powerful force in directing the social agenda. We liaise with the media to place tobacco control among the top 10 items on their agenda, both at local and national level. In Thailand, the media have played a key role during the past 10 years in promoting non-smoking norms and reinforcing political and legislative programmes. Press releases are not enough; we have to learn the nature of their programme or column and approach each of them on that basis. Since we do not have enough money to pay for television commercials, we build a network with talk show, games and drama programmes and encourage them to integrate non-smoking messages. We provide information, ideas or resources to help them make their programmes more interesting.

Community approach leads to change

A community approach not only serves to raise public awareness on tobacco but is an effective process that leads to change at the policy level. One case study that illustrates this is a campaign to oppose the plans of the Thai Tobacco Monopoly to produce a new brand of cigarette especially for women, announced in July 1996. We mobilized our networks and especially the media. We issued a press release, organized a press conference, wrote to some influential columnists, lobbied Members of Parliament, particularly female members, informed our networks and encouraged them to write to the Ministry of Finance which controls the Thai Tobacco Monopoly.

There was a great deal of support from the media. Some gave full-page coverage to the issue and criticized the plan as a 'dinosaur' or outdated plan, since we are now moving towards a non-smoking generation. The Ministry of Health sent a letter opposing the project to the Ministry of Finance, some Members of Parliament spoke out against it, and female film stars were interviewed. In September, just two months after their announcement, the Thai Tobacco Monopoly shelved its plans to produce the cigarettes.

What are the keys to success in a tobacco control programme?
Programmes and activities in tobacco control can vary from country to country, and the keys to success can be modified in different communities. Our experience shows at least four keys to a successful community approach.

Networking is the first key to success, as a tobacco control programme is a social movement. We need friends, we need supporters, we need cooperation, we need to motivate people to make change, so we must work with all sectors. Some may become active partners, while others give financial support.

The second key is having the media on your side. We can change public attitudes and behaviour and lobby for legislation if we work closely with the media.

The third key is to start with the young generation. I strongly believe that the tobacco industries target the same group we do. In 1990, when Thailand faced trade-related threats by the United States Government to open the cigarette market, we worried about how we could resist the tobacco industries' marketing strategies. Our colleagues from the United States suggested that we start with children. We are not only making the next generation smoke-free, but by working for them we also get public support for tobacco control. Moreover, children are clever in encouraging their parents to quit.

The last key is creative thinking to make campaigns effective. Anything is possible if you act with creativity and determination for a tobacco-free society.

Other important factors
Besides keys, we need resources, so that we can start, run and maintain a tobacco control programme. Both in the government sector and in non-government sectors, there are several important inputs. Information is essential. Today, it is much easier than 10 years ago to obtain updated information through computer networks. The UICC's Globalink is a good place to start.

A community-based programme requires funding. We started with only US$ 3000 in the first year. We work with a limited budget, but through our network we do many things that multiply by 10 what we have in our pocket. We are now funded by public and private donations. Having diverse funding sources ensures we can act without being pressured by one funding source or Government.

It is not necessary to have a large team, as long as it is effective. All bureaucracy should be eliminated and democratic principles used. The team needs speakers or leaders to represent the tobacco movement in the community or the country.

Learning from everybody and everything is a short cut to a tobacco control programme. Local and international friends, books, journals and web sites areall excellent resources of plans and activities. We must open our eyes and open our minds.

Conclusion
A tobacco control programme does not only prevent suffering and death, but it can also make you happy because you are doing a small thing in a small community that has an effect on the whole country and beyond. I strongly believe that we are making smoking a thing of the past. Some people may think that it is only a dream, but I think it is a possibility. I wish all of you joy and happiness in making smoking history.

Smoking intervention programme in the Mamre community, South Africa

K. Steyn, N.S. Levitt, J.M. Fourie, G. Reagan, K. Rossouw & M.N. Hoffman

Medical Research Council, Cape Town, South Africa

The Mamre community comprises 5000 working-class descendants of the inhabitants of a Moravian mission station 55 km north of Cape Town. A community-based tobacco control programme was initiated in response to a baseline survey in 1989 which found that 78% of the men and 48% of the women smoked tobacco. We have evaluated the impact on the prevalence of tobacco smoking and the community's response to a demonstration project in 1996.

The tobacco intervention programme was part of an overall programme to prevent the risk factors for ischaemic heart disease implemented over five years, with a high level of community participation. The intervention, with health promotion directed at the whole community, was coordinated from a blood pressure measurement station that served people with high risks for ischaemic heart disease. Volunteers from the community were trained and supervised by a clinical psychologist with extensive experience in running tobacco cessation programmes. Smokers identified at the blood pressure station were referred to this programme. The community was also targeted by means of posters and billboard messages and public activities during World No-Smoking Day, with schoolchildren and young people playing a major role. School art programmes planned around tobacco control were presented by an artist. A video programme was made of people in Mamre who had stopped smoking.

In a follow-up survey, a random sample of 974 subjects aged $\geq$ 15 years were interviewed to determine their sociodemographic characteristics, tobacco use, medical history, self-reported lifestyle and responses to the project. Provisional analyses suggest that the project was well accepted by the community: 55% quoted the project logo correctly and 14% quoted the tobacco control logo. The tobacco control aspects of the project were specifically referred to by 8.1% of the sample, without any prompting, while 60% of those who had ever stopped smoking did so after the baseline survey. Although the smoking rates decreased from 64% to 50%, they remained high; 71% of the non-smokers were exposed to environmental tobacco smoke in their homes and 10% at the workplace.

Smoking rates declined significantly. The programme was conducted at low cost, as tobacco control capacity was built by training volunteers to conduct most of the intervention.

The journal *Tobacco Front*, a cooperative project in building tobacco control networks

C. Holm

Skaraborg Institute, Skövde, Sweden

In 1993, the Skaraborg Institute, a World Health Organization (WHO) Collaborating Centre, resumed publishing the newsletter of a former non-governmental organization, Tobacco Front. The purpose was to establish a regular journal for people engaged in tobacco prevention in Sweden. At that time, the first networks of professionals against tobacco were formed. The members needed a common means of communication.

The first 'new' issue of *Tobacco Front* was distributed in 1993 to the members of the three existing organizations of professionals against tobacco: those of doctors, dentists and nurses. The National Institute of Public Health participated in forming a new editorial policy. *Tobacco Front* was to report on current events and experiences in tobacco prevention at local, national and international levels, cover activities within the national tobacco programme, comment on new literature and other material and review scientific articles. Two issues were published in 1993 and three in 1994, and the journal has been published regularly since 1995, four times anually.

The journal has developed into a major means of communication between tobacco control advocates in Sweden, whether they are active in non-governmental organizations or at governmental or county level. An editorial commitee with representatives from the

Skaraborg Institute and the National Institute of Public Health plans the content and the special feature issues. The professional networks participate in and contribute regularly to the editorial work. *Tobacco Front* now reaches approximately 5500 people. Most of the issues are sent out by subscription to four groups of professionals against tobacco, and each issue now also contains news from those organizations to their members. Special feature issues are printed in an additional number of copies for distribution at conferences and professional meetings, to schools, municipal public health boards and other centres. *Tobacco Front* contains no advertisements and is financed partly by the National Institute of Public Health and partly by subscription fees.

The Badvertising workshop

B. Vierthaler

The Badvertising Institute, Harpursville, New York, United States

The tobacco industry recruits children as 'replacement smokers', to replace the customers who have quit or died. Artist Bonnie Vierthaler takes a hands-on, no-nonsense approach to educating children about tobacco advertising. Pasting truthful images on deceitful tobacco advertisements shows how Badvertising can immunize children against the tobacco industry's powerful advertising and marketing campaigns. No preaching, no prohibition. By turning the advertisments against themselves, children learn how they are being deliberately targeted, seduced and manipulated. When they discover how they are being used, they are astonished. They feel foolish, ripped-off, indignant, perhaps even angry. Now their emotions are engaged; this shapes their desires and their resulting behaviour.

Bonnie Vierthaler began doctoring tobacco advertisements in 1986, to make them honest. Using her art to immunize young people against deceptive advertising, she created *The Joy of Smoking—A Spoof on Cigarette Advertising*, a travelling exhibit of 63 of her honest advertisments. She took the exhibit to schools, hospitals, libraries, shopping malls and even the Rotunda of the Russell Senate Office Building in Washington DC, at the invitation of a senator.

To make her work more broadly available, she made the images into a slide show and posters and called the resulting business 'The Badvertising Institute', as a spoof on The Tobacco Institute. Badvertising images have also been seen on billboards, bus cards, special television shows, videos, national magazines and professional journals. She has conducted hundreds of discussions with young people, physicians and health educators and is teaching educators how to offer Badvertising workshops as a means of prevention.

The Badvertising Institute's award-winning web site is reaching both young people and long-term tobacco addicts. Although there is no known way of measuring its effect on prevention, hundreds of 'thank you's' sent by e-mail have credited the images with saving lives, morivating people to quit their tobacco addiction and reinforcing their desire to quit. The Badvertising web site has been recognized for its leadership in quality and content.

At the Tenth World Conference on Tobacco or Health, the Badvertising approach was received enthusiastically as a unique, much-needed approach to the worlwide tobacco problem. This approach to cause and effect makes a profound and lasting impact and can be incorporated into any awareness programme in any culture.

Smoke-free sport—More than a banner!
Local activities in Birmingham, United Kingdom

P. Hooper

Smoke Free Birmingham, Southern Birmingham Community Health National Health Service Trust, Springfields Centre for Health Promotion, Birmingham, United Kingdom

Since 1993, Smoke Free Birmingham has supported a wide variety of sports organizations as part of an integrated tobacco control programme. The main sports that have been sponsored include football, basketball, cricket, women's volleyball (Smoke Free Birmingham have their own team), baseball, American football and swimming. The degree of involvement ranges from the provision of T-shirts to swimming clubs to full sponsorship of Premiership football matches around New Year's resolution time.

While the immediate effect of advertising at spectator sports is obvious, the long-term association of Smoke Free Birmingham with its sporting alliance partners has led to mutually beneficial developments. For instance, the growth in popularity of basketball among young people has been partly due to promotion of the sport in schools. Players from the City team (the 'Bullets') visit schools and train young people in basketball skills. By associating with the team and providing support to the players, 'smoke-free' messages are now imparted by these powerful role models.

Imaginative and creative promotions based on the databases of the Smoke Free Birmingham alliances have strengthened the association between sports and health. Other interactions have been encouraged. A newsletter has been produced which is targeted at young people and features sports activities and items of interest linked with the smoke-free message. The newsletter and other sponsored events have gone some way to countering the tobacco industry's use of sport to glamourize tobacco smoking and have encouraged young people to be involved in sport, both actively and as spectators.

Close relationships developed with high-profile sporting organizations have enabled the smoke-free message to be attached to events involving large numbers of people. We have also developed our own events for young people. These events, known as 'junior sports forums', provide an opportunity for young people to visit a sports ground, tour the facilities and then question their team idols. The events are hosted by a local sports radio personality, recorded by cable television and are wholly smoke-free.

During the annual Youth Festival, smoke-free events are frequently promoted, as are other cultural events with health-related themes. The added value of healthier alliances in sports sponsorship is especially apparent in the extent and nature of the media coverage obtained.

Competitions to win VIP seats at sports events are often featured on sports radio. This means that health messages are being sent to large numbers of people at a time when they least expect to receive them, and positive images of 'smoke-free' are imparted. Imaginative use of sporting connections can therefore be demonstrated to achieve value for money in health promotion.

Examples of our continued association with sports organizations can be found on our web site <www.smokefree.org.uk>.

Women

The role of public policy in reducing tobacco use among women

H. Selin

Policy Consultant, Smoking and Health Action Foundation, Ottawa, Ontario, Canada

Introduction

The tobacco epidemic in developed countries has followed a predictable pattern: smoking rates among men increase and peak and are followed by increased smoking by women while men's smoking declines. Men's smoking rates also tend to peak at a higher level than women's. Developing and recently industrialized countries are half-way into the epidemic. In many Asian, African and Middle Eastern countries, where men's smoking rates are very high, women's rates remain low in comparison, often below 10%. Still, women's smoking rates are increasing, signalling the beginning of a tobacco epidemic among females that could rival that of the developed world. This situation does not imply, as some have said, that we have not made progress in reducing women's tobacco use. In most developed countries, their use has declined because of improved tobacco control policies. Unfortunately, the tobacco industry has made greater progress. Having attracted men in many developing markets to their products, transnational tobacco companies have turned their attention to women. The marketing tactics they use are similar to those used in western countries decades ago.

Developed countries allowed an epidemic to occur among women, and tobacco transnationals would like a repeat performance in the emerging markets of Asia, eastern Europe and Africa. Their expansion will be minimized only if the health community uses the most effective strategies available. This will require approaches different from those often recommended in discussions of women and tobacco.

Past approaches to women and tobacco

Discussions of women's tobacco use often assume that the determinants of men's and women's smoking behaviour are different. The resulting solutions reflect this, focusing on educational and programming initiatives targeted specifically at women. Another common assumption is that women's smoking can be addressed only in combination with other issues such as stress, socioeconomic status and overall health. This has led to approaches that focus on the difficult task of improving women's lives generally. In these approaches, smoking behaviour is often pushed far into the background.

In reality, there are more similarities than differences in the reasons why men and women smoke, and women's smoking has often declined in response to tobacco-specific interventions, independent of other improvements in women's lives. The most successful and cost-effective approaches have been those that address the environment surrounding tobacco use rather than the environment surrounding women's lives. They also have been broad approaches rather than those targeted specifically at women. They include bans on tobacco promotion, warnings on tobacco packages, high tobacco taxes and restrictions on smoking (Emont et al., 1992; Brownson et al., 1995; Reid et al., 1995; Reid, 1996). Unfortunately, the importance of such measures is often left out of discussions on women and tobacco. Instead, the focus has remained on educational programmes, often implemented on a small scale or at great cost. These measures have minimal impact when used in isolation, particularly in the face of aggressive marketing by tobacco companies.

Legislative measures must be discussed as a key part of the solution to women's tobacco use because of their efficacy. But they should also be discussed because some have particular relevance to women, and because many can be better designed to address women's tobacco use. Some examples are discussed below.

Smoking restrictions

Many countries have recognized the value of restricting smoking in workplaces and public places, not only to protect non-smokers from environmental tobacco smoke but also to help change the acceptability of tobacco use. Smoking restrictions are extremely effective in reducing tobacco use (Emont *et al.*, 1992), but unfortunately tend to protect women last. Restrictions often occur first in professional, upper middle-class workplaces, which remain male-dominated. The last sector to be restricted is the female-dominated service sector, and particularly bars and restaurants.

In Canada, the smoking rates in the service sector are higher than in the general population. Over half the employees are female. The service sector also comprises more employees than any other single occupational category in Canada (Lowe, 1996), bans on smoking in service sector workplaces that are now weakly regulated, such as bars and restaurants, would therefore protect many female non-smokers from environmental tobacco smoke and would reduce smoking among large numbers of the female workforce.

In countries where women's smoking rates are very low and men's very high, protection from environmental tobacco smoke is particularly important, as it may present an aggregate health risk to women that is greater than that of direct smoking. This is true in Taiwan: Tsai *et al.* (this volume) show that the tobacco industry does not need to recruit women to smoke in order for women to die from their products. Although only 4% of adult females in Taiwan smoke, women comprise 30% of Taiwan's smoking mortality statistics. The reason? Eighty percent of women's tobacco-related deaths are due to passive smoking.

Clearly women are not adequately protected from environmental tobacco smoke, strategies around women and tobacco need to focus more on providing this protection. The ancillary benefits are a reduction in smoking and in the social acceptability of tobacco use.

Package warnings

Women, like all smokers, are generally under-informed about the nature and magnitude of the health risks of tobacco use. Figures 1 and 2 starkly illustrate this point (British Columbia Provincial Health Officer, 1996). An under-appreciation of the risks makes it more difficult to convince women of the need to change their behaviour. Women's belief that breast cancer is the leading cause of death explains why they often ask their doctors about mammographies and breast self-examination but rarely about smoking.

Figure 1. What kills women: Causes of death of women, British Columbia, Canada, 1994

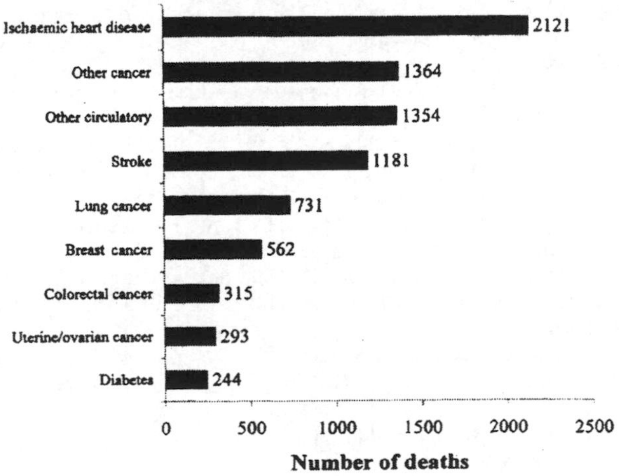

Figure 2. What women *think* kills women: Women's perceived causes of death of women, Canada, 1995 (% that named the disease)

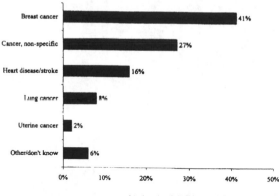

% deaths from named disease

Misperceptions of the role of tobacco in compromising health is perpetuated by the tobacco industry. Tobacco companies often support organizations that address diseases not known to be associated with tobacco use. For example, Shoppers Drug Mart, a sister company of Canada's largest tobacco company, regularly runs promotional campaigns on breast cancer research and prevention. Highlighting non-tobacco-caused illnesses heightens the perception that these illnesses are greater threats to health than those caused by tobacco products.

Sometimes the tobacco industry is supported by the medical community. Tobacco company directors are often affiliated with hospitals and medical schools. The chief lobbyist for the Canadian tobacco industry serves on the board of a leading women's teaching and research hospital. When a Canadian Cancer Society volunteer complained to the hospital about the inappropriateness of the situation, the female chair of the hospital board defended the lobbyist. She said he 'has always been a strong supporter of women's health issues' (Coutts, 1997).

One of the most cost-effective ways of correcting misperceptions about health risks is placing health warnings on tobacco packages. Evaluations of package warnings in Canada and Australia showed that even general information about health risks on the package influenced smokers to try to quit or to reduce consumption (Borland *et al.*, 1996; Tandemar Research Inc., 1996). Package warnings also detract from the allure of the tobacco package.

Despite the potential for package warnings to target population subsets (Figure 3), female-targeted warnings have not been implemented, except for warnings about the effects of smoking on pregnancy. In nations where little money is available for health education programmes and many women are hard to reach, targeted package messages represent a cost-effective education tool. In areas where illiteracy is a problem, word of mouth would help disseminate the information on tobacco packages. Visual messages could also be used.

Product modification

The relationship between smoking and weight control is a concern common to men and women, but the tobacco industry has exploited the weight control theme disproportionately with women. Tobacco companies have capitalized on the fashion industry-created desire in women to be thin that verges on obsession. Over several decades, tobacco products have been changed to meet the tastes of a variety of markets. Among the changes that have made the product more appealing to women are the

Figure 3. Targeted package messages

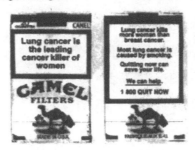

Package messages could help to correct the under-appreciation of smokers of the nature and magnitude of health risks due to tobacco use. In western countries, women commonly believe that breast cancer is the first cause of death among women, even though deaths from lung cancer are more common and deaths from heart disease surpass both.

development of filters, the lengthening of cigarettes and the 'slimming' of cigarettes. 'Slim' and 'luxury length' (100 and 120 mm) cigarettes are common brands marketed to women. Virginia Slims are perhaps the best-known, but numerous examples exist. These cigarettes recall the glamour days of smoking, when Bette Davis and other film stars smoked using long cigarette holders. The tobacco industry continues to modify and expand its product range to appeal to more consumers, including women. Reversal of this process should be a prime goal of people trying to reduce women's tobacco use.

Conclusion

The traditional focus of targeted programming and education strategies to reduce women's tobacco use will not suffice to combat the growing women's tobacco epidemic. It is important that interventions which do not specifically target women, such as broad-based policies, are not dismissed in discussions of women and tobacco. A policy that is effective with all men but only 20% of women is still preferable to a targeted intervention that affects only 1% of women. At the same time, the potential for broad-based policies to reduce women's tobacco use more effectively should be explored. The transnational tobacco companies have their strategy in place to recruit women, and they are implementing it successfully. The health community must have its strategy in place, quickly, to stem the epidemic. Unless this strategy includes the most effective tools at our disposal, we will fail.

References

Borland, R., Cappiello, M. & Hill, D. (1996) *Impact of the New Australian Health Warnings on Tobacco Products (draft)*, Canberra, Commonwealth Department of Human Services & Health
Brownson, R.C., Koffman, D.M., Novotny, T.E., Hughes, R.G. & Eriksen, M.P. (1995) Environmental and policy interventions to control tobacco use and prevent cardiovascular disease. *Health Educ. Q.*; **22**, 478–498
British Columbia Provincial Health Officer (1996) *A Report of the Health of British Columbians: Provincial Health Officer's Annual Report 1995*. Victoria: Ministry of Health and Ministry Responsible for Seniors
Coutts, J. (1997) Hospital body checks appointment. *The Globe & Mail*, 20 February
Emont, S.L., Choi, W.S., Novotny, T.E. & Giovino, G.A. (1992) Clean indoor air legislation, taxation, and smoking behaviour in the United States: An ecological analysis. *Tobacco Control*, **2**, 13–17
Lowe, G.S. (1996) *Workplace Smoking: Trends, Issues and Strategies*, Ottawa: Health Canada (Minister of Supply and Services)
Reid, D. (1996) Tobacco control: overview. *Br. Med. Bull.*, **52**, 108–120
Reid, D.J., McNeill, A.D. & Glynn, T.J. (1995) Reducing the prevalence of smoking in youth in western countries: An international review. *Tobacco Control*, **4**, 266–277
Tandemar Research Inc. (1996) *Cigarette Packaging Study: The Evaluation of New Health Warning Messages*, Ottawa: Health Canada

The International Network of Women Against Tobacco

M. Haglund

National Institute of Public Health, Stockholm, Sweden

Some of you might remember the exciting moment in Perth, Australia, more than seven years ago, at the Seventh World Conference, when 30–40 women from all continents met and discussed the possibility of a future network of women against tobacco. Our dream was to form a network of individuals who shared a common dedication to the importance of fighting against tobacco use by women. The International Network of Women Against Tobacco (INWAT) has since been founded and, what is even more important, recognized and accepted as an important partner in the tobacco control movement. INWAT is today a network of almost 600 members in 60 countries. Our main objectives are to counter the ruthless marketing and promotion of tobacco to women, to develop women-centred prevention and cessation programmes and to promote women's leadership in tobacco control.

As the newly elected President of INWAT at this conference, I should like to applaud the organizers' efforts to have women as almost 50% of the speakers, chairpersons and discussants. I hope that this conference will serve as a model for future world conferences. INWAT has arranged business meetings at the world conferences, and about 50 members attended our meeting at this conference, where several reports were made on progress during the past three years. One report was about the grant we have recieved from Centers for Disease Control and Prevention in the United States, which will make it possible for us to continue our efforts, including our worldwide newsletter, *The Net*, for at least the coming year. We also have released our first series of fact sheets on women and tobacco, which will be followed by fact sheets in languages other than English; the number of languages depends on our financial situation, so further grants are welcome!

The most important part of the meeting was a discussion of the development of INWAT's regional networks, since our members the main resource of our network. Like any other network, INWAT is as strong as its weakest link and, like a good-quality fishing net, INWAT will need strong knots and good links. Perhaps it should also be an extendable, flexible net, as we are quite often dealing with big fish. We heard many interesting reports on activities all around the world. I was amazed at the ideas and enthusiasm of our members, such as the Indonesian Women Against Tobacco, which has produced it's own leaflet and pins, despite limited resources. But money just can't replace enthusiasm, skill and ideas.

It was reported that the European Commission will fund a project to develop INWAT's activities in Europe, and since 4 September 1997, INWAT EURO has had an office at ASH Scotland with a part-time administrator. Since July 1997,we have had Alison Hillhouse as the project leader. The funding is for one year, but an application for the second year will be submitted to the European Commission. This development in Europe should be a pilot plan for other regions, so that INWAT will have more formal bases on every continent. The European branch of INWAT with the European Network for Smoking Prevention has published a report on current trends and an update on ongoing women-centred activities. A European conference on women and tobacco was scheduled for May 1998 in Paris.Finally, we had an interesting discussion on how to promote and develop INWAT further. The following suggestions were made:

- to follow Europe's example and arrange regional conferences on women and smoking elsewhere,
- to encourage women actively to submit abstracts to the World Conference in Chicago in 2000 and
- to make INWAT more visible at future world conferences and other important international meetings.

So, things are moving in the right direction and we are well on the road.

Beauties beating the beast: Working with women against tobacco in Sweden

M. Haglund[1] & A. Duckmark[2]

[1]*Tobacco Control Programme, National Institute of Public Health, Stockholm,*
[2]*Miss Sweden 1996, Boras, Sweden*

'Beauty and the Beast', the well-known fairy tale, inspired the name of our project to work with women against tobacco in Sweden. In 1946, only 9% of women in Sweden were smokers, compared with 50% among men, but since the Second World War this situation has changed dramatically and in 1996 23% of women and 21% of men were daily smokers. Today, Sweden is one of the very few countries in the world where women smoke more than men, and this is especially true in the youngest age groups. One explanation for the large increase in the prevalence of smoking among women is of course the increase in economic and social equality that occurred after the Second World War, but by presenting smoking as a symbol of liberation and sex equality, the tobacco industry has certainly accelerated the process! As a direct result of this tragic development, as many as 80% of all lung cancer patients in Sweden under the age of 44 are women.

Even though we knew for several years what was going to happen, most of our activities for women did not start until the beginning of the 1990s. As in many other countries, smoking in Sweden was for a long time seen as a male problem. Not until the lung cancer rate among women increased significantly did people start to wake up. Isn´t this the real dilemma of prevention: that things always gets worse before they get better?

Overall strategy

Tobacco control legislation has existed in Sweden since the beginning of the 1990s banning advertising and promotion, creating smoke-free public places and workplaces and prohibiting tobacco sales to persons under the age of 18; furthermore, the price of cigarettes increased by more than 40% during 1996, and Sweden has the highest price for cigarettes in Europe. During the last few years, we have chosen girls and women as the prime targets for our educational and information activities, the most important being young women with a low level of education.

The first and most important element of our strategy is to offer a broad variety of activities to make sure that every target group will be reached. The second element is the training of key professionals, which is often fundamental for achieving success in tobacco control, as many allies are needed. It is therefore important to identify those professionals who will best be able to influence specific target groups. In Sweden, we have identified the staff of antenatal clinics and child health clinics, teachers, school nurses and the staff of youth centres as our most important key groups. Since the beginning of the 1990s, many of these professionals, for example, 80% of those working in antenatal clinics, have been trained in how to initiate effective discussions on smoking and how to prevent and stop smoking. The training covers medical facts and methods of integrating smoking control into their daily work and information on the tobacco industry´s methods.

The third element of our strategy is to produce specific intervention guidelines for our key professionals. The idea is to develop in close cooperation with the professionals intervention programmes that are easy to use in their daily work situation. So far, we have produced programmes for the staff of antenatal clinics and child health clinics and for school nurses and staff of youth centres. The guidelines for the school nurses and the youth centre staff address how to initiate effective discussions about smoking with girls who have started to smoke or are at a specific risk of starting. We have also produced various self-help manuals, targeting, for instance, pregnant women, parents and girls aged 15–18 who want to give up smoking.

Offering supportive materials for each target group is the fourth element of our strategy. We have produced not only self-help manuals but also booklets about how to give up smoking without putting on weight and several supplements for popular young women's magazines, which are distributed as part of the magazines and are written and designed in exactly the same style. So far, we have cooperated with the largest magazine for girls aged 13–17, *Frida*, and the largest weekly magazine for women aged 15–35, *Vecko-Revyn*. In both these productions, the Institute of Public Health was responsible for the facts and the magazine editors for the layout, as they know best how to communicate with young women.

The fifth element of our strategy is cooperation with many different partners. The most important partners are teachers and staff in the health-care sector, but we also involve partners in the public sector, such as role models for girls, like television soap-opera stars, pop stars and models. The sixth element of our strategy is the involvement of the media. As the tobacco control programme has never been as well funded as programmes on AIDS and alcohol, we have had to rely on the interest of the media. To be successful in attracting media attention, one has to create good stories, such as our cooperation with the organizers of the Miss Sweden beauty competition. Last but not least important is that as many as possible of our activities are carried out by women. The Smoke-free Miss Sweden is one example of involving women.

Smoke-free Miss Sweden

The idea of making the Miss Sweden contest smoke-free was introduced in 1995 when Miss Sweden 1995, Petra Hultgren, was crowned. Petra was a smoker at the time but soon realized that her habit would be detrimental to her image in the media attention during her year as Miss Sweden. She became a non-smoker and contacted the Swedish National Institute of Public Health. Since 1996, all Miss Sweden candidates must be non-smokers and must tour their local schools with the smoke-free message for a minimum of four to six weeks.

Every year, the 28 candidates who have qualified for the semi-finals receive one week's education on tobacco control, including: how to work as an educator and how to bring the smoke-free messages to children aged 10–13; the health effects; various tobacco control strategies and the tobacco companies' methods. After the training programme, all candidates work with a partner from the local health district, who is responsible for scheduling school visits and contacts with the media.

So far, more than 30 000 pupils have met a Miss Sweden candidate, 10 000 during February and March 1996 and as many as 20 000 during the same period in 1997. Our goal for 1998 was 30 000 pupils. At first, the media and many others were somewhat suspicious about the campaign, but after more than two years the media are very supportive. The media attention that we received in February and March 1996 comprised 65 articles in local newspapers and items on 30 local radio programmes and 10 local television programmes. The Miss Sweden final is watched each year by almost 2 million viewers, one quarter of the Swedish population, and many of them are adolescent girls.

Many teachers were also sceptical at the beginning, but that changed radically after the candidates' visits. When we asked 340 teachers whether they regarded the visit as a good complement to the traditional educational activities, 90% responded positively. We also asked the teachers about their impression of the pupils' opinions; 60% reported that the visit had been extremely well received by the pupils, 34% said it was well received, and 1% said they were not sure. When asked whether a Miss Sweden candidate is a good role model for pupils, 90% of the teachers said they were good role models, 9% were not sure and only 1% said that they were not good role models. We also asked the teachers their opinion about using the Miss Sweden candidates in a smoke-free campaign. On a scale of 1–5 with 5 indicating 'extremely good', they gave the campaign a grade of 4.58. On a similar scale, they gave a grade of 4.20 for having the campaign repeated the following year. In the coming years, we shall develop the campaign further, and also involve parents.

Summary and conclusions

The lessons learnt from working with women in Sweden against smoking are:

- Be patient. It always takes a long time to get support for specific actions aimed at women.
- Train key professionals and key groups and take every chance to promote the message of the importance of stopping the tobacco epidemic among women.
- Offer a variety of actions: the broader the variety of activities you can offer, the better, as this increases the chances that you will influence your target groups.
- Be inventive, use your imagination in trying to find the right partners, methods and channels for your activities.
- Identify high-profile partners, perhaps not the organizers of beauty competitions, but try to identify and establish contacts with the best partners to promote your message in your own country.
- Involve the media; the more interesting partners you have, the more interest you will get from the media and the public.
- Have courage and be committed to your goals; otherwise, it can be difficult to survive in the tobacco control field. Even health educators are allowed to fail: if you don't dare to try something new, you will never know whether it's possible.

Our results with regard to smoking prevalence among women show a decrease in the prevalence of smoking among both men and women since the beginning of the 1980s. Another indicator of the effect of our activities is the falling trend in smoking among pregnant women. In 1992, when we started our nationwide training of the staff of all antenatal clinics, 25% of pregnant women were smokers, but in 1995 only 18% were smokers. An even more positive result is that the decrease is greatest in the youngest age groups.

Our women-centred activties in Sweden will continue, and in the end the beauty will beat the beast!

Women, low income and smoking:
Developing community-based initiatives

P. Gaunt-Richardson[1], A. Amos[2], E. Crossan[2] & M. Moore[1]

[1]Action for Smoking and Health (ASH) Scotland and [2] Department of Public Health Sciences, University of Edinburgh, Scotland

As the prevalence of cigarette smoking has declined in countries with the longest history of smoking, two patterns have emerged: the gap between smoking by males and females has narrowed, and smoking has become concentrated among people living in disadvantaged circumstances and on low incomes. The strong and growing interrelationship between sex, smoking, poverty and disadvantage raises important questions about the extent to which traditional approaches to tobacco control meet the needs of women on low incomes. We outline the approach that we have been taking to develop new and effective ways of addressing issues around women, smoking and low income in Scotland. Previously, few initiatives have been designed to meet the needs of women on low incomes, i.e. they fail to acknowledge the role that smoking plays in these women's lives and to develop ways of helping them that do not blame the victim. In particular, we focus on the processes that have been involved in generating interest in this initiative, and the range of projects that are being funded. The project is based in Action for Smoking and Health (ASH) Scotland, and it consists of two stages.

Stage 1 (Crossan & Amos 1994)
    This stage lasted nine months and involved examining a wide range of community-based projects and agencies to find out if they were doing any work on women and smoking, whether they were interested in developing such work and what was preventing

them from doing it. The findings of this telephone survey were reported and discussed at a national conference. There was a clear consensus at the conference that effective action can best be achieved within a comprehensive national tobacco strategy in which issues of inequality are addressed and measures to reduce tobacco consumption are implemented, including a ban on promotion. The specific recommendations were:

- A forum should be developed to facilitate the exchange of ideas, developments and problems around women living on low income and smoking.
- Multi-agency alliances should be developed to approach this issue in holistic ways that include consideration of sex and material deprivation at community, local and national levels.
- The issue of smoking should continue to be reframed in ways that are more sensitive to women's needs and day-to-day lives.
- Initiatives that are already growing in communities and are owned by local people should be given more recognition and support, and local people should be empowered to develop these initiatives further.
- The debates around issues such as criteria for evaluation and success should be continued and appropriate solutions developed at the community, local and national levels.
- An innovative Scottish project fund should be set up into which community-based individuals, projects and organizations could bid for grants to fund and evaluate new ways of addressing smoking among women living on low incomes.

After the conference, we were successful in getting funding from the Health Education Board for Scotland for a three-year project to start addressing these recommendations.

Stage 2

A three-year programme was started in April 1996 with the aims of setting up a database on community-based projects for women, low income and smoking; to provide funding and support to community groups in developing, implementing and evaluating innovative projects on women, low income and smoking; to explore various ways of evaluating such initiatives and to develop expertise in this new area and to disseminate the results of the project.

The programme has provided funding of up to UK£ 3000 for 20 innovative projects, each lasting up to a year. As the projects are still ongoing, it is too early to look at their success; rather, we briefly describe the types of projects that have been funded and how we generated interest in women, smoking and low income.

The projects are very diverse in terms of organizational location, including health, social work and educational settings, receiving State and/or non-State funding and based at national and local levels. They also differ in their participants and target groups, covering rural and urban populations, the young, pregnant women, single parents, homeless women, women who have suffered abuse, women with mental health problems, those dependent on drugs and/or alcohol, local residents and ethnic minorities.

The approaches used are of two types, although they overlap, comprising those that focus specifically on smoking and those that take a broader approach, in an attempt to address some of the underlying determinants of smoking. The smoking-specific approaches address:

- cessation, by individuals, groups and with peer support;
- assessments and surveys of community needs;
- drama;
- smoke-free policies;
- diversionary activities;
- new materials , such as videos, visual displays, leaflets and magazines;
- intersectoral alliance building and
- peer education.

The broader focus includes courses such as assertiveness, confidence building, stress reduction, relaxation, fitness and exercise for well women; health events and courses; body image; a smoke-free home environment and dependence on alcohol and drugs.

The approaches and processes used to generate awareness, interest and applications included networking at the national, regional, local and community levels. Contacts made during stage 1 were renewed, and materials were sent to statutory and voluntary health and social work agencies, practitioners who had access to community groups and umbrella organizations. We were concerned that some people would immediately throw away an application form when they saw the words 'smoking' and 'ASH', considering that the topic was either too narrow or irrelevant. We therefore developed information sheets and application forms which we pre-tested on community groups for their accessibility and relevance. We also emphasized that if people were interested they should telephone us for assistance in filling in forms. The selection criteria for the projects were put up front.

There were two waves of funding, which was important as some people take longer than others to develop ideas and disseminate. We could refocus in the second wave to encourage different types of projects and applicants from other parts of Scotland, giving the first applicants time to rework ideas and develop interagency proposals. Good support was provided (phone, visits, seminars, written) at all stages of the process. Many applicants were not used to filling in forms or putting their case, especially if they were local women. It was important for the project coordinator's background to be in community work, as this facilitated communication.

The selection criteria were broad, but all the projects had to have a clear link with smoking. The selection board was multidisciplinary. Additional information was obtained about, for instance, the viability and genuine interest of the applicants. The projects had to involve local women and be based on their needs.

Conclusions

We consider that we have been successful: we have not only generated 20 projects involving new ways of working on this issue but have also raised the issue of women, smoking and low income more widely throughout Scotland. We received over 120 applications for funding, and we could have funded many more projects if we had had more money. It is too early to comment on their success, but we have learnt at least one important lesson: working in this way requires considerable support and resources at all stages, from getting people interested in applying through to evaluating projects. This must be recognized and costed into similar programmes to develop bottom-up community-based approaches to tobacco control.

Reference
Crossan, E. & Amos, A. (1994) *Under a Cloud: Women, Low Income and Smoking*, Edinburgh, Health Education Board for Scotland

Involving women's organizations in tobacco control: What are the challenges?

A. Amos

*Department of Public Health Sciences, Medical School,
University of Edinburgh, Edinburgh, Scotland*

At the Fifth World Conference on Tobacco or Health, held in Winnipeg in 1983, women were identified for the first time as a group meriting 'special concern'. In the 'action policy' that was produced at a special session on women and smoking, women's organizations were identified as playing an important role in stopping the female epidemic. National and regional or local political and organizational aspects of the action policy were identified. "At the national level, all organizations concerned with smoking and health should designate an officer whose responsibility it would be to coordinate the women's programme, which should be complementary to other smoking and health initiatives, as well as women's health programmes. At the regional or local level, health, educational and consumer organizations should be encouraged to launch their own community activities and, where possible, to coordinate such efforts. Women's organizations, both traditional and feminist, should be involved."

The potential importance of involving national, regional and local women's organizations in tobacco control has since been echoed in numerous reports, policy statements and strategy documents around the world. While there has been some success in tackling the female smoking epidemic in some parts of the world, it is continuing to spread around the globe, and the numbers of deaths from smoking among women are rising dramatically. I have been actively involved in the United Kingdom in building alliances between the tobacco control movement and women's organizations at all levels, from community to national. I have only limited experience of this issue in other countries, however, and I have been struck not only by the diversity of experiences but also by notions of what constitutes a women's organization. For some, it is community or village educational groups; for others, it could be youth organizations, women's voluntary organizations or charities; for others, it is national bodies that advise governments and other agencies on policy and service provision. Views and opinions on the importance of involving women's organizations are likely to reflect not only experience in working with them but also cultural, social and political factors that affect the type of organizations that exist in a country and their role. I shall attempt to draw out a few key points from interviews I have held with colleagues around the world and whose names are listed at the end of this paper. My conclusions are bound to be influenced by my own experiences and values, i.e. those of a white, middle-class, middle-aged, British academic and activist living in Scotland, a country which has probably the highest number of smoking-related deaths among women in the world and where smoking is also a major cause of inequalities in health. I will consider four key questions:

1. What is a women's organization?
2. Why do we and should we want to involve women's organizations in tobacco control?
3. What are the challenges and barriers that people have faced in trying to get women's organizations involved?
4. Where do we go from here?

What is a women's organization?

Some of definitions that the people I interviewed came up with were: any organization for the advancement of women, any organization that addresses women's issues and any organization run by and for women. It was also recognized that there are other organizations which do not fall into these categories but could be viewed as 'tangential' women's organizations, for example, any organization whose purpose is to serve women but may also involve men; organizations most of whose members are women but whose focus is not necessarily on women; organizations all or most of whose members are women and which focus on topics that are considered to be traditionally women's areas of interest, e.g. family and children, and organizations that include women's issues in their overall remit.

Whatever the definition, there is considerable diversity between countries in the type of women's organizations that exist, their level, status, function, focus and ways that they work. They may be statutory, non-governmental organizations, voluntary, charities, ad-hoc, public or private. they may work at the international, national, regional or state, local, community or grass-roots level. Their function may be to provide services, networking, lobbying, education, empowerment, advisory, support, leisure or recreation; and they may focus on women in general or specific issues such as health or illness and social, environmental, occupational, political, legal, financial, family, religious and ethnic issues. Finally, their ways of working may be hierarchical or collective. In many countries, they play a crucial role at many levels in terms of policy development and in women's lives. This clearly has implications for their use in tobacco control but also in the action they could take or the support they could give.

Why do we want to involve women's organizations in tobacco control?

There is a range of possible reasons, which have implications for approaches and likely success. The first is to reach women about women and smoking in order to generate action and support to address a current problem or, when the prevalence of smoking among women is low, to prevent its emergence; and to gain access to women through membership. (For instance, half the Mongolian population are members of the Mongolian Women's Organization.) This may include key settings or groups such as nurses and flight attendants and community groups. Women's organizations are usually a credible source for women and are also a good way of reaching women leaders.

Another reason is to reach other groups—husbands and partners who may have much higher smoking rates, and children—in order to influence their behaviour and reduce their exposure to environmental tobacco smoke. In most families around the world, it is the women who are mainly responsible for children's upbringing. A third reason is to broaden the political base of support for tobacco control in general, that is, moving beyond the traditional health community. The fourth reason is to draw on their expertise in women's perspectives and experiences, needs assessment, ways of working and networking and alliance building.

In countries where attempts have been made to involve women's organizations, they have been motivated mainly by the first three reasons; yet, by ignoring the fourth reason the tobacco control movement will have limited success in involving women's organizations and will risk ignoring the expertise that is vital to developing effective ways of winning the battle against tobacco.

What are the barriers and challenges?

The people I surveyed, who have a long history of working on women and smoking in various countries, considered that there had been relatively few serious attempts to involve women's organizations in tobacco control, and none considered that the full potential for involving women's organizations had been achieved. They identified strikingly similar problems, irrespective of country, type of existing women's organizations or the level at which they were working. While some of these challenges are the same as those that are encountered when trying to involve any non-tobacco control organization, others are unique to women's organizations.

The range and diversity of organizations varies between countries but may be considerable, which has implications for the time and resources required. In addition, women's organizations may not be readily accessible, for instance at community level. Thus, in a project in Scotland supporting new ways of working at community level on smoking among women on low incomes, we had first to set up a database of community-based projects, as none existed at that time. Since organizations also have varied aims and functions, these must be examined in order to interest them in tobacco.

Smoking is not likely to be their main priority or, indeed, to be perceived as relevant to the interests of their constituency. They may consider that their main concern such as women's refuges, rape or reproductive choice, is more immediate and that other organizations are responsible for tobacco control, or they may consider that the tobacco control agenda conflicts with their own.

Lack of awareness and understanding of smoking as a relevant issue in general and for women is particularly important in countries where female smoking rates are low or deaths from smoking are much higher among men. Even in countries like United Kingdom and the United States, however, there is a perception in many organizations that breast cancer kills many more women than lung cancer. Even if smoking by women is recognized as a problem, it may be perceived to be a medical or health problem, not a women's issue, and its relevance to women's organizations may be unclear.

Many women's organizations, especially at the grass-roots level, have limited resources and struggle to survive. Many may feel that they have no extra resources to commit to tobacco control; even if they do, sustainability may be an issue. Many community groups exist for only a few years.

Because of the need for funding, some have accepted money from tobacco companies. For example, in the United States, Philip Morris spent US$ 3 million on women's causes between 1990 and 1995 and supported more than 100 women's groups in 1995 (Lerner, 1996). The Hong Kong branch of the International Women's Forum accepted sponsorship from Philip Morris for their 1996 conference.

Some see smoking as an issue of freedom of choice, whereas others, such as those working with women on low income, see it as one of the few strategies available to women for coping and are therefore hesitant to address it. Some women's organizations are highly critical of traditional health education approaches aimed at encouraging women either not to start or to try to quit smoking. They find these approaches individualistic, blaming the victim, inducing guilt, disempowering, unsupportive, stereotyping women and insensitive to why women start to smoke or find it difficult to quit. Some view the traditional approach as top-down, adopting a medical model and patronizing to women and women's organizations. While this approach may reflect the way in which some women's organizations work, it alienates many others.

Many women's organizations, particularly grass-roots and community-based groups, work in a collective, non-hierarchical or consensus way, and their membership may be fluid. Many of these organizations, whose focus is to push women's issues or voices higher up the agenda, adopt what they regard as a more empowering approach to their work. They may be unwilling or unable to engage in the tobacco control movement if it is seen as adopting approaches to smoking that are inimical to their ways of working.

The ways in which women and smoking issues are framed are often viewed as too narrow or irrelevant to women and/or their organizations. For example, in Scotland, when we consulted community organizations about action on women, low income and smoking, most said that they did nothing about smoking; when questioned further, however, many said they worked on some of the underlying determinants of smoking and would be willing to work on smoking if they could take a more holistic approach to women's smoking and did not blame the victim (Crossan & Amos, 1994).

The tobacco control movement has been successful in many countries in making alliances with a range of organizations to support policy and action. Depending on how these alliances are developed, however, there is a danger that they might, for example, sign a policy demand but do nothing more substantial, or be unidirectorial, in that no true partnership is developed. Perhaps, instead of asking 'Why aren't women's organizations interested in tobacco control', we should reverse the question and ask 'Why aren't tobacco control organizations interested in women's issues?' As argued by Lorraine Greaves, "... key to making these alliances work is the level of enthusiasm traditional tobacco control agencies show for women and women's issues, not just for smoking. Such a development will be crucial to collaborative efforts to develop meaningful and holistic programmes and policy for women smokers." (Greaves, 1996). Women's organizations will want to work with us only when they trust and respect us. This often means that we need well-placed, credible women to do networking. Time, skills and resources are needed in building any alliance, but we should perhaps change our expectations about the speed with which such links can be made and developed, perhaps by using different ways of working which require different skills and expertise.

Where do we go from here?

When listed together, these barriers may seem unsurmountable, but we can change the negatives into positives and the problems into possibilities. I shall end on an optimistic note. There are now quite a few examples from around the world in which these challenges have been recognized and addressed, and, as a result, women's organizations have become active in tobacco control in a range of ways which reflect their philosophy, values, remits, ways of working and resources. A few examples from industrialized countries are given below.

Japan: The Women's Action on Smoking group has, among its many activities, persuaded several women's organizations to lobby the Government about banning television advertising, provided a telephone hotline to give advice to smokers, mostly female, who were suffering from exposure to environmental tobacco smoke and encouraged women's magazines to cover smoking and health issues.

Sweden: The National Institute of Public Health has developed and implemented a series of training programmes for community and school nurses on women and smoking which take a woman-centred approach. Training is carried out by women who act as role models, thus promoting women's leadership role. Bridges were built with female Members of Parliament, who represent 50% of all Members of Parliament, from all parties, which led them to take the lead in enacting the legislation on banning tobacco promotion. Work with nurses has led to the establishment of the very active 'Nurses Against Tobacco' group.

United Kingdom: ASH Scotland in its 'Under a Cloud' initiative is funding 20 community-based projects on issues of women, low income and smoking. These include organizations which provide refuge for women who have suffered domestic violence, support for single homeless women and their children, support for women with mental health problems and community development groups for women living in deprived areas (Gaunt-Richardson *et al.*, this volume). In Northern Ireland, the Health Promotion Agency and the Women's Resource and Development Agency, a feminist organization which works in community development, formed a partnership to develop, run and disseminate a project for women smokers living in areas of social and economic disadvantage in Belfast (Barr, 1996).

United States: The American Medical Women's Association's Strategic Coalition of Girls and Women Against Tobacco was launched in 1994. Funded by the centers for Disease Control, its purpose is to reduce tobacco-related disease among women by educating and working with women's groups. It has trained women physicians and medical students to advocate tobacco control, produced the most comprehensive American resource on women, girls and smoking, held a women's leadership summit and worked with the media to generate coverage. Girls Inc. of Alameda County, California, designed the 'Josira Warriors' programme to educate young African–American girls about the tobacco industry's influence in their communities. The programme was designed to build self-esteem and empower the girls in decision–making skills. The National Organization for Women, a feminist organization, launched the 'Redefining liberation' campaign to educate its members about women and tobacco issues and to develop leadership on the subject. It used community-based strategies and developed an action guide and training video.

Conclusion
Involving women's organizations in tobacco control is possible, but it requires time, understanding and resources. It also requires an open mind, a willingness to learn and well-placed, credible women to make contacts. Colleagues who have worked with women's organizations around the world share the view that this experience leads to new ways of thinking about and working on tobacco control. Furthermore, when women's organizations have become involved, it is often based on the long-term, unacknowledged and un-resourced work of women, such as the ASH Expert Group on Women and Smoking in the United Kingdom, the Women's Action on Smoking in Japan and members of the International Network of Women Against Tobacco (INWAT) around the world. This work should be acknowledged, supported and resourced. We should go beyond getting women's organizations to sign up to our agenda. We must draw on their insight, experience and expertise and help them to attain their aims.

Acknowledgements
> Michele Bloch, United States
> Rhonda Galbally, Australia
> Margaretha Haglund, Sweden
> Alison Hillhouse, United Kingdom
> Deborah McLellan, United States
> Judith Mackay, Hong Kong
> Maureen Moore, United Kingdom
> Nobuko Nakano, Japan
> Teresa Salvador, Spain
> Patti White, United Kingdom

References

Barr, C. (1996) *Stopping For Me: Women, Disadvantage and Smoking*, Belfast, Health Promotion Agency for Northern Ireland

Crossan, E. & Amos, A. (1994) Under a Cloud: Women, Low Income and Smoking, Edinburgh, Health Education Board for Scotland

Greaves, L. (1996) *Smoke Screen*, London, Scarlet Press

Lerner, .S (1996) Tobacco stains. *Ms Magazine*, November/December, 47–55

Youth

Health-promoting schools and the prevention of tobacco use

R. Erben

Health Promotion and Mental Health, WHO Regional Office for the Western Pacific, Manila, Philippines

There is substantial evidence that the health of children and young people is a major factor in their capacity to learn. Similarly, the level of an individual's education influences his or her health. In fact, schooling alone has been proven to be the most effective public health intervention. The school is an extraordinarily effective setting in which to improve the health of students, staff, families and members of the community. Schools offer opportunities to achieve significant health and education benefits with the limited resources available to education and health agencies.

Much has been done to strengthen health through schools. Most schools around the world have some form of health education as part of their curriculum (Dillon & Philip, 1992–93). Many have educated their students about the dangers of tobacco use, but most had only limited impact with regard to prevention. The school's responsibility goes well beyond the narrow focus of increasing students' knowledge about health and reducing personal risk factors for disease, disability and death. as the school's responsibility includes translation of health knowledge into sound health practices, all resources of schools should be orientated towards health promotion, and the entire school should become a setting that promotes health (Erben, 1994).

WHO's Global School Health Initiative

In 1995, WHO convened an Expert Committee on Comprehensive School Health Education and Promotion to assess what is known about promoting health through schools. The Committee was made up of persons from ministries of education and health, nongovernmental organizations, universities and research institutions. It reviewed school health programmes and research in both developing and developed countries and concluded that, without question, school health programmes can simultaneously reduce common health problems (including tobacco use), increase the efficiency of the education system and thus advance public health, education and social and economic development in all nations (WHO, 1996a,b).

The Committee set out steps, which, if implemented, will enable schools throughout the world to become 'health-promoting schools' (WHO, 1996c). The goal of the Global School Health Initiative is to increase the number of institutions that can truly be called health-promoting schools. Although definitions and their implementation will vary among regions, countries and schools and according to needs and circumstances, a health-promoting school can be characterized as a school that is constantly strengthening its capacity as a healthy setting for living, learning and working.

WHO is implementing the Global School Health Initiative through three broad health promotion strategies:
- building capacity to advocate for improved school health programmes through technical documents designed to help international, national and local organizations to argue effectively to increased support for school health;
- mobilizing public and private resources to develop health-promoting schools. WHO's regional networks of health-promoting schools may represent the world's most comprehensive and successful international effort to mobilize support for school health promotion (WHO, 1996d). The first network was initiated by WHO's Regional Office for Europe, the Council of Europe and the Commission of European Communities. The network has grown in five years to include 34 countries (WHO, 1997). In 1995, networks for health-promoting schools were started in the Western Pacific Region,

and in 1997 each of the six WHO Regions should have established at least one network each.
- strengthening national capacity through the Global School Health Initiative, which collaborates closely with Regional Offices in support of national activities. WHO's 'mega countries' initiative, which aims at strengthening health promotion in the most populous countries in the world, including China, India and Indonesia, has a focus on school health.

Prevention of tobacco use as an integral part of health-promoting schools

The importance of preventing tobacco use in the development of health-promoting schools is demonstrated by the example of the Western Pacific Region and WHO's largest Member State, China. In 1995, 27 countries and areas expressed interest in working with WHO on the development of health-promoting schools in response to a project outlined in May 1995 for implementation of a regional policy document *New Horizons in Health*. This document identifies three themes for future work with Member States, namely, preparation for life, protection of life and quality of life in later years. The health-promoting schools have their most immediate application in relation to preparation for life, which focuses on health promotion relevant to infancy, childhood and youth. Fifteen countries now have health-promoting schools projects and mechanisms in place to develop them further, such as national coordinating committees for health-promoting schools, jointly staffed by the education and health sectors (Erben, 1997).

Regional guidelines for the development of health-promoting schools provide a framework for action (WHO, 1996e). They have been translated into many regional languages, including Chinese, Khmer and Lao. The English and French versions have been adapted for use in Pacific Island countries. The guidelines suggest actions in six broad areas, for which components and checkpoints have been developed: school health policies, the school's physical environment, the school's social environment, community relationships, personal health skills and health services. Prevention of tobacco use is an integral part of these areas, their components and checkpoints. For example, one component of school health policies is that schools be totally smoke-free and prohibit alcohol and illicit psychoactive substances in all activities, and the checkpoint indicates that the school has developed a strategy for phasing out smoking completely on its premises, with a deadline for being totally smoke-free: this policy applies to all staff, students and visitors. For a school to be recognized as a health-promoting school, a tobacco policy must be in place.

China is one country that has embraced the concept of health-promoting schools. It is about to issue a national strategy and adapted guidelines. It has many successful model projects, some of which are part of healthy city initiatives, for example, in Beijing and Shanghai. Of the 25 project schools in Beijing's Dongcheng District, five are already totally smoke-free. Efforts are under way to increase their number and to make all 120 primary and middle schools in the District smoke-free and health-promoting schools before the year 2000.

Prevention of tobacco use as an entry point for the development of health-promoting schools

Some schools have highlighted the importance of first addressing specific priorities in health and then moving towards a health-promoting school. Prevention of tobacco use is one of these entry points; others are control of helminths, prevention of HIV/AIDS and control of malaria and dengue fever. The Minister of Health of China launched the project 'Hundred no-smoking primary and middle schools' in May 1996 with the support of WHO.

Globally, WHO supports the use of entry points for the development of health-promoting schools through the WHO Information Series on School Health. One on prevention of tobacco use will provide useful guidance to all schools.

Conclusion

In order to develop lifestyles conducive to health and free of tobacco use, young people should experience health in the setting of everyday life: the home, the kindergarten, the school and the villages and cities in which they live. The school is an important setting. The extent to which a nation's schools become health-promoting schools will play a significant role in determining whether the next generation is educated and healthy.

References

Dillon, H.S. & Philip, I. (1992–93) Health in education for all: Enabling school-aged children and adults for healthy living. *Int. J. Health Educ.*, 11

Erben, R. (1994) Comprehensive school-based health promotion. In: Chu, C. & Simpson, R., eds, *Ecological Public Health: From Vision to Practice*, Nathan, Public Health Association of Australia and Institute of Applied Environmental Research

Erben, R. (1997) *Development of Health-promoting Schools in the Western Pacific Region of WHO*, Manila, WHO Regional Office for the Western Pacific

World Health Organization (1996a) *Improving School Health Programmes: Barriers and Strategies* (Document for the WHO Expert Committee on Comprehensive School Health Education and Promotion), Geneva

World Health Organization (1996b) *Research to Improve Implementation and Effectivness of School Health Programmes* (Document for the WHO Expert Committee on Comprehensive School Health Education and Promotion), Geneva

World Health Organization (1996c) *Promoting Health through Schools. The World Health Organization's Global School Health Initiative*, Geneva

World Health Organization (1996d) Health promoting schools. *World Health*, 4

World Health Organization (1996e) Regional Guidelines. Development of Health-promoting Schools: A Framework for Action (Health-promoting Schools Series 5), Manila, WHO Regional Office for the Western Pacific

World Health Organization (1997) *The European Network of Health Promoting Schools*, Copenhagen, WHO Regional Office for Europe

The European Network on Young People and Tobacco: Activities, experiences and interactions among networks in Europe

S. Ratte

Department of Epidemiology and Health Promotion, National Public Health Institute, Helsinki, Finland

General information

The Network was established in 1993, but the idea was first conceived in 1990 by Hein de Vries and discussed further with Anne Charlton, Ligia Lima and Alison Hillhouse. The original aims were to promote good practice and improve access to information among researchers and programme managers. The objectives were to collect information on current and recent European research and intervention projects, with particular focus on out-of-school projects, to set up a database and to recruit and support a network of researchers and programme managers. Additional goals were added at the request of the European Action Committee, such as good participation of all Member States, establishment of an agreed terminology to make the data comparable and organization of a conference. The network was hosted by ASH Scotland until 1996 and led by Cecilia Stephens and supported by a steering committee. For financial reasons, ASH Scotland was unable to take on the contract from then on. After a few months of collaboration between ASH Scotland and the National Public Health Institute of Finland, the Network moved to Helsinki in December 1996.

Drawing on the recommendations of the Edinburgh Conference, the evaluation report and the advice of the steering committee members, a new structure was agreed upon and the steering committee was replaced by an advisory board with representatives of the 15 Members States. The focus was slightly shifted from out-of school intervention. The project is financed to 80% by the Europe against Cancer Programme of the European Commission; the remaining 20% is provided by the National Public Health Institute.

Aims and objectives

The aims of the Network are to contribute to the reduction of smoking among young people by facilitating the exchange of information and know-how between organizations and disciplines involved in smoking prevention for young people in the European Community.

The Network is for people working in the fields of young people, tobacco and health, including programme managers, researchers, decision-makers and other interested parties.

The objective is to provide a transparent overview of all the organizations participating in the Network

The Network offers:

- access to relevant information through a classified directory of agents, a catalogue of initiatives and an information service;
- a regular bilingual newsletter (English and French), *Interaction*, with details of new initiatives and research; an opportunity for members to publicize their work, to advertise for collaborative partners and to make announcements;
- the opportunity to participate in an interactive network and to contribute to task forces on specific topics;
- the opportunity to participate in collaborative actions at the European level;

Tools

One of our tools is the database, which is now on Internet on our site. It is used to build up a mailing list , to develop the Network and monitor our progress for participants who may wish to identify individuals or groups with special interests and for background information for funders and policy planners who may wish to find reports on the incidence or effectiveness of particular actions. We can publish a directory of agents and a classified catalogue of initiatives, individual summary reports on initiatives and a list of initiatives under any broad classification.

The participants in the Edinburgh Conference made a few recommendation for the work of the Network. One of them was to set up task forces on various themes. The evaluation task force was set up in 1996, composed of seven researchers and programme managers. The efforts of the members resulted in guidelines for evaluation of smoking prevention programmes, which was published in *Interaction*, the Network newsletter. The next objective of the task force is to concentrate on definitions of smoking.

The 'Smoke-free class' competition is an idea first developed in Finland and now being implemented in several European countries. All the pupils of a class decide to refrain from smoking for a minimum of six months. The class that completes the six months can participate in a lottery with cash prizes. Evaluation of the competition in Finland showed that it delayed the onset of smoking. The first meeting of the task force was held in February 1997 in London. This meeting resulted in a joint application by seven Member States to EaC, which was successful. Meri Paavola is helping the participants to set up the competition in their own countries. Information on the competition has now been translated into English and French. The material is also available on Internet.

Another main tool for the exchange of information is the Network's newsletter, published twice a year in French and English. We also offer contributors the possibility of inserting other information and include articles in other languages. The newsletter is edited only slightly, for clarity. It is an open forum used for information exchange, requests for partnership to create collaborative actions, announcements and updates on smoking prevention activities in the field of young people and tobacco in the European coordination of all initiatives taken in smoking prevention for reasons of consistency and cost-efficiency. To this end, they have asked the European Network on Young People and Tobacco and the European Network on Smoking Prevention to regroup projects already submitted or to be submitted in the future. In an effort to satisfy this request, we are now asking people to send us their proposals, ideas and plans prior to submission to the Commission to try to ensure maximum geographical coverage across the Community, avoid duplication and double financing and ensure better coordination.

Greater collaboration with other international organizations is an area that needs to be developed. Our team is looking at ways to increase collaboration with organizations such as WHO in order to ensure that our work is not duplicating other people's efforts and that it fits into the global context of smoking prevention.

It has been proposed that we take full responsibility, including the financial responsibility, for all of the smoking prevention programmes for young people funded by the Europe against Cancer Programme. This new role raises a great number of questions about selection and the bureaucracy involved and is currently under discussion. The editorial of an issue of the newsletter *Interaction* addresses this topic. We will be pleased to get your comments on this role.

In 1996, Dr Ann McNeill and Dr Martin Raw evaluated the Network. Their report, 'Building a tobacco network', gave us a good insight and presented some valuable recommendations. I have selected some that might be useful for people contemplating setting up a network:

* choose a manageable number of objectives;
* define clearly the roles and responsibilities of different actors in the network (funder, manager, advising structure);
* pilot the use of certain tools (i.e. database before launching);
* use strategic thinking;
* take time to develop and maintain contacts.

More practically, there are areas where our experience can be of some use to others:

* identifying key people in various countries;
* creating and structuring a network covering 15 countries;
* building a database;
* analysing information from different countries in different languages;
* producing a newsletter and directories;
* facilitating collaboration and partnership;
* organizing a conference and
* setting up task forces.

Networking in Europe

The European Network on Young People can be described as a specialized network as it focuses on smoking prevention with one target group, i.e. young people, and seeks to promote good practice and exchange of information between professionals working in this specific field. The European Network on Smoking Prevention is an umbrella network that regroups other 'specialized' networks such as young people, smoke-free cities, hospitals and doctors. It has a wider remit and scope and looks at all aspects of smoking prevention. Collaboration between these two networks takes various forms. The European Network on Young People is a member of the European Network on Smoking Prevention, and the two ensure information exchange. One concrete and very pertinent example is our collaboration on the new role proposed by the European Commission. We discuss ideas, we agree or disagree, use each other resources and knowledge and try to find solutions to sometimes difficult questions. Perhaps the best example is that we both consider that networking with other networks is important.

Some benefits of networking are having more impact (when more people work with a similar aim), amplification and increased efficiency of work, validation of effort (feeling part of something larger), finding that being better informed it can be fun and very rewarding. This will increasingly be the way to work at local, regional and global levels.

Some realities of networking are that the share of resources (especially if they are scarce) can create obstacles in good networking; there are times when different organizations' pressures, priorities and outlooks make networking more difficult because everybody is not looking in the same direction; and networking across 15 countries with nine languages and varied cultures makes the task even harder.

Youth-centred tobacco control

W.D. Novelli

National Center for Tobacco-free Kids, Washington DC, United States

A focus on youth-centred tobacco control—whether national or international—has at least three important advantages in public policy, public action and public health. First, with respect to public policy, few people would disagree that it is simply wrong to market and sell tobacco products to young people. Politicians, celebrities, business leaders and even the tobacco industry must publicly agree that these products cannot and should not be sold to minors. Thus, a focus on youth in terms of influencing public policy is a powerful strategy. Next, regarding public action, our surveys show that establishing a national tobacco control plan that protects children is a high social priority. There is enormous public support for such a plan when the issue is framed in the context of protecting children from the tobacco industry's efforts to manipulate and take advantage of them. In a survey we conducted last March, more than half of 800 'consumer activists' in the United States placed the use of tobacco products by children among their top three concerns. One-third of them said that it was an issue in which they were likely to get involved. With regard to public health, tobacco addiction is fast becoming a paediatric epidemic of global proportions. While it is growing faster in some areas than in others, it is clear that smoking among young people has reached disturbingly high levels. Five million American children alive today will die prematurely because of tobacco use, if current trends are not reversed.

But we must not focus only on youth. It is important to reduce adult smoking levels as a means of reducing morbidity and mortality. Also, exclusive attention to smoking by young people may communicate to children that it is acceptable for adults to smoke. Since children want to emulate adults, this can create a 'forbidden fruit' desirability for tobacco products. Thus, a broad-scale effort is needed to 'de-normalize' tobacco—to make sure that it is no longer a normal part of everyday life, and to turn tobacco use into a socially unacceptable and offensive habit. We have identified six strategic areas for achieving this goal:

Price increases

This may well be what the tobacco industry fears most, since studies show that young people are highly responsive to differences in cigarette prices. The tobacco industry argues that tax increases are regressive and counterproductive over the long term, that is, that consumption and therefore tax revenues will decrease over time. They also argue that government should not play the role of 'nanny' by trying to discourage adults from making the personal choice to smoke. On this point, the American public seems to agree. Most people believe that adults who wish to smoke should be allowed to do so. But achieving price increases can be an important strategy for tobacco control among the young, at the state or provincial level as well as nationally, because the individual most likely to be affected by higher prices is the 'experimental' smoker—the child who has just begun to smoke or to consider smoking.

Youth access

The tobacco industry often appears to favour greater restrictions on sales of tobacco products to children. But, in our experience, its efforts are half-hearted and insufficient. Many sales clerks who are responsible for determining whether someone is old enough to buy cigarettes are inadequately trained, and not enough attention is paid by store owners and managers. Experts say that restrictions on the access of young people, if truly effective, can contribute substantially to smoking reductions.

Tobacco marketing

There are three reasons why we should work to restrict tobacco marketing. First, billboards, magazine advertisements and promotion are highly visible, and attacking them can generate media and public interest. Secondly, it is reasonable to assume that this can be a useful intervention. Various studies have shown that tobacco advertising and promotion have an impact on youth, both in taking up smoking and in the brands chosen. The third reason for pursuing tobacco marketing restrictions is that they are part of a comprehensive programme to de-normalize and de-glamourize tobacco and push it out of the mainstream of society. No one component is going to be successful on its own.

Public education

This strategy, also known as counter-marketing, would seem to have a better chance of success when tobacco marketing itself is restricted. In California, it is believed that the tobacco industry doubled its marketing spending in response to a massive public education campaign. There may soon be an opportunity for a national public education programme in the United States, if national tobacco-control legislation is enacted. Currently, there is no national campaign, and generations of American children have grown up without seeing a single anti-tobacco message, except perhaps occasionally in school.

Environmental tobacco smoke

Second-hand smoke makes children ill, and smoking by adults and peers, wherever children are exposed, provides negative role modelling. This is an important point for advocates: if adults are concerned about the health and welfare of their children, they have a responsibility to protect them from tobacco use. And they can't do that if they smoke near their children.

Product regulation

For the first time, the United States Food and Drug Administration has asserted jurisdiction over nicotine as an addictive drug and over cigarettes and chewing tobacco as drug delivery devices. We must label tobacco products for what they truly are if we expect to change the nature of the debate, both through policy and public opinion. The Food and Drug Administration's jurisdiction is currently being appealed. Court decisions and Congressional legislation will spell out our ability to regulate the manufacture of tobacco products and their ingredients and the concentration of nicotine in American tobacco products.

There are two additional areas of importance in the protection of children from tobacco. The first is youth advocacy—helping children become activists and thereby part of the solution, rather than simply a 'target audience' for the tobacco industry and the public health community. We are pursuing several ways to do this. One is 'Kick Butts Day', an annual anti-tobacco day for young activists that we sponsor. Thousands of children from all over America take part in activities such as lobbying, youth rallies and undercover buying operations. These activities have resulted in enormous media coverage, as well as the participation of President Bill Clinton, Vice-President Al Gore and Secretary of Health and Human Services Donna Shalala.

We have also begun a partnership with the Public Relations Society of America, in which public relations professionals teach children how to lobby, media relations and other skills. We also conduct a 'Youth Advocate of the Year' awards programme. Past winners have successfully lobbied for local anti-smoking ordinances, conducted undercover buying operations and had other positive impacts on local and state tobacco control policies.

A final area of importance is the United States entertainment industry. Children routinely see smoking portrayed as acceptable behaviour in movies, television and music videos. Actors and musicians can be attractive and seductive role models, and these messages are repeated innumerable times over the years, creating an impact on each successive generation. A decade ago, efforts were made to shift the image of alcohol from stumbling, drunken types of characters, and today alcohol use is rarely portrayed as something funny. This was accomplished by experts who developed guidelines and met with movie producers and others. This coincided with aggressive advocacy campaigns which together provided for a kind of 'good cop–bad cop' approach. These dual strategies may also be effectively applied to deglamourizing smoking.

In summary, tobacco control among young people can form the basis of a powerful political, public activist and public health campaign, made up of a number of strategies. But it should be seen as part of a total national and international tobacco control effort. Only then can it fully succeed.

How pupils themselves can work towards a tobacco-free society

I. Talu

Swedish Teachers against Tobacco, Stockholm, Sweden

As a teacher of social science who is interested in preventing the use of tobacco, I formed an idea about how pupils can learn in an effective way how society functions while at the same time forming opinions that lead to a tobacco-free adolescence. A project was carried out among junior high-school pupils (15 years old) in two schools in Uppsala, Sweden. Faced with the knowledge that 10 000 people die in Sweden each year as a result of tobacco use, that 600 teenagers start smoking every week, that the European Union gives US$ 1 thousand million in subsideies for tobacco production and only US$ 15 million to preventing its use and that the advertising of tobacco is widespread in Uppsala, the young people in the project asked why tobacco companies are allowed to target their marketing at children and young people and whether adults really care about the health of children and young people. They decided to show what they thought about this absurd situation, but were uncertain how to act in a democratic society. We discussed the various building blocks that make up a democratic society, including freedom of speech, freedom to express opinions, the right to hold meetings and how opinions can be spread by writing to the newspapers, by contacting people in positions of authority and by demonstrating.

European Union subsidies
On the subject of the European subsidies, the pupils started by writing letters to the newspapers in Sweden with the largest circulation. They were then contacted by an educational radio station and took part in a debate with a Swedish member of the European Parliament. They also wrote letters to European commissioners, Swedish members of the European Parliament and the leaders of the Swedish political parties. The European Union Commissioner Padraig Flynn visited Uppsala, and the pupils handed over an appeal from their friends.

Swedish Match Company
The pupils decided to demonstrate outside the place where the annual general meeting of the Swedish Match Company was being held in order to protest against the company's manner of marketing their products; the neighbourhood police officer informed the pupils about the regulations that apply to public demonstrations. The pupils also formed a media group, which visited the local newspaper offices, where they found out how and when the mass media can be contacted, how to formulate a press release and how to make an issue interesting to the mass media. The local television and radio stations and the newspaper covered the group's activities on the morning of the demonstration.

The pupils formulated their appeal in both words and pictures during Swedish, social studies and art lessons. They made placards and flyers and decided that the Company's shareholders should walk along a 'tar carpet' made of black plastic, rather than a red carpet, in order to enter the meeting place. Several shareholders praised the pupils' efforts. The action generated a great deal of attention from the mass media in the form of news coverage.

The pupils participated in the project only after their parents had given permission, and the parents were kept informed continually.

My aims in this project, as a teacher, were to demonstrate to the pupils that, in order to achieve a goal, they must seek information about how society is organized and functions; that the pupils worked on a subject that concerned them; that the pupils learned how to examine textual and visual material critically; that the pupils' interest in social issues was stimulated and that the pupils acquired the knowledge and skills needed to effect change in a democratic way.

Young people and tobacco: The Belgian experience of the 'Smokebusters' movement

F. Bourgeois

Association contre le Cancer, Brussels, Belgium

The Smokebusters movement, which started in the English-speaking world, came to Belgium in 1990 at the initiative of the Belgian Cancer Association. The movement currently has around 25 000 young Belgian members between 7 and 14 years of age, who share a commitment not to smoke and to lead a healthy life. Other clubs exist in Europe, and there are no doubt several organizers at this conference. The European Network on Young People and Tobacco gives the organizers in each country the opportunity to gather and to exchange knowledge and know-how at European meetings. The aim of this presentation is, first, to list the objectives of the movement and to outline by means of examples of practical action the methods we have used to achieve these objectives. The second part emphasizes the difficulties involved in assessing the efficiency of this action.

In Belgium, the percentage of regular tobacco consumption is on the increase within all age groups. Smoking starts at an early age: at the age of 11, 15% of boys and 7% of girls have already experimented with smoking. Girls catch up with boys at the age of 13 and overtake them at 15 in terms of experimentation and regular smoking. After the age of 15, the percentage of smokers continues to rise among boys, while it remains stable among girls. These figures show that our target age is justified. Since the first contact with tobacco is at the age of 11, children must be informed when much younger.

Quite apart from the importance of the transmission of knowledge, we are determined to go further with this initiative and to change certain behaviour patterns: to reinforce 'self-assertion', the possibility to say no; to develop attitudes unfavourable to the consumption of tobacco and favourable to a healthy lifestyle (sport, food vs. drugs, alcohol) and to help reduce the numbers of young people who smoke. The methods used to achieve these objectives include the widespread distribution of a health education newsletter, partnerships with schools around the country and activities in the field.

Smokebusters Info: The *club's health education newsletter*
This newsletter, which is sent out to members once every three months, was initially devoted entirely to information about tobacco. The problem of tobacco consumption was tackled from medical, psychological, economic and historical standpoints. Gradually, and against the background of the definition of health given by the World Health Organization (WHO), the newsletter opened up to encompass a number of other issues such as nutrition, sport and the environment. We always discuss issues in a

positive way: a healthy lifestyle is to some extent the slogan and driving force behind the club, rather than slogans that talk of fear, dire warnings and death.

We also invite researchers in education and teachers involved with children of the club's age group to participate in editing the newspaper. First, we get some ideas on the content of each issue, and the texts are then tested in the classrooms of our teachers. The desired feedback tells us how readable and interesting the texts are and to what extent they meet the expectations of our readers.On this basis, we decided to make the newsletter more readable, using graphics that are more appealing to a younger audience.

In general, the aim of this new approach is to create interaction at class and at individual level. At the individual level, we get feedback from the letters of readers varying in content from queries about health issues to drawings and poems. In addition, contests are organized on a regular basis to encourage the club members to be more active, responsible and committed.

Exchanges with schools

We decided to send *Smokebusters Info* to all the primary schools in the country to instigate lessons and discussions within the framework of the health education syllabus. This initiative led to requests for additional documentation on tobacco consumption and on the club itself and brought in new members. Some classes have organized independent health campaigns for pupils in other classes. *Smokebusters Info* publishes brief reports on these initiatives. Some schools call on our services to study issues more thoroughly in the form of a workshop or a visit to the Infomobile, a mobile information unit.

Activities in the field

Some of our field activities are meetings in a fun park, releasing European balloons during the European Week against Cancer and a petition to impose a total ban on tobacco advertising in Europe. The last initiative is a good example of young Belgian and European non-smokers taking action and assuming responsibility. The members received a petition form with the newsletter and were asked to collect signatures for a total ban on tobacco advertising in Europe. A total of 90 000 signatures were collected! This provided us with a fine media opportunity when we handed the signatures over to the President of the European Parliament at the World No-Tobacco Day on 31 May. The petition was officially registered by the European Parliament.

Evaluation

In 1992, our association solicited the opinions of the readers and their expectations from the club in a qualitative study. The young readers had a very positive view of the quarterly publication and even wanted it to be published every month. They were proud to belong to the club and wanted to play a more active role. A series of practical measures was implemented in 1992 to meet the expectations of the members.

The Belgian Cancer Association carried out a quantitative survey among its members in 1997. The suggested improvements to the newsletter concerned the colours used, more articles about tobacco and more games; they wanted more realistic graphics.

To what extent is the enhanced ability of young people to say no actually reinforced? At the end of the day, how efficient is the newsletter? Does it help reduce the number of smokers? A very broad-based survey should be carried out to demonstrate the efficiency of the club, but the cost of such a survey has made this project unfeasible. It would have to be carried out on a large scale and would have to involve at least 3000 respondents. When we follow up the participants four or five years later to see how many have started to smoke, we will have lost around 50% of the sample population because of mobility. We will also need a control group. Another problem is the possibility that former Smokebusters who have since started to smoke may feel guilty and refuse to respond at the time of the second survey.

This initiative has positive points but it also has its limits. The mail we receive, the queries from the schools and our surveys certainly reveal enthusiasm for the initiative, but this movement alone cannot combat the tobacco habit. It must be supported and relayed by education in the home, in schools and in sports clubs and by legal measures that are applied and respected. It is important to make the necessary adjustments on a regular basis to ensure that the movement meets the expectations and needs of young people with regard to health. That is precisely what we are trying to do.

Health education and changes in students' smoking habits at vocational institutions and senior secondary schools in Finland

A.-E. Liimatainen-Lamberg

National Board of Education, Helsinki, Finland

The purpose of this follow-up survey was to explain changes in the smoking habits, attitudes and related factors of 3129 first-year students at 30 vocational institutions and senior secondary schools in 1986–87. Students were surveyed at the beginning and end of the school year, and headmasters and physical education teachers were asked about the smoking culture, health education and its development.

More than 33% of the male students and 28% of the female students smoked daily, but the prevalence varied by type of educational institution: while almost 40% of the female students at the commercial institutions and male students at the vocational institutions smoked daily, only about 12% of the students at the senior secondary school smoked regularly, and the girls smoked a little more often than the boys. About 24 % of the students at the health-care institutions smoked daily. The students had adopted their smoking habits early, before entering these institutions. Few changed their habits during the first school year.

Their attitudes predicted their smoking habits, in that the most negative attitudes towards smoking were found among those who did not smoke, while those who smoked daily held the most positive attitudes towards smoking. Smoking was found to be so well established, that the attitudes at the beginning of the autumn semester predicted smoking during the spring semester, despite the fact that most of the students had circled the option, "I smoke now but intend to quit" as they entered the educational institutions.

The health education they received proved to give little information about health problems. About 85% of the students recalled that smoking had been discussed at least during one health education session, usually in those given by physical education teachers, and when visiting the school nurse. The emphasis had been on the health problems caused by smoking, while information about responsibility for and inquiry into smoking during employment had been almost non-existent. Most of the students considered that the smoking-related sessions had been important but ordinary. More male than female students felt that the sessions had been poor or boring. Over 70% of the students considered that relationships between smoking and various occupations should be discussed more than was being done currently at the educational institutions.

Opinions about how many employees in various occupations smoked varied according to which students were questioned. Students at the vocational and commercial institutions believed that their own future colleagues smoked a lot, while the students in the senior secondary school and those of the health-care institutions believed the reverse. These beliefs were strengthened during the school year and were reflected in the smoking habits of these students. Health habits are thus related to the development of an occupational identity.

Young people are criticized about their smoking and drinking habits as a group. In doing this, health education in Finland is not reaching its target group. Different kinds of students have different needs. How should we offer health education to students in a health-care institution who will become health educators themselves? How should we approach students at a commercial institution, a vocational institution or a senior secondary school? Attitudes may be affected through role modelling, examples and school practices. The quality of health education is of the essence. Students expect to receive professional teaching based on appropriate knowledge and skills especially designed for them.

Since students have quickly begun smoking early, the demand for health education during compulsory schooling, which lasts for 12 years, is considerable. Despite the fact that there is no such subject as health education in the school curriculum, the tasks of health education should be recognized. Attitudes towards health education reflect the attitudes of decision-makers towards health promotion among children and adolescents in Finland, which is a model country in the WHO programme of Health for All by the Year 2000.

Many educational institutions prepare students for various occupations, and the health behaviour of their students and institutional health education practices have hardly been investigated. The educational code of health promotion that would best support effective health education needs to be explored.

Intervention against smoking among boys in urban junior middle schools in China

H. Ma, Y. Hu & B-Y. Zhang

National Health Education Institute, China

The study

We conducted a study between April and October 1996 on the smoking behaviour of 3300 boys, selected by random cluster sampling, in junior middle schools in four cities in China. We divided the boys randomly into three groups: general intervention, high-intensity intervention and controls. The study consisted of three sessions of investigation, comprising individual interviews and small group discussions, and two stages of intervention. The procedure of practice–summary–re-practice–re-summary was adopted in order to find an effective intervention method. The data were analysed with Epi-Info and SAS software, and effectiveness of the intervention was evaluated by matched analysis.

Baseline survey

The smoking rate of the 3300 students was 4.0%; 26% had ever smoked. Most of the boys (60%) had smoked their first cigarette out of curiosity, 18% by imitation and 11% for emotional reasons. The age at which they had smoked their first cigarette was ≤ 10 years for 36% and 10–13 years of age for 57%; most of them (33%) had begun at 12–13, which is the age at which pupils leave primary school and enter junior middle school. The average score for knowledge was 37.6, and the average score for beliefs was 72.0.

Intervention

In the general intervention, small group discussions, drawing competitions, videos and specimens of lung tumours were used. It also involved establishment of a no-smoking class, a no-smoking school and writing letters to parents and teachers. In the high-intensity intervention, factors and misconceptions in taking up tobacco smoking, such as curiosity, socializing and being manly, were analysed; then, relevant counter-measures were sought to help the boys master refusal skills and to choose a healthy lifestyle without smoking.

The scores for knowledge and beliefs about smoking increased significantly ($p <$ 0.01) in both intervention groups, whereas those of the control group remained approximately the same or, for beliefs, even decreased. The rates of smoking were also reduced significantly ($p < 0.01$) in both intervention groups, from 3.5% before the general intervention to 1.5% afterwards and from 2.8% before the high-intensity intervention to 2.0% afterwards; however, that in the control group rose significantly ($p < 0.01$), from 3.4% before the time of the intervention to 4.5% after that time.

The results show that analysis of the factors that led the boys to smoke their first cigarette and teaching them counter-measures is an effective means of preventing them from smoking. On the basis of the results, we developed a set of practical health education materials to foster a new non-smoking generation. Steps must be taken in primary school to prevent children from smoking their first cigarette, and each school should undertake anti-smoking education.

A programme to prevent Indonesian youth from smoking

L.A. Hanafiah

Heart Foundation of Indonesia, Jakarta, Indonesia

The regulations issued by the Minister of Education and Culture and the Minster of Internal Affairs in Indonesia ban smoking in school communities, and non-governmental organizations, such as the Heart Foundation of Indonesia, are also playing a more active role in the prevention of smoking. Nevertheless, the prevalence of smoking in our country appear to be on the increase, especially among the young.

The emphasis of our programme is to prevent smoking. The target is high-school students, as young people are still easily influenced and searching for their identity. The programme was first tested on first-year students in 50 junior high-schools in Jakarta and is now part of the school curriculum in both public and private junior high-schools in that city.

The module was designed to give young people the right motivations for not smoking and to develop in them the skills to refuse smoking. The module was based on the assumption that young people start smoking because they are offered cigarettes or given the opportunity to smoke in places of recreation, in the homes of friends who smoke, at parties and in similar situations. The module can be given individually, although group study is preferable. The methods include interviews with smokers and non-smokers to determine the environments and situations in which cigarettes are offered, problem-solving and simulating situations in which cigarettes are offered. These methods help young people to internalize the information, to become aware of the dangers of smoking and to decide not to smoke.

In our study of junior high-school students, we found that their knowledge about the hazards of smoking and ways of resisting smoking had increased. Most of the students tried to quit, and some students tried to influence members of their families and their friends to stop smoking. The prevention of smoking cannot be limited to the provision of information but must also address behaviour. Factual information is necessary as part of the framework of changing smoking behaviour. The norms and values that accompany the smoking habot must be clarified, and the skills to make decisions must be developed. Our programme, which is orientated to resistance in situations where cigarettes are offered, has been effective in forming the right attitudes of young people towards smoking.

Life education: Prevention starts in primary school

M.M.H. Yu-Chan

Life Education Activity Programme, Hong Kong SAR, China

The Life Education Activity Programme (LEAP) is an international, school-based health awareness and drug prevention educational programme aimed at primary-school children aged 5–12. It originated in Australia and was introduced into Hong Kong in 1994, initially at English-language schools and later in local Chinese schools. Life Education is brought to schools in a mobile classroom equipped with state-of-the-art techniques such as audiovisual equipment, an illuminated human body model, electronic body system modules and Harold the giraffe, our mascot, who talks and sings to the children to reinforce our messages.

Life Education programmes include all of the components of drug education proved to be effective: close partnerships with participating schools, developmentally appropriate information about drugs, training in refusal skills, challenging adolescents' myths about drugs and interactive teaching techniques that emphasize student participation, group work and role play. Life Education is aware of the need for a partnership approach to school-based drug education. Research has shown that this approach consolidates student learning outcomes. In order to facilitate this approach, we provide a consultative service to schools before the visit of the mobile classroom as well as follow-up and ongoing support. We also provide adult education programmes for parents.

We believe, and this is supported by the results of a six-year study carried out at Cornell University Medical College in 1994 involving nearly 6000 students from 56 schools in New York State, that any prevention programme will be effective only if it is properly implemented over a long period. Because there are many competing demands on the school schedule, it is sometimes difficult to teach drug abuse prevention programmes in their entirety; studies show, however, that there is a direct relationship between how much of the prevention programme is implemented and its effectiveness. If prevention programmes are only partly implemented, they are not likely to prevent or reduce drug use. Drug abuse prevention programmes must be taught at least throughout the primary school years and preferably throughout high school. Prevention programmes that last only one year and do not contain two more years of booster sessions are not likely to produce sustained reductions in drug use. In fact, evaluations of prevention programmes that did not include booster sessions have shown that initial reductions in drug use decrease after a year and disappear totally after about two or three years. Life Education programmes run for seven consecutive years, from kindergarten to grade 6, and cover a multiplicity of age-appropriate health awareness and drug preventive programmes.

One of the main challenges in bringing Life Education to Hong Kong was its cultural adaptability and its conversion into a Chinese programme. Instead of a direct translation from the English, we made cultural adaptations to suit Hong Kong's needs. We use language that is appropriate to the local students and which reflects local popular culture, interests and lifestyles. Scenarios for discussion and role play are always realistic local situations which the students can relate to comfortably. Even with these modifications, however, we were still concerned about the acceptance of our methods by Chinese schools. They have a much tighter curriculum and employ a more conservative approach in their teaching methods than in many western countries. Our concerns were soon dispelled, however, when we demonstrated our programme to them. The response from the schools was overwhelmingly positive, and our first Chinese mobile classroom was fully booked on the first day of its introduction in 1995.

Our programmes for upper primary classes are particularly focused on smoking and alcohol. The uniqueness of the programme lies in its creative, highly communicative methods. Our educators act as facilitators in group discussions. Through constructed role-play situations, we help children develop the social skills to handle situations in which they are offered cigarettes or alcohol without losing face or friends. For example, in the Year 6 programme, we organize a camp-fire evening for the students in the mobile classroom. The excitement begins when the lights go out, the star ceiling is switched on and the kids are gathered around a bonfire on the video, creating a real-life yet awe-inspiring atmosphere. Through active discussion in relaxed atmospheres like this, we provide the children with social competency and strategies to resist peer pressure.

The educator employs a warm and genuine manner with the students, treating them with respect. This involves active listening, acceptance of their opinions, welcoming their questions and recognizing their contributions. Peer pressure, internal anxiety and stress are recognized, and social competency skills to withstand these pressures are emphasized throughout the programmes.

A segment of our Year 5 programme shows Tony, an adolescent smoker, who is handsome; many of the students think he looks cool. The story later shows how Tony is rejected by his girlfriend because of his bad breath and yellow, smelly fingers. Tony is not welcomed in many public places such as cinemas and restaurants. This material is effective because it brings out the more immediate concerns of adolescents about the negative side-effects of smoking. A 12-year old cannot relate to the remote possibility of cancer at the age of 30. Of much more importance are the cosmetic side-effects, not being accepted in public places and the fact that it drains them financially. Through a lot of fun and developmentally appropriate, interesting activities, we provide the students with factual information about the short-term and long-term consequences of smoking, environmental tobaco smoke, alcohol and other drugs. We teach the students that using tobacco and alcohol are not the norm among adolescents and correct the belief that 'everyone is doing it'.

Life Education is not just a one-off visit. The classroom teachers play a vital role in follow-up work, using our teachers' manual and student workbook to ensure that the programme is integrated into the school curriculum. We also conduct training at our centre for teachers from participating schools, to extend their knowledge of drugs and to provide them with Life Education strategies to develop their students' social competence. We also provide them with videos, books and teaching aids. We conduct sessions to involve parents in the programme and to show them how they can help at home. Some parents have told us that after their children had attended the Life Education class they warned them about the harmful effects of smoking and asked them to quit smoking or at least to protect the family by not smoking around them.

The performance and effectiveness of Life Education are carefully monitored through evaluations of teachers on a questionnaire which they are asked to fill in after each visit. The purpose is to ascertain their views on the programme, its components and their effectiveness and to elicit suggestions for alterations and improvements. The response of teachers and principals has been overwhelmingly positive. Our most recent evaluation showed that 92% of the teachers thought that the programme enhanced the social skills and needs of the students; 93% thought that Life Education extended the students' knowledge, and 84% thought that more frequent visits would be beneficial for the students.

LEAP is a privately funded nongovernmental organization. We have also received financial assistance and support from Government and community-minded organizations. LEAP now operates five centres targeting over 40 000 students.

No-smoking competitions for young people in Finland

M. Paavola, E. Vartiainen & P. Puska

National Public Health Institute, Helsinki, Finland

Two types of non-smoking competition have been organized for young people in Finland. The first, the 'Smoke-free class competition', has been organized annually since the school year 1989–90. The aim is to prevent the onset of smoking among pupils aged 13–14. Each class decides as a group if it want to be a smoke-free class for the next half year, from 1 October to 31 March. The classes in which all of the pupils refrain from smoking for six months can participate in a lottery with financial prizes. The two main prizes represent about US$ 2000 each. At the end of the period, every smoke-free class receives a diploma.

Classes make the decision to participate themselves. All the pupils must agree to participate and sign a commitment form not to smoke during the programme. Classes monitor non-smoking by their members by filling in a follow-up form. At the end of the competition, the forms are sent to the programme office for the lottery. The competition is based on mutual trust. If someone starts smoking during the competition and is not able to quit, the class drops out. The competition has been very popular, involving up to half of the pupils in the age cohorts, which means nearly 60 000 pupils. Only one-third of them, however, 'survive' to the end of the competition.

The classes have a contact teacher who helps them during the competition and also organizes health education sessions about smoking. The material is free for schools and partly designed to be used on the Internet (http://www.jyu.fi/no-smoking). It is available in English, Finnish, French and Swedish. Since 1997, some famous Finnish role models for young people, like stars of film, music and sport, have been supporting the competition in public. The Finnish competition is organized by five voluntary organizations and is financed by the Ministry of Health and Social Affairs. The competition was organized at the European level during the school year 1997–98, financed by the Europe against Cancer Programme of the European Commission. Seven regions—Denmark, Finland, France, Germany, Italy, Spain and Wales—participated at least regionally.

The competition was evaluated among pupils in the eighth grade, involving 1219 classes (23 012 pupils). Of these, 65 were randomly selected for the study. A control group of 30 classes was selected randomly from among those that did not enter the competition. Of the 65 participating classes, 28 finished the competition and 37 dropped out. Pupils in the classes filled in forms before, one month after and one year after the competition. Before the competition, smoking was more common in the control classes than in the classes participating in the competition, and smoking was almost as common in the classes that dropped out as in the control classes. The results showed that there was significantly less onset of smoking in those classes that participated in the competition. In a test for the difference between participants and controls by the regression analysis, the increase in smoking was similar between before the test and the second post-test. The main conclusion of the evaluation was that the competition at least delays the onset of smoking.

The second competition, the 'Non-smoking contest for young people', was tested for the first time during the school year 1996–97. The target group is 15–25-year olds. The contest is based on individual participation, with financial prizes in lotteries after one month and after half a year. About 100 000 application cards were sent to young people, mainly through schools, and a total of 18 060 returned the forms. Young people could participate either by remaining non-smokers (14 819) or by quitting smoking (3241). After one month, 40% of those who had tried to quit smoking were still non-smokers.

These two competitions have been popular in Finland, and the evaluation of the 'Smoke-free class competition' has shown that it prevents or at least delays the onset of smoking. It was therefore also tested at the European level to give us more experience on how it works in different countries.

Towards smoke-free schools

T. Fraser

Action on Smoking and Health (ASH), Auckland, New Zealand

In New Zealand, schools are not required by law to be smoke-free, and schools are not specified in the Smoke-free Environments Act, which covers offices specifically. Workplaces and schools fit within these categories. ASH is promoting the idea that all schools, including buildings and grounds, should be totally smoke-free, seven days a week, 24 hours a day. We believe that attitudes will be changed by pushing the message for smoke-free schools in the community.

In the Smoke-free Environments Act of 1990, schools are considered workplaces. As a workplace, a school must meet a number of minimum requirements. A staffroom can have a designated smoking area. If it is the lunchroom, 50% of the staffroom can be designated a smoking area. The areas in schools that can be legally designated as smoking areas are all offices with single occupation, the staffroom, enclosed areas occupied exclusively by staff who request smoking be permitted and school grounds

Smoke-free school projects in Wellington, 1994–96

Two smoke-free schools projects were undertaken by Hutt Valley Health and the Cancer Society (Wellington Division) which involved 215 schools. The initial project included 15 intermediate schools, and the second included 200 primary and secondary schools in the Wellington region. The intermediate project had two phases: the first covered policy and the second was smoke-free education for teachers. The project in primary and secondary schools was undertaken by Hutt Valley Health alone and was addressed to policy only.

The schools were visited to establish where they were between not complying with the Act and being totally smoke-free. The continuum line included not complying, complying, smoke-free buildings, smoke-free buildings and grounds and totally smoke-free. Officers and public health nurses worked with the schools towards becoming smoke-free.

By the end of the project, 112 schools had visible no-smoking signs compared with 110 before the project; 72 were complying with the Smoke-free Environments Act, compared with 41 schools before; 127 schools had written policies, compared with 121 before, and 60 schools were totally smoke-free, compared with 54 before the project.

Some problems were encountered in the project. One was that the schools were concerned about teachers' rights. Many believed that a human rights issue is involved and teachers have the right to smoke at school. Secondly, the public health nurses had to maintain a relationship with the pupils and were sometimes compromised in their work with schools for that reason. Shortage of funds means that schools often have to hire halls to groups with no restrictions on smoking. The schools were also concerned that the no-smoking policy would discourage parents from attending functions and meetings. Many schools have poor parental attendance at school events, and they worried that if smoking were banned the numbers of parents attending could drop further.

Although the results of the projects do not appear to be significant, the anti-smoking climate in New Zealand is increasing, and ASH is receiving regular reports of schools that are becoming totally smoke-free. The two projects have had some effect on these results. Since the projects were undertaken, two more schools have become totally smoke-free.

Recommendations

Smoke-free school projects should be undertaken on a regional basis and followed-up continuously. The law states that smoke-free policies should be reviewed annually. Independent advocates should push for legislation on totally smoke-free schools. Advocacy should be undertaken with the community, the education and health sectors and politicians. Surveys undertaken to provide evidence of the need to legislate show that many schools would find it easier if legislation were enacted; however, submissions for change in legislation must be accompanied by evidence that the change is required.

Options beyond smoke-free schools include monitoring local tobacco outlets. Schools may choose to include local tobacco outlets as part of their school policy, by contacting them and requesting them not to sell cigarettes to the students. A newsletter could be sent to parents, informing them of the policy, including monitoring of tobacco outlets. Parents could be requested to talk to children about smoking and to quit smoking themselves if possible, to support the school's smoke-free policy. Quit smoking courses and products should be provided for teachers and students, with counselling for students addicted to tobacco.

Reinforcing factors might include the Ministry of Health's guidelines for smoke-free schools and the Cancer Society's resources. Prosecutions under the Smoke-free Environments Act should be supported by the Ministry of Health. The Ministry is providing a supportive environment for taking prosecutions. No school has yet been prosecuted, but ASH believes that if the Ministry were presented with evidence of non-compliance, they would be prepared to take a case. This could have the effect of mobilizing other schools that are lagging in compliance.

Passive smoking is not covered by accident compensation. Boards of trustees consisting of volunteer parents, who are the employers at schools, could be sued in the future if a teacher or student suffered from a tobacco-caused illness. Increasing litigation overseas and recent papers on passive smoking from Australia and the United States make this a more likely scenario than ever before.

Smoking is finally starting to get the attention it deserves, and attitudes are changing. It is now time to make changes that would have been unacceptable a few years ago.

The present situation

ASH is promoting the concept of totally smoke-free schools at every opportunity. The Cancer Society has provided resources for smoke-free schools for all primary and intermediate schools. The Ministry of Health has developed a smoke-free guideline as part of their Healthy Schools document, which has been sent to all schools in New Zealand; it encourages schools to have a totally smoke-free policy. Several Crown Health Enterprises, which usually have public health units, have undertaken smoke-free school projects. The Health Sponsorship Council provides smoke-free signs to be displayed at the entrances of schools, and these are donated to schools that are totally smoke-free. The National Heart Foundation provides certificates to totally smoke-free schools, which are framed in silver and look very professional.

By the year 2000, all schools in New Zealand will be totally smoke-free. This will have been achieved by changes in legislation and health promotion strategies.

Youth are the leaders of today

D. Grande

American Cancer Society, Tucson, Arozona, United States

Background

In November 1995, a five-year, US$ 3.2 million grant from the Robert Wood Johnson Foundation was awarded to the Coalition for a Tobacco Free Arizona to develop a partnership of organizations in Tucson, Arizona, in order to design a prototype programme to help young people to quit smoking or not to start. National models such as those used for the American Stop Smoking Intervention Study for Cancer Prevention programme of the National Cancer Institute, were used to develop an operational framework, with lessons learned from other tobacco programmes and youth projects. Marketing principles were employed to develop a programme that would engage both the adult community and the adolescent population. A multifaceted plan incorporating a comprehensive tobacco control plan with community development was developed and implemented. The key ingredients were youth leadership, empowerment, adult–youth team building and innovative risk-taking which would allow all creative ideas to be considered.

Getting started

If the goal is only to affect tobacco use, the behaviour of adolescents with regard to tobacco will not be affected. Adolescents are facing a number of issues that go beyond tobacco use. A person working with youth must be sensitive to the place of adolescents in the community and how adults see them, for instance as a problem. The world of young people is relatively separate from that of adults, although there is coexistence. The needs, wants and desires of young people must be understood in order to affect their behaviour. They also have skills and talents that should be put to good use.

In Tucson, 'Full Court Press' served as a bridge between the adult and the young communities. This diverse group comprising both adults and young people could act as a 'full court press', a basketball term describing an all-out effort to beat the opposition.

Building trust

Adolescents with particular skills, talents and needs were identified by adults in the partnership. Others were recruited from among community service volunteers working at the American Cancer Society for high-school credits or for disciplinary reasons. Adolescents who lacked self-esteem or certain skills were also identified because they were considered to be in the best position to speak to their peers about high-risk behaviour.

The adults worked diligently with the young to engage them in the issue, using a process and vocabulary they could understand. Before jumping into the tobacco control agenda, the adults listened to the adolescents' concerns, asked questions about their experiences, treated them with respect and built trust.

Gaining knowledge

A community assessment was conducted to learn more about the environment and identify opportunities for raising awareness of the programme, creating changes in public policy and mobilizing various segments of the population of Tucson. One important opportunity for action was limiting the access of young people to tobacco products. The national focus on adolescent tobacco use, the emphasis of the programme on youth and the fact that Tucson had a history of restricting tobacco-vending machines directed us towards youth access. The Full Court Press partnership included a full-time police detective who was trained in conducting compliance checks and had years of experience of working with youth. We trained other adults and youth in the process, explored potential concern in the community and City Council and gathered information on the media perspective.

Relationships

Building relationships is the key to success in community action with youth or adults. A close relationship was built with staff of the State Health Department working on the media campaign and supported by tobacco taxes. This allowed us to coordinate efforts and benefit from media purchases that would have been prohibitive in the Full Court Press budget. Relationships were quickly established with the local media in

Tucson and with the Mayor and City Council, who would be instrumental in helping us to achieve our goals.

Throughout the process of building relationships and learning more about community expectations, adolescents were teamed with adults. This adult–youth collaboration provided a unique aspect to our programme and showed the community that we were serious about bridging the gap between the two worlds. The respect we showed the adolescents in business meetings reflected the standards of our programme and served as a model for other adults.

Early successes

Young people, like adults, want to have fun. They also want to be part of a winning team, so we were relentless in pursuing our first-year objectives, which were based on building strong community support for our programme and raising awareness of tobacco use among adolescents in order to create community action. The combination of youth–adult teamwork and the initial focus on young people's access to tobacco products proved to be a good combination.

The interns and adolescent volunteers went to 317 establishments to conduct compliance checks and succeeded in purchasing tobacco products in 34% of them. The young people gained valuable skills in following a protocol, investigating and observing tobacco advertising and product placement and filling in forms with the adult for the evaluation. Once the data had been compiled and the facts were ready, the media were invited to a press conference. Eight young people participated in the press conference, held in the police department's press room. Cigarette packs from the illegal sales were used to show the magnitude of the problem. We received over 22 minutes of air time during prime time over three days. Needless to say, the City Council was outraged when they heard the news.

The interns presented the results of the compliance checks at the next City Council meeting. They used video coverage to highlight and remind Council members of what their constituents had seen on the news. They stressed the need for action to protect young people from gaining easy access to tobacco. After the presentation, Full Court Press was assigned to work as technical advisors to draft an ordinance for full Council consideration.

Since we were pursuing a Government regulation, we needed to understand the internal dynamics of City politics. We met with a number of individuals in City government to hear their concerns and to achieve a better understanding of the issues and the Government process for licensing and issuing citations. The young people were involved throughout and offered advice and provided credibility.

We knew that one of our outcomes was a strong ordinance on access, but our main outcome was a skilled, informed group of youngsters who were empowered to affect political change and the ability of adults in leadership to respect them. Had we focused only on the ordinance and not on the process with the young people, we would not have the strength we have today.

Closing the deal

Through group discussions and networking, we identified key people in the community to whom both young people and adults listened, and we recruited them onto our team. Ten key community leaders either testified or wrote to City Council in support of passing an ordinance to license tobacco vendors and to ban self-service displays of tobacco.

Because the young people were involved in every step, from beginning to end, they had ownership. They recruited their friends to support the ordinance during the public hearing. The standing-room-only crowd consisted of an equal number of adults and young people.

Educating third-graders against smoking

A. Winder, M. Barnes & A. Geller

Boston University, Boston, Massachudetts, United States

Introduction

Educating third-grade schoolchildren (eight to nine years old) against smoking was conceived as an approach to counter the success of the tobacco industry's advertising targeted to young children The intervention involved a poster contest, a hands-on curriculum and evaluation. Many children in the United States begin smoking at the of age 10, in fourth grade. We designed our intervention for eight-to nine-year olds. We had two purposes. The first was to establish baseline data on the knowledge of third graders about the health effects of smoking, their attitudes towards smoking and their intention to smoke. The second purpose was to address and target third graders with educational materials developed specifically for them in order to change their knowledge, attitude and perceptions of smoking and their intention to smoke.

Method

The population was drawn from counties in Massachusett, including the City of Springfield, and the smaller cities of Chicopee and Holyoke. These three cities contain a large minority population. Hampden County also includes several affluent suburbs, while Hampshire County is predominantly rural. The final sample included 46 schools, 86 classes, all third grades and 1486 student. These break down into 37 urban classes, 28 suburban classes and 19 rural classes.

A learning packet on smoking and smokeless tobacco was prepared and distributed to all teachers involved in the project. The packet consisted of a teacher's guide, class demonstrations and games and extended activities. The demonstrations are especially appealing to third graders. The curriculum and evaluation instruments were delivered to the schools and the teachers were briefed and given a standardized procedure on their administration.

The evaluation instrument was prepared in two forms, a pre-test and a post-test. The forms were tested for readability and to make sure the questions elicited similar responses. The instrument measured knowledge about health risks from smoking, intention to smoke, attitudes towards smoking and perceptions of smokers.

Results

The pupils were given nine questions on knowledge, nine on attitude and three on intention to smoke; 71% gave correct answers to the knowledge questions; 66% judged the attitude questions to be unfavourable to smokers, and 83% did not intend to smoke.

In order to determine the effect of an educational intervention on the pupils' knowledge, attitudes, intentions and perceptions, we determined whether boys and girls differed in their total scores before and after the intervention. No difference was found. The only difference before and after the intervention was in knowledge, which improved appreciably. Significant differences were also found among urban, suburban and rural schools, the urban children having higher scores. Using factor analysis, we found two clearly identifiable factors: children's perception of smokers as possessing admirable traits and their perception of smokers as possessing undesirable traits.

Some limitations of this study were that there was a period of three to six weeks between the pre- and post-tests, and the large sample made it impossible to monitor the teachers' presentation of the curriculum. Some data were lost because teachers turned in only the pre- or post-tests, which might have affected the sample.

Discussion and conclusion

The baseline data reveal that third graders are fairly knowledgeable about the health effects of smoking. They are, however, less inclined to judge smoking negatively. Nevertheless, over two-thirds stated they would not become smokers; widespread advertising by the tobacco industry may explain the positive attitudes of a large minority. Finally, although our sample is large and diverse, it is drawn from only one state and may not reflect the rest of the country. In response to the curriculum, the only significant difference among the three sub-tests was on knowledge, which is not unexpected. Attitude questions are hard to write, and attitudes change more slowly than knowledge, which may have been responsible for the insignificant change before and after the intervention. No significant change in intention not to smoke was measurable since the great majority (82%) of the third graders stated that they intend not to smoke. More perplexing were the results of the factor analysis of student perceptions. Some students assigned admirable traits to smokers, and some assigned undesirable traits. This dichotomy may represent the emotional struggle that third graders face between conformity and rebellion.

A most significant result was that urban students had the greatest increase in total score, possibly because, in this sample, the urban students receive less health education and were therefore the most likely to benefit from a hands-on curriculum. In conclusion, therefore, urban and minority students need such interventions. This study demonstrates that a small, inexpensive effort can produce significant results.

'Staying safe': Smoking education for adolescents

L. Wiseman

Life Education Australia and Life Education Activity Programme (Hong Kong), Potts Point, New South Wales, Australia

Life Education Australia provides school-based drug education for 1.1 million primary-school pupils annually throughout Australia, using a nationwide network of more than 150 educators operating from 112 mobile and six static classrooms. Established in Sydney, Australia, in 1979, Life Education now operates over 200 classrooms in eight regions, including England, Hong Kong, New Zealand, Papua New Guinea, South Africa, Thailand and the United States. To fulfil its mission statement, 'excellence in drug education', Life Education Australia is implementing programmes on smoking, alcohol and marijuana in secondary schools throughout Australia.

Around 28 000 Australians die of drug-related causes each year: 20 000 (72%) from tobacco, 7000 (25%) from alcohol and 1000 (3%) from illicit drugs, mainly heroin. The direct and indirect costs of use of legal and illegal drugs in Australia is estimated to be around AUS$ 20 billion annually, due mainly to tobacco and alcohol use. Australia's triennial surveys of drug use in secondary schools and a national survey of drug use in households provide accurate data on the actual use among students. The three drugs used most commonly by secondary-school students are alcohol, tobacco and marijuana.

To determine what would most influence student smoking behaviour, bi-annual Quantum Harris Youth Monitor surveys and youth market research by leading Australian advertising agencies were used to probe issues such as the changing patterns of youth spending, use of leisure time, attitudes towards social and technological change, future priorities and popular fashions. In both the 1992 and 1995 surveys, the three major worries for 10- to 17-year olds were, in order, 'not getting a job', 'not being successful' and 'needing to make money'. It would therefore appear salient for many secondary students to stress that the most popular legal and illegal drugs are expensive. The market research also suggests that the idea of 'peer pressure', still found so frequently in drug education programmes, is not only rejected by most secondary-school students (as a put-down by parents and other adults) but is also dangerously out of date. Secondary-school students often belong to many peer groups, not just one.

Group activities may involve hanging out at the local mall, school band or sporting practice and dance or drama groups. Different behaviour may be adopted by these different groups, including that related to the opportunities to experiment with or use various drugs. It is useful to compare the features of the school drug education programmes preferred by students and teachers with the keys principles of school drug-education identified as effective in research literature. The common features of successful school-based programmes about which there is some consensus are described by Dusenbury and Falco (1995) and Botvin (1995). Recurrent themes in what young people want from school drug education included:

- fun, not fear,
- realism: 'show it how it is',
- honest, open discussion,
- opportunities to hear other young people's views,
- 'respect for our opinions' and
- 'hands-on stuff'.

In researching the means whereby students could best participate in programmes, an obvious choice was multimedia, which readily lends itself to 'situation learning', a case-based approach in which students view situations that act as a basis for realistic problem solving. In this experience-based approach to the learning process, pedagogical emphasis moves away from a didactic or teacher-centred mode and towards a more problem-based teaching mode, leaving room for increased student-to-student learning (Lewis & Treves, 1996). By using technology, the Life Education presenter is no longer the means by which information is conveyed but rather the facilitator of discussion, investigation, interpretation and problem-solving. In studies in other countries, multimedia have been shown to achieve significant improvements in student performance.

'Staying safe': Life Education's smoking education programme for students in years 7 and 8

In 1995–96, Life Education, with the cooperation of the Government, Catholic school systems and youth agencies, conducted focus groups with head teachers of personal development, health and physical education in eight Government and non-government, co-educational and single-sex schools. Evaluations were provided by 950 students who attended pilot alcohol and smoking sessions in year 7. Question times were conducted with more than 200 secondary-school classes in years 7 and 8. These focus groups helped to determine the smoking-related issues most salient to these students, the range of attitudes and the local situations, influences and potential harms most likely to engage junior secondary-school students and facilitate classroom discussion.

Having determined the content and direction of the smoking programme, Life Education employed Ruby Pictures, a small Melbourne film and video production company with flair and youthful energy, in collaboration with the Youth Research Centre of the University of Melbourne to research and produce a CD ROM entitled 'Dahtrooth about Cigarettes'. The CD ROM is shown on a multimedia projector to the whole class. During the Life Education sessions, students work with partners and in small groups of four to six. 'Dahtrooth about Cigarettes' provides maximum opportunities for student-centred learning, the audio-visual material being used to engage the student's attention. After each CD ROM 'page', the students discuss the information and situations depicted, look at alternatives, make decisions about hypothetical situations and participate in role plays based on local places and situations.

To support the programmes and assist teachers, Life Education Australia provides parent programmes, sessions for teachers, lesson plans for teachers, student workbooks and work-sheets and audiovisual aids. All resources are produced as curriculum-specific units of work to help ensure that the Life Education resources form part of an integrated, flexible programme that meets local student needs, Australia-wide curriculum requirements and various school cultures. The resources are developed in consultation and collaboration with governments, school systems, public and private drug education consultants and teachers and students in pilot schools.

References
Botvin, G.J., Baker, E., Dusenbury, L. & Botvin, E.M. (1995) Long-term follow-up results of a randomised
    drug abuse prevention trial in a middle-class population. *J. Am. Med. Assoc.*
Dusenbury, L. & Falco, M. (1995) Eleven components of effective drug abuse prevention curricula. *J.
    School Health*
Lewis, D.C. & Treves, J.A. (1996) The drug policy debate in the virtual classroom. *Int. J. Drug Policy*, 7

Swedish Teachers against Tobacco

C. Satterberg

Teachers against Tobacco, Stockholm, Sweden

Schools are the largest employer in Sweden, and every day, thousands of teachers work with hundreds of thousands of children and young people. Because of this daily interaction, teachers have a unique opportunity to influence students to choose a healthy lifestyle. 'Teachers against Tobacco' was organized in 1994 as a small, enthusiastic group of five teachers. Today we have 700 members and a board consisting of five members representing all levels in the Swedish school system. The aim of our organization is to unite all school personnel and support them in working for a tobacco-free school environment, including abstaining from tobacco use themselves and thereby acting as good role models for their pupils.

I have been working for many years as the leader of a project for a tobacco-free school in the County Council of Dalarna to promotes a school environment free from tobacco. The schools that have been most successful have used the following four cornerstones:

Information and agreement

In Sweden, the school culture is based on democratic principles, so that everyone can express an opinion on important issues. The school's principal must ensure that health issues are considered to be important. Together with the teachers, the students and their parents, the principal must draft a policy programme with a clear goal in which good health is the message and dealt with in the same way as other important issues. Information about the policy must be well communicated, so that everyone in the school is prepared for the actions to be taken; for example, aware that when school begins after the summer holidays, it will be smoke free.

Sanctions

It is important that non-observance of the new rules be sanctioned, for otherwise the students will ignore them. For example, student who break the rules should not be allowed to indulge in popular activities like working in the school cafeteria, playing on the football team or working in the computer room after school hours.

Methods

Working with tobacco issues is to a large extent a question of working with attitudes and values. Knowledge of facts is not enough to affect people's behaviour: they need to process their knowledge and practise taking a stand on important issues. Teachers should be offered training on health issues and on methods of working with students' attitudes and values.

Alternatives

The school should offer the students alternative activities to smoking. Instead of joining other students who are going to smoke during breaks, students should join each other in a positive activity such as gymnastics.

These are some examples of the work of Teachers against Tobacco. With the support of Government funding, we are trying to share our knowledge and ideas because, although no one can do everything, everyone can do something in this important issue for our children's health.

Sixteen years' experience of tobacco prevention among children in Sweden

G. Steinwall

A Non Smoking Generation, Stockholm, Sweden

The aim of the organization A Non Smoking Generation is to prevent children and adolescents from taking up the use of tobacco. It is the only organization in Sweden working exclusively with tobacco prevention among children. This non-profit organization, started in 1979, is completely independent of politics and religion and is financed through grants from county councils, industry, private people, local authorities, foundations and the Government. A pool of about 3000 companies supports us. Our annual turnover is about US$ 1 million. Our board members consist of well-known leaders in various industries, advertising, medicine, the law and culture.

Our work covers three areas: information (the school programme) and competitions, campaigns and opinion moulding. Our campaigns, conducted in the general media, are addressed to adults: politicians, decision-makers, opinion leaders and parents. The campaigns of the last three years have attracted huge attention, not only in Sweden but also internationally. The aims of our campaigns and opinion moulding are to reveal the methods of the tobacco industry, to instigate debate about tobacco and to make A Non Smoking Generation an interesting and credible provider of information to schools. The aim, therefore, is to bring about changes of behaviour in our main target group, children and young people aged 11–16.

Information and competitions

Our school programme has had 16 years' experience in tobacco prevention among children. According to a recent survey, the method that we use halves the number of smokers among schoolchildren. We do this by going to schools with a programme appropriate to this group, in order to reinforce the natural attitude against tobacco. The additional aim is to affect attitudes, awareness and involvement in the question of the use of tobacco products. The method involves studying the psychology, pattern of behaviour, values and attitudes of the children. We prepare young people for the day when they are offered a cigarette for the first time, by training them to say 'No, thank you' to tobacco.

In additional to class visits, we have organized school competitions, with information intended to influence attitudes. A total of 1 million children aged 11–16 have been invited over the past 12 years to these competitions, which are the largest in Sweden.

The cornerstones of our method are

- to use young people as sources of information and role models,
- to reach young people just before the age when they run the risk of smoking for the first time, by role play and various exercises in values, and
- to modify their attitudes to tobacco through discussions about lifestyle, self-confidence and peer pressure.

An important aspect of our method is that it is directed towards emotions, attitudes and values by concentrating efforts on behaviour reinforcement. Another important aspect is the role model concept, in which we use young people who have been recruited and trained in our method. When the message 'It is all right and cool not to smoke' is conveyed by a young person to a young person, and not by an adult to a young person, the message is free from adult values. The role models are regarded as slightly older classmates who do not smoke, and the schoolchildren see them as friends to look up to.

The role models must satisfy certain criteria: they must be young and outgoing, i.e not over 25; have completed a three-year high-school course; be firm non-smokers; be able to speak to groups; be ready to take initiatives; be excellent role models for young people, including former candidates for the Miss Sweden title, and be responsible.

The programme has been conducted successfully in Sweden since 1982. A Non Smoking Generation meets an average of about 70 000 schoolchildren in Swedish schools every year, mainly in classes 6 and 7 (ages 12 and 13). Over the 16 years that this work has been carried out, therefore, more than 1 million Swedish young people have been in contact with A Non Smoking Generation at some time during their school days.

Reactions, evalutions and conclusions

The reactions of pupils to our school visits are almost always positive, so that in many cases the role model becomes an idol, some being asked for their autograph after a class visit. This indicates the success of the mission in communicating the message and the possibility of providing a positive, tough, non-smoking role model for young people who is a much better example than the Marlboro Man or Joe Camel.

Annual surveys by an independent institute show that 37% of Swedish 15-year olds received most of their information on tobacco from A Non Smoking Generation. The reactions of teachers are also very positive, as 98.5% answered that it was good or very good on questionnaires handed to them by the role models. Out of a total of 700, none described it as bad.

On our behalf, the Chief Medical Officer of Sweden carried out a study of our method by examining about 40 national and international reports on tobacco prevention work among young people. Most of these studies recommended class visits. The aspects found to be most important were the use of young role models, the value of training young people in arguments against   tobacco and the timing of the information, in early adolescence. Others have identified the involvement that our method creates as an important element: young people are not passively forced into adopting an attitude; they take part and decide for themselves.

Independent surveys in the south of Sweden published in *The Swedish Medical Journal* show that the number of young people who smoke has decreased by 50% in areas in which A Non Smoking Generation has made class visits. Our own survey in Stockholm, based on 4000 answers to questionnaires, shows that a negative attitude to tobacco and tobacco advertising is much more prevalent among young people who have had a class visit than among those who have not. Most pupils wished to receive more information on tobacco in school. The survey showed that the effects were the same regardless of social group.

The visit of the role model usually lasts 80 min. This is of course far too short a time to keep the smoking issue alive in schools, and the role model gives the teachers a guide. More intervention is needed for a permanent effect on behaviour. In order to ensure an upbringing free from tobacco, stronger alliances must be forged with schools and parents, by providing supporting material to parents and educational material and training days for youth leaders, teachers and school managers. We plan to complement our method in this way in the next stage of our work. We are also developing our method to suit 10-year olds.

There is no political action programme on the tobacco issue in Sweden. The issue has never had political priority but is left to organizations like A Non Smoking Generation, the Heart and Lung Association and the Swedish Cancer Society. We have nevertheless achieved results: use of tobacco among young people in Sweden has decreased sharply over the past 20 years, from 44% of Swedish 15-year olds in 1971 to 21% in 1996. There is no doubt that the work of A Non Smoking Generation among children and young people in schools has contributed to this.

Engaging schools and families in tobacco prevention and control

T. Chen

Asia–Pacific Health Promotion and Development, Health Communications and Education Program, Department of Applied Health Sciences, Tulane University School of Public Health and Tropical Medicine, New Orleans, Louisiana, United States

Cigarette smoking is a learned behaviour reinforced by nicotine addiction which begins at an early age. The influences that contribute to the formation of this behaviour include those of parents, siblings, peers and role models, the latter usually exerted through the mass media. Parents who are smokers have children who are more likely to smoke, and nicotine predisposes a foetus at the very beginning of life. Smokers' children are likely to be influenced by their behaviour and become cigarette smokers as they grow up. Control and reduction of parental smoking is therefore crucial in the prevention of smoking by children (Department of Health and Human Services, 1989). Dr Gregory Tsang's paper, 'The family: The key to tobacco control' (this volume) proposes that the family should be targeted to reduce the prevalence of smoking among young people in China. This is in line with Confucious' teaching that one should correct one's own behaviour before correcting family behaviour and righting the wrongs of the world. In order to put Dr Tsang's proposal into effect, however, we need an effective method of stopping adults from smoking. Educating shildren at an early age to persuade their parents to stop smoking is clever and could work well in China, where there is a policy of one child per family and the health of that only child is highly valued by parents and other members of the family.

When children leave the family to enter the school environment, they spend an average of 8 h/day for more that 15 years away from home. During that long time, they learn, imitate and experiment with various positive and negative behaviours, including cigarette smoking. They also learn from books and exhibits designed by schools and outside schools. They learn by chatting with their peers and directly or indirectly modelling others whom they admire. Most smokers begin to smoke in elementary school and become confirmed smokers in junior high school. School is the captive setting in which these young people can be given doses of anti-cigarette smoking vaccine in the form of teaching. This approach is best made in the context of health promotion in which the risk of cigarette smoking is considered along with other major risk factors of health behaviour (Glynn et al., 1993). The successful example of 100 non-smoking schools in Beijing are an example of this approach. Ms Liao Wenke's description (this volume) of her experience of smoking control among students in China provides further insight into how this strategy can be implemented. Comprehensive school health education can be instrumental in building a healthy life for school children.

Young people are growing up in a media environment that is designed to lure them into all kinds of behaviour, many of which, including cigarette smoking, are unhealthy. The tobacco industry has long targeted young people with their advertising and sale promotion. The tobacco industry knows well that once these youngsters are lured they will become regular cigarette smokers, and many will be their customers until they die (Chen & Winder, 1990). Cigarette companies often use models for advertising and promotional purposes, to link cigarette smoking with being cool, beauty, athletics and strength, even though cigarettes represent the opposite. To counterbalance this media campaign, many health organizations have produced campaigns that stress the adverse effects of cigarette smoking, but the result is pathetic, as many such campaigns are not only out-spent by cigarette media campaigns but are also unattractive to young people (Reid *et al.*, 1995). Ms Kate Koplan's paper (this volume) describes the approach of the Centers for Disease Control, in which most of the health effects are down-played, being unathletic and unfit is emphasized and the anti-tobacco role models are chosen who appeal to adolescents' desire for self-expression and individuality. This is a social marketing approach designed with consonance to the needs and interests of young people.

Children and adolescents are the target of the tobacco industry and they are the future of humankind. They live and learn in the family, in schools and in communities. Those are the settings that should be the focus of anti-smoking activities. Tobacco prevention and control involve smoking cessation, cigarette taxation, litigation, education, media campaigns and advocacy; yet, the core of a tobacco-free campaign should be to address the problems of young people and their environment of family, school and the community.

References

Chen, T. & Winder, A. (1990) The opium wars revisited as US forces tobacco exports in Asia. *Am. J. Public Health*, **80**, 659–662
Department of Health and Human Services (1989) Reducing the Health Consequences of Smoking: 25 Years of Progress. A Report of the Surgeon General (DHHS Publcation No. (CDC) 89-8411), Washington DC: US Government Printing Office
Glynn, T.J., Greenwald, P., Mills, S.M.& Manley, M.W. (1993) Youth tobacco use in the United States: Problems, progress, goals, and potential solutions. *Prev. Med.*, **22**, 568–575
Reid, D.J., McNeill, A.D. & Glynn, T.J. (1995) Reducing the prevalence of smoking in youth in western countries: An international review. *Tob. Control*, **4**, 266–277

Restricting smoking among young students in global smoking control

W.K. Liao

Department of Physical, Health and Art Education, State Education Commission, Beijing, China

Young people are the future of the human race. Providing them with a proper education about the harm of smoking and dissuading them from smoking are important aspects of global smoking control. Surveys indicate that there are 5 000 000 young people among the 300 000 000 smokers in China, and the rate of smoking among young students has increased.

The Government has taken various actions to restrict the number of young smokers. A series of regulations on smoking have been issued, which have assisted national smoking control, created a good social environment and provided a sound social basis for no-smoking activity among young students. The State Education Committee has distributed a series of documents on smoking control activities and given clear instructions for smoking control in schools:
- Introduce smoking control into the work plans of schools.
- Ensure that responsible departments and teachers set good examples in smoking control.
- Introduce 'no-smoking' into middle and primary schools and strictly ensure that schools respect it.
- Prohibit smoking by middle and primary school students, dissuade college students from smoking and prohibit smoking in no-smoking areas.

- Designate no-smoking areas in each school on the basis of practical conditions and relevant rules and regulations to strengthen management.
- Place information on the harm of smoking to health in the health education curriculum of middle and primary schools and require that it be included in textbooks.
- Encourage schools to become no-smoking schools.

The requirements of the State Education Committee stipulate that regional educational administrative departments carry out smoking control measures and launch no-smoking activities. As there are more and more no-smoking schools, many stipulate that students who smoke cannot be considered excellent students, and classes with students who smoke cannot be considered excellent classes.

Effective restriction of smoking by young students is difficult and has a long way to go. We have made certain achievements, but have still not succeeded in slowing down the increase in the rate of smoking among young people. Controlling young students' smoking needs not only more effective work on the part of educational administrative departments and schools and continuing no-smoking activity among young students but also the cooperation and support of society.

The family: The key to tobacco control

G.Y. Tsang

Chinese Association on Smoking and Health, Beijing, China

The family is the basic social unit, and its members tend to love and protect one another. A family that is invaded by tobacco use suffers greatly, and a home free from tobacco is a better place to be. It is not surprising, then, that the best way to start tobacco control activities is with the family.

Tobacco control covers three main areas: prevention, cessation and control, tasks that can all start at home. Prevention is done primarily to avoid the onset of smoking by youngsters, so as to reduce the number of future smokers. Cessation applies to all smokers. The earlier they quit, the better. Control is setting limits to smoking, so that smokers cannot smoke conveniently and feel pressured to quit.

In a family, the task of prevention lies with the parents. Non-smoking parents constitute the best defence against their children's intention to smoke, whereas parents who smoke can hardly persuade their children not to. Smoking cessation is important to a family: when no smoker is present, everyone benefits. As family members interact readily, they can help the smokers among them to quit. Control of smoking is naturally a family concern: to smoke at home is to harm non-smoking members. As understanding of the dangers of smoking grows, the tendency to smoke, at least within the home, may decrease.

The family is also part of society. Events that can influence the home environment include governmental actions, school education, medical practice, work-site regulations and the mass media. How can such events affect attitudes and tobacco control in Chinese families? Governmental actions in tobacco control have accelerated recently, and several dozen major cities in China have banned smoking in designated public locations. In 1996, both the President and the Premier chaired a national health conference and stressed the importance of tobacco control. On 1 May 1997, six ministries jointly declared that all public transport and their waiting areas should be smoke-free. On 31 May 1997, 138 Chinese officials signed their names to a joint declaration promoting smoking cessation. President Jiang Zemin highlighted this World Conference by his presence on 24 August 1997. The official voice in tobacco control is clear, but the enforcement of regulations needs improvement. Economic progress in China has stimulated the sale and use of cigarettes, and the old practice of giving cigarettes as gifts and in the home is still prevalent. Maintaining a smoke-free environment is not an easy task.

The Chinese Association on Smoking and Health, established in 1990, is the leading organization for tobacco control in China, but as its funding and number of personnel are limited, its efficiency in tobacco control is limited. In high schools, students are forbidden from smoking anywhere on the premises, but many administrators and teachers are smokers and therefore cannot enforce the smoking ban effectively. Very few Chinese hospitals offer smoking cessation assistance, and about half of the male doctors are smokers themselves, providing a poor model for their patients. Some organizations in China have begun to establish smoke-free offices. Most non-smokers, however, do not realize that they have the right to refuse second-hand smoke; if they do, they hesitate to exercise such rights. The mass media can play an important role in tobacco control, but their involvement is still limited. The Chinese mass media are usually mobilized to campaign on a special issue at a chosen period, such as WHO's 'No Tobacco Day' on 31 May of every year. Once the event is over, the publicity is gone. It would be much better if the media could campaign for the cause of tobacco control on a more regular basis.

The overall picture of tobacco control in China is both promising and challenging. It is promising because it has come a long way in the struggle against the tobacco epidemic, and it is challenging because so much more remains to be done. Regardless of what happens in the larger environment, a determined and well-oriented family can still become smoke-free by its own choice. A family can advance towards becoming smoke-free, first, by all family members giving up smoking, not offering cigarettes to visitors, not allowing visitors to smoke in the house and advising and helping visitors to quit.

Helping smokers at home to quit requires teamwork with all members of the family. Outside assistance is also needed, including professional consultation, media publicity and use of nicotine patches. Once all family members are non-smokers, they can unite to stop guests from smoking. As this is difficult to do initially, Government officials and the mass media should help by publicizing the advantages and guidelines for a smoke-free family and urging people to respect this family wish. A well-designed symbol representing this idea should be created and widely distributed, so that people will know that a home is smoke-free as soon as they see the symbol.

Promoting a smoke-free family and home in China is an activity in which everybody can join and can benefit from. The Government and the mass media must take the lead by actively supporting this campaign. Smoke-free families and homes will then gradually become the norm. Safer and healthier families will emerge, to make a better society.

Youth and prevention: A comprehensive approach

C.A. Moyer[1] & C. Sutherland-Brown[2]

[1]Tobacco Reduction, Canadian Cancer Society, Toronto, and
[2]Office of Tobacco Reduction Programs, Health Canada, Ottawa, Ontario, Canada

Approach

During the 1980s, both Health Canada and the Canadian Cancer Society gave priority to school-based smoking prevention programmes, but towards the end of that decade, both developed strong concern about the value of their interventions. Health Canada had done some long-term evaluation of a peer-assisted learning programme for youth aged 11–13, aimed at the age at onset, which demonstrated, like other studies of similar programmes in the United States and Canada, that while the programme reduced smoking onset among boys aged 12–13, the effect wore off in a few years. It had no impact on girls. Meanwhile, the Canadian Cancer Society, with programmes based on the same concepts, evaluated its diffusion practices and discovered that its expensive materials disappeared into the void of the school system, where their use was unknown, or were being used incompletely, reducing the potential impact of the programme.

Both organizations were therefore disillusioned with their current programmes; both were still committed to prevention of smoking among young people; both were unsure of what to do next. Jointly they decided to undertake a survey across Canada to see which of the many programmes available were currently being used and where gaps existed. In Canada, education is under provincial jurisdiction, so each province and territory has responsibility for and control of its own educational system. Programmes were analysed against criteria for effective school-based programmes for preventing the use of tobacco among the young developed by Tom Glynn in 1989. We found that only 27.6% of Canadian elementary schools and 4.7% of secondary schools were using programmes that met the criteria and could influence behaviour. Many of these programmes were close to meeting all the criteria but showed some significant gaps. The survey also showed that provincial ministries were reducing the mandatory coverage of their health curriculum and that teacher training opportunities and other resources were being reduced. A separate Health Canada survey also showed that one-third of Canadian schools did not have a total ban on smoking. On the basis of the trends across the country and after consultation with provincial leaders, Health Canada decided on a four-pronged approach:

* to develop materials for students at the age of onset (11–13) to fill the common gaps in the most widely used programmes (i.e. to complement other programmes);
* to develop teacher training materials;
* to use a diffusion model that allowed each of the 12 provincial and territorial jurisdictions to develop its unique strategy and
* to develop a prevention programme for older adolescents to maintain the effect of the earlier programme.

Action by Health Canada on these decisions was facilitated by special three-year funding for tobacco control by the Federal Government, supported by a surtax on the tobacco industry. The two new curriculum units for students aged 11–13 were one for girls (to fill that gap in the earlier Health Canada programme) and one to encourage critical analysis of the tobacco industry and its marketing strategies.

The teachers' training component was implemented by positioning the programme within the comprehensive school health approach, which is popular in Canada's school health community. This approach stresses the need for four components: instruction for students, social support (role models, peer support, healthy public policy), support services (guidance, referrals) and the physical environment (e.g. ban on tobacco use in schools). It was also supported by emphasizing the need for linkage to other anti-smoking efforts and organizations in the community, such as coalitions working on by-laws for non-smoking public places and public health departments enforcing the ban on sales to minors. We also stressed the importance of long-term smoking efforts within schools, to continue until the adolescent left school. These materials for students and teachers were produced both as a CD-ROM and in print under the name *Improving the Odds*.

Diffusion

The planning and management team for the diffusion stage included Health Canada, the Canadian Cancer Society and the Canadian Association for School Health. Representatives of these organizations formed a national advisory group, which used a four-step diffusion model involving promotion and dissemination to increase awareness of the resource; adoption, when people agreed to act upon it; implementation and maintenance, with establishment of the programme, sometimes for a limited period.

Because of differences in the needs and structure of each of Canada's 10 provinces and two territories, each jurisdiction was allowed to develop its own plan to find funds to support implementation of the programme. Representatives of each jurisdiction from three areas, volunteer health agencies (usually the Canadian Cancer Society), the provincial health department and the provincial education department, were invited to a planning workshop in 1995, where they agreed on common criteria for their plans. They noted that although *Improving the Odds* was a gap filler and not a complete programme, it should be included in each plan; it should, however, be linked with another resource or resources to provide a complete programme. Its use should be linked to a comprehensive approach, and the intervention should be collaborative, involving the wide range of organizations necessary to provide the skills and resources for such an approach. The plan should include an evaluation, and a framework was provided by the national advisory group on the basis of the four stages of diffusion.

A small fund was provided to provincial and territorial teams to facilitate their planning activities in order to develop diffusion and proposals that would meet these criteria and regional needs. While working with 12 different teams meant that things did not move smoothly everywhere and at the same time, plans were eventually approved for each jurisdiction. Funding was provided through a contract with Health Canada and administered by the Canadian Cancer Society. In most jurisdictions, this funding was augmented by in-kind contributions from provincial and territorial ministries of education and health and volunteer organizations. The Canadian Cancer Society in turn contracted with a provincial agent, which was usually but not always the provincial division of the Canadian Cancer Society. National promotion of the programme was led by the Canadian Association for School Health, especially to educators.

Plans varied greatly with jurisdiction. For example, in the province of Saskatchewan, pilot sites in four communities diffused *Improving the Odds* and established youth and parent health committees to address the long-term, comprehensive needs. In the Province of Manitoba, individuals were trained at three workshops with *Improving the Odds* and a complete provincial resource guide. These trained people will in turn train teachers in smoking prevention programmes for schools. The Northwest Territories had a live phone-in television programme featuring students who promoted *Improving the Odds* and skits showing young people resisting peer pressure and provided cessation advice. Other provinces and territories provided direct training of teachers and held meetings of teachers and community leaders.

Results

Some of the provinces and territories are only now finishing implementation of the programme; however, some preliminary evaluation was undertaken because the funding of Health Canada ended in 1997. To that date, Health Canada spent CAN$ 1.9 million on the programme. Although it is hard to estimate the value of the contributions of the other partners at the Federal, provincial and local level, it was at least CAN$ 0.5 million.

We were moderately successful in expanding the range of activities from pure classroom programming. At least two-thirds of the provinces and territories undertook seven to eight types of activities identified in the comprehensive school health model. We reached over 9000 individuals and 572 organizations in some type of service or training situation throughout the country. About 2700 individuals were exposed to the programme at national conferences. So far, it is impossible to tell how much the programme was used in schools. A survey of teachers was premature, since many of them had just been exposed to the programme; indeed, some 1 workshops were held after the survey. Of those reached, however, 50% of those exposed to the content were likely to use it in 1997–98 school year. One of our most hopeful results was that 10 out of 12 of the provinces and territories reported that they planned to continue the programme in some way after their funding from Health Canada ended.

An evaluation expert has reviewed the detailed provincial and territorial plans to recommend what further evaluation would be cost effective. We have learned, first of all, that money helps: the funds motivated action and gave the collaborative teams some resources for both planning and implementation. Most of them were able to obtain more funds from other sources; despite the enthusiasm of most regions to continue without national funding, however, we expect to see some provinces and territories drop out. This expectation is particularly painful since, even where the programme was the most successful, prevention maintenance programmes are needed in higher grades for long-term effective prevention.

We are also aware of some major flaws. Throughout the process, we found it hard to communicate the need for a comprehensive approach and, when it was grasped, even harder to organize the type of coalition and resources needed to implement it over the long term. The time-pressured health workers often focused simply on distributing *Improving the Odds*.The fact that this publication was a 'gap filler' created difficulties, as it was extremely hard to maintain the understanding that the product was incomplete, and that the programme therefore needed to include complementary materials. The CD ROM version of the materials was expensive but could not compete un design with commercial products.

Our greatest problem has been to provide continuity of support at the national level in terms of resources. We benefited from having the same personnel involved in national advisory group throughout, but suffered from budget cutbacks which reduced the funding available to the provinces and territories and meant that Health Canada could not complete production and diffusion of a complementary prevention programme for older adolescents. We will continue some maintenance and evaluation activities, however, and will develop a set of recommendations for those considering diffusion strategies.

Smoke-free soccer, healthy kids, healthy communities

E.R. Forbes

*United States Department of Health and Human Services,
Washington DC, United States*

In 1996, the United States national women's soccer team captured an Olympic gold medal before a crowd of 76 500 in Athens, Georgia. The debut of women's soccer in the Olympics and the sport's growing popularity worldwide highlight the prominence of women's athletics both as spectator sports and as positive activities for young girls. Soccer is the world's most popular sport and represents a potentially powerful partner for the tobacco control community. During the summer of 1999, the Third Women's World Cup Soccer competition will be held in the United States. It is an opportunity for the tobacco control community to make 'Smoke-free soccer' an international campaign that links the tobacco control community in an alliance with the millions of girls worldwide who enjoy and participate in this most popular and egalitarian of sports.

Smoke-free kids and soccer

Smoking rates among adolescent girls have been rising in the United States. As part of a comprehensive strategy to address the problem, the Secretary of Health and Human Services announced in 1996 a new tobacco control campaign to promote participation in soccer to help adolescent girls resist pressures to smoke. Rather than merely talk about the adverse health effects of smoking, the programme encourages participation in soccer and, through such participation, works with coaches, parents and recreation officials to create environments that can help develop a healthy, smoke-free generation of young women. The programme was hailed by President Bill Clinton at a White House ceremony. "Young women are bombarded with billboards which suggest that smoking is cool and glamorous and a good way to stay thin," the President said. "The women of the US national soccer team know better. This spring and summer, they are going to make America proud when they compete in the Olympics. And just when thousands of young girls around the country are looking up to them, they are going to make it clear that smoking is not cool....It will make a real difference in people's lives."

'Smoke-free kids and soccer' is a collaboration between the Department of Health and Human Services, the women's national team and US Soccer, the governing body of American soccer. Credit for the original concept goes to the pioneering work of countries such as Australia and New Zealand which developed 'Smoke-free sport', but the United States emphasis on participation in a rapidly emerging women's sport is an important innovation.

The programme models the smoke-free lifestyle and success of national team members and encourages adolescent girls to participate in soccer to maintain fitness and resist pressures to smoke. Members of the team have agreed to bring the smoke-free message to millions of their young fans. They are personally committed to encouraging more girls to take up soccer and put down cigarettes. This unique partnership communicates the negative effects of tobacco use on athletic performance and promotes participation in soccer as a positive alternative to smoking.

In its first year, 'Smoke-free soccer' was introduced to more than 1 million children and adults through a combination of television, radio, posters, public events and an interactive web site. Components of the programme include: a 30-s television commercial featuring the United States players; a 60-s radio commercial featuring the team's assistant coach; three motivational posters; tips for coaches; a fact sheet on tobacco and soccer performance; tips for parents on how to encourage girls to play sports and a screen saver featuring images of the women's team in the Olympic games. The materials are distributed by the Department of Health and Human Services through state and local health departments, local chapters of the American Cancer Society, local soccer clubs, parent–teacher associations and an interactive web site [www.smokefree.gov].

During the inaugural year, materials were distributed in conjunction with the national team's schedule of international competition within the United States. Players and coaches from the team made public appearances at local elementary schools and emphasized the importance of playing soccer and staying smoke-free for success on and off the field. The events promoted public interest in women's soccer and helped to de-glamourize smoking.

One of the most prominent components of the campaign has been a series of motivational posters. Thousands of posters are now hanging proudly in the bedrooms of aspiring soccer players throughout the United States. The posters encourage young girls to participate in soccer and to make no smoking an integral part of their personal lifestyle. Messages such as "You don't get to be a champion by taking cigarette breaks" resonate with children and the adults who care for them. When presented by strong, attractive, confident role models, this is a positive, relevant and effective way of reaching children. Most importantly, it is a message conveyed by role models whom children can admire and, if they're lucky, will one day emulate on the soccer field.

Progress towards a smoke-free society is enhanced when the tobacco control community can form alliances with people committed to promoting physical activity through participation in sport, which, like avoiding cigarettes, is something to be learned when young. Through organized sport, children learn valuable lessons about competition, leadership, courage, confidence, fairness and health. The value of participation in sport for women has been documented in a series of research reports and a highly publicized television and print advertising campaign by a sporting goods company. For additional information on the health benefits for women and girls of participating in sport, see Canadian Association for the Advancement of Women and Sport and Physical Activity (1995) and The President's Council on Physical Fitness and Sports (1997).

Conclusion

For the women of the national team, the road to Olympic victory began in adolescence in cities and towns far from elegant athletic venues. Their athletic skills were developed by long hours of work and play in backyards and on community playing fields. Their commitment to fitness, health and a smoke-free lifestyle was nurtured by community-based groups of caring parents and other adults who volunteered their time to coach, mentor, organize and console. This 'soccer community' is a unique and sympathetic resource that can provide diversity and strength to community-based tobacco control strategies. It is a community present in any country that enjoys soccer and where participation in sport enriches the human experience.

References

Canadian Association for the Advancement of Women and Sport and Physical Activity (1995) *Evening the Odds (Tobacco, Physical Activity and Adolescent Women)*

The President's Council on Physical Fitness and Sports (1997) Physical Activity and Sport in the Lives of Girls, Washington DC, US Department of Health and Human Services

Tobacco art and children

K. Yavuz

Istanbul, Turkey

Action plans must be decided by discussing ideas openly and determining aims, and there should be collaboration with artists and representatives of the media who share the same views. As children all over the world love art and drawings, cartoons and drawings can be used to get the message about tobacco and its hazards across.

Cartoon art can express ideas that would be perceived as offending if expressed verbally

Just one cartoon may be powerful enough to replace many written pages or many spoken works. Cartoon art can express tenderness, humour and cynicism, and it has a universal language. Cartoons often call on the tolerance and understanding of people, as cartoonists may criticize mercilessly.

Anti-tobacco campaigns usually use graphs and tables. Tables with many numbers do not attract attention. Cartoons attract attention much more than graphs. If cartoonists were given information about the main topics in tobacco control in a particular year or for a campaign, they could prepared themselves. A cartoonist could draw cartoons during a meeting or conference to enliven the event.

The first step in tobacco control directed to children should be made in ante-natal clinics, where leaflets with cartoons explaining the health hazards of smoking could be distributed to prospective parents.

Development of cartoon art in countries where a democratic tradition is not well established and tolerance to ideas expressed by cartoons

When democracy is interrupted in a country, one of the first things that is severely affected is freedom of the press. Censorship is often not applicable to cartoons, and they become an important means of expressing opinions. They can become the mirror of the country. In countries without a long tradition of democracy, amateur cartoonists often gather in small groups in each city.

If the wit of cartoonists is used in anti-tobacco actions, the campaigns will be more powerful. The tobacco industry has not take any legal action against the cartoonists who have severely criticized them. Cartoon art requires only a pencil and paper. Cartoons can tell a lot in a short time.

Activities of cartoonists in tobacco control

The subject of tobacco and health hazards can be used during drawing lessons at school, and, with the permission of the municipality or owner, the walls of buildings can be used by children to express their views on tobacco. Competitions about tobacco could be organized.

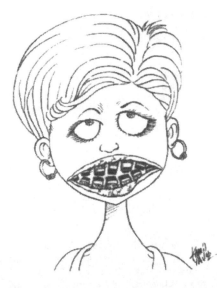

The tobacco industry spends huge sums of money on advertising and promotion in countries where effective anti-smoking campaigns are carried out. They organize prize draws in large shopping malls with the help of attractive young hostesses. A few years ago, one of the cigarette companies in Turkey promised to give a wheel-chair to the person who brought in 10 000 empty cigarette packs. But they never did.

Cigarettes are widely distributed, by many vendors and vans. During the Turkish Thoracic Society Meeting two years ago, I had organized a cartoon competition, and the cartoons were on display throughout the conference. Two of the cartoons that included the Marlboro logo were stolen from the exhibit, reportedly by a mobile Marlboro vendor. The report of this incident in the press did not elicit a denial from the Philip Morris Company.

Why children prefer drawings and cartoons

Instead of telling children repeatedly that tobacco is harmful, it would be better to use a form of education that is attractive to children. Celebrities and artists should be invited to schools to talk. I am organizing cartoon courses in nine schools at weekends, at which students can draw whatever cartoon they like on smoking, health, environment and sports. We also print a monthly magazine of cartoons and distribute it to schools. Even children in kindergarten can be given smoking as a subject for simple drawings.

They could be encouraged to write letters to cartoonists, asking them to draw cartoons for important dates like 31 May or 9 February. For example, Lucky Luke has quit smoking and now has a piece of straw in his mouth. This represents the action of anti-tobacco groups.

International group of cartoonists and other artists for tobacco control

Cartoons are used widely in the press all over the world. Several agencies buy or order cartons, but buying cartoons for tobacco control from an agency is costly. All amateur cartoonists follow the publications of the Federation of European Cartoon Organizations: if announcements of exhibitions and competitions on tobacco control were printed in these journals, large numbers of cartoons would be assembled in one place. If an international jury judged the entries in the presence of the press, the event could have a lot of coverage and the cartoons might be published in newspapers around the world. The cartoons could also be published in books or be used for postcards.

An educational anti-tobacco programme for preschool children: 'Clean air around us'

J. Szymborski[1], W. Zatonski[2], Z. Juczynski[1], T. Kowalczyk[1], M. Lewadowska[1], A. Dobrowolska[1] & N. Oginska-Bulik[1]

[1] *National Research Institute for the Mother and Child and* [2] *Department of Epidemiology, Cancer Centre and Institute of Oncology, Warsaw, Poland*

Children and young people have the right to protect themselves against smoking. They deserve the relevant education and health enhancement that will help them to resist the temptation of smoking and other uses of tobacco. The Polish Institute for the Mother and Child and the Institute of Oncology, under the auspices of the Ministry of Health, have together worked out 10 strategies to achieve this goal. The programmes were developed by two doctors (a paediatrician and an oncologist), educators, psychologists and a sociologist. They are conducted at various educational levels. The youngest group, six-year-old preschool children, is very important for anti-tobacco education, because they are at the age when they receive their first conscious impressions of smoking, in the outside world, at home and at school. We describe here the programme that was designed for this age group to create conscious anti-tobacco attitudes.

The programme

The programme is addressed to six-year-old children, the oldest preschool group. It is is intended to teach children how to protect themselves when people are smoking around them. The objectives of the programme are to help children recognize various sources of smoke, including tobacco smoke; to make them aware of the harmful effects of tobacco smoke; to raise their awareness of the consequences of smoking cigarettes; to tell them where they might encounter smoking and to make them assertive and self-assured in the presence of people smoking cigarettes.

Every educational programme should be addressed to the individual. A six-year-old child saya "I care about myself." Special emphasis is therefore placed on explaining terms to allow them to make responsible decisions about their own health, the effects of their decisions and activities on their health and how cigarette smoke influences their health. They are also concerned by their relationships with other people. The programme therefore raises awareness that the quality of a relationship influences health, the transmission of interpersonal standards an an introduction to assertiveness, to allow them to protect their own rights (to breathe fresh air) without encountering aggression from other people defending their rights. Another aspect of the individual is the relationship with the environment. The programme helps them to observe whether their environment is healthy, to determine the sources of threats to their health and to raise awareness of how they can influence their environment and take care of both it and themselves.

Teachers are free to choose a version suitable to their pupils' interests, depending on their age and knowledge. Each lesson focuses on stimulating one of the activities of a six-year-old child, such as group work or inventing or playing a game. The subjects of the lessons are:

A trip
What is smoking and why do some people do it ?
How do I feel around a burning cigarette?
What happens when a cigarette is smoked?
How can I avoid tobacco smoke?

The lessons are taught in a round-table setting, which gives children the chance to learn by experience. It includes activities that encourage children to test their knowledge, to think about their values and to learn how to recognize different sources of smoke and how to avoid them. The activities include a trip, drawing and writing to test their knowledge, 'brainstorming' about the causes of smoke. practice in breathing in various atmospheres, drama and singing. As the round-table setting means working in small groups, the children learn to cooperate with each other and teach each other. This allows shy children to increase their assertiveness. The teachers' role is to advise, coordinate and help the children but not attempt to control them.

Introduction of the programme

The programme has been introduced at a preschool in a town near Warsaw. The lessons have been conducted by an experienced teacher who is also the Director of the preschool in groups of 18 pupils, with the cooperation of the staff and parents. The programme appears to have attained its objectives.

For use in other schools, the requirements for each lesson is presented in a common scheme: objectives, required materials, estimated time and procedure. The teachers also receive educational and psychological notes on some aspects of the programme and health education materials such as posters, emblems and song lyrics. An information pack for parents is included, which describes the prevalence of smoking among children and young people and the reasoning behind the prevention programme. A letter is sent to preschool directors requesting that they take additional measures within the school, such as prohibiting smoking and exhibiting the children's work.

Anti-tobacco education programme for children and adolescents in Cuba

N. Suarez Lugo

Carlos J. Finlay National School in Public Health,
Ministry of Public Health, Havana, Cuba

Background

The prevalence of smoking in Cuba increased between 1960 and 1985, decreased between 1986 and 1990 and remained unchanged between 1990 and 1996. In the period 1984–95, however, 20% of youngsters smoked. The group aged 17–19 years was the only one that showed an increased prevalence between 1984 (11%) and 1990 (13%). They are also beginning to smoke earlier: children in Cuba start the experimentation phase at the age of 10 or before, although about 75% of smokers begin at the age of 19. The experimentation period increases with age, and the frequency is higher in boys than in girls (Table 1).

In 1985, the Government approved a programme for prevention and tobacco control. Its basic characteristics are its national scope, persuasion, social marketing, health promotion, a wide individual and social focus and a combination of education and legislation. The preventive strategy is directed to the majority of the population, which has not yet started to smoke. The general objective of the programme for 1996–2000 is to reduce the prevalence by 2% annually. The principal specific objectives are to stop the habit, reduce initiation and prevent smoking by children and young people.

Factors that contribute to initiation

Imitation and environment are considered to be the most important causes of initiation among Cuban smokers. The environment is favourable to smoking because Cuba is a tobacco-producing country, tobacco is accessible, smoking is socially and culturally acceptable, it is related to costume, traditions, music and folklore, and lack of legislation.

In Cuba, children know about cigarettes from a very young age and have a social image of smoking within their environment. The availability and price of the product

Table 1. Prevalence of starting smoking before the age of 19 in Cuba, 1990 and 1995

Age (years)	Boys (%)		Girls (%)		All (%)	
	1990	1995	1990	1995	1990	1995
< 10	11	5.4	10	5.1	11	5.1
10–14	24	31	24	29	24	29
15–19	44	45	37	41	42	41
Total	80	81	71	75	77	75

are factors that make it easy to obtain. They follow the patterns of their teachers (cited as the initiating influence by 83% of children), their brothers and sisters (62%), their friends (31%), their fathers (57%) and their mothers (35%). Various studies have shown that children whose parents smoke are more inclined to smoke; the attitude of their parents with regard to their children smoking is also an important factor. The finding that teachers are considered to be the most important influence is due to the fact that students in junior and senior high-schools in Cuba usually board at school. In addition, many work in the country for 15–45 days every school year accompanied by young teachers aged 25–30, and there is a close relationship between the teachers and students. The teachers are looked upon as older friends. This relatianship, together with their role as teachers, makes them very strong role models.

Preventive strategy

The legal measures for control include prohibition on sales of cigars and cigarettes to minors under 17, in automatic machines and in or near schools; prohibition on distribution of free samples and regulation of direct and indirect advertising in all mass media and at cultural and sports events. The educative actions include an educational programme in the school curriculum, teacher training, promotion, social events (sport and cultural) and special programmes on the mass media.

The anti-tobacco education programme is the initial attempt to change attitudes and behaviour and to increase knowledge about the risks of smoking. The programme is given before the first stage of adolescence, when addiction usually starts. The programme was designed on the basis of scientific research and introduced into the school curriculum of elementary and secondary education in 1992–93.

The general objective is to stop children from smoking and reduce the initiation rate. The specific objectives are to increase knowledge, change attitudes and behaviour and train the children to resist social pressure. The methods include:

- a package for teachers, giving the educational objectives, the method and techniques and material designed to be attractive for children and adolescents, like puppets, role and participative games, drawing competitions, plays and stories, films and traditional classes and lectures;
- guides to train teachers and promoters;
- guides to involve the family and community, based on material from the projects 'Latinoamerica against cancer', 'Tobacco, a multidisciplinary focus' and 'Tobacco and alcohol in the family and school'.
- instruments to evaluate the impact on attitudes, knowledge and behaviour.

The anti-tobacco education programme has been run annually since 1992. We found that it had increased knowledge markedly and changed attitudes among students. It also changed the smoking behaviour of teachers (95% were non-smokers after six months compared with 10% before the intervention) and of parents (65% non-smokers after the programme and 1% before). The age of initiation was increased by 1.3%.

In tobacco smoking control, the important factors are to increase knowledge about its ill-effects and achieve a favourable social environment for non-smoking. The two together will result in a new generation of non-smokers and allow us to build a new world free from tobacco.

Effect of a school-based smoking prevention programme on recruitment of smokers: A multi-level analysis

O. Jøsendal

Research Centre for Health Promotion, Norwegian Cancer Society, Universityof Bergeb, Norway

A representative, country-wide random sample of 94 secondary schools participated in a project launched by the Norwegian Cancer Society. A total of 195 classes and 4441 students started out in the project in November 1994. In an evaluation study, the Research Centre for Health Promotion at the University of Bergen followed the sample (cohort) through to graduation in spring 1997

The schools were systematically allocated to one of four groups: controls; smoking prevention intervention, comprising a classroom programme, parental involvement and courses given by teachers; a classroom programme and parental involvement but no courses; or a classroom programme and courses but no parental involvement.

Data were obtained at a baseline survey in November 1994 and at follow-up surveys in May 1995, March–April 1996 and April 1997. Analyses were performed with the SPSSwin programme. Data from the first and second follow-up surveys showed promising results: the adjusted odds ratios (logistic regression) were 0.5 in the group that received the full intervention, 0.68 in the group that received a classroom programme and parental involvement but no courses and 0.78 in the group that received a classroom programme and courses but no parental involvement, all $p < 0.05$.. These results were confirmed by multi-level analysis with the MlnWin programme, with four levels of analysis: measurements/occasion, person, classroom and school. The variance was significant at the individual and classroom levels.

The tobacco industry is not a popular sponsor among youth in Switzerland

V. El Fehri & H. Krebs

LINK Marketing Research, Swiss Association for Smoking Prevention, Bern, Switzerland

In Switzerland, about one-third of the population between the ages of 15 and 75 are smokers; 30% are women and 40% are men. Among youngsters, 10% aged 11–15 smoke at least once a week, while 25% aged 15–19 smoke every day. In the age group 20–24, 40% are daily smokers. The Swiss are thus heavy smokers, and Switzerland is at the top of the list of tobacco consumption per inhabitant.

Since 1992, a nationwide campaign known as 'New pleasure—non-smoking' has been in operation, targeted at young people aged 14–18. Its aim has been to promote a tobacco-free lifestyle among young people, partly by funding events for this age group, such as discotheques and sports competitions. The campaign has been well received by the public, and two-thirds of Switzerland's youngsters are aware of its existence: 63% are very positively disposed towards it, 24% think that it is 'not bad', and only 8% said that they 'don't really like it'. The strength of the campaign is its positive approach and the fact that it appeals to the target group by focusing on their lifestyle. LINK Marketing Research conducted surveys at various events sponsored by the campaign in 1994 and 1996, which provide an accurate idea of whether and how the public perceives the campaign.

Results of the 'International Roller & In-line Contest' in Lausanne, 1994

The survey showed that 70% of the 500 people aged 15–25 who were questioned were aware that the contest was partly sponsored by the campaign 'New pleasure—non-smoking', and that the campaign was listed sixth out of a total of 11 sponsors, ahead of Coca Cola! In response to the question 'Which sponsor would you prefer?', 63% preferred sponsorship by the campaign rather than the tobacco industry, 26% had no preference, while only 11% would have preferred the tobacco industry to have sponsored the event.

Results of a survey conducted at three types of event in one city, 1997

A survey was conducted at a street parade with 300 000 spectators, the Adidas 'Streetball challenge' with 2000 spectators and the 'Züri In-line' with 50 000 spectators. Samples of 200 persons aged 12–20 were selected at each event. The proportion of smokers varied from one event to the other. Relatively few smokers were among the participants in the Adidas 'Streetball challenge'; moreover, the average age of the spectators at this event was lower than at the other events. The campaign was recalled spontaneously by 6, 38 and 25% of the sample, respectively, at each event; the figures for prompted recall were 47, 88 and 82%. More smokers than non-smokers considered that the campaign was suitable for the respective events, except at the Adidas event, where equal numbers of smokers and non-smokers considered the sponsorship suitable. The majority of non-smokers had no preference about whether the event was sponsored by tobacco companies or the campaign, but most of the smokers preferred the sponsorship of the campaign.

Tackling smoking among 16–24-year olds through a large-scale art, design and fashion project

P. Hooper

Smoke Free Birmingham, Southern Birmingham Community Health National Health Service Trust, Springfields Centre for Health Promotion, Birmingham, United Kingdom

A long-standing relationship between Smoke Free Birmingham, a tobacco control alliance of the Health Authority, the City Council and others, and the University of Central England had previously led to the production of posters and other resources at low cost by graphic design students. This collaboration had included designs for a 12-month street poster campaign on a variety of health topics: food hygiene posters for Chinese caterers, pest control leaflets and other materials. Smoking-related products included designs for posters advertising a major scientific exhibit, temporary tattoos, interactive shopping centre displays for No Smoking Day and many others.

The initial concept of the project described here was to generate materials that would make smoking less 'fashionable'. This resulted in the idea of involving fashion and textiles students, which in turn led to it being set as a problem for second-year Bachelor of Arts students. A total of 120 students, including graphic design, video production and fashion specialists, were formed into 22 project teams. After a detailed brief presented by Smoke Free Birmingham, the teams were asked to produce original solutions for raising the smoking issue with 16–24-year olds. Numerous follow-up visits were made by health professionals, and the project was overseen by six course tutors.

It soon became clear that the project was not only the largest joint project of its kind attempted by the Institute of Art and Design, but also that some of the work was worthy of a wider audience. Certain teams were selected to develop their concepts further, while others continued to prepare for a major public showing of their designs.

At the end of the project period, numerous innovative solutions were presented. A major fashion show celebrated World No Tobacco Day, and other 'street events' were carried out. A touring exhibition of all the works was a major outcome of the project.

One of the concepts, 'Make history' was chosen to launch the City's new three-year smoking reduction programme and the event received considerable local media attention. Another concept 'Serial killer' was used as a focus for a summer street event and has since been developed into a form of theatre in health education .

It is estimated that a total of UK£ 10 000 was invested by the Health Authority and that the value of the creative and substantive product was at least UK£ 150 000!

These results prove that smoking issues can be exciting and made relevant to groups that are difficult to target. Considerable interest has been shown in the outcome of the project, both locally and nationally, and some of the innovative designs and fresh approaches will be developed into mainstream health promotion resources. Its success is a good example of creative alliance working.

Images from this project can be found on our web site <www.smokefree.org.uk>

Books on tobacco and smoking in the Danish education system

K. Trangbek

The Danish Council on Smoking and Health, Copenhagen, Denmark

Books about tobacco and smoking were produced for biology, social science, chemistry and geography classes during the period 1995–97. As 45% of Danish young people aged 16–19 study at 'gymnasia' or centres of higher education, the books are aimed specifically at this group, although they are also part of a larger campaign aimed at young people in general. The purpose is to provide students with knowledge about tobacco and smoking with a view to influencing their attitudes and behaviour. This is a cooperative project between the Danish Council on Smoking and Health, the Ministry of Education and the teachers' unions.

To make introduction of the books successful, it has been important to:
* ensure that the books are relevant to the classes,
* ensure a high standard of information,
* base the books on facts, not propaganda,
* design the books to resemble other books at school,
* include network and resource persons in the process and
* offer the books to schools for free

Smoking by adolescents: Three years later, there's an even larger revenue but little for prevention

C.M. Doran, A. Girgis & R.W. Sanson-Fisher

New South Wales Cancer Council Cancer Education Research Program, Newcastle, Australia

The purpose of this paper is to determine whether any changes occurred between 1990 and 1993 in the State Government revenue gained from the sale of cigarettes to minors and in the proportion of this revenue spent trying to prevent the uptake of this habit by adolescents. The method employed in this analysis is consistent with that of the 1990 study published in *The Australian Journal of Public Health* (19, 29–33), although some revisions were necessary. The prevalence of smoking by minors was extrapolated for the individual states from the prevalence for Australia, and estimates of annual cigarette consumption were coupled with the respective cost of cigarettes in each state to derive an estimate of the total revenue accumulating from cigarette consumption by minors.

From our analysis, 274 255 Australian children under the legal age to purchase cigarettes consumed approximately 14.6 million packs of cigarettes in 1993. We estimated that the State revenue from smoking by under-age children increased by 97%, from A$ 9.37 million in 1990 to A$ 18.45 million in 1993. State expenditure on anti-smoking campaigns (for the entire population) increased by 24%, from A$ 9.47 million in 1990 to an estimated A$ 11.75 million in 1993. When this expenditure is converted to a relative amount, relative State expenditure per under-age smoker fell by an estimated 10%, from A$ 4.40 in 1990 to A$ 3.98 in 1993. Thus, approximately 7.7% in 1990 and 5.1% in 1993 of State revenue from cigarette smoking by those under the legal purchase age was spent on discouraging adolescents from taking up this habit. These results suggest a growing inequity in the expenditure on anti-smoking activities in comparison with the revenues received from sales to minors.

This comparison was published in *The Australian Journal of Public Health* in 1998.

TOBACCO LEGISLATION
AND REGULATION

Legislation: A key component of a comprehensive tobacco control plan

G. Mahood

Non-Smokers' Rights Association, Toronto, Ontario, Canada

The global health response: too little, too timid, too late

It is important that the global health community look realistically at its past efforts to address the tobacco epidemic. It is difficult to determine where we are going if we have little understanding about where we have been. I think critics could develop a good case that the international tobacco control community, this speaker included, has been ineffective.

The tobacco epidemic is a growing rather than a shrinking problem. Between 1967 and 1996, world tobacco production doubled from 2.8 to more than 6 thousand thousand million cigarettes. The global health response has been too little, too timid, too late. Worse, we allowed tobacco consumption to expand rapidly at precisely the time that the scientific evidence about the risks of tobacco was building dramatically.

At the Seventh World Conference in 1990, I was among the plenary speakers when Richard Peto and Alan Lopez released the ominous World Health Organization prediction that the international tobacco industry would kill 500 million people from among the world's population—500 million victims! The magnitude of the predicted mortality is chilling. That is eight times the highest estimate for deaths, both military and civilian, during the entire Second World War. Our response to such an ominous threat has been too little, too timid, too late.

Some reasons why we have failed

First, with but a few exceptions, we have failed to focus on the vector of tobacco diseases, the tobacco manufacturers. Given the evidence, allowing tobacco manufacturers to promote tobacco use now is like allowing the promotion and sale of rats at the height of the bubonic plague, had officials of the time known the source of the plague. Comparison of the tobacco epidemic with the bubonic plague is perhaps appropriate, given the role that rats have played in both epidemics.

Second, we have failed to shift public opinion sufficiently with respect to the industry's 'legal product' argument. The industry contends that tobacco is a legal and, hence, legitimate product. But tobacco is not a legal product for children. Tobacco is legal only for adults and legally on the market because society did not know the risks when the product first came on the market. To argue now that the tobacco epidemic cannot be addressed because the product is legal is to argue, absurdly, that society will never be allowed to correct its mistake.

Third, we have failed to denormalize tobacco products and the tobacco industry. With the exception of the tobacco control media campaigns that are being run by the California and Massachusetts state departments of health, we have failed to strip respectability from tobacco products and to separate the tobacco industry from legitimate business.

Fourth, for too long, we have used a 'blame-the-victim' approach to tobacco control. Health agencies and government health departments have focused their campaigns on individual behaviour and personal responsibility. "It's the child's responsibility not to smoke and the adult's responsibility to break his or her addiction". Too often, in times of competing priorities, we have placed disproportionate stress on 'stop smoking' campaigns targeting individuals rather than on corporate behaviour and defective products that affect entire populations. This is not an issue of principle, of failing to show respect for individual life. It is a matter of practicality. Changing individual behaviour, one person at a time, is a slow and costly process. Focusing on changing group behaviour has the potential of protecting the lives of entire populations.

Fifth, until recently in the United States, we have failed to hold the manufacturers responsible for their criminal and civil misbehaviour and for products that kill one out of two of their long-term users.

Sixth, the tobacco epidemic is now recognized as a political rather than a medical problem. We have failed because, for the most part, human and financial resources have not shifted from curative approaches to the prevention of disease. We have not, as one British minister put it, changed emphasis from addressing tobacco diseases at the surgical table to prevention by decisions at the cabinet table. Signs of greater activism include suits by California health agencies and Australian consumer unions against governments, the tobacco industry and its friends. Another example is the intervention of the Canadian Cancer Society in the courts to defend Canada's tobacco legislation.

Seventh, huge financial incentives remain for the tobacco industry to make people ill. We have failed to persuade governments to remove those incentives and provide serious financial and legal disincentives for manufacturers who would undermine health policy or ignore the law. Our failures are especially glaring in developed countries where we could have had the human and financial resources to fight the industry, had we altered our priorities.

The challenge then is this: will developed countries finally start to introduce the serious measures needed to eliminate the ability of the tobacco industry to market its products? Will less developed countries make the same mistakes as Canada, Europe and the United States, where major changes have taken 30 years? There is room for hope. It took Canada and Australia three decades to obtain better tobacco package warnings. Yet it took Singapore, South Africa and Thailand only one or two years to catch up. Now, Poland seems ready to set the standard for package warnings in eastern Europe. There are many other examples of accelerated change after some jurisdiction has set the standard.

Comprehensive legislation is needed

Despite acceleration of this kind, the deaths predicted by Peto and Lopez will occur unless health interests force governments to act. Legislation is the key to implementation of comprehensive tobacco control plans. Fortunately, in comparison with other interventions, legislation can be inexpensive.

To be effective, legislation must provide governments with sweeping regulatory control over all aspects of the manufacture, import, marketing and use of tobacco products. Nothing less will do. An example of an attempt to secure comprehensive legislation is Canada's *Tobacco Act*, passed in 1997. This legislation gives our Government many of the necessary broad powers mentioned above which are needed to regulate the tobacco industry.

Model comprehensive tobacco control plans might include five elements.

1. Preventing the industry from reaching children

First, any plan must block the access of the tobacco industry to children. This will be easier if we try to reduce both demand and supply—reducing the desire of adolescents for tobacco while simultaneously making it more difficult for them to purchase tobacco. So far, legislators have not paid serious attention to reducing either.

In order to reduce supply and increase barriers to access, we must raise the age of purchase, decrease the number of sales outlets, ban vending machines, ban small packs, ban smokeless tobacco and require retailers or manufacturers or both to be licensed. Through licensing, we could hold retailers and manufacturers responsible if tobacco ends up in the hands of minors. Those who sell to children will have a real incentive to obey the law if the penalty is the loss of a license to sell or, for manufacturers, the de-listing of tobacco brands. Or jail.

At the same time, we must reduce youth demand. We must raise the price through government policy. We must 'de-normalize' tobacco products and show why they are not like other 'legal' products. We must transfer normal youth rebellion against authority from parents and teachers to the tobacco manufacturers. We must use social marketing campaigns to show adolescents how they are being exploited by the industry and focus health marketing on an industry that 'rips off' children. The California and Massachusetts state health campaigns have broken new ground in this critical area.

2. Informed consent

Improving information. The legal concept of informed consent between the buyer and manufacturer of a product requires that the consumer be fully informed about the nature of the risks associated with use of a product and the magnitude of those risks. This means that the tobacco manufacturers must tell consumers not only that cigarettes cause lung cancer but also that nearly 90% of people who get lung cancer die within one or two years.

A state of informed consent means that young people join the tobacco market with their eyes wide open. It means that existing users have sufficient information to be motivated to leave the tobacco market, that smokers have as much 'freedom of choice' as possible to quit smoking, given the constraints that flow from using an addictive product. Because risks are not taken as seriously by youth, the entire comprehensive plan discussed here must be implemented to create an environment in which children will not wish to risk becoming addicted to tobacco.

To encourage informed consent, it is necessary both to give better information to the public and to stop disinformation from the tobacco industry. Providing better information means:

- requiring better warnings on packages,
- introducing package inserts in order to expand package-based public education campaigns,
- forcing full disclosure of all toxins and all additives in cigarettes,
- improving warnings on existing advertisements,
- creating effective mass media campaigns,
- pressing for public inquiries into the activities of the tobacco industry and for disclosure of documents by legislative inquiries, criminal investigations and royal commissions.

Removing disinformation. Disinformation must be removed from tobacco marketing. Both tobacco brand advertising and tobacco sponsorship must be banned. Beautiful packages imply that the product inside is safe and is associated with desirable lifestyles. We therefore need legislation to implement plain packaging. Plain packs are packs of uniform colour, stripped of corporate design and graphics which carry the brand name in standardized typeface, warnings, lists of toxic constituents and other information required by law. Legislation must passed to prohibit false labelling, such as 'light', 'mild' and 'super light'. These labels falsely imply a tobacco product of lower risk.

3. Legislation to protect non-smokers

We need legislation to protect non-smokers from the harm caused by tobacco. Children and adults must be protected from environmental tobacco smoke. In addition, the techniques exist to manufacture fire-safe cigarettes, and this reform alone could save thousands of lives.

4. Product modification

Legislation should be passed to allow governments to control all aspects of cigarette manufacture, including control of additives and allowable levels of toxins. For years, the tobacco industry has been modifying cigarettes to make it easier for children to start smoking. Through product modification, we can reverse this process.

Cigarettes are dirty drug delivery devices. For those already addicted and who cannot quit, we must improve the techniques for delivering nicotine to the smoker without the poisons that are present when it is delivered by cigarettes. Legislation must be enacted to give regulators the power to ban certain categories of tobacco products and thus push consumption towards less hazardous nicotine delivery products.

At present, the tobacco industry has a virtual monopoly on nicotine maintenance. Cigarette nicotine delivery systems are the most harmful but are the least regulated. Nicotine replacement products, while less harmful and with great potential for reducing the amount of disease caused by tobacco, are the most heavily regulated. We must create a regulatory environment in which the manufacturers of less harmful nicotine delivery systems can break the monopoly of the tobacco manufacturers, so that less harmful options are available to currently addicted smokers. This must be done with sufficient regulation and care to ensure a net gain for public health.

5. Support for smokers

Finally, any comprehensive approach to tobacco control must include measures to help smokers break their addiction and to obtain compensation from the industry for the criminal and civil misbehaviour that has caused them harm.

Pressing for health reform

Legislation is critical because it is a powerful agent of social change. Peer group pressure is another important agent of change. Legislation designed to reduce exposure to environmental tobacco smoke is doubly valuable because it protects non-smokers and at the same time makes the use of tobacco products socially unacceptable. This activates peer group pressure.

Litigation can be another major agent of health reform. In view of the social change that will flow from the settlement talks in the United States, litigation should be given greater attention. Care must be taken in focusing on litigation, however, as many if not most of the proposed gains from the settlement have been achieved elsewhere by legislation, without trading away immunity or the potential for future tobacco reform. Public education is seldom very effective by itself, but public education campaigns combined with legislation can be very effective.

Principles of effective campaigning

In Canada, significant tobacco legislation has almost always followed a major battle. I have put together a number of rules for campaigning that have worked for us for 20 years. Many of the approaches involve embarrassing and pressuring governments, but such pressure must be balanced by an ability to work cooperatively and in partnership with governments. The skill lies in striking the right balance between pressure and partnership. We have worked closely with a number of health ministers. In most cases, we applied our pressure to the government as a whole to enable the Minister of Health to overcome resistance among cabinet colleagues to the reforms that the Minister and the health community wanted.

Not all of the principles for campaigning outlined below will work in all countries or will be right for all cultures.The principles are given to serve as ideas and as a possible campaign checklist. They should be modified to fit different countries and different budgets.

Principle 1: We all know the importance of good research, but it must be the right research. Economic, legal and policy research must be completed and ready to be provided to governments and the media.

Principle 2: Emphasize cost–effective legislation and other public policy initiatives that have the potential to keep thousands of children out of the market. Reduce emphasis on costly labour-intensive initiatives designed to persuade individuals to break their addiction to tobacco. The industry knows that it can bring children onto the market faster than well-intentioned health interests can persuade addicted smokers to stop smoking.

Principle 3: Transfer responsibility for the epidemic from individual behaviour to the behaviour of the industry. This will isolate and 'de-normalize' the industry, undermine its legitimacy and build support for legislation.

Principle 4: Build coalitions. Our campaigns have almost always been the result of team efforts. To be effective, agencies must set up procedures to cut bureaucracy and promote fast decision-making.

Principle 5: Remember that governments are often like footballs: they move up and down the field depending on how much force is applied to them and how hard they are kicked. They seldom move, especially on tobacco, without real pressure.

Principle 6: Don't take "No" for an answer. Remember that "No" is frequently an early stage of "Yes".

Principle 7: Campaign as if you were at war. The rates of mortality from tobacco-related disease approach those that occur during a war. And the industry has the children of the world under attack. Be as aggressive, as tough and as tenacious as the death rates suggest are necessary. Take risks, for our children.

Principle 8: Bring intensity to your campaign. Michael Pertschuk, former United States Federal Trade Commission Chairman and an articulate health spokesperson with the Washington-based Advocacy Institute, says, "the health lobby is large enough" but it lacks "intensity". We must bring greater intensity to our campaigns across the entire health community, and we must learn to sustain the intensity until the campaign objectives are achieved.

Principle 9: Remove blocks to legislation. Neutralization is a critical component of social change. When individuals or groups block tobacco reform, they are blocking attempts to reduce preventable deaths. You do not have to feel uncomfortable or impolite when you deal with these blocks. Make your opponents feel uncomfortable. Make legislators want to establish distance from those who support the industry.

Principle 10: Borrow good ideas from the tobacco industry's campaign manual. For example, the tobacco industry sets up organizations to achieve specific goals. We can too. When the tobacco industry organized artists to oppose the sponsorship provisions in Canada's new *Tobacco Act*, we organized 'Artists for Tobacco-free Sponsorship' and held news conferences to support the legislation.

In an earlier campaign, we decided to provide another perspective on the tobacco industry's claim that tobacco-related law reform will harm tobacco industry jobs. We organized a group, Relatives of Dead and Dying Smokers, to redirect attention to the industry's civil and criminal misbehaviour and to put a spotlight on the 45 000 tobacco-caused deaths each year in Canada and the harm done to their families.

Principle 11: Think strategically. Learn how to present your demands in a way that will fit in with government philosophy and public opinion. When Dr David Kessler was Commissioner of the United States Food and Drug Administration, he displayed brilliant strategic thinking. He spoke of the use of tobacco as a "paediatric disease". He knew that if he focused his reforms on helping to keep children off the tobacco market, the industry could not win support from the public.

Principle 12: Believe the impossible and then make the impossible happen. Despite the unacceptable speed of reform in the past, we are now in a period of accelerated change in tobacco policy. We have the research. Public opinion is beginning to come round. Everywhere we look, we see potential for major break-throughs. Stretch your imagination. Think of the reforms once thought to be impossible. Then work out a campaign plan to secure your goals. Don't take 'No' for an answer. Like Dr Kessler, make the impossible happen.

Trends over time and international variation in tobacco-control legislation: Experience of the European Union

A.J. Sasco[1], R. Ah-Song, I. Gendre & V. Bourdès

Unit of Epidemiology for Cancer Prevention
International Agency for Research on Cancer, Lyon, France

[1]Director of research at the Institut National de la Santé et de la Recherche Médicale, France. At the time of the conference, Dr Sasco was also Acting Chief, Programme for Cancer Control, World Health Organization.

Introduction

Tobacco use represents a major public health concern, as it has been causally linked to the occurrence of lung cancer and other tobacco-related malignancies, as well as a wide array of other serious health consequences, claiming a heavy toll in human lives and representing increasing health-related expenditure. The European Union, like most other parts of the world, is witnessing a continuous increase in the rate of mortality from diseases related to tobacco consumption (Pisani *et al*, 1993), in particular from lung cancer, the frequency of which is directly correlated with the prevalence and duration of smoking. Unfortunately, the forecasts for the decades to come are grim with regard to both the number of cases of lung cancer and the proportion attributable to smoking, which are still expected to climb (Parkin & Sasco, 1993). The situation therefore calls for the best strategies, including legislative measures, to withstand the aggressive lobbying of the tobacco industry and to lay down strict regulations under which tobacco products may be supplied and consumed. Legislative action is an efficient means of tobacco control and prevention, although not entirely sufficient by itself. Over the last decade, the legislative texts of the memberStates of the European Union have become increasingly restrictive towards tobacco use, giving hope to tobacco control advocates, although the battle is far from won.

Methods

The governments of the member states of the European Union were contacted individually in order to obtain their texts on tobacco control legislation. In addition, we carried out a systematic computer search and reviewed the *International Digest of Health Legislation* and the WHO database on tobacco. Once the original texts had been retrieved, they were translated (when necessary), and the contents were classified under topics such as control of advertising, restriction of smoking in public places, labelling of tobacco products, limitation of levels of harmful substances, protection of young people and education. The results were analysed at the International Agency for Research on Cancer (IARC). Several reports deriving from this study have already been published (Sasco & van der Elst, 1989; Sasco *et al*, 1992). An updated report is being prepared to integrate recent amendments and newly adopted laws and to take into account the legislative texts of the three new member States, Austria, Finland and Sweden, which joined the European Union in 1995.

Results and discussion

Legislation can intervene at two levels (Roemer, 1992): first by restricting the availability of tobacco products, for example through price policies and taxes, control of the composition of tobacco products offered for sale and control of advertising and promotional activities; and secondly, by regulating the demand side, which implies a progressive change in people's attitude through educational programmes and restrictive measures relating, for instance, to tobacco consumption in public places or in the workplace.

Between 1985 and 1995, there was a notable increase in the number of legislative measures on tobacco control in the countries of the European Union (Sasco & Bourdès,

1996), and most member States now have more or less comprehensive tobacco-control texts. Generally speaking, there has been a trend towards harmonization of the legislative measures taken with respect to tobacco control, the norm being increasingly restrictive. For instance, only one country out of the 12 members in 1985 had limited the tar content to 15 mg per cigarette, whereas 10 years later eight countries had adopted similar measures. Similarly, six out of 12 States had legislative measures regulating the advertising of tobacco products in 1985 as compared with 13 out of 15 States in 1995. The protection of non-smokers is addressed through coercive measures on tobacco consumption in public places. In 1989, the European Council and the ministers of health of the member States adopted a resolution to ban smoking in places open to the public, namely in enclosed premises and all means of public transport, while providing for the possibility of defining areas reserved for smokers. Some States have adopted even more restrictive texts than those enacted by the Council. The evolution of legislation in the European Union in this particular field is thus eloquent, not only qualitatively but also quantitatively. This can be regarded as an encouraging change in terms of the public health objectives to be attained, in view of the recent demonstration of the potential adverse effects of environmental tobacco smoke.

The rationale for having recourse to legislative action in tobacco control is the observed correlation between the number of anti-tobacco measures, including fiscal policies, and an effective reduction in tobacco use (Dalla Vorgia *et al.*, 1990). It is not enough, however, to enact legislative measures without ensuring that they are properly enforced and effective in practice and that adequate penalties are imposed against infringement of the laws (Sasco, 1993). This calls for regular evaluation of the measures, with amendments to existing texts whenever necessary, given that any deficiencies in legislation will be readily exploited by the tobacco industry. The potential public health benefits will be enhanced if coercive measures are coupled with comprehensive health promotion activities and educational programmes for the general population, and especially for high-risk groups such as the young, who are particularly vulnerable to tobacco marketing. Moreover, experience has shown that behaviour with regard to a harmful product can be changed profoundly with sufficient effort (Sasco, 1992).

Conclusion

Tobacco legislation constitutes the foundation on which a structured health promotion effort can be built. The trend observed during the past decade in the European Union towards harmonization of the legislative texts, which at the same time are becoming increasingly restrictive, can be regarded as encouraging in the perspective of a rational tobacco control programme.

Acknowledgments
This work was conducted within the EuroLego project, supported by the Europe against Cancer Programme of the European Union (Contract SOC 97 200385 05F02). During this work, Dr R. Ah-Song, Dr V. Bourdès and I. Gendre were supported by Special Training Awards in the Unit of Epidemiology for Cancer Prevention at IARC.

References
Dalla-Vorgia, P., Sasco, A., Skalkidis, Y., Katsouyanni, K. & Trichopoulos, D. (1990) An evaluation of the effectiveness of tobacco-control legislative policies in European Community countries. *Scand. J. Soc. Med.*, **18**, 81–89
Parkin, D.M. & Sasco, A.J. (1993) Lung cancer: Worldwide variation in occurrence and proportion attributable to tobacco use. *Lung Cancer*, **9**, 1–16
Pisani, P., Parkin, D.M. & Ferlay, J. (1993) Estimates of the worldwide mortality from eighteen major cancers in 1985. Implications for prevention and projections of future burden. *Int. J. Cancer*, **55**, 891–903
Roemer, R. (1992) Tobacco policy: The power of law. In: Gupta, P.C., Hamner, J.E. & Murti, M.R., eds, *Control of Tobacco-related Cancers and other Diseases*, Bombay: Tata Institute for Fundamental Research, pp. 329–339
Sasco, A.J. (1992) Tobacco and cancer: How to react to the evidence. *Eur. J. Cancer Prev.*, **1**, 367–373
Sasco, A.J. (1993) Comparative study of anti-smoking legislation in countries of the European Economic Community. *Tob. Alert*, **January**, 12

Sasco, A.J. & Bourdès, V. (1996) Tobacco legislation in the European Union from 1985 to 1995. In: *Smoke free Europe: Conference on Tobacco or Health.* Finnish Center for Health Education, p. 66
Sasco, A.J. & van der Elst, P. (1989) Anti-tobacco legislation in the countries of the European Economic Community. *Soc. Eur.*, **March**, 119–123
Sasco, A.J., Dalla-Vorgia, P. & van der Elst P. (1992) *Comparative study of anti-smoking legislation in the member states of the EEC* (IARC-EEC Technical Report No. 8) Lyon: International Agency for Research on Cancer

Strategies for successful legislation

C.H. Leong

Hong Kong SAR, China

If tobacco were to be introduced today, given all our knowledge about its harmful effects, it would be banned. Regrettably, our forefathers were not aware of the effects of tobacco and related products. Worse, for decades they were blindfolded by the tobacco industry, who now admit that they knew about the lethal effects of smoking but deliberately hid the truth. For years, the tobacco industry argued that there was no direct proof that smoking is related to lung cancer. Today, they confirm that they have had evidence of the link for a long time but withheld it from the public. For the first time, the tobacco industry has conceded that the nicotine in tobacco is addictive. What difference is there then between a cigarette and heroin? Why is heroin banned and cigarettes allowed to be glorified in beautiful advertisements? The harmful effects of tobacco and its products have not only resulted in unnecessary loss of life but have increased the health-care costs for chronic lung diseases, cardiovascular problems, cancer of the urinary bladder and many other conditions. In Hong Kong, an area of 1095 km^2 and a population of over 6 million, the direct health-care cost for smoking-related diseases amounts to HK\$ 670–970 million per annum, and the indirect cost, taking into consideration factors like loss of working hours and premature deaths, is HK\$ 1.33 thousand million.

But the wind is changing. Even in the land of Gold Virginia, tobacco leaves are losing their influence on Capitol Hill. The United States Federal Court has ordered the tobacco industry to pay some US\$ 370 thousand million within 25 years, including approximately US\$ 60 thousand million in lieu of punitive damage for past conduct. There is no doubt that this action will do much to reduce the activities of the tobacco industry and at the same time enhance the awareness of the public about the hazards of smoking, but it is not enough to bring the tobacco giants to their knees. Under the pretext that tobacco is still a legal product and in the face of increasing opposition in the western world, they are turning to the East, targeting the very young and the female non-smoker especially.

Anti-smoking activities have been fairly successful on a global scale, as the number of adult smokers is apparently declining, but adolescents are contributing increasingly to the ever-growing fortune of the tobacco industry. Among the means of tobacco promotion, nothing is more effective, more deceptive and more deleterious than tobacco advertising. The 'macho' effect of Marlboro, the manly effect of Camel, the cool, relaxing effect of Kent and Salem are irresistible to the immature. With Michael Chang standing in front of a Salem billboard holding a tennis racket, with Michael Schummacher driving to victory in a Formula 1 car splashed with 555, no wonder so many people fall prey to tobacco. Tobacco advertisements must be banned by proper legislation!

Tobacco industry lobbying tactics in Hong Kong

The tobacco industry, with its well-developed lobbying tactics and army of legal and human rights experts, have raised arguments targeted at all sectors of the public and legislators to deflect their determination to ban tobacco advertising in Hong Kong:

- They claim that banning of tobacco advertisments violates human rights and the principle of freedom of expression. After the Canadian experience and before the handover of Hong Kong to China, when a majority of legislators and the public feared that freedom of speech would be threatened by the return to Chinese sovereignty, this argument was very effective.
- They argue that tobacco is a legal product and Hong Kong is a free market economy. This argument is aimed at the business sector of legislators who are inclined to support free trade.
- They claim that the advertising industry and other businesses will suffer, thus shaking labour representatives.
- They claim that a ban will remove the lifeline for the small retailers and street hawkers who make most tobacco sales in Hong Kong. The cheap prices of illegally imported cigarettes have already removed much of the business of these small vendors, and the tobacco giants claim that their livelihood now depends on the few thousand dollars they receive in advertising fees. Labour representatives are further shaken and so is the public. As most of these small vendors are frail old grannies, emotions run high for the benefit of tobacco advertising.
- They threaten that support for sports and cultural activities will suffer. With no other means of support in Hong Kong, such a predicament does send a convincing message to sports and culture enthusiasts, some of whom are powerful community leaders.

A well-considered strategy must be in place before any assault on tobacco advertising is contemplated. I shall therefore share our experience in pushing through an anti-tobacco advertising bill in Hong Kong, a bill that is imperfect but is a step in the right direction.

Strategies for successful legislation

In the 1980s, the Hong Kong Government committed itself to the pledge of the Worlld Health Organization (WHO) Office for the Western Pacific that the Region would be a tobacco advertising-free zone by the year 2000. The Government made a good start by introducing a law to ban advertisments in electronic media, but little has been done since. The anti-tobacco groups in Hong Kong established the following strategy:

Have a bill ready: A proposal for a ban on tobacco advertising must first be placed before the Legislature. The relevant Government department has twice attempted to introduce such a bill, but on both occasions it was thrown out before being presented. To get around Government bureaucracy, I introduced a Member's Bill on the grounds that such advertisements are lethal. The legislators were in a quandary: they would find it difficult to pass such a radical bill but realized that they could not reject it entirely. The Government was embarrassed that an individual legislator and not themselves had introduced a bill that affected livelihood issues. They then introduced a much watered-down version of the bill, to 'control' tobacco advertisements. Well before introduction of the bill, a motion debate was organized in the Legislature in which the arguments for and against banning tobacco advertising were aired.

Make a well-documented, point-by-point attack on the arguments of tobacco lobbyists. The anti-human rights argument did not hold, because, according to the Hong Kong Bill of Rights, exemption is made when public health is at stake. Similarly, the claim of loss of revenue to advertising agencies was shattered, as experience in neighbouring countries showed the reverse. Our two major television corporations showed a health increase in revenue after tobacco advertisements were banned on electronic media.

Proper coordination of anti-smoking groups: Good coordination is essential. Anti-tobacco lobbyists round the world are usually volunteers, short of both financial and human support and sometimes naive about lobbying tactics.

Make use of the experience of neighbouring countries: Hong Kong was fortunate that by the time the bill was introduced, our neighbours—mainland China, Macao,

Singapore and Thailand—had already introduced advertising bans with positive results.

Give and take: As discussion of the bill proceeded, it became obvious that two provisions would not carry: the ban on sponsorship for sports and cultural activities and advertising at the point of sale for small vendors. Emotions ran high in their favour. I therefore introduced amendments to provide a grace period for the ban to take effect, citing the year 2000 as the date designated by WHO to achieve a tobacco advertisement-free region, to allow advertising at the point of sales of street hawkers and to relax restrictions for corporate sponsorship of sports and cultural activities. This may not have been a bad move, for the bill might otherwise not have been passed.

Result

With 'give and take', we passed the *Smoking (Public Health) (Amendment) (No. 2) Ordinance*, which:

- bans tobacco advertisements on billboards and displays, except at the points of sale of small vendors;
- bans tobacco advertising in printed media from 31 December 1999;
- requires designated no-smoking areas in restaurants and areas open to the public in supermarkets, shopping malls, banks and department stores;
- bans sponsorship with direct advertising of tobacco brand names (although tobacco brand names in association with non-tobacco goods are still allowed);
- bans gifts of tobacco products to all persons (not only minors) for the purposes of promotion or advertisement, in exchange for a token such as a prize, at a promotional discount, with any gift attached or attached to any non-tobacco product;
- requires more prominent health warnings on tobacco products and advertisements • bans the sale of tobacco products from vending machines.

This is only the first step. What is important is that the opinions of people and legislators have changed, and most are now convinced that tobacco is harmful and, although legal, could be lethal!

Measures to kick out and keep out transnational tobacco companies from a national market

R. Cunningham

Canadian Cancer Society, Ottawa, Ontario, Canada

Introduction

Since the 1960s, transnational tobacco companies have penetrated new markets in Latin America, Africa, Asia and central and eastern Europe. This has had an adverse impact on tobacco control. In contrast to former domestic tobacco monopolies, transnational tobacco companies market more aggressively and oppose government regulation more strenuously (Cunningham, 1996). Chaloupka and Laixuthai (1996) found that the entry of transnational tobacco companies into four Asian countries led to a per capita consumption in 1991 that was nearly 10% higher than it would have been if the markets had remained closed to United States cigarettes.

There are still some markets in which transnational tobacco companies have only a small presence, such as China and Thailand. This paper attempts to build on previous work by Connolly (1994) and Mackay (1989a,b) by presenting measures that will help in keeping these companies out of a particular market and in pressuring them to withdraw from a market.

Measures

1. Adopt a total ban on all forms of advertising and promotion, including sponsorships and other forms of indirect advertising. Without the ability to market their products, tobacco companies have a much more difficult time in gaining market share, a fact frequently advanced by the tobacco industry. In Thailand, where an advertising ban was in place when the transnational tobacco companies entered the market, they have obtained only 3% of the market. A ban on advertising and promotion should contain no loopholes and should be strictly enforced. The General Agreement on Tariffs and Trade (GATT, 1990) has ruled that an advertising ban is an acceptable measure, provided the law applies equally to domestic and foreign brands.

2. Adopt plain packaging. Plain packaging prevents the positive brand imagery associated with foreign brands from being exploited as a means of gaining market share. In Canada in 1994, Philip Morris, R.J. Reynolds and B.A.T Industries plc made written submissions to the House of Commons Standing Committee on Health when the Committee was conducting hearings on plain packaging. The companies argued that plain packaging was a protectionist measure. The President of Philip Morris International stated: "In time we would hope to develop our US brands in the Canadian market. However, plain packaging would make it virtually impossible to establish the brand recognition among Canadian consumers necessary to penetrate the Canadian market." (W.H. Webb, President and Chief Executive Officer, Philip Morris International Inc., letter to House of Commons Standing Committee on Health, 5 May 1994).

3. Adopt profit controls through maximum net-of-tax price controls, applied equally to all brands. In developing countries, foreign brands are typically much more expensive than domestic brands, partly because of higher costs. By controlling maximum profit levels through maximum net-of-tax prices, it might not be possible to sell foreign products profitably in a market, so that transnational tobacco companies would be prompted to abandon the market. Price controls could be adopted by national or sub-national governments. To prevent increased consumption resulting from lower manufacturer prices, governments should increase tobacco taxes on all brands.

4. Require mandatory public disclosure of additives and other product ingredients on a brand-by-brand basis. Manufacturers have fought hard to keep their product recipes a secret and might withdraw from a market rather than disclose the additives used. This happened in Canada in 1989 when Philip Morris stopped exporting products to avoid making reports to the Federal Government—reports that were not even going to become public.

5. Require mandatory disclosure of behavioural, market and product research. This would result in R.J. Reynolds, for example, being required to disclose all market research done in the country in question (or ideally anywhere in the world) for any brands (e.g. Camel, Winston) that the company wanted to sell in the country. Companies would be very unhappy about disclosing internal research and might withdraw from a market instead of complying with such a requirement.

6. Adopt effective anti-smuggling measures. There have been numerous examples where foreign cigarettes are denied access to a market but nevertheless appear in the country as contraband, with the full knowledge of the manufacturers. The presence of contraband, leading to lost tax revenue, puts pressure on governments to accept transnational tobacco companies into the market. Anti-smuggling measures can remove or reduce the pressure created by contraband.

7. Adopt tariffs and import quotas. Countries should maximize the tariffs and the use of import quotas to the extent permitted by the international trading agreements of which they are signatories.

8. Adopt a total ban on tobacco product imports and local manufacture of foreign brands. A total ban on foreign cigarettes is a direct way of preventing the presence of transnational tobacco companies, but since this measure is prohibited by GATT, it could be implemented only in countries that are not signatories of GATT (or of other agreements in which such a measure is prohibited).

Implementing the measures

To minimize the presence of transnational tobacco companies, health interests should recognize that the domestic tobacco industry is an ally, albeit an unusual one. For financial and employment reasons, domestic tobacco manufacturers, unions of tobacco factory workers and tobacco farmers do not want transnational tobacco companies to gain market share. These economic interests can be organized into a powerful lobby to persuade the government to implement appropriate measures to counter transnational tobacco companies. The combination of a tobacco lobby and a health lobby may be potent indeed, especially if there is a strong public campaign to mount popular opposition to transnational tobacco companies.

Health interests should seek assistance from tobacco control colleagues abroad, especially if the government in the home country of a transnational tonacco company (e.g. the United Kingdom and the United States) is exerting pressure to open up the market. This type of international collaboration was extremely effective when the United States Government was trying to open its market to American cigarettes.

Conclusion

The presence of transnational tobacco companies in a country has an adverse impact on tobacco control. To minimize the penetration of transnational tobacco companies in a particular market, countries should implement a series of counter-measures.

References

Chaloupka, F.J. & Laixuthai, A. (1996) US Trade Policy and Cigarette Smoking in Asia (National Bureau of Economic Research Working Paper 5543), Cambridge, Massachusetts: National Bureau of Economic Research
Connolly, G.N. (1994) Freedom from aggression: A guide to resisting transnational tobacco companies' entry into developing countries. In: *Building a Tobacco-free World. 8th World Conference on Tobacco and Health, Buenos Aires, Argentina*, American Cancer Society, pp. 125–158
Cunningham, R. (1996) *Smoke & Mirrors: The Canadian Tobacco War*, Ottawa: International Development Research Centre, Chapter 18, Exporting the epidemic
General Agreement on Tariffs and Trade (1990) Thailand: Restrictions on importation of and internal taxes on cigarettes. Report of the panel adopted on 7 November 1990 (GATT Document DS10/R, 46th sess., 37th suppl.), Basic Instruments and Selected Documents
Mackay, J. (1989a) Political and promotional thrusts in Asia by the transnational tobacco companies. In: Durston, B. & Jamrozik, K., eds, *The Global War. Proceedings of the 7th World Conference on Tobacco and Health, Perth, Australia*, pp. 139–141
Mackay, J. (1989b) Tobacco in the Third World: How to resist. *World Smoking Health*, 14 (3), 3–6

The Canadian set-back: Tobacco use in Canada, 1986–97

C. Callard

Physicians for a Smoke-free Canada, Ottawa, Ontario, Canada

A short-lived sense of victory

At the beginning of this decade, Canadians working in tobacco control claimed leadership on tobacco issues. At the Seventh World Conference on Tobacco or Health, a leading Canadian activist boasted that 'from 1983 to 1989, tobacco sales fell by 20% in absolute terms. The adult per capita fall was 29%. If there is another country with such a significant decline, we would like to learn more about that country's experience' (Mahood). The descriptor 'world precedent-setting' became hackneyed through overuse by justifiably proud anti-tobacco lobbyists to describe Canada's landmark 1988 legislation, its rapid tax increase on cigarettes in the late 1980s and its 1994 health warnings.

As recently as the last World Conference, Canadian Government officials continued to promote the view that Canada was an arena of active progress against tobacco use.

The Assistant Deputy Minister of Health Promotion came to inform the Conference that Canada had 'committed CDN$ 185 million to a new tobacco demand reduction strategy.' She promised a comprehensive programme that would target pregnant women and those who had given birth, encourage employers to adopt smoke-free workplace policies, deliver hard-hitting national advertising campaigns and conduct a panoply of research (Stanley, 1996). Other Canadian Government officials told the Conference that the national strategy to reduce tobacco use, established by the Federal and provincial governments, was 'well under way' to achieving its·overall mission of a generation of non-smokers by the year 2000, thanks to 'a comprehensive and cooperative approach that will help to ensure its success' (McElroy & Stephens, 1996).

As the decade and century draw to a close, the Federal Canadian Government and national public health advocates have more reason to feel humble. The CDN$ 185 million campaign has shrunk to only CDN$ 10 million a year. There are currently no advertising campaigns, hard-hitting or otherwise. Plans for new research and public programming have been suspended pending allocation of the CDN$ 10 million budget, promised in November 1996 but not yet authorized by August 1997. The group directing the national strategy to reduce tobacco use had not met for 10 months, and its future seemed uncertain even as its goal of a smoke-free generation within two years seemed certainly unattainable.

The 1988 'world precedent-setting legislation' was struck down by the Supreme Court in September 1995, with a blistering rebuke of Health Canada's defence. The replacement legislation, enacted in April 1997, has much less ambitious restrictions on promotion. The temporary tax reduction of 1994 now appears to be permanent, and cigarette prices are virtually the same as they were a decade ago. Promising new initiatives, such as plain packaging and the individual marking of cigarettes to protect against contraband, have been put to one side.

Public policy measures such as high cigarette taxes and bans on tobacco promotion are only the means—not the end. If tobacco use and mortality from tobacco-related causes continue to decrease at a satisfactory rate, despite the loss of these measures, then progress is still being made. Are there signs of progress against tobacco use? A number of indicators suggest otherwise.

Prevalence and consumption

Over the past decade, Canadians have continued to smoke less often and to smoke fewer cigarettes *per capita*, but aggregate measures of prevalence and consumption can mask some important movements in sub-populations. The prevalence of smoking among the young, as measured by Government surveys, is higher than it was in 1988 (28% versus 26%) and higher than it was during the mid-decade (21%) (Health and Welfare Canada, 1989, 1992; Statistics Canada, 1989, 1993). Smoking among young adults, as measured by the tobacco industry, has similarly returned to the level of a decade ago (33.4% in 1988 and 32.3% in 1996) (Figure 1; RJR Macdonald, 1997).

Accurate measurements of both prevalence and consumption during this period are made more difficult by the failure of the Federal Government to undertake consistent annual surveys and by the unreliability of manufacturing and sales data (due to high levels of smuggling between 1991 and 1993). Government statistics in both cases can now be supplemented by data provided by the smallest of Canada's three major tobacco companies, RJR Macdonald, a subsidiary of RJR Nabisco (Figure 2). Both industry and Government data suggest that there has been little change in *per capita* consumption since 1992. Industry data are available only for the years since 1990: we do not know whether their figures would also support the Government findings of a 29% decrease since 1986 (from 2483 to 1739 cigarettes per person).

The bottom line

During the past decade, cigarettes have become cheaper for Canadian smokers, a greater source of profits for the multinational corporations who sell them, and a diminishing source of revenue for governments. In 1994, the newly elected Canadian

Figure 1. Prevalence of smoking in Canada, 1988–96, among all adults and young adults aged 19–24

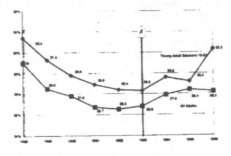

From RJR MacDonald. Prevalence of smoking in Canada as measured by the tobacco industry ('incidence') and by Statistics Canada. No data from national Government surveys conducted (if any) for the years 1987, 1988, 1992 and 1993 have been released. RJR Macdonald (a subsidiary of RJR Nabisco), has produced annual data and the only available data for 1996.

Government declared a price war on smugglers. Provinces were recruited to join the Federal Government in cutting taxes. As a result, in the five most populous provinces, cigarettes are now roughly the same price they were in 1986. In the five other provinces (with approximately 25% of the tobacco market), which have maintained a high-tax policy, cigarettes are approximately twice as expensive as in 1986. As a result of the tax reduction, Federal revenues from tobacco sales have declined significantly since the beginning of the decade, although they are marginally higher than in 1986.

In response to the reduction in tobacco taxes, the tobacco companies increased their profit margin on tobacco sales (Figure 3). This increased margin, together with increased sales, has resulted in significant gains in their earnings. The earnings of only two of Canada's three cigarette companies are reported publicly. Imperial Tobacco, the largest cigarette manufacturer, with 67% of the market share (based on wholesale shipment figures provided to Health Canada by manufacturers in 1996), saw its earnings grow by 339% since 1986, from CDN$ 208 million in 1986 to CDN$ 705 million in

Figure 2. Cigarette consumption in Canada, 1986–1996

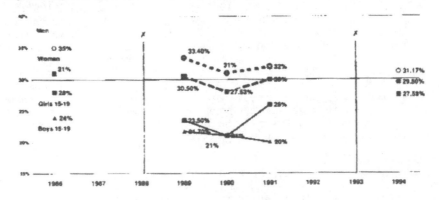

1996 (IMASCO annual reports, 1986–96). Rothmans, Benson & Hedges has seen its profits grow by an even more dramatic 468% (from CDN$ 21 500 000 to CDN$ 100 773 000) (Rothmans, Benson & Hedges annual reports, 1986–1996). The earnings of Canada's other cigarette company, RJR Macdonald, are not reported separately by its owner, RJR Nabisco.

Policy initiatives

Since 1986, Canadian public policy on tobacco has shifted a number of times. In 1986, the promotion and sale of tobacco products was governed for the most part by the tobacco industry voluntary code. By 1990, legislation providing for a total ban was on the statute books. By 1993, dramatic new health warnings were planned and cigarette taxes had risen to world levels; discussions about 'plain packaging' were beginning. By 1996, taxes had been slashed, the ban on advertising had been thrown out by theSupreme Court, and cigarette advertising had returned, governed by a tobacco industry voluntary code. In 1997, a new law banned direct advertising but allowed sponsorship advertising and other forms of promotion to continue, although some of these were to be banned at the end of 1998.

The chronology of policy decisions on tobacco issues (Table 1) reveals the vulnerability of policy gains to political change and the rapid pace at which legislative and tax decisions can be undone. The policy analysis and approach of Canadian governments and tobacco control advocates is consistent with those of international health communities, including WHO. An analysis of the changes in domestic Canadian policy over the past decade in comparison with tobacco policy measures proposed by WHO (Table 2) reveals that there have been significant policy changes towards WHO recommendations, but that progress towards meeting the WHO recommendations has been eroded since the beginning of the 1990s.

Conclusion

Canada has made enormous progress over the past 30 years against tobacco use and ultimately against tobacco-caused disease. Analysts of tobacco control should not, however, allow the achievements of the 1970s and 1980s to obscure the lack of progress over the past 10 years. The trends in smoking rates among young Canadians are particularly worrying. The temptation to perceive stalled progress as a reflection of a natural asymptote in the reduction of tobacco use should be resisted

The source of tobacco policy stagnation has not been identified, but a significant number of regressive policy decisions coincide with the election of the Liberal Government in October 1993. The restoration of established policy tools, such as a total ban on tobacco promotion and advertising and high cigarette taxes, should re-establish a reduction in tobacco consumption and smoking prevalence. The development

Figure 3. Tobacco profits in Canada. 1986–96

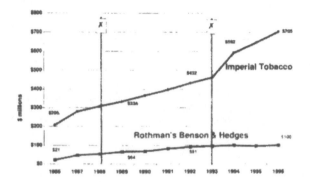

Table 1. Tobacco control in Canada: A chronology of public policy decisions, 1986–96

Date	Decision
1985	Federal government stops giving grants to amateur sports groups that accept tobacco sponsorship money
1986	Non Smoker's Health Act (Bill C-204) introduced. This private member's bill proposes to: • ban all tobacco advertising and promotion by including tobacco in the Hazardous Products Act • guarantee smoke-free workplaces for all Federally regulated workers • guarantee smoke-free travel on all Federally regulated carriers
1987	Tobacco Products Control Act (TPCA, Bill C-51) introduced. This government bill proposes to: • ban all tobacco advertising and sponsorship • require health warnings
1988	The TPCA becomes law (amended to allow existing sponsorship agreements) Smoke-free workplaces and public transport (when Federally regulated) Tobacco companies launch constitutional court challenge to TPCA Tobacco companies establish 'shell corporations' to circumvent ban on sponsorship advertising **Federal election. Conservative party returned with majority government**
1989	Tobacco taxes increased to CDN$ 4/carton
1990	Rotating health warnings effected
1991	Quebec Superior Court declares Federal ban on tobacco advertising unconstitutional Federal tobacco taxes increased by CDN$ 6/carton
1992	Lung cancer becomes the leading cause of cancer deaths among Canadian women
1993	Tobacco Sales to Young Persons Act (TSYPA) passed. Vendors may not sell cigarettes to children under 18 Contraband market peaks at 25–31% of total market **Federal Election. Conservatives defeated. Liberal majority government comes to power**
1994	Federal cigarette taxes cut as part of anti-smuggling initiative. The price of cigarettes is cut in half for 75% of Canadians Parliamentary Committee recommends adoption of 'plain packaging' Eight 'new and improved' health warnings on cigarette packages
1995	Supreme Court of Canada rules the TPCA unconstitutional Government introduces 'blueprint on tobacco control,' proposing to re-enact a total ban on tobacco promotion
1996	Government introduces Tobacco Act (C-71) which: • restricts direct advertising to direct mail, publications with 85% adult readership (this will include newspapers and most magazines) and bars • restricts sponsorship promotion to on-site promotion and the same distribution vehicles as direct advertising • gives the Government the authority to regulate retail displays, package labelling, cigarette manufacture • disallows promotion through clothing and other goods if they have youth appeal • bans mail-order sale of cigarettes • continues provisions of TSYPA
1997	Tobacco Act (C-71) is passed but restrictions on sponsorship are delayed until October 1998 Government announces plans to amend Tobacco Act to exempt motorsports from some provisions Government fails to pass regulations to put Tobacco Act in force: tobacco industry voluntarily complies with regulations established under previous legislation Tobacco industry launches court challenge to Tobacco Act. **Federal Election. Liberal majority government re-elected**

Table 2. Canadian Federal Government initiatives against tobacco use, 1986–96, compared with WHO recommendations

Policy	WHO recomm-endations	Tobacco Products Control Act as proposed	Tobacco Products Control Act as enacted	Blueprint on Tobacco Control	Tobacco Act as proposed including regulatory proposals	Tobacco Act as enacted, with regula-tions proposed to date
Ban advertising	Included	Included	Included	Included	Partly included	Partly included
Ban sponsorship	Included	Included	Partly included	Partly included	Not included	Not included

Table 2 (contd)

Policy	WHO recomm-endations	Tobacco Products Control Act as proposed	Tobacco Products Control Act as enacted	Blueprint on Tobacco Control	Tobacco Act as proposed including regulatory proposals	Tobacco Act as enacted, with regula-tions proposed to date
Ban promotion	Included	Included	Included	Included	Partly included	Partly included
Ban sales to minors	Included	Not included	Not included	Included	Included	Included
Increase tobacco taxes	Included	Not included	Included	Not included	Not included	Not included
Protect against passive smoking	Included	Partly included	Partly included	Partly included	Partly included	Partly included
Allocate tobacco tax revenue to health	Included	Not included	Not included	Not included	Not included	Not included
Health promotion, health education and cessation programmes	Included	Included	Included	Particularly strong measures	Included	Not included
Elimination of socioeconomic, behavioural and other incentives	Included	Not included	Not included	Not included	Not included	Not included
Health warnings on products	Included	Included	Included	Included	Included	Particularly strong measures
Health warnings on advertisements	Included	Not applicable	Not applicable	Not applicable	Included	Not included
Limits on toxic constituents	Included	Not included	Not included	Not included	Included	Not include
Reporting of toxic constituents	Included	Included	Included	Included	Included	Included
Economic alternatives to tobacco growing	Included	Included	Included	Included	Included	Included
Management and monitoring of tobacco issues	Included	Included	Included	Particularly strong measures	Included	Included

of new policy tools, particularly those designed for population sub-groups which show low resiliency to nicotine addiction, should be the focus of a reinvigorated tobacco control strategy.

References

Health and Welfare Canada (1989) *Smoking Behaviour of Canadians: A National Alcohol and Other Drugs Survey Report*

Health and Welfare Canada (1992) *Canada's Health Promotion Survey, 1990: Technical Report*

Mahood, G. Treating the tobacco epidemic like an epidemic, the road to effective tobacco control in Canada. In: *The Global War, Proceedings of the Seventh World Conference on Tobacco and Health*

McElroy, H. & Stephens, T. Tracking the progress of the national strategy to reduce tobacco use in Canada. In: *The Global War, Proceedings of the Seventh World Conference on Tobacco and Health*

RJR Macdonald (1997) Statistics produced in an internal memo dated 4 June 1997 to Rich Kauffeld, Chairman and CEO of RJR Macdonald from Lance Newman and Steve Wilson Stanley, K. Canada's tobacco demand reduction strategy. In: *The Global War, Proceedings of the Seventh World Conference on Tobacco and Health*, p. 129

Statistics Canada (1989) Surveys taken from *A Critical Review of Canadian Survey Data on Tobacco Use*

Statistics Canada (1993) *National Population Health Survey*

Tobacco control and Cuban legislation

N. Suarez Lugo

Carlos J. Finlay National School in Public Health, Ministry of Public Health, Havana, Cuba

The Cuban programme for prevention and control of tobacco use is described in another paper in this volume. Legal action is needed to support that programme, and the legislative actions taken are described here.

Cuban legislation: Actual situation

Smoking is currently regulated by State institutions through laws that are inadequate to protect human health, defend the right to breathe pure air and control tobacco advertising. The presence of direct and indirect advertising gives rise to the perception that smoking is acceptable, as otherwise the Government would ban it. A population survey showed that 78% believed that the existing restrictions were inadequate, and 76% said that bans on smoking in public places were not complied with. People are not protected from exposure to environmental tobacco smoke by law, and no conditions are created to make smoking socially unacceptable. The warning on cigarette packs is insufficient, as it is not strong enough and is always the same. Control of smoking by minors is poorly enforced, and the accessibility of tobacco and its social acceptability facilitate the initiation of smoking by young people.

Actions and results

The main actions undertaken within the programme in 1995–97 to improve Cuban legislation for tobacco control were to draw up a proposal for a law to change the warnings on packs and reduce nicotine and tar levels, propose a new price and marketing policy, control sales to minors, prohibit sales from vending machines and gradually prohibit and otherwise regulate smoking in public places. The principal results obtained in 1996 were:

- bans on smoking on domestic flights and in public transport, health and education centres, theatres, cinemas and shops;
- regulation of tobacco advertising through the Ministry of Public Health;
- an increase in the price of cigarettes between 1995 and 1997;
- a decrease in the nicotine and tar concentrations in popular cigarettes; and
- a proposed law on tobacco control.

The problems that remain to be solved are lack of controls on smoking in other public places, direct and indirect advertising, sales to minors, sale of loose cigarettes and the aggressive marketing of the Cuban–Brazil tobacco joint venture.

Proposed law for tobacco control

The proposal was drawn up by experts from the main Cuban organizations involved in tobacco control on the basis of a review of laws in other countries. They considered that the main targets of tobacco control are regulation of smoking in public places, reducing the access of young people to tobacco products and regulating the tobacco companies' marketing strategy. The proposed law will prohibit smoking in meeting places, health centres, educational institutions, public transport, sports centres, indoor cultural centres, recreation centres for young people and indoor public assistance centres. It will further prohibit sales of cigarettes to minors (< 17 years of age), from vending machines, in schools, at health centres and in recreation centres for young people. The warning on cigarette packs will be visible and rotating and approved by the Ministry of Public Health. The proposed law will also prohibit the distribution of free samples and regulate direct and indirect advertising in all mass media and at all sports and cultural events. The administrative authorities will be responsible for placing signs in all areas where smoking is prohibited and for determining the penalties that will be imposed for infractions of the regulations.

Conclusion

At the time of writing, the proposed law had been approved by the National Committee of the programme for tobacco control, the Ministry of Public Health and the Commission of the Cuban Parliament and had been presented to the Government for review, evaluation and approval. It was then to be presented to the National Assembly.

It is to be hoped that this activity will culminate in an act that supports the tobacco control progarmme and reduces the prevalence and social acceptability of smoking.

Legislation against tobacco smoking in France, 1996

G. Dubois

National Committee against Smoking, Versailles, France

Background

The scientific data on smoking are among the most extensive, consistent and wide-ranging to be found anywhere. It is difficult to teach epidemiology without using smoking as an example, since few factors are as consistent and forceful in their effects. Moreover, it is a risk factor that often meets the criteria of causality, as in the case of lung cancer.

One-third of people in France smoke: 40% of men and 27% of women. Smoking is an unparalled public health problem, since it is responsible for 60 000 deaths a year in France (3000 of them among women), equivalent to the crash of a Boeing 727 every day. If nothing is done, the death toll from tobacco will rise to 165 000 by 2025 (55 000 of them among women). Overall, there is no other product in common use that is addictive and has so many drastic and varied consequences as tobacco.

Principal obstacles to tobacco control

Tobacco is addictive. Although two out of three smokers want to stop, they often make several unsuccessful attempts before they succeed. Tobacco is a delayed-action killer and therefore a hidden one. Furthermore, the deaths are scattered by being classified under many headings whose common factor, tobacco, is not immediately obvious. It is brought into the open only in epidemiological surveys. Nevertheless, independent objective analysis of the data gives a clear verdict, beyond any reasonable doubt (to use a legal term).

In the meantime, the concerted, world-wide strategy of cigarette manufacturers has been:

- to force open markets with State monopolies;
- to make political parties, intermediate bodies and the mass media dependent on them as a source of funds;
- to finance research with a view to preventing its involvement with the tobacco issue or with a view to twisting data to create confusion or spread false information;
- to finance disinformation agencies, which are recognizable by their unlimited means and provision of information that is consistently truncated, incomplete or partial.

Principal methods

The World Health Organization and the European Union's programme 'Europe against Cancer' have laid down guidelines for effective action against smoking. This is based on two legal principles: recognition and protection of the individual's right to choose to live without exposure of tobacco and recognition of the right to frequent public places free from tobacco smoke. Five actions are proposed: to ban all direct and indirect tobacco advertising; to increase the price of all tobacco products; to protect non-smokers from other people's smoke; to inform and educate and to help smokers

The situation in France

The measures applied under the Act of 10 January 1991 (the Evin Act) have led to a decrease of 11% in cigarette consumption and a decrease of 8.5% in the consumption of all forms of tobacco. Between 1991 and 1996, this gave an overall reduction of 44 thousand million cigarettes when compared with the trend over the preceding 15 years, resulting in half of the 1991 consumption in 1996. This is a major success, although if the various means of action are examined separately, the picture is less uniform.

A ban on advertising in place since 1993 has eliminated all direct advertising and reduced indirect advertising by 95%. Illicit advertising continues, despite the fact that the three main cigarette manufacturers have been penalized by the courts 29 times in five years. They have continued to press for amendment of the Act, which shows how important advertising is for recruiting the 10 000 children and adolescents needed each week to maintain the level of tobacco consumption in France.

The increase in the price of tobacco made possible by removal of tobacco from the consumer price index was initially effective because it was done in steps of 10–15%. The cigarette manufacturers then obtained from the Ministry of Finance a joint price management system that provided insufficiently large price increases (6% in 1995 and 3% in January 1996).

Protection of non-smokers from other people's smoke was endorsed by 90% of the French population in 1994 (CFES Health Barometer), a higher proportion than in 1993 (84%). This figure included the support of 86% of smokers. In addition, the percentage of smokers in favour of fines for failure to comply with regulations increased from 39 to 53%, so it has become a majority view even among smokers. Today, two out of three people in France support fines, an endorsement most policies would be overjoyed to reach. Organized disinformation has so far prevented the law from being implemented, even in educational establishments. Reactivation of the effort is vital.

The level of provision of education and information on smoking is lamentable in France, as recognised by the Minister of Public Health and Health Insurance and a number of Members of Parliament. That did not, however, prevent them from maintaining the miserable FF 1.9 million allotted by the State to combating smoking in 1995 (FF 2.8 million in 1984), which should be compared with the FF 2 thousand million in tax revenue brought to the State by children and adolescents alone. Fortunately, other players such as the national employee health insurance fund (FF 8 million) are involved, but there is no funding commensurate with the problem.

Conclusion

If the prevalence of smoking in France is to decrease further, there must be ongoing political will and action on a broad front, encompassing the five strategies proposed in this paper. Although giving a good example on the advertising front, France is at the bottom of the class for health education. France had a difficult position from the start, since it has the largest proportion of young smokers in Europe. It must thus act promptly to cut down smoking as quickly as possible through the efficient use of effective means. Otherwise, the prospects are gloomy and the estimate of 165 000 smoking-related deaths by 2025 instead of the current figure of 60 000 is likely to be realized.

Movement for a people-friendly tobacco law in the Republic of Slovenia

E. Stergar[1], M. Bevc Stankovic[1] & S. Dizdarevic[2]

[1]*Institute of Public Health of the Republic of Slovenia, Ljubljana, Slovenia, and*
[2]*Free lancer*

The Republic of Slovenia is a central European country that became independent in 1991. The population is about 2 million. It is estimated that every year about 3500 people die from tobacco smoking-related diseases.

Before independence, legislation on tobacco advertising was included in a law on the health and nutritive standards of food and objects in common use. According to this law, which has been in force since 1978, advertising of tobacco products was forbidden. There were unwritten rules about not smoking in cinemas, in most theatres, on buses and in banks. There were areas for non-smokers on public transport, but there were no clear rules about smoking in other public places such as workplaces, schools and health-care centres.

Soon after our country became independent, the only tobacco factory in Slovenia began to advertise its products aggressively. In 1992, the Ministry of Health prepared a new law restricting the use of tobacco products, but it did not pass the three debates required by Parliamentary procedure and was removed in August 1993. A new proposal was prepared by two Members of Parliament, which was more favourable to the tobacco industry. A health-conscious Member of Parliament introduced the idea of exerting organized pressure on other Members for a law that would favour people's health and not the tobacco industry, and the 'Movement for a people-friendly tobacco law' was established in December 1994. Its only scope was to influence the so-called tobacco law in such a way that it would promote health rather than the tobacco industry's profits.

The members of the movement were 15 non-governmental organizations: the Heart Association, the Association for Health Promotion and Health Education, the Association against Cancer, the Association for Lung Diseases, the Non-smokers Association, the Association of Laryngectomized Persons, the Healthy Cities Maribor, Ljubljana, Celje, the Slovenian Ecological Movement, the Association of Patients with Cancer, the Scouts' Organization, the Red Cross of Slovenia, the Association for the Protection of Consumers and the Institute of Public Health. The core of the movement consisted of four persons. The movement had a small budget for only the most necessary expenditures.

A communications strategy was established and discussed at the start. The objectives were stated to be public sensitization to exert pressure on Members of Parliament to support amendments to the tobacco law. The target groups were thus Members of Parliament and the electoral body. We could not predict how long this would take; we knew there would be three phases from January 1995, before each discussion of the law in Parliament. Each phase consisted of analysis, media messages, visits to Members of Parliament, round-table discussions, street actions and feedback to the public. At the beginning it was estimated the exercise would last till summer 1995.

The general rules were to ensure a positive approach; to protect children from advertisements and environmental tobacco smoke; not to blame smokers; to act not aggressively but with energy; not to use children in media activities; to be clear and use facts and to be flexible and well prepared. The elements of the communication strategy were to use television spots, news and interviews; radio spots, news and talk shows, articles, contributions to correspondence columns, leaflets, posters and flyers; and to send letters to and visit Members of Parliament and to send letters seeking support from target groups such as teachers and parents.

Our aims were clearly set out from the beginning:
- a total ban on advertisements and promotion,
- a ban on smoking in public and at work places,

- a ban on sales to youngsters under 18 and sales only in tobacco shops,
- warnings on cigarette packs: 'Warning from the Minister of Health: Smoking kills! Smoking causes lung cancer! Smoking causes cardiovascular disease!"
- statement of nicotine and tar contents on packs and
- a fund for health promotion.

A further main objective was sponsorship for athletes and artistes who had been sponsored by the tobacco industry.

First phase: January –March 1995

Television and radio spots were prepared with statements from well-known persons such as athletes, actors and pop singers about their attitude towards smoking. A leaflet describing the movement's aims was printed, newspaper articles were prepared (mainly translations from the ASH bulletin), and thousands of letters were mailed asking for support from schools, health centres, kindergartens and university students. The day before the first discussion in Parliament, a press conference was held at which the movement was introduced to the public and the actions planned for the first phase were described. There was street action in various Slovenian cities on the day the law was discussed in Parliament, and more than 30 000 signatures in support of the people-friendly tobacco law were gathered in one day.

Second phase: end of March–November 1995

Amendments were prepared and submitted. Members of the associations wrote letters to Members of Parliament demanding a tobacco law that favoured children and health. New television and radio spots were presented. Two press conferences were held: one in September on the occasion of a no-smoking campaign for adolescents and the other in November, a day before the second reading of the law. An exhibit was prepared on indirect advertising and children's opinion about smoking and was shown in Parliament. Its removal after two days caused a scandal, and on the day of the second reading of the law, there were demonstrations in front of the Parliament building and street action in several Slovenian cities. When new tobacco campaigns were begun during the summer, denunciations were submitted, and tobacco advertisements were covered with graffiti. A booklet entitled 'What you should know about cigarettes ads' was printed and distributed to Members of Parliament and to the public.

Third phase: end of November 1995–8 October 1996

This was a phase during which the third discussion of the law was delayed—a very hard time for the movement. In January, the support of top athletes was sought for an article on the ban on promotion and sponsorship. Denunciations of the tobacco factory were made, letters to Members of Parliament were written and visits were paid to them to ensure that the law was placed on agenda. Tobacco advertisements were sprayed with paint. In May, the law on establishing a fund for tobacco or health was submitted to the first reading. In September, there was a press conference and street action demanding the third discussion of the law. The movement was present in correspondence columns throughout the year. On 2 October, the third reading was conducted in Parliament, and the law was passed. On 8 October, the law was discussed by the State Advisory Council and was accepted.

All but two of the movement's aims were achieved, as follows: banning sales to youngsters under 18 and sales only in tobacco shops and establishing a fund for health promotion. The law calls for a total ban on advertisements and promotion, forbids smoking in public and work places and requires warnings on cigarette packs, with nicotine and tar contents. The first part of the law came into force in November 1996 and the second in May 1997. Its implementation is strictly controlled by inspectors.

Results of a legislative approach to tobacco control: Thailand's experience

P. Vateesatokit

Action on Smoking and Health, Bangkok, Thailand

Background

Thailand is a rapidly developing country in South-east Asia with a population of 60 million. The Thai Government has owned and operated the Thai Tobacco Monopoly since the Second World War, but in 1991 the Thai cigarette market was opened to foreign imports. The prevalence of smoking among males is very high, over half of adult males being regular smokers, while the female smoking rate has remained low, at about 5%. The rate has decreased by about 1.4% per year among males but that for females has remained static. There were 11.2 million smokers in 1996, of whom 10.6 million were male and 0.6 million female.

Legislative developments in Thailand

Smoking control was initiated by the Thai medical community in the early 1970s, and it successfully lobbied the Thai Government to make the Thai Tobacco Monopoly print health warnings on cigarette packets. The first legislation for tobacco control was an ordinance issued by the Bangkok Metropolis in 1976, which banned smoking in cinemas and on buses. Another executive order banning cigarette advertising on the electronic media was issued in 1985, followed by a legislative ban on all forms of cigarette advertising and promotion in 1989. In 1992, two comprehensive tobacco control laws were enacted by the National Assembly. The *Tobacco Products Control Act* prohibits all forms of cigarette advertising and promotion, requires prominent health warnings and disclosure of ingredients and bans sales from vending machines and to persons under 18 years of age. The *Nonsmoker's Health Protection Act* bans smoking in almost all public places, including schools, throughout the country.

The Ministry of Public Health set up a Tobacco Consumption Control Office to coordinate the country's tobacco control activities, including surveillance and supervision of law enforcement. It has a budget of only US$ 750 000 and a handful of personnel to conduct all of its activities. Enforcement of the law therefore became a problem as soon as it went into effect. The Minister of Public Health then appointed officials from both central and local government departments to enforce the two laws, in addition to cooperation with the police.

Thai Action on Smoking and Health, a non-governmental organization, has assisted the Tobacco Consumption Control Office in the law enforcement effort by serving as a watchdog of law violators, and particularly the transnational tobacco companies, which frequently try to evade the law by advertising non-tobacco products, such as shirts and shoes carrying cigarette logos. The Tobacco Consumption Control Office initially adopted a rather lenient attitude towards law violators. In 1994, two years after the law was enacted, the Ministry issued 15 warnings to foreign cigarette companies, advertising agencies and publishers for violations of indirect advertising, and 11 warnings to owners of public places and establishments not complying with restictions on smoking in public places. Most of the advertising agencies and publishers alleged that they did not know about the provisions of the law with regard to indirect advertising. This may be true, since most of the violators did not commit the same offence, but new violations of the law are found constantly. Two publishers committed offences even though they had received warnings, and they were prosecuted. It is clear that foreign cigarette importers are behind these violations of the law. An employee of an advertising agency reported that the Thai subsidiary of a transnational tobacco company had tried to hire his agency to promote its products, despite the very strict Thai ban.

Violations of the *Nonsmoker's Health Protection Act* occur mostly in public places, and are committed mainly by owners of air-conditioned restaurants who fail to provide the no-smoking areas required by law. This occurs more commonly in the smaller provinces than in large cities. Although the Thai public is fully aware of the dangers of environmental tobacco smoke, complaints about violations of bans on smoking are common; however, individuals are rarely prosecuted. Officials appointed to supervise the law and the police have taken a passive role in enforcing the ban in public places and tend to view such violations as a minor offence. They check for compliance with the law only occasionally and usually take no action when they receive a complaint from the public. As even direct complaints to the police seldom see any legal action, they are infrequent.

A study of sales to minors carried out in 1995 involving 375 shops revealed that 99% of 10–15-year-old children could purchase cigarettes. Interestingly, 8.3% of these shops had signs saying 'No sales to minors' in front of their shops. In a second study in 1996 in another province covering 108 shops after an aggressive anti-smoking programme, 51% of 13–15-year-old children could purchase cigarettes. In the same study, out of 80 shopkeepers who knew of the law, 50 refused to sell tobacco to the children. Although the second study shows considerable improvement in compliance with the law, it is hard to know how long the effects of the campaign will last.

Our experience in the enforcement of the two tobacco control acts shows that many parties are involved, all of which must be informed about the law and, more importantly, be willing to cooperate to make the law work. The most problematic parties are the transnational tobacco companies, which constantly violate the law by using their big money to hire advertising agencies and influence publishers. One loophole in the Thai law is that it penalizes only the advertising agency that undertakes indirect advertising, while the tobacco company that hires the agency is not held responsible. This provision should be amended to make the tobacco companies responsible for indirect advertising violations.

The Ministry of Public Health is in the process of prosecuting the Thai subsidiary of one transnational tobacco company for arranging point-of-sale promotion through their retailers. While this is going on, point-of-sale promotion continues in many retail stores, organized by the subsidiary. It should be noted that the Thai Tobacco Monopoly never challenges the *Tobacco Product Contral Act*, since any employee who does so is challenging the State authority and risks losing his ot her job.

The third party in the law enforcement process is the smoking public. Although Bangkok's ordinance banning smoking in cinemas and buses has been in place since 1976, restriction of smoking in public places is new for the rest of the country, as smoking has been practised freely for over half a century. The limited budget of the Tobacco Consumption Control Office means that very little public information is made available about the content of the law. Many smokers therefore violate the no-smoking ban in public places through either ignorance or carelessness. The Ministry of Public Health's policy stresses the responsibility of the owner of any public place to provide and display no-smoking signs, as required by law. Little emphasis is placed on prosecuting smokers who violate the law, but when smokers are asked not to smoke in prohibited areas, almost all of them cooperate. We have carried out several projects aimed at making no smoking in public places the social norm. If this is sucessful, it will greatly facilitate the law enforcement processes.

Several lessons can be learned from the Thai experienec of enforcing the two tobacco control laws over the past five years. The most important element is the budget available for law enforcement. This must include funding for public campaigns for awareness of the law, training of law enforcement officials, rewards for law enforcement officers and campaigns for public compliance with the law. Commitment by policy-makers is crucial, for even if there are budgetary constraints, the Government-owned media could provide free time for campaigns against smoking and promote compliance with the smoking control laws.

Areas for improvement

Although the two tobacco control laws may appear to be comprehensive, there is room for improvement. The ban on the sale of cigarettes to young people may be difficult to enforce, but it sends a powerful health educational message to society: that smoking is really bad and that the law's intention is to protect children from becoming addicted to cigarettes. An earmarked tax, either strictly for tobacco control as in the states of California and Massachusetts, or to set up a health promotion foundation as in Victoria State, would not only strengthen smoking control globally but could be used to strengthen law enforcement. The tobacco settlement agreement concluded between state attorneys general, the tobacco industry and public health advocates in the United States has many provisions about funding of tobacco control law enforcement and clarifying the importance of the budgetary component of effective law enforcement.

Generic packaging will greatly reduce the value to the tobacco industry of using packs for direct advertising and brand stretching. A ban on sponsorship will eliminate its use by tobacco companies to promote their products and corporate image.

It is obvious that there are many problems in law enforcement in Thailand. This was predictable when the Ministry of Public Health was lobbying for passage of the law. Many conservative officials were reluctant to push for passage of the law, because they considered that Thai society was not ready for such an 'advanced' law and that it would be difficult to enforce. We argued that Asian countries should 'pass the law first and worry about the enforcement later'. We believe that no society will ever be 100% ready in terms of public acceptance, for a comprehensive tobacco control law. More importantly, delay in promulgating tobacco control laws may make it impossible to obtain good laws if the transnational tobacco companies are given time to build up their influence.

Although the value of legislation as a component of tobacco control is indisputable, it is difficult to distinguish its effect on tobacco control, especially quantitatively. Legislation is intricately linked with other components of tobacco control, such as health education, tax policy and smoking cessation. Because of limited resources, little effort has been made in Thailand to help smokers to quit. A health education campaign must be conducted to inform the public sufficiently before any meaningful legislation can be passed and especially before a tax can be raised for health.

Cigarette consumption in Thailand has increased slightly over the past decade in the face of rapid modernization and a threefold increase in per capita income. The Ministry of Public Health has been successful in lobbying for tax increases on three occasions, raising the excise tax from 55 to 68% and the price per pack of cigarettes from US$ 0.5 to 0.84. This has given the Government US$ 500 million more per year than a decade ago, while the total number of smokers has increased only slightly. The fact that the Government has received more income from tobacco by raising the tax for health reasons, as recommended by the Ministry of Public Health, means that the Government will be more receptive to the Ministry's tobacco control initiatives in the future. The Ministry of Public Health must win the Ministry of Finance's heart in order to obtain a brighter outlook for tobacco control.

Tobacco legislation in the Ukraine: Advertising and other issues

K. Krasovsky

Alcohol and Drug Information Centre, Kiev, Ukraine

Tobacco advertising was formally banned in the Ukraine in 1992, but enforcement of the law has been very poor. It has therefore become an issue to clarify the law on advertising.

The tobacco and advertising lobby, financed by Philip Morris and other transnational tobacco companies, persuaded the Parliamentary commission on the mass media to present a law with only some restrictions on tobacco advertising. They even prepared a document called 'Questions and answers on banning tobacco advertising in the Ukraine prepared for Members of Parliament by the associations of independent advertisers for the development of the Ukrainian tobacco industry'! This document stated that if advertising were banned the Ukraine would lose US$ 400 million. But the 'association' never existed, and the document was prepared by Philip Morris.

When the law was finally discussed in Parliament in March 1996, the health lobby was stronger, and Parliament voted for the ban. But the tobacco lobby spent an immense amount of money on a campaign against the law, and managed to persuade the President to issue a veto. The final decision, adopted in July 1996, was a compromise: tobacco advertising is banned on radio and television but allowed in printed media and on billboards.

At present, the health lobby is working on enforcement of some provisions in the law concerning public information and health warnings. We are using our experience of legislation against advertising for other legislation, such as increasing tobacco taxes with allocation of a portion of them for prevention work, restrictions on smoking in public places and health warnings on tobacco packs. Exchange of experiences with other countries on tobacco legislation will be valuable for all parties.

Analysis of tobacco policy in Viet Nam

D. Efroymson & D.T. Phuong

Programme for Appropriate Technology in Health, Ottawa, Ontario, Canada

In designing their response to the tobacco epidemic, tobacco control advocates often rely on legislative and policy measures, such as raising tobacco taxes, limiting advertising, and banning smoking in certain public places. These measures can be difficult to turn into law, and, once passed, they may not be enforced. In order to assist those making or advocating policy changes, it is helpful to study the policy environment and thus have guidance in making decisions about tobacco control. Policy analysis can be facilitated by a tool called PolicyMaker, a computer-based method of policy analysis designed by David Cooper and Michael Reich at the Harvard School of Public Health. The tool is a general method of policy analysis that can be used retrospectively or prospectively to study the chances of implementing a policy effectively, ways of improving those chances and ways of following the implementation process.

The method involves collecting information about people who will affect or are affected by the policy, including individuals or organizations like tobacco companies and ministries of health and finances, and smaller ones such as individual smokers and tobacco sellers. Documents and individuals can provide information about the power of these players and how they feel about the policy, what their interests are, how the policy will affect them, and so on. The tool also guides the examination of relationships among various players, such as who influences, cooperates with or is in conflict with whom and obstacles to and options for policies and strategies to increase the chances of success of a policy.

The Canadian Programme for Appropriate Technology in Health (PATH Canada) with support from the International Tobacco Initiative in Canada, used this method in Viet Nam. In addition, we conducted qualitative research to gain a better understanding of the public's attitudes towards various potential tobacco control measures and to examine people's understanding of the effect of tobacco on health and economics and their feelings about women smokers. The study revealed a number of possible supporters as well as existing opponents to tobacco control policies and several options for enhancing support by building on existing support and bringing groups working in health and credit into tobacco control. We also found that, while people have heard of the health risks of smoking, particularly of the risk of lung cancer, they often discount that risk or entirely disbelieve the information they hear. A typical comment would be "I have never heard of anyone who died from smoking." or "My grandfather smoked for many years and is old and healthy." In addition, very few smokers are aware of or concerned about the effect of their smoking on others.

Because of the lack of understanding of the reasons for tobacco control, both smokers and non-smokers are often intolerant of most moves by government to control tobacco use. These negative views are often shared by many people within the government who are responsible for formulating, implementing and enforcing policies. People consider that raising taxes would benefit only the government and tobacco sellers, without affecting smoking rates; that bans on smoking in certain areas, such as on public transport, would be impossible to enforce; that bans on selling cigarettes to minors would be laughable and useless; and that smoking is a free and independent right on which the government should not encroach. People believe that smoking is good for the economy and generally feel that any negative effects in terms of health are minor and too far off to worry about in comparison with the current pleasure of smoking and the income that is generated for farmers, producers, and sellers. People also feel that an increase in the price of cigarettes would help only the sellers, and an increase in tax would indicate that the Government is concerned with money, not with public health.

The negative views expressed by both men and women, smokers and non-smokers, towards a range of possible government actions indicates a need for greater understanding of tobacco as a health and economic issue in Vietnamese society; otherwise, measures are likely to be greeted with opposition and widely flouted. The study overall provided a clearer picture of the situation with regard to tobacco in Viet Nam, possible forms of intervention and the need for public education to accompany public policy.

We learned several things from using PolicyMaker. For us, it served more as a planning tool in our advocacy work, in deciding what areas to focus on and what sorts of education were needed for government officials and the public. It can be difficult to gather such information, particularly in countries with strong restrictions on the free flow of information. Potentially, PolicyMaker could be far more powerful in the hands of the people who habitually use it—governments and powerful organizations which influence policy directly. We believe that, with planning and understanding, it is possible to increase the chances of successfully implementing policies for tobacco control.

Smoking bans in domestic environments in South Australia

L. Roberts[1], C. Miller[1], M. Wakefield[2] & C. Reynolds[3]

[1]South Australian Smoking and Health Project, [2]South Australian Health Commission, Adelaide and [3]Law School, Flinders University of South Australia

In recognition of the adverse consequences of exposure to environmental tobacco smoke, many countries have called for a ban on smoking in all enclosed public places. In South Australia, there has been an unprecedented increase during the 1990s in the percentage of workplaces which have imposed bans on smoking, and legislation has been passed to ban smoking in restaurants from the beginning of 1999. These moves are important from the point of view of protecting the health of adult non-smokers, but they do little to limit exposure of children.

Much of the burden of illness caused by environmental tobacco smoke is incurred by children, especially young children, in the form of lower respiratory illness, asthma and sudden infant death syndrome. Domestic exposure to environmental tobacco smoke accounts for most of the total exposure of children. Recently in Australia, there have been calls to consider options for reducing the exposure of children to this hazard. In the same way that vehicles carrying young children are required by law to be fitted with child safety restraints, legal prohibition of smoking in vehicles carrying children is one option for consideration. In a climate of decreasing opportunities for smoking in public places, there is concern about the extent to which bans and restrictions on smoking in domestic environments, such as the home and car, might be applied.

Questions about domestic bans were included in the South Australian Health Omnibus Survey, which is an annual survey of South Australians aged 15 years and older about a range of health issues. The survey is based on a multistage, systematic, clustered-area sample of 4200 households. At each selected household, the person whose birthday is next is interviewed in person by a trained interviewer. Data were weighted by household size, age, sex and local government area of the South Australian population. The questions pertaining to domestic smoking arrangements were as follows: "Which of the following statements best describes the situation regarding smoking in your home?" The response options were: "Smoking is banned in my home"; "There is no ban, but no-one smokes anyway"; "Smoking is allowed on some social occasions"; "Smoking is allowed". For cars, the question was: "Which one of the following options best describes the situation regarding smoking in your car?" The response options were: "Smoking is banned in my car"; "There is no ban but no one smokes anyway"; "Smoking is allowed"; "Do not have a car". The sample sizes and response rates, respectively, for each year of the survey were: 1993, 3004 respondents, 72%; 1994, 3010 respondents, 72%; 1995, 3016 respondents, 74%; and 1996, 3009 respondents, 74%.

The reported prevalence of having a smoke-free home (first two possible responses) gradually increased from 60% in 1993 to 65% in 1996 (χ^2 for trend = 18.9; $p < 0.001$). Within this classification, people were more likely over time to say that they had a ban, rather than indicating that no one smoked anyway (χ^2 for trend = 26.9; $p < 0.001$). This reflects a more deliberate decision to impose a ban. Among those who had a car, the reported prevalence of having a smoke-free car (first two possible responses) did not change over time, although the percentage who deliberately imposed bans increased from 54 to 58% (χ^2 for trend = 23.3; $p < 0.001$). Thus, overall, the trend has been for people who do not usually smoke in their cars to take a stronger stand by imposing a ban.

Among the subgroup of respondents who reported themselves to be smokers and who were aged 25–40 years and thus most likely to have children, household smoking bans increased from 25% in 1993 to 31% in 1996 (χ^2 for trend = 4.6; $p = 0.03$), while bans on smoking in the car increased from 28% in 1993 to 35% in 1996 (χ^2 for trend = 5.4; $p = 0.02$).

These results suggest an increasing propensity for smokers and non-smokers alike to have smoke-free domestic environments and to formalize their decision by the deliberate imposition of a ban; nevertheless, there is much room for improvement.

Legislation prohibiting smoking in private vehicles carrying children would offer them some protection from the adverse health effects of environmental tobacco smoke. Such legislation would inevitably be criticized as an unwarranted intrusion into people's privacy, raising doubts about whether it could be enforced. Such difficulties should not deter legislators from considering this important public health initiative. We know very little about the difficulties of implementing and maintaining bans on smoking at home and what misperceptions parents may have about 'safe' ways of limiting exposure to environmental tobacco smoke. Ad-hoc comments from focus groups have suggested that parents may be under the impression that simply smoking in a different room or on the other side of a room from the child will suffice. These perceptions deserve further exploration in more formal studies, for use in educational programmes designed to minimize the greatest source of exposure of children to environmental tobacco smoke.

Public opinion in Australia about the adequacy of tobacco health warnings and information on tobacco-related harm, in the context of the introduction of stronger warnings on packs

R. Borland & D. Hill

Centre for Behavioural Research in Cancer, Anti-Cancer Council of Victoria, Carlton South, Victoria, Australia

Introduction

Informing the public about the risks associated with tobacco use is an important obligation of health authorities, governments and those in the community who promote its use (most notably, the tobacco industry). Understanding community views on the adequacy of the information given is one important consideration in deciding on strategies to modify existing methods of disseminating information. The introduction of new, more informative health warnings and product labelling on tobacco products provided the stimulus to explore public opinion about the adequacy of information on tobacco-related harm.

New warnings were introduced on packs manufactured in Australia from 1 January 1995 (Borland & Hill, 1997a). The law requires that one of six health warnings be displayed on the top 25% of the front of packs, with an elaboration of that warning and the telephone number of an information line on the top 33% of the back of the pack. One side of the pack is taken up with information about levels of tar, nicotine and carbon monoxide, plus a brief description of what each is and the harm it can do. All three components are required to be in black print on a white background. The requirements are far stronger than those they replaced—a warning in an area of 15% at the bottom of the front and back without requirements for contrast, and brief information on contents on one side. There is evidence that the warnings have improved community knowledge (Borland & Hill, 1997b) and stimulated increased concern about smoking (Borland, 1997).

Method

The participants in the December 1994 baseline survey were 510 smokers and 525 non-smokers, the latter comprising 183 ex-smokers and 342 who had never smoked. Of the non-smokers, 40% were male and 60% female, and among smokers 51% were male. The participants in the post-implementation (follow-up) survey in May 1995 were 512 smokers and 521 non-smokers (176 ex-smokers and 345 who had never smoked). Of the non-smokers, 39% were male, and among smokers 47% were male. Among non-smokers, there was a marginally significant difference in the age distribution across surveys ($p < 0.05$), with a greater proportion of 30–49-year olds in the follow-up sample. Among smokers, the age distribution was similar. There were no differences between the two surveys in the sex distribution of either smokers or non-smokers.

The two surveys were very similar, with no difference in the questions of relevance to this paper. As the order of questions was also the same, the context of asking about effects could not account for differences in the reports over time. The key questions of relevance here concerned opinions about the size and strength of the wording of warnings on cigarette packs and opinions about the adequacy of the information provided by both governments and the tobacco industry. In addition, we used indices of concern about health effects: strength of opinion about the veracity of the six health warnings and six other opinions about the harm of smoking, including some self-exempting opinions (e.g. "The dangers of smoking have been exaggerated."). The other question used was an assessment of the relative risk of smoking for smokers among six lifestyle-related risks (e.g. over-exposure to the sun, drinking too much, being involved in a car accident).

Results

Awareness of the new health warnings increased between baseline and follow-up from 28% to 91% among smokers and from 24% to 51% among non-smokers. (see Borland & Hill, 1997).

Opinions about the new Australian health warnings

Respondents were asked "In your opinion, is the amount of space on cigarette packs given over to health warnings too much, too little, or about the right amount?", followed by a similar question about whether the strength of the wording was too strong, too weak or about right. The results are presented in Table 1. For simplicity, to assess changes in perceptions of acceptability, "Can't say" responses were combined with "Right amount" responses. Smokers were significantly more likely at follow-up (as compared with baseline) to believe that the amount of space dedicated to warnings on cigarette packs was too much as compared with too little ($\chi^2_{M-H} = 125$; $p < 0.0001$) and that the wording was too strong as compared with too weak ($\chi^2_{M-H} = 68$; $p < 0.0001$). A large majority of smokers, however, did not consider that they took up too much space (75%) or were too weakly worded (86%). Most smokers saw the new warnings as reasonable.

Among non-smokers there was a similar pattern, although most of the shift was towards "Right amount" or "Can't say" for space ($\chi^2_{M-H} = 15$; $p < 0.001$) and for wording ($\chi^2_{M-H} = 31$; $p < 0.0001$). A sizeable minority of non-smokers (36% for space and 27% for strength of warning) continued to believe that the warnings should be strengthened further. We checked to see whether opinions at follow-up might have been affected by awareness of the changes to the warnings. We found no effect among smokers, but non-smokers who were aware of the new warnings were more likely to believe that the wording was too strong as compared with those who were not aware (3.8% vs 0.4%) and correspondingly less likely to believe it was too weak (22.3% vs 30.9%) ($\chi^2_{M-H} = 8.2$; $p < 0.005$). For opinions about the adequacy of the amount of space given to health warnings, there was a non-significant trend for non-smokers aware of the new warnings to think that the amount of space taken up by warnings was excessive.

We examined whether opinions about the health effects of smoking affected opinions about the adequacy of new warnings in the cross-sectional samples (see Table 2). There was a strong linear relationship between acceptance of both the warning-related smoking statements ($F_{(1464)} = 42$; $p < 0.0001$) and the non-warning-related statements ($F_{(1464)} = 28$; $p < 0.0001$) and opinions about the strength of the wording of warnings among those in the follow-up samples who were aware of the new warnings. Those who considered the warnings too strong were less accepting of the statements on health

Table 1. Opinions about the size and strength of wording of warning labels

Opinion	Smokers (%)			Non-smokers (%)		
	Baseline	Follow-up		Baseline	Follow-up	
		All	Aware only[a]		All	Aware only[a]
n	510	512	468	525	521	265
Warning space						
Too much	5	25	25	2	3	5
Right amount	53	56	58	33	39	51
Can't say	9	8	7	17	23	11
Too little	33	11	10	47	36	33
Warning wording						
Too strong	5	14	14	1	2	4
Right amount	62	71	73	38	50	63
Can't say	7	6	5	19	21	11
Too weak	26	9	9	42	27	22

[a]Those reporting being aware of the recent changes to health warnings

Table 2. Mean levels of acceptance of both warning and non-warning statements about health effects as a function of opinion on the adequacy of spacing and wording of health warning labelling among smokers in the cross-sectional follow-up sample who were aware of the new health warnings

Opinion	n	Warning opinions	Non-warning opinions
Wording			
Too strong	64	3.61	3.11
Can't say	23	3.44	3.11
Right amount	340	4.21	3.71
Too weak	41	4.39	3.83
Space			
Too much	117	3.69	3.16
Can't say	31	3.74	3.34
Right amount	272	4.24	3.74
Too little	48	4.58	4.11

Higher scores represent stronger acceptance of negative health effects.

effects. Similar results were found for opinions about the appropriateness of the amount of space taken up for warning statements ($F_{(1464)} = 60$; $p < 0.0001$) and non-warning statements ($F_{(1464)} = 55$; $p < 0.0001$).

Opinions about adequacy of provision of information about smoking

Respondents were asked two questions about the adequacy of the information provided. First, "Do you think the Government is doing too much or too little or about the right amount to inform people of the risks of smoking?", followed by a similar question about the activities of tobacco companies. The results are shown in Table 3.

At baseline, more smokers thought that the Government was doing too little than too much, and nearly eight times as many thought that tobacco companies were doing too little as compared with doing too much. Among non-smokers, these differences were even greater. At follow-up among smokers, more now thought that the Government was doing too much (30%) than too little (19%). By contrast, 47% thought they were doing the right amount. The difference between the surveys was significant for both Government ($\chi^2 = 17$; degrees of freedom [df] =2; $p < 0.001$) and tobacco companies ($\chi^2 = 8.6$; df = 2; $p < 0.05$). There were no significant differences between the surveys for non-smokers: most continued to believe that neither was doing enough.

Table 3. Perceived adequacy of information efforts of government and tobacco companies

Perception	Government (%)		Tobacco companies (%)	
	Baseline	Follow-up	Baseline	Follow-up
Smokers				
Too much	19	30	6	8
Right amount	50	47	42	47
Too little	25	19	47	38
Can't say	6	4	6	8
Non-smokers				
Too much	6	6	2	1
Right amount	45	51	23	26
Too little	43	38	69	66
Can't say	6	5	6	7
Weighted estimate for population				
Too much	9	12	3	3
Right amount/can't say	52	55	33	38
Too little	39	33	64	59

To assess whether opinions that too much information was being provided were related to knowledge of risks, in the follow-up survey we compared opinions about the adequacy of information among those who correctly identified smoking as the most harmful health-related behaviour from a list of six and those who did not ("Can't say" responses combined with "Right amount"). As can be seen from Table 4, those who had an appropriate understanding of the risk were about one-third as likely to believe that the Government was doing too much as those who were less well informed (χ^2_{M-H} = 22; $p < 0.0001$), and similarly they were about half as likely to believe that tobacco companies were doing too much (χ^2_{M-H} = 8.7; $p < 0.005$). Furthermore, those who reported being in the pre-contemplation stage of quitting at follow-up were more likely to say that the Government had been doing too much ($\chi^2 = 23$; df = 4; $p < 0.001$), but no such association was evident for the question about tobacco companies.

Discussion
With the introduction of new, larger, more informative warnings and contents labelling on packs, it is not surprising that the percentage of the population that thinks that the warning information and space was inadequate declined, with some increase in the minority believing they were excessive. Only 25% of smokers who were aware of the new warnings saw them as excessive. It is likely that this percentage will drop as the warnings become established. Non-smokers were far more likely to believe that the new warnings were insufficient. We can conclude that the changes were not of a magnitude that would threaten public support; indeed, it seems likely that many in the community would be prepared to accept even stronger requirements.

The finding that much of the opposition to stronger warnings among smokers comes from those who do not fully accept the adverse health consequences of smoking suggests that much of the opposition is based on false premises. Those who need the extra information most are those most likely to believe it is unnecessary. There is an obligation to inform this group better, even if they are not currently convinced of the need for it themselves. To convince the doubters, warnings should be commensurate with the known harm.

The finding of some reduction in the level of opinion that Government was doing too little to inform about the harm of smoking could be due to the fact that they are (correctly) seen as the impetus for the new warnings and other anti-smoking activity, such as a small-scale campaign that was staged to promote the introduction of the new warnings. Among smokers, tobacco companies may have got some credit for the new warnings, as the percentage that considered that they do too little fell a little. We are not aware of any other information disseminated by the industry that could be an alternative source of this change. Even given this small shift, there is still a strong community perception that tobacco companies are not doing enough. Opinions that

Table 4. Opinions of smokers about adequacy of information provided by Government and the tobacco industry as a function of whether they believe that smoking is the lifestyle factor likely to do them most harm (follow-up survey)

Opinion	Most harmful lifestyle factor (%)	
	Smoking ($n = 140$)	Other ($n = 372$)
Government doing:		
Too much	12	37
Can't say	3	4
Right amount	61	42
Too little	24	17
Tobacco industry doing:		
Too much	4	9
Can't say	6	9
Right amount	42	48
Too little	47	34

both governments and the tobacco industry were doing too much come predominantly from those who believe that other lifestyle risks are greater than those from smoking. Again this suggests that opposition to more being done is based on ignorance rather than a result of saturation with information.

For an activity like smoking which causes great harm, it is unconscionable for governments not to do all that their constituencies will allow to discourage use. In many areas, Australia is one of the leading countries in informing its population about the risks of smoking, but it clearly could be doing more. Since this survey, the Federal Government has forged an alliance with all states and some non-governmental organizations to produce the first truly active anti-smoking campaign in Australia. Governments should be encouraged to take a leading role in tobacco controlinstead of doing as little as they can get away with.

References
Borland, R. (1997) Tobacco health warnings and smoking-related cognitions and behaviours. *Addiction*, **92**, 1427–1435
Borland, R. & Hill, D. (1997a) The path to Australia's tobacco health warnings. *Addiction*, **92**, 1151–1157
Borland, R. & Hill, D. (1997b) Initial impact of the new Australian tobacco health warnings on knowledge and beliefs. *Tob. Control*, **6**, 317–325

Headmasters' views of the effectiveness of tobacco laws in vocational and commercial institutions

A.-E. Liimatainen-Lamberg

National Board of Education, Helsinki, Finland

I present the results of research we carried out in spring 1996 in vocational and commercial institutions to determine the practical implementation and effects of Finland's reformed tobacco law one year after it was introduced. The reformed tobacco law came into force in March 1995. An essential change, compared with the 1976 law, was to raise the age limit from 16 to 18. According to the law, providing students under 18 with smoking facilities is forbidden, as is the sale of tobacco products to persons under 18. Supervision of smoking on school premises is the responsibility of the institution. The main responsibility for general enforcement of the law lies with municipalities.

The study was carried out in 128 vocational and 72 commercial institutions, because institutions of this type have a large number of students under 18, that is those who are especially concerned by the new law. In almost 61% of the vocational institutes and 11% of the commercial institutes, the majority of students were under 18. The range of ages in the commercial institutions was wide, because they also provide adult education. The total number of students in the study was about 90 000. The respondents were the headmasters, who were sent a questionnaire; 98% of the headmasters in vocational institutions and 89% of those in commercial institutions answered the questionnaire.

Smoking by teachers and students and smoking restrictions
Teachers smoked considerably less than students. On average, slightly over 12% of all the teachers in vocational institutions smoked, whereas 35% of the students were smokers. In commercial institutes, the corresponding figures were 10 % and 28%. Very few institutions (3%) allowed smoking in a smoking room. An outdoors smoking ban was implemented in 39% of the vocational institutions but in only 5% of the commercial institutions

Half of the headmasters in vocational institutions and 33% of those in commercial institutions answered that local shops and kiosks sold tobacco to minors. In 95% of the vocational institutes, the school kiosk sold no tobacco, whereas in 41% of the commercial institutions there were tobacco products on sale in the school cafe or kiosk.

Attitudes towards measures required by the tobacco law and difficulties in observing the law

The staff in commercial institutes had a more positive attitude towards the law than those in the vocational institutions. This is understandable, because the law places fewer restrictions on commercial institutes than on vocational institutes, which had more under-age students to supervise. In vocational institutions, about one-third of the students had a positive attitude towards the law; in commercial institutions, the figure was 45%. A large majority of students in both institutions were indifferent to the law.

Of the teachers in vocational institutions, more than half had a negative attitude towards the supervision of smoking. The figure in commercial institutions was 36%. In both vocational and commercial institutions, one-third of teachers had a positive attitude towards supervisory responsibility.

Less than one-fifth of the teachers but 67% of the students had problems in observing the law, especially outdoors. Before the law was introduced, institutions had outdoor smoking places and the students were accustomed to them. When smoking in the school area was banned, students started going elsewhere in the neighbourhood for a smoke, which caused irritation and problems such as littering. The smokers also blocked streets and roads, which endangered traffic safety. As a result, the institutions received bad publicity in the press.

Influencing smoking by students

Over half of the headmasters in vocational institutions considered that the most effective way to reduce smoking was educational models at home. One-fifth mentioned health education and 12% raising prices as the most effective ways. Punishment was seen as the least effective means. The opinions of the headmasters in commercial institutions were similar.

The institutions had prepared for the new law by providing information at meetings organized by the headmasters. Students were invited to participate in planning measures to create a commitment not to smoke. Withdrawal courses were organized, and nicotine patches were provided. Almost 40% of the vocational institutions and about 30% of the commercial institutions received outside help in preventing smoking, mainly from public health nurses and doctos. Health inspectors also gave some support. The support received was mainly health education and information. In the headmasters' opinion, health education against smoking should be straightforward, reasonable and realistic. It should be based on objective information of the dangers of smoking. It should develop a sense of responsibility and raise self-esteem. The message should be appealing and stimulating to young people, and the expense of smoking should be emphasized

Changes in smoking after introduction of the law

Most of the headmasters thought that smoking by students during school hours had not changed; about one-third thought it had decreased. Of the headmasters in commercial institutions, 5% estimated that smoking had increased. Almost half of the teachers in vocational institutions and 39% of those in commercial institutions had reduced their smoking.

Conclusions

The reformed tobacco law was reasonably well implemented in educational institutions, but implementation was made difficult by lack of sufficient support from the community; for example, tobacco was still sold to minors in shops and questions of responsibility were unclear.

No single method, such as competitions and other once-in-a-school-year tricks is effective in reducing smoking. We need long-term cooperation of the whole community in promoting health and well-being, with an active role for students themselves. Some institutions would have liked a return to the old practice of allowing smoking in designated areas within the school premises.

Finland has perhaps the strictest tobacco law in the world. Still, Finnish 11–15-year olds smoke more than those in 20 other countries. The law should now be evaluated. Otherwise, a law that was meant to promote health will be watered down and people will slip into indifference in observing it.

Negotiating legislation to discourage the use of tobacco in a Pacific Island country

A. Vakacegu[1], Mrs Hong Tiy[1], Dr Brough[2] & Dr Phillips[2]

[1]*Ministry of Health and* [2]*Fiji School of Medicine, Suva, Fiji*

Negotiations were carried out in Fiji between the Ministry of Health, politicians and the tobacco lobby, which resulted in moderate legislation on tobacco control. This is likely to be enacted during 1997. We describe the nature and result of negotiations on restrictions on smoking in public places, prohibition of advertising of cigarettes and other tobacco products, prohibition of the sale of cigarettes and other tobacco products to young people and labelling of cigarette packs.

What is now proposed for Fiji is essentially a stronger piece of legislation, covering restrictions on tobacco advertising, stronger health warnings, limits on the concentrations of nicotine and tar in cigarettes, a ban on sales and the giving of free samples to children, the introduction of no-smoking areas in restaurants and a total ban on smoking in certain public places.

Early in the process, it was generally accepted that outdoor advertisements for tobacco would be banned and that advertisements in shops that sold tobacco should not be visible from outside the shop. A major issue was the sponsorship of sports by tobacco companies. Sports are very popular throughout Fiji society, and huge efforts are made to raise funds in support of sporting activities. It was therefore decided at the highest level that such sponsorship should be restricted rather than banned. The current bill permits such sponsorship but allows advertising only at the venue of the sporting event.

Under the bill, health warnings in three languages have become compulsory on cigarette packs, and the Minister of Health has the power to vary the warnings through regulations. The negotiations focused on the size and presentation of the warnings. They were complicated by the need to cover the three languages widely spoken in Fiji. The legislation also requires that cigarette packs bear a statement of the tar and nicotine content per cigarette, which must be within the limits set by the Government. The negotiations focused on the levels to be set. Further negotiations were held on the critical issue of phasing in the introduction of the various parts of the legislation. Lessons from this negotiation process may be useful to others.

Canadian legislators' support for tobacco control policies

J.E. Cohen, M.J. Ashley, R.G. Ferrence, D.A. Northrup, J.S. Pollard & D.L. Alexander

Ontario Tobacco Research Unit, University of Toronto and the Institute for Social Research, York University, Toronto, Ontario, Canada

Background: Because tobacco control policies are an important component of a comprehensive strategy to reduce tobacco use and its associated health consequences, and because legislators ultimately determine tobacco control policies, a study was undertaken to assess Canadian legislators' level of support for various tobacco control measures.

Methods: All 1044 Canadian Federal, provincial and territorial legislators were invited to participate in a 25-min, structured telephone interview. Ten of the 12 provinces and territories had response rates of at least 60%.

Results: At least two-thirds of respondents supported: regulating tobacco advertising, mandating plain packaging of cigarettes, instituting strong penalties for sales to minors, increasing the cigarette price by CAN$ 1, banning smoking in hockey arenas and restricting smoking in workplaces, restaurants and bars. Support for tobacco control policies showed bivariate associations with political party, smoking status and knowledge about the health effects of environmental tobacco smoke and the public health impacts of tobacco.

Discussion: This is the first systematic research to document Canadian legislators' knowledge of and attitudes towards tobacco. These findings can help guide the activities of health agencies, researchers and advocates.

Canadian legislators' knowledge of and attitudes towards tobacco and tobacco control

M.J. Ashley, N. A. de Guia, J. E. Cohen, R. G. Ferrence, D.A. Northrup, J.S. Pollard & D.L. Alexander

Ontario Tobacco Research Unit, University of Toronto, and the Institute for Social Research, York University, Toronto, Canada

Rationale: Tobacco control policies are ultimately shaped by legislators, but to date, there has been very little systematic study of legislators' knowledge about the health consequences of tobacco or their attitudes toward various tobacco control measures.

Methods: In 1996–97, computer-assisted telephone interviews were conducted with 438 provincial and territorial legislators across Canada, yielding a response rate of 59%. Because of a very low response rate among legislators from one province (Quebec), the analyses were restricted to 404 legislators from the other nine provinces and two territories of Canada, among whom the response rate was 65%.

Findings: Across all jurisdictions, 63% of the legislators supported a major Government role in discouraging young people from starting to smoke, but fewer (47%) supported such a role in encouraging people to quit smoking. The majority of the legislators (78%) thought that most smokers are addicted to nicotine and that it is very difficult for daily smokers to quit (67%). Although 59% indicated that environmental tobacco smoke can cause lung cancer, only 33% knew that tobacco causes many more deaths among Canadians than does alcohol. Support for policies ranged from 81% for the regulation of tobacco as a hazardous product and 77% for regulation of cigarette advertising to 36% for holding manufacturers liable for smokers' suffering and 33% for suing tobacco companies to recover health care costs. Most of the legislators supported strong penalties for selling to minors (70%) and price increases of 50 cents to CAN$ 1 per pack (65%), but only 49% and 45%, respectively, supported bans on smoking in workplaces and tobacco company sponsorship of cultural events.

Conclusions: These findings can guide the activities of health agencies, researchers and advocates in developing support for effective strategies to reduce the public health burden of tobacco use in Canada.

Legislation to prevent circumvention of bans on direct tobacco advertising

Z.M. Zain[1] & M.Assunta[2]

[1]Ministry of Health and[2]Consumers' Association of Penang, Malaysia

Introduction

Although prohibition of tobacco advertising is one of the most effective control strategies, arguments based on national economy have caused most countries to have only partial legislative bans on tobacco promotion. Incomplete restrictions are defective and provide opportunities for evasion. In Malaysia, direct tobacco advertisement in the local media is unlawful, but this does not apply to advertising at points of sale or advertisements in foreign publications circulated in the country. The legislation is also silent on other forms of tobacco promotion, hence giving alternatives to the industry to market their products. The use of tobacco brand names and logos on services and non-tobacco products is one of the best ways of disguising cigarette advertising.

Advertisements

A growing number of non-tobacco products and services now carry the insignia of cigarette companies—an effect of trademark diversification. This provides legitimate convenience for multinational and regional investors in the tobacco trade to continue marketing their actual commodity, using these false fronts. Cigarette substitutes are publicized throughout the nation, despite their limited access. Numerous prominent billboards, advertisements in the print media and frequent commercials on electronic media extend the distribution and availability of the products and services being advertised. The move to diversification is always begun by businesses associated with affluence, glamour and style, which are attractive to both smokers and non-smokers. Successful promotion schemes for these goods and services are also perceived favourably by the public, as goods with cigarette names and logos are generally considered to be quality materials.

Advertising companies working for tobacco industry clients exploit all possible channels to promote cigarette brand names and to optimize the potential of each of the mass media used. All indirect tobacco advertisements use seductive, fascinating themes and are aired on television during prime time at frequent intervals. Billboards carrying tobacco advertisements are often very prominent and situated at strategic sites, along busy, congested roads. The major tobacco companies in Malaysia also use their company vehicles, especially those for distributing cigarettes to retailers, as mobile advertising devices. Their trucks, vans and cars are attractively painted with cigarette brand names. Trolleys, rubbish bins, clocks and other surfaces are also used.

The most innovative approach, however, is getting society to be their advertising agents: enticed by the likelihood of winning prizes, members of the general public actively put up car stickers with indirect tobacco advertisements. Among the products and services used for tobacco 'brand-stretching' are clothing, adornment, travel, recreation, restaurants (the Benson & Hedges Bistro being the only one so far) and entertainment, such as music albums. Most tobacco companies invariably have t-shirts, caps, mugs, umbrellas, lighters and other paraphernalia with their names and logos on them. Some are given away free to guests at specific occasions, like sporting events, while many more are sold to the public from booths in major shopping complexes.

Advertisement at points of sale

Cigarettes are sold everywhere, from large shopping malls and duty-free shops to hawker stalls and small retail shops in rural areas. Quite often, tobacco companies provide these retailers with attractive display shelves and colourful posters. Since the prohibition of direct tobacco advertisements does not include points of sale, these places are full of cigarette advertisements. Direct cigarette advertising posters generally have the same pictures (i.e. in design, font, colour and models) as the indirect ones seen on television, billboards and newpapers, except for the cigarette boxes. As points of sale are everywhere, the industry has no problem in reminding the public that cigarettes are always the main motif. Satellite television and the Internet are the latest tools for the tobacco industry.

Sponsorship

Tobacco sponsorship is also legal, provided there is no link with direct cigarette promotion. Tobacco companies invest heavily in sponsorship of high-profile national events, particularly popular sports and entertainment, which receive wide media coverage.

Tobacco companies always want to be associated with sports, in spite of the fact that the two signify conflicting values. In Malaysia, the industry has become the primary sponsor for some of the most popular national sports. The best example is football: Dunhill has become almost synonymous with the game to its fans. Transnational tobacco companies are also involved in sponsoring the telecasting of major international sports to local viewers. Examples are the English Premier League, NBA basketball, tennis grand slams and even the tobacco-free Atlanta Olympics.

The involvement of tobacco companies in the entertainment industry has intensified recently and received mixed reactions from the public. Concern for the escalating magnitude of social ills among the young elicited protests from the community. Salem and Peter Stuyvesant have been responsible for sponsoring controversial concerts, which are heavily advertised on television and radio and in newspapers. These activities attract the interest of young people, mainly adolescents, and could contribute adversely to the growth and well-being of this vulnerable generation.

Foreign movies on television are almost always sponsored by tobacco companies. Television programmes such as the Dunhill Double, Dunhill Blockbuster Movies and Perilly's 25-Action Movies are those that draw many viewers.

The industry also uses miscellaneous tactics, such as hosting special events, competitions and others, to push their cigarettes. Cigarette companies often host fun-filled events when introducing new products to potential customers. When Kent came out with a new 'fresh' cigarette, the company organized a day-long event at one of Malaysia'a premier water theme parks, called the 'Kent Fresh Freakout'. There was nationwide promotion for more than a month before the event. Banners on lamp-post lined several main streets in Kuala Lumpur, and as part of the massive promotion a competition was set for young people. For the past two years, Benson & Hedges has been luring Malaysians to participate in their Benson & Hedges Golden Dreams programme, which involves acting out challenging activities based on the dreams of selected individuals. Their pursuit is taped and telecast in a programme with the same title.

Conclusion

The Government has authority to control tobacco by imposing laws to regulate the industry. Legal drafts must be made very stringent from the beginning, and there should be no consideration of any negotiations with the industry.

Tobacco advertising ban in Lithuania

T. Stanikas

Kaunas Medical Academy, Kaunas, Lithuania

As in other post-Soviet countries, the status of health in Lithuania is extremely poor and has fallen far behind that of the western world in the past two decades. Lithuania is also one of the States with the greatest increase in tobacco-related disease and mortality. Of its 3.7 million population, over 7000 die prematurely every year from diseases caused by smoking; that accounts for 20% of all mortality. About 50% of men and 15% of women are regular smokers. During the past decade, the prevalence of smoking increased dramatically among young women aged 25–29, from 7.9% in 1983 to 17.9 in 1993, which may be due to the virtually unrestrained tobacco advertising. Although the impact of advertising on smoking in Lithuania has never been examined, evidence from other countries with comprehensive tobacco control policies, including total bans on tobacco advertising, proves that an advertising ban cuts both tobacco consumption and the number of smokers. The aggressive marketing strategies of transnational tobacco companies will no doubt further spread tobacco addiction and increase the incidence of smoking-related disease. In order to stop this threat to the nation's health, comprehensive tobacco legislation in general and a total ban on tobacco advertising in particular are necessary.

In Soviet-controlled Lithuania, cigarette advertising was not allowed for nearly 50 years, as the State-run tobacco monopoly had no need of it. Although smoking has been established as a health risk factor for over three decades, very little was done at the State level to control tobacco use during that period. The first attempt to regulate tobacco use was made in 1980 when a decree on strengthening the fight against smoking was issued by the Soviet authorities. The anti-smoking campaign that followed the decree died soon, with no visible result. The only effective measure taken by the Government was a price increase in 1981 which caused a continuous fall in cigarette consumption, but this measure was not associated with the decree and did not have tobacco control as its object.

After the collapse of the Soviet Union, independent Lithuania started to create its own legislation. The draft law on tobacco control was prepared by professionals of the Kaunas Medical Academy, submitted to Parliament for hearing in 1992 and adopted at the end of 1995. The law was prepared in line with WHO recommendations and covered practically all spheres of tobacco manufacture, trade and use and prescribed a total ban on all kinds of direct and indirect advertising. Unfortunately, the law was very poorly implemented and caused much controversy in the mass media. The greatest criticism was levelled against the total ban on tobacco advertising, and it was not respected by advertising companies, since there was no proper enforcement. The Government itself was reluctant to implement the law, and its efforts to control advertising were formal and completely ineffective. Under the pressure of tobacco control activists, however, efforts were begun in June 1993 when the Government issued a decree on information about alcohol and tobacco, formally banning all kinds of advertising; but the ban has never been observed, since the law relating to the press, which anteceded the decree, did not ban advertising, and the mass media simply ignored the new ban. Later, a total ban on tobacco advertising was presented in two laws: one on the health system and one on tobacco control. The ban was to have come into legal force in July 1996, but just before that time the ban was suspended by the action of a large group of Members of Parliament who appealed to the Constitutional Court asking for a ruling on the constitutionality of such a ban. In February 1997, the Constitutional Court ruled that the ban was not counter to the Constitution, but despite the verdict, tobacco advertising continued to be unrestricted and the country remained flooded with all kinds of tobacco advertisements.

The State Tobacco and Alcohol Control Service, which is responsible for implementing the law, was founded in 1996; instead of enforcing the law, however, this agency, on the instructions of the Government, started to prepare amendments to the law. In June 1997, 17 amendments were submitted to Parliament. These amendments were aimed at changing the very essence of the law and making it favourable to the tobacco industry; for example, the suggested purpose of the law was formulated as "to regulate relations connected with tobacco growing, manufacture, sales, imports, advertising, and use of tobacco products" instead of "decreasing consumption of tobacco products and the harmful consequences to public health" in the existing law. The total ban on tobacco advertising would have been replaced by "regulation of tobacco advertising, sales and use of tobacco products" and indirect advertising not mentioned at all. The proposed article on tobacco advertising contained 25 points, many of which were real loopholes for advertising, like the "ban on cigarette advertising aimed at children or teenagers under 18", "ban on advertising demonstrating the relation between tobacco use and physical fitness or improved mental capacity" and also "demonstration of stimulating and healing action of tobacco", or even such a strange point as "the ban on positive demonstration of tobacco abuse". The amendments also suggested permitting television advertisements with certain limitations in time (a ban between 15:00 and 18:00). All of the amendments were approved almost unanimously by the ruling majority of the Parliament when voted chapter by chapter, but during the final nominal voting, which took place in July 1997 by a show of hands, the amendments were rejected by the minimal number of votes. Thus, the law on tobacco control remains in force, including the total ban on tobacco advertising; but, although it is in force, the ban is still not implemented, and many billboards, mostly without health warnings, still offer Marlboro, West, Prince and other brands.

From the judicial point of view, the current situation in Lithuania appears absurd: the total ban on tobacco advertising prescribed by the law and approved by the Constitutional Court is not observed and the Government is doing nothing to enforce the ban. On the contrary, the Prime Minister has publicly criticized the total ban as undemocratic and proposed a 'reasonable regulation of tobacco advertising' instead of the ban. It was to concretize this idea that the 17 amendments designed to weaken the law considerably was prepared. Although the amendments were voted down by Parliament, the position of the Government did not change. It is expected that the ban will not be implemented for another six months, when amendments to the law will again be submitted to Parliament. The tobacco industry will have enough time to strengthen the tobacco lobby and push the affair forward. If that happens, it will be a disaster for public health.

The conclusion can be drawn that the effects of smoking on health are poorly understood in this country, and the tobacco industry uses this situation to make profits from the citizens' ignorance and from the dishonesty of the authorities. To cope with the problem, it is not enough to have comprehensive legislation; continuous health education and firm community action are also necessary. As the health activists are also inadequately aware of the problem, inexperienced and underfunded, there are few grounds for expecting that Lithuania will become smoke-free soon.

In 1996, the Smoke-free Europe Conference held in Helsinki adopted a special resolution on the progress made in Lithuania and congratulated the Lithuanian Parliament on passing the law including a total ban on tobacco advertising. Regrettably, it made no impact on the Government. The resolutions of the present Conference may help our health advocates to convince the authorities that the health of the population of the country is more important than the profits of tobacco industry and that implementation of the existing legislation is necessary for the well-being of the nation.

Regulatory measures

Regulation of tobacco and nicotine

D.T. Sweanor

Smoking and Health Action Foundation, Ottawa, Ontario, Canada

Introduction

The diseases caused by tobacco products are well documented. While tobacco products are the agents of disease, they make their way to human beings through a mechanism other than the viruses and bacteria usually associated with disease. Transmission of these diseases is culturally determined, and the disease is driven by business goals. Tobacco products are created through the actions of a series of individuals and corporations who are seeking to maximize their own well-being at the cost of others' health. Like all disease vectors, the tobacco business resists attack and control.

A business-based disease agent operates in an environmental context, every bit as much as a viral or bacterial disease agent. But this environment is one of economics. The magnitude of the tobacco problem is due to many reasons, but an overwhelming factor has been the fact that tobacco products make extraordinary profits for their purveyors, even though the product represents a huge drain on the world's resources. This incredible profitability can be seen in a review of the financial reports of the major tobacco companies. Obviously, corporate entities that make massive annual returns on tobacco investments (often at a rate greater than 100% on the money invested in these businesses) present major obstacles to control.

The ability of tobacco companies to succeed as disease agents is circumscribed by the regulations to which these corporations must adhere, which specify what can be sold, how it can be sold and the conditions of use. The limitations will ultimately dictate the level of profitability of the industry and, hence, its success. By understanding the nature of the regulatory environment we can understand the economic environment of the tobacco industry and other potential suppliers of nicotine. From the standpoint of disease control, this is not essentially different from seeking to understand the workings of swamps in order to understand how best to control the mosquitoes responsible for the spread of malaria. In understanding the environment and considering how it could be changed, the future direction of a disease can be influences.

Regulation of tobacco and nicotine

The use of tobacco products can be ascribed to interrelated issues in psychology and sociology, yet the largest single issue appears to be addiction to nicotine. In understanding the regulation of tobacco products, it is therefore important to examine the regulatory framework of the drug that tobacco products administer. Such an analysis shows that regulatory regimes around the world treat nicotine in very different ways, depending on the form of administration. Essentially, the level of regulation of nicotine is most relaxed for the products of the tobacco industry, which are nicotine's deadliest delivery vehicles. The regulations are the most constraining for nicotine products that assist smoking cessation or could provide less hazardous nicotine to those who are addicted to tobacco products.

Regulation of nicotine in non-tobacco products

If nicotine is sold in a non-tobacco form, such as nicotine replacement therapy, it is invariably covered by the laws that govern pharmaceuticals. These laws give broad regulatory authority over any nicotine product used in the treatment or prevention of disease and over any drug marketed for the purpose of interfering with the normal operation of the body. Pharmaceutical nicotine delivery systems have been universally recognized as coming within these laws.

The laws governing non-tobacco use of nicotine are very broad and are permissive, meaning that it can be used only as specifically permitted. National drug laws typically prohibit the manufacture, sale, import or export of a drug except as specifically authorized. The result of this broad legislation is that there is an onus on the manufacturer to convince a government body why a specific nicotine product should be allowed on the market and what should be allowed in terms of distribution and marketing. This requires significant time and resources on the part of potential marketers of such products and greatly constrains the market. Years of preparation were required before existing nicotine replacement products were allowed on the market. Those that are allowed are subject to constraints on sales (often only through a pharmacist with a prescription from a medical doctor), how they can be made known to potential consumers (often with no direct advertising) and the purposes for which they may be sold (usually for assistance of short duration for cessation rather than longer-term use).

Products that are designed to provide an alternative source of nicotine on a maintenance basis are in a very precarious position. Although such products could greatly reduce the prevalence of diseases caused by tobacco-based nicotine delivery, they would almost certainly be found to be 'drugs' or drug 'devices'. As there is also a risk (albeit diminished) from use of such products, their use would be greatly restricted, if no banned, by drug laws.

Regulation of tobacco products

Tobacco products are subject to a regulatory system quite unlike those for other products. This is partly because the products were already on the market and sold in large quantities before their health and addictive qualities were recognized. If someone were to try to introduce such a product today, our laws governing drugs and hazardous products would virtually guarantee that it would never be legally sold. Tobacco smoking products are devices that administer an addictive drug. There is no safe level of consumption, and they will prematurely kill half of all long-term users when used exactly as intended. As a result, they would ordinarily be banned under consumer protection laws around the world.

As new laws have been designed to protect consumers, tobacco products have often been specifically exempted. Some of the lenient regulatory treatment afforded tobacco products may be based on pragmatic concerns about the impact on people who are dependent on the product. But fear of the impact of subjecting tobacco to other laws does not mean that it should be left largely unregulated. On the contrary, the great harm caused by tobacco should logically lead to specifically targeted, comprehensive laws to protect the public. A further reason for lenient treatment is that the tobacco industry has fought hard to prevent or out-manoeuvre any regulatory incursions that could affect its viability. To use the metaphor 'agent of disease' again, it is as if a virus not only found ways to mutate in order to evade control but could also retain counsel and influence politicians in order to prevent any effective viral control programme from being implemented.

In reviewing the template of key legislative measures needed for tobacco control set out by the World Health Organization in *Guidelines for Controlling and Monitoring the Tobacco Epidemic*, it is possible to discern how successful the tobacco industry has been in preventing effective control measures. In fact, very few of the recommended measures have been effectively enacted by more than a small number of countries.

The legislation that has been enacted on tobacco products is very different from that for pharmaceuticals. Rather than replicating pharmaceutical laws and prohibiting everything except what is allowed, the legislative frameworks that countries have developed for tobacco products typically allow uncontrolled manufacture, import, export, marketing, sales and use, subject to specifically enacted limitations. The result is that each control measure becomes a political fight, and the tobacco industry has the necessary financial incentive and resources to influence the debate.

Pressure to change regulations on nicotine and tobacco

The present regulatory systems for tobacco and for non-tobacco based nicotine result in an effective monopoly of the tobacco industry over nicotine maintenance. A person who wants or needs nicotine regularly, rather than as a short-term aid to cessation, has little choice but to use tobacco products. The regulation of 'drugs' and of drug delivery devices and the exclusion of tobacco products from these laws means that less hazardous forms of administering nicotine on a long-term basis are effectively kept from the market. Meanwhile, the entrenchment of traditional tobacco products within the legal system gives the tobacco industry many of the negative attributes associated with monopolists, including a disincentive for innovation. Tobacco products are protected from competition from novel nicotine delivery vehicles, and novel products from the tobacco industry are at risk of falling outside the regulatory exemptions given to tobacco products. The pressure to change this 'nicotine maintenance monopoly' is coming from many directions, including the growing body of scientific information on nicotine addiction, the development of new techniques for nicotine delivery, potential business opportunities, issues of consumer rights and a changing legal environment.

Scientific information on nicotine addiction

There is now a large body of scientific information on the extent of nicotine addiction and the role of tobacco products in maintaining that addiction. No longer can tobacco use be characterized as simply an issue of individual preference or even 'habit'. Those who use tobacco products are not suffering from a 'moral flaw' or lack of motivation. A large percentage of tobacco users would like to stop using it, and a large proportion each year attemot to quit, but the success rate is very low. Internal documents show that the tobacco industry has known this for decades. The health community has acquired this knowledge and the science underlying it only recently, and it is now difficult to ignore the possibility of less hazardous forms of nicotine delivery for those dependent on the drug.

New techniques for nicotine delivery

There are many ways to administer nicotine. An overview of the nicotine market by the tobacco company Philip Morris lists almost 100 nicotine delivery patents in the United States alone. An examination of these patents shows that the products being developed (whether by tobacco companies, pharmaceutical companies or others) fall into categories that are increasingly difficult to label as 'tobacco products' or 'pharmaceuticals'. As this distinction becomes ever more clouded, the existing regulatory mechanisms will become ever less adapted to deal effectively with the market.

Products that could reduce harm are put at a massive marketing disadvantage as soon as this news is made public. Most nations subject such products to much greater (and often insurmountable) legal hurdles. Under many national 'drug' laws, any product that could mitigate the diseases caused by tobacco would be prohibited if it injured health when used as intended. As a result, a substitute for existing tobacco products reported correctly by the maker to bring about a 95% reduction in the disease burden caused by smoking would probably be banned from the market.

Potential business opportunities

The global tobacco market comprises over 1 thousand million users who consume about 6 thousand thousand million cigarettes per year and spend more than US$ 400 thousand million annually. As a large percentage of these users would prefer not to smoke or would at least be willing to try a less hazardous delivery vehicle, there is a huge potential market for alternative forms of nicotine delivery. Since much of the price of tobacco products consists of excise taxes and there is no justification for applying such taxes to significantly less hazardous products, there are immense potential profits from such products. As new alternatives for nicotine maintenance are developed, there will be tremendous incentives for entrepreneurs to introduce them, and their economic potential would challenge the tobacco industry's nicotine maintenance monopoly in ways not previously encountered. The companies marketing these products would be able to save millions of lives while making thousands of millions of dollars.

Consumer rights

People who use nicotine maintenance have virtually no option other than tobacco products as a source of this drug. As a high proportion of users wish to discontinue their use, the failure to allow alternative products on the market is denying consumers a choice. This denial of choice is all the more important from the consumers' standpoint, given that there is clear evidence that these products could result in a massively reduced risk for disease and death.

The legal environment

A wide range of legal initiatives is leading to a potentially massive change in the regulatory structure for tobacco products. New tobacco control laws passed by various legislatures seek to subject tobacco products to much more rigorous control than before. Another initiative is application of existing laws, such as on food and drugs, to tobacco products. This may be done when an administrative body determines that there is sufficient information to warrant an extension of existing authority to tobacco products, as the Food and Drug Administration in the United States did in August 1996. In addition, litigation on issues such as products liability is putting increasing pressure on tobacco companies.

These legal issues interact in various ways, including the proposed litigation settlement agreement in the United States. In that agreement, the companies seek to avoid future litigation by agreeing to work towards less harmful products. The ability of the Food and Drug Administration to force product changes will thus be limited by the risk that contraband will supply dependent tobacco users. It should become increasingly obvious that less harmful products (nicotine replacement therapy) already exist but are kept from wider distribution and use by the Food and Drug Administration itself, but their influence to force tobacco product modifications will be increased if alternative forms of nicotine are allowed greater distribution and thus reduce the threat of contraband.

Potential forms of regulation

In order to achieve the greatest practical reduction in the harm currently associated with nicotine use, a few fundamental changes must be made in the regulation of nicotine delivering products. To begin with, less harmful products should not be placed at a marketing disadvantage. Indeed, there is a strong basis for establishing a competitive advantage for these products. An appropriate regulatory system should also seek to ensure that the potential reduction in harm is not just theoretical. The regulatory framework for the nicotine market should be designed to achieve the greatest practical reduction of harm.

Any system of health-orientated regulation of nicotine products would have to be in keeping with the approach to law in any particular jurisdiction; there are, however, some basic principles that should be be included in any legal framework:
• The legislation should deal comprehensively with all products that deliver nicotine (or essentially the same drug) at a pharmacologically active level. Inclusion of different nicotine delivery products (e.g. cigarettes and nicotine replacement therapy nasal sprays) in completely different legislative regimes invites inequity and could prevent an overall orientation towards the greatest practical reduction in the harm associated with nicotine dependence. Products with no significant quantity of an addictive agent (e.g. denicotinized tobacco) could be dealt with under separate legislation.
• All these products should be treated, as far as is possible, by the same criteria. The law should, for example, seek to ensure that any distinctions between 'pharmaceuticals' and 'tobacco' are based on science and health goals rather than perpetuating past

inequities. Subjcetion of products with similar pharmacological properties to unscientific standards within the law would not only create potential unfairness but could be increasingly difficult as hybrid products are developed. What, for instance, would we call a nicotine inhaler that was tobacco-based or a product with no tobacco?

• The aim should be the greatest practical reduction in the overall harm associated with nicotine-delivering products. While there is little likelihood of short-term elimination of the harm caused by nicotine-containing tobacco products, there is a clear opportunity to reduce the associated harm by developing alternative products. Other products could significantly increase the ease of cessation of nicotine use, which would achieve reduction of the harm associated with nicotine use.

• The regulatory regime must consider all aspects of the product and its marketing in order to ensure harm reduction. A product with technical attributes that could reduce overall harm might be marketed in such a way as to increase overall harm, for instance, by encouraging the uptake of nicotine by people who then move on to cigarettes. As with other consumer protection laws, there would have to be controls over import, manufacture, marketing and sale.

Conclusion

The regulatory systems that have evolved for tobacco products are very different from those for alternative nicotine delivery systems. The net effect of these systems has been to give tremendous marketing advantages to the most hazardous methods of supplying nicotine. Innovation has been stifled, and consumers have been effectively denied access to better products. This system of regulation, by creating a nicotine maintenance monopoly, has also enriched the tobacco companies, giving them both the incentive and the resources to oppose public health measures. The existing regulatory systems for nicotine have resulted in great health and economic costs worldwide. At the same time, a combination of pressures could lead to inevitable change. From a public health perspective, the key questions are the direction of the changes and the extent to which public health objectives can be met. As legislation is changed to adapt to scientific knowledge about nicotine and technical advances in its delivery, there are clear indications of the direction in which our laws should go in order to reduce the harm associated with nicotine use most effectively.

Dedicated regulation of nicotine use: It is time!

R. Borland

Centre for Behavioural Research in Cancer, Anti-Cancer Council of Victoria, Carlton South, Victoria, Australia

In March 1997, when I prepared the abstract for this talk, the title ended in a question "Is it time?". Since then, I have changed it to the statement "It is time". The talks between the tobacco industry, several states in the United States and tobacco control people and the tentative agreement they reached have changed our conception of what is possible. Some form of comprehensive tobacco control legislation is essential in all countries that do not have it. We have a historic opportunity to work towards a coordinated international response to the pandemic of tobacco-related harm. Legislation should control all aspects of nicotine use. The proposed 'settlement' in the United States places obstacles in the way of effective regulation. This major failing of the proposal has been highlighted by such key figures as Dr David Kessler, former Head of the United States Federal Food and Drug Administration, and Dr Everett Koop, former United States Surgeon General. Following the United States ideas, legislation can be funded from levies on the sale of nicotine products, as can health promotion and the costs of smoking-related illness. It could also include sanctions for failure to achieve targets of avoiding uptake of nicotine among the young.

Can the governments of the world, in all conscience, do only what the tobacco industry is prepared to concede? Indeed, most countries are currently doing less than the tobacco industry is prepared to agree to in the United States. We have an opportunity to shame governments into action, in the unlikely possibility that they don't act promptly. Governments can no longer deny that tobacco kills, that it is addictive and that the manufacturers have marketed it to the children of the world knowing what would happen to many of them. Can they afford to be in a position in which they offer their people less than the tobacco industry is (apparently) prepared to offer?

The aims of this paper are to consider the need for dedicated nicotine regulation, to outline key features and finally to discuss some issues of implementation.

Nicotine delivery devices come in a variety of forms, of which the cigarette is the most common A range of new products formulated to deliver nicotine for therapeutic reasons have been developed, along with new devices to deliver nicotine for recreational use. There is reason to believe that at least some of these products are safer than cigarettes, but they are typically more closely regulated. Lack of consistency in regulation is a barrier to tobacco control.

In exploring what form tobacco or nicotine regulations might take, we need to consider some basic facts about tobacco:

- Nicotine is highly addictive and harmful.
- Virtually all the harm is due to long-term use, which occurs because nicotine is highly addictive.
- Most of the harm comes from the tar and carbon monoxide, but nicotine is still harmful.
- Cigarettes and other products are typically used to optimize nicotine yield. Machine-based nicotine and tar yields may bear little relationship to the yields smokers achieve.
- New, potentially safer products are increasingly availablee, but their long-term effects cannot be known in advance, nor their patterns of use.
- In virtually all countries, use is too widespread to contemplate prohibition.

The goal of legislation should be the elimination of all harm associated with nicotine use, but the focus should be on minimizing the harm gradually, in ways that are acceptable to the community and which can be complied with by nicotine addicts. In most countries, an appropriate regulatory structure does not exist for a product such as nicotine when used for human consumption. Two regulatory models are often used to cover aspects of nicotine regulation: poisons laws, which focus on preventing ingestion of a product and on levels of contamination and are not designed to deal with products that are ingested by humans; and therapeutic goods, the aim of which is to benefit the user, such as products used to treat disease or promote health, which are regulated to prevent harmful use. By contrast, tobacco is designed to be ingested, and is demonstratively harmful when used in that way. It is also addictive (through nicotine), and is important to many of the world's economies. It does not fit into either regulatory mode. Nicotine must therefore be regulated as a drug. Nicotine replacement products are currently regulated as therapeutic goods, but they might be better regulated, at least in part, under dedicated nicotine regulation, if this facilitates appropriate use.

A critical feature of tobacco as a harmful product is that virtually all of the harm is due to long-term use. Until the product has been used for a long time, the harm per user cannot be estimated accurately, and the proportion of the population likely to use the product cannot be estimated until it has been on the market for a considerable time. Use patterns can also change over time. Put simply, this means that the total harm associated with any tobacco or nicotine product is unknown until it has been on the market long enough for those effects to be demonstrated. Data on toxicity and the composition of the product can be extrapolated to infer how dangerous the product will be for an individual user if it is used in the way for which it was designed: however, if such a product results in more use of nicotine products than would otherwise be the case, it can actually result in greater population harm.

'Mild' cigarettes should have been less harmful, but they were not as mild as they seemed: as smokers got more out of them than the machine-estimated levels, the harmfulness was not (markedly) reduced. Further, they may have facilitated uptake and led some smokers to use them rather than quit. As a result, a case can be made for the belief that that they may have actually increased harm.

Consider for a moment some of the possible outcomes of a new nicotine delivery device that is safer per user. Thus, for existing smokers, the worst possible scenario would be to continue to smoke as many cigarettes and to consume some of the new product as well, which could result in a mild increase in risk. All other scenarios for smokers suggest no effect or a reduction in risk: stay with cigarettes (i.e. no effect), change to the nicotine delivery device (reduction in risk) or use the device to quit (large reduction in risk). For ex-smokers, however, all the possible effects are neutral or negative: if they take up the device, they will have a small increase in risk and if they resume smoking cigarettes as a result of trying the new product they will have a large increase in risk. Similarly, for non-smokers all the potential effects are negative.

Estimating patterns of use in advance is not easy. Once a product is introduced into the marketplace, patterns of use become obvious, particularly if they are being carefully monitored. Obtaining this information and using it appropriately is a critical task for tobacco control.

While there remains a market for nicotine products, there is no simple solution. Neither the elimination of nicotine from cigarettes nor making nicotine delivery devices cleaner is clearly optimal. Less harmful nicotine delivery systems may encourage new use. Neil Benowitz and Jack Henningfield have argued that phasing out nicotine use, at least at addictive levels, may be a plausible strategy. It is certainly one that needs to be explored, but its viability is untested and it may not be feasible.

Less dangerous nicotine products are the other hope. Therapeutic products such as chewing-gum and patches may be less harmful, even if used in the long term. There is some evidence that smokeless tobacco may be safer than smoked tobacco, and there is also some evidence that non-inhaled smoked tobacco, as from pipes and cigars, may be less harmful than products like cigarettes, the smoke of which is inhaled into the lungs. As some forms of smokeless tobacco appear to be very harmful (i.e. those used with lime), broad generalizations should be avoided. It may be sensible to encourage existing smokers to move to non-inhaled products, but if this leads to new groups of users, the harm may be increased. The evidence from the United States and Sweden, where use of smokeless tobacco is quite common, suggests that it has attracted a largely independent market. There are still almost as many people smoking, but a new large group of people uses smokeless tobacco. Thus, far from replacing cigarettes, smokeless tobacco may be creating markets for new generations of addicts.

Given the large number of unknowns, the solution is to enact legislation that can change the regulatory requirements on particular products after they have been introduced into the market place on the basis of up-to-date information about their likely harm. In order to provide the control required, legislation on control is needed for all aspects of the manufacture and content of nicotine delivery devices. The legislation should be such that anything not specifically forbidden is banned. The tobacco industry has been infinitely creative in finding ways around attempts to legislate within a framework of prohibited activities. A framework in which anything not allowed is prohibited is one in which it is much more difficult to avoid the intent of the legislation. Some key features of such legislation should be:

- regulation of the content of all nicotine delivery devices, including tar, nicotine, carbon monoxide and additives;
- imposition of severe penalties for violations;
- raising funds to support all aspects of tobacco control;
- allowing for phasing out the most dangerous products when viable alternatives exist (The problems associated with creating black markets suggests that we must be very careful in ensuring that the short-term as well as the long-term needs of smokers, particularly addicted smokers, have been taken into account.) and

- allowing for graded classification of different products on the basis of total harm. This graded regulation would apply to packaging and labelling, distribution, sales, promotion and perhaps minimum requirements for restrictions on use. Such graded classification would be linked to such things as levels of nicotine and other active and/or potentially harmful ingredients, tar levels being an obvious indicator of the potential harm. There would be emphasis on additives and modifications that affect palatability, especially for children. Additives may play a particularly important role in facilitating uptake by girls and young women. Additives that might encourage increased use and make dangerous products seem less dangerous would either be banned or be subject to more stringent controls than similarly dangerous products without such masking. Products used for therapeutic purposes could have special requirements.

Such regulation will require built-in legislative mechanisms for altering the levels of classifications. These mechanisms must be open to public scrutiny but not allow extended delay by filibustering from vested interests. Of critical importance, determining and changing classification levels must be strongly linked to ongoing research on consequences, that is, the best available science.

The self-funding aspect of the legislation is critical if such laws are to be effective. In this regard, the United States settlement talks begin to give us a sense of how much might be required. The levy must fund the costs of regulation and the costs of enforcement. In particular, it must fund ongoing and special research on use patterns and health effects. If this information is not gathered in a timely fashion, then the capacity to change the classification of particular products will be held up and take longer than necessary; as a result, lives will be lost. The levy should also fund mass media public education, schools prevention programmes, cessation services and perhaps extra medical and other costs of use, particularly when existing tobacco taxes do not adequately compensate the medical system for those costs.

Such legislation could send a clear message to the community that the government has a strong view on the desirability of use. Using labels for classifications, such as 'accepted', 'tolerated', 'discouraged' and 'strongly discouraged' can help send a message about community views. The legislation begins with prohibition, then allows increasing levels of access. It should include limited release for research purposes. Such classifications further emphasize that control is being exercised, in a way that is based on reason, not whimsy.

Regulation imposed on a product must be real. It must be based on facts like the typical yields of product that users obtain or the maximum possible yields, given plausible use patterns. The measures used in many countries to assess the concentrations of tar, nicotine and carbon monoxide in products give values that are very different from those achieved by smokers using the product, who smoke to titrate the nicotine levels. If we continue to pretend that so-called 'milder', 'low tar', 'low nicotine' cigarettes are actually that, we will be deluding ourselves and the public and committing the gullible to premature death.

Much more thought and discussion are needed about what would be required at various levels of regulation, and indeed how many levels of classification are desirable or practical. I shall make some suggestions, which should be seen as examples rather than strong recommendations about what should happen. Decisions about what should happen should involve as broad a group as possible within the tobacco control community.

We may end up with a law that would prohibit products with tar levels, say, greater than 12 mg per cigarette, which would greatly reduce the tar levels in many countries. Some countries already have agreements or legislation limiting tar to similar levels, at least notionally. We do not have good information about whether the exposure of smokers is really limited to that level. Most regulation will apply to products that fall just below the prohibited criteria, such as generic packaging, with extensive warnings and sales restricted to special licensed premises. Lesser restrictions may be imposed on genuinely low-tar products and/or genuinely low-nicotine products. For example, we might indicate that we would be prepared to tolerate products with little addictive potential, shown not to be a conduit to the use of more dangerous products, and which, over their period of likely use, induce little or no demonstrable harm. Limited advertising might be allowed, and packaging might be unregulated except for warnings and information on contents. If some nicotine products became available that had demonstrable net benefits or no demonstrable harm, they might be accepted or in some cases even encouraged. It is unlikely that such products will appear, except for nicotine replacement therapy used as an aid to cessation of nicotine use. One result of the graded classification might be banning of cigarettes from public places but allowing nicotine chewing gum. Nicotine chewing-gum might be sold in convenience stores and cigarettes sold only by specially licensed tobacconists.

The centrepiece of this new model of regulation is that it is an evidence-based form of legislation. It would still require evidence of acceptably low toxicity and other such information before new products were released onto the market. This would be based on the premise that there was plausible evidence that the products were safer and would not attract new markets, unless they were so safe as to be acceptable for mass use, and were certainly not addictive. The novelty of the proposal lies in the need for systematic programmes of research once the product is on the market. These might start with limited-release trials to assess uptake and product transfer. The main focus of research would be studies to monitor use patterns of adults and minors, including uptake of nicotine use, and studies of the realization of harm, including long-term cohort studies. We must establish an adequate research base both for ongoing research and to allow for new ideas and special research projects. This research should not be owned or controlled by product manufacturers or governments. The results and data must be in the public domain, so that the public can have full confidence that the data are valid and be aware of what is known. Thus, they can have confidence that governments are acting responsibly on the basis of the weight of scientific evidence.

While the ideas I have presented might be desirable for individual countries, they would be even more useful if they were adopted internationally. The tobacco pandemic is an international problem demanding an international solution, and compatible legislation across the world would go a long way towards controlling the merchants of death. Countries with strong regulations might prohibit sales to countries without comparable regulation, except perhaps unless the products were sold under the same sort of requirements that apply in the country of origin. Less affluent countries could frame their legislation so that classifications could be revised on the basis of reviews in countries that can afford them and the cost of research. Thus, a smaller or poorer country could write into its legislation the possibility of review whenever other specified countries changed their regulatory requirements, with mechanisms for deciding whether they wished to do so. This would require international support to ensure that the necessary information is provided around the world and the resources are available to allow prompt revisions of regulatory requirement as necessary.

This proposal does not imply that every country has the same level of regulation. Countries with strong traditions of the use of particular products may continue to allow their use more freely than other countries. For example, the *bidis* of India, which have a very high concentration of tar, would almost certainly not be allowed in countries with no established market. But in India it would be impractical and arguably counter-productive to ban them outright. Strategies are needed in India to make *bidis* less dangerous. Similarly, the use of smokeless tobacco is banned in some countries, but in countries where its use is widespread, alternative strategies are needed. Adoption of compatible legislation would have the potential to stop the increased marketing of cigarette products in developing countries and in countries where sections of the population who do not smoke have been targeted for uptake.

Good public policy should encompass a problem, and litigation should be necessary only when the policy fails. A rational regulatory environment minimizes the possibility that people will be trapped into using products which are addictive and thus difficult to stop using, and ensures that resources are available to help them stop and to help the community cover the extra health cost associated with the use. In that case, it may not be reasonable, necessary or even desirable for those who suffer to have extra access to litigation. When the legislation is violated or illegal strategies are used to entrap people, litigation should still be available. I consider, however, that litigation is a very blunt instrument and that systematic regulation to ensure that harm is addressed is greatly preferable.

What will governments and the tobacco industry gain from adopting a proposal along the lines I have set out? Are they ready to accept it? For governments, it may provide a solution for a thorny problem: tobacco is the source of one of their greatest shames—that millions of people are being allowed to die without satisfactory attempts to do something about it. The attempts made to date have been piecemeal and made mainly under the pressure of health advocates. Legislation of this kind provides an opportunity for governments to take control and for debates about progress to be held relatively automatically, given that sensible, reasonable review processes are in place. The tobacco industry is open to change, as its representatives have demonstrated in talking to health experts in the United States. Stability and certainty are important in the business environment and are preferable to uncertainty and the threat of potentially enormous litigation.

With strong, flexible legislation, we will be equipped to reduce the harm associated with nicotine use. Such legislation must be comprehensive, prescriptive, flexible, research-based and self-funding. Even if such legislation is enacted, it will not guarantee results. Public health workers will have to redouble their efforts to develop and implement effective strategies to discourage use. The legislation should provide the framework and resources to help us do this more effectively.

In conclusion, the time for nicotine regulation is now. If we cannot move towards it now, when the industry has effectively admitted that it has been lying for many years and has been systematically targeting the young, it is unlikely that we will ever be able to obtain the essential international collaboration. We do not want a situation in which the affluent countries effectively protect their populations, only to see the problem being shipped to the less advantaged. We need a comprehensive perspective to help us cope with new possibilities. Tobacco control advocates must be involved in this process. We should be debating exactly what we want so that we can put coherent proposals to the world community for action. We cannot afford to let the moment slip away. The time for action is now.

Acknowledgments
The ideas presented in this paper come from a range of sources. The only part to which I lay claim is the synthesis. In particular, discussions with David Sweanor of the Canadian Non Smokers Rights Association have been responsible for some of the more novel ideas.

Smoke-free areas

Tobacco-free, healthy cities: Multi-city action plan

G.Pilati & E. Tamang

Centre for Health Education, Regional Documentation Service, Padua, Italy

In most cities of Europe, tobacco smoking kills more people than AIDS, alcohol, road traffic accidents, drugs, fires, suicides and murders put together. One of the most important steps that a city could take to ensure the future health of its citizens is to reduce smoking. The concept of the 'multi-city action plan' is based on the idea that groups of cities involved in the World Health Organization (WHO) Healthy Cities Project could work together to address common concerns which need priority consideration. The 'multi-city action plan' aims to encourage innovative action for health at the local level. It is a flexible framework for action that enables cities to work together on issues of particular importance to them, to share experiences, develop expertise and become models and resources for other cities. The cities involved in a multi-city action plan can gain political legitimacy and support from their alliance with other cities and from their international leadership role, in addition to shared ideas and knowledge.

History of the project

In 1990, seven cities interested in developing models of good practice in reducing tobacco use framed a multi-city action plan for tobacco-free cities. They took advantage of the major initiative of the WHO Regional Office for Europe, the Action Plan for a Tobacco-free Europe. The founding cities were Belfast, Dublin, Frankfurt, Glasgow, Gothenburg, Kaunas and Stockholm. At the first meeting, five key themes for intervention were identified: children, economic issues, local government, public places and health services. Belfast agreed to become the coordinating city for the multi-city action plan on tobacco and hosted the first business meeting, which concentrated on the five key themes and added a further one: adults in the community.

Each year, these cities meet to report on activities, exchange information and set up a new plan of action. The second business meeting in 1992 was hosted by Frankfurt, followed by Pécs in 1993, Padua in 1994, Bologna in 1995 and Kaunas in 1996. A survey was carried out in 1995 to examine the activities that were being carried out and the programmes being conducted in the member cities. (Figure 1).

The network has published *Working for Tobacco-free Cities* in the Smoke-free Europe series, which is also available in an Italian version. It has also produced 'Keep kids smoke-free' cards. A newsletter is also produced twice a year.

Figure 1. Tobacco prevention programmes in cities involved in the multi-city action plan for tobacco free cities

	Padua	Bologna	Gothenburg	Torun	Lodz	Warsaw	Kaunas	Belfast	Frankfurt	Gyor	Sumperk	Barcelona	Dublin
Hospital	◆	◆	◆		◆		◆	◆			◆	◆	◆
Schools	◆	◆	◆	◆	◆	◆	◆	◆	◆		◆	◆	◆
Smoke-free settings				◆			◆	◆					◆
Workplaces	◆	◆	◆	◆	◆			◆				◆	◆
Health-care centres			◆	◆		◆	◆	◆	◆	◆			◆
Primary health care	◆		◆	◆		◆		◆		◆		◆	

Third phase

During the meeting in Kaunas, it was decided to relaunch the multi-city action plan network with the third Action Plan for a Tobacco-free Europe for the period 1997–2001. A letter was to be sent to all core members of the Healthy Cities Project and cities participating in multi-city action plans against tobacco, alcohol and drugs, inviting them to join the next phase. In order to do so, all cities were asked to:

- send a letter to the WHO Tobacco or Health programme in Copenhagen, signed by an appropriate political authority and designating a technical focal point for the multi-city action plan;
- confirm their commitment to the guiding principles of the multi-city action plan;
- confirm their commitment to the principles and strategies outlined in the third Action Plan for a Tobacco-free Europe;
- confirm their commitment to the preparation and implementation of a city action plan to reduce tobacco use, along the lines of the guiding principles and the third Action Plan;
- confirm their commitment to the production of an annual report summarizing their activities and their attendance at the annual business meetings to present the report, share experiences and contribute to the development of the tobacco multi-city action plans.

The seventh business meeting was held in Vejle, Denmark, in 1997 in collaboration with the Vejle Non-smoking County Project. The cities currently belonging to the network are Barcelona (Spain), Belfast (Northern Ireland), Bologna (Italy), Dublin (Ireland), Ferrara (Italy), Gdansk (Poland), Geneva (Switzerland), Kaunas (Lithuania), Lodz (Poland), Pamplona (Spain), Pécs (Hungary) and Torun (Poland). The network is coordinated on behalf of the cities and WHO by the Centre for Health Education in Padua, a WHO Collaborating Centre for tobacco.

The potential competencies and responsibilities for tobacco control determined in Kaunas are to:

- ensure that tobacco action is incorporated into the municipal health strategy;
- ensure that tobacco control strategies are implemented as part of intersectoral strategies;
- provide staff and financial resources for tobacco control activities;
- use locally generated fines for tobacco control programmes;
- promote local networking for tobacco control activities;
- disseminate examples of good practice to non-municipal institutions and organizations;
- enforce existing legislation;
- implement national directives;
- advocate tobacco control policy at regional, national and international levels;
- enforce restrictions on sales to minors;
- control cinema advertisements;
- control advertisements on city-owned hoardings;
- control advertisements on city-owned properties, including public transport;
- provide educational and information programmes for schools;
- rovide educational and information programmes for the public;
- promote tobacco control policies and a non-smoking culture through city-owned media;
- implement non-smoking policies for municipal employees;
- advocate smoke-free workplaces;
- identify smoke-free public places;
- provide smoking cessation services;
- provide sponsorship for tobacco-free sports and arts.

The expected gains from a municipal action on tobacco are improved health for the population, improved economy for the municipality and an improved image with regard to public health action. The expected gains from joining the multi-city action plan on

tobacco are:
- networking and receiving ideas and experience from other cities;
- political support for tobacco control activities;
- facilitating fund-raising for tobacco control activities;
- allowing discussions of problems for which a forum is sometimes not available in the city;
- facilitating local lobbying based on international experience;
- enhancing the national and international image of the city;
- receiving documentation and publications, including one on community and municipal action on tobacco;
- receiving advice on evaluation;
- conducting common actions in other cities in the multi-city action plan.

The responsibilities of members of the multi-city action plan on tobacco are to:
- prepare a health strategy for the city;
- ensure that the health strategy includes action on tobacco;
- prepare a tobacco action plan for the city;
- make links with other tobacco networks at local and national levels;
- make links with other WHO networks at local and national levels;
- share experiences with cities in the Healthy Cities Project and others;
- help other cities to start tobacco action;
- be a vehicle for the ideals of the Healthy Cities Project;
- designate a focal point for tobacco control activities;
- designate financial resources to fund a city-based tobacco action plan;
- be committed to attend annual business meetings of the multi-city action plan on tobacco;
- prepare an annual report of activities to present to the 'multi-city action plan' tobacco business meeting.

The responsibilities of the coordinator of a multi-city action plan are to organize annual business meetinsg in association with WHO and a host city; to prepare and disseminate a report of annual business meeting and a newsletter and other information; to advise on problems; to represent the multi-city action plan at relevant meetings and networks and to investigate potential sources of funding.

The responsibilities of the WHO technical focal point are to disseminate information and resources, ensure links with other networks, provide technical support to citiess, work closely with the coordinator and ensure links with other health issues.

Attitudes and experiences of restaurant owners regarding smoking bans in Adelaide, South Australia

D. Turnbull[1], K. Jones[1], M. Wakefield[2] & D. Teusner[1]

[1]Department of Public Health, University of Adelaide, and [2]Epidemiology Branch, South Australian Health Commission, Adelaide, South Australia

Introduction

In Australia, as evidence for the adverse health effects of environmental tobacco smoke has become publicly accepted through legal rulings and civil liability payouts (Everingham & Woodward, 1991), efforts to ban smoking in public places have intensified, so that smoking bans are now the norm for South Australian workers who are employed indoors (Wakefield *et al.*, 1996a). Restaurants are an exception to this rule, however, so that both customers and staff are exposed to environmental tobacco smoke for extended periods. Efforts to introduce bans in restaurants have traditionally been met with vocal concern on the part of restaurateurs that such policies will lead to loss of business. This is despite the fact that several studies of the effect of local ordinances which ban smoking in restaurants show no adverse effect on business (Glantz & Smith, 1994; Centers for Disease Control, 1995).

While public opinion surveys in South Australia, as elsewhere, show very high support for smoke-free dining (Mullins & Borland, 1995; Wakefield et al., 1996b), restaurateurs grossly underestimate this level of support (Schofield et al., 1993) and have been slow to respond to community demand. In South Australia, efforts to restrict smoking in restaurants culminated in 1991 with the introduction of a voluntary code of practice whereby participating restaurateurs undertook to provide for separate smoking and non-smoking areas. The voluntary code was developed by a collaborative group comprising the hospitality industry, unions and public health representation. It required participating restaurants to provide at least one-third of their restaurant as smoke-free dining, increasing to two-thirds after one year. Under the code, customers were to be asked at the time of booking or entry which area they would prefer to be seated in. For each participating restaurant, window stickers and table signs were provided.

In 1996, given increasing community support for tougher restrictions and a perception that the voluntary code was not being complied with, it was decided to undertake a survey of restaurateurs with the aims of determining the status of no-smoking policies and the experience and attitudes of restaurateurs with respect to such policies. In particular, we sought to determine uptake of and compliance with the voluntary code and to assess the level of support for legislation that would ban smoking in restaurants.

Method

The sampling frame for the survey covered all restaurants and cafes in the metropolitan area of Adelaide which provide sit-down meals and that were listed in the telephone directory. A random sample of restaurants was selected, each of which was sent an introductory letter explaining the purpose of the survey, followed one week later by a telephone survey to restaurant owners or managers. Overall, 276 interviews were conducted, representing 70% of the eligible restaurants in the sample; 14% refused and 15% could not be contacted.

Results and discussion

Overall, 27% of the restaurants in the sample were totally non-smoking, 41% made some provision for non-smoking by providing separate smoking and non-smoking areas or allowing smoking only at restricted times after the main dining period was over, and the remaining 33% had no provision for non-smoking customers (Table 1). Among those which provided separate areas for non-smokers, only 34% made provision for more than half of the restaurant seating to be allocated to non-smokers. It was apparent that smaller restaurants (with seating for < 40 customers) had either no policy at all or a total ban, indicating their lack of structural ability to accommodate separate smoking and non-smoking areas.

The percentage of restaurants using the voluntary code was minimal: out of 186 restaurants that reported a ban or some provision, only 28 (15%) of those with a smoke-free area or premises had used the code to guide the development of their policy. Of the

Table 1. Non-smoking policies in Adelaide restaurants, 1996

Type of policy	No.	%
Total ban	74	26.8
Separate room provided	14	5.1
Permanent segregated area	89	32.2
Smoking allowed at restricted times	9	3.3
Non-smokers accommodated on request	23	8.3
No provision for non-smokers	67	24.3
Total	276	100

restaurants that had used the code, 36% were totally smoke free, but only 50% were complying with the requirement to provide at least two-thirds of seating for non-smokers, and 14% complied with the requirement.

We asked 90 restaurants with no provision for non-smokers, in an unprompted fashion, why they had no policy. Fear of loss of business was a prime concern (43%), followed by structural constraints (39%), a perception that there was no demand for provision of non-smoking areas (27%), a belief that segregation was ineffective in reducing exposure to environmental tobacco smoke (13%) and other reasons (21%), including a concern for 'smokers' rights' and not having thought about it.

Because we had anticipated that there would be substantial concern about loss of business, we also directly asked all those with no provision for non-smokers whether they expected that the introduction of a smoke-free area or premises would lead to a gain in business, a loss in business or make no difference. We were able to compare these responses with those of restaurateurs who had a policy, by asking them to report on the effect the introduction of the policy had actually had on their business (Table 2). Of those with no provision for non-smokers, nearly half expected that the introduction of such a policy would incur a loss in business. By comparison, only 12% of those with a total ban and 6% of those with some other provision for non-smokers reported that the provision had been associated with a loss of business. In the main, bans and restrictions had meant no change in the level of business, although one-quarter of those with total bans had experienced an increase in business, which they attributed to the ban. These results show a clear mismatch between the expected and actual effects of introducing bans and restrictions on smoking in restaurants.

Although many restaurateurs feared loss of business, however unsubstantiated, there was a high degree of support for restrictions and bans, 84% agreeing that restaurants should provide smoke-free areas and 50% agreeing that the Government should introduce a ban (Table 3). It was of interest that 45% of those with no provisions thought there should be a Government ban, perhaps indicating that these restaurants are waiting for Government intervention before they will act.

Table 2. Reported and perceived effects of non-smoking policy on business, by type of policy

Effect	Reported (%)		Perceived (%)
	Some provision (n = 109)	Total ban (n = 74)	No provision (n = 90)
No difference to business	69.7	52.7	31.1
Gain in business	14.7	25.7	2.2
Loss in business	6.4	12.1	46.7
Don't know/can't say	9.2	12.1	20.0

Table 3. Percentages of respondents in agreement with statements about smoking in restaurants

Statement	Agreement with statement (%)			
	No provision (n = 86)	Some provision (n = 111)	Total ban (n = 73)	Overall total (n = 270)
Restaurants should provide smoke-free areas	64.0	93.7	91.8	83.7
Banning smoking in all restaurants and cafes will have a negative effect on the restaurant industry	60.0	55.9	35.6	51.7
Should be a Government ban on smoking in all restaurants and cafes	45.3	46.8	61.6	50.4

Conclusions
We conclude that the voluntary code of practice made an insignificant contribution to adoption of non-smoking policies, both uptake and compliance being poor. This is consistent with evaluations of voluntary arrangements elsewhere. While loss of business is frequently expressed as a reason for not introducing non-smoking policies, most restaurateurs who have introduced a policy have found that this simply does not happen. Most report no change or an increase in business, which they attribute to the policy. Despite these fears, there was a high degree of support for restrictions and bans, half believing there should be a Government ban on smoking in all restaurants and cafes.

These are encouraging results and formed part of a briefing given to the South Australian Government in late 1996. Subsequently, as part of a package of tobacco control reforms, legislation was passed to ban smoking in all indoor dining establishments. This legislation will come into effect from the beginning of 1999. We will continue to monitor the experiences and concerns of restaurateurs when the bans come into force and to monitor the exposure of restaurant staff to environmental tobacco smoke through surveys involving measurements of cotinine in saliva. It is important for the legislation to be subject to evaluation, in order to reassure restaurateurs and Government policy makers that bans offer real benefits, which ought not be eroded by the vocal and biased concerns of forces complicit with the tobacco industry.

References
Centers for Disease Control (1995) Assessment of the impact of a 100% smoke-free ordinance on restaurant sales: West Lake Hills, Texas, 1992–1994. *Morbid. Mortal. Wkly Rep.*, **44**, 370–372
Everingham, R. & Woodward, S. (1991) *Tobacco Litigation: The Case against Passive Smoking: AFCO vs TIA*, Sydney: Legal Books
Glantz, S.A. & Smith, L.R.A. (1994) The effects of ordinances requiring smoke-free restaurants on restaurant sales. *Am. J. Public Health*, **84**, 1081–1085
Mullins, R. & Borland, R. (1995) Preference and requests for smoke-free dining. *Aust. J. Public Health*, **19**, 100–101
Schofield, M.J., Considine, R., Boyle, C.A. & Sanson-Fisher, R. (1993) Smoking control in restaurants: The effectiveness of self-regulation in Australia. *Am. J. Public Health*, **83**, 1984–1988
Wakefield, M., Roberts, L. & Owen, N. (1996a) Changes in the prevalence and acceptance of workplace smoking bans among indoor workers in South Australia. *Tobacco Control*, **5**, 205–208
Wakefield, M., Roberts, L. & Kent, P. (1996b) *Smoking Restrictions in Restaurants: A Re-assessment, Quit Evaluation Report No. 4: 1992–1995*, Adelaide: South Australian Smoking and Health Project

Are the bars in Glasgow, Scotland, ready to ban smoking?

D. McIntyre

Glasgow 2000, Glasgow, Scotland

The bar setting is of particular interest to Glasgow's health promotion programmers, as it is the last setting in the City to address the issue of smoking. In general, 75% of the city's workplaces restrict smoking, all of its health-care facilities are smoke-free, as are most of its education and public transport facilities. These long-established smoke-free policies, coupled with a sustained effort to promote cessation and discourage uptake of smoking, helped Glasgow's smoking prevalence to fall from 44% in 1983 to 32% in 1995. The leisure setting is important in the public health effort, both because of the amount of time people spend there, whether as workers or customers, and because of its significance to young people: the social norms in the leisure environment have a large impact on young people's aspirations and behaviour. Two studies were therefore undertaken to explore issues affecting the introduction of smoking restrictions in bars in Glasgow, in order to provide information on this aspect of health promotion strategy and programme development.

The first study was a cross-sectional descriptive study designed to estimate the extent of unrestricted smoking in Glasgow's bars and to identify the factors that inhibit the restriction of smoking in that setting.

First study: Objectives

The objectives were to estimate how many bars in Glasgow restrict customers' smoking, to explore physical or operational factors that might affect the provision of smoke-free areas in bars, to estimate smoking rates among workers in bars and to explore workers' concerns about passive smoking in bars.

A structured telephone interview survey was carried out with staff members from 100 bars randomly chosen from Glasgow's 481 bars; the response rate was 82%.

First study: Findings

Only 6% of bars in Glasgow imposed restrictions on smoking by customers; none offered completely separate areas. Circumstances associated with favourable attitudes towards restricting smoking were admitting children, serving food and an interest in offering customers a choice. None of the bars with restrictions reported problems with enforcement, stating that adequate signs and support from staff and other customers were sufficient to encourage observance of the rules. The protection of children's health was felt to be a particularly strong argument for overcoming the few objections they received from customers.

Regular smoking was reported by 45% of bar workers. Most of them were heavy smokers, consuming ≥ 20 cigarettes per day. Most of them had tried to quit smoking before or were currently trying to do so. Almost all the bar workers estimated that the prevalence of smoking among their customers was considerably higher than the known rate for Glasgow adults, a third believing it to be 80% or more. The actual rate was 34%.

Many bar workers did not perceive passive smoking as a current or serious problem for staff or customers.

The bar workers were most interested in the practical, commercial and ethical issues of restricting customers' smoking. Many Glasgow bars have more than one public room: 44% of those in the study had two rooms and 9% had three rooms, but there was no variation in the response pattern from staff in different-sized establishments. Customer type and the recreational nature of the setting, which is strongly associated with a spirit of free choice, were seen as more important. One practical issue affecting the restriction of smoking was a local government licensing condition requiring a smoke-free room for children. This condition was not, however, always met.

The bar workers perceived little or no demand from customers for restrictions on smoking and felt that legislation would be needed to force change. Several said they would restrict smoking if compelled by law but would be very unhappy about the prospect and did not believe it would work in practice. Among the staff overall, there would be a moderate preference to work in smoke-free bars, but a significant proportion, even of non-smokers, would not prefer this. There was some feeling that tobacco smoke is an essential element of the bar atmosphere

Overall, there was little variation between the opinions of smokers, non-smokers and ex-smokers within this occupational group.

First study: Recommendations
Short term:
- The health effects of passive smoking on bar workers should be fully researched.
- Further research should be undertaken to establish the level of demand for smoke-free facilities among present and potential bar customers.
- Existing environmental health and licensing regulations could usefully be exploited to maximize current provision of smoke-free environments.
- Bars should be offered practical guidance on how to introduce restrictions on smoking in ways appropriate to their special circumstances.

Long-term:
- Bar workers should be targeted as a homogeneous occupational group for health education about smoking issues. They are major sufferers from the problem of passive smoking, they are opinion leaders in the setting and they are essential agents of change.
- General public education should be undertaken to increase understanding of the risks of passive smoking.
- General public education should be undertaken to encourage smokers to consider the effects of their smoking on others, particularly on workers in the leisure settings they use. It should be framed in the context of the need to balance individual freedom against public health concerns.

The second study was a response to the recommendation for further market research among bar customers, to detect the extent of public interest in smoke-free areas. This, along with practical issues, had emerged in the first study as the main issue for managers who simply did not believe that their customers would be interested.

Second study: Objectives

The objectives of this study were to ascertain public awareness of the dangers of passive smoking, to explore the role of smoking in people's decision to visit a bar, to discover whether the prevalence of smoking is higher among bar users than among non-users and to determine the level of support for smoke-free areas in bars.

A street sampling approach was used to recruit and interview 490 respondents over a two-week period. The sample was structured to include four groups of particular interest to bar staff: people who were regular customers of their local bar, users of bars with a more transient customer base (i.e. people who travelled into particular social centres in the city), older working-class men (seen by bar staff as an important but difficult group) and students.

As bar staff are most interested in people who use bars often, the results were analysed both on this basis and according to smoking status.

Second study: Findings and conclusions

No significant difference in smoking prevalence was found in relation to bar use patterns (Table 1). The overall smoking prevalence of bar customers, even regular customers, seems to be no greater than that of the general population. This suggests that bar workers have a very inaccurate perception of their customers' smoking rates, which is likely be one of the factors in workers' anticipation of a low demand for restrictions.

In an analysis of places where tobacco smoke is encountered most often, bars were the main source of exposure to smoke, even for smokers (Table 2).

Overall, 85% of respondents considered that passive smoking is generally damaging to health. The lowest levels of awareness were among people > 60 (75%) and the lowest socioeconomic groups (78%). Smokers were least likely to regard passive smoking as damaging to health: 74% compared with 89% of ex-smokers and 95% of non-smokers. The most commonly identified health risk was an increased risk for cancer. Despite these high levels of awareness of health risks, respondents showed rather less personal concern about passive smoking (Figure 1). The results obtained when the

Table 1. Prevalence of smoking by frequency of visiting bars

Smoking status	Frequency (%)			
	Weekly	Monthly	Less often	Never
Smoker	46	38	41	35
Ex-smoker	22	29	21	30
Non-smoker	32	34	38	34

Table 2. Places where tobacco smoke is encountered most often (%)

Place	All	Smokers	Ex-smokers	Non-smokers
Bars	41	42	35	44
Own home	20	36	8	9
Restaurants	8	3	10	11
Friends' homes	8	4	13	10
Work	8	7	10	8
Never	5	2	6	7
Street or malls	4	2	6	4
Transport	4	2	8	3
Other	2	1	3	3

same question was analysed by frequency of bar visiting are shown in Figure 2, which illustrates clearly that large numbers of the customers who are probably of most interest to bar staff, i.e. frequent bar users, feel at least some discomfort from passive smoking.

Another aspect to customer demand is personal assertiveness, as bar staff seem to be relying on customers to make their feelings known. Non-smokers are often reluctant to make a fuss about a smoky atmospheres, particularly in social settings. In spite of the high level of discomfort found in this survey, the usual reluctance to complain was also observed (Figure 3). The commonest reason given for doing nothing was being a smoker, although many non- and ex-smokers stated that they just put up with it or were reluctant to complain. Overall, 21% of customers reacted by leaving. Respondents were also asked whether they ever cut short or avoided social occasions because of a smoky atmosphere: 37% of the sample said they did. Of that group, 50% said they regularly or occasionally did so when visiting friends, 66% in bars and 73% in restaurants.

Another indicator of customer demand is their tendency to ask spontaneously for smoke-free facilities. In this survey, 49% asked at least sometimes and 51% never did

Figure 1. Responses to the question 'How much does passive smoking bother you?'

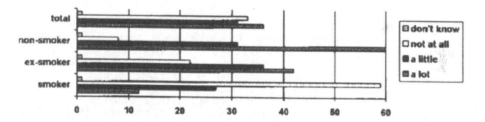

Figure 2. Responses to the question 'How much does passive smoking bother you?' in relation to frequency of bar visiting

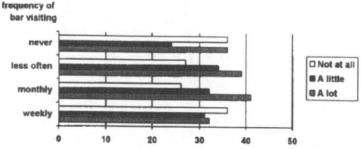

Figure 3. Responses to the question 'What do you do when a bar gets smoky?'

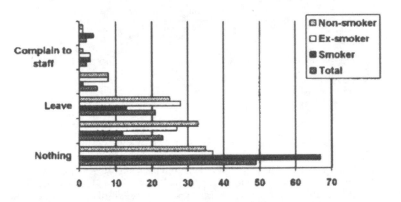

so. Non-smokers were much more likely to ask. More women (56%) than men (42%) asked, and asking was commonest among people in the highest socioeconomic grouping. Common reasons for asking were while eating, when accompanied by children, being pregnant or being with a pregnant woman and knowing that an area was available.

The last set of questions addressed bar managers' fears that introducing restrictions on smoking would result in lost custom. Respondents were asked to speculate about what they would do if offered a choice of smoking and non-smoking areas in bars, and what might be the effect on the atmosphere (Table 3). The findings were conclusively positive: a net gain of 22% in customers and a net gain of 19% in length of stay were projected. Both of these effects would occur particularly among women and in the higher socioeconomic groups, which currently form desirable new market segments for the licensed trade.

Overall conclusions

Bars were the commonest situation in which people spent time in a smoky atmosphere. Since passive smoking does bother people and is seen as a threat to health, the findings suggest that a smoky atmosphere has a negative effect on attitudes towards and use of bars among a significant proportion of customers. At present, the only alternatives are to put up with it or leave, and a number do take the latter course.

There is popular endorsement of the provision of choice of smoking and no-smoking areas in bars. A majority would use no-smoking areas at least occasionally, and smokers showed no opposition to their introduction. A less smoky atmosphere would improve the environment for non-smokers in particular and would be likely to lead to increased

Table 3. Projected effects of introduction of non-smoking areas in bars

Effect	Response (%)			
	All	Smokers	Ex-smokers	Non-smokers
Frequency of visiting				
More often	24	5	35	41
Same	74	92	62	59
Less often	2	4	3	
Time spent				
Longer	20	4	26	37
Same	70	96	72	63
Less	1	1	2	
Atmosphere				
Improve	48	22	61	70
No effect	48	72	36	27
Spoil	4	6	3	3

trade. These commercial issues, combined with the already compelling evidence of the health effects of passive smoking on bar workers, offer convincing reasons for bars to start restricting smoking on their premises.

Will Birmingham become the United Kingdom's first smoke-free city?

P. Hooper

Smoke Free Birmingham, Southern Birmingham Community Health National Health Service Trust, Springfields Centre for Health Promotion, Birmingham, United Kingdom

Birmingham is the largest provincial city in England, with a population of 1 million. Smoking has been identified as the first priority for improving the health of the inhabitants of the City of Birmingham by the local Health Authority. Following on from the successful activities of Smoke Free Birmingham and the City's Health Promotion Units, the vast majority of the current 1997–98 health promotion budget was allocated to smoking prevention. A three-year tobacco control programme was designed, which closely followed and expanded the national Tobacco Control Alliance Strategy. The main elements are described here.

Support for high taxation and duty on tobacco: This is a central Government function, but it requires popular support at a local level.

Effective enforcement of illegal sales: The law is enforced by trading standards officers working for the local Council. The Health Authority provides practical support to ensure that the activity continues and encourages publicity of any legal action that is taken.

Dealing with promotion and advertising by the tobacco industry: A close watch is kept on tobacco advertising to ensure that breaches of the current voluntary code are reported. Other tactics are exposed in the media. Counter-advertising and sponsorship, particularly of sport, is undertaken. Young people are involved at every opportunity.

Promoting non-smoking as the norm in public places and workplaces: Statutory bodies provide for almost completely smoke-free public places and workplaces, but the public sector is still some way behind. Assistance is given to organizations that wish to implement new policies on their premises. Awards are given to restaurants that provide smoke-free facilities, and a guide is published to help people find smoke-free environments.

Providing effective cessation advice: Events such as No Smoking Day and New Year's resolutions provide a focus for cessation campaigns, and this is underpinned by the training of health professionals such as health visitors, midwives and pharmacists to provide 'staged-based' advice to their clients. The local campaign is supported by free-phone Quitline services.

Media advocacy: The whole programme is supported by media profiling of smoking issues and by involving key opinion formers and other players in the tobacco control movement.

Birmingham is already recognized as a leading smoke-free city in the United Kingdom. Smoke Free Birmingham works closely with other successful alliances, regionally, nationally and internationally. The outcome of Birmingham's bold strategy for a 'Smoke-free City by the Year 2000' is being monitored by other organizations which may follow Birmingham's lead. Although most of the funding will be from the Health Authority, the programme also relies on the support of the City Council and other organizations, including leading sports clubs, commerce, industry and the media.

The City has a number of research projects focusing on both cessation and prevention that will both assist in the success of the Birmingham programme and provide valuable data for others. Linking closely with nationally organized campaigns, the City-wide programme reflects the cultural, religious, racial and socioeconomic diversity of the City. Its ultimate success will be measured by the supplementary added value and by its progress towards national targets.

Effectiveness of Thailand's non-smokers' rights protection law in restaurants

C. Supawongse

Department of Health, Ministry of Public Health, Thailand

Abstract

Thailand has implemented its Non-smokers' Rights Protection Act since mid-1992. The law restricts smoking in designated public places, but air-conditioned restaurants are public places in which smokers' rights are easily violated. This survey addressed the situation in four towns to determine the opinions of people exposed to second-hand smoke.

Restaurants were chosen randomly, and 1744 respondents, including restaurant owners, waiters, waitresses, policemen, inspectors and customers were selected systematically. About 29% of the smokers smoked in restricted areas. Almost all of the respondents had adequate knowledge. One-third of the customers reported that many restaurants did not have no-smoking zones. The majority reported that the weakness of responsible officers was the primary cause of ineffective enforcement. Many recommended stringent enforcement, a strong public campaign and extension of restricted areas from the current 50% to 75% of the area.

Introduction

The *Non-smokers' Health Protection Act* in Thailand has been effective since October 1992. Its aims are to protect non-smokers' health in public by designating public places into four categories. The first is totally smoke-free zones such as public buses, taxis, air-conditioned passenger trains, public boats, domestic flights, passenger elevators, school buses and cinemas. The second is zones that are totally smoke-free except for private rooms in such places as schools, museums, art galleries, libraries, nurseries and air-conditioned passenger boats. The third is zones that are totally smoke-free except for private rooms and designated smoking areas in such places as hospitals, university buildings and air-conditioned department stores, trade centres and trade exhibitions. The last category is areas that must be at least 50% smoke-free, such as air-conditioned restaurants and non-air-conditioned passenger trains. The *Act* includes punishment for any offender who smokes in a smoke-free zone and for any restaurant owner who does not provide a smoke-free zone and a no-smoking sign.

To evaluate the effectiveness of the *Act*, only well-known restaurants with air-conditioned rooms were selected. Five sample groups were chosen, consisting of restaurant owners, waiters or waitresses, inspectors, police authorities and customers.

Objectives and methods

The objectives of this study were to ascertain whether the *Non-smokers' Health Protection Act* has been enforced in restaurants where air-conditioned rooms are provided and to determine the knowledge, attitudes and practice of respondents towards the *Act*.

The survey was implemented with five types of questionnaire used to determine the knowledge, attitudes and practice of 1744 respondents in five sample groups in four regions, in one province in each region.

Opinions

All five groups were well aware of the hazards of smoking, both to smokers themselves and to people nearby. Most of them obeyed the *Act* and often berated offenders. All of the respondents knew about the content of the *Act*, 49% from television, 19% from posters and leaflets and 10% from radio. Most of the respondents agreed that smoke-free zones should be extended to 75 or 100% of the whole area of a restaurant, as shown in Table 1. In the five sample groups, 92% of all respondents agreed that all non-air-conditioned restaurants should provide customers with a smoke-free zone, and 96% of the respondents agreed that an offender who smoked in a smoke-free zone should be punished.

Inspectors and police authorities

The *Act* assigned 'officers in charge' or inspectors to inspect and supervise restaurant owners, but 40% of them reported some difficulties in implementing the *Act*, such as lack of authority, cooperation and assistance from the police and little attention from the Ministry of Public Heath. Although the *Act* assigned police authorities to investigate violations and inflict penalties, they could not fully implement the *Act* because of other, much more important assignments. It may therefore be concluded that inspectors and police authorities were ineffective in implementing the *Act*.

Recommendations

The Ministry of Public Health should:
- set up policies to implement health protection for non-smokers;
- inform the public about the hazards of smoking and publicize the *Act* continuously through mass media and especially television, to which most people have access;
- allocate a budget for non-governmental agencies that dedicate themselves to campaigning effectively on non-smoking and health protection; and
- review its declaration on smoke-free zones in air-conditioned restaurants and insist that non-air-conditioned restaurants provide smoke-free zones that comprise at least 50% of its area.

The Provincial Health Office should:
- develop a mechanism to inspect, supervise and follow up air-conditioned restaurants continuously;
- develop a mechanism to ensure that inspectors and police authorities are aware of the essential aims of the *Act*;

Table 1. Opinions on the provision of smoke-free zones in restaurants in Thailand

Group	Smoke-free zone										Total no.
	Extension from 50% to				Maintaining at 50%		Reduction from 50% to				
	100%		75%				25%		0%		
	No.	%	No.	%	No.	%	No.	%	No.	%	
Restaurant owners	10	18.9	27	50.9	11	20.8	5	9.4	0	0	53
Waiters or waitresses	82	23.6	160	46.1	71	20.5	21	6.1	13	3.7	347
Customers	192	38.0	224	48.0	64	12.0	7	1.0	2	1.0	489
Inspectors	46	29.1	91	57.6	18	11.4	3	1.9	0	0	158
Police	161	24.6	263	40.0	171	26.0	62	9.4	0	0	657
Total	491	28.8	765	44.9	335	19.7	98	5.8	15	0.8	1704

- cooperate with police authorities in examining samples, punishing offenders and disseminating the results of their work through the mass media at regular intervals;
- support the public involved in clubs, societies and associations in running anti-smoking campaigns, calling for consumer rights and strengthening surveillance in the community by allocating a budget and providing essential information on technical matters, if needed.

People should:
- cooperate by notifying the authorities or the mass media when they observe offenders;
- refuse to patronize air-conditioned restaurants with no separation of smoking and non-smoking areas;
- form clubs societies or associations to protect consumer's rights to health.

Creating smoke-free facilities

L.L. Fairbanks[1], R.D. Hurt[2] & B. Watanabe[3]

[1] *Arizonans Concerned about Smoking, Mesa, Arizona, United States;*
[2]*Nicotine Dependence Center, Mayo Clinic, Rochester, Minnesota, United States;*
and [3]*Tobacco Problems Information Center, Tokyo, Japan*

"Diseases related to smoking are an important cause of premature deaths in the world, both in developed and developing countries. Eliminating smoking can do more to improve health and prolong life than any other measure in the field of preventive health." Director, Pan American Health Organization, 1992

"Smoking is slow motion suicide and slow motion homicide toward others." Takeshi Hirayama, director of large-scale Japanese cohort studies on passive smoking, World Conference, Paris 1994

"Public smoking is not a right." John F. Banzhaf, III, Professor of Law

"Americans who've made the choice not to use tobacco products should not be put at risk by those who choose to smoke." William Jefferson Clinton, President of the United States of America

Health damage and preventable deaths due to both active and passive smoking must be kept in focus as health issues. Much of the progress made on the road toward tobacco control in the United States and in other countries has come from the non-smokers' rights movement and the widespread reporting of the hazards of passive smoking from studies such as the large-scale prospective cohort studies of Takeshi Hirayama. If healthier, smoke-free workplaces and other smoke-free facilities of all types are to be achieved in a community, leadership by the health-care community is needed. When hospitals and clinics totally ban smoking both inside and outside buildings, a clear message is sent to all that smoking is a health issue, which provides a positive example for others in the community (workplaces, schools, restaurants, sports arenas) to follow.

One of the most successful weapons in the non-smokers' rights movement in the United States was 'strategic embarrassment', or publicity that exposed physicians and other health-care officials who smoked as negative role models, who had to choose whether to quit smoking and start to support smoke-free workplaces and smoke-free public places or lose all credibility as healers, teachers and leaders.

The steps in creating a totally non-smoking facility involve leadership commitment, gathering data on smoking, educating people about the hazards of smoking, obtaining participation and involvement, planning an implementation strategy, communicating the policy, setting a timetable and evaluation.

In order to change health facilities from smoke-filled to smoke-free areas, one should start by inciting physicians, nurses, other staff and administrators to be leaders and role models.

Smoking indoors should be banned in a first phase, and then smoking outside near entrances and on the grounds around hospitals and clinics. Ashtrays should be removed wherever smoking is restricted, as they are a non-verbal signal that smoking is permitted. 'Smoking breaks' for all employees should be termed 'rest breaks'. The first areas to be made smoke-free should be out-patient centres and offices, and then 24-h in-patient hospitals. Substance abuse and mental health treatment centres require special planning, but no addiction treatment is complete without including nicotine addiction.

The message should be presented with understanding and sympathy but with'no-nonsense' firmness. Smoking is 'slow-motion suicide' for both smokers and others, exposed to environmental tobacco smoke. Despite rationalizations to the contrary, 'designated smoking areas' are really designated negative role modelling, disease-causing, cancer promotion areas. Money spent to build smoking shelters on the grounds of medical facilities is inappropriate use of limited patient-care funds and gives the wrong message to everyone, especially our children and those who must pay for the high cost of preventable tobacco-related diseases. The temptation to cope with the embarrassment of continued staff smoking by simply trying to hide the location of sanctioned smoking areas should be resisted. The message for positive health promotion and disease prevention at every health facility should be very clear.

Supportive smoking cessation programmes should be offered. Failure to offer help to smokers who are trying to quit is medical malpractice. Smoking by health-care staff destroys their credibility when they offer help to pregnant women and other smokers to quit. Accordingly, adherence to a smoke-free premises policy, which has been a condition of future and continued employment at Mayo Clinic-affiliated clinics and hospitals in the United States since 1993, should become the standard everywhere. This is necessary if we want to help our children 'say no to drugs', including nicotine, and to curb tobacco-related disease and death. As advocated by the Director General of the International Hospital Federation, hospital accreditation requirements should include a smoke-free premises standard.

Public smoking is not a right. Public smoking in airspace which others must share is a wrongful act against one's neighbour. If necessary, we must add legislation and legal action to education about the harmful effects of tobacco use and ensure that no one is forced to become a captive involuntary smoker.

Tobacco-free venues

S.B. Cohen

Atlanta, Georgia, United States

The tobacco-free venue is an emerging concept that is simple, clear-cut and unambiguous. Simply stated, this means that tobacco in all forms is proscribed in designated areas in a manner similar to that for illicit drugs and alcohol. One major difficulty in creating a clean indoor environment is the endless bickering by the tobacco industry about when, where and how much consumption of tobacco products is to be allowed or encouraged. The industry thrives on the publicity attached to this pseudo-issue. Those trying to protect the health and welfare of the public are forced to spend a significant portion of their meagre resources of time and manpower battling the industry.

The principle that no tobacco use is allowed in circumstances where it will negatively affect others is well accepted. No one disputes the fact that children, pregnant women and the sick deserve total and absolute protection, but few argue the proposition that other non-smokers deserve similar protection. No one denies the authority of businesses to forbid smoking on their premises. Likewise, no civil libertarian has argued that convicted felons, deprived of ordinary rights such as voting, are entitled to smoke, sniff or chew in a penal institution. Problems arise when arbitrary locations are set up to allow the use of tobacco products, so that those entitled to protection are forced to run a gauntlet of smoke at building entrances. Corporations and taxpayers may be forced to pay for attempts to create smoking havens in public facilities.

Ambiguity arises when attempts are made to accede to tobacco industry pressures with the designation of smoking areas. This has produced corridors of smoke at the entrances of smoke-free buildings such as hospitals and offices. Workers waste their own valuable time and that of their employers going back and forth for smoke breaks. Prisoners are permitted to indulge their most pleasurable addiction. Another major problem with the designation of smoking areas is that there are always people who try to be provocative by smoking or chewing in a forbidden zone, sometimes leading to serious consequences such as fire.

The concept of tobacco-free venue offers an unambiguous way to cut through this Gordian knot. A purely tobacco-free venue means quite simply that tobacco products are not allowed on any part of the venue operated by that particular organization. Those who use, work in or visit such facilities will see signs similar to those used by Kimball Physics, Inc.:

Welcome

Kimball Physics Inc.

Visitors' Entrance

Please note: For the protection of everyone, this is a tobacco-/tobacco residue-free facility. No smoking (or other tobacco use) in buildings, entryways, parking lots, vehicles, or on grounds. No tobacco paraphernalia (cigarettes, etc.) are to be brought into the building at any time.

Please do not enter if you have used a tobacco product within the past 2 hours or are otherwise tobacco-contaminated.

If you require assistance, please push night bell.

The policy was established by an employees' committee at Kimball Physics, a producer of electron optics. Signs such as these provide ample precedent for such a technique.

Resistance to change

Although we all acknowledge that we live in a rapidly changing world, personal behaviour, particularly that associated with drug dependence, changes with glacial speed. Perhaps because individuals are giving up autonomy in so many areas, their determination to hang on to a pleasurable addiction looms as an even more important right to be assiduously held onto. Likewise, as institutions make major changes, they hang on to their institutional addiction (Cohen, 1986).

Practical implementation

Dire warnings to the contrary, the implementation of clean indoor environments has proceeded with little fanfare and insignificant consequences. Smoking aboard commercial airlines is so rare as to rate news headlines and is usually perpetrated by inebriated passengers who also engage in other inappropriate behaviour. Hospitals, including psychiatric facilities (Cohen, 1990), and prisons have implemented smoke-free policies, again without significant problems. Indeed, repeated experience has shown that, when properly implemented, these are virtually non-events.

If the experience of Kimball Physics is any guide, significant problems would be virtually nonexistent. That company has taken the position that it does not have to be a policeman, and, as long as people create no incidents, they will be left alone. They report that since the policy was written in 1993 there have been no complaints from any employees and virtually none from anyone else.

Every day, thousands of citizens walk the streets with contraband material such as alcohol, illicit drugs and concealed weapons. Unless their behaviour is aberrant in some way, they are left undisturbed. Likewise, we can expect the vast majority of public and private facilities to take a similar approach. In the absence of a confrontational attitude, such as smoking or flaunting tobacco, no one will know or care if someone is in possession of a tobacco product. Even then it is expected that a simple reminder will suffice to resolve the issue.

Perhaps the best analogy is that many normal activities are out of place in particular venues. Just as no one thinks of throwing a baseball in the corridors or having sex on the grounds of an office building, hospital or prison, in the future they will not even entertain the notion of bringing tobacco products into designated tobacco-free venues.

References
Cohen, S.B. (1986) Institutional tobacco withdrawal symptoms. *J. Med. Assoc. Georgia*, **75**, 261–263
Cohen, S.B. (1990) Tobacco-free psychiatric facilities: Achievements, resistances and prospects. In: Durston, B. & Jamrozik, K., eds, *Tobacco and Health 1990: The Global War*, East Perth: Organising Committee of the Seventh World Conference on Tobacco and Health, pp. 476–478

A completely smoke-free university?

P. Schioldborg

Institute of Psychology, University of Oslo, Norway

In 1995, the Academic Senate of the University of Oslo agreed to make the University completely smoke-free, with stepwise closure of existing smoking rooms within three years, starting on 1 July 1997. A survey among students, professors and employees in autumn 1995 showed that 52% were for the resolution, 36% against and 12% undecided. Daily smokers were clearly against it, with 46%, while non-smokers were 63% for it.

To explore the strength of the attitudes for and against the resolution, a second survey was conducted in spring 1996, emphasizing two context conditions: one describing the University as an institution of freedom and democracy and the other describing it as a research institution with extensive knowledge of the hazards of smoking. No effect of context was observed among smokers, while the agreement of non-smokers with the resolution decreased significantly from 63 to 47% within the freedom context.

Youth access

A comprehensive approach to reducing the supply of tobacco to children in Western Australia

D. Sullivan & T. Jackiewicz

Smoking and Health Program, Health Promotion Services, Health Department of Western Australia, Perth, Western Australia, Australia

Introduction

In Australia, tobacco accounts for 18 000 avoidable deaths each year (English *et al.*, 1995) and is responsible for 72% of all drug-caused deaths (National Drug Srategy, 1994). In Western Australia, tobacco kills over 1400 people a year (Health Information Centre, 1997). Cigarette smoking is a major risk factor for disabling and fatal conditions such as cardiovascular and lung diseases and some cancers. In addition, men and women are at risk of developing a number of sex-specific health problems due to smoking (i.e. reduced fertility). There is also increasing evidence of health risks for non-smokers exposed to tobacco smoke (Winstanley *et al.*, 1995).

Smoking and young people

While the prevalence of smoking among adults in Western Australia has steadily declined in the past decade, there has been relatively little change in the prevalence of smoking among young people. In 1996, 20% of schoolboys and 27% of schoolgirls aged 15 reported that they were current smokers (i.e. they had smoked during the past week) (Health Promotion Services, 1994).

Most adults start smoking in adolescence and most before 18 years of age. Research shows that the younger people are when they start to smoke, the less likely they are to quit and the more likely they will be to become heavy smokers, suffer from smoking-caused health problems and die prematurely (Single & Rohl, 1997).

Many factors influence a young person's decision to smoke or not to smoke, including smoking by family and peers, parental attitude to smoking, the cost and availability of cigarettes, exposure and attitude to cigarette advertising (Single & Rohl, 1997). While all of these factors cannot be controlled, strategies for reducing the availability of tobacco to young people can at least inhibit if not prevent the start of smoking by young people and progression from experimentation to regular smoking and addiction. Strategies for reducing the availability of tobacco to young people are considered an important component of a comprehensive approach to tobacco control.

The comprehensive approach is applied to the tobacco control programme of the Health Department of Western Australia as a whole and also to key components. The Department's strategy for reducing the availability of tobacco to young people is therefore comprehensive, integrated and collaborative. The activities include legislation, enforcement, prosecution, the fostering of key alliances with other regulatory authorities, retailer education, community mobilization and research and evaluation.

Legislation

Although it has been an offence to sell tobacco to children in Western Australia since 1917, until the passage of the *Tobacco Control Act 1990*, the practice of selling tobacco to persons under 18 was widespread, the penalty for such offences was very small and there were no recorded prosecutions. The *Tobacco Control Act 1990* bans the sale or supply of tobacco to children under 18 and makes it an offence to permit minors to obtain cigarettes from tobacco vending machines. Penalties for the sale or supply of tobacco to minors range from a maximum of AUS$ 5000 for an individual to AUS$ 20 000 for a corporate body. The maximum penalty doubles for subsequent offences. Under this *Act*, it is not an offence for a child to purchase or possess tobacco products, but it is an offence for a child to sell or supply tobacco to another child.

Enforcement

While enactment of the *Tobacco Control Act* strengthened tobacco control legislation in Western Australia, for the legislation to be effective it must be fairly and rigorously enforced. This message was brought home within the first 18 months. In 1992, a sample of retailers within the Perth metropolitan area was surveyed to measure their willingness to sell tobacco to young people. The results were startling, with 89% of retailers showing that they were willing to sell tobacco products to minors involved in the survey (Health Department of Western Australia, 1996).

The Health Department's approach to enforcement is both proactive and reactive. As a proactive measure, routine inspections of retail outlets are conducted by the Department's investigative staff in order to check compliance with the *Act* and the display of mandatory signs. During inspections, signs and information materials about the *Act* are distributed, checks are made to ensure that retailers fully understand the *Act* and their responsibilities and that training is provided to new staff. Inspections also provide an opportunity for retailers to discuss issues relating to the application of the *Act* with Department representatives. More cordial and cooperative relationships with tobacco retailers have developed over time as a result of regular contact. They are more aware and understanding of the Department's role in monitoring and enforcing the *Act*, are more likely to contact the Department if they have enquiries about its application and in some instances report potential breaches to the Department.

The Health Department also responds to complaints from parents, schools and community members concerned about the selling practices of retailers in their local areas. Most complaints are investigated within 48 h. Investigation of a complaint usually involves meetings with the retailer, complainant and juveniles involved and, sometimes, surveillance of the retail outlet. A decision will be made on whether the *Act* has been breached and whether a warning or recommendation to prosecute is the most appropriate action.

Prosecution

While enforcement of tobacco control legislation is vital, it is unlikely to achieve compliance unless the threat of prosecution for breaches is real. The Department has prosecuted 42 retailers for selling tobacco to minors. Fines for the sale or supply of tobacco to minors have ranged from AUS$ 50 to AUS$ 2500, although the size of fines has been erratic rather than steadily increasing, suggesting that more work needs to be done to impress on the magistracy the seriousness of sales to minors and the strength of community feeling about the sale or supply of tobacco to children.

The Health Department also issues media releases publicizing successful prosecutions. These achieve a number of purposes: they raise awareness of the *Tobacco Control Act 1990* and the Health Department's role in its enforcement; they remind retailers that the risk of prosecution for the sale or supply of tobacco to minors is real and that the penalties are substantial; they reinforce community feeling about the seriousness of the offences and they encourage media coverage of the issue.

Fostering key alliances

In Western Australia, there are over 4000 tobacco retail outlets, and the support of other regulatory authorities and regional health authorities is therefore vital to ensure effective enforcement of the *Act*, as the Department's resources are limited. We have therefore fostered alliances with police services, local government and regional health authorities. The support provided by other regulatory and health agencies includes monitoring compliance with the *Act*, reporting and investigating breaches, distributing information on the *Act* to retailers in their area and raising community awareness of the *Act* and the importance of strategies to reduce the availability of tobacco to young people.

A pilot programme conducted in 1996 involving four local government authorities showed that environmental health officers can play a role in monitoring compliance with the *Act* with minimal disruption of their normal duties. All regional health authorities throughout the State have also established programmes to reduce the availability of tobacco to young people in their communities.

Retailer education

Education of retailers helps to raise awareness of the *Act* and of their responsibilities under the Act and encourages compliance. Such training is done during inspection of retail outlets for compliance with the *Act*. The Department also produces and distributes a range of information material, signs and stickers on the *Act* to retailers; 'advertorials' and advertisements are placed in trade journals from time to time; and the Department liaises regularly with the tobacco and retail industries to ensure that they have up-to-date knowledge and understanding of the *Act* and to resolve issues concerning its application.

Community mobilization

Community involvement is essential to the effectiveness of strategies for reducing the availability of tobacco to young people. Community support for such measures has been consistently high: 95% of respondents in the 1993 and 1995 National Drug Strategy Household Surveys supported measures to restrict the availability of tobacco to young people (Single & Rohl, 1997).

As a means of maintaining community awareness and support for measures to restrict the availability of tobacco to young people, the Health Department has also produced a community action guide, entitled *Choke the Supply*, for the use of parents, schools and community groups; tobacco and youth smoking issues are covered in community drug education programmes conducted by the Department, which also publishes articles on tobacco and youth in school health journals and community newspapers from time to time.

Research and evaluation

Research and evaluation conducted by the Department include biennial retailer compliance surveys and triennial surveys of tobacco consumption by school pupils aged 12–17 years. Retailer compliance surveys have been conducted since 1992 to measure the willingness of retailers to sell tobacco to young people, the effectiveness of retailer education on the *Act*, the types of retail outlets and areas where sales to minors are more likely to occur and the variables that influence the sale of tobacco to minors (e.g. sex of the seller and the purchaser). The surveys show that there has been a 78% reduction in the willingness of retailers to sell tobacco to young people since 1992, down from 89% in 1992 to 20% in 1996. While these results show improved compliance with legislation banning the sale or supply of tobacco to minors, it is of concern that one in five retailers is still willing to sell to young people, indicating a need for further retailer education and action on this issue.

Surveys of tobacco consumption by secondary-school pupils have been conducted since 1984. The surveys provide data on the prevalence, consumption, knowledge, attitudes and beliefs about smoking and on the availability of and ease of access to tobacco for young people. A comparison of the 1993 and 1996 surveys shows a significant reduction in the proportion of respondents reporting that they themselves had last purchased their cigarettes (down from 42% in 1993 to 33% in 1996); however, there were significant increases in the proportions of respondents reporting that they had last obtained their cigarettes through other people, such as friends and family (up from 58% in 1993 to 67% in 1996), or from vending machines (from 2% in 1993 to 6% in 1996).

The results of retailer and consumption surveys conducted since the enactment of the *Tobacco Control Act 1990* indicate that retailers are less willing to sell tobacco to young people and that young people are finding it more difficult to purchase cigarettes from retail outlets. Problem outlets and areas have also been identified and subjected to intensive monitoring and retailer education, resulting in improved compliance.

Where to next?

The influences on young people to smoke are diverse and often not within the control of health professionals and regulatory authorities. Furthermore, even within a comprehensive programme, it is difficult to achieve an appropriate balance because of resource constraints, environmental influences and competing priorities. Research and evaluation of measures implemented by the Health Department of Western Australia to reduce the availability of tobacco to young people have highlighted priorities for the future. They include the need to become more proactive in our approach and to address other major sources of supply and the need to extend our public education programmes to involve the broader community in measures to reduce the sale and supply of tobacco to young people. Maintenance of a comprehensive approach to tobacco control that is intersectoral and collaborative, robust and sustainable and complemented by strategies to reduce the supply of tobacco to children will in the longer term move us towards our vision of a smoke-free generation.

References

English, D., Holman, C.D.J., Milne, E., *et al.* (1995) *The Quantification of Drug Caused Morbidity and Mortality in Australia*, Canberra: Commonwealth Department of Human Services and Health
Health Department of Western Australia (1996) Fewer retailers sell tobacco to children. Media statement
Health Information Centre (1997) *The Impact of Tobacco Smoking on Health in Western Australia 1984–1995*, Perth: Health Information Centre, Health Department of Western Australia
Health Promotion Services (1994) *Cigarette Consumption among Western Australian Secondary School Students in 1993*, Perth: Centre for Behavioural Research in Cancer and Health Promotion Services, Health Department of Western Australia
National Drug Strategy (1994) *Drug Caused Deaths in Australia, 1991 and 1992. Statistical Update, March 1994*, Canberra: Department of Human Services and Health
Single, E. & Rohl, T. (1997) *The National Drug Strategy: Mapping the Future. A Report Commissioned by the Ministerial Council on Drug Strategy, Canberra 1997*, Canberra: Commonwealth of Australia
Winstanley, M., Woodward, S. & Walker, N. (1995) *Tobacco in Australia: Facts and Issues*, 2nd Ed., Melbourne: Victorian Smoking and Health Program

Reducing young people's access to tobacco: An evaluation of policies and laws in New South Wales, Australia

K. Purcell, L. Burns, B. O'Hara & C. O' Neil

Tobacco and Health Unit, Centre for Disease Prevention and Health Promotion, NSW Health Department, North Sydney, New South Wales, Australia

It is widely acknowledged that reducing young people's access to tobacco products is an important component of an effective strategy for reducing their tobacco use. It complements tobacco tax increases, mass media campaigns and school-based education programmes (Department of Health and Human Services, 1994). The 1992 survey 'Drug use by NSW secondary students' indicated that the prevalence of smoking among the young had increased since 1989 (Cooney *et al.*, 1993), that a large number of young people obtained cigarettes by purchasing them (Hill *et al.*, 1995) and that most indicated that obtaining tobacco was easy or very easy. It was also found that over half of those students who were occasional or regular smokers and who had tried to purchase cigarettes had never been asked for proof of age (Bauman *et al.*, 1997).

At around the same time, compliance surveys were undertaken to assess the rate of illegal sale of tobacco to minors, in which young people attempted to purchase tobacco from a retail outlet under the supervision of an adult. In one such survey, conducted in 1992, 12–13-year-old children could purchase tobacco 39% of the time. After publicity about the compliance monitoring survey and warning letters, illegal selling rates were reduced by 29% (Chapman *et al.*, 1994). Other studies in New South Wales (NSW) indicated that in some areas the selling rate was as high as 60% (Andrews et al., 1994; Schoenmakers et al., 1997).

Comprehensive programme for New South Wales

In response to the rise in smoking prevalence and the ease of tobacco purchase by young people in NSW, a comprehensive programme has been put in place since 1994, which focuses on the following key elements:

Strengthening legislation: Under the NSW Public Health Act (1991), it was illegal to sell tobacco products to people under the age of 18. This Act was amended in 1996 to tighten the defence available to retailers, to introduce proof of age for tobacco purchases which included an identification with a photograph and to ensure that the holder of the tobacco licence or the employer could be held liable if an offence were committed.

Development of policies and procedures for enforcement of legislation: A policy and procedure manual was developed for area health services in NSW which describes how to monitor compliance and enforce the legislation. NSW Health defines compliance monitoring as the process of measuring the proportion of retailers who comply with the relevant legislation. It is undertaken by young volunteers who enter shops and attempt to purchase cigarettes while under the supervision of a responsible adult. The NSW policies also include training and consent procedures for young people, provision for sending warning letters for a first breach and prosecution for a second breach and suggestions for involving the community at the local level.

Prosecutions: Prosecutions are regarded as the final option in achieving compliance and necessary as a deterrent to retailers who continued to sell despite warning notices. Since 1991, there have been 38 prosecutions of retailers for the illegal sale of tobacco to minors. Before 1994, only two prosecutions were undertaken by the police in NSW.

Comprehensive training programme: A training programme for health workers developed in 1994 included training in compliance monitoring, working with young people, court procedures and preparation of evidence. The Health Department also consulted with the police and provided assistance in developing police policies and training programmes.

Community and retailer education and community action: A community education strategy and a retailer education strategy were developed which included point-of-sale materials and television, radio and press advertising. The public relations strategy included a public information telephone line, and a community education kit was developed for parents, schools and community groups.

Evaluation

An evaluation is being conducted to determine the effectiveness of these policies and procedures for reducing young people's access to tobacco. Compliance monitoring was conducted in 750 shops in Sydney. In the initial sample, 42% of shops sold tobacco to minors, a compliance rate of 58%. The preliminary results suggest that the rate of sales to minors depends on the type of shop, however, there is no significant difference between the sex of the seller and the rate of sales to young people, and there is no difference between the sex of the purchaser and ability to purchase cigarettes.

In an audit of area health service compliance monitoring activities in 1995–96 before and during implementation of the policies and procedures, 57% of the health services had undertaken compliance monitoring, visiting an average of 180 shops and issuing an average of 63 warning letters per area health service.

The next steps will be a qualitative survey of health workers, young people, parents and retailers and further compliance monitoring. In addition, the results of the 1996 school survey will be analysed for smoking prevalence and information about proof-of-age requests, refusal of service and ease of purchase.

Conclusions

We are not yet in a position to report on the overall effectiveness of this approach, but feedback from area health services and local compliance surveys has been encouraging. For example, a study conducted on the Central Coast in New South Wales indicated a significant reduction in the illegal sale of tobacco after compliance monitoring and well-publicized prosecution, from 39 to 19%. NSW Health believes that the programme will be effective in reducing young people's access to tobacco. We believe that easy access to tobacco is important in establishing and maintaining nicotine addiction and that if this access is curtailed we can improve the future health of our community by having fewer smokers.

References

Andrews, B., McKay, E., Hahn, A. & Stephenson, J. (1994) Cigarette sales to juveniles: Retailer compliance in Dubbo, NSW. *Health Promot. J. Aust.*, 4
Bauman, A., Phongsavan, P.H., *et al.* (1997) Access and availability of tobacco and alcohol among New South Wales teenagers in 1992. NSW Health Department (draft)
Chapman, S., King, M., Andrews, B., McKay, E., Markham, P. & Woodward, S. (1994) Effects of publicity and a warning letter on illegal cigarette sales to minors. *Aust. J. Public Health*, 18
Cooney, A., Dobbinson, S. & Flaherty, B. (1993) *1992 Drug Use by New South Wales Secondary Students*, Sydney: NSW Health Department
Department of Health and Human Services (1994) *Preventing Tobacco Use among Young People: A Report of the US Surgeon General*, Atlanta, Georgia: Public Health Services, Centers for Disease Control and Prevention, National Center for Chronic Disease Prevention and Health Promotion, Office on Smoking and Health
Hill, D., White, V. & Segan, C. (1995) Prevalence of cigarette smoking among Australian secondary school students in 1993. *Aust. J. Public Health*, 19
Schoenmakers, I., Nyhuis, A., Rissel, C. & Chapman, S. (1997) The role of ethnicity in sales of cigarettes to minors. *Health Promot. J. Aust.*, 7

Measurement of retailers' compliance with legislation on tobacco sales to minors in Canada

J. King & M.J. Kaiserman

Environmental Health Directorate, Health Protection Branch, Health Canada, Ottawa, Ontario, Canada

Abstract

As part of a strategy for reducing the demand for tobacco, Health Canada, with the assistance of a Federal and provincial working group, undertook a study of the compliance of retailers with respect to the *Tobacco Sales to Young Persons Act*, provincial legislation on sales to minors and requirements about advertising signs under the *Tobacco Products Control Act*. Measurements were made over four weeks during the summer of 1995 and released later that year, and figures for 1996 were collected over the corresponding period one year later and released in January 1997.

In one of the largest studies of its kind to be undertaken in Canada, teams of one adult and one minor attempted nearly 10 000 cigarette purchases over a two-year period. The study was conducted in 25 cities across Canada, in at least one city in each of the 10 provinces.

The most significant finding was an increase in the level of compliance, from 48 to 60%, between 1995 and 1996. Also, the percentage of retailers who refused to sell to girls increased from 35 to 53% in one year. Although there are still differences between sales to boys and girls, the gap decreased significantly.

Objectives

The primary objective of this study was to compare the compliance of retailers with requirements concerning tobacco sales to minors over two years. Between the 1995 and 1996 surveys, key provisions of the *Tobacco Products Control Act*, including a ban on advertising, were found to be unconstitutional by the Supreme Court of Canada. Shortly thereafter, in January 1996, the Canadian tobacco industry resumed product-specific advertising. In order to determine the effect of this advertising at the retail level, information on various promotional items at points of sale was collected in 1996.

Methods

Under contract to Health Canada, ACNielsen sent research teams consisting of one minor and one adult observer into retail establishments selling tobacco products in 25 cities across Canada, in at least one city in each of the 10 provinces. The same cities were visited in both years. A separate random sample of about 5000 shops was selected for each year. Retailers in five classes of trade were sampled: grocery supermarkets, convenience chains, small independent groceries and variety shops, drug stores and service stations with convenience shops.

The team members entered the establishments independently. The minors were instructed to attempt to buy a pack of cigarettes. They carried no identification and made no effort to disguise their appearance. Nevertheless, if asked, minors were instructed not to give their actual age. Under no circumstance did the adolescents actually purchase tobacco. If an offer to sell was given, the adolescent had instructions on how to back out of the transaction. The minor would approach the tobacco counter and ask for a pack of du Maurier Regular 20s or Players Light Regular 20s, two brands that are popular with young people. If the shop carried neither of these brands, the minor would ask for any other brand displayed.

During the attempted transaction, the minors made no misleading statements except if they were asked their age. If they were asked their age, they were not truthful but rather claimed to be 18 or 19 years old, depending on the minimum age requirements of that province. If the retailer appeared willing to sell them cigarettes, they checked their money, indicated that they did not have enough to buy the cigarettes and casually left the premises. If the retailers offered to sell a smaller or broken pack for the money available, the minors said that they preferred a full pack and left. If the retailers refused to sell the cigarettes, the minors politely thanked them and left.

The adult observers were responsible for supervising the minors and for collecting information on compliance with sign requirements under the legislation and the items on display in each retail outlet. In particular, the adults had to verify the proper posting of tobacco age and hazard warning signs at entrances and/or on windows. The adults entered the shops and proceeded systematically up and down each aisle searching for point-of-sale tobacco advertising in any form. They then proceeded to each tobacco counter and discreetly verified the presence of signs, properly posted, in compliance with the Tobacco Act or corresponding provincial legislation. After leaving the shop, the minor and adult would meet and record their observations before going to the next retailer on their list.

Key findings

The key findings of this study were that compliance with provisions on sales to minors was 60% in 1996 and 48% in 1995. The results by province are given in Table 1. Improvements in compliance were widespread. Retailers were less likely in 1996 to attempt to sell cigarettes to girls than to boys: sales were made to 57% of boys in 1995 and to 66% in 1996 and to 35% of girls in 1995 and to 53% in 1996. While retailers remained more likely to refuse a sale to boys than to girls, the gap in compliance was

Table 1. Compliance with legislation on sales to
minors, Canada, 1995 and 1996

Province	Compliance (%)	
	1995	1996
All	48	61
Newfoundland	33	58
Prince Edward Island	90	34
New Brunswick	89	85
Nova Scotia	76	90
Quebec	24	29
Ontario	62	73
Manitoba	57	77
Saskatchewan	30	78
Alberta	60	69
British Columbia	69	74

much narrower in 1996 than in 1995. Compliance decreased as the age of the minor
increased in both years (Table 2). Compliance also improved among retail clerks of
every age and in three of five classes of retail trade. Younger adolescents were thus
more likely than older ones to be denied a sale, and younger sales clerks (those about
the same age as minors) were generally more willing to sell cigarettes to minors than
older ones. Only in service station shops and grocery convenience chains did compliance
fall, although the decrease was not general across regions.

In 1996, the percentage of retailers who asked for identification rose to 59%, up
from 45% the year before. Of those who did, 96% in both years refused to sell, indicating
a strong relationship between willingness to ask for proof of identity and refusal.

Conclusions

The results of this study lend support to the hypothesis that if compliance levels are
to increase enforcement must be visible and continuous. In 1995, Health Canada had
been enforcing legislation on sales to minors for about one year, and during this first
year enforcement officers spent much of their time explaining the new law to retailers.
During the second year of enforcement, many more retailers were charged with offences
under the legislation, and, as can be seen, compliance increased.

Table 2. Compliance with legislation
on sales to minors, Canada, 1995 and
1996, by age of minor

Age (years)	Compliance (%)	
	1995	1996
All	48	61
15	68	70
16	39	56
17	36	42

New Zealand cigarette manufacturers compete on nicotine and price for young smokers

M. Laugesen

Health New Zealand, Waiheke Island, Auckland, New Zealand

Abstract

In 1996, shopkeepers and adolescents were interviewed, manufacturers' returns were analysed and the amount of nicotine in cigarettes was tested. In two research contracts and further analyses, it was shown that cigarettes in New Zealand in 1996 contained 40% more nicotine than those in Canada or the United States; the cheapest packs, of 10 cigarettes, preferred by young adolescents, contained 17% more nicotine per gram of dry tobacco than packs of 20 and 25 cigarettes of the same brands; 67% of Rothmans had a high level of nicotine (> 1.2 mg), 70% of Wills' had a medium level (1.0–1.2 mg) and 69% of Philip Morris' had a low level (< 1.0 mg). The volume sales of the 10 top brand variants were highly correlated with nicotine yield and content ($r =$ 0.79 for both) in 1996.

After advertising was banned in 1990, companies competed mainly on nicotine, price and brand name. Publication of the nicotine content of brands that are popular with youth resulted in considerable publicity, encouraging regulation. The reporting required by the 1990 law provided vital data for lobbying for changes in 1997.

Introduction

How did New Zealand cigarette manufacturers maintain inter-firm competition after tobacco advertising was banned in 1990? Three lines of investigation were followed.

Method

In 1996, a medical student interviewed Wellington retailers and students aged 11–13 in one school about their attitudes to buying packets of 10 cigarettes. In 1996 and 1997, a Crown research institute tested unburnt cigarettes for nicotine content and concentration. Testing content is cheaper than testing smoke for yield. Manufacturers tested 95 brand variants by the smoke test of the United States Federal Trade Commission for nicotine yield, and the manufacturers' returns for 1994–96 were analysed by brand for nicotine yields and sales.

Results

The 11–13-year-olds interviewed were extremely cost-conscious. Retailers reported that over 80% of young smokers asked for (cheaper) packets of 10 cigarettes. In response, manufacturers launched new brands of 10s; thus, there were none in 1991 but 15 in 1995, reaching 6% of the market share in 1996. Sales of high-nicotine brands predominated. Cigarettes in New Zealand in 1996 contained 0.5–1.5 mg of nicotine, which was 40% higher than in Canadian or United States cigarettes. Of the manufactured cigarettes sold, 49% had a high smoke yield of nicotine (> 1.2 mg), 25% a medium concentration (1.0–1.2 mg) and 24% a low concentration (< 1.0 mg).

The companies each focused their sales in a different segment of the nicotine market, whereas this was not the case for tar. Of the Rothmans cigarettes sold in 1996, 67% were high in nicotine; of the Wills cigarettes, 71% had a medium level of nicotine; of the Philip Morris cigarettes, 69% had low nicotine. The nicotine sales-weighted average yield also varied by company: Rothmans, 1.21 mg; Wills (British–American Tobacco), 1.10 mg; Philip Morris, 0.89 mg. Rothmans sold 98% of high and two-thirds of low nicotine cigarettes.

Cigarettes sold in packs of 10 contained 17% more nicotine per gram dry weight than the same brands of 20 or 25 cigarettes. Of 20 brand variants tested, the five brands with more than 2.0% nicotine dry weight were in packs of 10. Smoke-test yields gave no indication of these differences.

The manufacturers' sales varied directly with the nicotine content. The yield in the smoke of the top 10 selling brands in 1994, 1995 and 1996 was highly correlated with their sales volumes ($r = 0.76$).

Discussion

The manufacturers' youth marketing strategy in New Zealand from 1990 to 1997 appears to have been to launch and display new brand names, priced and named to appeal to youth; to provide major brands in packs of 10 and advertise their low price at the sales counter; and to insert extra nicotine in cigarettes in packs of 10, enabling smokers to maintain addiction from fewer cigarettes.

Conclusion

Tobacco companies, which are banned by law from advertising, continued to compete for young customers through nicotine and price. Publication of the results of testing the nicotine content of brands popular with youth produced considerable publicity, encouraging regulation. The reporting requirements built into the 1990 Act generated data useful for lobbying for stronger controls in 1995–97.

Acknowledgement

Dr Sharmila Veerasinghe, Wellington School of Medicine, interviewed adolescents and shopkeepers in 1996; and Dr Tony Blakely, Dr Bob Symons and Dr Kevin Fellows were co-authors for nicotine content.

Community context of minors' access to tobacco in 20 communities in the United States

D. Sharp, P. Mowery, J. Myllyluoma, G. Giovino, T. Pechacek & M. Erilsen

Office on Smoking and Health, Centers for Disease Control, Atlanta, Georgia

Five million children and adolescents under 18 years of age in the United States will die prematurely from smoking-related diseases if current patterns of smoking persist. The commonest source of tobacco for minors is the retail store. We designed a large study to evaluate the community context in which tobacco sales to minors occur. We asked 16-year-old girls to attempt to buy tobacco in 725 stores in 20 communities and conducted telephone surveys with 579 store managers, 449 clerks and 151 community leaders to assess knowledge, attitudes and practices regarding tobacco sales to minors.

The sales to the minors varied by community, from a low of 7.1% to a high of 84%, and by type of store, from 29% in convenience stores to 58% in grocery stores. Decreased sales were correlated with older clerks, female clerks, asking for proof of age, warning signs, previous enforcement checks in the store or in other stores in the neighbourhood and increased community support.

Our findings support the effectiveness of having and enforcing laws that require retailers to ask for proof of age. In addition, strong community support increases enforcement of minors' access laws and decreases illegal sales.

ECONOMIC MEASURES TO CONTROL TOBACCO USE

Annual submission to the Ministry of Finance by the Tobacco Control Alliance in the United Kingdom

P. White[1], K. Aston[1] & L. Joossens[2]

[1]Health Education Authority, London, United Kingdom; and
[2]European Union Liaison Office, Brussels, Belgium

Abstract

We examine ways of influencing Government to increase taxes on tobacco products as part of an overall tobacco control strategy. We give advice on how to promote submissions to the Government Treasury Office most effectively, including strategic issues around various tax structures.

Background

Fiscal policy has long been acknowledged as a prime component of a comprehensive tobacco control policy in the United Kingdom. Advocates aim to promote the role of tax in reducing tobacco consumption through a number of activities, including an annual submission from the United Kingdom Tobacco Control Alliance, an informal grouping of about 50 national organizations. In this submission, it asks the Treasury to increase the tax on tobacco products to as high a rate as possible during its annual Budget review.

Action on Smoking and Health and other organizations had been writing separately to the Treasury each year for a number of years to request tax increases on tobacco products. In 1993, a small group of tobacco control advocates recognized the opportunity to develop this initiative and to influence further the thinking behind the Government's Budget decisions. It was recognized that the impact was likely to be maximized by working in partnership through the Tobacco Control Alliance, particularly at a time when increasing price was the Government's preferred method of reducing consumption. They agreed to produce a detailed argument in favour of tax increases on tobacco products over and above the current rate of inflation. The document would contain a list of supporting organizations in health and other sectors, including children's organizations and women's groups, and would be sent with a covering letter asking for a meeting with the Treasury.

The document and letter

Timing was critical if the document and letter were to have any impact. In the United Kingdom, the annual Budget is normally published in November, but the key meeting that determines its content is held in July. It was absolutely essential that the document reach officials and politicians well in time for the July meeting. The next thing to take into account was the audience. It was agreed that the document was meant primarily for officials as opposed to politicians, as it was unlikely that politicians would have either the time or motivation to read a somewhat detailed case for increasing tax on tobacco products. As tobacco control advocates, we were used to working with health officials and making our case on health grounds. Now, we had to remember that we were targeting officials whose primary interest was finance, not health, and the style and tone needed to reflect that. The style was therefore very plain and the document looked rather like one received from a bank. It had no pictures of children or healthy people, which are common features of many health reports. The tone and content appealed on economic grounds, rather than the more emotive issues associated with health and welfare, as we knew that officials would be using finance as their criterion in making recommendations to politicians. The covering letter, however, was designed to target the politicians. It was short, to the point and specifically asked for a meeting with the Treasury Minister.

The meeting delegation
Once we had secured a meeting, we agreed that it was essential to keep the delegation small and of a high level. The five organizations selected were the two main cancer charities in the United Kingdom, the British Medical Association, Action on Smoking and Health and the Health Education Authority. Each organization nominated one of its leaders, such as the chief executive or chair, so that the Treasury would be assured of the importance that the health lobby attached to this initiative.

Our job as tobacco control advocates was to make sure that the delegation was well briefed. It was agreed that the meeting was the right time to make the case for health, partly because of the delegates' status in the health field, but also because the economic case had already been made in the document. The health case included highlighting the Treasury's role as part of Government's collective responsibility for health.

Strategic use of the document
Even though the main purpose of the document is to ask for an increase on the tax on tobacco products, it also provides an opportunity to highlight structural issues, such as the difference in the tax rates on manufactured and hand-rolled cigarettes. Over the past few years, this annually prepared document has been used to explore various aspects and themes of fiscal policy. Issues that have been examined in detail include tax policy options for tackling smuggling of tobacco and consideration of the impact of a regressive tax on poor smokers. The document also provides an opportunity to engage in and influence the dynamic process of anticipating changes in the tax structure and to highlight new ideas.

The submission also has significant political strength. It lets Treasury officials and politicians know that there is a large constituency that supports and justifies an increase in the tobacco tax. It must be remembered that the tobacco industry will also submit well-prepared documentation to the Treasury, bring in top economists and other experts and will probably also be successful in securing a meeting at the Treasury. The tobacco industry may also go to some lengths to secure the support of tobacco retailers who claim that increases in tax will put them out of business.

It works!
During the past decade, the prices of cigarettes in the United Kingdom have been among the highest in Europe. Both the Government and health advocates have used high price of cigarettes to send a health message to smokers. The Chancellor of the Exchequer now regularly makes reference to the high cost of tobacco for health when he annolunces changes in taxes in his Budget speech. Tobacco consumption in the United Kingdom continues to show a healthy decline.

We are confident that the high price of tobacco products is linked at least in part to our strategic, high-level representations to the Treasury each year and to our willingness to support and advise officials on any initiatives they wish to take forward.

Smoking in disadvantaged communities:
Assessing motivation and ability to quit

G.B. Hastings[1], M. Stead[1], D.R. Eadie[1], A.M. MacKintosh[1] & P. Graham[2]

[1]*Centre for Social Marketing, University of Strathclyde, Glasgow, Scotland;*
[2]*Department of Management, The University of Newcastle, Callaghan,
New South Wales, Australia*

For several years, tobacco control organizations have advocated price manipulation by raising taxes on tobacco products as a strategy for promoting smoking cessation.

Data from several countries have shown a direct correlation between price and consumption (e.g. European Bureau for Action on Smoking Prevention, 1992; Townsend *et al.*, 1994): when prices rise, consumption decreases, and *vice versa*. Recent evidence suggests, however, that price rises may be ineffective among the poorest smokers (Marsh & McKay, 1994). The decreases in prevalence that have occurred in all other sections of the population have not occurred in the poorest groups, who continue to smoke at the same rate as 20 years ago (Figure 1).

It has been argued that low-income smokers not only fail to give up smoking when prices are raised but also become poorer, because a greater proportion of their income than previously is spent on tobacco; as a result, tobacco price manipulation may actually contribute to the disadvantages and ill-health already experienced in low-income communities (Marsh & McKay 1994). Tobacco control organizations in the United Kingdom are increasingly addressing this problem through research and interventions to address the barriers to cessation among disadvantaged smokers and provide appropriate support. This study, by the Centre for Social Marketing at the University of Strathclyde in Glasgow and funded by the Cancer Research Campaign, is one such attempt

A number of studies have addressed the enabling factors of and barriers to cessation (e.g. Prochaska & DiClemente, 1985; Graham, 1993, 1994; Rose *et al.*, 1996; Shadel *et al.*, 1996; Stronks *et al.*, 1997), but greater understanding is needed of why low-income smokers specifically find it difficult to quit. Furthermore, there is a need for basic information about the level of low-income smokers' motivation to quit. Although several surveys (e.g. NOP Omnibus Services, 1992; Lennox & Taylor, 1994; Kaplan *et al.*, 1993) have been made of how general populations are distributed with regard to the 'stages of change' of smoking cessation (Prochaska & DiClemente 1983, 1985), there appears to have been no study in the United Kingdom of whether low-income smokers are distributed in a similar way. Intuitively, one might expect that a greater proportion would be at the 'pre-contemplation stage' in a community where smoking is normal, majority behaviour. People planning interventions in disadvantaged communities must understand the smokers' motivation and readiness to quit in order to tailor support accordingly.

The study

The objectives of the study are:
- to identify and explore the barriers to cessation in disadvantaged communities;
- to assess the level of readiness to quit in disadvantaged communities and to estimate the distribution of the population in stages of change in relation to smoking status;

Figure 1. Prevalence of smoking according to income, United Kingdom, 1976–90

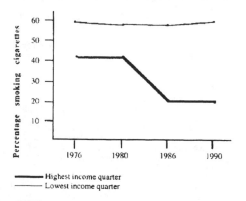

From Marsh & Mackay (1994)

- to identify and compare the factors and characteristics associated with different stages of smoking behaviour change in low-income communities and
- to identify appropriate methods for research on smoking in disadvantaged communities.

The research is being conducted in three stages. The first involves a review of the literature to ensure that the results will build on existing understanding of cessation and smoking in disadvantaged communities. We are examining information on the distribution of populations in general and low-income communities, in particular across the stages of change; the factors and characteristics that have been found to predict or correlate with cessation and the range of existing cessation interventions, with emphasis on their effectiveness in low-income groups. The second stage is a developmental phase of qualitative research to confirm and elaborate on the findings from the literature review. This stage involves focus groups in disadvantaged areas, comprising female non-smokers aged 18–24, male non-smokers aged 25–44, women aged 25–44 and men aged 18–24 in the 'action' or 'maintenance' stages, women aged 18–24 and men aged 25–44 in the 'contemplation' or 'preparation' stages and women aged 18–24 and men aged 25–44 in the 'pre-contemplation' stage. Smoking status was based on definitions used in a survey in California, United States (Kaplan et al., 1993).

The third stage of the research is a pilot questionnaire survey of 300 individuals to measure the distribution of a disadvantaged population across the categories of pre-contemplation, contemplation, preparation, action, maintenance and non-smoker. We shall also measure factors and characteristics and their relationship to smoking status, with the aim of identifying those factors associated with moving towards successful cessation. It is hoped to test three different methods of administering the questionnaire: postal, face-to-face in the home and face-to-face in a central local venue such as a community centre. The three methods will be compared for response rate, quality of data generated, cost–effectiveness and ease of administration, taking into account factors such as security and interviewer safety.

All of the primary research is being conducted in eight areas of Glasgow that have highly deprived populations, as calculated from a combination of variables in the 1991 Census: overcrowding, male unemployment, low social class and no car (McLoone, undated); in which less than 5% of households are owner-occupied and which have a population of over 5000 (General Register Office Scotland, 1994).

On the basis of the results of this pilot study, final amendments will be made to the questionnaire and method, where necessary. Should funding be provided for the second year of the study, a full survey of 2500 individuals will be conducted with the most appropriate of the three methods tested. This will be followed by a final phase of qualitative research, comprising 12 focus groups, to explore the smokers' responses to and experiences of a range of potential support options for cessation.

References

European Bureau for Action on Smoking Prevention (1992) *Taxes on Tobacco Products: A Health Issue*, Brussels

General Register Office Scotland (1994) *1991 Census Monitor for Postcode Sectors in Strathclyde*, Edinburgh: Government Statistical Service

Graham, H. (1993) *When Life's a Drag: Women, Smoking and Disadvantage*, London: Her Majesty's Stationery Office

Graham, H. (1994) Gender and class as dimensions of smoking behaviour in Britain: Insights from a survey of mothers. *Soc. Sci. Med.*, **38**, 691–698

Kaplan, R.M., Pierce, J.P., Gilpin, E.A., Johnson, M. & Bal, D.G. (1993) Stages of smoking cessation: The 1990 California Tobacco Survey. *Tob. Control*, **2**, 139–144

Lennox, A.S. & Taylor, R.J. (1994) Factors associated with outcome in unaided smoking cessation, and a comparison of those who have never tried to stop with those who have. *Br. J. Gen. Pract.*, **44**, 245–250

Marsh, A. & McKay, S. (1994) *Poor Smokers*, London: Policy Studies Institute

McLoone, P. (undated) *Carstairs Scores for Scottish Postcode Sectors from the 1991 Census*, Glasgow: Public Health Research Unit, University of Glasgow

NOP Omnibus Services (1992) *Smoking Habits 1991*, London: NOP

Prochaska, J.O. & DiClemente, C. (1983) Stages and processes of self-change of smoking: Toward an integrative model of change. *J. Consult. Clin. Psychol.*, **51**, 390–395

Prochaska, J.O. & DiClemente, C.C. (1985) Common processes of self-change in smoking, weight control and psychological distress. In: Shiffman, S. & Wills, T.A., eds, *Coping in Substance Use*, San Diego, California: Academic Press, pp. 345–363

Rose, J.S., Chassin, L., Presson, C.C. & Sherman, S.J. (1996) Prospective predictors of quit attempts and smoking cessation in young adults. *Health Psychol.*, 15, 261–268

Shadel, W.G., Mermelstein, R. & Borrelli, B. (1996) Self-concept changes over time in cognitive-behavioural treatment for smoking cessation. *Addict. Behav.*, 21, 659–663

Stronks, K., van de Mheen, H.D., Looman, C.W.N. & Mackenback, J.P. (1997) Cultural, material and psychosocial correlates of the socio-economic gradient in smoking behaviour among adults. *Prev. Med.*, 26, 754–766

Townsend, J., Roderick, P. & Cooper, J. (1994) Cigarette smoking by socioeconomic group, sex and age: Effects of price, income and health publicity. *Br. Med. J.*, 309, 923–927

The case for profit control of the tobacco industry

R. Cunningham

Canadian Cancer Society, Ottawa, Ontario, Canada

Introduction

Profit is the driving force behind the tobacco epidemic. The pursuit of profit explains industry behaviour: profit is the reason why manufacturers have sought to recruit new adolescent customers and have vigorously opposed tobacco control interventions. It follows that reductions in profit would have the potential fundamentally to alter industry behaviour in favour of public health.

Recent examples demonstrate how a threat to profit can change the industry's perspective. Litigation costs, in terms of legal fees and potential damage awards in the courts, prompted the Liggett & Myers tobacco company to agree to an unprecedented settlement of litigation with a number of state governments in the United States. Subsequently, the other major American cigarette companies agreed to a national settlement. In both cases, the pressure on profit brought the industry to the bargaining table and resulted in concessions that a few years earlier were considered to be unthinkable.

There are two ways of reducing profit: to increase costs, as in the above examples, or reduce revenues, as is proposed in this paper.

Implementing profit control

Profit control is best implemented through price control, that is by controlling the net-of-tax price charged by tobacco manufacturers and importers. A manufacturer might charge US$ 6 per carton of 200 cigarettes before taxes for all brands. Government could control this price, such as by setting a maximum of US$ 6 per carton, thus reducing the manufacturer's price by US$ 2 per carton. The government could then step in to increase tobacco taxes by the same amount, US$ 2 per carton. The result is that while the retail price to the consumer is unchanged (and thus has no impact on consumption or the threat of smuggling), the government gains the revenue instead of the tobacco companies. An option for government is to earmark part of the new revenue for funding tobacco control initiatives.

One method for curbing industry profit is a surtax on the profits of tobacco companies, a measure currently in place in Canada. This option, however, has its limitations. Tobacco companies can increase their prices to derive enough additional revenue to ensure that their after-tax profit remains unchanged.

Benefits of price control

Price control reduces the profit potential for tobacco companies, thereby decreasing the companies' financial incentive to recruit new smokers, to discourage existing smokers from quitting, and to fight anti-tobacco initiatives. When the potential annual profit per smoker falls to only US$ 30 instead of US$ 100, for instance, there is less economic motivation to maximize the number of smokers. From a health perspective, that is a good thing. Some may hypothesize that less profit per smoker means that companies will more aggressively seek to maximize the number of smokers to protect existing profit levels, but such a hypothesis can be dismissed as simply inconsistent with financial analysis and business practice. The greater the potential profit at stake, the more aggressively companies behave.

Price controls could lead to a very significant increase in government revenue as the reduction in manufacturers' net-of-tax prices is replaced by an equivalent increase in tobacco taxes. In Canada, the total amount of money to be obtained in this manner could exceed CDN$ 500 million per year. In the United States, at least several thousand million US dollars could be obtained annually in this way.

Dramatically reduced revenue would put huge pressure on the industry to reduce costs, given that cutting costs may be the only way to increase profit. The result would be significantly decreased marketing expenditures, which are largely discretionary.

Price controls would reduce the financial attractiveness of a particular market, thereby giving manufacturers an incentive to withdraw from, or not to enter, the market. In many developed countries, foreign brands are priced much higher than brands of domestic manufacturers. By putting a net-of-tax price ceiling on cigarettes, the profit potential might be too low for transnational tobacco companies to operate in the country in question.

Price controls can benefit most national economies by reducing the amount of money that transnational tobacco companies take out of the country through dividends.

Price controls place government in a powerful negotiating position with the tobacco industry, given that the government determines the industry's profit level. Here is what one tobacco company executive had to say (Kluger, 1996):
"...to overcome suffocating price controls, [Philip Morris International] executive Walter Thomas recalled how, on more than one occasion, 'I had to knock on the French finance minister's door, get down on my knees, and tell him how poor a company Philip Morris was and how badly it needed a price increase'."
With tobacco companies begging for a price increase, the tobacco control concessions that the government could obtain in return would undoubtedly be extremely important.

Profit controls remove the injustice whereby manufacturers earn profits at the expense of individuals who fall prey to disease and death. It is simply unfair that manufacturers should enjoy returns on investment so much higher than those of other industrial sectors. In Canada, Imperial Tobacco Ltd consistently has a pre-tax return on assets of about 90% per year, far more than other industries. This level of profit, resulting from the pricing power of an oligopolistic industry, should not be allowed to continue.

Profit controls partly allocate tobacco-related health-care costs from government to the source responsible, the tobacco industry, without any need for litigation. Litigation takes time and money to pursue, while price controls can be implemented immediately through legislation.

Price controls might encourage competition to make a safer tobacco product. If manufacturers cannot compete on promotion (because of a legislated ban) or price (because of legal controls) or distribution (because of legislated controls or because all companies essentially have products in all shops), then the only major competitive avenue is product. In order to differentiate their products from those of their competitors, companies will seek to develop product innovations.

Are profit controls politically achievable?

In many countries, profit controls are definitely achievable. Indeed, price controls are already in place in some markets (Philip Morris Companies Inc., 1997), although the number of countries in which this is the case does not appear to have been well documented outside the tobacco industry. Admittedly, in some countries such as the United States, profit controls may be a longer way off, given the prevailing political culture.

In most countries there are many examples in which the price of certain goods and services is already subject to government regulation: cable television, local telephone services, public transit, postal rates, electricity, water and other utilities, doctors' fees, funeral services and prescription drugs. In Canada, there have been restrictions on the price of nicotine patches, resulting in reduced prices, but there are no price controls on tobacco products containing nicotine.

Price controls are typically introduced into sectors where the free market has failed or would fail to bring about competitive price levels. The classic example is a monopoly. In the case of the tobacco industry, an oligopoly, the free market has failed in many countries, leading to unreasonable rates of return on investment.

A ruling pursuant to the General Agreement on Tariffs and Trade (1990) states that price controls are an acceptable government measure, provided that domestic and foreign companies are treated equally.

Conclusion

Controlling the profits of the tobacco industry is an important component of a tobacco control strategy and should be implemented by national and subnational governments, as appropriate, and depending on a country's constitution. Profit control will radically influence the behaviour of tobacco companies, which in turn will result in lower rates of smoking. Although profit control has received little consideration in the past (Cunningham, 1993, 1995, 1996), it deserves to be given priority by tobacco control advocates in the future.

References

Cunningham, R. (1993) *Evaluation of Federal and Provincial Legislation to Control Tobacco*
Cunningham, R. (1995) *Addressing the Lack of Competition in the Canadian Tobacco Industry. A Report Prepared for the Non-Smokers' Rights Association*
Cunningham, R. (1996) *Smoke & Mirrors: The Canadian Tobacco War*, Ottawa: International Development Research Centre, pp. 251–252
General Agreement on Tariffs and Trade (1990) Thailand: Restrictions on importation of and internal taxes on cigarettes (Report of the panel adopted on 7 November 1990, GATT Document DS10/R, 46th session, 37th suppl.), Basic Instruments and Selected Documents (1991) 200
Kluger, R. (1996) *Ashes to Ashes*, New York: Knopf, p. 531
Philip Morris Companies Inc. (1997) *Quarterly report pursuant to Section 13 or 15(d) of the Securities Act of 1934 for the quarterly period ended March 31, 1997*, p. 31

Socio-epidemiological data underlying the programme for control of tobacco use in Romania, 1997–2000

C. Didilescu & C. Marica

National Institute of Pneumophtisiology, Marius Nasta, Bucharest, Romania

When elaborating a strategy for the programme to control tobacco use in Romania for 1997–2000, we took into account epidemiological data gathered within the last few years. Thus, the proportion of the population using tobacco increased from 26% in 1989 to 28% in 1995, representing an increase of 2%. The difference is due to the increasing percentage of women using tobacco in the same period, from 11 to 15%.

A study undertaken in 1995–96 on a sample of approximately 9000 pupils in 10 crowded towns showed that the prevalence of tobacco use was 2.8% at 14 years of age, 12% at 16 years and 28% at 18 years. The study also showed that the prevalence of smoking was 39% among boys and 22% among girls. In a large university centre (Cluj-Napoca) in 1994, the percentage of smokers among physicians was 59%.

On the basis of these data, the programme for control of tobacco use will be focused mainly upon young people, pregnant women and categories of persons such as physicians and teachers who because of their profession serve as behavioural examples to others.

Economic aspects of tobacco smoking in Romania

C. Marica & C. Didilescu

National Institute of Pneumophtisiology, Marius Nasta, Bucharest, Romania

In Romania during 1989–95, the national production of tobacco (expressed in thousands of tonnes) decreased from 27.5 in 1989 to 13.3 in 1995, and the national production of cigarettes and cigars decreased from 33 000 tonnes in 1989 to 25 000 tonnes in 1995. The decrease of interest in tobacco production can be explained by the increased use of imported cigarettes, obtained either legally or illegally.

These data cannot be dissociated from the fact that Romania has been an attraction for the penetration of the large tobacco producers onto the central and eastern European markets during the past few years,. At the same time, Romanian exports of cigarettes have decreased drastically, from 1532 tonnes in 1990 to 78 tonnes in 1995.

A series of Governmental norms have been aimed at controlling the imports more efficiently. Thus, there is a customs tax on imported tobacco which varies with country of origin, the type of tobacco and the way in which it is manufactured. In order to control illegal imports, as from 1995 cigarettes packs, whether produced domestically or imported, must have a special stamp on them.

Effect of cigarette advertising bans and warning labels on cigarette packs: Evidence from aggregate and individual data

H. Saffer

National Bureau of Economic Research, New York City, New York, United States

Introduction

Cigarette advertising is a public health issue if it affects total consumption rather than simply affecting brand choice. Some public health advocates claim that cigarette advertising results in increased use. The cigarette companies claim that their advertising affects only brand choice. Over the past 25 years, a number of econometric studies have been conducted on this issue and on the whole have provided little evidence that advertising increases total consumption. One of these studies (Hamilton, 1975), presented at the Third World Conference on Smoking or Health, showed no effect of advertising bans on cigarette consumption. This paper updates Hamilton's work with newer data and newer econometric techniques.

Specification

The usual approach to estimating the effects of advertising is to specify a demand curve and include an advertising variable. The advertising coefficient is a measure of the effect of a small change in advertising on consumption. One reason why many previous studies failed to find an effect of advertising is the approach they used to measuring advertising. Advertisers have found that they can maximize their effect by using a technique known as 'pulsing', which is the use of comparatively short bursts of advertising in a few markets at a time, rather than running a steady but weaker schedule of advertising simultaneously in many markets. These pulses are run in different markets at different times. If advertising is measured at a highly aggregated level, such as at the annual national level, there will be little variance in the data, but if advertising is measured at a disaggregated level, such as at the monthly market level, the variance in the data will be larger.

Most commonly in empirical studies, advertising is measured by annual national expenditure. Studies of this type show no effect of advertising on consumption because there is little variance in the data. At a disaggregated level, the variance in advertising is relatively larger, and a study using this type of data may find an effect of advertising.

In another category of econometric study, the effects of advertising bans on consumption are examined. A ban in itself will not reduce the demand for advertising, and substitution of other media and other forms of marketing is likely. As the remaining media are used more intensively, the marginal products of these media will fall. This results in a lower average product for a given level of advertising. The industry may compensate by increasing advertising, depending on the expected response by rivals. Some previous empirical studies showed that bans reduce consumption (Laugesen & Meads, 1991), but others did not (Stewart, 1993).

Data

In the study reported here, two international data sets were used to test the effects of cigarette advertising bans. One was an aggregate data set and the other an individual set. The aggregate data set is a time series of cross-sectional data for 22 countries of the Organisation for Economic Co-operation and Development (OECD) for the years 1960–92. The dependent variable is per-capita annual consumption of cigarettes, which has been transformed into a logarithmic specification. Seven dichotomous cigarette advertising ban variables and two variables for cigarette pack warnings were defined. The variables for advertising bans are for television, radio, cinema, outdoor advertising, print, point of sale and sponsorships. The variables for warnings are those on cigarette advertisements and on cigarette packs. Additional variables were the real price of a pack of 20 cigarettes, real income, unemployment and the percent of cigarettes that are filtered.

The individual data set is a cross-section for 12 countries of the European Union in 1989. A dichotomous variable for cigarette participation was defined as being equal to 1 for people who smoke. Two of the advertising bans, warning labels and price data, are the same as in the aggregate data set. The following variables were also included: income, marital status, education, age, sex, unemployment and number of children.

Results

The results for the aggregate data show that advertising bans reduce consumption by about 6% and the price elasticity is about –0.3. The results for the individual data show that advertising bans reduce consumption by about 2–3%, and the price elasticity is about –0.09.

Acknowledgements
This study was funded by the National Cancer Institute (United States).

References

Hamilton, J. (1975) The effect of cigarette advertising bans on cigarette consumption. In: *Proceedings of the Third World Conference on Smoking and Health*, Washington DC: US Department of Health, Education, and Welfare

Laugesen. M. & Meads, C. (1991) Tobacco advertising restrictions, price, income and tobacco consumption in OECD countries, 1960–1986. *Br. J. Addict.*, **86**, 134–154

Stewart, M. (1993) The effect on tobacco consumption of advertising bans in OECD countries. *Int. J. Advert.*, **12**, 155–180

Taxation and pricing

Price, tobacco control policies and smoking among young people in the United States

M. Grossman[1] & F.J. Chaloupka[2]

[1]City University of New York and National Bureau of Economic Research, New York City, New York, and [2]University of Illinois at Chicago, Illinois, and National Bureau of Economic Research, New York City, New York, United States

We examine the effectiveness of several cigarette control policies in discouraging smoking among people aged 12–17 in the United States. These policies are cigarette excise taxes, which result in higher prices; restrictions on smoking in public places and private work sites; and limits on the availability of tobacco products to youths.

It is not surprising that current anti-smoking initiatives in the United States and other countries focus on curtailing smoking among young people. Numerous studies show that 90% of all smokers begin the habit as adolescents. Each day, approximately 6000 young people try a cigarette, and about half of them become daily smokers. Among persons who have ever smoked daily, 82% began smoking before the age of 18. Thus, cigarette control policies which discourage smoking by adolescents may be the most effective way of achieving long-run reductions in smoking in all segments of the population.

The sensitivity of adolescent smoking to cigarette prices has been addressed in only two published studies (Lewit et al., 1981; Wasserman et al., 1991). Lewit et al. reported that adolescent smoking was quite sensitive to price. They found that a 10% increase in price would reduce the total number of young smokers by 12% and would reduce daily consumption by young people who smoke by 2%. This total price response is two to three times larger than the corresponding price response among adults. Wasserman and his colleagues, however, found much smaller price effects and indicated that adolescents are no more responsive to price increases than adults. The applicability of these two studies to the current cigarette policy debate is limited because they are both based on fairly old data. Lewit et al. used a survey conducted between 1966 and 1970, while Wasserman et al. used a survey conducted between 1976 and 1980. In addition, the generalizability of the study by Wasserman et al. is limited because of its small sample of slightly less than 2000, whereas 5300 people were used by Lewit et al.

The study that we summarize in this paper overcame these shortcomings by using the 1992, 1993, and 1994 surveys of pupils in the eight, tenth and twelfth grades conducted by the Institute for Social Research at the University of Michigan as part of the 'Monitoring the future' project. Altogether, these nationally representative samples included about 150 000 adolescents. We added cigarette prices and tobacco control policies in the respondents' counties of residence to these surveys, as cigarette prices vary widely among areas of the United States due mainly to the very different rates at which they are taxed by states. Currently, the excise tax ranges from 2.5 cents a pack in Virginia to US$ 1 a pack in Alaska. The other tobacco polices at issue in our research also differ considerably among cities and states.

We found large price effects: a 10% increase in price would lower the number of young smokers by 7% and would lower consumption among smokers by 6%. We also found that strong restrictions on smoking in public places would reduce the prevalence of smoking among young people, and limits on smoking in schools would reduce average cigarette smoking among young smokers. Limits on the access of young people to tobacco products appeared, however, to have little impact on cigarette smoking among the young, probably because of the weak enforcement of these laws.

Our results underscore the effectiveness of increases in cigarette excise taxes and other policies to raise the price of cigarettes in the anti-smoking campaign. The Federal excise tax on cigarettes, currently 24 cents a pack, will rise to 39 cents a pack by the year 2002 as part of the recently enacted Balanced Budge Legislation. If this 15-cent tax increase is fully passed on to consumers, the price of a pack of cigarettes would rise by approximately 8%. According to our estimates, this would result in almost 1 million fewer smokers in the current cohort of 0 to 17-year olds and over 300 000 fewer smoking-related premature deaths in this cohort. Larger price increases would result in even larger reductions in the number of young smokers and the number of premature deaths. It has been estimated that the proposed settlement of the Medicaid lawsuits brought against the tobacco industry by the attorneys general of most states would raise the price of a pack of cigarettes by approximately 34%. This would reduce the number of adolescent smokers by approximately 24%, which would almost reach the goal of a 30% reduction in five years called for by President Clinton in September 1997. The decline in the number of adolescent smokers would translate into over 1.3 million fewer smoking-related premature deaths in the current cohort of 0 to 17-year olds.

These are short-run effects. A tax or price increase would, if it were maintained in real terms or adjusted for inflation, continue to discourage smoking by successive generations of young people and would gradually affect the smoking rates of older cohorts as those discouraged from smoking move through the age spectrum. Accordingly, the effect would be much greater in the long run.

References

Lewit, E.M., Coate, D. & Grossman, M. (1981) The effects of government regulation on teenage smoking. *J. Law Econ.* **24**, 545–569
Wasserman, J., Manning, W.G., Newhouse, J.P. & Winkler, J.D. (1991) The effects of excise taxes and regulations on cigarette smoking. *J. Health Econ.*, **10**, 43–64

Cigarette taxation in China:
Lessons from international experiences

T.-W. Hu

University of California, Berkeley, California, United States

China is the largest cigarette-producing and consuming country in the world. Cigarette smoking is harmful to health, and smoking has increased health-care costs and contributed to loss of productivity due to early death and illness. This paper is a discussion of the economic feasibility of raising the existing tax on cigarettes in China, drawing upon the experiences of other countries.

Current international data and published Chinese data indicate that there is some leeway for raising the tax on cigarettes. Using estimated price elasticity of demand for cigarettes in China, this paper gives a sensitivity analysis of the impact of tax revenue. There could be a negative economic impact on the cigarette industry and the tobacco farming sector. It is suggested that part of the increased revenues could be allocated for tobacco control programmes, financing health care among the poor and subsidizing tobacco farmers and the tobacco manufacturing industry, to allow for possible conversion of tobacco production to alternative crops or products.

Empirical analysis of the output effects of cigarette taxes in South Africa and the regional impact

R. van der Merwe & I. Abedian

University of Cape Town, Cape Town, South Africa

Cigarette excise taxes declined in real terms in South Africa over the period 1970–95. We have attempted to quantify the effects on output and employment that would occur if real tax rates had been maintained over that period. The analysis suggests that the net effects on employment would have been positive if expenditure on tobacco had been switched to other industries. We have also analysed the regional effects of maintaining real excise taxes over the same period. The effects on prices, consumption and government revenue were analysed for the southern African region, in particular South Africa and Zimbabwe.

In the empirical analysis described in the paper, we used multivariate regression analyses and co-integration.

An empirical analysis of cigarette taxes and advertising in South Africa, 1970–95

I. Abedian & N. Annett

University of Cape Town, Cape Town, South Africa

Cigarette excise taxes in South Africa declined in real terms over the period 1970–95. We have attempted to quantify the consequences of not maintaining real taxes from the point of view of public finance and anti-smoking activities. We conclude that the decline in real tax rates halved the potential excise tax revenue from cigarettes. The econometric analysis also suggests a positive impact of advertising on cigarette consumption. These findings imply that declining tax rates and the absence of controls on cigarette advertising stimulated cigarette consumption during the period under study.

The empirical analysis was performed by multivariate regression analysis with particular emphasis on co-integration tests.

Global approaches to active tobacco taxing and pricing: Initiative for standardization

N. Krstic

Mikroklima Clearinghouse d.o.o, Ljubljana–Menges, Slovenia

Active tobacco taxing and pricing is a highly effective tool for smoking control; the term 'active' is used to indicate that annual tobacco price indexes are higher the indexes of personal incomes and inflation. This model was created and implemented in the developed world, however, and may not be directly applicable in countries with a small gross national product and the associated problems, such as high unemployment, high inflation rates and latent or obvious socioeconomic crises. Smoking control policies must be adapted to local circumstances, and each country should develop its own strategy to counteract the domestic and international tobacco lobbies.

The most crucial aspects of a smoking control strategy are to create a bridge between the available options and their concrete application and to evaluate active tobacco taxing and pricing for countries with a gross national product of US\$ 20 000 *per capita* and those with only US\$ 200, i.e. to standardize this policy. Each country must establish its own priorities and their balance within a smoking control policy. This would be facilitated by the availability of a comprehensive global analysis and relevant standardization. A global view leads rapidly to the conclusion that socioeconomic crises are more frequent in developing parts of the world. If we are proposing greater use of active tobacco taxing and pricing, information is needed about situations in which this policy has been used during such crises.

As I reported in Buenos Aires in 1992, active tobacco taxing and pricing can be extremely dangerous for developing regions in that situation. In the former Yugoslavia, this policy was implemented during a period of hyperinflation because of financial shortages, as is usually the case in socioeconomic crises. Although the model was considered to be appropriate, the result was a sudden, complete sub-systemic implosion owing to the existent social turbulence. In this case, active tobacco taxing and pricing aggravated an already complicated situation, resulting in total disintegration.

When visiting the Chinese subcontinent, it might be concluded that this huge country is heterogeneous, but in fact some regions are economically dynamic and prosperous and large parts are underdeveloped with more or less obvious signs of socioeconomic turmoil. China is in a stage of development when such phenomena are to be expected. Another main characteristic is a strongly centralized mode of government. If active tobacco taxing and pricing were implemented intensively throughout China, what would happen in the less-developed regions with latent or perhaps obvious socioeconomic problems but with very large populations? It might liberate negative centrifugal social energy, which might be dangerous in a situation in which the gross national product is only several hundred US dollars *per capita*..

Active tobacco taxing and pricing remains an important weapon for a comprehensive smoking control policy, but it must be adapted for use in the developing world, for states with a low gross national product. An international collaborative centre could be set up to design, develop, support and coordinate global implementation of such policies.

It is clear that care must be taken in implementing this policy in situations of latent or obvious socioeconomic crisis, where the average personal income may be decreasing. The extent to which it results in an 'invisible' increase in tobacco prices must be estimated. There may be economic mechanisms that have the same result as active tobacco taxing and pricing, and no simple conclusion can therefore be drawn about whether active tobacco taxing and pricing should be used in socioeconomic crises.

APPROACHES TO CESSATION

Pharmacological methods

Pharmacological approaches to smoking cessation

M.J. Jarvis

ICRF Health Behaviour Unit, Department of Epidemiology and Public Health,
University College, London, United Kingdom

Introduction

It is widely recognized that because many millions of people already smoke, progress in reducing smoking-related disease in the next few years will depend mainly on increasing the rate of smoking cessation. Within the spectrum of policies and interventions aimed at promoting cessation, pharmacological approaches have an important part to play, and indeed have seen major advances in the past decade.

It would be unwise to expect too much from pharmacological treatments. Firstly, we need to remember that they can only ever be adjuncts: people are not cured of smoking by drugs; what drug treatments can do is to ease the process of translating the desire to give up into reality. Secondly, although cigarette smoking is now recognized as a form of drug addiction, as with other drug dependencies, pharmacological factors are only part of the problem. Personal, family and broader social influences generally outweigh drug dependence in determining cessation (Jarvis, 1997). Drug dependence may be the aspect that is most amenable to intervention, but not the most important determinant of outcome. That being the case, it may be hard to improve substantially on the current success rates from state-of-the-art interventions of about 30% sustained one-year abstinence.

How might pharmacological treatments help? Four potential routes can be envisaged: by replacing the effects of nicotine, they could reduce withdrawal symptoms and craving; alternatively, they could block smoking rewards, making cigarettes less attractive; they could make smoking aversive; or they could not target nicotine mechanisms directly, but have non-specific effects on mood state (e.g. anxiolytic effects), making it easier for smokers to cope. All of these approaches have been explored. Among the drugs examined, nicotine itself has been overwhelmingly the most thoroughly studied and the most successful.

Nicotine replacement therapy

Nicotine replacement therapy aims to provide some of the nicotine that smokers previously got from smoking, but for a limited period and in an inherently safer way. A number of products have been tested in randomized trials with rigorous research protocols. They vary from the patch, with the slowest rate of absorption and no accompanying behavioural ritual, through chewing-gum, lozenges and inhalers to the nasal spray, which has the fastest absorption and a complex behavioural ritual. None provides the bolus characteristic of inhaled cigarette smoking, but conclusions concerning efficacy are broadly similar for the different products. I shall focuses on the most recent products: patch, spray and inhaler.

About 20 trials of the patch have now been published, most showing significant effects (Fiore et al., 1994). Overall, success with active nicotine patches is approximately doubled in comparison with placebo. While higher absolute quitting rates are reported in trials with more intensive behavioural support, the doubling of success rates is similar for brief and intensive interventions (Stapleton et al., 1995).

The nasal spray has been tested in three trials, each conducted in specialized smokers' clinics with intensive support (Sutherland et al., 1992; Hjalmarson et al., 1994; Schneider et al., 1995). The results are again consistent, each trial finding a significant advantage for active sprays. Taken together, the rate of successful outcome is more than doubled in relation to placebo.

The inhaler, which is most like cigarettes in its appearance and use but not in nicotine absorption, has also been tested in three trials (Tonnesen et al., 1993; Schneider et al., 1996; Leischow et al., 1997). Only one found a significant effect after one year, but the trials together again indicate more than a doubling of sucessful outcome rate over placebo.

The tobacco addiction module of the Cochrane Collaboration gives clear evidence of efficacy for each nicotine replacement product, largely independent of the setting or intensity of additional support (Silagy et al., 1997). Nicotine replacement therapy is therefore well suited to widespread application in brief interventions in primary care, permitting many smokers to be reached, with a valuable public health impact. Studies in real settings confirm this evaluation. The findings for elderly smokers prescribed patches in the United States (Orleans et al., 1994), people attempting to quit who did or did not purchase the patch in California (Pierce et al., 1995) and over-the-counter customers in Denmark (Sonderskov et al., 1997) are consistent with those from the randomized trials.

Of course, each nicotine replacement product has its own drawbacks. All give rise to side-effects which may compromise compliance with effective use; however, these effects are mainly local and people soon adapt. There is potential for some transfer of dependence, which is least marked with the patch and most likely when the product permits self-dosage coupled with a behavioural ritual. This is a problem for only a small minority of users, usually the most dependent smokers. Also reassuring is the safety profile: very few serious adverse events have been reported among the millions of users of nicotine replacement therapy. Direct examination of the cardiovascular risk presented by these products indicated a benign profile (Benowitz & Gourlay, 1997).

Numerous issues remain to be explored in nicotine replacement therapy, including whether there is a dose–response relationship between the extent of replacement and outcome and whether more intensive support justifies its extra cost by promoting higher cessation rates. In the only trial in which smokers were randomized to different levels of support, no advantage was found for more support at follow-up (Jorenby et al., 1995). The issue of whether more nicotine replacement can give better outcomes has been studied by varying the dose of a particular product and by combining several products (Kornitzer et al., 1995). In the multi-centre CEASE trial across Europe, in which 3600 smokers were randomized to placebo or to two doses of nicotine patch, there was a clear dose–response effect.

Other drugs: mecamylamine, clonidine, bupropion

Numerous other drugs have been tested, many of which gave no clear evidence of efficacy (buspirone, ondansetron, naltrexone, anxiolytics); some indications of efficacy for moclobemide in a single trial need following up. More data are available on mecamylamine/nicotine combination, clonidine and bupropion.

Concurrent administration of agonist/antagonist has been proposed as a potentially effective means of promoting cessation, as it would block drug reinforcing effects as well as alleviating withdrawal (Rose & Levin, 1992). A preliminary trial of a combination of nicotine and mecamylamine has shown evidence of efficacy, and further trials are under way (Rose et al., 1994).

Clonidine has been tested in a number of trials, with mixed results (Gourlay et al., 1997). This is an agent marketed as an anti-hypertensive which has also been used in alcohol and drug withdrawal. There is some evidence of efficacy, but negative results wer obtained in short-term trials. A major reason for not giving this drug priority is its unacceptable side-effects.

Bupropion, which has been licensed as an anti-depressant for some years, was recently licensed as an anti-smoking aid in the United States. It is an atypical anti-depressant, unique in its class, but there is no indication that its value in smoking cessation stems from its anti-depressant action. In animal models, it appears to act somewhat similarly to amphetamine and cocaine, but potential dependence is not a concern in humans. Two large multi-centre trials have been conducted, the first on dose–response and the second looking at a combination of bupropion with the nicotine patch. The first trial found improved rates of cessation at doses up to 300 mg per day that were significantly better than with placebo and were sustained up to one year (Hurt et al., 1997). In the study of the combination with patch, only short-term outcomes are currently available (Nides et al., 1997). Both patch and bupropion were significantly better than placebo, and bupropion was more effective than patch; their combination showed added efficacy. If these results are confirmed, they will have implications both for improving the outcomes of pharmacological interventions and for understanding more about the mechanisms in the brain underlying nicotine addiction.

References

Benowitz, N.L. & Gourlay, S.G. (1997) Cardiovascular toxicity of nicotine: Implications for nicotine replacement therapy. J. Am. Coll. Cardiol., 29, 1422–1431

Fiore, M.C., Smith, S.S., Jorenby, D.E. & Baker, T.B. (1994) The effectiveness of the nicotine patch for smoking cessation: A meta-analysis. J. Am. Med. Assoc., 271, 1940–1947

Gourlay, S.G., Stead, L.F. & Benowitz, N.L. (1997) A meta-analysis of clonidine for smoking cessation. In: Lancaster, T., Silagy, C. & Fullerton, D., eds, Tobacco Addiction Module of the Cochrane Database of Systematic Reviews, Oxford: The Cochrane Collaboration

Hjalmarson, A., Franzon, M., Westin, A. & Wiklund, O. (1994) Effect of nicotine nasal spray on smoking cessation: A randomized, placebo-controlled, double-blind study. Arch. Intern. Med., 154, 2567–2572

Hurt, R.D., Sachs, D.P.L., Glover, E.D., et al. (1997) A comparison of sustained-release bupropion and placebo for smoking cessation. New Engl. J. Med., 337, 1195–1202

Jarvis, M.J. (1997) Patterns and predictors of unaided smoking cessation in the general population. In: Bolliger, C.T. & Fagerstrom, K.O., eds, The Tobacco Epidemic (Progress in Respiratory Research, Vol. 28), Basel: Karger

Jorenby, D.E., Smith, S.S., Fiore, M.C., et al. (1995) Varying nicotine patch dose and type of smoking cessation counseling. J. Am. Med. Assoc., 274, 1347–1352

Kornitzer, M., Boutsen, M., Dramaix, M., Thijs, J. & Gustavsson, G. (1995) Combined use of nicotine patch and gum in smoking cessation: A placebo- controlled clinical trial. Prev. Med., 24, 41–47

Leischow, S.J., Nilsson, F., Franzon, M., Hill, A., Otte, P.S. & Merikle, E.P. (1996) Efficacy of the nicotine inhaler as an adjunct to smoking cessation. Am. J. Health Behav., (in press)

Nides, M.A., Jorenby, D.E., Leischow, S. & Rennard, S. (1997) Paper presented at annual conference of Society for Research into Nicotine and Tobacco, Nashville, Tennessee, June 1997

Orleans, C.T., Resch, N., Noll, E., et al. (1994) Use of transdermal nicotine in a state-level prescription plan for the elderly. A first look at 'real-world' patch users. J. Am. Med. Assoc., 271, 601–607

Pierce, J.P., Gilpin, E. & Farkas, A.J. (1995) Nicotine patch use in the general population: Results from the 1993 California Tobacco Survey. J. Natl Cancer Inst., 87, 87–93

Rose, J.E. & Levin, E.D. (1992) Concurrent agonist–antagonist administration for the analysis and treatment of drug dependence. Pharmacol. Biochem. Behav., 41, 219–226

Rose, J.E., Behm, F.M., Westman, E.C., Levin, E.D., Stein, R.M. & Ripka, G.V. (1994) Mecamylamine combined with nicotine skin patch facilitates smoking cessation beyond nicotine patch treatment alone. Clin. Pharmacol. Ther., 56, 86–99

Schneider, N.G., Olmstead, R., Mody, F.V., et al. (1995) Efficacy of a nicotine nasal spray in smoking cessation: A placebo-controlled, double-blind trial. Addiction, 90, 1671–1682

Schneider, N.G., Olmstead, R., Nilsson, F., Mody, F.V., Franzon, M. & Doan, K. (1996) Efficacy of a nicotine inhaler in smoking cessation—A double-blind, placebo-controlled trial. Addiction, 91, 1293–1306

Silagy, C., Mant, D., Fowler, G. & Lancaster, T. (1997) The effect of nicotine replacement therapy on smoking cessation. In: Lancaster, T., Silagy, C. & Fullerton, D., eds, The Tobacco Addiction Module of Systematic Reviews, Oxford: The Cochrane Collaboration,

Sonderskov, J., Olsen, J., Sabroe, S., Meillier, L. & Overvad, K. (1997) Nicotine patches in smoking cessation: A randomized trial among over-the-counter customers in Denmark. Am. J. Epidemiol., 145, 309–318

Stapleton, J.A., Russell, M.A.H., Feyerabend, C., et al. (1995) Dose effects and predictors of outcome in a randomized trial of transdermal nicotine patches in general practice. Addiction, 90, 31–42

Sutherland, G., Russell, M.A.H., Stapleton, J., Feyerabend, C. & Ferno, O. (1992) Nasal nicotine spray: A rapid nicotine delivery system. Psychopharmacology, 108, 512–518

Tonnesen, P., Norregaard, J., Mikkelsen, K., Jorgensen, S. & Nilsson, F. (1993) A double-blind trial of a nicotine inhaler for smoking cessation. J. Am. Med. Assoc., 269, 1268–1271

Improving the effectiveness of the transdermal nicotine patch: A multicentre study

J. Gonzàlez Quintana, D. Marín Tuyà, M.J. Consuegra Manzanares & A. Garcia Baena

Unit of Smoking, Corporacío Sanitària Clínic, Barcelona, Catalonia, Spain

We conducted a multicentre study simultaneously in four smoking cessation clinics, in Bilbao, Majadahonda (Madrid), Virgen de las Nieves (Granada) and the University Clinic Hospital in Barcelona, which was the coordinating centre for this study. The aim of the study was to improve the effectiveness of the 24-h transdermal nicotine patch in a clinical setting with psychological support, and with rigid selection criteria for participants.

Methods

A smoking history was obtained for each candidate, and qualitative data were collected on motivation, smokers in their environment, desire to change their habit, previous attempts to quit, psychological dependence and health questionaire. The nicotine dependence level was evaluated by the Fagerström test (Fagerström & Schneider, 1982). Data were also collected on such objective variables as weight and height and concentration of carbon monoxide. Each subject also completed a questionnaire based on that of Horn and Russell, which was adapted and validated for the Spanish population by our team (Marín & González-Quintana, 1998).

The inclusion criteria were the physiological nicotine dependence level, smoking > 10 cigarettes per day during the previous six months, more than one attempt to give up smoking, a score of ≥ 6 in the physiological scales ('addictive', 'sedative' and 'stimulation') of the questionnaire and motivation level and quality (Marín & Salvador, 1987; Salvador *et al.*, 1988; Agustí *et al.*, 1991). The exclusion criteria were mental disorders, addiction to other drugs and subjects who had low or weak motivation, high scores in the four psychological scales ('automatic', 'hand or mouth activity', 'indulgent' and 'psychological image') of the questionnaire or contraindication to the patches.

The treatment involved two phases during a total of 10 visits. The intensive phase involved one visit per week, and the follow-up phase involved one visit after 15 days, one visit after the first, second and third months and a final visit in the sixth month. Weight and carbon monoxide concentration were measured at every visit. According to their nicotine dependence, subjects received 24-h 'Nicotinell' patches releasing 21 mg (81%) or 14 mg (19%). Group therapy was given to 80 subjects and 19 had individual therapy

The participants were 99 volunteers; 71% were women, which may reflect the growing sensitivity among women in our country to the dangers of smoking. The average age was 39 (± 2) years, they smoked an average of 29 (± 2) cigarettes per day and had made an average of 1.1 (± 0.1) previous attempts to give up smoking. Their average carbon monoxide concentration was 28 (±4) ppm. The average score in the Fagerström test was high, 7.6, indicating the high nicotine dependence of the subjects.

Results

The success rate was 81% in the first week and up to the end of the first month. By the third month, when the patch treatment was stopped, the success rate had decreased to 72%. At the the study, in the sixth month, 53% of the participants were still not smoking. These results are better than other published results with the transdermal nicotine patch (Abein *et al.*, 1989; Buchkremer & Minneker, 1989; Transdermal Nicotine Study Group, 1991; Silagy *et al.*, 1994). Verbal reports of abstinence were always checked by seeing whether the carbon monoxide concentration was ≤ 8 ppm, as accepted internationally (Jarvis *et al.*, 1986; Martín *et al.*, 1988); all the subjects told the truth.

We found no statistically significant differences in the success rate with age, sex, previous cigarette consumption, group therapy versus individual treatment or centre, and no difference was found between subjects who started with 21 mg of nicotine for six weeks and those who started with 14 mg for four weeks.

An association ($p < 0.004$) was found between short- and long-term treatment success and proper use of the patch: a new patch every morning and completion of treatment, and an association ($p < 0.001$) was found between the number of cigarettes smoked before treatment, score in the Fagerström test and use of the high-dose transdermal nicotine patch.

The final weight of those who succeed was increased by an average of 3.0 kg. This increase was already observed during the first month, and correlates with the findings of other published studies (Weekley *et al.*, 1992; Perkins, 1993).

Conclusions

Proper selection of smokers optimizes the efficacy of the transdermal nicotine patch. The long-term (six months) success rate is significantly higher than those reported in other published studies with transdermal nicotine patches. This may be due to our rigid selection criteria and the specialized psychological intervention, but also to the experience of the professionals who work in the centres where this study was conducted. The cost–efficacy of this kind of treatment is important in the present climate of lack of funds for public health in our country.

References

Abelin, T., Buehler, A., Muller, P., Nenasen, K. & Imhorf, P.R. (1989) Controlled trial of transdermal nicotine patch in tobacco withdrawal. *Lancet*, i, 7–10

Agustí, A., Estopà, R., González-Quintana, J., et al. (1991) Estudio multicéntrico de la deshabituación tabáquicq con chiclé de nicotina en personal sanitario. *Med. Clin. (Barcelona)*, **97**, 526–530

Buchkremer, G. & Minneker, E. (1989) Efficiency of multimodal smoking cessation therapy combining transdermal nicotine substitution with behavioral therapy. *Meth. Find. Exp. Clin. Pharmacol.*, **11**, 215–218

Fagerström, K.O. & Schneider, N.G. (1982) Measuring nicotine dependence: A review of the Fagerström tolerance questionnaire. *J. Behav. Med.*, **12**, 159–182

Jarvis, M.J., Belcher, M., Vesey, H., et al. (1986) Low cost monoxide monitors in smoking assessment. *Thorax*, **41**, 886–887

Marín, D. & González-Quintana, J. (1998) Tabaquismo ¿cómo ayudar al fumador? Rol de enfermería. *Formación Continuada*, **234** (Suppl.), 1–30

Marín, D. & Salvador, T. (1987) *Determinación de los Factores Psicológicos y Fisiológicos Implicados en el Abandono de la Dependencia al Tabaco*. Thesis, Autonomous University of Barcelona

Martin, I.J., Clark, E., Crombie, I., et al. (1988) Evaluation of a portable measure of expired-air carbon monoxide. *Prev. Med.*, **17**, 109–115

Perkins, K.A. (1993) Weight gain following smoking cessation. *J. Consult. Clin. Psychol.*, **61**, 768–777

Salvador, T., Marín, D., González-Quintana, J., et al. (1988) Tratamiento del tabaquismo: Eficacia de la utilización del chicle de nicotina. Estudio a doble ciego. *Med. Clin. (Barcelona)*, **90**, 646–650

Silagy, C., Mant, D., et al. (1994) Meta-analysis on efficacy of nicotine replacement therapies in smoking cessation. *Lancet*, **343**

Transdermal Nicotine Study Group (1991) Transdermal nicotine for smoking cessation. *J. Am. Med. Assoc.*, **266**, 3133–3138

Weekley, C.K., Klesges, R.C. & Reylea, G. (1992) Smoking as a weight control strategy and its relationship to smoking status. *Addict. Behav.*, **17**, 259–271

Review of nicotine replacement therapy in helping people to stop smoking

J.-L. Tang[1] & J.L.Y. Liu[2]

[1]Department of Community & Family Medicine and [2]Centre for Clinical Trial and Epidemiological Research, The Chinese University of Hong Kong, Shatin, New Territories, Hong Kong SAR, China

Nicotine replacement therapy is probably the most effective of the many methods available to help people to stop smoking (Law & Tang, 1995). Four major forms of nicotine preparations are now available: chewing-gum, patch, inhaler and nasal spray. Chewing-gum and patch have been the most extensively studied in randomized controlled trials, but the four preparations probably have very similar effectiveness: 10–15% of people give up smoking as a result of the treatment (Tang et al., 1994). The effectiveness is highly dependent on the provision of instructions for use and the choice of smokers. Nicotine replacement therapy is also recommend for patients with coronary heart disease and pregnant women since the benefits of treatment well outweigh any harm it may induce. We review the evidence from randomized controlled trials and systematic reviews, raise some issues with regard to the use of nicotine replacement therapy and point out potential ways of increasing the benefit–harm ratio of this therapy.

Nicotine replacement therapy works fairly well in smokers who are motivated to give up and is most effective in smokers who are highly nicotine-dependent (Silagy et al., 1994; Tang et al., 1994). Smokers who are voluntarily looking for assistance in smoking cessation can usually be considered as motivated. Nicotine dependence can be assessed by asking a smoker a few brief questions about his or her smoking habits (Heatherton et al., 1991). Chewing-gum containing 4 mg is more effective than that containing 2 mg nicotine, and both are more effective in highly nicotine-dependent smokers. When used by these smokers, the 4-mg preparation can enable one-third of them to give up. The nicotine patch is probably most useful for moderately nicotine-dependent smokers (Yudkin et al., 1996). There is a lack of data on the effectiveness of nicotine inhalers and nasal sprays in relation to the level of nicotine dependence.

The four forms of nicotine differ considerably in route of administration, dose, efficiency of nicotine delivery, convenience of use, side-effects and long-term dependence on nicotine replacement therapy. Each form of nicotine is therefore most suitable for a certain type of smoker and by itself cannot achieve maximum efficacy. A combination of preparations may be desirable, but this deserves more research. Combined approaches could be used to maximize effectiveness and cost-efficiency and/or to reduce side-effects or long-term dependence. For example, a trial has shown that the combined use of chewing-gum and patch is more effective than either alone (Kornitzer et al., 1995).We suggest that the following factors be taken into account in designing combinations of preparations: convenience of use, efficiency of nicotine delivery, side-effects, long-term dependence and cost.

Convenience and side-effects affect compliance, which in turn affects efficacy. Correct chewing of gum is important: many people chew the gum too quickly and/or swallow air or saliva while chewing. This reduces its effectiveness and causes most of the side-effects, including hiccoughs, flatulence, indigestion and nausea. Although the effects are seldom severe enough to stop use of the gum, they may reduce the amount consumed. The patch offers greater convenience and minimal need for instruction. It causes only mild, local skin reactions in people with normal skin, which rarely require stopping its use, and long-term dependence is very rare. In one study, 25% of tobacco abstainers were still using chewing-gum after one year, while 43% were using the nasal spray. The irritating effects of the nasal spray affect nearly all users.

The efficiency of nicotine delivery is measured in relation to that of smoking cigarettes. Nicotine preparations that can produce the rapid surge and steady-state concentrations of nicotine in blood similar to those produced by smoking cigarettes are more likely to alleviate craving for cigarettes and offer greater effectiveness. Inhalers and nasal sprays are the most efficient in this respect and patches the least. The preparations that produce changes in blood nicotine similar to those of smoking cigarettes are also more likely to cause long-term dependence. Accordingly, use of the nasal spray or inhaler for one or two weeks followed by the patch or chewing-gum for another two to three months by those who have abstained, for example, might reduce side-effects and long-term dependence and increase compliance and efficacy. This claim is supported by the finding that those who manage to stop during the first week of treatment are most likely to benefit from continuing use of nicotine replacement therapy (Yudkin et al., 1996).

References

Heatherton, T.F., Kozlowski, L.T., et al. (1991) The Fagerström test for nicotine dependence: A revision of the Fagerström tolerance questionnaire. Br. J. Addict., 86, 1119–1127

Kornitzer, M., Boutsen, M., Dramaix, M., et al. (1995) Combined use of nicotine patch and gum in smoking cessation: A placebo-controlled clinical trial. Prev. Med., 24, 41–47

Law, M. & Tang, J.L. (1995) An analysis of the effectiveness of interventions intended to help people stop smoking. Arch. Intern. Med., 155, 1933–1941

Silagy, C., Mant, D., et al. (1994) Meta-analysis on the efficacy of nicotine replacement therapies in smoking cessation. Lancet, 343, 139–142

Tang, J.L., Law, M. & Wald, N. (1994) How effective is nicotine replacement therapy in helping people to stop smoking? Br. Med. J., 308, 21–26

Yudkin, P., Jones, L., Lancaster, T. & Fowler, G.H. (1996) Which smokers are helped to give up smoking using transdermal nicotine patches? Results from a randomized, double-blinded, placebo-controlled trial. Br. J. Gen. Pract., 46, 145–148

Smoking cessation programme with nicotine patches for employees of a teaching hospital

T.E. Jones

The Queen Elizabeth Hospital, Woodville, South Australia

Introduction

Tobacco smoking by employees of teaching hospitals reflects poorly on the institutions and health professions and negates the important health message that patients should quit the habit. Smoking by staff also increases the running costs of the institution because of the combined effects of increased absenteeism that smokers incur and the need to provide a safe workplace environment. At the time the 'Stop Smoking Service' was introduced, transdermal nicotine patches were available only on doctor's prescription in Australia, which contrasted sharply with the ready availability and attractive outlets for cigarettes. Prior to the introduction of the programme, The Queen Elizabeth Hospital did not provide any support for employees who smoked cigarettes, although smoking was known to be commonplace and was forbidden in hospital buildings.

Methods

The 'Stop Smoking Service' is run by the Clinical Pharmacist attached to the Respiratory Unit of this 400-bed teaching hospital. It operates from a convenient, 'one-stop shop' location in the main hospital block, where a friendly, non-clinical environment is fostered. Competitively priced transdermal nicotine patches are provided on a weekly basis, with brief support sessions. The programme is individualized for each smoker: the strength of the patch and duration of its use are determined by the number of cigarettes smoked at commencement, the degree of difficulty in quitting and the adverse effects experienced. Smokers complete a questionnaire (based on the Fagerström questionnaire) at weekly intervals, and success is assessed by self-reports and routine determinations of exhaled carbon monoxide.

The price charged for the nicotine patches is substantially less than that charged by community pharmacists and is less than the cost of smoking 20 cigarettes per day.

Results

In the first 18 months of operation, 111 employees had attended the service at least once. Twenty-one were lost to follow-up at the first assessment (three months), when 29 of the remaining 90 were not smoking. At the next assessment (six months), 20 out of 25 who completed the period were not smoking; and at 12 months, 13 out of 16 who had completed the period were not smoking.

There appeared to be a relationship between success in not smoking at three months and the number of cigarettes smoked at the start of the programme (Table 1), but the trend did not reach statistical significance.

Of the 61 smokers who were not successful in quitting at three months, 25 (41%) attended on only one occasion. The reason most often quoted for not returning by these smokers was that they were not ready to quit and had not used any patches; seven smokers nevertheless experienced adverse effects (chest pain, sweaty palms, migraine, skin irritation, rashes, nightmares, vomiting and diarrhoea), which resulted in discontinuation of patch use before the end of the first week. Although rarely described as distressing, dream disturbances were reported by 33/90 contacted at three months. These disturbances were often reduced or abolished by removing the patch before retiring to bed.

After the inital assessment, the average period of support was 4.75 weeks (range, 1–56). The time taken for the initial interview averaged 45 min, and subsequent follow-up interviews lasted an average of 15 min. Assuming that all who were lost to follow-up returned to smoking, the approximate cost for each known successful quitter (based on salary plus 30%) at three months is thus AUS\$ 180.

Twenty five smokers who were either unsuccessful initially or who resumed smoking after an initial period of success returned to the programme at least once. Eleven returned more than once (range, 2–5 times). Insufficient data are available at this time to report the success rates of these smokers.

Discussion

This report describes the success of a medium-intensity stop-smoking service in a 400-bed teaching hospital. In a voluntary survey of > 2200 hospital employees conducted after 18 months' operation of the Service, regular cigarette smoking was reported by 12% of employees. This figure is lower than those for the area surrounding the hospital (27%; B. Smith and M. Nitschke, personal communication) or nationally (24%; Australian Bureau of Statistics, 1996) and is due in part to the success of the Service.

Our results are comparable to those quoted for other medium-intensity stop-smoking services. We believe that the community atmosphere of the hospital and the attractive price are factors that promote success.

Employers in the health sector should be more aware of the addictive nature of tobacco smoking than employers in other business sectors and should therefore be at

Table 1. Success in stopping smoking at three months according to number of cigarettes smoked at entry

No. cigarettes per day	Stopped	Not stopped
< 10	4	3
11–20	12	19
21–30	10	26
> 31	3	12

Chi-squared = 3.67; $p = 0.055$

the forefront in providing opportunities for employees to quit. Because of their dual roles as educators and role models, it is of paramount importance that hospital employees do not smoke. We believe that the 'stop smoking service' described herein is affordable and should be replicated by other health units for their employees. Barriers to stopping smoking should be reduced, and, in particular, nicotine patches should be more readily available than they are currently in Australia. Because counselling has been shown to increase success rates (Silagy et al., 1994), nicotine patches may best be provided through selected retail pharmacies where specially trained pharmacists could receive a counselling fee rather than the traditional profit from sale.

References

Australian Bureau of Statistics (1996) ABS Catalogue No. 4392.0, Canberra
Silagy, C. et al. (1994) Lancet, 343, 139–142

Pharmaceutical approach to smoking cessation: Public health benefit of over-the-counter nicotine medications— The experience in the United States

G.M. Quesnelle[1], S.L. Burton[1], K.E. Kemper[1] & J. Gitchell[2]

[1]SmithKline Beecham Consumer Healthcare, East Kowloon, Hong Kong SAR, China
[2]Pinney Associates, Bethesda, Maryland, United States

Tobacco-related morbidity and mortality remain the primary causes of disability and premature death in the United States. Prevention of smoking is an important policy focus, as demonstrated by the Food and Drug Administration's Tobacco Regulation (Department of Health and Human Services, 1996a). Providing effective and easily accessible treatments for smokers to help them quit is another important need, and was recommended by the United States Surgeon General in 1990 (Department of Health and Human Services, 1990). Nicotine medications, the smoking cessation pharmacotherapies with the longest records of safety and efficacy, have been available in the United States by prescription since 1984 and in other countries as non-prescription aids. In April 1996, Nicorette chewing-gum was launched as the first nicotine medication available without a prescription (over-the-counter; equivalent to general sale status); two nicotine patches, including NicoDerm CQ, followed in July and August of 1996.

The greater access to these products has been accompanied by large-scale promotional efforts and indications of significant public health benefit:

- Consumer-focused marketing and promotion have delivered strong smoking cessation messages while appropriately managing expectations and reminding smokers that to use the medications effectively they must be 'committed quitters'. As a result, demand for and use of the products has risen steadily and continues to be strong, as opposed to the strong surge followed by a rapid decline that marked the prescription marketing of nicotine patches in 1992.
- Manufacturers have established partnerships with public health agencies such as the American Cancer Society. An impressive example of the results of these partnerships was SmithKline Beecham Consumer Healthcare and the American Cancer Society's co-promotion of the 'Great American Smokeout' in November 1996. In an article on the 1996 campaign, the Centers for Disease Control and Prevention concluded that "Marketing and promotion efforts designed to promote attempts to quit, along with OTC availability of nicotine medications, are a useful part of a national strategy to decrease the prevalence of smoking' Centers for Disease Control, 1997).
- Promotion of smoking cessation to health-care professionals has increased, rather than declining as was feared by some, since manufacturers have worked hard to motivate and train pharmacists, physicians, and other health-care providers to encourage their patients to quit smoking. A useful tool in this process was the 1996

release of the Agency for Health Care Policy and Research's Smoking Cessation Guideline (Department of Health and Human Services, 1996b).

• The expansion in reach, access and use of nicotine replacement therapy does not appear to have been accompanied by an increase in problems. Surveillance has not found shown evidence of significant misuse or abuse of the products by adult smokers, use by adolescents or use by non-smokers.

In summary, the availability of nicotine medications over the counter in the United States demonstrates that responsible, committed marketers of nicotine medications, working in partnership with the public health community, can significantly increase access to and use of effective smoking cessation therapies. It is believed that other countries could benefit from the lessons learned in the United States.

References

Centers for Disease Control (1997) Impact of promotion of the Great American Smokeout and availability of over-the-counter nicotine medications, 1996. *Morbid. Mortal. Wkly Rep.*, **46**, 867–871

Department of Health and Human Services (1990) *Health Benefits of Smoking Cessation. A Report of the US Surgeon General*, Washington DC: US Government printing Office

Department of Health and Human Services (1996a) *Regulations Restricting the Sale and Distribution of Cigarettes and Smokeless Tobacco to Protect Children and Adolescents; Final Rule* (21 CFR Part 801 et seq.), Washington DC: Food and Drug Administration

Department of Health and Human Services (1996b) *Clinical Practice Guideline: Smoking Cessation* (AHCPR Publication No. 96-0692), Washington DC: US Government Printing Office

Continuously up-dated systematic reviews of nicotine replacement therapy: The latest evidence of effectiveness

C.A. Silagy[1] & T. Lancaster[2]

[1]*Department of General Practice, Flinders Medical Centre, Bedford Park, Australia*
[2]*Department of Primary Care, University of Oxford, Oxford, United Kingdom*

Aim: To update previous systematic reviews of nicotine replacement therapy in the light of the results of a substantial number of recently completed randomized clinical trials of the various forms of nicotine replacement therapy (chewing-gum, transdermal patches, nasal sprays and inhalers). In particular, to determine whether combinations of nicotine replacement therapy are influenced by the clinical setting in which the smoker is recruited and treated, the dose and form of the nicotine replacement therapy used or the intensity of additional advice and support offered to the smoker.

Methods: A systematic review (incorporating a meta-analysis) was undertaken under the auspices of the Cochrane Tobacco Addictions Group. Randomized clinical trials in which nicotine replacement therapy was compared with placebo or no treatment or in which different doses of nicotine replacement therapy were compared were included in the study, providing that they reported cessation rates at a follow-up of six months or more. Two authors abstracted data independently. The principal outcome measure was abstinence at 6–12 months, and we performed meta-analyses with a fixed-effects model.

Results: Of the 76 trials identified (23 more than in the largest published meta-analysis), 47 trials were of nicotine chewing-gum, 22 of transdermal nicotine patches, three of intranasal nicotine sprays and two of inhaled nicotine. In two trials, combinations of two forms of nicotine therapy (patch and chewing-gum) were compared with patch or chewing-gum alone. The odds ratio for abstinence with nicotine replacement therapy relative to control was 1.8 (95% confidence interval, 1.6–1.9). The odds ratios for the various forms of nicotine replacement therapy were 1.6 for chewing-gum, 2.0 for patches, 2.4 for nasal sprays and 2.4 for inhaled nicotine. These odds were largely independent of the intensity of additional support provided or the setting in which the nicotine replacement therapy was offered.

Conclusion: Nicotine replacement therapy is an effective component of cessation stategies for heavier smokers. It should be offered routinely. The type of nicotine replacement therapy chosen will depend on individual circumstances.

Overview of nicotine replacement therapy

M.A.H. Russell, J.A. Stapleton & G. Sutherland

National Addiction Centre, Institute of Psychiatry, London, United Kingdom

Regular tobacco use is a form of drug addiction caused by the behavioural and pharmacological effects of nicotine. Rapid neuroadaptation, including development of tolerance to aversive effects, sensitization (i.e. enhancement of response) at so-called 'pleasure centres' of the brain and an increase in the number of nicotine receptors in the brain of smokers may help explain why so many smokers have difficulty in giving up smoking and why as many as 90% of teenagers who smoke more than three or four cigarettes for psychosocial reasons go on to become regular smokers as adults.

Nicotine chewing-gum, transdermal nicotine patches and, more recently, a nicotine nasal spray and nicotine inhaler have been developed as aids to smoking cessation. All have been shown effectively to reduce the severity of withdrawal symptoms and to double the rates of long-term cessation when compared with placebo or supportive psychological and behavioural methods alone. Their therapeutic value in various settings and various kinds of smokers is related to their ease of use and rate of nicotine absorption. Patches, for example, have been shown to have dose-related efficacy with brief support in non-specialist settings. In contrast, nasal sprays from which nicotine is rapidly absorbed are more difficult to use, but in a specialist clinic setting have been shown to be four to five times more effective than placebo in highly dependent smokers. More recent work has been conducted on their use in combination with each other and with other drugs such as mecamvlamine, bupropion and moclobemide.

Treatment is indicated only for individuals and populations of smokers well motivated to quit.

Real-world efficacy of computer-tailored smoking cessation material as a supplement to nicotine replacement

S. Shiffman[1], J. Gitchell[2] & V. Strecher[3]

[1]University of Pittsburgh, Pittsburgh, Pennsylvania, [2]Pinney Associates, Bethesda, Maryland, and [3]University of Michigan, Ann Arbor, Michigan, United States

Making effective smoking cessation programmes widely available is a public health challenge. The efficacy of printed materials is limited because they cannot take into account individual smokers' needs. We examined the efficacy of the 'committed quitters' programme, which evolved from the programme marketed with prescribed NicoDerm patches and consisted of written materials tailored by computer algorithms to smokers' stated needs and demographics. 'Committed quitters' is available by enrolment to purchasers in the United States of Nicorette chewing-gum, which is packaged with a quit-smoking booklet. To test the programme, 3627 'committed quitters' enrollees consented to be randomized to three conditions: no materials (received no additional assistance), standard 'committed quitters' programme or enhanced 'committed quitters' programme (standard plus a counselling telephone call). The participants' smoking status was determined by telephone interview after 6 and 12 weeks.

At six weeks, the 28-day continuous quit rates among the subjects reached were 25% for those who received no materials, 36% for those who received the standard 'committed quitters' programme and 36% for those given the enhanced programme. The 'committed quitters' programme was thus associated with significantly higher quit rates (odds ratio, 1.7; 95% confidence interval, 1.4–2.2); adding a telephone call had no incremental effect. At 12 weeks, similar results were obtained. The study demonstrates that low-cost, tailored printed materials can have significant impact on cessation, even among smokers who are already receiving nicotine medication and basic written behavioural advice.

Determining who will benefit from nicotine replacement therapy and choosing a product

A. Hjalmarson

Smoking Cessation Clinic, Sahlgren's University Hospital, Gothenburg, Sweden

We have compared data from three randomized, placebo-controlled trials to evaluate the efficacy of nicotine chewing-gum, nicotine nasal spray and the nicotine inhaler, respectively, as smoking cessation aids. The studies were all of the same design and had similar numbers of subjects (206–248) who were given the same type of group support as adjunctive therapy. Nevertheless, the studies were conducted at different periods.

In all three studies, the long-term success rates were significantly better with nicotine than with placebo, but the three products appeared to be equally effective, with success rates ranging from 27 to 29%. Given such similar success rates, other factors associated with the three nicotine products become important in selecting which treatment to recommend to patients. We therefore compared the side-effects, withdrawal symptoms and weight gain associated with the three products. Dependence and other background factors correlated with successful cessation were also compared.

The most important factors to consider when choosing between the various nicotine products are their adverse effects and the smoker's personal preferences.

Determination of concentration of cotinine associated with smoking cessation

M. Abe, E. Midorikawa, T. Takubo, K. Yoshino, A. Nagai & K. Konno

Internal Medicine 1, Tokyo Women's Medical College, Tokyo, Japan

Introduction

In nicotine replacement therapy, relapse remains a major problem (Fiore *et al.*, 1992; The Smoking Cessation Clinical Practice Guideline Panel and Staff, 1996). There are two critical difficulties in medium-term cessation: one is relapse just after stopping smoking and beginning nicotine replacement therapy and the other is relapse weeks or months later. Some people undergo persistent stress due to lack of nicotine, even on nicotine replacement therapy (Ashton & Stepney, 1982; Hatsukami *et al.*, 1993). In order to decrease the stress, we propose that the optimal nicotine concentration be maintained during the early stage of therapy for some patients, in order to prevent relapse. In the study reported here, we investigated the concentrations of cotinine in plasma in patients who had and had not relapsed.

Subjects and methods

We studied 68 patients who had stopped smoking for at least 10 days and were on nicotine replacement therapy; 38 of them had smoking-related diseases. The mean age was 53 years, and 20 of the patients were women. The Brinkman index (amount smoked x years of smoking; Akiba, 1994) was 1035. Plasma cotinine concentrations were measured before and after cessation by gas chomatography with mass spectrometry (Feyerabend et al., 1985; Fiore et al., 1992). The first sample was taken at the time of the first visit to our out-patient department and the second on the third or eighth day after starting nicotine replacement therapy. After six months, the patients were divided into two groups on the basis of whether they had relapsed.

The values were determined as means and standard deviations; differences at $p < 0.05$ were considered significant.

Results

There was no significant difference in the baseline parameters of the two groups; the mean cotinine concentration was 243 ± 119 ng/ml. By six months, 48 (70%) of the subjects had not relapsed; 20 had relapsed. In the early stages of replacement therapy, the mean cotinine concentration of patients who subsequently relapsed was significantly lower than that of patients who succeeded in quitting: $38 \pm 24\%$ of the original concentration in those who relapsed and $62 \pm 27\%$ of the original concentration in those who succeeded. Patients who had previously experienced strong withdrawal symptoms (Shiffman & Jarvik, 1976; The Smoking Cessation Clinical Practice Guideline Panel and Staff, 1996) were seen to need higher cotinine concentrations for successful smoking cessation.

Conclusion

Measurement of plasma cotinine before and after cessation is useful for determining the replacement dose of nicotine for therapy. Higher cotinine concentrations are predictive of easier smoking cessation, especially in patients who have previously experienced strong withdrawal symptoms.

References

Akiba, S. (1994) Analysis of cancer risk related to longitudinal information on smoking habits. Environ. Health Perspectives, 102, 15–19

Ashton, H. & Stepney, R. (1982) Smoking Psychology and Pharmacology, New York: Tavistock Publications

Feyerabend, C., Ings, R.M.J. & Russell, M.A.H. (1985) Nicotine pharmacokinetics and its application to intake from smoking. Br. J. Clin. Pharmacol., 19, 239–247

Fiore, M.C., Jorenby, \D.E., Baker, T.B., et al. (1992) Tobacco dependence and the nicotine patch: Clinical guidelines for effective use. J. Am. Med. Assoc., 268, 2687–2694

Hatsukami, D., Huber, M. & Callies, A. (1993) Physical dependence on nicotine gum: Effect of duration of use. Psychopharmacology, 111, 449–456

Shiffman, S. & Jarvik, M.E. (1976) Smoking withdrawal symptoms in 2 weeks of abstinence. Psychopharmacology, 50, 35–39

The Smoking Cessation Clinical Practice Guideline Panel and Staff (1996) The Agency for Health Care Policy and Research Smoking Cessation Clinical Practice guideline. J. Am. Med. Assoc., 275, 1270–1280

Urinary cotinine: An indicator for smoking cessation therapy

L. Martinez-Rossier, J. Villalba-Caloca, R. Montes-Vizuet, S. Flores-Sanchez &
L. Teran-Ortiz

National Institute of Respiratory Diseases, Mexico City, Mexico

Introduction

Nitrogen compounds represent 0.5–5% of the chemicals in tobacco leaves (International Agency for Research on Cancer, 1986). Of these, nicotine is the most important, as it is the cause of physical dependence on tobacco (Pool et al., 1985). The main metabolite of nicotine is cotinine, which results from oxidation of the pyridine ring in the liver. Cotinine is very stable and has a half-life of 19 h, in comparison with 30 min for nicotine. Quantitative measurement of cotinine in blood, urine and saliva has therefore been used as an indicator of tobacco consumption (Jarvis et al., 1984), cessation of tobacco use and exposure to environmental tobacco smoke (Biber et al., 1987).

We carried out a study to test the validity of quantitative measurement of cotinine in urine in order to evaluate objectively the success of our smoking cessation programme.

Material and methods

We carried out an observational, comparative, prospective and experimental study in an immunotechnology department in collaboration with the smoking clinic of the National Institute of Respiratory Diseases in Mexico City, involving 59 moderate to heavy smokers. The subjects first completed a questionnaire that included questions on daily cigarette consumption and were then given 4–12 mg nicotine in chewing-gum daily for 12 weeks; they then received cognitive–behavioural restructuration therapy. The questionnaires were applied again after 12 weeks of treatment to ascertain the rate of cessation. The results were compared with those for a group of 20 smokers who were not treated and 50 non-smokers. None of the subjects had renal insufficiency or consumed barbiturates or isoniazid during the study period.

Cotinine was measured in samples of early-morning urine at the beginning and end of the cognitive–behavioural therapy. The method used consisted of adding 4 nmol sodium acetate, 1.5 mol potassium cyanide, 0.4 nmol chloramine T and 78 nmol barbituric acid to the samples, mixing for 10 s and incubation at room temperature for 15 min. The reaction was stopped by addition of 1 mol sodium metabisulfide. Absorption was read at 490 nm against a water blank and compared with that of a cotinine standard of known concentration. The results were analysed statistically with the test for comparing means of homogeneous samples.

Results

The mean age of the subjects in the experimental group was 40 years, and that of both control groups was 35 years; the male:female ratio was 1 for all three groups, and all of the subjects were of middle socioeconomic status. The mean cotinine concentrations were 60.9 µmol/L (range, 16.6–210; SD, 53.8) for the control smokers and 3.92 (0.3–12.4; SD, 2.97) for the control non-smokers. At the beginning of the cognitive–behavioural therapy, the mean urinary cotinine concentration of the experimental group was 67.0 µmol/L (13.1–246; SD, 44.2); at the end, it was 9.8 µmol/L (1.2–82.1; SD, 11.6). This difference was statistically significant ($p < 0.001$).

There was a significant difference between the mean cotinine levels of the treated smokers at the end of therapy and those of the non-smokers, because some of the treated smokers had concentrations similar to those of the untreated smokers, although 75% of the treated smokers had cotinine levels similar to those of the non-smokers. The subjects with higher cotinine levels were found at the final questionnaire interview not to have stopped smoking.

Conclusions

The barbituric acid method of direct quantitative analysis of urinary cotinine is reliable for validating the success of cognitive–behavioural restructuration therapy for smoking cessation and can be used to classify smokers and non-smokers. The 25% of smokers who did not stop smoking after therapy should probably undergo individual therapy.

References

Biber, A., Scherar, G., Hoepfner, L., Adlkofer, F., Heller, W.D., Haddow, J.E. & Knight, G.J. (1987) Determination of nicotine and cotinine in human serum and urine: An interlaboratory study. *Toxicol. Lett.*, **35**, 35–52

International Agency for Research on Cancer (1986) *IARC Monographs on the Evaluation of Carcinogenic Risks to Humans*, Vol. 28, *Tobacco Smoking*, Lyon

Jarvis, M., Tunstall-Peedoe, H., Feyerabend, C., Vesey, C. & Salloojee, Y. (1984) Biochemical markers of smoke absorption and self-reported exposure to passive smoking. *J. Epidemiol. Community Health*, **38**, 335–339

Pool, W.F., Godin, C.S. & Crooks, P.A. (1985) Nicotine racemization during cigarette smoking. *Toxicologist*, **5**, 232

Behavioural methods

Behavioural approaches to smoking cessation

K. Slama

International Union Against Tuberculosis and Lung Disease, Paris, France

Tobacco advertising is an example of an attempt to influence behaviour. Whether it or any other approach influences people to change their behaviour depends on a number of factors, including the way the individual perceives the approach and whether or not opportunities arise for change to occur. Behavioural interventions focus on the environment and the individual's thoughts and actions in relation to the environment. Behavioural approaches based on social learning theory stem from the observation that behavioural change is difficult: environment influences lifestyle choices, while at the same time lifestyle choices influence the environment (Orlandi, 1996).

In behavioural approaches to smoking or other tobacco use at the individual level, the environment is seen as providing both cues to action and consequences of action that influence the choices that a person makes. Inability to stop using tobacco is seen as a complex web of dysfunctional thinking and acting that is influenced by those cues and consequences that make up the context of smoking (Enright, 1997). This takes into account the pharmacological effects of nicotine and also conditioning and other environmental factors.

In parallel to individual differences in the perception of the pharmacological effects of smoking (Perkins, 1995), people can be more attentive to aspects of their surroundings that reinforce the act of smoking, to perceptions of the value of smoking and choosing friends to share in this behaviour (Slama, 1997). In this way, behavioural choices limit the extent to which negative aspects of tobacco use or positive aspects of quitting are included in what a smoker perceives.

Taking up smoking or other forms of tobacco is a social phenomenon. If some people smoke, others may start. Whatever the psychological make-up or situations that provoke smoking, the choice for most people is possible only if smoking is already part of known modes of activity. Like an epidemic, tobacco uptake can rise and fall depending on the environment, as can be seen by looking at men's and women's maximum rates of tobacco smoking over 70 years in the United States (Giovino *et al.*, 1995).

But what about stopping smoking? Tobacco contains nicotine, and nicotine is a dependence-producing drug. Can behavioural approaches to cessation be of interest? Behavioural approaches can help in interventions because smoking cessation is also a social phenomenon: if many people are stopping, more people will stop. If we consider a model prevalence curve, as shown in Figure 1, we see that prevalence of smoking rises when there is more uptake than quitting, that maximum rates occur when there is equilibrium between starting and quitting (or dying) and that rates decline when the numbers quitting or dying are increasingly greater than the numbers who are starting. Low prevalence occurs when there is low uptake but also high ex-smoking rates (Slama, 1997). Whatever the psychological make-up of smokers, whatever the situations they are in, stopping smoking becomes a considered action as more and more of those around them do it (Fisher *et al.*, 1990). The environment can be a force that combats tobacco use, just as it can reinforce it.

Whereas nicotine replacement is used to counteract the pharmacological dependence created by smoking and to help smokers to stop smoking by reducing their withdrawal symptoms and, in terms of motivation, reducing the fear of quitting (Haxby, 1995), behavioural approaches work on weakening conditioned urges (the urges to smoke that come from thinking about and reacting to situations) (Pechacek & Danaher, 1979; Giovino *et al.*, 1995; Perkins, 1995). In treatment settings, the results of the combination of behavioural change strategies and nicotine replacement are better than either alone (Parker & Lenfant, 1986; Agency for Health Care Policy and Research, 1996), but the

Figure 1. A model prevalence curve

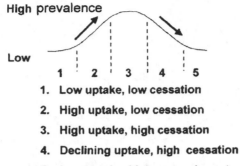

1. Low uptake, low cessation

2. High uptake, low cessation

3. High uptake, high cessation

4. Declining uptake, high cessation

5. Low uptake, high ex-smoker rate

From Slama (1997)

effects overlap rather than add together. In low-income areas particularly, where resources for individual treatment are scarce, nicotine replacement products may not be a feasible element of treatment. Cognitive and behavioural strategies can be useful for low-cost cessation treatment but should also be considered in community tobacco-control efforts. Behavioural approaches have already shown potential in other kinds of public health initiatives in low-income countries (Elder, 1987).

Cognitive and behavioural techniques are used in behavioural approaches to cessation in order to change the context and perceptions of smoking. Because of addiction, perceptions of withdrawal and behavioural responses to withdrawal are included in these strategies.

In a behavioural approach, we first assess the environment, by answering the questions:
• What behaviour is perceived to be possible?
• What are the signals and pressures to smoke or not to smoke?
• What are the consequences of smoking or not smoking?
Treatment consists of finding appropriate strategies to respond to the questions:
• How can we change the perceptions surrounding smoking?
• Can we change the signals to smoke or our responses to them?
• Can we arrive at the desired consequences by a behaviour other than smoking?

Helping people to stop smoking or using other forms of tobacco by cognitive and behavioural strategies means that smokers identify their environment and the way they react to it and then change the stimuli (cues to smoke) or their perceptions of or reactions to them, change the way they perceive the consequences (the reasons for smoking) and go about seeking the consequences not by smoking but in a different way, such as relaxation strategies to manage stress and urge-reduction strategies to manage craving.

Cognitive change approaches include health education and cognitive skills training. Health education involves relating information about smoking-related disease, the risks of smoking and risk reduction upon quitting. In cognitive skills training, people are helped to redefine themselves, their behaviour and their attitudes, in order to cope better with their environment and to succeed in changing (Roskies & Lazarus, 1980). These elements are often included in multi-component programmes for self-selected smokers, but their effect is now considered to be appropriate to smokers who are not yet ready to stop, in interventions to increase motivation or in health promotion campaigns (Nolan, 1995).

Behavioural approaches to cessation include self-management (self-control) strategies, stimulus or response substitution and aversive techniques. Self-control involves understanding the situational prompts to a behavioural response, so as to be able to vary that response. Self-control depends on the accuracy of evaluation of the prompts that cue the behaviour one wishes to change (Kalish, 1981). The long-term success rate of self-management is 15–30% (Roskies & Lazarus, 1980). Artificial stimuli or responses disturb the normal stimulus response sequence, so that the original stimulus produces a different response and/or the original response is cued by a stimulus that does not occur normally (Kalish, 1981). Stimulus or response substitution rarely attains 25% long-term cessation (Raw, 1978). Aversive techniques increase the amount of smoking beyond pleasurable limits under controlled conditions, to produce an aversive reaction which carries over to the prompts to smoke. These treatments are generally combined with self-management strategies. Multi-component interventions that include aversive techniques, such as rapid smoking, satiation or focused smoking, have shown up to 60% successful cessation, but the results are often difficult to replicate (Frederiksen & Simon, 1979).

The results of a large number of experimental trials of behavioural approaches to smoking cessation were published in the 1970s and 1980s; the techniques grew in sophistication as various treatments were compared, control groups were added and longer follow-up times were included. In the 1980s, researchers began uniformly to measure results at least one year after the end of treatment, because relapse occurs throughout the first year of abstinence and beyond. Behavioural treatments sometimes doubled or tripled the cessation rates found with other treatments or control group rates, and generally produced a cessation rate of around 25% among participants (Schwartz, 1987). Self-help guides based on cognitive–behavioural strategies were considered to have the potential to aid about 5% of smokers (Davis et al., 1984).

Even though cognitive–behavioural strategies were producing better results than placebo, there was still dissatisfaction: On an individual basis, few people out of the millions who smoked were clamouring for help, and not enough of those who did were helped to stop successfully. Adding more time or more techniques, or letting patients choose the most appropriate techniques were not improving results. On a larger scale, the process itself was being subverted by society, as it was very difficult to change a pro-tobacco environment beyond the treatment setting, showing the necessity for community-wide or national tobacco control policy.

Research and theory have, however, led to new cognitive–behavioural approaches. The concept of readiness to change was popularized by the adoption of a simplified version of a model of change called the 'transtheoretical model', developed by Prochaska and DiClemente (1983), which defined discrete steps in the process of cessation. On the basis of observational and prospective studies of smokers, the stages of change hypothesized in this model provided explanations for the puzzling failure to quit by smokers who had been warned about the health risks and given strategies for change. If smokers are at different stages of readiness to stop smoking, cognitive strategies can get them moving forwards, but they are of less use when the smokers are closer to action. Strategies that are useful to someone who is attempting to quit are of no help to someone who is for the most part satisfied to be a smoker.

The simplified stages of the model are (Velicer et al., 1995):
- pre-contemplation: no current plans to stop smoking;
- contemplation: the smoker is ambivalent, but is thinking of trying to stop in the next six months;
- preparation: the smoker plans to try to stop very soon, within the next month;
- action: the smoker has recently stopped (< 6 months);
- maintenance: the smoker has been abstinent for between six months and one year (or more). After that, the ex-smoker is considered to have moved beyond the stages of change and to have become a confirmed non-smoker.

In studies of the proportions of smokers at each stage in South Australia and in Rhode Island, California and health maintenance organizations in the United States (Kaplan et al., 1993; Velicer et al., 1995), no important difference were found in the proportions of men and women in the same settings. An estimate of the stages of readiness of smokers in the United States showed that 40% were in the pre-contemplation stage, 40% in the contemplation stage and about 20% ready either to quit on their own or to be helped to quit (Velicer *et al.*, 1995). That percentage may be lower in areas where smoking is a newer phenomenon or where there are fewer anti-smoking norms.

Readiness to change depends on personal motivation and confidence and the opportunity to consider alternative behaviour. The way behavioural approaches try to help is by augmenting individual knowledge and skills and by changing the environment so as to make it more conducive to cessation. With 80% or more of all smokers currently undecided to stop smoking, in effective individual interventions one must first determine whether the smoker is ready for the strategies and techniques that have been developed to help quit and avoid relapse. According to these measures, the challenge lies in increasing the motivation of a majority of smokers and in creating an environment that can be perceived to be conducive to change. Indeed, motivation should be considered an important intermediate outcome of cessation interventions (Abrams & Biener, 1992). In a cognitive–behavioural approach, motivation (or lack of motivation) is seen as a state that is influenced by the degree of perceived self-efficacy (personal control), the balance between perceived advantages and disadvantages of quitting, the perception of addiction and the degree of awareness of discrepancies between life goals and current behaviour.

The concept of motivational interviewing (Rollnick, 1996) has become an important tool in determining the readiness of individual smokers to stop, and aiding those in the early stages of readiness to recognize and resolve their ambivalence to stop. This consists of a non-judgmental discussion, which allows the smoker to reveal both the advantages and disadvantages to change, the interviewer reinforcing the advantages as a negotiator. Steps in a simple motivational approach for counselling by general practitioners, for example, include (Botelho, 1996):

*   identification of smoking behaviour;
*   assessment of the level of readiness;
*   provision of information;
*   externalization of the smoker's ambivalence (In responding to ambivalence, the interviewer encourages closer examination, to restructure the assessment of the possibility for change (Haynes & Ayliffe, 1991));
*   negotiation of the smoker's response to the new assessment (The motivational interview helps smokers to arrive at an informed decision that success is possible (Haynes & Ayliffe, 1991));
*   follow-up.

Barriers to change exist at every level of readiness. Smokers can be ready to change if there is motivation and an environment conducive to change. But smokers are not ready to change if there is no motivation, strong negative perceptions and reactions to withdrawal, no confidence either in themselves or in the consequences of quitting or an environment that does not prompt or sustain readiness (Cohen *et al.*, 1994). The issue of cessation goes beyond the individual, however, to look at the community and the social environment in terms of the development of a tobacco control policy. The majority of smokers are not yet ready to stop, and it can take up to 10 years for low-readiness smokers to move towards cessation (Haynes & Ayliffe, 1991). When so many people are stopping smoking that a change is visible in society, this generates a supportive environment for others to stop (Schelling, 1992).

We want to move from a situation that encourages relapse (Figure 2) to one in which the environment encourages maintenance of non-smoking (Figure 3).

Conclusions

If we want to help individuals to change, we must make it possible for them to change (Stott *et al.*, 1994), in an environment that limits tobacco company tactics to influence behaviour, an environment that permits or provides a sense of personal worth independent of tobacco use and includes non-smoking as a positive value.

Figure 2. Environmental barriers to cessation

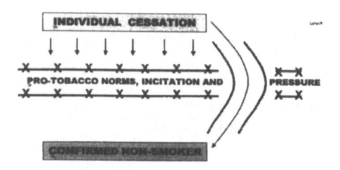

Figure 3. Environment conducive to cessation

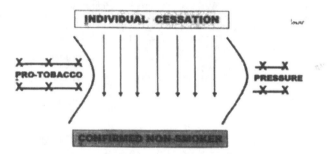

Behavioural approaches encourage change towards cessation by encouraging a re-evaluation of the stimuli and consequences surrounding smoking, by encouraging new responses and by making the environment more conducive to cessation. These strategies can help individuals, especially when they are supported at the community and national level.

References

Abrams, D.B. & Biener, L. (1992) Motivational characteristics of smokers at the workplace: A public health challenge. *Prev. Med.*, **21**, 679–687

Agency for Health Care Policy and Research. Smoking Cessation (1996) Clinical practice guideline. *J. Am. Med. Assoc.*, **275**, 1270

Botelho, R.J. (1996) When 'quit smoking' advice doesn't work: Use motivational approaches. In: Richmond, R., ed., *Education Medical Students About Tobacco: Planning and Implementation*, Paris: International Union Against Tuberculosis and Lung Disease

Cohen, S.J., Halvorson, H.W. & Gosselink, C.A. (1994) Changing physician behavior to improve disease prevention. *Prev. Med.*, **23**, 284–291

Davis, A.L., Faust, R. & Odentlich, M. (1984) Self-help smoking cessation and maintenance programs: A comparative study with 12-month follow-up by the American Lung Association. *Am. J. Public Health*, **74**, 1212–1217

Elder, J.P. (1987) Applications of behavior modification to health promotion in the developing world. *Soc. Sci. Med.*, **24**, 335–349

Enright, S.J. (1997) Cognitive behaviour therapy—Clinical applications. *Br. Med. J.*, **314**, 1811–1816

Fisher, E.B., Haire-Joshu, D., Moregan, G.D., Rehberg, H. & Rost, K. (1990) Smoking and smoking cessation. *Am. Rev. Respir. Dis.*, **142**, 702–720

Frederiksen, L.W. & Simon, S.J. (1979) Clinical modification of smoking behavior. In: Davidson, D.S., ed., *Modification of Pathological Behavior*, New York: Gardner Press

Giovino, G.A., Henningfield, J.E., Tomar, S.L., Escobedo, L.G. & Slade, J. (1995) Epidemiology of tobacco use and dependence. *Epidemiol. Rev.*, **17**, 48–65

Haxby, D.G. (1995) Treatment of nicotine dependence. *Am. J. Health-Syst. Pharm.*, **52**, 265–281

Haynes, P. & Ayliffe, G. (1991) Locus of control of behaviour: Is high externality associated with substance misuse? *Br. J. Addict.*, **86**, 1111–1117

Kalish, H.I. (1981) *From Behavioral Science to Behavior Modification*, New York: McGraw-Hill

Kaplan, R.M., Pierce, J.P., Gilpin, E.A., Johnson, M. & Bal, D.G. (1993) Stages of smoking cessation: The 1990 California Tobacco Survey. *Tobacco Control*, **2**, 139–144

Nolan, R.P. (1995) How can we help patients to initiate change? *Can. J. Cardiol.*, **11** (Suppl. A), 16A–19A

Orlandi, M.A. (1996) The challenge of changing health-related behavior. *Prev. Med.*, **25**, 51–53

Parker, S.R. & Lenfant, C. (1986) Educational and behavioral approaches to the prevention and control of lung disease. In: Murray, J.F. & Nadel, J.A, eds, *Textbook of Respiratory Medicine*, New York: Saunders

Pechacek, T.F. & Danaher, B.G. (1979) How and why people quit smoking. A cognitive–behavioral analysis. In: Dendall, P.C. & Hollon, S.D., eds, *Cognitive–Behavioral Interventions—Theory, Research and Procedures*, New York: Academic Press

Perkins, K.A. (1995) Individual variability in responses to nicotine. *Behav. Genet.*, **25**, 119–132

Prochaska, J.O. & DiClemente, C.C. (1983) Stages and processes of self-change of smoking: Toward an integrative model of change. *J. Consul. Clin. Psychol.*, **51**, 390–395

Raw, M. (1978) The treatment of cigarette dependence. *Res. Adv. Alcohol Drug Problems.*, **4**, 441–485

Rollnick, S. (1996) Behaviour change in practice: Targeting individuals. *Int. J. Obesity*, **20** (Suppl. 1), S22–S26

Roskies, E. & Lazarus, R.S. (1980) Coping theory and the teaching of coping skills. In: Davidson, P.O. & Davidson, S.M., eds, *Behavioral Medicine: Changing Health Lifestyles*, New York: Brunner/Mazel

Schelling, T.C. (1992) Addictive drugs: The cigarette experience. *Science*, **255**, 430–433

Schwartz, J.L. (1987) *Review and Evaluation of Smoking Cessation Methods: The United States and Canada, 1977–1985* (NIH Pub. No. 87-2940), Washington DC: Government Printing Office

Slama K. (1997) L'addiction à la nicotine et la dépendance psychologique. In: Martinet, Y. & Bohadana, A., eds, *Le Tabagisme—De la Prévention au Sevrage*, Paris: Masson

Slama, K. (1997) *Tobacco Control and Prevention. A Guide for Low-Income Countries*, Paris: International Union Against Tuberculosis and Lung Disease (in press).

Stott, N.C.H., Kinnersley, P. & Rollnick, S. (1994) The limits to health promotion. They lie in individuals' readiness to change. *Br. Med. J.*, **309**, 971–972

Velicer, W.F., Fava, J.L., Prochaska, J.O., Abrams, D.B., Emmons, K.M. & Pierce, J.P. (1995) Distribution of smokers by stage in three representative samples. *Prev. Med.*, **24**, 401–411

Self-efficacy theory, locus of control and smoking cessation among Asians

W.C. Andress

Health Promotion/Wellness, Hong Kong Adventist Hospital, Hong Kong SAR, China

A universal dilemma associated with smoking cessation programmes is the fairly high rates of recidivism. While some interventions may boast of 70, 80 and even 90% success rates at programme end-points, repeated assessments at three-month and six-month follow-up generally show a high degree of recidivism. As much as 40% of the relapses may occur within the first week after treatment (Cummings *et al.*, 1985). More than 100 years ago, the American humourist Mark Twain recognized this problem when he declared, "Stopping smoking is the easiest thing in the world. Why, I've done it a thousand times." Twain's innuendo demonstrates the physiological and psychological addictiveness of tobacco. The tobacco industry has known this for years, and hence its advertisements have been multi-faceted, targeting not only the cognitive domain but the physiological, behavioural and psychological dimensions as well. The industry's powerful advertisements accentuate sexuality, femininity, masculinity, pleasure, romance, financial success, social popularity and, yes, even health.

Unfortunately, anti-tobacco interventions have too often been focused almost entirely on cognition, assuming that if the smoker is given enough data on morbidity and mortality he or she will quit. A bland black-and-white warning label declaring "Smoking is deadly and may cause heart disease, cancer, and a host of other problems for you, your spouse, and your kids" cannot compete affectively (nor effectively) with an attractively designed package or a billboard displaying a four-colour image of masculinity, excitement, success, fame and glamour, no matter how bold the print.

It is now known that the process of quitting smoking involves several stages. Smokers go from pre-contemplation to contemplation, from contemplation to action, and from action to either maintenance or, much too often, relapse (Department of Health and Human Services, 1989). In 1980, Marlatt and Gordon described a theoretical model to predict reactions to relapse in addictive behaviour (Figure 1) According to the model, relapse is most likely to occur when addicts are confronted with high-risk situations in which they lack the skills or the knowledge to deal with the situation. A critical finding was what they termed 'the abstinence violation effect'. When an initial 'slip' occurs, if the overwhelming guilt and sense of lack of willpower produced combine with the perceived positive effects of the substance, a full-blown relapse is practically guaranteed.

Application of the paradigm to smoking shows that primary relapse prevention should be directed towards providing the smoker with the coping mechanisms needed to deal with high-risk situations. A person who is capable of not smoking, even in high-risk situations, has increased self-efficacy, thereby minimizing the chances of relapse; if coping skills are lacking or ineffectual, self-efficacy decreases, thereby heightening the probability of using tobacco 'just this once'. At this point the 'abstinence violation effect' becomes operational. The ex-smoker begins to have feelings of guilt and remorse. If at the same time some personal satisfaction is received from the cigarette, in all probability a complete relapse will occur. Thus, self-efficacy can be crucial in determining whether or not a smoker will be successful in quitting.

Self-efficacy and locus of control

The self-efficacy theory was developed within the framework of social-learning theory by Albert Bandura (1977) at Stanford University (United States). According to the theory, outcomes are largely determined by personal expectancies, which to a great degree determine how much effort people will expend and how long they will persist in the face of obstacles and aversive behaviour. Researchers have attempted to develop a self-efficacy tool that would predict the likelihood of future relapse among smokers. The premise is that if such individuals can be identified, appropriate individualized strategies can be provided, thereby heightening the probability of a reduction in recidivism during the first year after treatment. Several studies (e.g. Condiotte & Lichtenstein, 1981; DiClemente, 1981; Prochaska et al., 1982; Brod & Hall, 1984; DiClemente et al., 1985; Yates & Thain, 1985) consistently demonstrated the robustness of the construct of the self-efficacy theory. When administered at programme end-points, self-efficacy scales can assist in predicting abstainers and relapsers up to several months after treatment. Successful quitters consistently report higher self-efficacy than do non-quitters.

Figure 1. Cognitive behavioural model of the relapse process

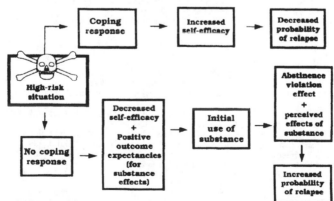

From Marlatt & Gordon (1980)

In the mid-1980s, while I was a graduate student in public health, I conducted a study to test whether the usefulness of self-efficacy theory as a predictor of future relapse could be generalized cross-culturally to a homogeneous population that was collectivist, rather than individualistic. The study, conducted on 48 Japanese smokers, failed to demonstrate this hypothesis (W.C. Andress, unpublished data). This does not necessarily mean that self-efficacy is invalid as a measurement tool for use in Japan or other parts of Asia, although that is possible. The method contained several possible confounders including a small sample size, a confidence questionnaire in which the five-point Likert scale was probably too narrow and indications of an 'overconfidence bias' on the part of some participants. It is probably more significant that a measurement for 'locus of control' was not included in the study.

'Health locus of control' was introduced by Rotter (1966) to describe how expectations are under the control of oneself or of others. 'Internal control' is the belief that one is responsible for or has control over influences on health. In contrast, the externally controlled person believes that fate or the influence of powerful others controls his or her destiny. Some investigators suggest that cessation is related to internal locus of control (James *et al.*, 1965; Chambliss & Murray, 1979). Prochaska *et al.* (1982) suggested that since relapsers have a tendency to depend on the social environment, those who are successful in the long term have a stronger internal locus of control. Studies based on locus of control scales have consistently shown that oriental Asians (Dyal, 1984; Smith *et al.*, 1995), in particular Japanese (Bond & Tornatzky, 1973; McGinnies *et al.*, 1974; Parsons & Scneider, 1974; Evans, 1981), score more externally than do their American counterparts. This being the case, it may be that western approaches to cessation will not be as effective in Asian societies.

A Johari window comparing locus of control with self-efficacy suggests that those with high self-efficacy and an internal locus of control will be most successful in quitting smoking, while those with low self-efficacy and an external locus of control will be most prone to relapse. It remains for further research, especially among Asian populations, to determine if indeed this is true in practice. In the meantime, scales of efficacy and locus of control can assist the health-care provider in designing and implementing cessation strategies that are client-specific and thereby improve long-term outcomes of cessation programmes.

References

Bandura, A. (1977) Self-efficacy: Toward a unifying model of behavioral change. *Psych. Rev.*, **84**, 191–215

Bond, M.H. & Tornatzky, L.G. (1973) Locus of control in students from Japan and the United States: Dimensions and levels of response. *Psychologia*, **16**, 209–213

Brod, M.I. & Hall, S.M. Joiners and non-joiners in smoking treatment: A comparison of pyschosocial variables. *Addict. Behav.*, **9**, 217–221

Chambliss, C. & Murray, E.J. (1979) Cognitive procedures for smoking reduction: Symptom attribution versus efficacy attribution. *Cognitive Ther. Res.*, **3**, 91–95

Condiotte, M.M. & Lichtenstein, E. (1981) Self-efficacy and relapse in smoking cessation programs. *J. Consult. Clin. Psych.*, **49**, 648–658

Cummings, K.M., Jaen, C.R. & Giovino, G. (1985) Circumstances surrounding relapse in a group of recent exsmokers. *Prev. Med.*, **14**, 195–202

Department of Health and Human Services (1989) *Reducing the Health Consequences of Smoking: 25 Years of Progress. A Report of the Surgeon General* (DHHS Publ No. (CDC) 89–8411), Washington DC: Public Health Services, Centers for Disease Control, Office on Smoking and Health

DiClemente, C.C. (1981) Self-efficacy and smoking cessation maintenance: A preliminary report. *Cognitive Ther. Res.*, **5**, 175–187

DiClemente, C.C., Prochaska, J. & Gibertini, M. (1985) Self-efficacy and the stages of self-change of smoking. *Cognitive Ther. Res.*, **9**, 181–200

Dyal, J.A. (1984) Cross-cultural research with the locus of control construct. In: Lefcourt, H., ed., *Research with the Locus of Control Construct*, New York: Academic Press, Vol. 3, pp. 209–306

Evans, H.M. (1981) Internal–external locus of control and word association: Research with Japanese and American students. *J. Cross-cultural Psychol.*, **12**, 372–382

James, W.H., Woodruff, A.B. & Werner, W. (1965) Effect of internal and external control upon changes in smoking behavior. *J. Consult. Psychol.*, **29**, 184–186

Marlatt, G.A. & Gordon, J.R. (1980) Determinants of relapse: Implications for the maintenance of behavior change. In: Davidson, P.O. & Davidson, S.M., eds, *Behavioral Medicine: Changing Health Lifestyles*. New York: Brunner/Mazel

McGinnies, E.I., Nordholm, C., Ward, C.D. & Bhanthumnavin, D. (1974) Sex and cultural differences in
    perceived locus of control among students in five countries. *J. Consult. Clin. Psychol.*, **42**, 451–455
Parsons, O.A. & Schneider, J.M. (1974) Locus of control in university students from eastern and western
    societies. *J. Consult. Clin. Psychol.*, **42**, 456–461
Prochaska, J.O., Crim, P., Lapsanski, D., Martel, L. & Reid, P. (1982) Self-change processes, self-efficacy
    and self-concept in relapse and maintenance of cessation of smoking. *Psychol. Rep.*, **51**, 983–990
Rotter, J.B. (1966) Generalized expectancies for internal versus external control of reinforcement. *Psychol.
    Monogr. Gen. Appl.*, **80**, 1
Smith, P.B., Trompenaars, F. & Dugan, S. (1995) The Rotter locus of control scale in 43 countries: A test
    of cultural relativity. *Int. J. Psych.*, **30**, 377–400
Yates, A.J. & Thain, J. Self-efficacy as a predictor of relapse following voluntary cessation of smoking.
    Addict. Behav., **10**, 291–298

Quitline®

P. McCabe

QUIT, London, United Kingdom

Introduction

QUIT is a British non-governmental organization dedicated to helping smokers quit. It was formed in 1926 as the National Society of Non-Smokers. It has a proud history of pioneering new initiatives in tobacco control and smoking cessation. Today, QUIT's focus is providing practical services to smokers who want to quit. We are not a 'finger-wagging' organization: we don't believe in lecturing people. Instead, we offer support, understanding and practical help.

QUIT's flagship service is the Quitline®, our telephone help-line, staffed by qualified counsellors fully trained in smoking cessation. Quitline® was launched in 1990 and received 10 000 calls in its first year. The Health Education Authority in England used the Quitline® number to support its television advertisements featuring the well-known British comedian John Cleese from January to March in 1993, 1994 and 1995. Over those three-month periods, the volume of calls increased from 13 000 in 1993 to 22 000 in 1994 and 39 000 in 1995: an increase of over 200% in three years.

Independent evaluation of the Quitline® service demonstrated high customer satisfaction rates and significant changes in smoking behaviour. The service came under criticism, however, because it was available only on a London number, which callers had to pay for. This meant that the service was expensive for callers in other parts of Britain and could not be afforded by many smokers with low incomes.

Development

In 1995, our partners, the Health Education Authority, took the important decision to fund Quitline® as a free phone service and to fund it all year round. The free phone number was promoted on new television advertisements between December 1995 and March 1996, with a dramatic effect on the number of calls. During the 1996 campaign, 184 000 calls were answered in three months, an increase of 378% in only one year. Thus, during its first year Quitline® received 10 000 calls, and on No-Smoking Day in 1996 we answered more calls than that in one day alone! In 1994, we were concerned that we were able to answer only 50% of the calls made; in 1997, despite the massive increase in calls, we improved that performance to over 90% of calls.

The increase in demand continues to grow. Quitline® received nearly 500 000 calls in 1997, making it, we think, the busiest smoking cessation help-line in the world. We knew we were achieving recognition when *The Sun*, a popular tabloid, ran a cartoon about Quitline®.

Training

Improving the quality of the training we offer our counsellors is of vital importance in continuing to develop the service. QUIT employs over 100 fully qualified counsellors whom we train in smoking cessation. This year, we launched the QUIT Certificate in Smoking Cessation and Telephone Counselling. The course consists of 17 training modules consisting of lectures given at Guy's Hospital Medical School in London by leading experts from the United Kingdom and overseas. The lectures given are on the health consequences of smoking (Professor John Moxam, Professor of Respiratory Medicine, King's College, London), smoking addiction (Professor Robert West, St George's Hospital Medical School, London), smoking among children and adolescents (Dr Anne Charlton, Professor of Cancer Health Education, University of Manchester), smoking and pregnancy (Anthony Kennedy, Consultant in Obstetrics, St Thomas' Hospital Medical School, London), nicotine withdrawal (Gay Sutherland, Maudsley Hospital Smokers' Clinic, London), smoking cessation methods (Dr Peter Hajek, Head of Psychology Section, The London Hospital Medical College, London) and nicotine replacement therapy (Karl Olov Fagerström, Scientific Information, Pharmacia and Upjohn, Sweden). The QUIT Certificate is awarded on successful completion of the course, a written examination and a case study and 300 supervised hours of smoking cessation telephone counselling.

New initiatives

On the basis of evaluations that have shown consistently high consumer satisfaction, the Health Education Authority has committed itself to continued funding of the service. The success of Quitline® gave us the impetus to pilot two further services.

There are numerous minority groups in the United Kingdom, including, for example, 1.3 million people originating from Bangladesh, India and Pakistan. The prevalence of smoking in many minority groups is higher than the national average: for example, 40% of Bangladeshi men are regular smokers. Many people in these communities cannot reach existing smoking cessation services because of cultural and language barriers. With support and advice from the minority communities themselves, QUIT is launching Quitline® in Bengali (Sylheti), Gujurati, Hindi, Punjabi and Urdu. This initiative is being funded by the British Heart Foundation—an excellent example of two non-governmental organizations working in effective partnership. QUIT has also successfully tested a Cantonese phone line, and we are raising funds to provide the service for free.

The second new initiative is our Pregnancy Quitline®. In the United Kingdom, one-third of pregnant women smoke. Only one in four succeed in stopping during pregnancy, and most of those start again after the birth. Pregnancy Quitline® will offer a dedicated, one-to-one smoking cessation service. By agreement with the pregnant women, our specially trained counsellors will help them to quit and call them regularly throughout and after their pregnancy. The service offered will be flexible, personal and accessible and will provide positive, empathetic help. This project is being tested over two years in the Doncaster Health Authority in the north of England. The service is funded by Cosatto Cots and the Doncaster Health Authority and is a good example of a partnership between the private, public and voluntary sectors.

Both of these intiatives will be evaluated formally, and we will be glad to share the results with colleagues in the future. We have been pleased to welcome colleagues from many countries who have come to see Quitline® operate, and on each occasion we have learnt a great deal from each other.

Quitline in Thailand

B. Ritthiphakdee & S. Suwanrasami

Action on Smoking and Health Foundation, Bangkok, Thailand

Ring 1600 from anywhere in Thailand, and you'll reach Quitline. Operated by the Action on Smoking and Health Foundation, Quitline is Thailand's only telephone counselling service for people who want to quit smoking. Quitline started as a dedicated service in 1993 and receives about 5500 calls a year. It employs trained counsellors and a telephone answering machine for callers out of hours.

The service is anonymous if the caller so wishes, but if he or she wishes to receive a 'quit kit' or other information, the name and address must be given. Callers who leave their names and addresses are followed up one month later and encouraged to describe their experience in giving up, the problems thay faced and their success. Those who have given up are rewarded with a congratulatory card, a certificate and a non-smoking key chain. Those who were less successful are sent cards of encouragement to cheer them along as they try to quit.

We have found that those who are 100% committed to giving up when they call us are the most successful. Not everyone has such strong will power, and many require further encouragement and follow-up. Quitline has helped many Thais to stop smoking. The best advertisement for Quitline is word of mouth from successful ex-smokers themselves.

Tabac Info Línea: Implementation and first results

T. Marín, A. Garcia & J. Gonzàlez

Catalan Association for Smoking Prevention, Barcelona, Catalonia, Spain

Catalonia is an autonomous Spanish community with a democratic Government represented by a parliamentary monarchy. The official languages are Catalan and Spanish. Spain is the fourteenth largest producer of tobacco in the world and the fourth in Europe, producing 7650 million cigarettes per year. The daily consumption of cigarettes in Spain is 150 million; 36% of the Spanish population smokes, representing 48% of men and 25% of women. The prevalence of smoking among women has risen to 28% in Catalonia. The annual cost of smoking is equivalent to US$ 800 million in Catalonia and US$ 4 thousand million in Spain.

The Catalan Association for Smoking Prevention is a private, independent, non-profit association registered in Barcelona in May 1996 and presented to the Spanish public in March 1997. It is made up of specialists and multidisciplinary professionals such as psychologists, doctors, nurses, lawyers, journalists, economists and teachers in an intersectorial alliance, working towards comprehensive tobacco control. The Association was created in order to conduct research and development and to spread information about effective tobacco control. The main objectives are to prevent tobacco use, especially among children, adolescents and pregnant women, and to provide protection from environmental tobacco smoke and Help for Smoking Cessation. Another aim is to promote collaborative, coordinated activities at national and international levels. The first sponsored project was Tabac Info Linea, with the objective of monitoring progress towards our goals.

Tabac Info Línea (+34 02 11 38 30)

This is the operational tool for communication between people and the Catalan Association for Smoking Prevention. It consists of a telephone line answered by well-trained staff who speak both official languages. Smokers, non-smokers and passive smokers can call and receive realistic information and materials by telephone, fax, mail or e-mail at no cost. The line offers information and proactive personalized attention, filtering and clarifying the most appropriate and effective answers to questions on the stated objectives of the Association: prevention (counselling and programmes), protection (advice on legislation) and cessation (existing public and private services and treatment by telephone). Information on cessation is requested by 85% of callers, information on prevention by 13% and protection by 2%. Telephone treatment for cessation is given in 63% of cases, and public or private services are recommended in 22% of cases. The average age of the callers is 40 years, a time at which the negative consequences of smoking become problematic.

Tabac Info Línea is the service with the lowest cost-effectiveness relationship for tobacco control in all of Spain. It was publicized by a press release in March 1997 and followed-up through mass-media contacts. Two publications have been issued, and Governmental and non-governmental institutional networks have been established.

Results of evaluation at three months

Between March and May 1997, there were more than 2000 telephone calls. The average time spent with the callers was 5 min. Of the callers, 51% were men and 49% women. Of smokers who used Tabac Info Línea as a quit line, 85% smoked a daily average of 25 cigarettes and had previosuly tried to quit once to three times. They showed high nicotine dependence and reported various health disorders linked to smoking. People called from all over Spain, but mainly from the north and the islands.

Conclusions

Tabac Info Línea is a welcome tool, especially for middle-aged people, women and highly addicted smokers. It has allowed the creation and improvement of networking between institutions, the mass media and the Catalan Association for Smoking Prevention. Despite the early stage of development of the Association, we have observed a gradual but large improvement in awareness and acceptance of this initiative. Knowledge of this local success could stimulate actions at other levels. The significant decline in smoking prevalence among men and young people of each sex provides encouragement to pursue our efforts, although we must not forget that the prevalence of smoking in Spain is still higher than in other western European countries.

Smoking cessation programme in Catalonia, Spain: A 10-year retrospective study

D. Marín Tuyà, J. Gonzàlez Quintana & M.J. Consuegra Manzanares

Unit of Smoking, Corporació Sanitària Clinic, Barcelona, Spain

Background

We evaluated relapse rates among people who had followed our smoking cessation programme for 10 years. The programme combined group therapy, nicotine chewing-gum and behavioural assistance. Each group consisted of 15–20 people, with no preselection except for the exclusion of people with drug dependence and other mental disorders. Before the group sessions were begun, the amount of chewing-gum that would be needed was determined by the Fagerström test and from answers to a questionnaire based on that of Horn and Russell and validated for the Spanish population by our team. Variables such as motivation, smoking environments, previous attempts to quit, psychological dependence, weights, carbon monoxide concentration, sex and age were also registered. The behavioural assistance included recommendations on diet, new habits and relaxation and discussion of advantages, strategies and the prevention of relapse. Each group met 10 times per year.

The programme was considered to have been successful for people who were not smoking at the end of one year.

Subjects and methods

A total of 903 people of an average age of 45 years were treated between May 1983 and January 1993 in 62 therapy groups. Their average cigarette consumption was 30 cigarettes per day. Of the total, 530 (58%) were men and 376 (42%) were women. The rate of succesful quitting was 45% (406 people).

After one year, the participants were telephoned at various hours on various days and asked to respond to one of two questionnaires, depending on whether they had relapsed or not. The questionnaire for people who had not relapsed included questions on positive changes, health habits and quality of life, whereas the one for people who had relapsed included questions on attempts to give up smoking, health, quality of life, relapse situations and whether they still wished to quit. The response rate was 53%, with a similar distribution of men and women as in the original sample. The main reasons for non-response were no answer, changed telephone number and change of residence.

Results

The main results are that 43% were no longer smoking, although the treatment had been considered successful for 48%. Of people for whom the treatment had been successful, 31% had maintained their abstinence and 17% had relapsed; 12% of the participants for whom the treatment had been considered unsuccessful had given up afterwards and were not currently smoking. Of the current smokers, 85% said they still wanted to give up smoking, but 20% needed help, 19% said they 'couldn't quite' give up and 29% said they couldn't because the time was not right, they had family problems or were working.

With reference to quality of life, 59% reported that it had improved since they had stopped smoking, 10% felt more fit, and 9.3% had experienced positive changes in their lifestyle.

Discussion

We found a relationship between successful treatment and abstinence one year later. The quality of life of the non-smokers had improved, and 85% of the relapsed smokers still wished to quit. The last-named group should be the main target group of therapy.

Evaluation of a multi-component behavioural programme for smoking cessation in Spain after 36 months' followup, with survival analysis

E. Becoña[1], F.L. Vázquez[1] & A. Montes[2]

[1]*Faculty of Psychology, Department of Clinical Psychology and Psychobiology and* [2]*Faculty of Medicine, Department of Preventive Medicine and Public Health, University of Santiago de Compostela, Santiago de Compostela, Galicia, Spain*

Abstract

The aim of this study was to apply the method of survival analysis to a sample of 175 smokers who smoked ≥ 10 cigarettes per day, in order to describe and evaluate treatment outcomes and to identify critical periods for intervention. Ex-smokers were followed for 36 months. In addition, subgroups of individuals who relapsed during various high-risk periods were identified and compared to determine any relationship with individual factors (demographics and smoking history). At the end of treatment, the rate of abstinence was 69%. The median 'survival time' was 4.94 months. Only consumption before treatment was related to relapse.

Introduction

The consumption of tobacco is considered to be like the use of any other drug and continues to be the leading cause of premature morbidity and mortality in Spain (Peto *et al.*, 1994). Although smoking is an addictive behaviour, the techniques of cessation treatment have improved the rates of abstinence considerably. Nevertheless, there have been few studies of the efficacy of behavioural smoking cessation programmes based on long-term follow-up (Glasgow & Lichtenstein, 1987; Vázquez & Becoña, 1996). This is due partly to the practical difficulties posed by long-term follow-up studies, whether on smoking or any other behaviour. In the case of smoking cessation, however, long-term follow-up is particularly important, in view of the known tendency to relapse, as we still do not understand this process in ex-smokers in the long term. Moreover, 37% of smokers who are abstinent for 12 months may, at some stage in their life, eventually relapse (US Department of Health and Human Services, 1990).

The aim of this study was to apply the methods of survival analysis to smoking cessation, to describe and evaluate treatment outcomes and to identify critical periods for intervention with a multi-component behavioural package.

Method

The sample consisted of 80 men (46%) and 95 women (54%), who were participating in the smoking cessation programme at the University of Santiago de Compostela, Spain. They were recruited by press and radio advertisements. The mean age was 32.3 years (SD, 9.4; range, 19–64 years). The average consumption of cigarettes before treatment was 27.3 per day (SD, 10.0; range, 10–55 cigarettes), and the self-monitoring baseline rate was 19.4 cigarettes per day (SD, 9.3). The mean nicotine intake per cigarette was 1.06 mg (SD, 0.14; range, 0.7–1.4 mg).

The smokers were offered a multi-component behavioural programme (Becoña, 1993) which included a motivational contract (a signed contract of their rights and duties and a refundable deposit), self-monitoring, information on smoking, nicotine fading (in which subjects changed their brands each week to ones containing progressively less nicotine, with 30% reduction per week for three weeks), stimulus control procedure, avoidance of withdrawal symptoms and physiological feedback (knowledge of amount of carbon monoxide in expired air).

Before beginning treatment, the participants completed a form giving demographic information (e.g. sex, age) and measures of smoke intake (cigarettes smoked per day, expired carbon monoxide). They were then randomly placed into one of 17 treatment groups and attended six 1-h sessions over six weeks of a smoking cessation programme run by two experienced therapists.

After finishing the treatment, the subjects were contacted in person at 6 and 12 months. Abstinence was corroborated with a Smokerlyser EC 50 expired carbon monoxide indicator (Bedfont Instruments, Sittingbourne, Kent, United Kingdom) with a cut-off point of 9 ppm. At 36 months' follow-up, all subjects were interviewed over the telephone, and abstinence was corroborated from the reports of informants.

Survival analysis was used to describe the relapse function. The life-table method was used to calculate the cumulated probability of being abstinent at the time *t+1* at the start of study and the hazard function (conditioned probability by unit of time of relapse at moment *t* if the subject was abstinent until the previous moment). The Kaplan-Meier procedure was used to determine differences in relapse by demographic variables and smoking history. Cox regression analysis was used to model an equation to explain the relapse curve as a function of the chosen variables.

Results

At the end of treatment, the abstinence rate was 69% ($n = 120$). The life-table analysis of the cumulated probability of being abstinent and the hazard function are showed in Table 1. The probability of relapse was increased at months 11, 23 and 35 of follow-up, i.e. 1, 2 and 3 years after quitting. When sex, age and initial consumption were introduced into a Cox regression analysis, only consumption was related to relapse, as shown in Table 2. Kaplan-Meier analysis for initial consumption is showed in Figure 1. The pattern of relapse is similar in all groups but is related to initial consumption. The critical period for relapse is the first six months in each category of consumption.

Table 1. Life table of cumulated probability of not smoking

Interval start time	Proportion surviving	Cumulative proportion surviving at end	Probability density	Hazard rate
0.0	0.8326	0.8326	0.1674	0.1826
1.0	0.8283	0.6897	0.1430	0.1878
2.0	0.8902	0.6140	0.0757	0.1161
3.0	0.9041	0.5551	0.0589	0.1007
4.0	0.8939	0.4962	0.0589	0.1120
5.0	0.8983	0.4458	0.0505	0.1071
6.0	1.0000	0.4458	0.0000	0.0000
7.0	0.9245	0.4121	0.0336	0.0784
8.0	1.0000	0.4121	0.0000	0.0000
9.0	0.9796	0.4037	0.0084	0.0206
10.0	1.0000	0.4037	0.0000	0.0000
11.0	0.8750	0.3532	0.0505	0.1333
12.0	1.0000	0.3532	0.0000	0.0000
13.0	1.0000	0.3532	0.0000	0.0000
14.0	1.0000	0.3532	0.0000	0.0000
15.0	1.0000	0.3532	0.0000	0.0000
16.0	1.0000	0.3532	0.0000	0.0000
17.0	0.9524	0.3364	0.0168	0.0488
18.0	1.0000	0.3364	0.0000	0.0000
19.0	1.0000	0.3364	0.0000	0.0000
20.0	1.0000	0.3364	0.0000	0.0000
21.0	1.0000	0.3364	0.0000	0.0000
22.0	1.0000	0.3364	0.0000	0.0000
23.0	0.8500	0.2860	0.0505	0.1622
24.0	1.0000	0.2860	0.0000	0.0000
25.0	0.9412	0.2691	0.0168	0.0606
26.0	1.0000	0.2691	0.0000	0.0000
27.0	1.0000	0.2691	0.0000	0.0000
28.0	1.0000	0.2691	0.0000	0.0000
29.0	0.9688	0.2607	0.0084	0.0317
30.0	1.0000	0.2607	0.0000	0.0000
31.0	0.9032	0.2355	0.0252	0.1017
32.0	1.0000	0.2355	0.0000	0.0000
33.0	0.9286	0.2187	0.0168	0.0741
34.0	0.9615	0.2103	0.0084	0.0392
35.0	0.7857	0.1652	0.0451	0.2400

Survival time in months

Table 2. Cox regression model of reasons for relapse

Variable	Instant hazard rate	95% confidence interval	
		Lower	Upper
Pre-treatment consumption (cigarettes per day)			
< 12	1	–	–
12–21.9	1.82	1.07	3.10
≥ 22	2.78	1.56	4.96
Sex			
Female	1	–	–
Male	1.27	0.83	1.95
Age (years)			
≤ 25	1	–	–
26–30	1.10	0.61	1.97
31–38	1.25	0.071	2.18
> 38	1.20	0.66	2.21

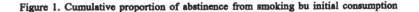

Figure 1. Cumulative proportion of abstinence from smoking bu initial consumption

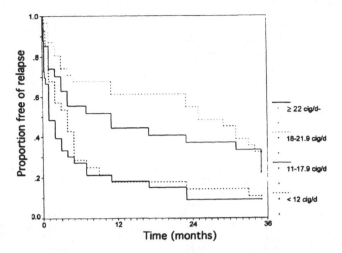

Discussion

The results of this study are similar to those of previous studies (e.g. Glasgow & Lichtenstein, 1987). Our results are particularly encouraging in view of the predominance of heavy smokers in the sample (mean number of cigarettes per day before treatment, 27.3); as is well known, smoking cessation programmes are usually less effective for such subjects, particularly in the long term.

In our study, the first six months were a critical period for relapse: more than half of those who had quit at the end of treatment resumed smoking during this period. Only consumption before treatment was inversely related to relapse. Although it is clear that the relapse curve decelerates, relapse continues to occur beyond six months' follow-up, in contrast to the findings of Hunt and Bespalec (1974). We also observed, as did Glasgow and Lichtenstein (1987), an empirical relationship between initial cessation and long-term success. Participants who had not achieved abstinence by the end of the intervention programme did not become abstinent over the follow-up.

The need for longer-term follow-up becomes more pressing as initial outcomes improve. Long-term abstinence may be a moot point in treatments in which minimal abstinence is obtained at short-term follow-up, but treatments that achieve good initial results should be closely monitored to assess the durability of the effect.

References

Becoña, E. (1993) *Programa para dejar de fumar* [Smoking cessation programme], Santiago de Compostela: Servicio de Publicaciones de la Universidad de Santiago de Compostela

Glasgow, R.E. & Lichtenstein, E. (1987) Long-term effects of behavioral smoking cessation interventions. *Behav. Ther.*, **18**, 297–324

Hunt, W.A. & Bespalec, D.A. (1974) An evaluation of current methods of modifying smoking behavior. *J. Clin. Psychol.*, **30**, 431–438

Peto, R., López, A.D., Boreham, J., Thun, M. & Heath C. (1994) *Mortality from Smoking in Developed Countries 1950–2000*, Oxford: Oxford University Press

US Department of Health and Human Services (1990) *The Health Benefits of Smoking Cessation. A Report of the Surgeon General*, Rockville, Maryland

Vázquez, F.L & Becoña, E. (1996) Los programas conductuales para dejar de fumar. Eficacia a 2–6 años de seguimiento [The behavioural smoking cessation programmes; Efficacy at 2–6 years follow-up]. *Adicciones*, **8**, 369–392

Smoking cessation intervention with a multiple-component programme for the general population of Gran Canaria, Spain: Evaluation after six months' follow-up

A. López[1], M. López[1], J.R. Calvo[1], M.Torresi[1], J.M. Segura[1], M.C. Navarro[1], J. Calvo[1], M.P. García[2], C. Jiménez[3], A. Ramos[3], O. Rojas[3] & S. Solano[3]

[1]University of Las Palmas de Gran Canaria, [2]University of La Coruña, [3]Hospital de la Princesa, Madrid, Spain

Introduction

After publication of the first report of the United States Surgeon General in 1964, the role of tobacco in the aetiology of a wide range of illnesses became firmly established. The magnitude of the problem has grown, and today smoking is considered to be the main cause of preventable diseases and premature deaths in developed countries. According to R. Peto, 40 000 deaths in Spain are estimated to be caused by tobacco. In the Canary Islands, smoking kills more than 600 people every year only from tobacco-related cancers. Approximately 70% of smokers report that they would like to quit smoking, and one-third of these say they have tried at least once during the previous year, yet the prevalence of former smokers in Spain is 15%.

In Spain, 36% of the population aged ≥ 16 smokes. Of these, 48% are male and 25% female, but the increase is most evident in the female population. In the Canary Islands, 37% of men and 26% of women smoke (Encuesta Nacional de Salud, 1993). The University of Las Palmas de Gran Canaria has therefore been organizing smoking cessation courses aimed at the general population since November 1995. A multiple-component method including progressive reductions in nicotine and tar levels was chosen because of the excellent results obtained by other authors and because it can be used in populations in which other methods are contraindicated. Our objectives were to adapt the programme to our population and to assess the results six months after the beginning of the programme.

Materials and methods

The Unit has treated 68 people, with a six-month follow-up. The participants were recruited by responding to posters placed in pharmacies, which were brought up to date for each course, or to advertisements in the local press and on several radio stations which we approached to explain our activities. There were no previous selection criteria, and all people who stated that they wanted to quit smoking were accepted. Before the first session, they complete a questionnaire eliciting sociodemographic variables, smoking habits and behaviour, consumption and a clinical report.

The mean age of the participants was 40 (range, 21–67); 26 were men (38%) and 42 women (62%); 63% considered themselves to be middle-class, 24% upper-middle class, 8.8% lower-middle class and 4.4% did not know. The mean consumption of tobacco at the beginning of the treatment was 28.3 cigarettes per day.

The treatment is organized in five weekly 1-h sessions. In the first session, an 18-page support manual explaining the main contents of each session is given to the participants. They then talk about why they want to quit smoking and the situations in which they feel the need to smoke. They are trained to fill in self-monitoring reports, in which they record each cigarette they smoke, the situation in which they do so, the time and the pleasure they experience, on a scale of 0–5. These reports help them understand their own smoking habit. In the second session, the participants are trained in techniques to avoid the withdrawal syndrome. They are also taught how to deal with their psychological dependence and how to control their stimuli. The main topic of the third session is physical improvement as a result of the treatment, with regard, for instance, to breathing and fitness. The aim of the fourth session is to make the participants ready to quit definitively. In the fifth session, the participants are trained to prevent relapse.

All the sessions include carbon monoxide monitoring of exhaled air to assess progress towards quitting and to check abstinence. Nicotine and tar intake is reduced by decreasing the number of cigarettes smoked and changing the brand of cigarettes smoked each week to those with less nicotine and tar.

After the treatment is finished, follow-up is carried out by telephone at 1, 3, 6 and 12 months. The follow-up does not include any therapeutic intervention.

Results

By six months, 38 (55.9%) had changed their habit: 17 (25%) had quit and 21 (31%) had reduced their cigarette consumption. No change was reported by 19 (28%), and 11 (16%) were lost to follow-up.

Conclusions

More women than men attended the courses, the typical participants being women aged about 40 who smoked an average of 28.3 cigarettes per day. A high percentage of participants changed their smoking behaviour. More intensive follow-up techniques would achieve longer abstinence periods in the long term.

Effectiveness of a five-day plan to eliminate the smoking habit in France

R. Romand

Ligue Vie et Santé and Laboratoire de Neurobiologie Université Blaise Pascal, Aubière, France

Summary

The effectiveness of a five-day plan for eliminating nicotine dependence was tested in relation to the Fagerström tolerance questionnaire. The plan was used by 137 adult smokers of each sex who were attempting to quit, and their success in quitting was evaluated one year later with the questionnaire. About 30% succeeded in quitting. Of those who succeeded, 87% were in the moderate and high categories of dependence.

The proportion of people who stopped smoking corresponded closely to other results reported for behavioural therapy. Comparison of the groups with moderate and high dependence showed that they had a similar ability to quit. The results argue against the assumption that the five-day plan works mainly for people with a low degree of dependence.

Introduction

The most effective behavioural techniques correspond to elements of behavioural modification therapy that allow better understanding of the environmental and physical cues to smoking, to enable smokers to modify their responses to these cues. On the basis of this information, smokers analyse their fears and the difficulties involved in abstinence from smoking and can therefore prepare adequate non-smoking strategies for coping (Kottke *et al.*, 1988; Hirsch *et al.*, 1994).

The five-day plan involves psychological group therapy designed to cope with the addictive behaviour and withdrawal symptoms associated with dependence on smoking. The main goal of the strategy is to reinforce motivation to stop smoking through behavioural and cognitive procedures in order to reduce withdrawal symptoms rapidly. Controlled trials have shown that the success rate of the plan is about 30% after one year (Romand, 1995), which corresponds well to the rates achieved by other smoking cessation methods (Schwartz, 1987). Despite the success of the five-day plan, it is sometimes argued that such group therapy is effective only for smokers with a low degree of dependence and with less severe withdrawal symptoms, i.e. people who have less difficulty in quitting. In order to test this assumption, we studied the dependence of a group of smokers using the plan to quit smoking.

Methods

A group of 137 people of each sex who wished to stop smoking attended daily group therapy sessions lasting about 2 h for five days. Their success in quitting was evaluated one year later, and evaluated in relation to their degree of dependence as measured by the Fagerström tolerance questionnaire at the beginning of therapy; the categories are mild, moderate, high and very high dependence. The responses were collected mainly by telephone, some by personal visits and a few by mail. People who had unsuccessful attempts were pooled with those that were impossible to contact. The relationship between success in smoking cessation and level of dependence was analysed statistically by the chi-squared test.

Results

The proportion of participants who had stopped smoking after one year was 30%. The distribution of dependence according to the Fagerström tolerance questionnaire showed that the majority of the participants were moderately (about 33%) or highly dependent (about 55%) before therapy. The distribution corresponds well with previous reports on larger groups. Similar proportions in these two categories were found among the participants who succeeded in stopping smoking. Statistical analysis of smokers who quit and those who did not after therapy showed that the degree of dependence did not affect the likelihood of quitting. As few of the smokers were mildly or very heavily dependent, no definite conclusion can be drawn for these two categories; but comparison between those with moderate and high dependence showed no difference in the ability to quit smoking.

Conclusion

This study provides evidence that the five-day plan is an effective aid to smoking cessation, with a success rate of about 30%. Moreover, it is effective in helping smokers with various levels of dependence on nicotine.

References

Hirsch, A., Slama, K., Alberisio, A., Fowler, G., Lagrue, G., Malvezzi, I., Manley, M., Molinard, R. & Tonnesen, P. (1994) Smoking cessation methods: Recommendations for health professionals. Advisory Group of the European School of Oncology. *Eur. J. Cancer*, **30A**, 253–263
Kottke, T.E., Battista, R.N. & DeFriese, G.H. (1988) Attributes of successful smoking cessation interventions in medical practice. A meta-analysis of 39 controlled trials. *J. Am. Med. Assoc.*, **259**, 2883–2889
Romand, R. (1995) A cognitive strategy for stopping smoking. The Five Day Plan. In: Slama, K., ed., *Tobacco and Health*, New York: Plenum Press, pp. 813–816
Schwartz, J.L. (1987) Review and Evaluation of Smoking Cessation Methods: United States and Canada, 1978–1985 (DHHS Publication No. 87-2940), Washington DC: Department of Health and Human Services, Public Health Service, National Institutes of Health

Seven years of smoking cessation campaigns in The Netherlands

G. Zeeman

Dutch Foundation on Smoking and Health (Stivoro), The Hague, The Netherlands

In 1989, the Dutch Foundation on Smoking and Health, with the support of the Ministry of Health, developed a framework for a smoking cessation campaign. A working party of experts and representatives of key organizations was set up to advise. After a regional pilot study, the first national campaign was conducted in 1991. The campaign appeared to be effective, because the number of smokers who quit smoking during the three-month period doubled. It was decided to continue campaigns in accordance with this framework and to develop and refine elements of this approach. In subsequent years, we conducted two small and four moderate-sized campaigns.

The campaign strategy is based on three essential points. The first is that mass media campaigns can affect behaviour only if the target group already has a favourable attitude and intention to change. 'Contemplators'—people intending to quit within six months—were selected as the target group, representing about 30% of the smokers in the Netherlands. In developing the communication, motivation to quit was thus taken for granted, and we did not give arguments to give up smoking but focused on the process of change: 'Each moment is a good moment to quit' and 'Quit smoking together'. We gave a cue to action and stimulated smokers to quit: 'Come on, quit'.

The second point was to make the campaign more effective by combining it with strategies aimed at creating interpersonal communication. To do this, we involved regional and local public health organizations, health-care workers and companies to promote activities. The idea was that the closer you get to the skin of the smokers the more impact you have and the more their smoking behaviour will be affected.

The third point was to offer concrete behavioural alternatives and plans for action to improve the effectiveness of public health information campaigns. This is especially important in the case of a behavioural problem like smoking dependence. We developed written information on how to quit smoking and organized help in the form of smoking cessation clinics. A telephone line was provided for moral support, advice and information about available forms of cessation assistance.

During the campaign, 20–25% of smokers each year made an attempt to quit. In 1991, when we had a particularly intense campaign, the percentage was twice as large. In 1996, a year with a campaign of moderate intensity, we found that 1 million of the 4.4 million smokers had made an attempt to quit. Research on the 1991 campaign showed that about 10% of the attempts were successful. This observation made us change the focus of the campaigns, with the aim of not just generating attempts but improving their quality.

We looked at the target groups we reached: of every 1000 smokers, 70% are 'pre-contmplators' (no intention to quit within the coming six months), 23% are 'contemplators' (intention to quit within six months), and 7% are 'preparers' (intention to quit within one month). Of those who were still abstinent after one year, 17% had been preparers, 13% had been contemplators and 5% had been pre-contemplators at the start of the campaign. This indicates that cessation campaigns aimed at contemplators can also affect pre-contemplators.

During the years of these campaigns, the alliances with regional and local organizations resulted in a firm, skilled smoking cessation network. Their activities had a low intensity, however, because of lack of funds. To make this network more productive, we must convince regional and local policy-makers to give smoking cessation higher priority. We think this is necessary to bring stimulus to change and support to the smoker. General practitioners were the first group we tried to involve in cessation activities, and the percentage of interventions by these professionals increased substantially. It is difficult and time-consuming to involve health-care workers in smoking cessation interventions; nonetheless, we think this is important for motivating large groups of smokers and creating high-quality cessation support on a large scale. We are developing interventions for a broad range of health-care workers to support patients who are quitting as well as strategies to implement these innovations.

Smoking cessation clinics are available to the public in almost every region of the Netherlands, but use of this and other forms of assistance is low: More than 80% of smokers who quit use no assistance, while of the 20% of smokers who try to quit each year only a few succeed. Incorporation of effective forms of assistance that can be used on a large scale and good marketing strategies to get smokers to use this assistance are needed. With these improvements, future campaigns will gain considerable potential effect.

Quit and Win contest for daily smoking mothers of children 0-6 years of age in Stockholm County, Sweden

P. Tillgren[1,3], L. Eriksson[2], K. Guldbrandsson[2], A. Reimers[2], M. Spiik[2], T. Ainetdin[1,3] & M.-L.Stjerna[3]

[1]*Stockholm County Council, Department of Social Medicine, Sundbyberg,*
[2]*South West Health-care Region, Department of Public Health and Public Relations Unit, Huddinge, and* [3]*Karolinska Institute, Department of Public Health Sciences, Division of Social Medicine, Sundbyberg, Sweden*

Introduction

A 'Quit and Win' contest strategy was implemented as a method to assist smokers to stop smoking. This method was developed in the United States at the beginning of the 1980s in three programmes for prevention of cardiovascular disease in the population. It was first introduced in Europe in 1986 in the North Karelia Project in Finland (Tillgren, 1995). The basis for this population-directed model is that most tobacco users wish to quit, and the use of a contest involving attractive prizes has been shown to be an effective method for stimulating and supporting tobacco users to quit. Quit and Win contests have been held in Sweden both nationally and locally since 1988.

The prevalence of smoking has decreased during the past decades in Sweden and several other western countries. In 1995, 22% of men and 24% of women in Sweden were daily smokers (Statistiskå centralbyrån, 1996). While a substantial decrease in smoking has occurred among men, the decrease among women has not been as striking.

One fifth of Sweden's population of 9 million live in the metropolitan area of Stockholm County, and the prevalence of daily smokers is similar to the figures for the rest of the country. One of the nine health-care regions in the Stockholm County Council is in the south-west, with about 255 000 inhabitants. This region has the highest proportion of young people in the County and the highest proportion of people with short education and immigrant background; persons who are socioeconomically underprivileged are thus over-represented in this region.

Two of the goals set for this health-care region in preventive health are a decrease in tobacco use and improvement of women's health. A contest for quitting the use tobacco was held between autumn 1995 and spring 1996, with the goal of encouraging daily smoking mothers to quit.

Material and method

The target group was women living in this health-care region who had at least one child aged 0-6 years. Of the nearly 18 000 women who met the criteria, about 25% were daily smokers (Sydvästra sjukvårdsområdet, 1995). The final group consisted of approximately 4500 women with children aged 0-6 years who smoked daily. The main recruiting strategy was personally addressed letters enclosing a contest folder sent to each individual in the target group (Eriksson *et al.*, 1997) derived from the national registry of vital statistics. The addressing and mailing of the envelopes was carried out by a firm. Further information about the contest was published in the local newspaper, which is distributeds to all households in the region, and in a brochure placed in general, child and maternal health-care centres, pre-schools and pharmacies. The information in the brochure was given in Swedish, Spanish, Turkish and Arabic.

In order to be eligible to win a prize, the women had to have remained free from tobacco for seven months. Two individuals were required to certify in writing that the person in question had in fact not smoked during the period stipulated by the contest. The first three prizes were trips for three persons to Legoland in Denmark. The winners were required to undergo carbon-monoxide testing to verify that they were in fact free from traces of smoking. In order to help them to remain free from tobacco, a brief information letter was sent on five occasions. Furthermore, the participants were invited to a get-together six weeks after the day of quitting tobacco. Additional support was given on two occasions on which the participants were given the opportunity to contact a smoking cessation hot-line with a trained cessation counsellor. Nicotine substitutes were allowed.

Evaluation

The Quit and Win contest has been evaluated for process, cost-effectiveness and outcome among tobacco-free individuals. In this paper, we focus on process and outcome evaluation on the basis of information from the participants' application forms which included number of years of smoking, daily cigarette consumption, mailing address, age, profession, number of children and motive for quitting tobacco use. The process evaluation was carried out mainly to study the channels used for disseminating information, namely brochures, mass media and two interviews with the participants (Stjerna & Tillgren, 1997). The interviews dealt with the types of aids used for support and how the participant felt about the contest as a method for quitting smoking.

In order to determine the proportion who remained tobacco-free, questionnaires were sent out after 1, 6 and 12 months, to elicit supplementary information on earlier smoking habits and civil status. A telephone interview was carried out with drop-outs in the first two follow-up studies. The rates of participation in the three follow-up studies were 96, 90 and 75%.

Results

A total of 238 women qualified to participate in the contest. Most (80%) were 25–39 years of age, 13% were > 40 years and 6% were 19–24 years. Nearly half of the women (49%) had two children, 29% had one child, 17% had three children and 5% had four to five children of various ages. The majority of the women (60%) had been smokers for 11–20 years, 22% had smoked for ≥ 21 years and the remainder (18%) had smoked cigarettes for 1–10 years. Most of them (67%) smoked 11–20 cigarettes per day, 18.5% smoked ≤ 10 and 13.5% smoked > 20 cigarettes per day.

The majority of the participants (78%) had signed up for the contest after receiving the application form in the mail. This corresponds to about 5% of the total target group of tobacco consumers. The application form in the local newspaper had been used by 8% of the participants, and the remaining 14% had joined up at a day-care centre, pharmacy, health-care centre or some other channel. The motives given for wishing to stop smoking were: for their own health (32%), their children's health (15%), to set a good example for their children (13%) and for economic reasons (9%). The main support factors in quitting smoking identified by the interviewers were: meeting others in the same situation (get-togethers), information and counselling, the possibility of winning a prize and receiving encouraging letters. The second interview focused on the efficacy of the method and the way in which the campaign was carried out. Some mothers thought that more support should be given by the contest organizers, but the attitudes of those who succeeded in quitting smoking and those who relapsed differed.

At the one-month follow-up, 43% of the women were still tobacco-free; at the time of the survey, a further 7% were still tobacco-free, giving a point estimate of 50%. The corresponding numbers for the six-month follow-up were 27 and 7%, with a 34% point estimate. After one year, the corresponding proportions were 14 and 24%, respectively.

Conclusion

All smoking women with children under the age of seven were reached by the direct-mail technique, and about 5% were recruited into the contest for smoking cessation. An important factor in their willingness to participate was their own health and that of their children. The method was shown to have a long-term effect, with 14% still tobacco-free after one year, comparable to several other minimum intervention smoking cessation programmes. Whether these measures are also cost-effective will be evaluated in later studies.

References

Eriksson, L., Guldbrandsson, K., Reimers, A., Spiik, A., Tillgren, P., Stjerna, M.-L. & Ainetdin, T. (1997) *En rapport om "Fimpa tjejer"—en rökslutstävling för småbarnsmammor i Sydvästra sjukvårdsområdet 1995–1996* (A report on 'Women Quitting Smoking'—A smoking-cessation contest for mothers with small children within the south-west Health-care Region, 1995–1996), Huddinge: Sydvästra sjukvårdsområdet, Hälsoenheten (in Swedish)

Statistiska centralbyrån (1996) *Undersökningar av levnadsförhållanden* (Annual Survey of Living Conditions), Stockholm: Statistiska centralbyrån (in Swedish)

Stjerna, M.-L. & Tillgren, P. (1997) Tävling som metod för att sluta röka. Utvärdering av tävlingen "Fimpa tjejer" ur ett deltagareperspektiv genom telefonintervjuer med tävlande. (A contest as a method to quit smoking. Evaluation of the contest 'Women Quitting Smoking' from the perspective of the participants obtained through telephone interviews) (Grön rapport 356), Sundbyberg: Karolinska Institutet, Institutionen för folkhälsovetenskap, Avdelningen för socialmedicin (in Swedish)

Sydvästra sjukvårdsområdet (1995) Folkhälsorapport 1995. En rapport om hälsoutvecklingen i Sydvästra sjukvårdsområdet (Public health report, 1995. A report on developments in health within the south-west Health-care Region), Huddinge: Sydvästra sjukvårdsområdet, Hälsoenheten (in Swedish)

Tillgren, P. (1995) *'Quit and Win' Contests in Tobacco Cessation. Theoretical Framework and Practices from a Community-based Intervention in the Stockholm Cancer Prevention Program (SCPP)*. Doctoral dissertation, Sundbyberg: Karolinska Institutet, Department of International Health and Social Medicine, Unit of Social Medicine

Effectiveness in Poland of the second international 'Quit and Win' anti-smoking campaign

W. Drygas, A. Kowalska & E. Dziankowska-Stachowiak

Department of Social & Preventive Medicine, Medical University, Lodz, Poland

Mass anti-smoking campaigns seem to be an effective method for discouraging the use of tobacco, especially in countries with a high prevalence of smokers (Drygas *et al.*, 1996; Korhonen *et al.*, 1997; Przwozniak *et al.*, 1996; Puška, 1996; Tillgren *et al.*, this volume). Two regions of Poland, Lodz and Kalisz, participated in the second international 'Quit and Win' campaign in 1996, organized under the auspices of the National Health Institute in Helsinki, Finland. As few trials have been carried out in central and eastern Europe (Kamardina & Zaikin, 1996; Kvasha *et al.*, 1996; Przwozniak *et al.*, 1996), our experience is of particular interest.

As compared with the previous campaign, more emphasis was placed on social marketing of the activities and mass-media participation. In order to organize the campaign in Poland, we contacted 160 companies, organizations and foundations. Above 20 firms and organizations in the public and private sector offered us financial help. With this support, we printed about 100 000 attractive entry forms and offered valuable prizes for winners.

In Lodz, 25 000 entry forms with a letter about quitting smoking were mailed to households, and the campaign was supported by local newspapers, radio and television. The press sponsor of the competition, *Dziennik Lodzki*, published the entry form and competition rules four times. The preliminary data from the health behaviour survey demonstrated that the campaign was highly visible and may have influenced community knowledge, attitudes and behaviour. More than 2200 smokers declared their willingness to stop, representing 0.3–0.4% of the target population.

To evaluate the outcome at 12 months, a follow-up study was performed on a random sample of 1700 men and women. The response rate was 82%. Among 1388 responders, 942 (68%) had smoked before the campaign, and 446 (32%) had quit smoking several weeks or months previously. During the first month of the campaign, 74% of these smokers had quit smoking and more than 21% had reduced their consumption; only 2% of the participants had been unable to change their smoking habit. Data were missing for 2.4%. The sustained abstinence rate after one year was 30% and that after 14 months was 29% (considering all non-responders as smokers). The preliminary results of our study thus demonstrate the high effectiveness of the intervention.

References

Drygas, W., Kowalska, A. & Sapinski, W. (1996) II International 'Quit & Win' antismoking campaign in Poland—Success and failures. In: *Smoke Free Europe, Helsinki, Finland*, 168 (abstract)

Kamardina. T. & Zaikin, E. (1996) Smoking cessation effectiveness in 'Quit & Win' campaign in Russia. In: *Smoke Free Europe, Helsinki, Finland*, 103 (abstract)

Korhonen, T., Kamardina, T., Salto, E., *et al.* (1997) Quit and Win Contest 1994: Evaluation in three countries. *Eur. J. Public Health* (in press)

Kvasha, E., Smirnova, I., Gorbas, I. & Davidenko, N. (1996) The first experience of conducting the international antismoking campaign 'Quit & Win' in Ukrainia. In: *Smoke Free Europe, Helsinki, Finland*, 102 (abstract)

Przewozniak K., Jaworski M. & Zatonski W. (1996) The 'Stop smoking together' campaign in Poland. In: *Smoke Free Europe, Helsinki, Finland*, 37 (abstract)

Puška, P. (1996) Smoking in central and eastern Europe. In: *Smokefree Europe. A Forum for Networks*, Helsinki, Finland, 138

A study of smoking cessation in Egypt: Perspective for success

H.M. El Shahat, A.A.M.T. Mobasher, L.A. Zaki, M.H. Fawzy & E.I.D. Nour

Faculty of Medicine, Zagazig University, Cairo, Egypt

Abstract

We investigated the effects of smoking cessation treatment with acupuncture, transdermal nicotine patches or the antidepressant fluvoxamine in 29 patients with chronic obstructuve pulmonary disease, six subjects with chronic non-obstructive bronchitis and five healthy subjects. Respiratory symptom score, psychological score and pulmonary function were determined before and after treatment. Acupuncture resulted in the highest rate of cessation, followed by fluvoxamine for depressed persons and, lastly, nicotine replacement therapy. Health motivation, education, urbanization and low nicotine dependence appeared to predict successful smoking cessation. Respiratory symptoms and pulmonary function were significantly improved after cessation of smoking.

Introduction

Cigarette smoking is the main avoidable cause of premature death and morbidity (Crofton, 1990), and developing countries clearly need to take their own action against tobacco (Mackay, 1991). Age, sex, motivation, education and many other variables are associated with the success of smoking cessation treatment (Gourlay *et al.*, 1994).

Numerous clinical trials have shown that transdermal nicotine patches help people to quit smoking by separating physical and psychological withdrawal into two phases: learning to live without cigarettes and learning to live without nicotine (Abelin *et al.*, 1991). Smokers who quit who have pre-existing depression may experience exacerbation of their depression, which is alleviated by a return to smoking (Jaffe, 1991), indicating that treatment for clinical depression may increase the rate of cessation (Hurt *et al.*, 1992). Acupuncture is becoming increasingly popular as an aid to smokers who wish to quit, as it inhibits the abstinence syndrome and is economical, simple and easy to accept (Aiping & Meng, 1994).

As smoking cessation is the most important approach to management of chronic obstructive pulmonary disease (Petty, 1991), we evaluated the success rate of various methods of smoking cessation, the predictors of success and the effects on respiratory symptoms and pulmonary function.

Subjects and methods

The study involved 40 smokers in three groups: 29 patients fulfilling the American Thoracic Society's (1987) definition of chronic obstructuve pulmonary disease, six subjects with chronic non-obstructive bronchitis and five healthy subjects. Before treatment, a detailed history of smoking was obtained from each subject, and level of education (El Sherbini & Fahmy, 1985), urban or rural residence and respiratory symptom score (Medical Research Council, 1960) were recorded. Nicotine dependence was evaluated by the Fagerström tolerance questionnaire, low dependence being considered a score < 7 and high dependence a score > 7 (Fagerström, 1978). Psychological status was assessed on the basis of symptoms suggesting depression (Weller & Weller, 1991) and classification of depression on the Zagazig depression scale (Fawzy *et al.*, 1983). Pulmonary function was assessed by measuring expiratory flow volume in 1 s (FEV_1) and 25–75% of forced expiratory flow predicted (FEF_{25-75}).

Three methods of smoking cessation were used. Acupuncture was used for 23 subjects of a mean age of 46.3 (SD, 15) years. The subjects were asked to stop smoking at the onset of treatment. They then received stainless-steel needles into *shenmen* points on the ear linked to the liver, stomach and lung (Aiping & Meng, 1994), which were fixed and covered; they were changed to the opposite ear each week, for a total of four weeks of abstinence (Choy *et al.*, 1983). Transdermal nicotine patches ('Nicotinell TTS', Ciba-Geigy) were used in seven subjects of a mean age of 47.5 (SD, 16) years. The subjects were asked to stop smoking at the onset of treatment. A fresh patch was applied every morning at locations rotated to different parts of the arm for three months (Abein *et al.*, 1989). Fluvoxamine was given to 10 subjects of a mean age of 47.4 (SD, 17) years with depression, at a dose of 50 mg per day at bedtime for up to two weeks. The smokers were then asked to stop smoking, and the treatment was maintained for three months.

For all subjects, a withdrawal symptom score was determined daily, each symptom being rated as absent (0), mild (2), moderate (4) or severe (8). The mean weekly score was then calculated (Hurt *et al.*, 1993). Supportive psychotherapy was given to all subjects weekly, and self-reported abstinence, defined as no smoking within the previous seven days, was recorded (Fiore *et al.*, 1994).

Three months later, respiratory symptom score, pulmonary function (Paoletti *et al.*, 1993) and the presence of depressive symptoms were re-evaluated, and the results were analysed statistically (Armitage, 1983).

Results and discussion

The highest success rate was found with acupuncture (65%). This rate is lower than those found in some other studies: 88% (Weller & Weller, 1991), 90% (Yang, 1984, quoted by Aiping & Meng, 1994) and 95% (Cheung, 1987, quoted by Aiping & Meng, 1994), perhaps because the other rates were reported one month after quitting, while we reported the rate after three months, and the effect of acupuncture on abstinence decreases with time (Aiping & Meng, 1994). Our rate was, however, higher those reported six months after quitting: 15% (Martin & Waite, 1981), 41% (Fuller, 1982) and 18% (Chwartz, 1992).

The success rate with transdermal nicotine patches was 43%, similar to those of other studies after three months of use: 47% (Hurt *et al.*, 1995) and 36% (Muller *et al.*, 1990). The lower success rates reported by other investigators (21%: Martin & Robinson, 1995; 6.7%: Gourlay *et al.*, 1995) may be due to lack of psychotherapy.

The rate of success among depressed subjects treated with the antidepressant drug was 60%. As the symptoms of nicotine withdrawal and depression are similar, antidepressants ease withdrawal. Higher rates were found in other studies in which different drugs were used (78%: Edwards et al., 1989; 68%: Bassuny, 1990).

The success rate among patients with chronic obstructuve pulmonary disease was 62%, that among patients with chronic non-obstructive bronchitis was 83% and that among healthy subjects was only 20%, in accordance with the finding that concern about health and fear of imminent death are strong motives for quitting (Manley *et al.*, 1992). Slightly more men than women succeeded in quitting (Table 1), in accordance with other studies (Fiore *et al.*, 1990; Norregard *et al.*, 1994). There was little difference by age, in accordance with the study of Kivz *et al.* (1995), but Gourlay *et al.* (1994)

Table 1. Characteristics of subjects who succeeded and failed to stop smoking

Characteristic	Succeeders		Relapsers	
	No.	%	No.	%
Sex				
Male	23	60.5	15	39.5
Female	1	50	1	50
Age (years)				
14–243	75	1	25	
25–44	13	72.2	5	27.8
45–64	5	41.7	7	58.3
≥ 65	3	50	3	50
Educational level				
High	10	66.7	5	33.3
Secondary	9	75	3	25
Primary or preparatory	3	60	2	40
Illiterate	2	25	6	75
Residence				
Urban	17	74.4	6	25.6
Rural	7	41.2	10	58.8
Dependency level				
High	10	52.6	9	47.4
Low	14	66.7	7	33.3

reported that successful cessation attempts were associated with increased age. In our study, those who succeeded tended to be more educated and to live in cities, also in accordance with other studies (Bassuny, 1990; Fiore *et al.*, 1990; Manley *et al.*, 1992).

More of those who succeeded had a low level of nicotine dependence and thus did not need the intensive counselling required by smokers with a high level of dependence (Fagerström, 1991). Furthermore, the severity of withdrawal symptoms during the first week among all the subjects in the study was significantly related to the level of nicotine dependence, as reported earlier (Fagerström, 1991). The lowest severity was found with acupuncture, as seen previosuly (Fuller, 1982), and the greatest severity with the transdermal nicotine patch; the difference was significant.

We assessed the success of smoking cessation after three months, since that is the period during which most relapses occur (Hughes & Miller, 1984); furthermore, the longest duration of nicotine replacement therapy is three months (Abelin *et al.*, 1989). A third reason was that partial recovery of mucociliary transport has been observed in cigarette smokers after cessation for three months, so that improvement can be expected in respiratory symptoms (Wanner, 1990). We found a highly significant improvement in FEV_1 and FEF_{25-75} three months after cessation in the whole group. Other studies have demonstrated beneficial effects of smoking cessation on FEV_1 (Buist *et al.*, 1979; Sherrill *et al.*, 1994), indicating that there is a reversible component to the effect of smoking on pulmonary function, in addition to permanent changes that may be due to emphysema (Sansores *et al.*, 1992). We also found a significant improvement in respiratory symptoms after cessation, as reported elsewhere (Gross, 1990).

References

Abelin, T., Muller, P., Buehler, A., *et al.* (1989) Controlled trial of transdermal nicotine patch in tobacco withdrawal. *Lancet*, i, 7

Abelin, T., Ehrsam, R., Imhof, P., *et al.* (1991) Clinical experience with a transdermal nicotine system in healthy nicotine dependent smokers. In: Withelmsen, L., ed., *Smoking As a Cardiovascular Risk Factor—New Startegies for Smoking Cessation*, Lewiston, New York: Hogrefe & Huber, p. 35

Aiping, J. & Meng, G. (1994) Analysis of therapeutic effects of acupuncture on abstinence from smoking. *Trad. Chin. Med.*, 14, 56

American Thoracic Society (1987) Standards for the diagnosis and care of patients with chronic obstructive pulmonary disease (COPD) and asthma. *Am. Rev. Respir. Dis.*, 136, 225

Armitage, P. (1983) *Statistical Methods in Medical Research*, Oxford: Oxford Scientific Publications

Bassuny, M.M. (1990) *A Comparative Study of the Therapeutic Effect of Imipramine versus Acupuncture in Smoking Cessation,* MSc Thesis, Neuropsychiatry, Zagazig University

Buist, S.A., Nagy, J.M. & Sexton, G.J. (1979) The effect of smoking cessation on pulmonary function. *Am. Rev. Respir. Dis.,* **120**, 953

Choy, D.S.J., Lutzker, L. & Meltzer, L. (1983) Effective treatment for smoking cessation. *Am. J. Med.,* **75**, 1033

Chwartz, J.L. (1992) Methods of smoking cessation. *Med. Clin. N. Am.,* **76**, 451

Crofton, J. (1990) Tobacco and the third world. *Thorax,* **45**, 164

Edwards, N.B., Murphy, J.K., Downs, A.D., *et al.* (1989) Dozepin as an adjunct to smoking cessation. *Am. J. Psychiatr.,* **146**, 373

El Sherbini, A.F. & Fahmy, S. (1985) Determining simple parameters of social classification for health research. *Bull. High Inst. Public Health,* **5**, 95

Fagerström, K.O. (1978) Measuring degree of physical dependence to tobacco smoking with reference to individualization treatment. *Addict. Behav.,* **3**, 241

Fagerström, K.O. (1991) How to measure nicotine dependence. In: Wilhelmsen, L., ed., *Smoking As a Cardiovascular Risk Factor—New Strategies for Smoking Cessation,* Lewiston, New York: Hogrefe & Huber, p. 25

Fawzy, M., El-Maghraby, M., El-Amine, H., *et al.* (1983) *Zagazig Depression Scale,* Cairo: El-Nahda, p. 1

Fiore, M.C., Novotny, T.E., Pierce, J.P., *et al.* (1990) Methods used to quit smoking in the United States. *J. Am. Med. Assoc.,* **263**, 2760

Fiore, M.C., Kenbord, S.L., Jorenby, D.E., *et al.* (1994) Two studies of the clinical effectiveness of the nicotine patch with different counselling treatments. *Chest,* **105**, 524

Fuller, G.A. (1982) Smoking withdrawal and acupuncture. *Med. J. Aust.,* **9**, 28

Gourlay, S.G., Forbes, A., Marriner, T., *et al.* (1994) Prospective study of factors predeicting outcome of transdermal nicotine treatment in smoking cessation. *Br. Med. J.,* **309**, 842

Gourlay, S.G., Frobes, A., Marriner, T., *et al.* (1995) Double blind trial of repeated treatment with transdermal nicotine for relapsed smokers. *Br. Med. J. Middle East,* ii, 12

Gross, N.J. (1990) Chronic obstructive pulmonary disease: Current concepts and therapeutic approach. *Chest,* **97**, 195

Hughes, J.R. & Miller, S.A. (1984) Nicotine gum to help stop smoking. *J. Am. Med. Assoc.,* **252**, 2855

Hurt, R.D., Dale, L.C., Meclain, F.L., *et al.* (1992) A comprehensive model for the treatment of nicotine dependence in a medical setting. *Med. Clin. N. Am.,* **76**, 495

Hurt, R.D., Dale, L.C., Offord, K.P., *et al.* (1993) Serum nicotine and cotinine levels during nicotine patch therapy. *Clin. Pharmacol. Ther.,* **54**, 98

Hurt, R.D., Dale, L.C., Offord, K.P., *et al.* (1995) Nicotine patch therapy for smoking cessation. *Addiction,* **90**, 1541

Jaffe, J.H. (1991) Drug addiction and drug abuse. In: Gilman, A.G., Rall, T.W., Nies, A.S. & Taylor, P., eds, *Goodman and Gilman's The Pharmacological Basis of Therapeutics,* 8th Ed., New York: McGraw Hill, p. 522

Kivz, F.J., Clark, M.A., Crittenden, K.S., *et al.* (1995) Age and smoking behaviors. *Prev. Med.,* **24**, 297

Mackay, J. (1991) Tobacco:The third world war. *Thorax,* **46**, 153

Manley, M.W., Epps, R.P. & Glynn, T.J. (1992) The clinician's role in promoting smoking cessation among clinic patients. *Med. Clin. N. Am.,* **76**, 477

Martin, P.D. & Robinson, G.M. (1995) The safety, tolerability and efficacy of transdermal nicotine (Nicotinell TTS) in hospitalized patients. *N.Z. Med. J.,* **108**, 6

Martin, G.P. & Waite, P.M. (1981) The efficacy of acupuncture as an aid to stopping smoking. *N.Z. Med. J.,* **93**, 421

Medical Research Council (1960) Aetiology of chronic bronchitis. Standardized questionnaire for respiratory sumptoms. *Br. Med. J.,* ii, 1665

Muller, P.H., Abelin, T.H., Ehrasm, R., *et al.* (1990) The use of transdermal nicotine in smoking cessation. *Lung, Suppl.,* 445

Norregard, J., Tonnesen, P. & Peterson, L. (1994) Causes of relapse during attempted smoking cessation using nicotine or placebo plasters. *Ugeskr. Laeg.,* **156**, 7692

Pauletti, P., Tonnesen, P. & Roisin, R.R. (1993) CEASE (Collaborative European Anti-Smoking Evaluation). A challenging multicenter trial organized by the European Respiratory Society. *Chest,* **103**, 1317

Petty, T.L. (1991) Chronic onstructive pulmonary disease. In: Mitchell, D.M., ed., *Respiratory Medicine (5),* Edinburgh: Churchill Livingstone, p. 79

Sansores, R.H., Pare, P. & Abboud, R. (1992) Effect of smoking cessation on pulmonary carbon monoxide diffusing capacity and capillary blood volume. *Am. Rev. Respir. Dis.,* **146**, 959

Sherrill, D.L., Holberg, C.I., Enright, P.L., *et al.* (1994) Longitudinal analysis of the effects of smoking onset and cessation on pulmonary function. *Am. J. Respir. Crit. Care Med.,* **149**, 591

Wanner, A. (1990) The role of mucus in chronic obstructive pulmonary disease. *Chest,* **97**, 11s

Weller, E.B. & Weller, R.A. (1991) Mood disorders. In: Lewis, M., ed., *Child and Adolescent Psychiatry, A Comprehensive Text Book,* Baltimore: Williams & Wilkins, p. 646

Implementation of a smoking cessation programme for adolescents in Israel: Lessons learnt

S. Gan-Noy, M. Blitner, A. Aizick-Kelem & M. Michaeli

Information & Education Department, Israel Cancer Association, Givatayim, Israel

An experimental smoking cessation programme for youngsters was implemented when a number of students requested assistance to stop smoking in a smoking prevention programme by peer counsellors, prepared by the school staff in collaboration with the Israel Cancer Association. In Israel, 28% of the adult population smokes, representing 32% of the male population and 25% of the female population. The highest rate of smoking is among people aged 25–44. People with a higher level of education smoke less than those with a lower level of education. The rate of daily smoking among youngsters aged 16–17 is 11% for boys and 10% for girls. More than 25% of students aged 12–17 have tried smoking at least once.

Planning the project

The management of a religious boarding-school approached the Israel Cancer Association, which conducts smoking cessation projects for adults, to request an experimental programme for adolescents. Preparation and coordination meetings were held between school staff members, including the principal, the school nurse, the school counsellor, the head counsellor and the social worker, and representatives of the Association comprising a clinical psychologist and the head of the information and education department. The parents were notified about the programme. The students at the school comprise new immigrants, mostly from Ethiopia, children from families with socioeconomic problems and children from families with no obvious problems.

The objective of the programme was to design an effective smoking cessation group programme, based on behaviour modification and the cognitive–behavioural approach, adapted to the needs of children in a boarding-school.

The group

The group consisted of 18 adolescents, 16 boys and two girls, aged 15–18. Twelve had been born in Ethiopia, two boys had been born in Morocco and two boys had been born in Israel. Seven were 16 years of age, seven were 17, three were 15, and one was 18. The average age at which they had begun to smoke was 13; three had begun at < 10, one at 12, six at 13, four at 14 and four at 15 years of age.

The programme

The programme consisted of six 1-h group meetings each week at the school and emphasized aspects that were relevant to the children, such as advertising, social pressure and relations with the educational system. The meetings were led by the clinical psychologist, whose expertise is smoking cessation, and evaluation questionnaires were distributed at the beginning and end of the programme. The participants were students who had expressed a wish to stop smoking.We had planned to hold a reinforcement meeting five months later, after the summer holiday, but because of the large turnover rate of the students, this was not feasible.

The meetings included: acquaintanceship with students from other classes, determining the students' objectives and expectations from the workshop, why they started and continued to smoke and why and how they should stop smoking. They were asked to make a detailed record of their habit, so that we could identify the relevant reinforcements and rewards for each participant in order to enhance motivation to change their habit. The students learned alternative behaviour, especially under pressure, such as hobbies, sports and doing something with their hands, and learned which situations led to smoking and how to prevent or cope with those situations. Another element was strengthening their self-efficacy, so that they could believe in their ability to change their habit and stand up to pressure and temptation. At the end of the programme, the group worked on their ability to continue without smoking and take personal responsibility.

Results

Eight students, all boys, completed the workshop; six were Ethiopian and two Israeli-born. The others stopped because of conflicting school activities, of their own accord or because they left the school. Of those who completed the programme, one stopped smoking, four reduced their daily consumption, one smokes from time to time and two rarely smoke. They recommended the workshop to friends who smoked; seven found that the workshop had been interesting, and five felt that it had helped them. The parts of the programme they had found most appealing were the open discussions, information on the dangers of smoking, coping methods and advice on how to stop smoking.

Conclusions

The lessons we learnt that will help us plan and implement effective workshops are:
• to start at the beginning of the school year, so that 12 sessions can be held, contact will be maintained and reinforcement provided;
• to appoint a member of the school staff to coordinate meeting times, the participation of the students and communication between the students, the school management and the group coordinator;
• to involve only students in the same grade, in order to ensure homogeneity;
• to ensure positive reinforcement of success by the school management in order to maintain a high level of motivation.

A randomized controlled trial of smoking cessation in Government out-patient clinics in Hong Kong

C.L. Betson[1], T.H. Lam[1], T.W.H. Chung[2] & S.F. Chung[1]

[1]*Department of Community Medicine, The University of Hong Kong, and*
[2] *Department of Health, Hong Kong SAR, China*

Introduction

A review of the smoking cessation pattern in Hong Kong in 1984–90 reveals that the role of doctors remains static. Only 25% of smokers quit on a doctor's advice (Lam *et al.*, 1994). Very few facilities such as smoking cessation clinics and self-help materials (e.g. booklets and leaflets) are available, and those which are available are limited and their effectiveness has not been evaluated. In addition, the Government clinics in Hong Kong are extremely busy, so that doctors spend an average of 3–5 min with each patient and often see nearly 100 patients a day.

The aim of this study was to examine the effects of an intervention in which doctors gave simple advice and/or a self-help booklet on smoking cessation to patients visiting Government out-patient clinics in Hong Kong.

Methods

Doctors working in Government out-patient clinics were recruited through their regional service heads. Although there was no special requirement for the recruitment of doctors, those who did not volunteer to participate in the study were not recruited. Each doctor participated for about three weeks. All the participating doctors were briefed by the researchers, with both verbal and written instructions, questionnaires and intervention materials, so that they all understood their role and the procedure of the study.

Chinese-speaking patients aged ≤ 65 who had smoked cigarettes for a month before attending one of the clinics during the three-week study period were included. The patients had also to be available in Hong Kong during the six months following the intervention and to have consented verbally to be contacted by telephone. Those patients who voluntarily asked for information on smoking cessation before randomization or who had illnesses that led the attending doctors to consider that it would be unethical not to advise them urgently on smoking cessation were excluded.

Each doctor was given a set of sealed envelopes with serial numbers. Each envelope contained a brief questionnaire and identification of one of the four intervention groups: control, i.e. no intervention (the doctor filled in the questionnaire); the doctor gave a self-help booklet on smoking cessation; the doctor gave simple advice on smoking cessation; or the doctor gave both the booklet and advice. The subjects were allocated to an intervention group according to a table of random numbers. The self-help smoking cessation booklet, produced by the American Cancer Association, was translated into Chinese, with permission. The standardized advice was an abridged adaptation from recommendations of a National Cancer Institute programme (Glynn & Manley, 1989). It took the doctor about 1 min to give the standardized advice. The doctors could also provide treatment and other advice to patients in their usual practice.

The patients were contacted by trained interviewers for a telephone interview one week, three months, six months and one year after the intervention. The interviewers asked about their smoking status and additional demographic information at one week (as only limited information was available from the questionnaire filled in by the doctors). The interviewers did not know the intervention group of the patients during subsequent follow-up.

Three quit rates—point prevalence abstinence, consecutive abstinence and sustained abstinence at one year—were used as the outcome measures of success. Point prevalence abstinence is self-reported abstinence from smoking during the 24 h before the follow-up interview. Consecutive abstinence is self-reported abstinence for the 24 h before the interview and at all previous follow-ups. Sustained abstinence is continuous abstinence from after the intervention until the time of interview. In this study, sustained abstinence was defined as not smoking at the three-month follow-up and continuously up to the one-year follow-up. Relevant quit rates were also assessed at one, three and six months to examine the short-term effect of the intervention.

All smokers who claimed not to have smoked for at least 24 h at the one-year follow-up were invited to submit a urine sample for a urinary cotinine test.

The study was a 2 x 2 factorial design. The three intervention groups were compared with the control group, and the data were also analysed as booklet versus no booklet and advice versus no advice (Russell et al., 1979, 1987). For the latter comparison, it was conservatively assumed that 4% of smokers in the intervention group and 1% in the control group would quit. The sample size was determined to be 383 per group, or 766 in total.

Results

There were 59 Government out-patient clinics in Hong Kong in December 1994; 42 doctors from 15 of these clinics were recruited to participate in the study. A total of 865 smokers (796 men and 63 women) were included in the trial. Data were available from 88% at the one-week follow-up, 71% at three months, 68% at six months and 64% at one year. As the data were analysed by intention-to-treat, subjects were assumed to continue to be smoking if data were not available. Table 1 shows that the characteristics of the four groups were similar. Their age ranged from 15 to 65, with a mean age of 43.1 years. Daily smoking was reported by 662 patients (89%), and 62% had previously attended the clinics.

Table 2 shows that at one year the point prevalence abstinence was 17%, consecutive abstinence was 2.9%, and sustained abstinence was 3.1%. The quit rates in the three intervention groups were not significantly different from those in the control group. Table 3 shows that this was true even when the groups were collapsed to compare

Table 1. Characteristics of subjects in various intervention groups

Characteristic	Controls (n = 241) %	Booklet only (n = 181) %	Advice only (n = 213) %	Booklet and advice (n = 230) %	All (n = 865) %
Sex					
Male	93	92	92	94	93
Female	7	8	8	6	7
Age					
< 21	5	6	3	6	16
21–44	47	60	49	49	51
≥ 45	49	34	47	45	44
Education					
≤ Primary	42	37	50	40	42
Secondary	53	58	45	55	53
≥ Tertiary	5	6	5	5	5
Monthly income (HK$)					
≤ 4999	31	24	34	27	29
5000–4999	35	34	36	38	36
≥ 10 000	35	42	30	34	35
Age started smoking					
< 16	25	22	27	20	24
16–20	53	53	48	57	53
≥ 21	23	25	25	23	24
No. of years smoked					
≤ 10 years	29	31	21	30	28
> 10 years	71	69	80	70	73
Smoking status					
Daily	89	89	89	89	89
Occasional	12	11	11	11	11
No. of cigarettes per day					
< 11	55	57	45	50	52
11–19	16	17	22	17	18
≥ 20	30	26	33	34	31
Reasons for consultation					
Common chronic illness	34	21	30	26	28
Acute or rare chronic illness	54	65	60	65	61
Other	12	14	10	9	11
No. consultations in past 6 months					
< 6	76	78	71	71	74
≥ 6	25	23	30	29	27
Type of case					
New	37	44	32	39	38
Old	63	56	68	61	62

p values for comparison among four groups: all > 0.05

those receiving the booklet with those not receiving the booklet, and those receiving advice with those not receiving advice; nevertheless, 5.6% of subjects who received advice only had stopped smoking continuously for one week after the intervention. This was significantly higher than the 2.1% for those not receiving advice.

Table 4 shows the smoking cessation rates of people who had previosuly attended the clinic in the different intervention groups. The proportion of consecutive abstinence in the group that had received both the booklet and advice was significantly higher than that in the control group at one year (5% versus 0%), and all three quit rates were significantly higher than those of the controls at the short-term follow-up. The point prevalence and the sustained abstinence rates in the group that had received advice only were also significantly higher than that in the controls at one week.

A total of 147 (17%) former smokers claimed not to be smoking at the one-year follow-up. Only 16 of them agreed to come forward for a urinary cotinine test. One admitted that he had smoked again just before coming for the test. No urinary cotinine was detected in 12 of the remaining 15; one subject was found to have a high cotinine level which indicated recent smoking, and the other two had trace amounts of cotinine which might have been due to recent smoking or exposure to environmental tobacco smoke.

Table 2. Smoking cessation of all subjects in four intervention groups

Measure of cessation	Controls (n = 241) %	Booklet only (n = 181) %	Advice only (n = 213) %	Booklet and advice (n = 230) %	All (n = 865) %
Point prevalence abstinence					
at 1 week	10.4	11.0	14.1	13.0	12.1
at 3 months	7.9	8.8	9.9	12.2	9.7
at 6 months	10.4	11.0	8.5	11.7	10.4
at 1 year	16.2	19.3	14.1	18.7	17.0
Consecutive abstinence					
at 3 months	4.1	2.8	4.7	4.8	4.2
at 6 months	2.5	2.8	3.3	3.9	3.1
at 1 year	2.1	2.8	3.3	3.5	2.9
Sustained abstinence					
at 1 week[a]	2.5	1.7	5.2	6.1	4.0
at 1 year[b]	3.3	2.8	2.3	3.9	3.1

[a]Not smoking continuously for past week
[b]Not smoking at 3-month follow-up, then continuously to 1-year follow-up

Discussion

We found that the smoking cessation rate of patients who received doctors' advice with or without a self-help booklet, was not significantly different from that of the controls after one year; however, doctors' advice did significantly help patients to stop smoking in the short term. Doctors' advice was found to be effective in helping patients seen previously to stop smoking at one year. A pre-established doctor–patient relationship (i.e. trust) may have augmented the effect of the doctors' advice, especially in a busy clinic setting. This association and the possible effect of follow-up advice for patients who stopped smoking in the short-term must be examined further.

The limitations and constraints of this study in comparison with other studies are as follows. This study included only patients aged ≤ 65 attending general Government out-patient clinics. The patients who attend these clinics are generally older, of lower social class and have more chronic problems than those visiting private practitioners (Census and Statistics Department, 1992; Department of Health, 1994) and include a higher proportion of smokers (Health Care Providers' Liaison Subcommittee, 1994). As about 70% of patients in Hong Kong consult private practitioners, these results cannot be generalized to them. Although the response rate of 64% at one year is low, it is compatible with those of similar studies elsewhere, in which the rates were 61–73%

Table 3. Smoking cessation of all subjects given booklet vs no booklet and advice vs no advice

Measure of cessation	No booklet vs booklet		No advice vs advice	
	(n = 454) %	(n = 411) %	(n = 422) %	(n = 443) %
Point prevalence abstinence				
at 1 week	12.1	12.2	10.7	13.5
at 3 months	8.8	10.7	8.3	11.1
at 6 months	9.5	11.4	10.7	10.2
at 1 year	15.2	19.0	17.5	16.5
Consecutive abstinence				
at 3 months	4.4	3.9	3.6	4.7
at 6 months	2.9	3.4	2.6	3.6
at 1 year	2.6	3.2	2.4	3.4
Sustained abstinence				
at 1 week[a]	3.7	4.1	2.1	5.6*
at 1 year[b]	2.9	3.4	3.1	3.2

Booklet vs no booklet, advice vs no advice: * $p < 0.05$
[a]Not smoking continuously for the past 1 week
[b]Not smoking at 3-month follow-up, then continuously to 1-year follow-up

Table 4. Smoking cessation of previous cases in four intervention groups

Measure of cessation	Controls (n = 149) %	Booklet only (n = 100) %	Advice only (n = 143) %	Booklet and advice (n = 140) %
Point prevalence abstinence				
at 1 week	4.7	8.0	14.7**	15.7**
at 3 months	6.0	7.0	10.5	14.3*
at 6 months	8.7	11.0	9.8	14.3
at 1 year	13.4	20.0	15.4	22.1
Consecutive abstinence				
at 3 months	0.7	0.0	4.9*	6.4**
at 6 months	0.0	0.0	2.8	5.0**
at 1 year	0.0	0.0	2.8	5.0**
Sustained abstinence				
at 1 week[a]	0.0	1.0	4.9**	9.3***
at 1 year[b]		1.3	3.0	2.8 5.0

Each intervention group compared with controls: * $p < 0.05$, ** $p < 0.01$, *** $p < 0.001$
[a]Not smoking continuously for past week
[b]Not smoking at 3-month follow-up, then continuously to 1-year follow-up

(Stewart & Rosser, 1982; Fielding, 1985; Dermers *et al.*, 1990; Wilson *et al.*, 1990; Department of Health, 1992).

The merit of this study was the true randomization of subjects. In most studies in the literature, true randomization was not used, especially in those with large sample sizes (Russell *et al.*, 1979, 1987; Wilson *et al.*, 1990; Slama *et al.*, 1995). The smoking cessation intervention used in this study is simple, brief, one-off and involves no specific follow-up for the patients. The brief advice given to the patients lasted < 1 min. 'Brief' advice in other studies ranged from 2 to 5 min (Wilkin *et al.*, 1987; Dermers *et al.*, 1990; Gilbert *et al.*, 1992). Although the advice given by the doctors to eligible patients has the advantage of being standardized and easily reproducible and could be adopted by physicians in clinical practice, doctors might find it unnatural to read from a pre-established set of instructions, and the formality of the approach might affect the effectiveness of the advice.

Use of various quit rates in different studies was often not explained. Point prevalence abstinence is a common measure of cessation but indicates only smokers who have stopped smoking at a particular time; it usually overestimates actual long-term cessation by including people who have relapsed between assessments. Sustained abstinence can be measured as continuous abstinence since the intervention or as prolonged abstinence (i.e. continuous abstinence for a prolonged period before assessment but not necessarily starting at the time of intervention). Sustained abstinence is more stable over time than the point prevalence rate (Wilkin *et al.*, 1987). Whereas prolonged abstinence is more commonly used than continuous abstinence because it also includes those who take delayed action to quit after receiving the intervention; however, sustained abstinence relies on self-reporting and cannot be validated biochemically. Consecutive abstinence is less commonly used but can be a useful indicator of smoking cessation, especially if point prevalence abstinence is validated by biochemical testing. Repeatedly validated point prevalence, although costly, may provide supplementary data to sustained abstinence when biochemical validation is not practicable or may be used as a proxy for sustained abstinence.

In this study, the consecutive abstinence rates, but not the point prevalence or sustained abstinence rates, for previous clinic patients were significantly higher in the group given advice than in the controls. It is not uncommon to have different findings for different outcome measures in the same study. Slama *et al.* (1995) found that the proportion of sustained abstinence, but not point prevalence, in the intervention group was significantly greater than that in controls at one year. They concluded that their interventions were effective. It is possible that some researchers use only the outcome measures that show significant results and do not present non-significant findings.

Only 10% of the subjects who claimed to have stopped smoking agreed to come forward for a test. When Russell *et al.* (1987) invited former smokers by post to undergo urinary cotinine analysis, 75% turned up. Biochemical validation was performed in only 23 of 2138 smokers initially recruited in another study by Russell *et al.* (1979).

In our study, most of the point estimates of quit rates in the intervention groups were higher than those in the controls, but only a few of these differences were statistically significant, possibly because of inadequate sample size and the unexpectedly high quit rates among the controls. The latter could have been due to the repeated follow-up interviews.

Acknowledgements

We wish to thank the Health Services Research Committee for funding this project, the doctors and patients for their participation, Professor E.D. Janus and the Clinical Biochemistry Unit, The University of Hong Kong, for the cotinine assays and Mrs J Cheang for research assistance.

References

Census and Statistics Department (1992) *Health Status of the Population in Hong Kong (Special Topics Report No. 10)*, Hong Kong Government

Department of Health (1992) *Report on Survey of Doctors Consultation* (Internal report), Hong Kong Government

Department of Health (1994) *Survey on Disease Surveillance at GOPC* (Internal Report) Hong Kong Government

Dermers, R.Y., Neale, A.V., Adams, R., Trembath, C. & Herman, S.C. (1990) The impact of physicians' brief smoking cessation counseling: A MIRNET study. *J. Fam. Pract.*, 31, 625–629

Fielding, J.E. (1985) Smoking: Health effects and control. *New Engl. J. Med.*, 313, 491–498, 555–561

Gilbert, R.J., Wilson, D.M.C., Sunger, J., et al. (1992) A family physician smoking cessation program: An evaluation of the role of follow-up visits. *Am. J. Prev. Med.*, 8, 91–95

Glynn, T.J. & Mamley, M.W. (1989) *How to Help Your Patients to Stop Smoking: A National Cancer Institute Manual for Physicians* (NIH publication no. 89–30640), US Department of Health and Human Services, Public Health Service, National Institutes of Health National Cancer Institute

Health Care Providers' Liason Subcommittee (1994) The potential of opportunistic screening of risk factor and patient education—A one day risk factor survey in Kwun Tong District Health System. *Hong Kong Pract.*, 16, 622–626

Lam, T.H., Betson, C.L. & Hedley, A.J. (1994) Pattern of smoking cessation in Hong Kong, 1984–90. *J. Smoking Relat. Dis.*, 5 (Suppl. 1), 283–287

Russell, M.A.H., Wilson, C., Baker, C. & Tayor, C.D. (1979) Effect of general practitioner advice against smoking. *Br. Med. J.*, ii, 231–235

Russell, M.A.H., Stapleton, J.A., Jackson, P.H., Hajek, P. & Belcher, M. (1987) District programme by reduce smoking: Effect of clinic supported brief intervention by general practitioners. *Br. Med. J.*, 295, 1240–1244

Slama, K., Karsenty & Hirsch, A. (1995) Effectiveness of minimal intervention by general practitioners with their smoking patients: A randomised, controlled trial in France. *Tobacco Control*, 4, 162–169

Stewart, P.J. & Rosser, W.W. (1982) The impact of routine advice on smoking cessation from family physicians. *Can. Med. Assoc. J.*, 126, 1051–1054

Velicer, W.F., Prochaska, J.O., Rossi, J.S. & Snow, M.G. (1992) Assessing outcome in smoking cessation studies. *Psychol. Bull.*, 111, 23–41

Wilkin, R., Hallam, L., Leavey, R. & Metcalf, D. (1987) *Anatomy of Urban General Practice*, London: Tavistock Publications

Wilson, D.H., Wakefield, M.A., Steven, I.D., Rohrsheim, R.A., Esterman, A.J. & Graham, N.M.H. 'Sick of Smoking': Evaluation of a targeted minimal smoking cessation intervention in general practice. *Med. J. Aust.*, 152, 51? 609

Stop-smoking contests in Japan

T. Kinoshita & M. Nakamura

Department of Cancer Prevention, The Osaka Cancer Prevention and Detection Center, Osaka, Japan

Our centre has been conducting stop-smoking contests every year since 1988, in order to develop effective and efficient approaches to reach a number of smokers at a time. Participation is open to all smokers who want to quit smoking. They are recruited mainly through the mass media and take on the challenge of stopping smoking using self-help cessation materials sent to them by mail. The contest is held in two phases. In the first two weeks, the participants prepare to quit by monitoring their smoking behaviour, making sure of their reasons for quitting, checking their nicotine dependence and so on. The following four weeks are used for complete cessation, by checking the advantages of quitting and self-efficacy for maintenance. To be eligible for a contest prize, participants must have abstained completely from all forms of tobacco use during the four-week abstinence period. Quitters are asked to sign a 'Declaration of success in quitting smoking', with two witnesses.

During 1988 and 1996, a total of 22 034 current smokers participated in the contests, and 4493 succeeded in quitting. The overall short-term success rate was 22%.

Stop-smoking contests can result in many cases of quitting at a time and also serve as campaigns for raising awareness about smoking cessation. Contests could play a significant role in reducing the prevalence of smoking in Japan.

Smoking cessation for patients with heart disease

H. Nurkkala, U.-R. Penttilä & M. Romo

Finnish Heart Association, Helsinki, Finland

Smoking is the major cause of cardiovascular disease, and stopping smoking greatly reduces the risk for myocardial infarct and death from coronary heart disease. The North Karelia Project showed, however, that over 50% of patients continue to smoke after a heart attack. This suggests that patients do not receive enough support to stop smoking. Our aim was to create and evaluate a smoking cessation programme for patients with cardiovascular disease, to be given by health-care staff in hospitals, health centres, occupational health centres and the private sector.

Method

Two groups of smokers were included: all patients hospitalized within a six-month period for myocardial infarct and 159 out-patients with previous diagnoses of coronary heart disease. The patients were invited to the intervention and to follow-up after one year. Their smoking status and stage of change were determined at 3, 6 and 12 months. The criteria for inclusion were having been born in 1921 or later, smoking and having coronary heart disease.

The intervention consisted of counselling by a nurse, supported by a physician, through face-to-face and telephone contacts. Each smoking patient seen by a physician or nurse in any health-care unit was given the opportunity of receiving individual guidance if they expressed readiness to stop smoking. The intervention was continued in the patient's own health-care unit if it had begun in hospital. The smoking cessation programme for each patient included two personal visits and three phone contacts, continuing for six months after the patients had decided to quit smoking. Patients were invited for an extra visit if they needed more support or resumed smoking.

The model of individual guidance is an application of the stage of change model, based on the theory of Prochaska. In our application of this model, the patient's readiness for change is divided into four stages: pre-contemplation, contemplation, preparation and action and maintenance. Guidance is started at the first visit by determining the stage of readiness to stop smoking. Smoking cessation is then maintained with booklets and education.

The programme was launched on 1 October 1996. The results will be available shortly.

Short-term effectiveness of a multi-media smoking cessation programme for pregnant women

M.J. Bakker & H. de Vries

Maastricht University, Department of Health Education, Maastricht, The Netherlands

Introduction

Pregnant women are a special target group for smoking cessation interventions for several reasons. First, smoking during pregnancy can cause serious damage to the unborn child. Examples of complications that might occur during or after pregnancy because of smoking are low birth weight, prematurity, spontaneous abortion and perinatal mortality. Secondly, pregnancy can be a good moment for women to quit smoking because of the harmful effects of smoking for their baby. A study by Hill (1988) showed that pregnant women are more motivated to quit smoking because of the unborn child. Thirdly, pregnancy could be a window of opportunity to discuss smoking cessation with pregnant women, who are in regular contact with a health-care provider during this period of their lives. It is possible to develop effective smoking cessation programmes for pregnant women (Floyd *et al.*, 1993; Walsh & Redman, 1993). Walsh and Redman (1993) concluded that cognitive behavioural smoking cessation programmes are effective, but none of the studies examined in their review fulfilled the criteria necessary for a programme to be incorporated into routine care.

The aim of the study described here was therefore to develop a programme to be provided by usual care providers which can be adopted easily, once it has been shown to be effective. Since in the Netherlands approximately 45% of deliveries are supervised by midwives (10% general practioners, 45% gynaecologists), we decided to train midwives in providing the programme to their pregnant clients.

Methods

Midwifery practices were randomly assigned to either experimental or control conditions, the latter being standard prenatal care. The programme consists of a video, self-help guide, partner booklet, relapse prevention booklet and a health counselling protocol. A total of 318 women were included in the study after signing an informed consent form at the midwife's office. A randomized pre-test–post-test control group design was used to evaluate the programme. Pre-test data were gathered at the first consultation with the midwife; post-test data were collected by means of a structured telephone interview six weeks after the first consultation. Quitting was not validated biochemically, but a 'bogus pipeline' procedure—telling the women that biochemical samples might be taken—was used to enhance the validity of self-reports (Windsor & Orleans, 1986).

The questionnaire elicited information on educational level, number of weeks pregnant, number of pregnancies and age. The smoking behaviour of the women was measured by determining the age at onset of smoking, the number of cigarettes smoked per day before becoming pregnant and at the time they started the programme, the number of attempts to quit after the first consultation and if they were still non-smokers. The smoking behaviour of the partners was also assessed.

Results

The response rate to the telephone interviews was 94% (300 women), 136 women in the experimental condition and 164 controls. The age of the women ranged from 15 to 40 years, with a mean of 28.5. On average, the women were 12.9 weeks pregnant at entry into the programme. Most of the women were pregnant for the first (50%) or second (28%) time. More women in the control branch had a lower educational level (62%) than those in the experimental branch (15%). Before becoming pregnant, the women had smoked about 18 cigarettes per day; at the beginning of the programme, the rate had been reduced to 9.09 cigarettes for women in the experimental branch and 7.07 for controls. The women had started to smoke at an average age of 15 years. On average, 63% of the partners smoked.

Attempts to quit were made by 38% of the women in the experimental branch and 26% of controls (chi-squared(1) = 4.91; $p < 0.05$). Six weeks after the intervention, 19% of women in the experimental branch and 7.9% of controls claimed to be non smokers (chi-squared(1) = 8.23; $p < 0.01$). Multiple logistic regression analysis showed that significant predictors of trying to quit were assignment to the experimental branch (odds ratio, 1.9; 95% confidence interval, 1.1–3.4; $p < 0.05$) and age at onset of smoking (1.1; 1.0–1.3; $p < 0.05$). Strong predictors of remaining a non-smoker were being in the experimental branch (3.1; 1.4–6.9; $p < 0.01$) and having a partner who smoked (2.5; 1.2–5.6; $p < 0.05$). A significant inverse relationship was seen with the number of cigarettes smoked at the beginning of the programme (0.84; 0.76–0.93; $p < 0.01$).

Discussion

The results of the first post-test measurement indicate that the programme was more effective than standard prenatal care in initiating attempts to quit among pregnant women in their first trimester. Furthermore, more women in the experimental branch successfully quit. Follow-up measurements will be conducted six weeks and six months *post partum* in order to estimate whether the programme is also effective in preventing relapse at that time.

Acknowledgement
This research was financed by a grant from the Dutch Cancer Society, the Dutch Heart Foundation and the Prevention Fund.

References
Floyd, R.L., Rimer, B.K., Giovino, G.A., Mullen, P.D. & Sullivan, S.E. (1993) A review of smoking in pregnancy: Effects on pregnancy outcomes and cessation efforts. ??, **14**, 379–411
Hill, A.E. (1988) Considerations for smoking advice in pregnancy. *Ulster Med. J.*, **57**, 22–27
Walsh, R. & Redman, S. (1993) Smoking cessation in pregnancy: Do effective programmes exist? ??, **8**, 111–127
Windsor, R.A. & Orleans, C.T. (1986) Guidelines and methodological standards for smoking cessation intervention research among pregnant women: Improving the science and art. ??, **13**, 131–161

Smoking and smoking cessation among men whose partners are pregnant

M. Wakefield[1], Y. Reid[2], L. Roberts[3], R. Mullins[2] & P. Gillies[4]

[1]*South Australian Health Commission, Adelaide, South Australia;* [2]*Victorian Smoking and Health Program, Victoria, Australia;* [3]*South Australian Smoking and Health Project, Adelaide, South Australia;* [4]*Department of Public Health and Epidemiology, University of Nottingham, United Kingdom*

Introduction and method

Smoking among partners of non-smoking pregnant women has been linked to adverse pregnancy outcome, including low birthweight. Paternal smoking also increases the risk of infant respiratory infections and sudden infant death syndrome, irrespective of maternal smoking status. Furthermore, men's smoking habits are probably one of the strongest influences on the extent to which women are able to quit smoking in pregnancy and maintain cessation after the birth.

In four focus group discussions in Adelaide, South Australia, male smokers whose partners were pregnant discussed their beliefs about passive smoking in pregnancy, the barriers they perceived to quitting during the pregnancy and their preparedness to support maternal cessation. The aim of the present study was to explore these issues, in order to assist the development of messages and strategies that might influence change in paternal smoking habits during pregnancy.

Main themes from focus groups

'The pregnant woman's attitude to smoking will influence the partner's smoking.' The most frequently reported concern about passive smoking was the discomfort or level of annoyance caused to the person who did not smoke. The rule of thumb seemed to be that if the pregnant woman did not mind, then it was acceptable to smoke near her: "I wouldn't smoke in a room with a pregnant woman unless she said it was all right. It's annoying and irritating, but it's not going to kill anyone." "As long as she doesn't mind, I'm not really worried about it."

Men with pregnant partners who smoked had made very few changes to their own smoking habits, and most continued to smoke inside the home. In contrast, most men who lived with women who were non-smokers or who had quit during pregnancy, now smoked outside the home or the car. For many men, their partner was the major instigator of this change: "I smoke in another room or outside now. The woman nags if I smoke inside." One man suggested that the best way of getting the message to fathers to stop smoking was to "... tell the women, and then they hound us."

'Passive smoking is not perceived to be important if the pregnant woman is herself a smoker.' Very few men had even a vague understanding about the effect passive smoking might have on people in general or on pregnant women in particular. Many men did not accept that their smoking had affected their own health and thought that it was illogical that passive smoking could affect others' health: "I've smoked for a long time and I'm not very fit, but it hasn't affected me, so why would it affect someone sitting on the other side of the room?" "If you think about it, by the time it's been in my lungs and into the atmosphere and then into someone else's lungs, there isn't much chemicals left (*sic*)."

Many men related instances of people they knew who had smoked 'all of their lives' without any apparent ill effects, and women who had smoked in pregnancy and delivered normal babies: "I myself don't think it has any effect. I come from a family of six kids and my father smoked right through the whole of us (*sic*) ... it didn't do anything to us." "My wife's just lost a baby a couple of months back, but I don't think it was because of smoking."

'Doctors rarely give advice about smoking to partners.' When asked about information or recommendations about smoking, the usual experience was that only women were questioned about their smoking habits and sometimes advised to quit: "They mention smoking to the female but not to the male." "They ask you if you smoke, and that's the end of it. They don't ask 'do you want some help stopping?'"

'Concern about smoking cessation increases stress and marital discord.' The stress experienced when going without cigarettes was commonly cited as a barrier to successfully quitting smoking: "My wife gave up smoking, but her moods were unbelievable. I told her just to have a few to stop the arguments."

This, on top of the irritability and mood swings attributed to the pregnancy itself, made the concept of quitting smoking too much to cope with. As one man explained, "They get grumpier than they already are." Some acknowledged that smoking around their partner contributed to the difficulty she experienced in quitting. When men were asked what they would do to support their partner in giving up, the usual response was that they would offer words of encouragement. Only a few said they would be prepared to quit as well. The general consensus was that 'one stressed out person' in the home was bad enough, without there being two: "I'd support her and say you can have one if you want, but I'd try to talk her out of it. But if she was getting stressed out about it, I'd give her a cigarette."

'*More explanation is needed as to why passive smoking is harmful.*' What men wanted to know was 'what it does, not just that it harms them (unborn children)'. Those who were more receptive to smoking cessation messages thought that advertising which showed in detail the damage that smoking can cause was the most effective, while others wanted information about 'exactly how' smoking harms your health: "There's no point in just saying 'don't do it', they've got to say why: that anything that goes into the mother goes to the baby." "Tell us the real story, what it really does to people."

'*Acknowledgement that smoking reduces fitness.*' One aspect of smoking that most men acknowledged as applying to them personally was reduced fitness, manifested by shortness of breath, persistent phlegm and 'wheeziness': "It slows you down if you want to do something physically, I feel it there."

Recommendations for smoking cessation intervention among partners

- Encourage pregnant women to ask their partners to quit or to smoke outside. Provide smoke-free home and car stickers to pregnant women.
- Encourage medical and nursing staff to enquire about partner's smoking habits and offer appropriate assistance to quit.
- Explain to pregnant women and partners how passive smoking is harmful, perhaps by explaining that inhalation of tobacco smoke reduces the oxygen-carrying capacity of the maternal blood supply to the foetus, so that the baby's source of food for growth is reduced.
- Give smoking cessation advice and reinforcement when motivation is strongest, perhaps when partners accompany pregnant women to the routine ultrasound appointment.
- Remind men that they need to maintain their fitness to make the most of being a father. Smoking cessation will increase their fitness.

A dental office intervention for cessation of use of smokeless tobacco

H.H. Severson, J.A. Andrews, E. Lichtenstein & J.S. Gordon

Oregon Research Institute, Eugene, Oregon, United States

The goal of this project was to evaluate the effectiveness of dental hygienists in advising their patients to quit use of smokeless tobacco and/or smoking. Seventy-five private practice dental offices in western Oregon were randomly assigned to give usual care or a minimal or extended intervention. Over 34,000 patients (average age, 45; 93% Caucasian; 60% female) were enrolled in the study. Of these patients, 30,136 did not use tobacco, 632 used smokeless tobacco, 4029 smoked and 100 used both smokeless tobacco and cigarettes (Andrews et al., 1998).

Smokers received usual care or the minimal or extended intervention, but owing to the relatively small number of users of smokeless tobacco, these received the extended intervention or usual care. The minimal intervention consisted of four steps: determination of the patient's tobacco use from charts and enrolment form; an oral examination; direct advice to quit in relation to the results of the examination; and giving the patient a package of written materials including pamphlets on health problems due to tobacco use and how to stop using tobacco and a quit kit comprising a cup filled with items to help cessation. Smokers and smokeless tobacco users in the extended intervention received the same four steps and three additional components: asking the patient to set a date for quitting within two weeks of the visit; giving the patients a motivational video and calling the patient within two weeks to give support and encouragement.

The programme was not effective in convincing smokers to stop but was effective for chewers. Assuming that those lost to follow-up were chewers, the results indicate that the intervention was very effective for users of smokeless tobacco at both 3 months (18 versus 8.8%, $p < 0.01$) and 12 months (16 versus 8.8%, $p < 0.01$). In addition, significantly more smokeless tobacco users who received the intervention quit at 3 months and had not resumed chewing by 12 months (10%) than smokeless tobacco users receiving the usual care (3.3%; $p < 0.001$) (Severson et al., 1998).

The results suggest that advice on cessation of smokeless tobacco use is effective when delivered by dental professionals in the context of a dental hygiene visit. This study replicates our similar study in prepaid dental clinics (Stevens et al., 1995) and demonstrates the consistent effect of providing a low-intensity intervention to dental patients who use smokeless tobacco. Since 50% of tobacco users see their dentist each year, the public health implications of this programm are significant, even if the actual cessation rate is modest. The relative effectiveness of cessation advice to smokeless tobacco users, as compared with smokers, could be due to the fact that the effects of smokeless tobacco on oral health are readily observable (e.g. oral lesions), dental staff are more comfortable and committed to providing advice to users of smokeless tobacco and/or smokeless tobacco users are more receptive to information on cessation.

References
Andrews, J.A., Severson, H.H., Lichtenstein, E. & Gordon, J.S. (1998) Relationship between tobacco use and self-reported oral hygiene habits. J. Am. Dental Assoc., 129, 313–320
Severson, H.H., Andrews, J.A., Lichtenstein, E., & Gordon, J.S. (1998). Using the hygiene visit to deliver a tobacco cessation program: Results of a randomized clinical trial. J. Am. Dental Assoc., 129, 993–999
Stevens, V.J., Severson, H.H., Lichtenstein, E., Little, S.J. & Leben, J. (1995) Making the most of a teachable moment: A smokeless tobacco cessation intervention in the dental office. Am. J. Public Health, 85, 231–235

Multi-faceted treatment of tobacco addiction in a group of health professionals

L. Sanchez-Agudo[1], J.M. Carreras-Castellet[1], M.P. Jiménez-Santolaya[2] & F.J. Iñigo-Barrera[2]

[1]Servicio de Neumología, Centro de Investigación Clínica, Instituto de Salud Carlos III, Madrid; [2]Sección de Neumología, Hospital San Pedro, Insalud, La Rioja, Spain

Introduction

Health professionals are a reference for a healthy lifestyle in the minds of the public. Thus, health professionals who do not smoke influence the public not to smoke and contribute to the understanding that tobacco damages health. Those who smoke counteract measures designed to control the epidemic of addiction to tobacco. Health professionald should be conscious of the example they give. We therefore developed a specific tobacco cessation programme directed to this population group.

The objective of the study reported here was to evaluate the motivations of a group of health professionals to give up smoking, to treat them with a multi-component programme and to compare the results with those of non-health professionals treated similarly.

Material and methods

A group of 105 health professionals, including physicians, nurses, pharmacists and veterinarians, who applied for tobacco cessation treatment were sent a questionnaire eliciting information on their dependence (determined by the Fagerström test; Heatherton et al., 1991) and motivation. It was correctly completed and returned by 50, but 12 of these were excluded because they had a low dependence on nicotine and had made no previous attempt to quit. The characteristics of the group are shown in Table 1; 75% had previously made at least two serious attempts to stop smoking.

The treatment consisted of a 7–10-day preparation period, during which they recorded the number of cigarettes they smoked, their motives for smoking and why they wanted to give up; a one-month period of intensive treatment during which they did not smoke; and follow-up treatment of 8, 12 and 24 weeks. The treatment consisted of nicotine replacement therapy with patches and chewing-gum, the dose being decreased progressively over 12 weeks, and eight 2-h sessions of group therapy with behavioural support, with five sessions during the intensive treatment and the other three during the follow-up. At each session, anxiety state (Spielberger et al., 1970), withdrawal symptoms and expired carbon monoxide were measured.

People were considered to have become non-smokers if they had not smoked for 12 weeks and had less than 6 ppm carbon monoxide in expired air.

Statistical significance was determined from the relative risks, odds ratios and chi-squared values in comparison with a group of 111 non-health professionals with similar characteristics submitted to the same treatment.

Results

The most frequent reasons given for wanting to stop smoking were tobacco dependence (92%), prevention of illness (87%), family pressure (53%), giving a good example to children (34%), social pressure (29%) and respect for non-smokers (26%). The abstinence rates among the health professionals were 92% after four weeks, 87% after eight weeks, 79% after 12 weeks and 76% at six months; while those among the non-health professionals were 83, 77, 68 and 55%, respectively.

Similar proportions of health and non-health professionals (about 68%) attended a minimum of six treatment sessions. One of the patients refused to use nicotine replacement. No serious side-effects were seen: only four subjects had a local cutaneous reaction to nicotine patches, and the dose was replaced by chewing-gum.

Discussion

As in the general population (Ministerio de Sanidad y Consumo, 1992), the main reasons given by this group for giving up smoking were to escape dependence on tobacco and to prevent ill health; they were, however, more sensitive to these issues than other segments of the population. It is noteworthy that their role as health professionals was not one of their reasons for wishing to quit.

The efficacy of behaviour modification (Schwartz, 1987) and nicotine replacement therapy (Fiore et al., 1994) for smoking cessation is widely confirmed, as is the absence of adverse secondary effects. The percentage of non-smokers after this treatment is usually 30–50% after six months; in our group, the percentage was significantly higher. As the only difference was the fact that they were health professionals, we may conclude that this is the reason for the better result. Although health professionals are sometimes

Table 1. Characteristics of participants

Characteristic	No.	Standard deviation
Sex		
Male	14 (36.8%)	
Female	24 (63.2%)	
Mean age (years)	40.6	6.6
Degree of dependence	6.6	2.2
Mean age at starting to smoke (years)	19.1	3.9
No. of cigarettes smoked per day	26.3	10.4
Expired carbon monoxide (ppm)	41.2	19.2
Anxiety state	18.1	10.5
Anxiety trait	21.9	9.2

sceptical about this type of treatment or reluctant to use it, we believe that good results can be achieved with suitable selection of candidates.

The good performance of this treatment in health professionals is especially important in view of their capacity to affect use of tobacco in the general population.

References

Fiore, M.C., Smith, S.S., Jornby, D.E. & Baker, T.B. (1994) The effectiveness of nicotine patch for smoking cessation: A meta-analysis. *J. Am. Med. Assoc.*, **271**, 1940–1947

Heatherton, T.F., Kozlowski, L.T., Frecker, R.C. & Fageström, K.O. (1991) The Fagerström test for nicotine dependence: A revision of the Fagerström tolerance questionnaire. *Br. J. Addict.*, **86**, 1119–1127

Ministerio de Sanidad y Consumo (1992) *Estudio de los Estilos de Vida de la Pobalcíon Adulta Española*, Madrid

Schwartz, J.L. (1987) *Review and Evaluation of Smoking Cessation Methods: The United States and Canada, 1978–1985*, Washington DC: Department of Health and Human Services

Spielberger, C.D., Gorsuch, R.L. & Lushene, R.E. (1970) *STAI, Manual for the State–Trait Anxiety Inventory (Self Evaluation Questionnaire)*, California: Consulting Psychologist Press, Inc.

Multi-component smoking treatment in a pneumological unit: Method, results and predictors of success

L. Sanchez-Agudo, J.M. Carreras-Castellet & B. Maldonado-Arostegui

Servicio de Neumología, Centro de Investigación Clínica, Instituto de Salud Carlos III, Madrid, Spain

Introduction

In Spain, there are few treatment units for smoking cessation and little social sensitivity about the hazards of smoking. It has been 10 years since we first introduced a multi-component treatment for smoking cessation in our Service, using previously described methods. This paper gives the results obtained in the smokers who were treated in the unit during a 12-month period. The objectives were to analyse the sociodemographic characteristics and tobacco dependence of the subjects, to evaluate the treatment results and to analyse the differences between smokers who achieved six months' abstinence and those who failed to do so in order to identify the variables that predict successful treatment.

Material and methods

Between January and December 1995, 111 people, 49 men (44%) and 62 women (56%) requested treatment for smoking. Their sociodemographic characteristics and tobacco consumption are shown in Table 1. The men were significantly ($p < 0.05$) older than the women, and most of the participants had finished intermediate or higher studies. The men had started to smoke at a significantly earlier age than the women and had a significantly higher baseline concentration of expired carbon monoxide.

The treatment consisted of an initial interview, an intensive treatment period and follow-up. The first, individual visit involved questioning about medical and smoking history, administration of the Fagerström questionnaire to determine nicotine dependence (Heatherton *ett al.*, 1991), measurement of expired carbon monoxide (with a calibrated Mini-Smokerlyzer after a 15-s apnoea), an inventory of anxiety state and traits (Spielberger *et al.*, 1970) and training for compliance. This was followed by a preparation period of 7–10 days, when the participants recorded the number of cigarettes they smoked, their motives for smoking and why they wanted to give up.

The four-week intensive treatment period included five 2-h group therapy meetings of 12–16 people, which were directed by a pneumologist and a nurse. The first was held the day before the participants were to give up smoking, the second 24 h after abstinence and the three others one, two and four weeks after smoking had been stopped.

Three further group therapy sessions were held after 8, 12 and 24 weeks. At each meeting, anxiety state, withdrawal symptoms and expired carbon monoxide were measured. Beginning on the day they gave up smoking, participants were given nicotine patches that release 0.7 mg/cm^2 for 16 or 24 h. Subjects with a Fagerström score of $\geq$ 7 received 30, 20 and 10 mg/cm^2 for three consecutive periods of 28 days, and those with a score of 5 or 6 received 20 mg/cm^2 for 56 days and then 10 mg/cm^2 for 28 days. Patches of 24-h duration were used for subjects who smoked their first cigarette during the first half-hour after waking and for people working on shifts; the remainder received the 16-h patches. Chewing-gum containing 2 mg nicotine was added on demand, up to a maximum of seven sticks per day. In 15 subjects (14%), nicotine supplements were contraindicated for medical reasons (e.g. coronary accident) or because of intolerance on previous attempts.

People were considered to have become non-smokers if they had not smoked for 12 weeks and had less than 6 ppm carbon monoxide in expired air.

Statistical significance was determined from the relative risks, odds ratios and chi-squared values.

Results

The abstinence rates were 93% at 24 h, 91% at one week, 83% at four weeks, 77% at eight weeks, 69% at 12 weeks and 55% at 24 weeks. We observed a significant decrease in daily cigarette consumption between the first visit and the first group meeting, from 27.1 to 22.5 cigarettes per day ($p < 0.05$) and in expired carbon monoxide, from 42.0 to 29.4 ($p < 0.001$). Furthermore, the recording of cigarette consumption and motives for smoking during this period is a good indicator of smoking cessation, as of the 81 subjects who completed this requirement, 52 remained abstinent for six months ($p < 0.05$).

Table 2 shows the characteristics of the subjects who had and had not remained abstinent for 24 weeks. The only meaningful differences were found for level of education, Fagerström score and having made one to five previous attempts to stop smoking.

Of the 111 subjects, 33 failed to stop smoking completely during the first week; of these, only nine (27%) were still abstinent at six months. Of the 78 who did stop smoking during the first week, 52 (67%) were still not smoking at six months ($p < 0.0005$). Inability to stop smoking in the short term was more marked among women in our group than among men ($p < 0.05$), but no significant difference was seen at six months. Subjects who were unable to give up in the short term also had a greater score for anxiety state (22.8) than those who did (14.0; $p < 0.005$); again, these differences were not seen after six months.

No serious side-effects were seen. Ten of the subjects who used nicotine patches had a local cutaneous reaction, and the dose was replaced with chewing-gum. The dose of one subject had to be reduced after bouts of dizziness.

Table 1. Sociodemographic characteristics and tobacco consumption of participants

Characteristic	Men	Women	All
Number (%)	49 (44.1)	62 (55.9)	111
Mean age (SD)	46.2 (11.5)*	40.1 (9.2)	43.3 (10.4)
Primary education (%)	9 (18.4)	5 (8.1)	14 (12.7)
Intermediate studies (%)	18 (36.7)	32 (51.6)	50 (45.5)
Higher studies (%)	21 (42.9)	25 (40.3)	46 (41.8)
Cigarettes/day (SD)	29.1 (13.4)	25.4 (9.5)	27.1 (11.4)
Fagerström score (SD)	6.5 (2.3)	5.9 (2.1)	6.3 (1.9)
Expired CO (ppm) (SD)	50.7 (32.8)*	35.2 (19.9)	42.0 (27.2)
Previous attemps to quit (SD)	2.9 (3.1)	2.7 (3.0)	2.8 (3.2)
Age at starting smoking (SD)	18.5 (3.2)	20.8 (5.1)	19.8 (4.5)
Pack-years (SD)	39.8 (24.7)**	25.9 (13.6)	32.1 (20.4)

* $p < 0.05$; ** $p < 0.001$

Table 2. Differences in characteristics of abstinent and non-abstinent smokers after six months

Characteristic	Abstinent	Non-abstinent
Number (%)	61 (54.9)	50 (45.1)
Male (%)	28 (57.1)	21 (42.9)
Female (%)	33 (53.2)	29 (46.8)
Higher education (%)	30 (65.2)*	16 (34.8)
Age (SD)	43.9 (10.7)	42.5 (10.2)
Fagerström score (SD)	5.5 (2.2)*	6.6 (2.0)
CO (ppm) (SD)	38.8 (11.7)	45.6 (29.9)
1–5 previous attempts (%)	52 (85.3)*	32 (64)
< 1 or >5 previous attempts (%)	9 (14.7)	18 (36)

* $p < 0.05$

Discussion

The abstinence rates after six months or one year with various treatment methods have been reported to be 30–50%, both internationally (Linchestein & Danaher, 1976; Raw & Russell, 1980; Schwartz, 1987) and nationally (Salvador *et al.*, 1988; Becoña, 1992), generally in controlled studies. Our results are similar and were obtained without conducting a controlled study, indicating that this treatment can be incorporated into clinical practice with equal efficacy. Nicotine replacement therapy has been shown to be effective (Tonnesen *et al.*, 1991; Fagerström *et al.*, 1993; Fiore *et al.*, 1994).

The preparatory phase was shown to be useful for reducing the number of cigarettes smoked, as confirmed by expired carbon monoxide. Like other authors (Gourlay *et al.*, 1994; Kenford *et al.*, 1994; Rice *et al.*, 1996), we found that the ability to stop smoking was related to the baseline nicotine dependence and the number of previous attempts to cease smoking (≤ 5) and a higher level of education. The ability to stop smoking within the first week also predicted maintenance of abstinenece up to six months, as noted elsewhere (Westman et al., 1997), indicating that specific methods should be used for the first week of treatment among certain subjects.

References

Becoña, E. (1992) La técnica de ingestión de nicotina y alquitrán: Una revisión. *Rev. Esp. Drogodep.*, 10, 92

Fagerström, K.O., Schneider, N.G. & Lunell, E. (1993) Effectiveness of nicotine patch and nicotine gum as individual versus combined treatment for tobacco withdrawal symptoms. *Psychopharmacology*, 111, 271–277

Fiore, M.C., Smith, S.S., Jornby, D.E. & Baker, T.B. (1994) The effectiveness of nicotine patch for smoking cessation: A meta-analysis. *J. Am. Med. Assoc.*, 271, 1940–1947

Gourlay, S.G., Forbes, A., Marriner, T., Pethica, D. & McNeil, J.J. (1994) Prospective study of factors predicting outcome of transdermal nicotine treatment in smoking cessation. *Br. Med. J.*, 309, 842–846

Heatherton, T.F., Kozlowski, L.T., Frecker, R.C. & Fagerström, K.O. (1991) The Fagerström test for nicotine dependence: A revision of the Fagerström tolerance questionnaire. *Br. J. Addict.*, 86, 1119–1127

Kenford, S.L., Fiore, M.C., Jorenby, D.E., Smith, S.S., Wetter, D. & Baker, T.B. (1994) Predicting smoking cessation. *J. Am. Med. Assoc.*, 271, 589–594

Linchestein, E. & Danaher, B.G. (1976) Modification of smoking behaviour. A critical analysis of theory, research and practice. In: Herse, M., Eisler, R.M. & Miller, P.M., eds, *Progress in Behaviour Modification*, New York: Academic Press, pp. 79–132

Raw, M. & Russell, M.A.H. (1980) Rapid smoking, cue exposure and support in the modification of smoking. *Behaviour*, 18, 363–372

Rice, V.H., Templin, T., Fox, D.H., Jarosz, P., Mullin, M., Seiggreen, M. Lepczyk, M. (1996) Social context variables as predictors of smoking cessation. *Tobacco Control*, 5, 280–285

Salvador, T., Marín, D., González-Quintana, J., et al. (1988) Tratamiento del tabaquismo: Eficacia de la utilización del chicle de nicotina. Estudio a doble ciego. *Med. Clin. (Barcelona)*, 90, 646–650

Schwartz, J.L. (1987) *Review and Evaluation of Smoking Cessation Methods: The United States and Canada, 1978–1985*, Washington DC: Department of Health and Human Services

Spielberger, C.D., Gorsuch, R.L. & Lushene, R.E. (1970) *STAI, Manual for the State–Trait Anxiety Inventory (Self Evaluation Questionnaire)*, California: Consulting Psychological Press, Inc.

Tonnesen, P., Noregaard, J., Simonsen, K. & Säwe, U. (1991) A double-blind trial of a 16-hour transdermal nicotine patch in smoking cessation. *New Ebgl. J. Med.*, 325, 311–315

Westman, E.C., Behm, F.M., Simel, D.L. & Rose, J. E. (1997) Smoking behaviour on the first day of a quit attempt predicts long-term abstinence. *Arch. Inter. Med.*, 157, 335–340

Community-based smoking cessation

P. Tvaermose

Center for Smoking Cessation, Copenhagen Health Services, Copenhagen, Denmark

Background

The city of Copenhagen in Denmark offers free smoking cessation groups for all citizens. Smoking cessation groups are operated at the workplaces, in five local neighbourhood settings and at the Center for Smoking Cessation. The groups are led by part-time facilitators who are trained in an intensive three-day course and are supervised by the Center for Smoking Cessation. Since 1995, more than 200 facilitators have been trained. In 1997, around 100 of them were available for public smoking cessation activities. The activities have been increasing steadily since the start, from 35 cessation groups in 1995, to 61 in 1996 and 123 in 1997.

The group sessions consist of five 2-h sessions over six weeks. Cessation of smoking is scheduled after the second session for all participants. Each session comprises five elements: individual attention, information, group discussions, carbon monoxide monitoring and homework. As an introduction to nicotine replacement, the participants are offered a free nicotine product for one week.

The content of the smoking cessation course is (i) presentation of participants and course format and recording of smoking history and profile; (ii) determination of nicotine dependence and withdrawal symptoms and introduction of nicotine replacement; (iii) cessation day; (iv) relapse prevention, with stress mangement and relaxation techniques; (v) explanation of the health benefits of smoking cessation and information for avoiding weight gain; (vi) maintenance and evaluation of the course.

Results

A sample of 22 smoking cessation groups comprising 328 persons was followed for one year from January 1997. Each group consisted of an average of 15 persons. As 208 personens attended two or more sessions, the attendance rate was 63% with an average of nine participants per group.

The cessation rate one month after the quit date was 54%. Smoking status after treatment was validated by monitoring carbon monoxide at the last session.

After three months, 208 participants were mailed a follow-up questionnaire and were invited to follow-up sessions. The overall reponse rate was 78%; 33% came to the follow-up sessions and their smoking status was validated by carbon monoxide measurements; 46% returned the questionnaire by mail. The quit rate at three months was 41%. At the six-month follow-up, all participants were mailed the questionnaire again. The combined response rate was 77%, with 32% attendance and carbon monoxide validation and return of the questionnaire by 45%. The quit rate was 32%.

The results of the 12-month follow-up were not available at the time of writing.

Effectiveness of teaching advice on smoking cessation

L.C.Y. Tsang

*Training and Education Center in Family Medicine, Department of Health,
Hong Kong SAR, China*

Objectives

In a comparison of the effectiveness of brief, intensive smoking cessation advice with no advice, it was concluded that although giving advice is effective, it would have to be provided to 35 smokers to result in one quitter. As smoking cessation advice may not be appropriate for all smokers, we designed an approach that includes consideration of the readiness of smokers to quit, based on the five stages of change in the integrative model of Prochaska and DiClemente (1983): pre-contemplation, contemplation, action, maintenance and relapse. We report here an evaluation of the effectiveness of teaching this approach to health-care workers.

Method
Groups comprising a total of 88 nursing colleagues attending a structured refresher course in February, June and October 1996 were given a 30-min description of an approach based on the model of Prochaska and DiClemente and strategies to help smokers stop smoking. Anonymous questionnaires were sent out in March 1997 to evaluate the perceived effectiveness and usefulness of the approach; 37 questionnaires (42%) were returned.

Results
The three groups gave consistent results. Most (> 75%) had not heard about the approach previously; but, by March 1997, they could remember only some of the suggested strategies. Most of the nurses graded the approach as 4 out of 5 on a linear scale, 1 being the lowest, for perceived effectiveness and usefulness. Suggestions for improving teaching of the approach included distribution of prepared notes at the end of the course and more suggested strategies for each stage of change.

Discussion and conclusions
Theoretically, smoking cessation advice is worth while, with a high potential for health gain. Although giving such advice is an important part of the daily practice of health professionals, we are often not taught how to give it. This can result in giving advice to people who are not ready to receive it or spending time with someone who is already decided. The result could be rejection of good intentions, deflated egos and inefficient use of time. Greater effectiveness and client satisfaction could be achieved by taking people's readiness into account.

From an educational point of view, taking home prepared notes may improve retention and fulfill a cultural expectation. Another strategy might be to repeat the information in varying detail periodically. This could be done formally in refresher courses or informally in educational newsletters or at regular group meetings.

The effectiveness and usefulness of the approach will now be evaluated in randomized controlled trials of outcome in the community.

Acknowledgements
The author would like to thank the tutors and Principal of the School of Public Health Nursing, Department of Health, for their assistance in conducting the evaluation, all the nursing colleagues for their comments and participation and clerical colleagues at the Training Center for assistance in preparing the report.

Reference
Prochaska, J.O. & DiClemente, C.C. (1983) Stages and processes of self-change of smoking: Toward an integrative model of change. *J. Consult. Clin. Psychol.*, 51, 390–395

Workshop in smoking cessation

A. Carr & R. Hayley

Allen Carris Easyway (International) Ltd, London, United Kingdom

Allen Carr's Easyway To Stop Smoking was first established in the United Kingdom in 1983, and there are now over 30 clinics worldwide. The method consists of a verbal delivery by one therapist to about 10 smokers in sessions lasting about 4.5 h. Two back-up sessions lasting about 2 h each are offered for people requiring them. No substitutes, pharmaceutical or other, are used. The focus of the talk is on why smokers smoke, not on why they should not smoke. By hearing about the way nicotine addiction operates, smokers are drawn to the realization that smoking provides them with no genuine pleasure and does not serve as a crutch. They therefore realize that they will not be making any sacrifice when they quit and need not feel deprived. On the contrary, they will make only marvellous, positive gains. The result is that they need not miss or crave cigarettes afterwards. Simple instructions are given to overcome the very minor physical withdrawal symptoms, which are easy to deal with once the correct frame of mind has been attained.

Preliminary evaluation of the method has yielded the following results: In Spain in 1996, 75–80% of 125 Schweppes employees quit after attending the course and were still non-smokers after 18 months. In 1997, 80% of 40 Transfesa employees quit and were still non-smokers after four months. In the United Kingdom in 1997, 70% of 45 employees of Middlesborough Council (a Government agency) quit and were still non-smokers after three months. Also in 1997, 52% of 44 employees of Easington Health Authority (another Government agency) quit and were still non-smokers after three months. In The Netherlands in 1993, 70% of 23 Levi Strauss employees quit and were still non-smokers after 18 months.

A money-back guarantee is given at all clinics whereby smokers are entitled to claim a full refund of their fee if they do not stop smoking for at least three months after having attended three sessions. An audit at the London Clinic (United Kingdom) confirmed that only 2.5% of 6862 smokers who had attended that clinic before 1 January 1996 had requested a refund. The refund rate at all clinics consistently averages less than 10%.

The book *Allen Carr's Easyway To Stop Smoking* is by far the most successful book on stopping smoking ever published. It has been a Penguin bestseller in the United Kingdom every year since its publication in 1987, reached the number one best-selling spot for non-fiction paperbacks in Germany in 1997 and was number five non-fiction bestseller in The Netherlands in 1996 and 1997. It has been translated into 20 languages and has sold over 1 million copies. Video, audio and CD-Rom versions of the method are also available.

Using diffusion research for participatory tobacco cessation

A.B. Lund

Communication Studies, Rosklide University, Roskilde, Denmark

On the basis of theoretical work by DiClemente, Gilbertini, Prochaska and Rogers, the Danish health authorities have experimented with participatory methods, such as focus groups, workshops and direct mailings, to involve smokers actively in the design of tobacco cessation programmes.

The evaluation showed that 57% of Danish smokers consider stopping smoking during a random period of a programme, but that only a small fraction of heavy smokers succeed in doing so. A number of social barriers have been detected. Consequently, it is concluded that health education should not be based primarily on health knowledge directed at cognitive and behavioural aspects of the motivation of an individual.

As an alternative, a diffusion model for social intervention has been developed, which focuses on how stages of change can be communicated persuasively. This research-based model is being tested in regional settings, and tentative results will be presented.

A stepped-care plus matching model of community smoking cessation

R.S. Niaura & D.B. Abrams

Center for Behavioral and Preventive Medicine, The Miriam Hospital, Providence, Rhode Island, United States

The use of a stepped-care model to treat smoking and prevent relapse is proposed. Population-based cessation efforts for adult smokers should involve four steps to smoking cessation at the community level. First, general community-level interventions are used to increase motivation to quit. Then, only when smokers are ready to quit, should they be evaluated for individual factors that would complicate cessation efforts, such as: past history of quit attempts and severity of withdrawal symptoms; degree of nicotine dependence; and co-morbid factors including substance abuse, mood disorders, especially depression and weight gain among women smokers.

The answers to these questions result in assignment to one of three levels of treatment. These three levels (or steps) differ substantially in their intensity, cost and requirement for professional qualifications, e.g. the training of specialists in treatment of nicotine dependence. The levels therefore range from self-help materials with no special counselling treatment (least costly, least intensive and most easily disseminated to large numbers of smokers) to the highest level of specialist training (the most costly, intensive and least accessible). The three steps are therefore: self-change materials; brief treatments, individual or group cessation programmes with volunteer counsellors with or without nicotine replacement; and referral to a formal clinic, staffed by specialists in behavioural medicine and trained physicians who can provide a full range of nicotine replacement and psychiatric pharmacotherapies. For more details on the approach, see Abrams *et al.* (1996).

Reference

Abrams, D.B. et al. (1996) Integrating individual and public health perspectives for treatment of tobacco dependence: A combined stepped-care and matching model. *Ann. Behav. Med.*, **18**, 290–304

A new, effective smoking cessation programme based on the Internet

Y. Takahashi

Yamato-takada City Hospital, Nara, Japan

Introduction

In spite of the increasing social awareness of the hazards of smoking, the prevalence of smoking among Japanese is still very high: statistics show that 58% of men and 14% of women are smokers. Since September 1994, we have been holding a smoking cessation clinic for patients with various diseases. For instance, although smoking is an important risk factor for complications of diabetes, diabetic patients often fail to stop smoking for fear of gaining weight and poor control of diabetes after cessation. Between September 1994 and November 1995, 29 male diabetic patients aged 35–80 years visited our clinic and were advised to ingest a lot of cold water, hot Japanese tea, seaweeds, sliced tangle and boiled vegetables. The one-year cessation rate was 72% (21/29); none of the patients gained more than 2 kg of body weight and haemoglobin alkalinity was lowered. As a p.rt of our counselling to help people quit smoking, we designed a programme based on Internet mailing list capability to reach people. It was first introduced in June 1997.

Method

By signing up for this two-month programme, applicants are registered on a closed mailing list and are offered the official 'Guiding Mail', which contains medical information and tips for avoiding smoking. The advice is given a few days before the participant stops smoking and then almost daily for two months. Participants can choose one of four versions of 'Guiding Mail' tailored for: heavy smokers, moderate smokers, female smokers and smokers who are not certain they want to quit. Our goal is to make them avoid smoking for two months and, ideally, help them retain the status of non-smoker. Participants can exchange mail within the mailing list, providing ideas, tips, experiences and encouragement to other participants. They can call for help and advice at any time and are answered by our medical staff within a day or two.

Results

We introduced the first 'Internet quit-smoking marathon' in June 1997, and 205 male and 23 female smokers aged 21–65 (mean, 40.8; standard deviation, 9.1) applied. They smoked 5–100 cigarettes per day (mean, 29.9; standard deviation, 14.4). At the end of the two-month period, 142 participants reported that they had completed the programme; the 86 applicants who did not report were considered to have failed. Of the 142 who completed it, 95 had not smoked for the entire two months and 23 had begun to stop smoking at some time within this period, giving an overall cessation rate of 51.7%.

Discussion

This success rate was considered to be high, largely because of the flexibility of the mailing list system. The exchange of mail among people who share the same goal helps to create a bond. Mutual encouragement was the best aid to resisting the temptation to smoke, and medical information from our staff through the mailing list system was also very helpful.

Tobacco control measures and smoking cessation therapy: Different strategies for different types of smokers

R. Schoberberger & M. Kunze

Institute of Social Medicine, University of Vienna, Vienna, Austria

It is obvious that some smokers have little difficulty in stopping and others have great difficulty or even do not succeed. Nicotine dependence, as assessed by the Fagerström test, has been studied in several countries among random samples of smokers. These studies show a statistically significant correlation between the prevalence of smoking and scores for nicotine dependence. The probable explanation for this finding is that tobacco control measures result in smoking cessation among smokers with low dependence on nicotine.

Our analysis shows that significantly fewer very highly dependent smokers report attempts to quit (32–45%) in comparison with those who have intermediate or low dependence, and seldom achieve even short-term success; 61% of highly dependent smokers could not stop smoking for even a short time, in comparison with 43% of those with intermediate or low dependence, even when using nicotine replacement therapy. Smokers with low dependence had a good success rate even without nicotine replacement therapy, but such therapy appears to be essential for highly dependent smokers even to initiate a quit attempt.

Nicotine dependence thus has a strong influence on smoking cessation. Prescription of nicotine replacement therapy on the basis of a pre-treatment diagnosis is effective for smokers of intermediate and heavy dependence. Those with low dependence can be motivated by tobacco control measures and have a better chance of quitting without external help.

Experiences with alternative means and indirect cessation

A. Lund

Roykfritt Miljo Norge, Oslo, Norway

Traditional means give traditional results—results that are visible only as small percentages in big polls. Should we be content with that? I'm not. I believe that all of us want to see sensational results in our work, but to do that we must be willing to develop and use untraditional means. I suppose that health workers must choose their means within certain professional limits. I am not a health worker, so that I can use a wider range of means and arguments.

We should start by considering the words we use. Words are our weapons and should be chosen with great care. Nobody would call him or herself a 'non-alcohol user' or a 'non-drug user', but unfortunately the word 'non-smoker' is well established. This is regrettable becaue 'non' is a negative prefix. As smoking became more and more common over the years, the impression was created that smoking was normal behaviour. Most smokers seem to believe this. Adoption of the word 'non-smoker' implies that we are an unusual minority. This is of course incorrect, but by continuing to use the word we unconsciously contribute to the preservation of this illusion. This common view gives an advantage to the tobacco industry, and we should try to eliminate that advantage. The process will be long, but things should be said in a way that indicates that smokers are different and everybody else is normal. We must remember that the industry itself has stated that the battle for the social acceptability of smoking is the issue that will determine the future of tobacco in the long run. Personally, I prefer to call myself a normal person.

Another word that could cause problems is 'dependence'. We all agree that nicotine causes dependence, but if a smoker is told that quitting is very difficult, it becomes more difficult. People with enough willpower and who consider it a challenge have good chances; most ex-smokers have broken their habit without help. Unfortunately, heavy smokers, one of our most important target groups, are less easy to influence. Many do their best to avoid information and sometimes do not understand the information that reaches them; they resent interference in their private lives. These people see little difference between 'difficult' and 'impossible', which means for them that there is no use in trying to quit. Many of them do not even believe what doctors say. Those who ask for advice and help should receive it, but I think that focusing on dependence benefits only those who make a profit from quitting courses and remedies. By keeping our knowledge about dependence to oursleves, we could make it easier for the most important and difficult target group to quit.

It is useful to point out that tobacco can't make decisions; only a human being can. Success or failure in quitting depends on the decision that the smoker has made. Those who decide to try quitting have little chance of success; those who decide to quit do quit. People who seem to be allergic to information about tobacco can be reached in different ways. They may stop reading a text the moment they discover that it's about smoking, but such information can be included as part of other literature of possible interest to smokers. They will read it unwittingly and cannot avoid learning something.

Most people in tobacco control consider that their main task is to prevent children and youngsters from starting to smoke. This group is under many influences of various kinds, much of it being pressure to smoke. Who can counteract that, with smokers everywhere? Common courtesy ought to be enough to stop most people from smoking. Polite smokers refrain from smoking the moment they realize that it is disagreeable to someone else. Unfortunately, most smokers are not always polite. We need an army of angry people demanding more smoke-free environments. It is particularly important to demand consideration for children. Smoke-free environments have many good effects. Each time smokers are forced to smoke elsewhere than usual, their smoking becomes more conscious and their attitude to smoking changes. With limited possibilities for smoking, consumption must go down. Many smokers will quit simply because it is too difficult to find a place to smoke. With more smoke-free environments, the change in public opinion will accelerate and gradually become the main influence on young people. Smoke-free environments are cost-effective and even save money for employers and for society. It is smoking that is expensive.

As smoking is not a rational activity, rational arguments often have little effect. Fortunately, we have other methods. The best of all is humour, but it is also the most difficult. Professional entertainers could do miracles if they were convinced of the usefulness of their talents. Rewards, unexpected arguments and shock can be useful. In difficult situations, when normal arguments have no effect or have lost their value because of repetition, shock can effective. If smokers are told something quite different from what they expect, they might be distracted from their firm conviction and become interested in further conversation. For instance, one might say, "OK, smoke as much as you like, I don't mind. But do it somewhere else, please." When I was a taxi driver with a smoking ban in my car, one of my passengers told me that she had tried vainly to make her husband understand that his smoke bothered her. She was on her way to her son's house, where nobody smoked, and she dreaded returning home. I advised her to write to her husband, telling him that she would stay at her son's house until he stopped smoking. She took to the idea immediately. When I met her again by chance several months later, she told me, "It worked!" The toughest approach I have used so far is to say, "Smoke as much as you like. The world is already overpopulated."

We can all make gestures to change our environment: Turn down an invitation, explaining that you are certain someone there will be smoking, or take the time to find a smoke-free place to eat when travelling and explain why you are taking the time to do so. Thirty years ago, when guests lit up in my home, I moved from a chair down to the floor, explaining that the air was better there. In the beginning it caused a lot of laughter, but gradually our guests began to smoke outside, and our home has been smoke-free ever since.

Future of smoking cessation

M. Kunze

Institute for Social Medicine, University of Vienna, Vienna, Austria

A systematic approach to smoking cessation involves a complex system of services. Primary prevention is usually regarded as the most desirable goal, but primary prevention programmes have not proved very effective, and it would take 30–40 years before any major effects on health are seen. Although traditional smoking control measures, such as health education and legislation, have had moderate success, smokers in countries with low smoking prevalences such as the United States may have higher scores for nicotine dependence than those in countries where smoking is more prevalent, like Austria and Poland. This is because most conventional measures help smokers with low dependence scores, who can quit easily, resulting in an increase in the relative proportion of highly dependent smokers.

There are two possible strategies for risk reduction in this group: modification of tobacco products and reduced consumption. We in the tobacco control field must concentrate on the second. Conventional smoking control measures have a limited impact on the incidences of cardiovascular disease and lung cancer, which are correlated with a high nicotine dependence, and additional measures are needed, with two possible end-points: cessation (the ultimate goal) and reduction in risk (or harm). A variety of pharmacological and psychological smoking cessation strategies has been developed to assist smokers who want to quit. High nicotine dependence can be managed with improved diagnosis and more intensive treatment. Diagnosis is important because as nicotine dependence increases, self-help becomes less effective, and professional support is needed. Nicotine replacement medications combined with behavioural advice can provide effective treatment.

Recent findings on the 'nicotine pre-abstinence syndrome' should be taken into consideration in designing smoking control measures. This term addresses one of the most interesting questions in smoking behaviour and cessation: What happens before a smoker actually stops smoking, and how can this phase be used or modified? Part of the answer can be found in the differentiation of smokers into consonant (attitudes and behaviour in agreement) and dissonant (attitudes and behaviour not in agreement). Data from Austria show that only 29% of dissonant smokers want to quit, while the majority want to reduce smoking (57%) or switch brands (14%). Since consonant smokers accept the risk of their behaviour, many smokers are experiencing the nicotine pre-abstinence syndrome and have the following options: quit, reduce their consumption, continue smoking, switch brands or product or move to long-term nicotine replacement. Nicotine replacement therapy may play a role in the nicotine pre-abstinence syndrome as it motivates smokers to quit, especially if available over the counter. It is preferable to allow smokers to try different nicotine preparations and select the one they feel to be most helpful for them. Although none of the existing medications is more effective than the others, long-term compliance is likely to be better if individuals feel comfortable with their chosen preparation. As complete cessation cannot be achieved by all smokers with heavy nicotine dependence, reducing smoking is of great importance.

One of the most important tasks ahead of us is to include cessation techniques in the health-care system and establish nicotine dependence as a disease, which must be disgnosed and treated according to established scientific standards. On the other hand, self-help should be stressed more than it has been until now, with nicotine replacement therapy freely available without having to contact the health-care system.

Public policy as a smoking cessation tool: A framework for discussion

H. Selin

Smoking and Health Action Foundation, Ottawa, Ontario, Canada

Introduction

Tobacco control often is divided into the goals of prevention, cessation and protection of non-smokers. We pay lip service to the notion that progress toward each of these goals is best achieved through a comprehensive approach comprised of policy and legislation, education and programmes. Yet differentiation of primary approaches to each goal persists. Cessation has been discussed almost exclusively outside the realm of public policy, and yet policy approaches are the most effective way of achieving broad-based reductions in tobacco use. The result is that progress in cessation has been much slower than it could and should be. If we are to make significant future gains in cessation, a broader view of the interventions that affect cessation must emerge. This paper is an attempt to stimulate discussion of new perspectives on how we help smokers quit.

Influences on cessation

Much of the literature on cessation focuses on educational and counselling techniques. While medical professionals and others involved in cessation are encouraged to get involved in community initiatives against tobacco, the focus remains on influencing individual smokers, one by one. Although the success rate of formal interventions is significantly higher than that of unaided quit attempts (Lando & Gritz, 1996), because few smokers use formal programmes, the vast majority quit on their own. It is therefore as important to identify the determinants that increase motivation to quit as to discuss which programming strategies are most effective.

Smokers are motivated to quit for a variety of reasons: family pressure, health concerns, cost or an inability to smoke in the workplace. Some factors are easily influenced; others are not. Ironically, the factors most often discussed are those that are difficult, impossible or expensive to control. The literature focuses on individual differences such as socioeconomic status or the presence of family members and friends who smoke. Environmental factors common to all smokers in a given jurisdiction often are not discussed or are mentioned only peripherally. These include the affordability of tobacco, restrictions on tobacco promotion and restrictions on smoking in workplaces and public places. Yet these are powerful influences on consumption. They are also within the ability of the health community to change. It is important to ensure that the cessation interventions that are available are as effective as they can be, but this should be secondary to shaping an environment that encourages more smokers to use those interventions or to quit on their own. The most cost-effective way of doing this is through public policy.

Case study: How tobacco package labelling affects motivation to quit

The policies mentioned above and other public policies have a well-documented impact on consumption and should be vigorously pursued. Tobacco package labelling is discussed here as just one example of how public policy affects the quitting process.

Package messages: Smokers do not adequately appreciate the nature and magnitude of the risk of tobacco use. Package warnings increase this knowledge. They also, as preliminary evaluations of package warnings in Canada and Australia suggest, dissuade tobacco use through prompting quitting, preventing uptake or reducing the amount smoked (Borland *et al.*, 1996; Tandemar Research Inc., 1996). In Canada, 19% of smokers surveyed said that the warnings influenced them a lot (11%) or a little (8%) to try to quit. Smokers in both Canada and Australia also said that the warnings influenced them to reduce their consumption. While these percentages may seem low, the resulting impact is huge. Every smoker sees package warnings, and 19% of smokers in Canada represents 1.2 million smokers. If just 10% successfully quit, 120 000 smokers quit because of the warnings. The warnings in both Canada and Australia had a greater impact on younger smokers. This finding points to a potential antidote to the difficulty of recruiting young people to cessation programmes and the lack of success of cessation counselling. It should encourage research into youth-targeted package messages.

Package messages could potentially have an even greater impact if they specifically provided cessation advice and pointed smokers towards cessation options. A toll-free number could be advertised, as could referral to specific organizations ("Call your local lung association. They run programmes in your area," or "Your physician can help you design a quitting programme that works for you."). Cessation messages would increase smokers' confidence in their ability to quit. Just as tobacco advertising serves as a daily comforting reminder of the social acceptability of tobacco, package cessation messages could keep quitting to the forefront of the mind. ("Thousands have quit. You can too. We'll show you how."). Such a constant antidote to other factors that erode smokers' confidence could only be of benefit.

Misleading labelling: Mandated package messages do not operate in a vacuum. They must compete with other elements of the package, many of which deter quitting. The most pervasive misleading and deterrent information is descriptive terminology: qualifiers such as 'light' and 'mild'. These terms have gained increased legitimacy because they are loosely based on flawed government-mandated testing systems for tar and nicotine yields. The reported yields do not reflect smokers' actual intake, and much of the difference between brands is illusory (National Cancer Institute, 1996). Most variation in yield. is due to smoking behaviour rather than to cigarette brand.

For years, governments (often supported by the health community) have actively advised switching to lower-tar cigarettes for health benefit. While this is now much less common, the continued use of tar categories on packages and advertisements tacitly sends smokers the message that there are safe alternatives to quitting. Smokers seem to have received this message. Many believe that so-called 'light' cigarettes have fewer health risks (Ferrence *et al.*, 1996). There is ample evidence that this misunderstanding keeps smokers in the market who might otherwise quit (Imperial Tobacco Ltd, 1978; R.J.R.–MacDonald Inc. v. Canada, 1989; Ferrence et al., 1996; National Cancer Institute, 1996). Removing much of the false perception of product choice through better testing systems and removal of misleading language would result in a significant increase in attempts to quit.

Absence of information: The package omits much information that smokers should have. Tobacco manufacturers are rarely required to reveal the contents of tobacco products or tobacco smoke to the public. Where ingredients are required to be released to the government, the tobacco industry has fought hard to ensure that the information remains inaccessible to the public. Seeing arsenic, formaldehyde, benzene and lead listed on a tobacco package would undoubtedly give some smokers pause. The absence of an adequate ingredient list on packages allows them to avoid the discomfort of knowing the specific poisons in cigarettes and cigarette smoke, making it less likely that they will be compelled to quit.

Replacing misleading package information with health messages would greatly increase attempts to quit and would recruit more smokers to cessation programmes. Packages could place cessation information in the hands of every smoker, every day, indefinitely. This would occur at a fraction of the cost of posters and pamphlets, and the tobacco industry would bear that cost. This potential is too great for cessation interveners to ignore.

Reorientating cessation approaches

A first step toward greater progress in cessation is reorientation of discussions to incorporate both programmes and policies. But this alone is not sufficient. Changes must occur in the way money is spent, if an environment conducive to quitting is to be built. This will require the leadership of professional associations and health organizations. Currently, most put far more resources into cessation education and programming than into advocacy. Resolutions calling for healthy public policy on tobacco are not always backed by resources for activities that achieve policy change: professional media campaigns, lobbying and research to support policy initiatives. Leadership backed by resources sends a message to other organizations, governments and the public that an issue is important to an organization.

Change will depend also on an increased role of cessation interveners as advocates. Recognizing the potential for policies to motivate quitting, clinicians, programmers and educators must also see themselves as advocates to a much greater degree. Those who work directly with smokers bring added credibility to the debate. It is very powerful for individual programmers to inform politicians that their activities are undermined by lack of political action. This course of action does not amount to lobbying by cessation programmers for the elimination of their jobs. While redistribution of resources may, in the short term, result in a shrinking of cessation activities, in the long run it will greatly increase demand and resources for cessation programmes.

Conclusion

Public policy has an enormous impact on smoking cessation. It could do much more to motivate cessation and recruit smokers to cessation assistance. Recognition of this should compel a reorientation of the way in which cessation interventions are viewed and how resources are directed. A move away from individual counselling to a public health approach will create population-based smoking reduction due to quitting, something that cessation programming alone has been unable to achieve.

References

Borland, R., Cappiello, M. & Hill, D. (1996) *Impact of the New Australian Health Warnings on Tobacco Products* (draft), Canberra: Commonwealth Department of Human Services & Health

Ferrence, R.G., Kozlowski, L.T., Ashley, M.J., Cohen, J., Pederson, .L.L, Poland, B. & Bull, S. (1996) The meaning of 'light' and 'mild': What smokers and non-smokers believe and how they respond. Paper presented at the Second National Conference on Tobacco or Health, Ottawa, Canada, 30 October–2 November

Imperial Tobacco Ltd (1978) *Response of the Market and of Imperial Tobacco to the Smoking and Health Environment* (Exhibit AG-41 in *R.J.R. MacDonald Inc. v. Canada (A.G.)*, 2

Lando, H.A. & Gritz, E.R. (1996) Smoking cessation techniques. *J. Am. Med. Women's Assoc.*, **51**, 31–34

National Cancer Institute (1996) *The FTC Cigarette Test Method for Determining Tar, Nicotine, and Carbon Monoxide Yields of US Cigarettes. Report of the NCI Expert Committee* (Smoking and Tobacco Control Monograph No. 7), Bethesda, Maryland: National Cancer Institute, National Institutes of Health, Public Health Service, US Department of Health and Human Services,

R.J.R.-MacDonald Inc. v. *Canada (A.G.)*, Vol. 4, 27 September 1989, 507

Tandemar Research Inc. (1996) *Cigarette Packaging Study: The Evaluation of New Health Warning Messages.*, Ottawa: Health Canada

Methods for young people

Call for a new approach to tobacco 'cessation' programming among youth

J.J. Librett & H.R. Borski

Utah Department of Health, Salt Lake City, Utah, United States

Thirty years of focus on the prevalence of adult smoking has left a shortfall in our understanding of the treatment of adolescent addiction to nicotine. This gap, combined with the reported desire of young tobacco users to quit, warrants research, so that effective tobacco cessation programmes can be developed for this group. The literature indicates several areas for programme development and evaluation. Several studies indicate principles for effective tobacco cessation among adolescents, including the Surgeon General's report, *Preventing Tobacco Use among Young People* (Department of Health and Human Services, 1994); a report from the Institute of Medicine, *Growing-up Tobacco Free* (Lynch & Bonnie, 1994); and the Clinical Practice Guideline, *Smoking Cessation* (Department of Health and Human Services, 1996). All conclude that there is a paucity of research in the area. While many questions remain unanswered, however, we believe there is sufficient information on adolescent tobacco use and school programme development to establish preliminary national guidelines for programme development and evaluation.

Base adolescent tobacco cessation or reduction programmes on research on adolescents

Despite the absence of convincing evidence to support an adult model (Hitchcock, 1990), virtually all programmes for tobacco cessation among children and adolescents have been developed on the basis of theories, principles and materials used in programmes for adults. In fact, our recent review showed that none of the 30 adolescent tobacco cessation programmes reviewed, including national programmes, had developed appropriate methods for adolescents. In addition, they do not appear to include comprehensively the recommendations already existing in the literature on adolescent tobacco cessation for development, implementation and evaluation.

Measure outcomes by precursors of change, not just cessation

The literature on prevention and cessation of tobacco use among adolescents and major theories of behavioural change clearly state that outcome-dependent variables such as changes in knowledge, attitudes and intentions, social and refusal skills, resilience and behaviour including involvement in high-risk environments and peer groups should be measured to assess the efficacy of the programmes (Hulbert, 1979; Glanz *et al.*, 1997). The development, evaluation and reporting of current programmes should include these precursors of risk and protective factors in outcome evaluations. Furthermore, to improve the development and dissemination of effective prevention and treatment programmes, agencies extract the principles of effective programmes rather than searching for those applicable to culturally diverse groups. In our literature review, we determined 14 critical principles for increasing the effectiveness of adolescent tobacco cessation programmes:

- Design a continuum of programmes, matching use level, age, sex and culture.
- Develop interventions specifically tailored to adolescent populations.
- Improve recruitment by increasing motivation and incentives to attend class.
- Assess participants' use level.
- Focus on immediate health consequences.
- Reinforce the immediate health benefits of reduction and cessation.
- Reward even small successes.
- Assess stages of change and belief structures.

- Include relevant training techniques for life skills (not related to tobacco).
- Address tobacco-related cognition, beliefs and behaviour.
- Make appropriate use of peers.
- Include a parent or family component.
- Use maintenance components to increase programme effectiveness.
- Assess broad outcome measures of programme effectiveness.

The 'Ending Nicotine Dependence' programme

A multidisciplinary team in Utah developed a tobacco cessation curriculum for adolescents based on these recommendations. During three years, the team reviewed over 50 articles on adolescent tobacco cessation, published between 1977 and 1996; conducted and summarized the results of interviews with a limited number of key informants; reviewed over 30 existing programmes for tobacco cessation among adolescents; reviewed research on theories of adolescent development and behavioural change; and surveyed the attitudes towards tobacco use and quitting of hundreds of adolescent tobacco users in Utah.

The resulting programme, 'Ending Nicotine Dependence' (END), was specially designed to meet the needs of adolescents and help them reduce and quit tobacco use. The programme not only builds skills and knowledge about tobacco use, but also focuses on developing a wide variety of social skills, including communication, stress management, decision-making, goal-setting, nutrition and physical activity. The modules consist of techniques to influence the knowledge, attitudes, intentions, beliefs, self-awareness and self-efficacy of adolescent tobacco users. END is appropriate for implementation in schools, community agencies and juvenile court districts and is designed for use with junior and senior high-school students.

The curriculum consists of a wide variety of developmentally appropriate teaching techniques, including videos on the health effects of tobacco and personal accounts by young people about their experiences in tobacco cessation; interactive demonstrations of the health effects of tobacco; pages on which students process elements of tobacco use, tobacco addiction and tobacco cessation skills; and skill-building activities to improve social skills through role practising, communication and problem-solving skills, practising stress management techniques and making healthy food choices. END consists of eight comprehensive modules: (i) health effects of tobacco; (ii) nicotine addiction, coping with recovery symptoms, how and why participants use tobacco and quitting methods; (iii) short-term and long-term consequences of tobacco use, personal financial costs of tobacco use, causes of stress and stress management techniques; (iv) communication skills, refusal skills and social support; (v) problem-solving skills, coping with triggers, alternative activities to tobacco use and goal-setting skills; (vi) chewing tobacco use and time for review of any previously covered topics; (vii) nutrition and physical activity; and (viii) maintenance and dealing with relapse.

We must move beyond the current 'adult model' of cessation and redesign tobacco cessation programmes for youth. We intend to provide insight for consideration when reviewing and developing programmes. We hope that these principles will be further expanded, refined, tested and operationalized by individuals designing, implementing and facilitating local programmes.

References

Department of Health and Human Services (1994) *Preventing Tobacco Use among Young People: A Report of the Surgeon General*, Washington DC: Government Printing Office

Department of Health and Human Services (1996) *Clinical Practice Guideline No. 18: Smoking Cessation*, Washinton DC: Government Printing Office

Glanz, K., Lewis, F.M. & Rimer, B., eds (1997) *Health Behavior and Health Education Theory, Research, and Practice*, San Francisco: Jossey Bass Publishers

Hitchcock, J. (1990) *Questions and Answers About Smoking Cessation Programs. Update Details*, 14

Hulbert, J. (1979) Cessation among Youth: Experiences in Selected Secondary School in Iowa. Obtained from Centers for Disease Control, Office on Smoking and Health

Lynch, B. & Bonnie, R., eds (1994) *Growing up Tobacco Free: Preventing Nicotine Addictions in Children and Youths*, Washington DC: Institute of Medicine, National Academy Press

Adolescent smoking cessation: A multi-level approach

S. Thomas & E. Choi

*American Lung Association of San Francisco and San Mateo Counties,
San Francisco, California, United States*

To be effective, programmes for smoking cessation in schools should address two key issues. The first is that young smokers vary greatly in their readiness to quit smoking. The second is that schools differ in their ability to offer administrative support for cessation programmes. We have found that by having five programme levels to choose from, we can provide the best match for both smokers and schools. The levels are described below.

The first level is a brief intervention conducted near a school or at a school health fair. The second level provides cessation information to smokers during tobacco education presentations in health classes with both smokers and non-smokers.The third level is a cessation awareness workshop for smokers who are ready to think about quitting but not ready to change their behaviour. The fourth level is a two-part workshop in which smokers agree to make a quit attempt between the first and second meetings. The fifth level is a multi-session class in which smokers join to stop smoking.

The effectiveness of the first two levels has been measured by the immediate response of the smokers. In both the brief and health-class interventions, the majority of smokers request self-help quit packets to learn more about quitting. The other three levels are evaluated by questionnaires and tests before and after the intervention. In the cessation awareness workshops, 90% of 115 participants indicated an increased commitment to quit, and 88% indicated an increased belief in their ability to quit.The two-part quit workshops have just begun. Early data show that approximately 60% are making a quit attempt, and 50% are reducing their daily cigarette consumption. The multi-session classes have produced an average cessation rate of 36%.

School staff have responded positively to the availability of five levels of smoking intervention. This has been demonstrated by our ability to work with more than 25 schools. We have also trained more than 100 teachers, counselors and peer educators in these methods.

'Quit because you can': The Western Australian 'Young women and smoking' campaign

D. Sullivan & C. Thompson

Smoking and Health Program, Health Promotion Services, Health Department of Western Australia, East Perth, Western Australia

Abstract

While smoking is a major public health concern across all social, sex and age groups within a community, the prevalence of smoking among young women in the late 1980s and early 1990s provided strong justification for interventions specifically targeting this group. In 1991, 25% of the Western Australian adult population smoked, but the prevalence of smoking among women aged 18–29 was significantly higher, at 33%. In response to this finding, the Health Department of Western Australian launched a comprehensive, four-year campaign targeting young women in October 1991. The campaign initially aimed to demonstrate to young women that a healthy, smoke-free lifestyle was fashionable and that smoking was no longer attractive or the cultural norm. In 1993 and 1994, the campaign focused on raising awareness of the short- and long-term consequences of smoking that are most relevant to young women.

This paper describes the progress of the 'Young women and smoking' campaign from 1991 to 1994. It describes the campaign's target group, objectives and strategies and the effectiveness of the campaign in motivating and encouraging young women to quit smoking. Maintenance of the campaign and the results of more recent qualitative research are also discussed.

Introduction

Smoking among young women has been a key public health issue for some time. In 1991, the prevalence of smoking among Western Australian adults was 25% (27% for males and 23% for females), but that among women aged 18–29 was 33% and that among women aged 25–29 was 36% (Health Promotion Services, 1997). Cigarette smoking is a leading cause of premature death and disease among Western Australian women, with over 400 women dying each year from tobacco-caused illnesses (Unwin & Thompson, 1996). In addition to the risks of all smokers for lung cancer, heart disease, stroke and other diseases, women who smoke are also prone to a number of sex-specific health problems, such as an increased risk for cervical cancer, reduced fertility, earlier menopause, problems related to use of the contraceptive pill, menstrual problems and difficulties with pregnancy and childbirth (US Surgeon General, 1980). Recent research also indicates a significant link between parental smoking and sudden infant death syndrome (Klonoff-Cohen et al., 1997).

In 1991, the Health Department of Western Australia initiated a four-year campaign targeting young female smokers, because of their higher prevalence of smoking and the additional health risks to women who smoke. This decision was further justified by the growing body of literature supporting interventions specific to particular segments of the population to achieve maximum effect (World Health Organization, 1992; Walsh et al., 1993).

Target group and objectives

Extensive research was conducted during the planning of the campaign to determine the most appropriate target group, objectives, approach and strategies. The research included a review of the literature and of interventions targeting women implemented in other states and countries as well as formative research on young women who smoked. The research conducted by the Health Department of Western Australia provided information on young women's knowledge, attitudes and beliefs about smoking, their smoking behaviour and factors that may predispose, enable or reinforce young women's intentions to quit or to continue to smoke (Table 1). The research highlighted the fact that while many young women express a desire to quit smoking, they often lack confidence in their ability to do so and social support for their attempts.

The target group selected for the campaign was 16–29-year-old women, with an emphasis on those with lower levels of formal education, because of the higher

Table 1. Motivators and barriers to quitting smoking for young women

Motivators	Barriers
Health and fitness	Nicotine addiction and withdrawal
Costs, potential savings	Fear of weight gain
Pregnancy, other major life changes	Smoke to relax, cope with stress
Self-control, willpower	Smoke to feel at ease in social settings
Desire to quit	Lack of confidence in ability to quit and
Awareness of health effects	social support for quit attempts
	Belief that will quit some time in the future
	Low awareness of sex-specific health problems

Social settings
Pressure from others
Perception of social norms

prevalence of smoking within that sub-population. The campaign primarily focused on young women who were contemplating or attempting to quit smoking (67% of the target group) (Health Promotion Services, 1997).

On the basis of the research, the primary objectives of the campaign were:
- to increase awareness of the health effects of smoking, in particular the sex-specific health problems caused by smoking,
- to motivate and encourage young women to quit smoking, and
- to counter the rationalizations suggested by young women as barriers to quitting smoking.

The campaign also aimed to encourage and reinforce young women's confidence in their ability to make positive health and lifestyle choices and to take control of their lives, as well as promote positive images of a non-smoking lifestyle.

The campaign

The statement selected for the campaign was 'Quit because you can', as it best encapsulated the aims, objectives, tone and approach of the campaign, which was to be empathetic and encouraging. The campaign was implemented in three phases over four years. Each phase was supported by a comprehensive range of strategies, which included mass media advertising, public relations, community and school education initiatives, the production of publications and merchandise, sponsorship of women's sports and sporting organizations and support for smoking cessation services. The campaign (media schedule and community-based strategies) was run for four weeks of each year of the campaign, although publications and sponsorship and smoking cessation support were available throughout the year. The focus of each phase of the campaign differed. The first phase, implemented in 1991 and 1992, aimed to demonstrate to young women that a healthy, smoke-free lifestyle was fashionable and that smoking was no longer attractive or the cultural norm. The second and third phases, implemented in 1993 and 1994, focused on raising awareness of the short- and long-term consequences of smoking that are most relevant to young women.

Mass media advertising: The media used for the campaign included television, radio, press and outdoor advertising. All advertising was statewide. New advertising was developed to support the communication objectives specific to each phase of the campaign. Television advertising used in phase 1 of the campaign aimed to boost young women's confidence in their ability to quit, while radio advertising developed for the campaign, which featured a prominent female comedian, used humour to counter rationalizations suggested by young women for not quitting smoking.

In phase 1 of the campaign, the Department, in partnership with other state and territory tobacco control agencies, participated in a project in a national women's magazine that aimed to raise awareness of the health effects of smoking for young women and to encourage smoking cessation and reinforce the resolve of non-smokers to stay non-smokers. The project, which ran for nine months from September 1991 to May 1992, featured advertisements and supporting editorials in magazines with a high readership among young women.

Outdoor advertising was also used in phases 1 and 2 to highlight the negative short-term cosmetic effects of smoking, which was cited as a motivator for quitting smoking by young women in the focus group research.

Media strategies developed for phase 2 aimed to guide young women who smoked through the stages of quitting. New television advertising developed for the campaign used humour to highlight the irony of why women smoke, while the radio advertising provided tips to avoid weight gain when quitting smoking and encouraged young women to 'have a go' at quitting.

Television advertising for phase 3 of the campaign placed particular emphasis on sex-specific health effects, such as cervical cancer, menstrual problems and complications during pregnancy, and on the short-term cosmetic and financial benefits of quitting smoking. Radio advertisements developed for this phase of the campaign focused on stress and weight gain issues and provided practical and supportive quit tips and advice. Press advertising was also used for the third phase of the campaign. Two advertisements in the style of a cartoon story were placed in major State newspapers. The first story provided advice on how to avoid weight gain during a quit attempt, while the second story gave tips on stress management and quitting smoking.

Public relations activities: Additional media coverage for the campaign was generated through a range of public relations activities, which included media launches involving prominent personalities in the promotion of the campaign and its health messages and radio station promotions and give-aways. An initiative of phase 1 of the campaign was a series of public relations activities linking fashion with a positive, healthy, smoke-free lifestyle. The activities were staged at a large metropolitan shopping centre and included fashion parades (supported by fashion retailers) and encouragement of smoke-free policies in retail stores. A Quitter's Day and Kid's Day were also run to complement the fashion parades and to gain additional media exposure for the campaign and its health messages. The fashion parades aimed to promote the benefits of quitting and a smoke-free lifestyle through a medium that appeals to young women; however, care was taken to ensure that the models involved in the parade were non-smokers, that their looks were healthy and down-to-earth, and that no element of the parades promoted unattainable images for young women.

Community-based strategies: Community support and involvement were important for the success of the campaign. Community involvement provided an additional means of raising awareness of the campaign and its health messages. It also encouraged social support for young women contemplating or attempting to quit smoking. Groups invited to support the campaign included health professionals, women's organizations, schools, tertiary education institutions, fashion retailers and regional health education officers. Health professionals were considered important for the campaign because they are in a unique position to provide direct encouragement and support to smokers. Letters and campaign resources were sent to over 4000 health professionals throughout the State, including general practitioners, dentists, pharmacists, physiotherapists, community, child and school nurses and antenatal and parenting educators. A letter and supporting publications were also sent to major women's organizations, all Government and non-government secondary schools, colleges and universities.

A strategy involving fashion industry retailers was piloted in phase 1 of the campaign. Metropolitan and rural retailers who were interested in participating received a campaign kit which comprised a window sticker promoting their support for a smoke-free policy in their stores, campaign posters and merchandise items such as emery boards, notepads and lapel stickers with the campaign image and logo to be distributed to customers. A prominent fashion chain also participated in a joint promotion in which customers took part in a competition to win AUS$ 1500 worth of clothing. Grants and campaign publications and merchandise were also made available to the Health Department's regional health education officers, who were encouraged to support the campaign through local initiatives.

Publications and merchandise: A range of new and existing publications and merchandise were produced and distributed to support the campaign. These were designed to inform health professionals and other groups about the campaign and to provide information and assistance to young women in their quit attempts. All resources carried the campaign image and logo. The resources included fact sheets, posters, 'quit tip' note pads, T-shirts, emery board packs, stickers, pens, lapel stickers and refrigerator magnets.

Four new publications that were core resources for the campaign included:
- a resource kit for young women which provided tips on quitting and staying smoke-free, highlighted health risks specific to women who smoke and addressed some of the rationalizations suggested by young women as barriers to quitting;
- *Don't Get Weighed Down—Dealing with Weight and Stress When You Quit Smoking.* This booklet was an adjunct to the resource kit and addressed myths and fallacies about diet and food, presented facts about nutrition and provided tips on diet management and quitting smoking and healthy snack recipes and ideas.

- *Smoking and Pregnancy.* This pamphlet discussed the effect of smoking on unborn and new babies, fears and fallacies about smoking and pregnancy, the effects of smoking on breast-feeding, passive smoking and quit tips.
- *Girls Talk About Smoking.* This resource addressed the health risks associated with smoking and use of the contraceptive pill in a question-and-answer format. The publication was designed as a tear-off pad, and was distributed to general practitioners and pharmacists.

Sponsorship: Awareness of the campaign and its health messages was also extended through sponsorship of women's sports (basketball, netball and baseball) and women's sporting organizations. Sponsorship funding was provided through the Health Promotion Foundation of Western Australia (Healthway).

Counselling and referral: Quit counselling and referral to support agencies was promoted and provided through the campaign to young women seeking assistance in quitting smoking. Quit information and resources were available through the 24-h Quit line and telephone counseling support through the Alcohol and Drug Information Services. Referrals were also made to other services, such as the National Heart Foundation and the Australian Medical Association, for young women seeking information on organized courses or alternative therapies.

Evaluation

Evaluation was an important component of all phases of the campaign, but the focus was on the effectiveness of media strategies. Process and impact were evaluated to measure awareness of the media campaign, the credibility of the campaign messages and the target group's response to the media advertising in self-reported attitudinal and behavioural changes. Surveys were conducted before and after phase 1 of the campaign and after phases 2 and 3. The media concepts for all phases of the campaign were tested before production. Community involvement in the campaign was measured by the number of agencies supporting the campaign (by mail), demand for campaign resources and media coverage.

High awareness of the campaign strategies was seen in all phases (Table 2). Over 4500 health professionals, Government and community agencies and businesses were contacted during the campaign, and demand for resources was high, with over 70 000 resources distributed in phases 1 and 2 of the campaign and over 115 000 during phase 3. All regional health education officers implemented local programmes to extend awareness and involvement in the campaign.

Table 2. Process evaluation by women aged 20–29 after the 'Young women and smoking' campaigns

Process	% positive responses after campaign		
	1991–92 (*n* = 212)	1993 (*n* = 300)	1994 (*n* = 224)
Unprompted recall of seeing or hearing something about quitting aimed at young women during the campaign	42	89	83
Recognized television advertisement(s)	67	91	83
Recall of radio advertisement(s)	53	47	48
Recall of one or more elements of the campaign	86	99	95
Believability of the television/radio advertisement(s)	ND	81 (television and radio)	83 (television)
Personal relevance of television/radio advertisement(s)	ND	58 (television and radio)	62 (television)

The sample for phase 1 of the campaign comprised 20–29-year-old smokers with year 12 or less formal education and who indicated some desire to quit. The samples for phases 2 and 3 comprised 20–29-year-old smokers and recent quitters (within the last month) with year 12 or less formal education. The phase 3 sample was extended to include 16–19-year-old smokers and recent quitters.
ND, not determined

All phases of the campaign stimulated thoughts about quitting in at least 50% of the survey respondents (Table 3). Awareness of the sex-specific health effects of smoking increased between the end of the 1993 and the 1994 campaigns. Encouragingly, in the 1993 and 1994 campaigns, about 45% of the sample attempted to quit or reduced the number of cigarettes smoked per day, while approximately 30% claimed they had successfully quit smoking.

This campaign is but one component of a comprehensive approach to tobacco control. The campaign was strongly supported by the implementation of new tobacco control legislation in 1991 banning the advertising and promotion of tobacco, installing real increases in taxes on tobacco and the retail price of cigarettes, providing school education on drug issues and growing community support for smoke-free policies. State population surveys on tobacco consumption also showed a 16% decline in the prevalence of smoking among young women (from 33% in 1991 to 28% in 1994). While we cannot attribute the decline in the prevalence of smoking among young women to the campaign, the reduction in their prevalence of smoking is a positive change that is consistent with the campaign activities.

Maintenance

Although funding constraints and competing public health priorities do not allow continuation of a separate mass media campaign targeting young women, the Health Department of Western Australia continues to target this group through community-based and health professional strategies developed through its smoking and health programmes. In 1996–97, a series of workshops was conducted at colleges in the metropolitan area, which targeted 16–20-year-old women and aimed to boost their confidence in their ability to make positive health and lifestyle choices. The workshops did not specifically focus on smoking but covered a range of issues, including body image, self-esteem, diet and stress management. Prominent role models, including media personalities and 1996 Olympians, took part in the workshops. The department is currently developing a resource kit based on the workshops for the use of health professionals and community organizations.

Qualitative research was conducted in 1997 to provide more up-to-date data on the health beliefs and behaviour of young women with regard to smoking and appropriate ways of communicating to young women the desirability of quitting smoking (Donovan Research, unpublished). While the research did not suggest that there had been any major changes in the knowledge, attitudes, beliefs and behaviour of young women since 1991, it did highlight the need for further segmentation when developing

Table 3. Impact evaluation of the 'Young women and smoking' campaign by women aged 20–29

Impact	% positive responses after campaign		
	1991–92 (n = 212)	1993 (n = 300)	1994 (n = 224)
Impact of television advertisement(s) on thoughts about quitting	67	54	60
Whether the campaign had affected how they felt about smoking	64	40	72
Knowledge of at least three female-specific health effects of smoking	ND	56	71
Attempts to quit during the campaign	ND	14	23
Attempts to reduce during the campaign	ND	30	22
Successful quit attempts during the campaign	ND	2	3
Successful reduction attempts during the campaign	ND	26	25

The sample for phase 1 of the campaign comprised 20–29-year-old smokers with year 12 or less formal education and who indicated some desire to quit. The samples for phases 2 and 3 comprised 20–29-year-old smokers and recent quitters (within the last month) with year 12 or less formal education. The phase 3 sample was extended to include 16–19-year-old smokers and recent quitters.
ND, not determined

communication messages and strategies. Many of the younger group (16–24 years) were likely to smoke out of rebellion and to belong to a social group and described their smoking as an expression of self-determination and freedom of choice. This group also expected eventually to quit: smoking was seen as a phase that would end with a lifestyle change such as marriage, pregnancy or getting a job. The older group (25–29 years) were more concerned about the negative cosmetic effects of smoking (i.e. ageing) and more freely acknowledged their addiction to nicotine. This group was also concerned by how long they had been smoking, when challenged, and by the realization that they had passed whatever elastic and arbitrary 'quit' deadline they had set when younger. They were also likely to recognize shifts in the social acceptability of smoking and express feelings of discomfort about smoking in social settings.

There has been a steady decline in the prevalence of smoking among young women since 1991, which runs counter to the overall adult trend of no change; it is still a matter of concern, however, that 32% of young women who smoke are not contemplating quitting smoking (Health Promotion Services, 1997). Interventions targeting young women will continue to be a priority for smoking and health programmes of the Health Department in the foreseeable future.

Acknowledgements
The authors acknowledge the work of Lisa Wood, Rita D'Adamo and Sue Leivers, who played key roles in the development, implementation and evaluation of the Young Women and Smoking Campaign from 1991 to 1995.

References
Health Promotion Services (1997) *Smoking and Health in Western Australia, 1996 Resource Book*, Perth: Health Department of Western Australia
Klonoff-Cohen, H., Edelstein, S., Lefkowitz, E., Srinivasa, I., Kaegi, D., Chang, J. & Wiley, K. (1997) The effect of passive smoking and tobacco exposure through breast milk on sudden infant death syndrome. *J. Am. Med. Assoc.*, **273**, 795–798
Unwin, E. & Thompson, N. (1996) *Cigarette Smoking, Life Expectancy and Premature Death in Western Australia* (Health Statistics Western Australia, No. 9), Perth: Epidemiology and Health Statistics Branch, Health Department of Western Australia
US Surgeon General (1980) *The Health Consequences of Smoking for Women: A Report of the Surgeon General*, Maryland: US Department oh Health & Human Services
Walsh, D.C., Rudd, R.E., Moeykens, B.A. & Moloney, T.W. (1993) Social marketing for public health. *Health Affairs*, **12**, 104–119
World Health Organization (1992) *Women and Tobacco*, Geneva

Tobacco use cessation among children and young people

T.J. Glynn

National Cancer Institute, Bethesda, Maryland, United States

Tobacco use among children and youth is increasing in all parts of the world. While most young people who use tobacco say that they could stop at any time, data suggest that this is not the case and that most children and young people who try to stop using tobacco have great difficulty in doing so.

Most research on tobacco use among children and youth has focused, quite correctly, on prevention. There are few programmes and little research that can help determine the most effective ways of helping children and young people stop their tobacco use once they have started. Yet, intervening as early as possible may make the cessation process easier for children and youth and have a significant effect on future rates of prevalence of tobacco use.

Existing treatments and research, specific programmes, policy and research needs and the global effects, now and in the future, of the continuing rise in tobacco use by children and youth are reviewed in this paper.

HEALTH EDUCATION

Health promotion in tobacco control: Widening our horizons

D. Tan

University of the East College of Medicine, Manila, Philippines

Health promotion is the process of enabling people to increase control over and to improve their health. This positive concept combines personal, social, political and institutional resources to fight against health hazards caused by tobacco. Using diverse and/or complementary methods and approaches against tobacco hazards, health promotion directs action on the cause of ill-health—tobacco—rather than focusing on people at risk from specific tobacco-related diseases. Health promotion should be applied to all aspects of tobacco control.

Health promotion in tobacco control means building public policy on tobacco, creating a supportive environment, strengthening community involvement and action, developing personal skills, and reorientating health services. Building a public policy on tobacco requires putting health on the agenda of all policy-makers while accommodating certain realities that can obstruct full implementation of these health policies, such as the nature of the political system in a country, the level of education and problem awareness and competing demands on limited resources. The policies include advertising bans, increased taxes for health and not fiscal reasons and strong, effective tobacco warnings, among others. Creating a supportive environment involves enforcing measures such as smoke-free homes and workplaces, banning the sales of cigarettes to minors, banning the use of vending machines to sell cigarettes, banning advertisements with images of tobacco or smoking that make non-smoking the norm. Success in creating the environment can encourage reciprocity of a uniform policy of tobacco control among communities, nations, regions and the world.

Strengthening community involvement includes encouraging medical associations and non-governmental organizations to form coalitions, to draw upon available human and material resources and to access information on tobacco-related research so that priorities, decisions, strategies and action plans against tobacco can be implemented. Developing personal skills involves enabling individuals to make decisions on non-smoking and environmental safety on the basis of facts. It involves giving individuals access to tobacco-related information such as the hazards of smoking and how the industry and its allies undermine public health. Reorientating health services entails moving health practitioners to go beyond clinical and curative services. It includes integrating tobacco and health-related issues into medical curricula, training and research.

Successful health promotion has the following prerequisities:
- advocacy: Leaders, policy-makers and legislators should be pressured to act in support of health and not tobacco. Advocacy generates public interest and demand for health, places tobacco high on the public agenda, creates a supportive environment favourable to tobacco control and mobilizes alliances for action.
- empowerment: People have the right to a safe, supportive environment, free access to truthful information about tobacco and opportunities free from pressure to make non-smoking decisions.
- alliances and social support systems: Alliances with non-governmental organizations having complementary interests can serve as a channel for actions and people's pursuit of health.

The purpose of health promotion is to inform, to convince, to empower and to mobilize.

The African experience: Present difficulties and future possibilities

Y. Saloojee

National Council Against Smoking, South Africa

One definition of insanity is 'to keep doing the same things over and over again and to expect different results'. Given the continued expansion of the tobacco industry into the developing world, the global tobacco control movement needs to change its way of working or face a charge of insanity. One particular aspect of concern is the relationship between developed and developing countries. With the notable exception of the International Tobacco Initiative and, to a lesser degree, the Swedish International Development Agency, no international donor agencies are active in tobacco control in Africa. African representation at international policy-making meetings is minimal. To get 'different results', we will need to enter into dynamic new health promoting partnerships. This paper examines the choices that have been made in Africa about tobacco, why those choices were made and what choices are likely to be made in the future.

Tobacco use in Africa

The African region has the lowest rates of tobacco consumption in the world. In 1963, it is estimated that just under 400 cigarettes per adult per year were sold; by 1990, that had risen to about 580. This compares to a 1990–92 global average of about 1660. There are, of course, large variations in tobacco use from country to country in Africa. In 1990–92, consumption was highest in Mauritius (1830 cigarettes per adult), Tunisia (1750) and South Africa (1720) and lowest in Niger (170), Sudan (150) and Ethiopia (90).

Africa is thus the only World Health Organization (WHO) region in which primary prevention of the unfolding global tobacco epidemic is possible. The 1993 World Development Report estimated that in 1990, 2 million of the 8 million deaths in Africa occurred among people over the age of 30, and about 90 000 of those could be attributed to smoking. In contrast to some developed countries where tobacco causes one in every five or six deaths, in Africa it causes only one in every 84 deaths. And yet, only time separates Africa from the rest of the world. In middle-income countries such as South Africa, smoking-related diseases are already a common and important health problem. If African countries follow the trend of developed countries, its tobacco epidemic can be expected to peak in the middle of the next century. Very rarely do we have the ability to predict an epidemic so far into the future and also have the knowledge of how to prevent it now.

Why are smoking rates so low?

It is paradoxical that poverty and sexual inequality have protected Africans from harm by cigarettes. The smoking rates among men remain low because of a lack of consumer purchasing power. The rates among women are even lower because women, on average, have even less disposable income than men and because social, religious and cultural prescriptions preclude women from smoking, particularly in public.

The low smoking rates and even lower levels of smoking-related morbidity mean that tobacco control is not a priority in most countries. In 1993, fewer than 30% of the governments in the WHO Africa Region had introduced any tobacco control legislation. For most countries, economic development, job creation, housing, AIDS and other communicable diseases are higher and more urgent priorities. The reluctance to give priority to disease prevention through tobacco control in Africa reveals a lack of advocacy on this issue. There is a very small core of tobacco control experts in the Region. This undermines their ability to mobilize interest on policy issues around tobacco and also means that Africa benefits less from the global momentum for tobacco control. The international lessons of tobacco control are not being applied in Africa.

Future possibilities

The task before us, however, is not to explain why we cannot do better, but to set about the job of making improvements. If we maintain the current status quo, we will maintain the current level of performance.

Africa is a more inviting prospect to the multinational tobacco companies than is immediately apparent, for several reasons. It is beginning to lose its image as a continent riven by conflict, poverty, famine and corruption. The last few years have witnessed a revival of business interest in Africa, and the outlook for tomorrow's Africa has changed. Its economies are becoming increasingly equity-financed rather than debt-driven. The flow of direct foreign investment into Africa is picking up. In 1996, Africa's economy turned in its best performance for years, according to the African Development Bank. Africa's overall growth in gross domestic product last year was 4.8%, up from 2.8% the year before. And although violent upheavals continue, the United Kingdom Foreign Office estimates that 39 of the 53 African countries now enjoy a freely elected government.

The implications of political stability and economic growth are startlingly clear. The industry predicts that between 1994 and 2000, cigarette sales will increase in selected African countries by 1–6%, and it expects that the number of cigarette consumers in all markets in Africa will rise. The reasons for this are the following:

- Increasing affluence will make cigarettes more readily affordable. The World Bank estimates that an increases in income of 10% will result in a 7% increase in consumption in low- income countries and a 13% increase in even lower-income countries.
- Africa has a very young population. At least half the population in most countries is under 19 years of age. This cohort of what the industry euphemistically calls 'potential young adult smokers' represents a great opportunity for long-term cigarette sales.
- Women smokers represent another vast untapped potential market.
- Africa has the world's highest rates of population growth and urbanization. So, even if the prevalence of smoking remains at the present rates, more smokers will enter the market.
- Populations are switching from traditional forms of tobacco to manufactured cigarettes.
- Community awareness of the tactics of the tobacco industry is generally poor. As a result, there are no marketing restrictions and no hostile environment for the industry in most African countries.

Recent years have seen the entry of British and Japanese tobacco companies into South Africa. Philip Morris too is preparing to enter southern Africa as it tries to get out of local licensing agreements. R.J. Reynolds has procured a manufacturing plant in the United Republic of Tanzania.

In order to obtain enactment of tobacco control measures, we must convince policy-makers of the many reasons for controlling tobacco. These include the negative balance of trade in tobacco, with a vast majority of African countries importing far more than they produce. There are also the environmental effects of heavy pesticide use associated with tobacco growing and deforestation in countries where tobacco is cured with wood as fuel. Finally, the industry cannot be allowed to continue to enjoy the cosy consensus it has with politicians and the media, and community outrage at being targeted by an industry which 'sells death for profit' must be harnessed.

Africa remains the last unconquered frontier for the tobacco industry, and the struggle to keep it that way must continue.

The shifting tobacco paradigm and the role of the American Cancer Society

D.G. Bal, J. Cook, R. Todd, M. Morra, N. Lins & H. Eyre

American Cancer Society, Atlanta, Georgia, United States

We shall illustrate how we undertake health promotion and how we go beyond the limits of traditional health promotion in order to be truly effective. Today's health promotion must keep pace with the shifting tobacco paradigm, or we will just cease to be effective.

The Global Burden of Disease, published by the Harvard School of Public Health on behalf of the World Health Organization and the World Bank, notes that "By 2020, tobacco is expected to kill more people than any single disease surpassing even the HIV epidemic." Tobacco kills half a million women worldwide every year and, in many countries, including the United States, lung cancer has overtaken breast cancer as the leading cause of death among women. In my native India, oral cancer (a direct consequence of chewing tobacco with areca leaf and betel nut) is more common than breast cancer. Tobacco has mutagenic effects in pregnant women (in addition to its carcinogenic, atherogenic and other effects) and the gradual increase in tobacco use among women and girls, even in countries where tobacco use is steadily declining among men, indicate that this is a rapidly evolving and lethal women's issue.

The root societal cause for this explosion of tobacco use in the developing world is a cabal between governments in less-developed nations and the multinational tobacco conglomerates, based mainly in the United States and Europe. Just as the tobacco industry has made addicts out of users of tobacco, they have equally cleverly made large governments fiscal addicts of tobacco money. We understand the competing needs of balancing the budget and health and other social priorities, but we equally strongly posit that the fiscal bureaucrats and finance ministers involved in short-term financial balancing acts do not understand the enormous downstream societal costs of these Faustian bargains.

The American Cancer Society is a nationwide, community-based, voluntary health organization dedicated to eliminating cancer as a major health problem by preventing it, saving lives and diminishing suffering from cancer through research, education, advocacy and service. The involvement of the American Cancer Society in tobacco control began with a focus on cessation, moved to emphasis on prevention and public education, shifted to social and environmental change and then to our current aggressive advocacy stance. We shall inevitably be drawn into eradication, because the growing evidence on environmental tobacco smoke and the addictive nature of nicotine lead to zero-tolerance logic. The next long-range project is therefore to address the financial consequences of a decline in tobacco use, especially for small shopkeepers, small businesses and small farmers, which have unwittingly become progressively more dependent upon tobacco sales for an ever-increasing percentage of their cash flow and their profits. This is an area of great significance to developing nations, where the small retailer is the principal provider of tobacco. We urge the Federal and state governments to increase the tax on cigarettes and use the resulting revenue to fund small shopkeepers to phase out their tobacco business over time. The current phase of the Society's activities, advocating for a change of the societal norm of acceptance of tobacco, requires the setting up of local and state programmes funded by additional taxes on tobacco. More recently, we have encouraged national efforts in the public and private sectors, such as the rules of the Food and Drug Administration and the 'Center for tobacco-free kids'.

Anti-tobacco advocates took some time to understand the immensity of the task and the carefully designed barriers set up by the tobacco industry. They saw the necessity of interacting with larger societal constituencies within and without the public sector to achieve common ends. The American Cancer Society (and the American Lung Association and the American Heart Association) began to play a more prominent role

In this bridging of public and private sectors. They acted especially where Government had been ineffectual; for instance, some of the most successful state programmes on tobacco use prevention and cessation (most notably in Arizona, California and Massachusetts) would not have been conceived if those organizations had not bypassed tobacco-supported state legislatures and gone directly to the electorate.

The increasing stridency of the American Cancer Society on this issue over the years has had a considerable cost. As the Society is dependent on its fund-raising efforts to finance its cancer control and research programmes, it did not wish to alienate either the considerable minority of the United States population that smokes or people directly or indirectly involved in the large economic infrastructure created by the tobacco industry. The volunteer and staff leadership of the Society determined, however, that tobacco was a core priority. In view of the decreasing prevalence rates, the market for tobacco in the United States will eventually dwindle to nothing. Although we are not extremists, we consider that eradication is inevitable. This will mean planning for progressive scaling down of the economic infrastructure dependent on tobacco. We must act to make the production, marketing and sale of tobacco unprofitable for economic, social, moral, medical and legal reasons. Ken Warner (this volume) has concluded that tobacco accounts for an overall economic loss to the United States as a whole. Even though 136 000 people are employed in tobacco farming in 23 states and nearly 50 000 are employed in manufacturing tobacco products at 114 tobacco factories in 21 states, many of these jobs are being exported, as the costs of growing, production and manufacture are lower elsewhere. Thus, the potential impact of eradication of tobacco could be lower than anticipated. Similarly, the huge amounts spent by the tobacco industry on advertising and promotion will be a net loss to the advertising and public relations industries but a net gain for society, and the ostensible loss of tax revenues will be more than offset by cost savings in medical care and loss of productivity due to illness.

The American Cancer Society stands ready to help its international partners. As a world community, we must resist the lure of tobacco money. Otherwise, the United States 'global' settlement will merely sanction the companies to do business elsewhere. We must think globally or we are destined to fail.

Cost–benefits of health promotion

J.R. Terborg

Lundquist College of Business, University of Oregon, Eugene, Oregon, United States

Health promotion programmes at work involve: the periodic or continuing delivery of materials and activities for educational and/or behavioural change that are designed to maintain or improve the workers' fitness, health and well-being; and changes in organizational practices and policies conducive to health promotion. Cost–effectiveness analysis and cost–benefit analysis suggest that such programmes can provide financial benefits to work organizations through reduced health-care costs, occupational injuries and absenteeism, and through increased worker productivity (Fries et al., 1993; Pelletier, 1993; Kaman, 1995).

Work-site programmes for hypertension and tobacco are the most effective, followed by programmes for weight control and stress management and then by programmes on nutrition, cholesterol, alcohol and exercise. Programmes on health risk appraisal and HIV/AIDS are the least effective (Wilson et al., 1996). Once the effectiveness of programmes has been established, cost-effectiveness analysis and cost–benefit analysis can be used to examine their effects in financial terms. Cost–effectiveness analysis examines the economic cost associated with producing a unit measure of change.

Cost–benefit analysis examines the economic benefits that might be expected per economic unit of programme cost. A cost–benefit ratio of 1/3.5 means that for every US$ 1 in programme cost there are US$ 3.50 in benefits. Generally, the results of cost–benefit analysis are presented as a ratio of benefits divided by costs. Policy-makers would choose to support the programme with the highest benefit to cost ratio as long as the ratio is greater than 1.00.

In the United States, workers with five or more risk factors have annual health-care costs that are 25–75% higher than those of workers with no risk factors (Kaman, 1995). The incremental cost for each high-risk worker can range from US$ 200 to over US$ 1000 per year. As the economy becomes more global and competitive, firms and nations that can avoid preventable illness and disease will have an advantage in costs of production.

Absenteeism is defined as failure to report for work or to remain at work as scheduled. In the United States, absenteeism costs can easily exceed US$ 100 per worker per day. Health promotion programmes at workplaces have been shown to reduce absenteeism due to illness and injury (Kaman, 1995; Wilson et al., 1996). Companies with low absenteeism rates have lower production costs, on average.

Growing evidence suggests that employees with numerous health risk factors have lower productivity than employees with few or no heath risks (Kaman, 1995). Workers who smoke on the job may waste 15 min or more per day of scheduled work time smoking instead of working. This represents a potential 3% decrease in productivity in an 8-h work day. Workers who abuse alcohol and drugs have been reported to be as much as 25% less productive than those who do not. Finally, there is evidence linking diet to mental performance. Considering these factors, a difference in performance between healthy and unhealthy workers of 1–5% is a reasonable, and perhaps conservative, estimate.

In a study of one United States company, the incremental costs associated with poor worker health in was estimated to be US$ 3419 for each unhealthy worker. Use of a computer simulation showed that excess medical costs accounted for 10–25% of these costs, while excess absenteeism and reduced productivity accounted for 75–90%. This means that even in countries with national health care, there is a substantial financial reason to hire and keep healthy workers. Cost–benefit analysis suggested that for every US$ 1 spent on health promotion, the company received back US$ 3.75 in benefits (Terborg, 1995).

Hiring smokers and allowing smoking at work add substantial costs to a company. When compared with non-smokers, smokers have higher rates of absenteeism, higher medical costs, more accidents and more injuries. Allowing workers to smoke at work increases property damage and depreciation, increases building and equipment maintenance and increases the cost of insurance, Exposure to environmental tobacco smoke by non-smokers also affects the health and absenteeism of those workers, which costs the company more money. It has been estimated that the total direct and indirect cost per smoker per year in the United States is US$ 2853. This figure does not include the value of time lost on the job because of smoking. When that is added, the total cost is over US$ 5000 per smoker per year (Cascio, 1991). The direct costs of delivering a smoking cessation programme at the work site are estimated to range from US$ 100 to US$ 1000 per ex-smoker, assuming a 10–20% success rate. Given the high costs of smoking, implementation of no-smoking policies at work combined with smoking cessation programmes would appear to result in financial benefits that would greatly exceed the costs.

Smoking during pregnancy is associated low birth weight, and low-birth-weight babies have more health problems (Rasmussen & Adams, 1997). For women workers who smoke, this means higher medical costs, higher absenteeism rates associated with caring for a sick child and reduced productivity resulting from care for the sick child. Smoking by pregnant women also has long-term implications for the labour force of the next generation. Low-birth-weight babies show long-term deficits in general intelligence. A prenatal programme that targeted smoking, alcohol and drug use and nutrition in a United States company reduced the annual medical costs associated with childbirth by over US$ 800 000 in just three years (Jacobson *et al.*, 1996). Work-site health promotion programmes that target women workers who smoke will save the company money.

In today's highly competitive global market, companies continuously search for ways of increasing productivity and reducing costs. Providing health promotion programmes at work is not a priority in developing countries. Companies and nations which take this view, however, are making a mistake. Short-term financial gains obtained by exploiting cheap labour and ignoring workers' health will eventually lead to long-term declines in overall competitiveness. Economic development requires investment in human resources and technology. Technology places high value on cognitive and mental abilities, education and performance. Healthy workers have the potential to be more productive than workers who follow unhealthy lifestyles.

References

Cascio, W. (1991) *Costing Human Resources: The Financial Impact of Behavior in Organizations*, Boston : PWS-Kent.

Fries, J.F., Koop, C.E., Beadle, C.E., Cooper. P.R., England, M.J., Greaves, R.F., Skolow, J.J., Wright, D. & Health Project Consortium (1993) Reducing health care costs by reducing the need and demand for medical services. *New Engl. J. Med.*, **329**, 321–325

Jacobson, M., Kolareck, M.H. & Newton , B. (1996) *Business, Babies and the Bottom Line*, Washington DC: Washington Business Group on Health

Kaman, R., ed. (1995) *Worksite Health Promotion Economics: Consensus and Analysis*, Champaign, Illinois: Human Kinetics Publishers

Pelletier, K.R. (1993) A review and analysis of the health and cost effectiveness outcome studies of comprehensive health promotion and disease prevention programmes at the worksite: 1991–1993 update. *Am. J. Health Promot.*, **8**, 50–62

Rasmussen, K.M. & Adams, B. (1997) Annotation: Cigarette smoking, nutrition, and birthweight. *Am. J. Public Health*, **87**, 543

Terborg, J.R. (1995) Computer simulation: A promising technique for evaluation of health promotion programmes at the worksite. In: Kaman, R., ed., *Worksite Health Promotion Economics: Consensus and Analysis*, Champaign, Illinois: Human Kinetics Publishers

Wilson, M.G., Holman, P.B. & Hammock, A. (1996) A comprehensive review of the effects of worksite health promotion on health related outcomes. *Am. J. Health Promot.*, **10**, 429–435

Soul City: A health promotion initiative against tobacco

S. Goldstein, G. Japhet, S. Usdin, P. Esterhuysen & T. Shongwe

Soul City, Institute for Urban Primary Health Care, Houghton, South Africa

Soul City is an multi-media health promotion initiative. The project is unique in that instead of responding to one particular issue (such as HIV/AIDS) and developing a specific 'one off' media intervention around it, Soul City is a powerful media vehicle that can be used to confront a variety of issues on an ongoing basis. Soul City 1 was screened in 1994 and repeated in 1996. Soul City 2 began in August 1996. We describe this initiative and the process used to place tobacco as an issue, with a brief summary of the results and messages developed.

Many tobacco education initiatives have as their cornerstone the desire to empower people through knowledge and changed attitudes that enable them to make positive, informed decisions about their lives. The mass media is the most powerful communication tool at our disposal, with far-reaching influence; unfortunately, those influences are most often negative. The media in both the developing and the developed world depict lifestyles that are generally unattainable and unhealthy; they promote the use of tobacco, alcohol and unhealthy foods and represent health as a subject for individual behavioural change, with no attention to the environmental and socio-political determinants (Hynd, 1990; Wallack, 1990).

The multi-media health promotion strategy positively promotes health and development through three forms of mass media: television, radio and newspapers. The strategy embraces the concept of 'edu-tainment' (Piotrow *et al.*, 1990; Lettenmaier *et al.*, 1993), in which social messages are creatively woven into drama programmes. The print medium supplements these programmes, providing in-depth information to complement the dramas. Three points are critical for the media to achieve their maximum potential. The first is popularity; each medium should be used in its most popular form. For the electronic media, this means having access to 'prime time' and using a genre that is accessible. The difference in the size of the audience for prime time and off-prime time television in South Africa is huge: up to 3 million viewers compared with about 500 000 people. The second important point is that different media reach different audiences and if people have access to more than one medium the information and messages received are reinforced (Wallack, 1990). One of the most important determinants of successful media education is careful formative research on the target audience. This is often the most neglected area of communications strategy. The messages should be developed with the target audience and pre-tested to ensure they are received as designed (Wallack, 1990).

The Soul City strategy was born at the Alexandra Health Centre and became a project of the Institute for Urban Primary Health Care. We describe here the tobacco messages in the Soul City mass media vehicle.

Background

Thirty-four percent of adult South Africans smoke, with 52% of men and 17% of women, for a total of 7 million people. The overall figures have increased by 1% per year since 1992, and the increase was greatest among the coloured population, who have the highest overall smoking rate, 59%. There is at least one smoker in 48% of households, so that exposure of non-smokers and children to cigarette smoke is a major health hazard (Yach *et al.*, 1995).

The Government of National Unity has begun legislative reform with regard to tobacco. Although the Tobacco Products Control Act of 1993 has imposed restrictions on advertising and enforced health warnings on cigarette packs and advertisements, little has been allocated to public awareness or education campaigns or campaigns to popularize the new legislation. Clinics and health personnel may intend to educate but have inadequate resources, personnel, time and training to embark on face-to-face education or cessation assistance and a real scarcity of printed materials.

Despite the inequities of apartheid, the media infrastructure in South Africa is relatively well developed. Previous attempts to reach poor, rural and illiterate people were successful, particularly during the voter education campaign of 1993. An evaluation of the campaign by the Community Agency for Social Enquiry showed that 80% of Africans (i.e. Negroid South Africans: although we are against any form of racism, the various racial groups in South Africa must be described to ensure that past inequities do not go unnoticed) listen to the radio and 58% watch television three times a week or more (Everatt *et al.*, 1994). Although the people of South Africa are not all literate, many use the newspapers for information. In a survey by the Matla Trust, one-third of rural respondents said that they used daily newspapers as a source of political information. South Africa has the highest rate of media penetration in Africa, with one television set per 11 people, one radio for every six people and a daily newspaper circulation of 41 per 1000 people (SABC Radio, 1993)[1]. The Community Agency for Social Enquiry found that the main reasons why people listened to the radio and watched television were to be entertained and informed rather than to be educated (Everatt *et al.*, 1994).

The combination of poor health education resources and skills, very poor health indicators and relatively good mass media penetration was the basis for the Soul City intervention.

Soul City

Drama captures people's imaginations like no other television genre. 'Soul City', our television drama, has a prime-time slot on SABC 1, the most popular channel, and is produced in a series of 13 half-hour episodes. It has attracted a large and loyal audience. In its second week, it was the second most popular television programme nationwide. A daily, 15-min, 60 part drama also called 'Soul City' follows a similar story line. It is aired on nine of the country's vernacular radio stations, with a potential audience of 12 million listeners.

While the electronic media effectively convey broad messages, they cannot deal with specifics and maintain audience interest. Soul City therefore uses newspapers to provide detailed information to supplement the health messages in the electronic media. Thus, 36-page high-quality colour booklets are illustrated with characters from the television series and are serialized in newspapers in the same three months that the television and radio series are broadcast. Ten major national newspapers participate, and the complete booklet is inserted in the papers at the end of the period of serialization.

We recognize that the mass media can raise awareness, generate discussion and increase knowledge. They can also play a part in shifting attitudes and behaviour, but to be most effective, they should be backed up by face-to-face communication. We are therefore building on the popularity of the Soul City vehicles by combining them into education packages of audio and video tapes and written material. These materials are designed to facilitate learning in a variety of formal and informal educational settings.

The four media are coordinated in a carefully thought out strategy to popularize the dramas and booklets and to raise further awareness of the issues they raise. This is achieved through a public relations campaign that places the programmes and their issues on the public agenda in editorials, competitions and a range of programmes in the media.

The first series of Soul City was broadcast in 1994 and concentrated on a number of crucial issues in mother and child health, within broader development concerns such as community mobilization and the empowerment of women. The second series of Soul City dealt with tobacco, HIV/AIDS, tuberculosis and healthy housing. Both series were made available to an increasing number of countries in Africa, currently Kenya, Namibia, Zambia and Zimbabwe.

Formative research

The core of Soul City is commitment to vigorous research on each topic, including tobacco. In this process, a local and international literature review is commissioned, and the major players in the field are consulted about what they consider to be the major national messages on the topic. On the strength of this information, focus groups are conducted with members of the target audience. All the information is then brought to a message design workshop attended by material developers and the major players who were consulted. We agree together on a national message for the topic, and a written brief is drawn up for our material developers. The creative team, the consultants, the researchers and the Soul City team meet in a creative workshop to develop ideas for the series. The material developers then draw up an outline of the series and the first drafts of the written material.

The outlines and each episode are pre-tested: we send copies of the first drafts to consultants nominated at our message design workshop and pre-test the drafts on focus groups of members of our target audience. On the strength of the feedback, the material developers re-work the scripts and written material. These steps are repeated until we are happy with the final draft, and the material is then produced. After national dissemination, an impact evaluation is conducted.

Key issues arising from research on the target audience

When girls and boys below the age of 25 years, in and out of school, were interviewed, the key issues that arose were:

- peer pressure: Young people felt helpless in the face of pressure from peers to smoke; their perception of the extent of the pressure was exaggerated, as they thought that many more of their contemporaries smoked than really did. The peer pressure was particularly strong among boys.
- weight loss: There is a lot of pressure on young girls to conform to a western ideal of thinness, extensively portrayed in the media. Girls felt that smoking was an easy way to control their weight.
- independence: There is still a fairly strong taboo on girls smoking in South Africa, and it was seen by almost all the girls as a sign of independence, freedom and taking on western values.
- confusion among messages: Some young people were confused by the information they were getting about tobacco. Although most knew that tobacco causes cancer, they were not sure whom they should believe: those who encouraged them to smoke (the industry) or those who discouraged them (the anti-tobacco lobby).
- boredom: Some young people said that they smoked from boredom. Recreation and school facilities are bad in most poor urban and rural areas, and young people are often out of school by 11:00, with the rest of the day stretching ahead.
- ease of access to tobacco: In South Africa, there is a thriving informal sector which sells single cigarettes, so that young people can afford cigarettes almost anywhere.

The issues for adults were somewhat different. Almost all those interviewed knew that tobacco is harmful, although the details of the harm were somewhat vague, but they had little knowledge about the effects of passive smoking. Most adults said that they wanted to give up but mentioned a number of barriers. Many felt helpless and didn't know how to give up; some said that they had tried, with no success. Some felt that it was cheaper to smoke than drink and had therefore opted for smoking. Some said that they couldn't give up as all their friends smoked. Others said that giving up would make them feel sick

Tobacco messages

The results of the research were combined with other results, and the messages for the series were developed in a workshop with key stakeholders.

The messages for young people were: "Don't start smoking; once you start, it is difficult to stop." and "You are being duped into smoking."

Smoking is not cool.

Smoking interferes with sports and decreases performance.

Smoking doesn't increase your independence, it enslaves you.

The community action messages were: "There should be community support for the ban on sales to people under 16 years." and "Smoking in public places should be restricted."

Adults can and do play a definitive role in the access that young people have to cigarettes.

Non-smokers have a right to clean air.

The messages to adults were: "Giving up smoking is both beneficial and possible." and "Most people who smoke want to give up."

If you give up smoking, it will improve your quality of life, by decreasing your chances of debilitating illnesses. It will also prolong your life.

If you give up smoking, it will prevent passive smoking which is especially damaging to children's respiratory health.

If you give up smoking, it saves you money.

Smokers who are giving up need support from their family and friends.

Conclusion

The use of a multi-media 'edutainment' vehicle to carry anti-tobacco messages is unique in South Africa. The development of the messages and the development and distribution of the materials was an exciting interactive process which brought messages to an audience previously untouched by anti-tobacco information. The success of the intervention is discussed in a separate paper in this volume.

References

Everatt, D., De Castro, J., Tshandu, Z., Orkin, M. & Stevens, C. (1994) Reaching the voters: Voters, voter education needs and mass media. Prepared for the Independent Forum for Electoral Education. Community Agency for Social Enquiry

Hynd, S.W. (1990) Do decision-makers have the capacity to make the strategies work? *World Health Forum*, 11, 155–156

Lettenmaier, C., Krenn, S., Morgan, W., Kois, A. & Piotrow, P. (1993) Africa: Using radio soap operas to promote family planning. *Hygie*, 12.

Piotrow, P.T., Rimon, J.G., II, Winnard, K., Kincaid, D.L., Hunington, D. & Convisser, J. (1990) Mass media family planning promotion in three Nigerian cities. *Stud. Family Planning*, 21

SABC Radio (1993) *Reaching Critical Mass*

Wallack, L. (1990) Two approaches to health promotion in the mass media. *World Health Forum*, 11, 143–154

Yach, D., Reddy, P. & Weitz, A.M. (1995) MRC/HSRC Survey: Key National Findings

Evaluation of Soul City: A multi-media health promotion initiative against tobacco

S. Goldstein, G. Japhet, S. Usdin, P. Esterhuysen & T. Shongwe

Soul City, Institute for Urban Primary Health Care, Houghton, South Africa

We describe an evaluation of the impact of Soul City, the South African multi-media intervention against tobacco, in terms of audience, popularity, discussion of the issues, knowledge, attitudes and behaviour. The project itself is described in another paper in these proceedings.

The objectives of the evaluation were to establish the overall penetration of the vehicle, including demographic profiling and the loyalty of the audience, and to determine the impact of the series in terms of: message retention, increase in knowledge, change in attitude and reported behaviour and the ability of the material to catalyse interpersonal communication

Methods

The study took place over six months, with a baseline study in July 1996 and a post-intervention survey in November 1996. 'Soul City' was broadcast over three months, from 6 August to 29 October. Four sites were chosen as typical of where previously disadvantaged South Africans live: New Brighton Township in the Eastern Cape, a metropolitan area of 85 000 people; Eatonside in Gauteng, an informal settlement of 5000 people; Motwabeng in the Free State, a small town and Belfast in Mpumulanga, a rural area with a population of 6000.

At each site, 200 people were surveyed before the mass media intervention in July 1996 and afterwards, in November 1996, for a total of 800 respondents. In-depth interviews were held with key informants before and after the mass media intervention, and eight focus groups were held after it. The quantitative material was analysed by the SSPS program, and verbatim transcripts were analysed qualitatively.

Results

'Soul City' reached substantial numbers of people and particularly the target audience. The audience ratings for the entire South African population over all four channels were 11.3–15.2 for adults and 17.0–21.3 for children. These ratings showed that it was in the top three rated programmes for 11 out of the 13 weeks it was on air. The rates for our specific target groups, Sotho- and Nguni-speaking people, were even higher, ranging from 21.3–32.6. The lowest values were recorded for a week in which there was a television black-out in many parts of the country.

'Soul City' reached 61% of the respondents, comprising 59% of women and 61% of men, and 70% of all 16–24-year olds. Of people with no schooling, 51% accessed 'Soul City', 40% of them through radio. 'Soul City' was especially popular in the urban informal settlement Eatonside, where 78% of respondents had seen or heard it. In the rural area of Belfast, 63% of respondents had accessed 'Soul City'.

Smoking was a popular and engaging issue: 86% said that they liked the information about smoking, 90% said that they believed the messages, and 49% of those who discussed 'Soul City' discussed smoking issues.

There was an overall increase in knowledge, as concluded from the answers to four questions asked of people who accessed 'Soul City' and those who did not. The increase was greatest for those who had accessed two types of Soul City medium, followed by television. Although the increase was not as great among those who had heard the programme on the radio, these people were less well educated than those who did not hear it, and the knowledge gains may still be large. Knowledge about passive smoking increased: 95% of those who accessed two types of Soul City medium gave the correct answer, while 85 % of those who had access to two types of medium but did not see or hear 'Soul City' got the answer correct. Again, television was more effective than radio. The qualitative data illustrate some of the gains in knowledge: A young man in Motwabeng said, "With me it taught me not to smoke because it is bad to lungs." One in Eatonside said, "The other lesson is about how one can quit smoking." A middle-aged woman in Eatonside said, "I've got a mother who smokes cigarette. Since we saw 'Soul City', we ask her not to smoke in front of us especially children though she shouts at us but we do and we also try to discourage her, we tell her that smoking is dangerous to her.", and women in Motwabeng said, "I think that a person who smokes must do so outside the house lest he affect the children." and "In my family my children do not allow any visitor to smoke inside the house." Another person in Motwabeng said, "Pertaining ¬moking I have learned to avoid smokers near me because I too will inhale the smoke."

Attitudes also shifted after the Soul City intervention. For instance, many more people who accessed 'Soul City' disagreed very strongly with the statement "Its cool to smoke.", and more people who had access to 'Soul City' agreed with the statement "It's never too late to stop smoking." than those who did not.

As was expected, the study could not show any changes in the numbers of people who smoke. At baseline, 25% smoked every day, 6% smoked some days and 69% did not smoke. At the time of the evaluation, 23% smoked every day, 7% smoked some days and 70% did not smoke. Behavioural change is a process, and a lag phase can be expected between an increase in knowledge, changes in attitudes and an actual change in behaviour. The qualitative research showed, however, that a few people claimed that their behaviour had changed directly because of the intervention.

Conclusion

The Soul City multi-media health promotion initiative achieved its objectives in raising awareness of tobacco-related issues, getting people to discuss tobacco, increasing knowledge about the health effects of tobacco and changing attitudes towards tobacco. Its messages reached a substantial number of people in South Africa, representing 61% of the identified target audience. Although no quantitative change in smoking behaviour can be demonstrated, people mentioned both quitting smoking and smoking outdoors to prevent passive smoking. The evaluation continued into 1997 with two further quantitative surveys and follow-up of knowledge, attitudes and smoking behaviour.

Giving smokers what they want: Certainties, not probabilities

T. Cotter¹, D. Hill², J. Watt¹ & J. Boulter²

¹Victorian Smoking and Health Program and ²Centre for Behavioural Research in Cancer, Anti-Cancer Council of Victoria, Melbourne, Australia

In preparation for Australia's first national campaign on smoking, a comprehensive review of published and unpublished literature on smokers' attitudes and behaviour was undertaken. The results showed consistently that smokers want clear, strong, convincing information about the health effects of smoking and not other motives for quitting. Using new health insights, the campaign has focused on the certain consequences of smoking rather than on the probabilities as the mechanism for making giving up smoking number one on the list of priorities for every smoker.

Most anti-smoking advertising campaigns warn smokers that they are at risk of ill health or death. Of the 124 000 deaths that occurred in Australia in 1992, 18 920 were attributed to smoking (English *et al.*, 1995). We have rightly called this an epidemic and concluded that the public needs to be informed about the huge risks they take when they smoke. Tobacco control advocates have quoted figures like those of Peto *et al.* (1994) on tobacco-related mortality, which show that one-quarter of all deaths among middle-aged males are caused by smoking, or the calculation of Doll *et al.* (1994) that people who continue to smoke have a 50% chance of dying from tobacco-related disease. Such calculations provide the rationale for extensive action to reduce smoking in our community. People, however, are notoriously bad at understanding and acting on information about risk; they distort and objectify the hazard and 'self-exempt' themselves with various rationalizations (Borland, 1997). They are much more concerned about the risk at the moment than the risk for the future. Smokers translate warnings about the risks of their habit into statements like, "Smoking is like buying a ticket in a lottery that's drawn when you are 70....I'll take a chance on that." Smokers must be made to understand that disease is not like a lottery, but is building a pathway from imperceptible early damage to serious disease.

In Australia, there was a decline in the prevalence of smoking in the 1980s, but in the 1990s smoking rates have flattened out, with 25% of the adult population continuing to take the chance on smoking tobacco (Mullins *et al.*, 1995). In preparation for Australia's first national tobacco campaign, smokers were asked what would motivate them to quit and what type of information they wanted. In addition, a comprehensive review was made of the relevant published and unpublished literature on smokers' attitudes and behaviour, and the psychological basis of changing individual behaviour was analysed.

The majority of smokers intend to quit at some time and most commonly give 'health' as the reason why they would quit (Mullins *et al.*, 1995). Ex-smokers also give this as the reason why they quit. When asked what kinds of messages would help them to quit, smokers most commonly called for graphic portrayals of the health damage (Morand & Mullins, 1996). Many smokers also want to know exactly what smoking does inside their body.

A representative sample of Victorian smokers was asked, "If an advertisement was going to make you more likely to stop smoking, what sort of ad would it be?" Half (50%) said they wanted graphic material showing the impact of their smoking. Typically, their responses were, "Show the harm it does to you.", 'Show a pair of lungs dripping with cancer.", "Ads that look real" and "Concentrate on health." Other strategies, such as encouragement to quit, effects on others and the benefits of quitting, were mentioned by only 17%; the remainder were evenly divided between those who thought nothing would work and those who did not have any opinion (Morand & Mullins, 1996).

Thus, many smokers are interested in what happens to them as individuals and want the doctor's eye view: they want to know what happens to their heart and their lungs. They want something strong, but the challenge is to give them something that does not allow them to say, "That's not me." Focusing on what happens every time you smoke closes these escape hatches and rules out the response "That's too far in the future." and the lottery response "That may not happen to me." Unlike traffic accidents, where people can see the cause and effect, the serious consequences of smoking are only an abstract concept to most smokers. They know the long-term effects of smoking only because they have been told what scientists have discovered about it. Unlike the traffic accident, there is no immediate fear associated with the behaviour. Given that we all learn best from experience, the communication challenge is to translate the scientific knowledge about smoking into experience.

We describe here some of the thinking that went into Australia's National Tobacco Campaign. One of the first steps was to arrange meetings between scientific and medical experts and creative people. The product was an informed creative agency, a panel of experts and a clear, creative direction for the campaign. The process of concept development, testing, re-testing and final production took seven months. Three commercials were produced, on lungs, arteries and tumours, all within the following framework: Each commercial opens with an empathy device, a typical moment in which smokers can recognize themselves doing something that only smokers do. The next scene is a conditioning device, in which a close-up of the cigarette follows the smoke through the mouth, down the throat and into the lungs. This is where we bridge the gap between the action of smoking and the disease process. Once inside the body, the viewer receives the new health information, presented in a realistic manner. The commercial ends with the camera following the smoke out of the lungs, to a shot of a smoker, oblivious to the damage that is happening inside. The final frame simply states, "Every cigarette is doing you damage." and gives the Quitline number for further information.

Early research on the advertisements indicates that the campaign was approved by smokers, who said that the advertisements were thought-provoking, believable and relevant. What better positive reinforcement, however, than this quote from one of Australia's best-known sporting heroes, after a match in which he played particularly well. The headline read, "Walters fires up in new role with healthy outlook", and the quote was "I wasn't a heavy smoker by any means, but I saw the ad on television and I thought they could be my lungs. I went cold turkey."

This communication gives real health information that focuses on the individual and is personally relevant, a communication that looks at the certain consequences of smoking—not at what might happen. It is perhaps most importantly a communication that is unforgettable and confrontational, with the ability to evoke an emotive response that can be stored in the memory and used as a psychological tool to assist in quitting.

References
Borland, R. (1997) What do people's estimates of smoking related risk mean? *Psychol. Health*, **12**, 513–521
Doll, R., Peto, R., Wheatley, K., Gray, R. & Sutherland, I. (1994) Mortality in relation to smoking: 40 years of observations on male British doctors. *Br. Med. J.*, **309**, 901–911
English, D.R., Holman, C.D.J., Milne, E., Winter, M.G., Hulse, G.K., Codde, J.P., Bower, C.I., Corti, B., De Klerk, N., Khulman, M.W., Kurinczuk, J.J., Lewin, G.F. & Ryan, G.A. (1995) *The Quantification of Drug Caused Morbidity and Mortality in Australia*, Canberra, Commonwealth Department of Community Services and Health
Morand, M. & Mullins, R. (1996) *Evaluation of the Excuses Campaign: Results of a Telephone Survey Conducted Immediately after the 1996 Media Campaign*, Victoria, Centre for Behavioural Research in Cancer, Anti-Cancer Council of Victoria
Mullins, R., Morand, M. & Borland, R. (1995) Key findings of the 1994 and 1995 Household Surveys. *Quit Eval. Stud.*, **8**, 1–25
Peto, R., Lopez, A.D., Boreham, J., Thun, M. & Heath, C., Jr (1994) *Mortality from Smoking in Developed Countries 1950–2000: Indirect Estimates from National Vital Statistics.*, Oxford: Oxford University Press

Health education and smoking cessation

R. Sadek, S. Mostafa, M. Dydamony & L. Zarief

Epidemiology Department, Minia University, Minia, Egypt

Abstract

The main aim of this study was to increase awareness about the hazards of smoking and to help smokers stop smoking. The subjects were male workers at a cotton gin. We found no significant relationship between the residence of workers and their smoking status but a significant relationship with the type of work they did and with their level of education. Of those who followed a health education programme, 8.8% quit smoking, and there was a significant increase in the mean score of knowledge about the hazards of smoking. The most effective variable for quitting or reducing smoking was level of education.

Introduction

Smoking-related diseases are by definition associated with a particular behaviour, which is susceptible to change by health education. In this study, a health education programme was used which was designed to increase awareness about the hazards associated with smoking and a practical strategy was proposed to help smokers to quit.

Subjects and methods

The subjects were male workers at the Nile Cotton Ginning Company in Minia, Egypt. The study was performed in three stages. During the first two months, all of the workers were screened to identify smokers. In the second stage of four months, health messages were given to the smokers in group discussions and personal interviews, with pamphlets and audiovisual aids describing the hazards of smoking and how to quit smoking. In the third stage, which lasted three months, we evaluated our programme.

Results

The total number of workers screened was 645; of these, 321 (50%) were smokers. About half were urban and half rural residents. The highest percentage of smokers (52%) was found among manual workers, followed by clerical workers (51%), and the lowest percentage (39%) was found among professional workers. A relationship was seen with level of education, 53% of smokers being among those with the lowest level of education, 48% among those with intermediate education and 38% among those with a higher educational level.

Of the 62 smokers who attended health education sessions, 8.8% quit, while 46% reduced the number of cigarettes they smoked daily by at least 50%; 1.8% quit but subsequently relapsed. The highest percentage of quitters (10%) was found among those who had smoked < 10 cigarettes per day, and none of those who smoked > 40 cigarettes per day quit; 13% of men who had smoked for < 20 years quit smoking, while only 6% of those who had smoked for 20–40 years were able to do so.

We measured the men's knowledge about smoking hazards before and after the health education programme. A significant improvement in the mean score was seen both among smokers who had quit smoking and those who reduced their smoking ($p <$ 0.001); even smokers who did not change their smoking habit showed improved knowledge, although the difference was not significant. The most effective determinants for quitting or reducing smoking are shown in Table 1.

Discussion

Screening of workers at the Nile Cotton Ginning Company showed that the prevalence of smoking among male workers was 50%, while WHO has estimated that 33% of Egyptian men are smokers. We found a significant association ($p = 0.002$)

Table 1. Effects of various determinants on quitting or reduction of smoking among 62 men in Egypt

Independent variable	β	p value
Education	0.24	0.2
No. of cigarettes per day	0.14	0.6
Duration of smoking	0.13	0.9
Occupation	0.11	0.5
Age	0.10	0.9
Residence	0.04	0.8
Marital status	0.03	0.8
Age at starting to smoke	0.01	0.9

$r^2 = 0.28$

between the type of work and the smoking status of these men, with the highest prevalence among manual and clerical workers and the lowest prevalence among professional workers, in agreement with the findings of Austoker et al. (1994). In our study, the prevalence of smoking among the less well educated men was 72% higher than that in the best educated group, figures similar to those reported by Macaskill et al. (1992).

The quit rate in our study is similar to that reported by Salive (1992) and better than those achieved by Macaskill et al. (1992) and Warnecke et al. (1992). There was a significant relationship between the number of cigarettes that the person had smoked per day and the response to the health education programme: the majority of those who stopped completely or reduced their consumption had previously smoked fewer than 10 cigarettes per day. Warnecke et al. (1992) also found that light smokers were more likely to quit after an intervention. Our study showed a significant increase in the mean score for knowledge among men who quit or reduced smoking, and this agrees with the report of Wynder (1993). The level of education was the most predictive variable for quitting or reducing smoking.

We succeeded in improving the knowledge of these men about the hazards of smoking, and some of the participants quit. Health education is therefore an important tool in smoking control.

References

Austoker, J., Sander, D. & Flower, G. (1994) Cancer prevention in primary care. Smoking and cancer: Smoking cessation. Br. Med. J., 308, 1478–1482

Macaskill, P., Pierce, P., Simpson, J.M., et al. (1992) Mass media anti smoking campaign can remove education gap in quitting behavior. Am. J. Public Health, 82, 96–98

Salive, M.E. (1992) Predictors of smoking cessation and relapse in older adults. Am. J. Public Health, 82, 1368–1370

Warnecke, R.B., Langenberg, P., Wing, S.C., et al. (1992) The second Chicago televised smoking cessation program: A 24 months follow up. Am. J. Public Health, 82, 835–840

Wynder, E.L. (1993) Towards a smoke free society: Opportunities and obstacles. Am. J. Public Health, 83, 1204–1205

A systematic approach to setting up a health promotion organization in Thailand

B. Supakorn

Task Force for the Health Promotion Fund Project, Health Systems Research Institute, Ministry of Public Health, Nonthaburi, Thailand

Introduction

As in other dynamic societies, in Thailand public health has been affected by multiple social, economic and environmental changes. The Ministry of Public Health is the infrastructure primarily responsible for securing basic health care, although other Government agencies implement vertical programmes serving their constituencies. Most existing programmes are designed to provide preventive services, such as immunization and maternal-and-child care, and only trivial attempts with small budgets have been made to mobilize the potential sources within society to act together for good health. The lack of effective coordination among the vertical programmes has become the primary limitation to the promotion of good health in the community.

In April 1996, Thailand's Ministry of Finance initiated a 'Master plan for social development through financing measures', which incorporates a health promotion fund project, as proposed by the Health Systems Research Institute. The proposed fund is modelled on Australia's health promotion foundations. Although legislation for the establishment of the fund had not been completed at the time of writing, a number of lessons have been learnt from advocacy while awaiting the approval of the Ministry of Finance for the fund.

Situation analysis

Each year, more than 70 000 Thais die prematurely, mainly from cardiovascular disease, accidents and cancer. These diseases result in health-care expenditures that represent 5.5% of Thailand's gross national product. The country spends much more on health care then neighbouring countries, and this high expenditure partly reflects inefficiency within the health service system.

Thailand thus faces two major health problems: high preventable mortality and morbidity rates and inefficient health care. The former can be tackled primarily through effective promotion of good health and preventive measures, i.e. health promotion. Theoretically, health promotion would be less effective in rectifying the inefficiency of the health-care system, but solving the first problem could lead to large public savings.

The Ministry of Public Health has been successful in providing essential preventive services to the population in community-based programmes: immunization, nutrutional supplements, family planning, maternal-and-child health and dental health. Two departments are responsible for monitoring and support services, while the programmes are implemented through another department. A further department organizes programmes for the control of non-communicable diseases, i.e. cardiovascular diseases, accidents and cancer, including tobacco-related diseases. These vertical programmes are also delivered through provincial administrative offices and hospitals. The centralization, bureaucratic compartmentalization and rigid budgetary system present obstacles to interdepartmental collaboration.

Collaborative efforts are hindered to an even greater extent when it comes to 'diseases of modernization' such as prevention of tobacco use, accidents and HIV/AIDS. There is no mechanism to ensure the commitment of partners to work collaboratively on projects. Indeed, any collaboration that does exist depends to a large extent on the personality of the officers in charge.

The inefficiency ofthe public bureaucracy has been recognized by the Government for a number of years, and a move has been made to decentralize the civil service. Meanwhile, the Ministry of Finance has developed its 'Master plan for social development through financing measures', which aims to achieve financial decentralization and empowerment of the community's organizations for local development. To achieve these two goals, the Ministry has devised fiscal and monetary measures including selective taxation, loans for community development and efficient administrative agencies.

Over the past two decades, non-governmental organizations have contributed significantly to health improvement, despite limited resources. Outstanding examples include organizations for family planning, tobacco control, consumer protection, community pharmacies, self-care, child health and rural health services. Nevertheless, they have little opportunity to collaborate with Government agencies.

Problem

There is thus ample room for improvement in health development in Thailand. To unlock that potential, health promotion must be reorientated to meet the following challenges:

- changes in disease patterns and determinants that require action beyond the existing preventive services;
- rising expenditure on health care and high social costs due to preventable ill health;
- the structural rigidity of the Government bureaucracy that hinders multisectoral interventions;
- trends towards greater decentralization of the public sector and
- increasing public awareness of health and potential community involvement.

These five forces indicate that the existing health promotion infrastructure should be reorientated towards a greater capacity for social mobilization. If nothing is done, the existing structures will become increasingly inadequate for curtailing the disease burden, resources will continue to be used inefficiently and potential partnerships and non-governmental resources will not be realized.

A health promotion fund

The main areas for improvement are therefore resource allocation for partnerships and effective coordination among multiple vertical interests. This idea led to the design of a new infrastructure similar to Australia's health promotion foundations, which aim to promote health efficiently. Their key features are statutory organization, limitation of their functions to funding and managing and not implementing vertical activities and financing from the Government budget (i.e. tobacco excise tax).

Since 1990, Thailand has established four organizations that structurally resemble Australia's model. Three are research institutes and one is a regional university. Sample legislation therefore exists. The Health Systems Research Institute has concluded that Australia's health promotion foundation model is the most promising, as it provides not only funding but also an organizational base. This structure allows the setting of national priorities, proactive management, comprehensive programming and accountability. The links to the Government enhance its acceptance by ministerial departments, while flexibility is maintained.

The main characteristics of Thailand's health promotion fund (tentatively called 'ThaiHealth') are that it is a statutory agency linked loosely to the Ministry of Public Health through legislation; the Government provides the financial support; it has proactive management and a small office for mobilization and enabling, but not for implementation.

The objectives to be achieved are to further effective health promotion, to reorientate the social attitude to 'good health' and to strengthen the capacity of civic movements and encourage an active role in health promotion. Under the Ministry of Public Health, there is a policy steering board consisting of representatives from six ministries and 12 distinguished persons; an evaluation board consisting of representatives from four ministries and eight experts; a director, who is appointed for a five-year term by the policy steering board; 10 administrators and 20 programmers.

Lessons learnt

Development of the fund represents a case study of organized approaches to health promotion. The first lesson learnt was to start with a good example. The advocacy started with the premise that the existing infrastructure was inadequate. A preliminary review was conducted and identified an excellent model in Australia: VicHealth, which has gained experience and recognition during its 10 years of operation. The advocacy was thus based on a real example and not on a quixotic proposal. This has generated credibility.

The second lesson was to accommodate current reforms. The approach was based on the existing policy process and current trends, namely the master plan of the Ministry of Finance and public sector reform. This feature is critical for establishing ThaiHealth as part of a trend and not as a new entity.

Thirdly, it is supported by research. While the approach adhered fundamentally to the policy process, essential information was anticipated and planned for. Research was carried out in a timely manner to support the policy formulation and to respond to all questions asked.

Finally, we gained international support. Examples are crucial for policy formulation. The delegation from the Ministry of Finance heard first-hand testimony when it visited Australia and New Zealand. Most critical was a meeting with high-ranking administrators of Victoria's Ministry of Finance, who strongly influenced opinions about a dedicated tobacco tax. The support of the World Health Organization also provided a credible environment for the advocacy.

Rural community health promotion for tobacco control in Thailand

N. Charoenca[1] & S. Hamann[2]

[1]*Mahidol University and* [2]*Rangsit University, Bangkok, Thailand*

A one-year smoking control campaign funded by the World Health Organization (WHO) was undertaken in Sanarmchaikait, Chachoengsao Province, Thailand, in 1995. The purpose of the project was to demonstrate the feasibility, methods and effects of forming a rural community coalition against tobacco use in Thailand.

We first identified community participants, conducted training and tobacco control activities and established a working team of active community members. We assessed the interest and readiness of the community with the assistance of the community physician, two community health nurses and a health-centre leader. We focused on launching a campaign which would generate pride and enthusiasm and was relevant to the existing social patterns and channels of community activity. To do this, we conducted a survey and elaborated 'sociograms' of community relationships to identify the main social patterns. The research team took the time to visit, confer with, question and encourage representatives of the three main areas of community life in rural Thailand: the *wat* (temple), the school and the hospital, which provide support, encoragement and hope.

After the initial community assessment, a discussion with the abbot of the *wat* resulted in a community gathering to present and discuss the need to involve the community in tobacco control. After several planning meetings, materials and gifts were presented to the *wat*, establishing it as a tobacco-free *wat*. This occurred at a community festival attended by about 300 people.

At the elementary school, the principal and several teachers were visited on several occasions, resulting in a school assembly at which a noted tobacco control leader from Bangkok gave information about the use of tobacco and its dangers to 400 pupils. Awards were given to several well-known adults in the community, including one teacher who had recently quit smoking. A follow-up activity was participation of the school in World No Tobacco Day activities in Bangkok involving 80 schools.

Because of the community assessment, involvement and individual empowerment, the project achieved wide exposure and general acceptability. The most important indication of the success of the project is the sustainability of the coalition. A year after the project's last formal activity, the coalition continues to plan and carry out activities in the *wat* and the school.

Formal assessment of this small community project included quantitative measures of participation, cohesion and satisfaction and qualitative measurements of needs, leadership, management, organization and resource mobilization (Butterfoss *et al.*, 1996; Nakamura & Siregar, 1996). The results showed increased participation, group identity and cohesion and satisfaction with the project. The qualitative results showed substantial progress in needs assessment and resource mobilization. This study establishes the feasibility and several important elements of rural community coalitions for tobacco control, which include the importance of perceived needs, community social patterns, subgroupings and pace of rural life as well as health development goals. Careful attention to establishing the relevance and community ownership of this health promotion function is crucial to sustaining progress in tobacco control.

References

Butterfoss, F.D. *et al.* (1996) Community coalitions for prevention and health promotion: Factors predicting satisfaction, participation, and planning. *Health Educ. Q.*, **23**, 65–79
Nakamura, Y. & Siregar, M. (1996) Qualitative assessment of community participation in health promotion activities. *World Health Forum*, **17**, 415–417

Changes in adult smoking prevalence after a three-year community health education: the Nose Town Project in Japan

M. Nakamura & S. Masui

Osaka Cancer Prevention and Detection Center, Osaka, Japan

The Nose Town Project is a pilot study of community-based smoking intervention to examine the feasibility and the effects of a three-year community-wide activity for smoking prevention and cessation. The smoking cessation activities included individual counselling at out-patient clinics and health check-ups, smoking cessation classes at health centres and a quit contest. The smoking prevention activities include school-based and family-based interventions involving family members. Comprehensive evaluations were made of the impact and process. The evaluation of the impact of the intervention on adult smoking behaviour was based on analysis of data from two cohort surveys conducted before and after the intervention.

During the three-year intervention period, 38% of all adult smokers in Nose received smoking cessation counselling or encouragement through family-based interventions. Of these, 11% quit smoking, and 40% tried to quit or intended to quit. Intervention programmes combined with routine activities such as out-patient visits and health check-ups reached a larger fraction of the smoking population and yielded more quitters than 'active recruitment' programmes such as cessation classes.

This community-wide intervention project proved to be feasible and showed promise in reducing the prevalence of smoking within a relatively brief period. We are planning to conduct a controlled study with a matched reference area to examine the effects of the intervention.

Awareness initiatives on the negative effects of smokeless tobacco

C. Grant

Chinook Health Region, Fort Macleod, Canada

In the summer of 1992, the Chinook Health Unit Dental Programme undertook a survey of 1859 students in junior and senior high-schools. These schools are located in the most southwestern corner of Alberta in the First Chinook Health Region. The survey revealed that 40% of all students had tried chewing tobacco, and the average age of experimentation was 11–12 years; 11% of the boys were regular users, and 47% of these users chewed three or more plugs daily. The 1994 Teen Health Survey in this same region revealed similar information: 10% of teenage boys were users and half of these also smoked cigarettes. The original survey also showed that 29% of the male students who tried chewing tobacco took up the habit. The Canadian Cancer Society estimated that the incidence of oral cancer in males in Alberta was 13:100 000 in 1996. Similar data in 1988 revealed the incidence rate to be 4: 100 000.

The lack of public awareness about the long-term negative effects of smokeless tobacco use prompted the Oral Health Services to initiate a multisectoral approach to reducing the use of chewing tobacco. The group initially decided to focus on public awareness and research, with future plans for education and cessation programmes. The awareness phase has included the production and airing of a 30-s television commercial, development of a display for rodeo events and production of a sticker to be handed out by local western-wear retailers.

Having determined that the use of chewing tobacco is initiated at a young age, our region will continue to explore the issue by looking at the psychosocial aspects of initiation and use as we implement education and cessation strategies.

A survey of sportsmen's attitudes to tobacco

J. Talmud

Basque Association against Smoking, Toki Eder Medical Centre, Cambo les Bains, France

In the Basque region, 39% of 4123 children of school age smoked, but there was a statistically significant association between practising sports and nicotine addiction, since club permit-holders smoked less. A mass socio-epidemiological survey, involving administration of an anonymous questionnaire with 107 questions, was undertaken among 7002 permit-holding sportsmen of all ages and levels, civilians and servicemen; 56 subjects were interviewed. The mean age was 24 years, and they smoked an average of 9.9 cigarettes per day.

Four groups aged 18–24 were studied in detail: school attenders in 1994 and sportsmen and sportswomen and a military battalion in 1997. The smoking rates were as follows:

	School attenders	Sports participants	Military
Smokers (%)			
Men	36.4	23.0	20
Women	42.9	20.3	None
No. of cigarettes per day			
Men	18.3	9.7	8.6
Women	17.7	8.6	None

Permit-holding sportsmen thus smoked fewer than 10 cigarettes per day. Those involved in individual sports and/or with high energy expenditure smoked less than those participating in team sports: triathlon, 0%; rowing, 4.5%; cycling, 5.1%; boxing, 7.2%, and gymnastics, 8.6%; but football, 37%; volley-ball, 37% and rugby, 40%. Whatever the sport practised, however, all sportsmen consumed the same amount, 10 cigarettes per day. Otherwise, the higher the level of competition, the less they smoked. Prevention through sports is therefore important, rather than sport used as an alibi. The prevention effort must be pursued at the youngest possible age.

LITIGATION

Litigation by individuals against the tobacco industry

J. Banzhaf

Action on Smoking and Health, Washington DC, United States

During the last 40 years, American tobacco companies have killed almost 20 million Americans and disabled tens of millions more, yet they have never been forced to pay one penny, one farthing, one fen in compensation. But that is now changing, and lawsuits against American cigarette companies on behalf of individuals are now a major threat to the tobacco industry. Indeed, lawsuits by individuals—as well as the class actions and state lawsuits they inspired—were the principal reason why American cigarette makers were forced to offer an unprecedented deal in the United States in the hope of obtaining immunity, and have now settled two for over US$ 10 thousand million. I will briefly explain the most important factors responsible for those changes, how and why we are now beginning to win individual suits in the United States and how similar legal actions could be brought in other countries under other legal systems.

During the first wave of lawsuits in the United States, beginning around 1967, plaintiffs relied on four major legal theories, or what lawyers call causes of action:
* breach of express warranty: failure to keep promises made in advertisements;
* breach of implied warranty: producing products less safe than expected;
* negligence: not being careful enough to discover the dangers of cigarettes and
* deceit: lying or other deliberate deception.

The second wave of lawsuits in the United States, beginning in the mid-1980s, added two more legal theories:
* failure to warn: not telling users about the dangers and
* strict liability: holding manufacturers of dangerous products responsible for the harm they cause, even if they did nothing wrong.

None of these suits succeeded. Some failed because of problems of proof. Some failed because the courts decided that placing the health warning that the Government required on cigarette advertisements was all that the cigarette makers had to do. More information about these legal theories and the cases, including the full text of most of the major judicial decisions and many major legal complaints, can be found on the Internet web site maintained by my organization, Action on Smoking and Health (ASH).

But the biggest problem was not legal. It was that the tobacco companies were willing to spend millions or even tens of millions of dollars on a single suit, filing motion after motion, getting delay after delay, until the individual plaintiffs and their lawyers were worn out or ran out of money or both. The other big problem was the tobacco company argument that smokers were responsible for their own illnesses because they voluntarily continued to smoke even though they knew the risks. This legal defence is called 'assumption of risk'.

This losing streak is now changing. In Florida, a jury awarded a smoker with lung cancer US$ 750 000. A case in Indiana was lost only because of that State's law; under the law of Florida or New York and many other states, the plaintiff would have won. Industry lost a further two cases which involved the dangers of cigarette filters rather than cigarettes, and another in which huge costs forced the plaintiffs to give up even after winning an initial verdict.

We are finally beginning to win, or to force the industry to settle, for four major reasons. The first is that in newer cases, plaintiffs' lawyers are arguing that nicotine is addictive. Thus, they say, most smokers do not really choose voluntarily to continue smoking and so should not be held solely responsible for their illnesses. The second reason is that, in contrast to earlier cases, lawyers acknowledge that smokers may bear some responsibility, but argue that the industry must also bear some responsibility, not only for marketing a deadly, addictive product but also for covering up and even lying about the addictive properties of nicotine. The third reason is that in these arguments they are aided by thousands of previously secret documents which show that tobacco industry executives not only knew that nicotine was addictive, but also discovered and apparently used techniques to make it more addictive and routinely manipulate the levels of nicotine in cigarettes. Seeing and reading these documents make jurors angry and more likely to compensate victims and to punish tobacco companies by awarding punitive damages. The fourth reason is that one lawyer is no longer forced to take on the tobacco industry all alone, as was frequently the case in the past. Instead, many lawyers are cooperating, and a number are beginning to specialize in this area and to develop the expertise necessary to provide very effective representation.

The important question is whether such lawsuits could be brought in other countries, so that their citizens, governments and entities such as insurance companies can begin to recover the thousands of millions of dollars that smoking costs them individually and through taxes, as well as uncover and publicize the underhanded tactics of the tobacco industry by findings documents and with testimony. I think the answer is "Yes" for at least three reasons.

A number of other countries are already starting to bring suits against tobacco companies. The tiny nation of Costa Rica will shortly file a legal demand against two tobacco companies to cover the cost of smoking-caused diseases to the State's social security system over the past decade, estimated to be over US$ 500 million. Government officials in Israel are also planning to sue, for about US$ 8 thousand million. Recently, the Government of British Columbia, Canada, introduced legislation to help individuals or governments sue the tobacco industry for health damages caused by smoking. Other countries that have expressed interest in suing tobacco companies, including some which have already met with United States plaintiffs' attorneys or anti-smoking organizations, include Belgium, Brazil and the United Kingdom. If countries with such very different legal systems can bring such suits, it is very likely that similar suits could be brought in many other jurisdictions.

My legal colleagues in other countries tell me that their judges often look to and follow decisions of courts in the United States. This is true not only in countries which, like us, follow the English common law, such as some provinces of Canada and Australia, but even those whose legal system is based on the French Napoleonic Code and other systems, including those of Malaysia and Singapore. In short, if courts in the United States start forcing tobacco companies to pay thousands of millions of dollars in damages, it is likely that many other countries will conclude that their citizens are likewise deserving of at least some compensation.

Suppose a company came to your country and began to advertise heavily and to sell a new food. The food became very popular, but people soon found that once they had begun to eat it regularly, they could not stop, even when they learnt that it was likely to kill them. The company denied that the food contained an addictive drug or that it was dangerous, but company documents proved that they were lying. Soon the food was killing at least half of all those who had started using it. Unless your courts say that such conduct is perfectly proper and acceptable, they should be willing to hold the companies liable for at least some of the deaths or disability they cause. And the only way you will know for sure is to try. Here, perhaps for the first time in many countries, is an opportunity for your lawyers and law professors to become as much involved in the anti-smoking movement as doctors have been. Here, perhaps for the first time in their lives, they can actually do well by doing good. And when you sue for and recover thousands of millions of dollars, believe me, you are doing very well as well as doing a lot of good. In short, to use an American phrase which has become ASH's motto, you too should 'Sue the bastards' as we are now doing. All of the information you need to get started, including the judicial decisions and many of the actual complaints, is available on ASH's Internet site: ash.org. I therefore invite you to make an ASH of yourself by taking hard-hitting legal 'Action on Smoking and Health'.

Legal protection for child victims of adult smoking: A call for action

M. Whidden

The Association for Nonsmokers' Rights, Binfield, Berkshire, United Kingdom

The most innocent victims of tobacco smoke are children.

People all over the world love young animals, especially furry ones, and a lot of people get terribly upset when seal cubs are clubbed to death, especially because they can see the blood in the snow and imagine the pain the animals suffered. Many people are also horrified enough to take radical action when they see a young calf in a crate, doomed to a short life in a tiny, uncomfortable prison. Situations like this result in a huge outcry. It is difficult, however, for people to visualize the suffering of young humans, who are the most vulnerable to the effects of other people's smoking. For instance, a victim of sudden cot death, brought on by parental tobacco smoke, doesn't look like a little skeleton, a starving Rwandan or Zaïrian refugee baby. A cot death victim looks quite healthy, and yet children whose health is damaged and who may even die because adults expose them to tobacco smoke are surely more urgently in need of our protests than are seals or calves, however appealing those animals may be.

I never call myself a 'passive smoker'. I am not 'passive' about environmental tobacco smoke. But very young children are passive smokers, and they suffer for it. Sometimes the price of being the child of a smoker is the ultimate price. A very unusual visual demonstration of what other people's smoking can do to a child is the silhouette of a little girl, the clean area left behind on her bed when a fireman lifted her dead body out of a bedroom that had been on fire. The child had been asphyxiated. One of her parents had accidentally dropped a lighted cigarette onto a sofa or bed and the smoke of the resulting fire had killed the young child.

Every year in the United Kingdom, somewhere between 180 and 280 people die in cigarette-related fires. One in 10 of those people is a child. Two thousand or so people are injured in fires started because of smoking. One in six of those people is a child. Remember, these figures refer just to the United Kingdom. I wonder if we are taking cigarette-related fires seriously enough. Governments certainly aren't. They need our views about legislating to make it mandatory for all cigarettes to be 'fire-safe', which is quite feasible, by the way. The tobacco industry has known for 30 years how to make cigarettes that would not ignite furniture fabrics. The numbers of people who die in fires started by cigarettes are tiny, however, when compared with the numbers of children who die every year simply because their parents smoke.

"Some people commit child abuse before their child is even born." I didn't invent that slogan. It is the caption of a hard-hitting television advertisement shown in the 1980s by the American Cancer Society. Where are the environmental protesters when it comes to pollution of the womb and forcing unborn babies to do what amounts to smoking? The dose of tobacco poisons delivered to the foetus is more like the dose from active smoking than that from 'passive' smoking.

60% of cot deaths could be avoided if parents did not smoke.

British scientists have estimated that 60% of cot deaths could be avoided if parents did not smoke (Blair *et al.*, 1996). I don't need to bore you with lists of other adverse health effects that passive smoking has on children; they range from acute to chronic, short-term to long-term, minor to fatal. Yet, even in the western world, where we have known for a long time about the health hazards associated with environmental pollution of all kinds, we keep on smothering children with tobacco fumes. In Scotland, for instance, 51% of children grow up in homes where at least one person smokes. This lack of action will not change unless we do something effective.

Tobacco smoke contains polonium-210 and facilitates the clustering of radioactive pollution in the air. Why should parents be allowed to blow radioactive tobacco smoke over their children? When the Perrier company found tiny amounts of benzene in some of its bottled water, it withdrew every bottle of Perrier in the world. And yet our actions (or lack of action) show that we think it is acceptable to bombard children in our homes with tobacco smoke which contains benzene.

We in the clean-air movement have had good success in many countries in banning or limiting smoking in the workplace, by banding together and taking planned, concerted action. We've had so many successes that smokers are now feeling like outcasts, victims. Even on their own, adults can take action to achieve clean air. It's not so simple for children. Very small children remain as helpless as seal pups or veal calves. There are laws in most countries against physical abuse and neglect of children. Parents and others responsible for children's welfare are subject to court action if they beat or kick their children, or if they leave them alone and thus subject them to danger. In London in March 1997, a father was ordered to pay large damages to his teenage daughter because she had been left alone in her father's apartment when she was aged only four, and her clothing had been set on fire when she moved too close to a gas heater. She suffered terrible, disfiguring burns. If someone can be taken to court because of this kind of neglect of a child, surely a parent or other adult can be considered liable to prosecution under the law if he or she causes damage to the child through other carelessness, such as exposing a child to the potentially lethal poisons found in tobacco smoke.

Of course there is sometimes a fine line between a damaging assault and a smack that is a light punishment which might sometimes act beneficially. But there is no question about tobacco-smoke: it is never good for a child. So why don't we include in the legal term 'child abuse' the act of smoking in the air children have to breathe? Why not make it an offence to smoke in the home or to smoke while pregnant? Or, in very cautious, very tradition-bound societies where smoking has been a norm for many years, why not at least make it an offence to smoke in a car when children are present? In 1992 in England and Wales, about 90 children died because of one kind of abuse or another, as traditionally defined. During the same period several hundred children died of cot deaths attributable to smoking in their homes. If we include the 7500–10 000 babies that are aborted or stillborn or die within the first weeks after their birth because of parental smoking, then child abuse by smoking is on a vast scale, although not intentional. We must have the courage to tackle this huge problem.

Asking a parent to quit smoking for the sake of a child is not 'blaming the victim', as many people suggest. Children are the real victims. Parents' duties, which involve protecting their children from harm, are the same in regard to tobacco hazards as they are in relation to other risks or dangers. Laws concerning child neglect and abuse are difficult to enforce. Nevertheless, it seems wise to have such laws. Just the existence of such laws allows people to understand better the boundaries of good and bad behaviour. The existence of laws to give specific protection to children from environmental tobacco smoke would provide legal backing for extreme cases of damage to a child's health. I do not anticipate that offenders would be automatically prosecuted. Such laws would tend to act as deterrents, to give relief to large numbers of children now subjected to smoky atmospheres at home and elsewhere. Other types of intervention (individual and public education through television, for example) might succeed more readily if people became aware of the existence of laws to protect children from environmental tobacco smoke.

Courts have already intervened, in the United States in particular, to separate some children from deliberately abusive smokers. Many adoption agencies make rules to keep children from being placed in families with smokers. Politicians should follow these leads and provide legislative protection for children from the harm done to them by a selfish habit.

Reference

Blair, P.S., Fleming, P.J., Bensley, D., Smith, I., Bacon, C., Taylor, E., Berry, J., Golding, J. & Tripp, J. (1996) Smoking and the sudden infant death syndrome: Results from 1993-5 case–control study for confidential inquiry into stillbirths and deaths in infancy. *Br. Med. J.*, **313**, 195–198

Litigation by states against the tobacco industry

R.A. Daynard

Northeastern University School of Law, Boston, Massachusetts, United States

By late June 1997, 39 of the 50 states of the United States had sued the tobacco industry, seeking reimbursement of the medical expenses they had paid for their indignant citizens and orders requiring the industry to stop lying and stop targeting children and adolescents. On 20 June 1997, representatives of most of these states, together with private attorneys who had brought class actions against the tobacco industry, reached a tentative settlement with the industry. Under the agreement, the industry would pay US$ 368.5 thousand million over 25 years. As part of the settlement, the industry would also consent to a variety of tobacco control measures long sought by public health advocates. At the time of writing, the agreement was contingent, however, on Congress enacting legislation that would make it harder to regulate or to sue the industry in the future.

While many public health advocates are sceptical about the merits of the proposed settlement, it is nonetheless clear that the agreement demonstrates the power of tobacco litigation, especial by the states, to force major concessions from the tobacco industry. What I describe here is, first, how we arrived at this point in the United States; second, exactly where litigation in the United States stands today; third, the probable effects of the proposed settlement; and finally, what this means in terms of the possibilities for tobacco litigation in the rest of the world.

How we got here

It wasn't easy. There have been three waves of tobacco litigation in the United States. Both the first (1950s and 1960s) and the second wave (1980s and early 1990s) were made up of individual cases, brought by smokers or their families, seeking compensation for their losses and their suffering resulting from tobacco-caused diseases. These first two waves never reached the shore, largely because they were unable to get past three barriers which the tobacco industry erected. The first barrier was the 'personal responsibility' or 'blame the victim' defence, which implies that "anyone stupid enough to believe us when we tell them that smoking our products will not cause disease deserves to get the diseases that our products cause". The next barrier was financial and strategic. The tobacco industry poured disproportionate legal resources into the litigation, burying the plaintiffs' lawyers in legal papers and ancillary legal proceedings. In the words of an R.J. Reynolds lawyer, "the way we won the cases, to paraphrase General Patton, is not by spending all the Reynolds' money, but by making the other son-of-a-bitch spend all of his". The final barrier consisted of a series of inhospitable judicial rulings, perhaps reflecting the judges' concern that, with hundreds of thousands of new tobacco victims each year, to allow them justice would simply overwhelm the courts.

The third, and current, wave of tobacco litigation began in the spring of 1994. It was initiated by the announcement in February 1994 by Dr David Kessler that the Food and Drug Administration was considering classifying nicotine and cigarettes as drugs. Part of his reasoning was that he had learnt from tobacco industry documents, found during the second-wave *Cipollone* case, that the industry itself thought of nicotine and cigarettes in just those terms. Three days later, the ABC television network broadcast the results of an investigation which led it to conclude that the industry was actually manipulating the amount of nicotine in cigarettes, presumably for the purpose of keeping its customers hooked. Later that spring, millions of people around the world watched tobacco executives swear at televised congressional hearings that they didn't believe nicotine was addictive, while, at the same time, leaked industry documents and the testimony of former industry scientists were proving the contrary. Suddenly, many of the people who had previously dismissed tobacco litigation on the basis that smokers had chosen their own poison began to consider the possibility that tobacco companies were villains and smokers their victims.

This change in public understanding of the relationship between the tobacco industry and its customers, this 'paradigm shift' from 'blaming the smokers' to 'the tobacco industry as corporate drug dealers', encouraged lawyers and public officials to consider ways of making tobacco companies pay for the harm they cause. Some lawyers worked out ways of bringing the old-style individual lawsuits more efficiently and inexpensively, so that the industry's tremendous advantage in legal resources and firepower would no longer determine the results. They sought court orders providing for prompt trials, allowing several cases to be heard at the same time ('consolidations'), and for the possibility of obtaining 'punitive damages' if they could convince a jury that the industry had behaved in a grossly improper fashion. Other lawyers joined together to file class actions—cases in which one or only a few named plaintiffs filed suit on behalf of all other people 'similarly situated'. The prospects of winning a multi-thousand-million dollar damage and of sharing in an award of attorneys' fees proportional to those damages induced plaintiffs' attorneys to pool their resources, enabling them to fight complex procedural battles with the industry without being outgunned.

But the most important legal development was the decision by public officials, principally state attorneys general working with private attorneys, to sue tobacco companies for the damage they caused to the Government itself. In the United States, state and local governments pay for the medical expenses of their poorest citizens through a programme known as 'Medicaid'. Studies have shown that 6–7% of these expenses are used for treating cigarette-caused diseases. In most states, that amounts to a burden of at least US$ 100 million per year that the industry and its products have imposed on the state's taxpayers.

The lawyers for the states developed a number of legal theories requiring the companies to reimburse the states for these expenses. Some were based on the idea that the companies' misbehaviour and their unreasonably dangerous products were responsible for cigarette-caused diseases, and hence for the expense of treating them. Since the states had paid money that the companies were morally and legally obligated to pay, the companies had been 'unjustly enriched' at the states' expense, and the states were entitled to reimbursement. A variant of this idea treated the states' Medicaid funds like bystanders injured in an automobile accident: the defendants, in this case the tobacco industry, should have known that their reckless behaviour would cause economic injury not just to their direct victims, here the smokers, but to the Medicaid funds as well.

Another legal approach was that the tobacco companies have violated various statutes that were designed to control corporate behaviour in general. In the United States, the anti-trust laws prohibit anti-competitive conduct such as agreeing to raise prices or, as with the tobacco companies, to refrain from doing research on the dangers of their current products or to develop and market safer ones. Similarly, consumer protection laws prohibit 'unfair or deceptive' commercial practices. In most states, these laws give the state 'standing' to sue to recover its own losses.

As the cases progressed, the states' lawyers began to realize that their damage claims were not limited by the losses that the states themselves had suffered. The states, after all, represent not only their own interests but those of their citizens as well. Both anti-trust and consumer protection laws frequently permit the state to sue as *parens patriae*, on behalf of all of their citizens who were victimized by the unlawful practices. The citizens' losses may include the price they paid for cigarettes, on the theory that the industry's unfair and deceptive practices tricked them into becoming addicted consumers.

The latest legal theory to be used these cases is that the industry and its various organizations constitute a 'racketeer-influenced corrupt organization' under either a Federal or similar state statute. These statutes were passed to control narcotic drug traffickers, who make huge profits from selling addictive drugs and use them to infiltrate and purchase otherwise legitimate businesses. Does that sound familiar? In addition to criminal sanctions, the 'racketeer-influenced corrupt organization' statutes provide a large range of civil remedies, including confiscation of the profits that the defendants have made through their illegal schemes.

Finally, in all 39 of the state cases, the state has sought from the tobacco industry not just money but also specific changes in behaviour ('equitable relief'). Court orders requiring the end of the infamous Joe Camel and of other marketing campaigns aimed at children and adolescents, dissolution of the fraudulent Council for Tobacco Research, public disclosure of internal inudustry files documenting their scientific research and marketing strategies and the end of lying as the industry's basic public relations strategy, are among the relief that these state cases demand.

Where are we now?

In the field of tobacco litigation, much more had been accomplished in the previous three years at the time of writing than in the 40 years before that. In terms of numbers of cases pending in the United States, the expansion of litigation has been exponential. For example, one company, the R.J. Reynolds Tobacco Company, recently reported that it had 68 cases of all sorts pending against it in July 1995, 302 cases in July 1996 and 448 cases as of 7 August 1997. Class actions are now pending on behalf of most smokers in the United States, who are seeking tobacco industry funding of trust funds to pay for assistance in quitting and for monitoring the smokers' medical conditions. There are also class actions on behalf of smokers who have contracted tobacco-caused diseases and the class action on trial in Miami, Florida, on behalf of 60 000 non-smoking flight attendants.

Three state suits against the industry were on file by the end of 1994, five by the end of 1995, 17 by the end of 1996 and 39 by 20 June 1997. Furthermore, about 15 cities and counties have sued the tobacco industry, making legal claims similar to those being asserted by the states. In the last few months, class actions have been filed in 20 states on behalf of hundreds of labour-management health and welfare funds seeking reimbursement for the tobacco-caused health care costs that they have been paying for their members. These quantitative changes have been accompanied by qualitative changes, including the reception that courts are giving to the plaintiffs' legal claims. Despite strenuous efforts by the tobacco companies, none of the state cases has been dismissed.

The industry has defended these cases by asserting that, while states are free to sue for reimbursement of their Medicaid payments, they have to do so under the doctrine of 'subrogation', which puts the state in the legal position of the Medicaid recipient. If the industry were right, the state would have to show which brand was smoked by each Medicaid recipient for whose expenses it is seeking reimbursement, the exact cause of that recipient's disease and the proper apportionment of responsibility between the recipient and the cigarette manufacturer for the recipient's beginning and continuing to smoke. The states, on the other hand, would like to proceed on the basis of epidemiological and other statistical data, both because that would lead to more accurate estimates of their total tobacco-caused expenses and because doing it the industry's way, under the subrogation doctrine, would cost the states more than they could possibly recover.

Fortunately, the states have won this argument each time the defendants have made it, at least with respect to some of the claims being asserted. Thus, it appears likely that the states will be able to prove their allegations of anti-trust, consumer protection and 'racketeer-influenced corrupt organization' by statistical data. Courts have considered, however, that the subrogation procedure is the proper one for 'bystander'-type claims, and judicial opinions have differed as to whether the 'unjust enrichment' claims are appropriate at all. Furthermore, the courts all seem receptive to the states' 'equitable' claims, those seeking court orders to change industry practices. While we do not yet know which unfair, deceptive or anti-competitive industry practices the courts will be willing to prohibit, at least they listen to evidence of industry misbehaviour and explore the practical and legal possibilities for stopping it.

This new receptiveness of United States courts to claims against the tobacco industry, and especially to the innovative state cases, is due in part to the fact that many of the new plaintiffs, such as states, cities and union-management health and welfare funds, unlike the smoker plaintiffs, cannot be blamed for choosing to smoke in the face of public health warnings. It may also be due in part to a sense by the judges that the flood of tobacco cases is now inevitable and they might a well deal with it efficiently. But it is also due importantly to the paradigm shift I discussed earlier: the fact that judges and the public in general now view the tobacco companies as outlaws that must be controlled and punished.

Probable effects of the proposed settlement

One effect of the agreement on 20 June 1997 has been totally positive. In early July, on the eve of the first trial of a state case against the tobacco industry, the industry reached an unconditional settlement with the State of Mississippi worth US$ 3.6 thousand million over 25 years. This figure, which was four times the amount Mississippi had been seeking for its past damages, was based on the schedule of payments that had been negotiated as part of the proposed national settlement. The industry also agreed to reimburse the State's lawyers for up to US$ 12.5 million in expenses, plus additional attorneys' fees in amounts to be determined by a panel of arbitrators.

What Mississippi had asked for and did not receive in the settlement of its case were agreement by the industry to stop marketing to children, disclosure of its internal documents and the other tobacco control measures included in the proposed national settlement. This allows the proponents of the national settlement to argue that, even if all states were to settle with the industry under the same, favourable financial terms, the public health benefits promised by the national settlement would still not be achieved. However, the State of Florida, which had been scheduled to begin its trial against the industry in September, signalled that it would not settle its case unless the industry also agreed to convert many of the proposed public health measures in the national settlement into legally binding commitments. This was, in fact, achieved, and the industry agreed to remove all tobacco billboards, transit advertising and vending machines from the State and release hundreds of incriminating internal documents as a requirement of the settlement ending Florida's litigation on 28 August 1997.

By settling the cases of Mississippi and Florida, the industry has abandoned its 40-year-old strategy of winning cases by out-spending the other party. The strategy finally failed because the State of Mississippi and the wealthy attorneys who were litigating its case were able to respond effectively to all the industry's legal manoeuvres without running out of money. But this binding settlement, for four times the amount originally sought, will probably serve as a magnet for plaintiffs' attorneys, encouarging them to bring suit on behalf of the countless other victims of the tobacco industry, unless the proposed national settlement is enacted into law.

From the perspective of tobacco control in the United States, the proposed national settlement is a gamble. As the American Medical Association noted in its analysis of the settlement, it would largely destroy the litigation that has brought the tobacco companies to the point where fear of bankruptcy is motivating their behaviour. All pending class actions would be 'settled', including classes not represented at the negotiating table, and no new class actions would be permitted.

All of the state cases and the cases brought by cities and counties would be 'settled', despite the fact that the Attorney General of Minnesota, who at the time of writing was scheduled to go on trial, was objecting vociferously, and the cities and counties will get nothing out of the deal. Even more important, no cases filed after 9 June 1997 on behalf of any entity seeking reimbursement for having paid the medical expenses of smokers will be permitted to proceed on any basis other than subrogation, which means, in practice, that they cannot proceed at all. Thus, other private medical insurance plans will not be able to follow the example of Blue Cross and Blue Shield of Minnesota, which joined with the State in suing the industry, and most of the cases brought by labour-management health and welfare funds would have to be dropped. Nor could the Federal Government sue the industry for the huge medical expenses for tobacco-induced disease that it pays on behalf of elderly citizens (the 'Medicare' programme), military personnel or veterans.

Theoretically, suits on behalf of individual smokers or of non-smokers with diseases caused by exposure to environmental tobacco smoke could continue to be brought. But the industry's overwhelming strategic advantage in these cases would be restored. The efficiency gained by combining these cases into classes, or even trying smaller groups of similar individual cases together, would be lost. Attorneys representing existing smokers may not seek punitive damages. In practice, there would be little incentive for the few law firms that have the resources to match the tobacco industry in court to devote those resources to pursuing individual cases, each of limited value.

Finally, just in case the tobacco industry miscalculated the dampening effect that the settlement would have on law suits against it, the proposed settlement also includes a future annual ceiling that rises from US\$ 2 thousand million per year initially to US\$ 5 thousand million after six years. Since the agreement provides that the industry can deduct 80% of its future liability cost from the other amounts that it would owe under the settlement, its actual disbursement ranges from US\$ 400 million to US\$ 1 thousand million annually. At a maximum of about 5 cents per cigarette pack sold, this effectively eliminates any residual deterrent effect that tobacco litigation could have on future industry misbehaviour. The gamble, then, is that the public health gains from the other provisions of the settlement would more than make up for the near-total destruction of litigation in the United States as a tobacco control strategy.

Possibilities for litigation against the tobacco industry outside the United States

The incriminating documents and testimony emerging from the United States cases generally concern transnational tobacco companies such as Philip Morris, British–American Tobacco and R.J. Reynolds. Many of these documents are currently available for use in any case in the world, and more will soon become available.

With worldwide media attention on the revelations of industry misconduct coming out of the litigation in the United States, the paradigm shift in the public understanding of the relationship between the transnational tobacco companies and their customers, begun in the United States, is spreading. As in the United States, judges elsewhere who used to see the issue as one of personal choice by smokers are likely to be increasingly open to reformulating the issue as one of industry misconduct. As the experience with the first two waves of litigation demonstrated, judges and juries in the United States were hardly more receptive to litigation against the tobacco industry than judges elsewhere, as long as they believed that it was the smokers' fault. With spread of the new paradigm, receptiveness to litigation should also spread.

The willingness of the industry to spend US\$ 368.5 thousand million to settle and terminate cases in the United States, which it has insisted were 'worthless', will increase the credibility of current and future cases throughout the world. Furthermore, the willingness of the industry to agree as part of the proposed settlement to a series of public health measures, which the industry has successfully fought for years, should encourage tobacco control advocates throughout the world to place litigation against the tobacco industry at the top of its list of strategies for achieving a wide range of public health goals.

International implications of the United States 'global settlement' of tobacco litigation

B. Fox, J. Lightwood & S.A. Glantz

Institute for Health Policy Studies, University of California, San Francisco, California, United States

Introduction

Litigation against the tobacco industry has exploded in the United States and is spreading worldwide. On 20 June 1997, a 'global settlement' of this litigation was announounced that had been negotiated by some state attorneys general and the tobacco industry. This settlement is neither 'global' in the sense that it applies only to the United States nor a 'settlement' in that it is not a binding agreement that resolves legal disputes among the parties in the litigation. The agreement raises a complex array of issues for public health and public policy and legal and economic issues. It was intended to be a blueprint for national tobacco control legislation that would end the most important current and potential litigation against the tobacco industry. As with most complex legislation, the deal, after it was announced, underwent a great deal of scrutiny and criticism. Many public health and policy groups analysed it in whole or in part in order to provide guidance for those who wished to distil the essential elements and implications. (A complete report on the proposed resolution of United States tobacco litigation by the same authors is available on the World Wide Web at http:// galen.library.ucsf.edu/tobacco/ustl/.) While many have pronounced the original deal to be 'dead' as a result of this criticism, it remains the fundamental framework around which most proposals for Federal legislation on tobacco has been based. As a result, a careful analysis of the terms and implications of the original deal remains worthwhile.

The tobacco industry is probably willing to enter into a deal with public health forces in the United States so that it can remove the financial uncertainties associated with litigation and clear the way for international expansion. The fastest growing segment of the American companies' profit base is foreign markets. As eastern Europe and Asia open their markets wider to foreign cigarettes, these manufacturers are expected to participate more and at great profit. Delegates to the Tenth World Conference on Tobacco or Health reflected an international consensus that any national tobacco control policy, including that of the United States, should take steps to assist international tobacco control efforts. The deal, however, fails to address international issues in any manner.

Current United States efforts to control tobacco are of worldwide significance

The ongoing litigation and tobacco control efforts in the United States assist the international tobacco control efforts in the same way that they benefit public health. The uncovering of tobacco industry documents and behaviour can assist countries in their efforts to control tobacco. By watching the experience of the prosecution of the lawsuits in the United States, countries can learn ways of holding the tobacco companies responsible for the damage caused by tobacco in those countries. Since the deal was announced, several other countries have indicated interest in filing suits to recover tobacco-induced costs; some of these actions would involve United States courts and would be precluded by the deal. Finally, other countries can work with United States tobacco control advocates and policy-makers to make a coordinated response to international tobacco issues. The United States cannot pretend that its actions have no influence on international events.

A standard has been developed by an international body which can assist the United States in its review of the proposed deal. At the Tenth World Conference on Tobacco or Health, the following resolution was adopted:

"The Conference recommends governments consider the international implications of tobacco control policies or settlements with the tobacco industry, to ensure that:

"i.   such measures do not contribute to an increase in the worldwide epidemic of tobacco-related death and disease;

"ii.   the legal rights of those not party to any agreement or policy are fully protected;

"iii.   such measures do not inhibit full public scrutiny of the past, present and future activities of the tobacco industry; and

"iv.   the tobacco industry pay the costs of damage caused by tobacco."

This resolution embraces a model that looks beyond the impact of a lawsuit or settlement on its participants. The United States is at the forefront of private and public lawsuits against the tobacco companies, setting important precedents both domestically and internationally. If these lawsuits are eliminated, international tobacco control efforts will be hindered. Similarly, because the United States is the home of many of the world's most dominant tobacco companies and of the second largest number of smokers, any regulatory measures taken could have a ripple effect internationally.

The deal fails to address the United States tobacco problem effectively

If the deal addressed the domestic tobacco problem effectively, it could be argued that omission of international issues from the deal was of limited relevance. The deal could be said to both present the maximum solution that could be adopted by the United States and act as a model for other countries. The deal, however, fails to present a reasonable public health solution for the United States. First, it is greatly underfunded in comparison with both what the tobacco companies can afford to pay and the damages caused by tobacco products. This is directly contrary to item iv of the World Conference resolution: that the tobacco companies be held liable for the full measure of damages caused by tobacco.

Because of the deal's financial inadequacy, it will have limited effect on the profits of the tobacco companies. With their profits protected, they will be able to accelerate the marketing of their products both domestically and internationally. The fact the deal 'resolves' many of the contentious issues within the United States, such as litigation and regulation, will also free the industry of distractions from selling their wares elsewhere.

Second, the public health measures in the deal are inadequate. The measures can be seen as neither good enough for the rest of the world to use as a model nor strong enough to explain the need to omit international issues.

The deal will result in increased international tobacco sales

Although the deal is insufficient, it may make the United States market less hospitable than those of other countries. This situation will encourage worldwide expansion. The drafters of the deal could have avoided this problem by expanding the application of the restrictions to all foreign markets. For example, under the deal, the new warnings need to be applied only to packs of cigarettes sold in the United States. They are not required on packs manufactured in the United States or overseas and sold overseas. In fact, the deal specifically restricts Food and Drug Administration controls on 'products sold in US commerce'. Similarly, any Food and Drug Administration requirements regarding advertising, ingredient disclosure, less hazardous products and lower nicotine products will apply only to the United States.

Increased inequity between the market controls in different jurisdictions will increase the incentive for the tobacco industries to expand into less restrictive markets. This result of the deal, combined with guaranteed tobacco industry profitability, specifically contravenes point i of the World Conference resolution, because the deal would probably contribute to increasing the sale of cigarettes around the world.

The deal will encourage overseas corporate expansion

The deal will encourage American tobacco companies to establish overseas corporations. The only entities that are subject to the terms of the deal are those that sell on the United States market. Accordingly, if the American tobacco companies were to move offshore, or to create foreign subsidiaries while eliminating United States sales, they would be immune from the terms of the deal. It can therefore be argued that one effect of the deal would be to force the United States problem out of the country while ignoring what happens to the rest of the world. By pursuing the litigation, United States plaintiffs are seeking compensation for damages, not to establish international tobacco control policy. Nevertheless, under the deal, the United States Government would be making the conscious choice of encouraging overseas expansion while limiting the tobacco companies' domestic liability. The tobacco companies would be out of the United States market and therefore not subject to market and civil liability controls, and the Government would abdicate from its regulatory authority.

The deal affects the legal rights of non-United States entities

The protections for the tobacco industry against litigation provided by the deal will almost certainly preclude the filing of lawsuits by foreign governments in United States courts. Although such cases may prove to be difficult, if not impossible, to maintain for procedural reasons, elimination of the possibility of these suits is unnecessary. Should a government otherwise meet the appropriate requirements of United States courts, it should not be precluded from proceeding because of the deal. The deal, however, eliminates all suits by governmental entities and all class actions and severely restricts actions for civil liability related to tobacco and health. As a result, all original cases from foreign governments would be precluded.

Lawsuits by private entities in United States courts would similarly be restricted. If allowed to proceed, they would probably be subject to the same restrictions on civil liability as those faced by United States citizens. The problem with this is twofold. First, the civil liability fund is based on the number of possible United States litigants. Should this fund be additionally taxed by satisfying claimants worldwide, all litigants would suffer the risk of insufficient compensation for damages. Second, United States citizens are theoretically sacrificing some of their rights because they are able to benefit from other aspects of the deal. Non-United States persons will not be similarly benefitted.

Besides the restrictions placed on original suits, it is possible that provisions of the deal could be used as a defense by the tobacco companies against efforts to domesticate foreign judgements. Given that many of the assets of the American tobacco companies remain in the United States, plaintiffs who are successful in other countries may still need to pursue assets in the United States. The deal could act as a barrier to such efforts.

In sum, the deal could foreclose the possibility of foreign governments recovering against the tobacco companies and could place serious restrictions on private suits. At best, foreign judgements are likely to be subject to the litigation restrictions accounted for in the deal, limiting their overall effectiveness. Thus, the deal fails to meet the second provision of the World Conference resolution because it limits the legal rights of those not participating in the settlement.

The deal could prevent full disclosure of tobacco industry documents

The deal also fails to meet the third requirement of the World Conference resolution, because it does not require complete disclosure of tobacco industry documents and information, but instead develops a complicated procedure that will probably delay, if not eliminate, the need for complete industry disclosure. Because many important tobacco industry documents are in the United States, this process may preclude dissemination of the information worldwide.

The deal could stop future efforts by the United States to influence international tobacco control

The deal also eliminates the United States' ability to develop a coordinated international tobacco control policy. By embracing a dual-tiered system, which applies one set of standards to the United States and another to international community, the United States loses whatever moral authority it has to influence international tobacco control efforts. It is ignoring the health of non-United States citizens. Furthermore, by restricting the ability of the Food and Drug Administration to affect international sales of tobacco products, the United States would be giving the American tobacco companies assurance that their overseas actions will be protected. In the past, the United States has often used a two-stage regulatory process, first regulating domestically and then regulating overseas sales. For example, pesticides and hazardous consumer products are sometimes outlawed in the United States first, and then the sale or 'dumping' of these products overseas is proscribed. The deal apparently legitimizes tobacco use and seems to preclude the application of the terms of the deal to any international markets, precluding the possibility of ever taking the second regulatory step.

Acknowledgements

Supported in part by National Cancer Institute Grant CA-61021 and the University of California Tobacco Related Diseases Research Program Grant 6FT-0105, this paper is an excerpt from a larger report 'A Public Health Analysis of the Proposed Resolution of Tobacco Litigation' by B. Fox, J. Lightwood and S. Glantz (University of California, San Francisco Institute for Health Policy Studies), which is available on the World Wide Web at http:/galen.library.ucsf.edu/tobacco/ustl/.

LOBBYING, ADVOCACY AND USE OF MASS MEDIA FOR TOBACCO CONTROL

Lighting up locally and not burning out:
Tobacco control activism in a tobacco industry town

C. Farren

South West ASH and GASPSmoke Free Solutions, Bristol, United Kingdom

Introduction

In 1979, as a new health promotion officer in Bristol, I was given the task of running the smoking education programme. Bristol is the home of W.D. and H.O. Wills, one of the oldest and richest tobacco companies in the world and part of the Imperial Tobacco Company. I had no idea of the deviousness and cunning of the tobacco industry! Instead I thought like a recent ex-smoker and started promoting non-smokers rights. It was later, when the wrath of the tobacco barons descended on my activities, that I began really to challenge the tobacco industry's hold on Bristol. I am now of the belief that an activist knows when he or she is on the right track—when the tobacco industry starts fighting back. The Chairman of the Health Authority arrived at my office one day to ask me to stop my anti-tobacco industry activities as Bristol depended on tobacco for its wealth. I answered that Bristol used to depend on slavery for its wealth and thankfully we had got rid of that. We now needed to rid Bristol of the tobacco industry. The battle commenced in earnest in the form of a range of creative and energetic pressure groups and campaigns. They fought back in the press and through their powerful friends.

Since that time, the Wills Tobacco Company, with the largest cigarette factory in western Europe, has moved from Bristol to combine with another factory. It is now impossible to find a cinema or bus where smoking is allowed, and the local Member of Parliament, who was the former Conservative Minister of Health, lost his seat to an anti-smoking Labour candidate. This paper outlines a selection of the local tobacco control activities and summarizes our successes and their applicability to others situations.

The main strategy has been to use memorably-named pressure groups and media-led campaigning on a wide range of issues. The pressure groups were:

- GASP, Group Against Smoking in Public, a non-smokers' rights group campaigning for smoke-free areas;
- AGHAST, Action Group to Halt Advertising and Sponsorship by Tobacco, which campaigned to stop tobacco advertising and sponsorship of arts and sports events by tobacco companies;
- COUGHIN, Citizen's Organisation Using Graffiti for Health In the Neighbourhood, inspired by Australia's BUGA UP, a group that drew graffiti on tobacco advertisements, and
- South West ASH, Action on Smoking and Health, a branch of the national registered charity that campaigns to introduce national and local policies for comprehensive tobacco control. It involves chest physicians, public health specialists and other health professionals and is seen as much more respectable than the other groups.

GASP and South West ASH still exist.

Our priorities and activities included promoting non-smokers' rights, price rises on tobacco, stopping illegal sales of tobacco to children under 16 years of age, banning tobacco promotionm advertising and sponsorship, and lobbying and public education.

Promoting non-smokers rights

GASP did grassroots campaigning to demand more smoke-free areas in public places. The campaign strategies included surveys, direct action, publications and health promotion publications and awards.

We surveyed the customers of five well-known local restaurants and cafes, with the permission of the managers. The results showed massive support for smoke-free dining, and three out of the five managers quickly introduced smoke-free areas. We attracted press coverage and wrote letters to all restaurant managers urging them to follow suit. We subsequently surveyed the managers of restaurants with smoke-free areas to confirm customer satisfaction. Surveys were also carried out at cinemas, banks, workplaces and public transport. Publicity and changes in policies always resulted.

While researching smoke-free restaurants in order to publish a smoke-free guide to Bristol, we found out that the prestigious 'Harvey's of Bristol' restaurant not only did not provide a no-smoking section but also gave cigars to diners after meals. GASP decided to create a 'GASPing Gourmet Gas Mask Award in recognition of the fine wine, fresh foods and foul air' for Harvey's. We also awarded a 'Good Air Garland' to a totally smoke-free restaurant. The event was reported nationally, especially as the award, a gas mask sprayed gold and mounted on a plinth, was given to the manager of Harvey's restaurant by the GASPing gourmet 'Chuck Foulair'.

To support the campaign, GASP produced a series of simple illustrated leaflets and resources which included a leaflet on passive smoking, fact sheets, posters and visiting cards requesting smoke-free areas and a GASP guide to smoke-free areas in Bristol. GASP attracted national interest and duplication when its successes were published in various newspapers. One of the projects won a national health education award.

Price rises on tobacco

Every year, the tobacco industry fights rises in the real price of tobacco products. While South West ASH cannot compete with the resources of the tobacco industry, we have managed to 'sabotage' or use the industry's anti-tax rise campaigns to promote health. Examples includecountering a national tobacco industry petition in tobacco outlets and full-page advertisements encouraging smokers to sign. South West ASH, with the help of medical students, surveyed public attitudes to tobacco tax and found that a majority supported an increase when they were given the information that a rise in price would discourage young people from smoking. To obtain maximum publicity for our survey results, we attended the tobacco industry press conference and presented our own results. As all the national press was there, our findings received more coverage in the media than the tobacco companies' campaign.

South West ASH mounted a giant petition on the side of a van and toured supermarket carparks, inviting parents to sign a petition supporting an increase in tobacco prices in order to reduce smoking. This giant petition was delivered to the Chancellor of the Exchequer just before presentation of the budget. In other years, we have prepared cartoon campaign postcards for constituents to send to their Members of Parliament, lobbying for an increase in tax. We distributed these with fact sheets to help people write their own messages.

Each year, ASH publishes ready-made press comments suitable for the tobacco tax entry in the national budget. It also includes thenumbers of lives saved by each penny of increase. We provide a press release to the local media either supporting the Government action or criticizing it for not doing enough.

Illegal sales of tobacco to children under 16 years of age

Although it is illegal to sell cigarettes to children under 16, we know that children are spending over US$ 1.5 million per year on cigarettes. Reducing access would discourage them from starting to smoke. South West ASH asked four children aged 10–13 to visit 100 randomly selected tobacconists; 92 sold cigarettes to these children. A week later, the tobacconists were approached and asked a set of questions about the law and their compliance with it. Almost all knew the law, and most claimed that they never sold cigarettes to children. Press coverage and subsequent follow-up surveys have reduced sales significantly but not completely. We have tried to support the tobacconists and not always be seen to be attacking them. We have carried out surveys of shopkeepers' attitudes to illegal sales and publicized the findings.

Because the trading standards officers of the local authority are charged with monitoring the laws on illegal sales, South West ASH has contacted all of the relevant officers to identify good practice and remind the others of their role. Good practice is publicized.

Tobacco promotion, advertising and sponsorship

Banning tobacco advertising and promotion is one of the key aims of any comprehensive tobacco control programme. At the local level, South West ASH and AGHAST used a wide range of strategies to campaign for a ban. A group of local activists picketed and demonstrated outside all local tobacco-sponsored arts and sporting events, using irony and wit to highlight why the sponsorship was inappropriate. We distributed leaflets to those attending the events, explaining our reasons for being there and what they could do.

Local Members of Parliament are visited regularly and sent letters to support action to ban tobacco advertising. One of the more creative means was presentation of a giant birthday card showing a map of the constituency with photographs of all tobacco advertisements to a local Member who was also Health Secretary. More radical activists took inspiration from the Australian activists and started a graffiti campaign on billboards. Photographs of the graffiti were published in two best-selling books and in many newspapers.

South West ASH's surveys have been published in journals such as *The British Medical Journal* and *The Health Education Journal*. These include a survey of tobacco advertising on post offices and three surveys of public attitudes.

Lobbying and public education

South West ASH routinely lobbies policy-makers and uses the media to keep smoking and health issues in the news. With the publication of Government figures on tobacco-related deaths by local area, we organized a wreath-laying ceremony outside the Imperial Tobacco Company for local people who had died from smoking and erected a memorial stone outside the Wills Memorial Building.

Before the last election, South West ASH sent all parliamentary candidates a questionnaire to elicit information about their support for tobacco control. We routinely write letters to the press on national and local issues related to tobacco. South West ASH responded quickly when the Imperial Tobacco factory displayed an illuminated Santa Claus who was smoking and carrying a sack of cigars. We picketed with our own Santa Claus who threatened to boycott Bristol unless the smoking Santa was switched off. When Wills held a 200th birthday party for all its staff, we responded with a black-edged birthday card, reminding the city of how many Bristolians had been killed in 200 years by smoking.

Conclusions and lessons for others

The experiences of our small but dedicated group of tobacco control activists have some important lessons for others involved in local campaigning:
- using media advocacy as the most cost-effective strategy for local tobacco control;
- staying focused on the main issues: in our case, non-smokers rights, tobacco advertising and promotions, price, access by minors and reminding the public and policy-makers how bad smoking is;
- being opportunistic and creative: some of our activities were planned in advance, but the most successful campaigns were often those in which we responded to local issues in the news, reacting while the story was still fresh;
- humour and wit: although there is nothing funny about smoking-related deaths and disease, humour attracts publicity and public interest; humour is also an excellent way of showing up the fake respectability of the tobacco industry, keeps up the spirits of the activists and shows the press a positive side;
- keeping it local: even when a story was a national one, we would put a local aspect

on it either by our actions or by finding local statistics and case studies; even when we had no local story, we would research local statistics such as the number of legs, lungs and larynxes lost through smoking;
- Pictures speak 1000 words: thinking visual and using photo opportunities provide more opportunities for the press and television; photographs always attract more interest and impact; simple props such as placards state the case clearly and props such as coffins, wreaths and funeral garb still attract the press; anything larger than life works, including giant cigarettes, petitions and letters on T-shirts or boards spelling out demands.
- using other news or being seasonal: when there is no real news about tobacco, it can be created by linking the risks due to tobacco to existing news stories or seasonal issues such as New Year, Valentine's day or the budget;
- pressure groups: even though most of our activists were health professionals, the creation of pressure groups with memorable names had far more impact than enlisting health spokesmen. Pressure groups and a campaign make more of an issue for the media.
- 'turning tables' on the tobacco industry: our focus for attack was always the tobacco industry and smoking and not smokers; one must counter the tobacco industry's promotions and show them up for what they are;
- surveys and small-scale research: surveys are likely to attract press coverage; thus, if you want to publicize some angle of tobacco control, do some research, such as attitude surveys, visual surveys (e.g. the position and number of advertisements), behaviour surveys and numbers, such as point-of-sale promotions for children; the findings must be presented simply and visually.

Role of a national cancer society in lobbying for tobacco control legislation: A case study from Canada in the campaign for the 1997 Tobacco Act

K. Kyle

Office of Public Issues. Canadian Cancer Society, Ottawa, Canada

Introduction

By jumping fully into the lobbying game in 1986, the Canadian Cancer Society, Canada's largest charitable organization, initiated important gains for public health. A year earlier, its national Public Education Committee had held a workshop to determine whether the Society should become involved in public policy advocacy. It was agreed that it was 'time to recognize officially a policy of advocacy to control cancer'. It was at this workshop that the phrase, now famous in the Canadian Cancer Society, was coined: "It's time to wake the sleeping giant". The Board of Directors later agreed to establish a national public issues committee with staff support. Other comments made at the workshop were that the Society should 'proceed with care into grey areas, but we can't be timid on clear-cut issues' and 'unless we have had our wrist slapped, we haven't gone far enough'.

In analysing its strengths and weaknesses, the Canadian Cancer Society quickly determined that it could not do advocacy—particularly tobacco control advocacy—by itself. We soon became coalition partners with a variety of groups interested in tobacco control, although some waxed and some waned in the intensity of their efforts over time and depending on the particular tobacco issue. In addition to the Canadian Cancer Society, the other key groups were the Canadian Council on Smoking and Health (now the Canadian Council for Tobacco Control), the Canadian Lung Association, the Canadian Medical Association, the Heart and Stroke Foundation of Canada, the Non-Smokers' Rights Association and Physicians for a Smoke-free Canada. To paraphrase a statement made in the House of Commons by a Member of Parliament, Lynn McDonald, in 1988, when you combine grassroots conservative organizations like the Cancer Society, the Heart and Stroke Foundation and the Lung Association with the missionary zeal of Physicians for a Smoke-free Canada and the Non-Smokers' Rights Association, 'you get a dynamic combination'.

The Tobacco Act

Following the trend of 'two steps forward and one step back' that has characterized tobacco control in Canada, a major movement forwards in public health and cancer control took place on 25 April 1997, when Royal Assent was given to Bill C-71, Canada's new *Tobacco Act*. The national tobacco control coalition, the National Campaign for Action on Tobacco, had been lobbying for new national regulatory framework legislation to replace the *Tobacco Products Control Act*, the important sections of which had been declared unconstitutional by a one vote majority judgement of the Supreme Court of Canada in late 1995. The new law:

* creates the authority to regulate tobacco products and smoke constituents;
* prohibits tobacco advertising, except for advertisements containing information about tobacco products in publications with primarily adult readership, in direct mailings and in premises where young people are prohibited by law;
* prohibits sponsorship and promotional materials containing tobacco brand names, except in publications with primarily adult readership, in direct mailings, on the site of the sponsored event and in premises where young people are prohibited by law. On-site promotional materials will be subject to restriction on size and duration (For example, brand names and logos can appear only on the bottom 10% of the display surface).
* prohibits self-service displays and requires photo identification to confirm minimum age;
* prohibits the use of tobacco brand names or logos on non-tobacco products orientated to youth; and
* re-establishes the legislative requirement for package health warning messages, except that now there will be an optional attribution to 'Health Canada'.

I shall address the unique opportunities and challenges of tobacco advocacy for many voluntary cancer societies around the world and tips that can be taken from the Canadian Cancer Society's experience in dealing with them.

In the war against the marketing aggression of the tobacco industry, health and medical groups in Canada had for many years been 'conscientious objectors', for a variety of reasons. One was simply the 'medical model': as David H. Hill, a former Vice-President of the Canadian Cancer Society, stated in a lecture on controlling cancer through political means, Canadian health organizations ". . . have been dominated by professionals whose orientation is the search for the biological causes of illness, rather than the social factors at the root of the problem. Both health professionals and volunteers involved with charitable organizations have a desire to be perceived as 'nice guys' and have, therefore, tended to avoid the controversy that is a part of hard hitting advocacy." In many charitable health organizations around the world, money has been available only for activities that do not cause controversy, such as medical research.

Opportunities

In a very real sense we are in a protracted war with the tobacco industry. One of the world's foremost military experts, B.H. Liddell Hart, explained, "The principles of war ... can be contained into a single word—concentration. But for truth this needs to be amplified as the concentration of strength against weakness". What are the strengths that cancer societies can bring to tobacco control advocacy campaigns?

1. Credibility: The first on everyone's list would certainly be the credibility of a cancer society with the public and government. This might be expected of Canada's largest voluntary organization and largest funder of cancer research, and the Canadian Cancer Society's positive image has been borne out by survey research. In March 1996, Environics Research Group in Toronto released the results of a survey funded by the Heart and Stroke Foundation of Canada, the Canadian Cancer Society and the Canadian Lung Association, which concluded that most Canadians seeking information about tobacco issues have confidence in health charities (67%), doctors and other health practitioners (52%) and professional organizations (50%). Fewer than one in 10 said the same about the Federal and provincial governments (9%) and tobacco companies (4%). Canadians also want health groups to do advocacy. Nine in 10 Canadians strongly (64%) or somewhat (25%) agreed that health charities such as the Heart and Stroke Foundation, the Canadian Cancer Society and the Canadian Lung Association should attempt to influence government health policy issues such as tobacco control. Only one in 10 strongly (5%) or somewhat (5%) disagree. When Canadians were of the existence of evidence that certain kinds of government policy can have a significant effect on changing behaviour such as tobacco use, 66% said that this information did not affect their opinion that health charities should play a role in influencing government health policy. Of the three in 10 who would change their opinion, most would want health charities to play a role (30%).

These results and other factors were helpful in establishing a small group within the National Campaign for Action on Tobacco, to convince senior volunteers in the Heart and Stroke Foundation, the Canadian Lung Association, the Canadian Cancer Society and the Canadian Medical Association who were reticent about being associated with other groups which they saw as more radical, to put additional resources into the campaign for the new bill and work together on a select number of lobbying activities. The credibility of such groups is particular important when their names are cited as endorsing advocacy advertisements in daily newspapers. Coalitions of this type are useful, as they naturally lend themselves to a 'good cop–bad cop' tactic, in which charities play the good guy and the typically more aggressive non-smokers' rights groups can play 'the heavy'.

Credibility also creates opportunities to give awards to politicians where it really counts: in public. For example, a Federal election was called shortly after the bill was passed. Just before the election, the Canadian Cancer Society sent congratulatory letters about the work of Members of Parliament who had supported us to the editor of every community newspaper within their electoral districts. We did the same for the Health Minister. Many of these letters were published.

2. Resources: Human (both volunteer and staff) and financial resources are typically more plentiful in cancer societies than in groups like ASH, although many of the staff are chronically overworked. Volunteers of all kinds and politics typically join cancer societies. As they are from all over the country, they can give their politicians a regional view of our lobbying efforts.

The Canadian Cancer Society lays emphasis on recruiting lawyers, rather than physicians, since volunteer advocacy has paid off. For example, some have convinced their own firms to provide full or partially free legal advice in cases that go to the courts. Large firms often have a policy of doing a certain percentage of this kind of work. On a number of occasions, the National Public Issues Committee has decided that the fight would be advanced by obtaining formal intervenor status in the courts in defence of tobacco bills under constitutional challenge by the industry. In our meeting in 1997, a group consisting mostly of lawyers convinced the National Public Issues Committee to proceed on this course of action; the Board then petitioned a judge to give us intervenor status, and this was granted. This course of action also meant the commitment of a significant sum.

Professional volunteers can also assist in writing letters to the editors of newspapers and magazines. We received excellent feedback from an article by Dr Gerry Bonham, a physician and retired senior Health Ministry official, reminding Canadians of other areas where legislation had advanced public health: seat belts prevent traffic fatalities, the addition of vitamin D to milk prevents rickets, requiring salt be iodized has annihilated goitre and cretinism and safe packaging laws have reduced fatal poisoning of small children. With financial resources provided by the national Board of Directors of the Society, we were able to hire Rob Cunningham, author of *Smoke and Mirrors: The Canadian Tobacco War*, to assist with the campaign. In one project, he exposed the sham of the industry's voluntary code by documenting 90 violations of the code on advertising practices in the Ottawa area in summer 1996 and filed a submission to the industry-appointed committee that supervises compliance. The upholding of these complaints by the Committee became a major national news item and showed many that the industry could not be trusted to police itself and that legislation was the only viable recourse. The industry admitted that it had broken one of its rules, advertising cigarettes within 200 metres of a school, but instead of complying with its code, it announced that it would modify the code to permit this in the future. The industry explanation was that it had made an error by not specifying in the code that the rule was to apply only to outdoor advertising such as billboards.

Many cancer societies have a medical and health research arm. In Canada, the National Cancer Institute, our research-orientated sister agency, has been extremely helpful in providing research expertise, especially behavioural research and assistance in evaluating our activities. These research scientists are often the first to point out to boards of directors that a political solution of cancer control is faster and can do more good in the long run than research or clinical trials.

3. Geographical distribution: As stated by a former Speaker of the United States House of Reprentatives, "All politics is local." This is also true for Canada. Local staff and grassroots volunteers can, for instance, assist with local media events and visit Members of Parliament in their home districts. The best example in our campaign of the benefit of having volunteers and staff all over the country occurred at a particularly sensitive stage in the bill's progress. The host of a radio show in Montreal who was a friend of the tobacco industry gave the Prime Minister's telephone number and convinced 300 listeners to phone the Prime Minister's Office directly to oppose the bill. We faxed our divisions and volunteers across the country pleading for 1000 phone call and e-mails to support the bill, within 24 hours. The Prime Minister's Office later confirmed that while the majority of callers were opposed to the bill on the first day, on the next day 90% of callers supported the bill. The final report was that two-thirds of the 2000 callers were supportive. Prime Minister Jean Chrétien even announced his personal support for the bill. We also asked our people across Canada to e-mail the Prime Minister. In this kind of situation, e-mail is a comparative advantage for health coalitions, as few workers in tobacco factories have access to e-mail, while health professionals generally do.

Challenges

We should not minimize some of the real challenges inherent in advocacy work in a cancer society. The first is our federated structure. In a number of countries, national cancer societies are really a federation of local, state or provincial cancer organizations. This can be problematic if urgent action is needed at a critical time, as the national organization has little power to channel resources spread across the country. In Canada, we encouraged our provincial divisions to agree to nationally decided strategies. Working in a federation is, however, excellent preparation for working in a coalition. Many of the principles of success are exactly the same, including respect for the other person's point of view and common courtesy. Just as a successful marriage requires constant attention, it takes real work to keep a coalition healthy and productive. One would think that a large, federated structure would impede rapid decisions, yet our advocacy experience over the last 11 years has taught us the value of structuring to allow for quick decision-making. The terms of reference of the National Public Issues Committee include 'special authority', a mechanism that permits overnight decisions on matters comprised in previously agreed general Board policy. Such a decision can be taken by two of three senior volunteers: the National President, the Chair of the National Public Issues Committee or the Honorary Solicitor. As everyone in the organization knows that the 'special authority' exists, we can proceed quickly without unintentional slowing down by other components of the Society that also have an interest in the issue.

A second challenge is competing internal priorities, which is a regular problem for health volunteer organizations. So many worthwhile causes need resources, including research on breast cancer and advocacy of examinations for prostate cancer. When I first joined the Canadian Cancer Society, it was customary at budget time for each department to try to increase resources in its own area by criticizing projects from other departments. The absence of data on the relative merits of various types of interventions made this almost inevitable. We prevented the eroding of resources for advocacy by stating the fact uncovered by the 1996 Environics poll that Canadians think that health charities spend much less than they should on lobbying: 33% of Canadians even said that more than 40% of the budgets of health charities should be spent on trying to influence government health policy. While I must exercise caution here, as half of the respondents did not answer this question, the amounts suggested were certainly more than the infinitismal amount most of these groups now spend on public policy advocacy. This kind of information helps in defending the budget line.

The third challenge is planning overkill. Large volunteer organizations usually have many academically qualified professionals who like to spend time planning. Of course, we must do serious planning, but, as Nigel Gray stated at an advocacy workshop, "Planning is the enemy of opportunity.' The most important aspect of planning is to ensure the resources necessary to make use of lobbying opportunities when they occur.

Conclusion

The most important lesson that the Canadian Cancer Society has learnt is, "... we have the power. If we are willing to learn the political ropes and mobilize our volunteers to exercise their political clout, our organizations can bring about significant legislative change that can reduce disease, that can prevent deaths and, in the long run, do more than all the hospitals put together. And in the final analysis, isn't that what we are really all about?"

Smokeline: Australia's Internet library

P. Markham[1] & C. Hilder[2]

[1]*Australian Council on Smoking & Health, Subiaco, Western Australia, and*
[2]*QUIT Vic, Carlton South, Victoria, Australia*

Getting the facts straight is essential for tobacco control. We should leave inaccuracy to the tobacco industry. Most tobacco control organizations have a reference library, small or large, for their own or for public use. The Australian Council on Smoking and Health (ACOSH), which is involved primarily in advocacy and research and is based in Perth, Western Australia, has built up a considerable reference library over many years. The library contains books, reports, surveys, journal articles, acts of parliament and conference proceedings. It provides in-house information for ACOSH and also for students, researchers and the public. All of the papers in the library are allocated to major subject areas such as cessation, legislation, economics and the workplace and given key words which best describe their contents. The library is organized into the following subject areas relevant to tobacco control:

Aboriginal and indigenous
Attitudes
Campaigning
Cancer
Children (and adolescents) and smoking
Cigarette advertising/marketing
Cigarettes: low tar/special type
Costs
Developing countries
Economics
Education
Heart/vascular disease
Legal
Legislation
Mortality
Other conditions
Other drugs
Passive smoking
Respiratory
Returned ex-service personnel
Smokeless tobacco
Smoking and sport
Smoking cessation and addiction
Smoking control general information
Tobacco industry
Trends
Women and smoking
Workplace

ACOSH puts the publication details—author, title, journal and publication date—on a database and allocates up to six of 140 possible key words related to tobacco control, such as passive, tax, cancer, adolescents and legal. ACOSH also prints out an author index and a subject index from the database to make daily use of the library easier. Many library users find these sufficient and do not need a database search.

This library with its database is called Smokeline. It has over 5000 papers at present and is growing at around 500 papers a year. This is far from being a large collection on a world scale. By comparison, in the 1970s the US Surgeon General cited 50 000 references, and between 1990 and 1996 a Medline search came up with 21 954 references on smoking or tobacco. ACOSH cannot compete on size, but information is useless if it is inaccessible.

Smokeline is accessible, quick and specialized in tobacco control; it is specialized for Australia, health and advocacy, with less emphasis on detailed medical information, which is available elsewhere; it also has a subject and key word system that can be adapted for use elsewhere.

Geography and finance took the library a step further. Perth is an attractive, pleasant city but very isolated from the rest of Australia and the world. ACOSH is a small non-governmental organization, and the library is only a part-time effort, The library costs ACOSH a good deal of time, as the papers must be collected and details allocated, filed and maintained. To make it more useful to interstate users, some years ago ACOSH started a subscriber service to supply printed indexes and send copies of papers as requested. While this increased the usefulness of the library significantly, it took time, was expensive and was used by a very limited number of other tobacco control organizations. With the rise of the Internet, the resources at Quit Victoria and generous assistance from the Commonwealth Department of Health and Family Services, we have made Smokeline increasingly accessible to people working in tobacco control in

Australia. Moreover, we have been able to improve the way people use Smokeline. By putting this information into a searchable database, we have now made the service a fast and convenient means of finding articles in specific areas of tobacco control. An example of search results is shown in Figure 1.

The Smokeline web site is intended to assist Australian tobacco control organizations and advocates to locate references which for the main part are available in their own city (or even in their own library!) but could not otherwise be found easily. While ACOSH will provide copies of papers not found elsewhere, it is not intended to run an 'on-demand' supply service, owing to the burden of cost and time this would place on ACOSH. In time, we may be able to extend this information source beyond Australasia and may be able to share it with tobacco control advocates throughout the world.

Smokeline is an extensive, comprehensive information resource. By putting Smokeline on the Internet we have significantly changed the form it takes to improve the accessibility and usability of this excellent resource. In this paper, we hope to inspire thoughts about new ways of using available information in conjunction with people in your region and to encourage use of information in new ways according to developments in technology.

As tobacco companies concentrate their efforts on developing countries, we hope that exchanges of information such as this among tobacco control organizations will help combat these efforts. The Smokeline story provides a useful example of how collaboration between such organizations in different places can work. It also provides a model of a tobacco control library and website.

Figure 1. Smokeline Web search results

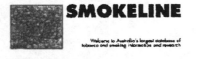

Welcome to Australia's largest database of
tobacco and smoking information and research

Reference Number: 1699
Category: AA
Author: Dadour T.
Title: Independent opinions from Queens Counsel on major objections to 1983 Bill
Publication: Dr Dadour MLA. To Mr Old MLA, WA Parliament
Publication Details: Subiaco: Electoral Office, 10 November 1982.
Resource Type: Correspondence

Countering Philip Morris in The Netherlands

B. de Blij

Dutch Foundation on Smoking and Health (Stivoro)

The Philip Morris campaign

Philip Morris is the world's largest cigarette manufacturer and includes Marlboro among many other brands. It sells cigarettes in almost every country of the world, and in most countries it is among the three top sellers. Its largest factory outside the United States is in Bergen op Zoom, The Netherlands.

In the early summer of 1996, Philip Morris Europe, based in Switzerland, decided to launch a European campaign to counter growing public concern about environmental tobacco smoke. A number of European governments had decided to place limitations on smoking in public and at the workplace, with the aim of minimizing the health risk of tobacco smoke for non-smokers. Philip Morris tried to stop such government regulation of smoking by showing that all concern about environmental tobacco smoke was unfounded. The Philip Morris campaign had two parts: The first was a 'scientific' study conducted by Professor Jeffrey Idle that concluded that "there exists insufficient evidence to endorse the view that environmental tobacco smoke is a primary lung carcinogen." The second consisted of four full-page advertisements in most daily newspapers in which the public was 'shown' the scientific evidence that environmental tobacco smoke is not more dangerous than drinking chlorinated tap-water, using pepper or eating a biscuit made with rapeseed oil. For the first time ever , by the way, the tobacco industry admitted that active smoking is a risk factor for several diseases. The campaign was launched in the European countries in which Philip Morris has a considerable market share. In The Netherlands, the advertisements were those shown in Figure 1. They looked 'scientific', with a lot of text. Their message was: "Philip Morris is going to educate you on something very complicated."

What we did

As the Philip Morris campaign started in the United Kingdom, we in The Netherlands were warned in advance; for instance, we were able to attend the press conference at which the Dutch campaign was presented. Some Dutch scientists, including a reputed cancer epidemiologist and a professor specialized in asthma in children, were also warned in advance and prepared themselves to counter the false reasonings in the campaign. They confirmed to the press that environmental tobacco smoke is harmful to the health of the population and causes discomfort, especially for children and people with asthma. Idle's report was effectively discredited as a tobacco-funded, biased piece of research by relatively little-known scientists. A Dutch participant in the study, a professor at Leyden University, distanced himself from the study group during the first days of publicity.

From the beginning of the campaign, it was attacked in the media. The judgement of health experts, such as a representative of the Union of Epidemiologists, was solicited frequently and was invariably negative. Most members of the public had read about the campaign before they saw it. Even the media, which are usually friendly to 'big tobacco', judged the Philip Morris campaign 'stupid', and most considered that they would have argued the case for the innocuity of environmental tobacco smoke in a much more subtle way. The way in which it was done gave the impression that a big tobacco company was telling the public what to think, and the public didn't like it. Of course, a few people admired Philip Morris for standing up to public opinion.

In addition, a complaint was made to the Advertising Control Board by the Asthma Foundation, the Clean Air Now action group and producers of tap-water and spices. The highly respected Minister of Health condemned the campaign at a very early stage as 'misleading'.

Figure 1. Philip Morris advertisements against the dangers of environmental tobacco smoke

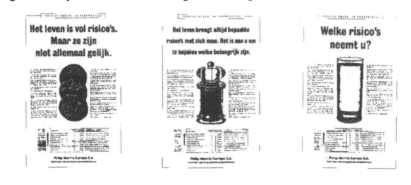

The immediate result was that Philip Morris ended the campaign prematurely, with the pretext "We have created enough discussion about this issue". Later, the company was convicted by the Advertising Control Board in unusually fierce terms, as this body is usually friendly to the industry. They confirmed that the campaign was misleading. As Philip Morris did not appeal this verdict, it stands uncontested.

Philip Morris intended the campaign to decrease public support for greater provision of non-smoking areas. The campaign did not achieve this goal. By chance, Stivoro had commissioned an opinion poll from the Dutch survey Institute NIPO about passive smoking in the first quarter of 1996, a few months before the start of the campaign, and the survey was repeated in the fourth quarter with the same questions. The surveys were based on a representative sample of the adult (> 15 years) population, consisting of more than 6000 people. Philip Morris succeeded in one respect: the percentage of people who thought that passive smoking is harmful to health had fallen by 1% (not statistically significant) to 73%, and significantly fewer people thought that environmental tobacco smoke causes lung cancer.

The ultimate goal of the Philip Morris campaign was not achieved, however, as more people thought that separate areas for smokers and non-smokers should be provided in public buildings (from 75% before the campaign to 85% afterwards), more people thought that smokers should ask permission to light up a cigarette (74% to 79%), and more people thought that employees should be able to work without being bothered by cigarette smoke (80% to 84%).

Conclusion

The Philip Morris campaign did not achieve its ultimate goal of convincing the Dutch people that environmental tobacco smoke does not warrant more regulation by the authorities. It also showed that big tobacco companies can make mistakes in their public relations and that such mistakes can be used to counter them effectively.

The 'reality check': A way to make tobacco shareholders aware

G. Boëthius[1], Y. Bergmark-Bröske[2], B.-M. Lindblad[3], G. Steinwall[4] & I. Talu[5]

[1]Doctors Against Tobacco, [2]Nurses Against Tobacco, [3]Swedish Cancer Society, [4]A Non Smoking Generation and [5]Teachers Against Tobacco, Stockholm, Sweden

To make the public in general and shareholders in particular aware of the true character of tobacco companies is an important part of a comprehensive tobacco control strategy. This report describes an activity carried out in May 1997 at the annual shareholders' meeting of the Swedish Match company. We owe the idea to an Australian 'Tobacco Company Alternative Report' of 1987.

Swedish Match used to be a respected company, producing and selling matches world-wide. Today, it has 80% of the cigarette market in Sweden. The largest shareholders are banks, insurance companies and pension funds. The annual report for 1996 contained the usual figures on production, sales, profits, a generous dividend as well as promises of expanding markets in eastern Europe and Asia.

Doctors and nurses in white coats and others handed out a 'reality check' to all those attending the annual shareholders' meeting. This alternative report contained other figures, such as '5700 people died from Swedish-made cigarettes in 1996', and public health comments on citations in the company report. For instance, the company's statement, "Many of the Group's markets are mature .... New and expanding markets in eastern Europe and Asia are our next priority" caused us to comment, "These markets are also mature—with respect to smoking among men, that is. So what is new and expanding? What can generate growth? Smoking among women and children, of course." Our report also identified the largest shareholders and their dividends in 1996. It concluded by encouraging shareholders to consider their ownership from the ethical point of view: "Swedish Match has an extremely generous dividend policy. Now you know why."

A debate article was published in a major newspaper before the event, and two of us made statements at the meeting. Press coverage was excellent, including all the television channels, radio and the major newspapers. Within three weeks of the event, two major insurance companies announced the sale of their shares, for ethical reasons. Follow-up letters and the 'reality check' have been sent to board members of other major shareholders. We have indications that discussions are taking place in boardrooms. We have also made use of the alternative report to influence various organizations not to become involved in sponsorship with Swedish Match: "You don't want to be in bad company!"

We conclude that the 'reality check' has fulfilled its purpose very well: it has made the shareholders aware of the true character of the company and what it stands for. The debate on ethical ownership has come to stay!

A framework for using the media for tobacco control

R.J. Donovan

Marketing and Health Promotion and Evaluation Unit, Graduate School of Management and Department of Public Health, University of Western Australia, Nedlands, Western Australia

Introduction

Well-designed and well-implemented mass media campaigns based on sound communication principles and developed with close cooperation between health and media professionals have had substantial impact, both in health and in other social areas (e.g. Donovan & Leivers, 1993; Egger *et al.*, 1993; Reid, 1996). Similarly, the effectiveness of the media in tobacco control, via both publicity and paid advertising, is now well established (e.g. Pierce *et al.*, 1990; Elder *et al.*, 1996). In this paper, we present a framework for using the media in tobacco control that combines the three main ways of using the media with the three major roles or objectives of media campaign components.

Methods

The media can be used in a number of different ways for health promotion (Egger *et al.*, 1993). This paper focuses on the three main methods: advertising, publicity and 'edutainment'.

Advertising is the paid placement of messages in various media vehicles by an identified source. We include here the voluntary placement by the media of messages for social change that are clearly in the form of paid advertisements (called community or public service announcements).

Publicity is the unpaid placement of messages in the media, usually in news or current affairs programmes, but also in feature articles and documentaries. Publicity involves attracting the media to run a particular story or cover a particular event in a way that creates, maintains or increases the target audience's awareness of or favourable attitudes towards the organization's products or message, or towards the organization itself. Many campaigns now involve press conferences with celebrities and staged events, supported by activities such as providing the media with press releases, videotapes, feature articles and photographs and by making experts available for interview on radio and television.

A third, increasing use of the media for health promotion is the deliberate inclusion of socially desirable messages in entertainment vehicles such as television soap operas, to achieve social change objectives. For example, the Harvard alcohol project in the United States approached television writers to introduce actions and themes into highly rated television programmes that would reinforce and encourage a social norm that drivers don't drink (DeJong & Winsten, 1990).

The decision to use advertising, publicity or edutainment or some combination of these in any health promotion campaign is determined by the objectives of the campaign, the budget, the relative effectiveness of the various modes in reaching and affecting the target audiences, the complexity of the message, time constraints, relations with the media and the nature and types of media and media vehicles available.

Roles of the media in health promotion campaigns

The media appear to have three major roles, two of which apply primarily to the targeting of individual behavioural change and one to the achievement of socio-political objectives.

The two primary objectives of the media components of most campaigns that target individual behavioural change, whether via paid advertising, publicity or edutainment, are (Donovan, 1991) to inform (or educate) and to persuade (or motivate). The distinction between these two roles is blurred, in that the provision of information is generally not intended for its own sake but to lead to desired behavioural changes. While information alone can arouse emotions and motivate some people to cease an unhealthy practice, it is clear, for example, from the public health literature that information in itself is insufficient to bring about desired behavioural changes in most individuals.

Most uses of the mass media in health promotion have been directed towards changing individual risk behaviour, but the mass media have also been used to advocate and achieve socio-political environmental changes that affect health (Chapman & Lupton, 1994). The quit-smoking lobby is the most professional health advocacy group successfully using the media. They have used them to redefine smoking as a public health issue of concern to all and to attack the morals and motives of tobacco companies' marketing techniques. The subsequent arousal of public opinion has been used to support direct lobbying of legislative changes, such as restricting the advertising of cigarettes and the sponsorship of sporting and arts events by tobacco companies.

Each of the methods—advertising, publicity and edutainment—can be used in conjunction with any of the overall objectives to educate, motivate and advocate. The two objectives of individual and socio-political change should be combined in any comprehensive health campaign; in some cases, however, it is likely that campaigns targeting the individual must first have some impact on beliefs and attitudes towards the recommended behaviour, before socio-political advocacy objectives can be achieved. For example, it is unlikely that efforts to frame smoking as a public health issue would have been as successful without prior quit campaigns that emphasized the health effects of smoking. Similarly, efforts to control smoking indoors were undoubtedly facilitated by increasing awareness of the effects of passive smoking.

References

Chapman, S. & Lupton, D. (1994) *The Fight for Public Health: Principles and Practice of Media Advocacy*, London: BMJ Publishing Group

DeJong, W. & Winsten, J.A. (1990) The use of mass media in substance abuse prevention. *Health Affairs*, Summer, 30–46

Donovan, R.J. (1991) Public health advertising: Execution guidelines for health promotion professionals. *Health Promotion J. Aust.*, 1, 40–45

Donovan, R.J. & Leivers, S. (1993) Using mass media to change racial stereotype beliefs. *Public Opin. Q.*, 57, 205–218

Egger, G., Donovan, R.J. & Spark, R. (1993) *Health and the Media: Principles and Practices for Health Promotion*, Sydney: McGraw-Hill

Elder, J.P., Edwards, C.C., Conway, T.L., Kenney, E., Johnson, C.A. & Bennett, E.D. (1996) Independent evaluation of the California tobacco education program. *Public Health Rep.*, 111, 353–358

Pierce, J.P., Macaskill, P. & Hill, D. (1990) Long-term effectiveness of mass media-led antismoking campaigns in Australia. *Am. J. Public Health*, **80**, 565–569

Reid, D. (1996) How effective is health education via mass communications? *Health Educ. J.*, **55**, 332–344

Family smoking campaign:
Evaluation of a mass media campaign in England

L. Owen, D. McVey, A. McNeill, J. Stapleton & K. Bolling

Health Education Authority, London, United Kingdom

The family smoking campaign

In July 1992, the British Government presented its 'white paper', 'The Health of the Nation', which outlined various targets for smoking and health, one of the main ones being to reduce the prevalence of cigarette smoking among men and women aged 16 and over to no more than 20% by the year 2000. At that time, 33% of the adult population amoked cigarettes regularly, and the highest prevalences were among 16–44-year olds, people in manual jobs and the unemployed. In response to this challenge, the Health Education Authority of England launched a 'Family smoking campaign'. It was designed as a trial to test the effectiveness of mass media alone versus mass media with local activities on the attitudes, knowledge and smoking behaviour of manual workers and unemployed adults, especially those who were parents.

The purpose of this paper is to outline the development and evaluation of the campaign. The evaluation was conducted over two years to test the effectiveness of mass media (television), to establish the optimum amount of television advertising required to bring about a change in smoking behaviour and to see whether there was any added value in supporting the campaign by local activities.

A trial was designed involving three regions in the north of England and a fourth region which was used as a control. The key test region was West Yorkshire, which received a double weight of television advertising and support from a very active local tobacco control network. Tyne Tees and the rest of Yorkshire had a double weight of television advertising but no local network attached to the campaign; Granada had a single weight of television advertising and no local support. Central served as the control, with no television advertising and no funding for any local network activity. 'Double' and 'single' weighting refer to the number of times the advertisements were shown in each region. Thus, in the first year of the study, people in the regions with double weight were likely to see the advertisements 40 times in the three-month campaign, while those in Granada were likely to see them 20 times.

The television advertisements consisted of 14 different commercials starring a well-known comedian, John Cleese. The advertising was supported by a national telephone help line (Quitline), on which smokers who wanted to quit could receive advice and support; the Quitline number was given in all of the television advertisements and in other publicity initiatives. In West Yorkshire, a local tobacco control alliance was supported and funded by the Health Education Authority to generate as much unpaid publicity on smoking and health as possible and to support health professionals by providing appropriate resources and training, for instance in cessation methods and use of the media. Finally, there was a comprehensive programme of research and evaluation, including surveys of the general population, pre- and post-testing of the television advertisements, a process evaluation of the local activity network, evaluation of the telephone help line and monitoring of unpaid media coverage.

Qualitative research conducted before the campaign indicated that it should show understanding of the difficulties smokers face when trying to give up, that it should try to motivate smokers to attempt to quit, that it should build confidence in their ability to quit and that it should support smokers in their attempts to quit. It also showed that specific messages should be included that highlighted the short-term benefits of giving up and the effects of parental smoking on children. This and other qualitative research showed that use of a celebrity was the best way of delivering the messages; John Cleese, an ex-smoker, agreed to take part in the campaign.

Until this campaign, most of those conducted in England had focused on reducing smoking among children and adolescents. We included adults on the basis of the evidence that attempts to reduce smoking among adolescents are likely to fail unless the prevalence among adults is reduced. Changes in smoking behaviour and attitudes were measured in a large-scale panel survey, one carried out before the campaign and two about 6 and 18 months after each television campaign. People were selected randomly in each region and asked to give a face-to-face, structured, 25-min interview in their own homes.

Results

The campaign appeared to have an effect on the prevalence of smoking. A clear dose–response relationship was seen, in which the region with the greatest input showed the greatest change. Thus, the prevalence in West Yorkshire, which received a double weight of advertising and was supported by a local network, fell by 3.5% over the two-year period. The region that received double weight of advertising but no local support showed a smaller reduction in prevalence, and the region that had only single weight advertising showed no evidence of an overall change . These findings are provisional, as they have not been adjusted for the effect of factors independent of the inervention on the behavioural change, which is necessary since individuals could not be allocated randomly to the interventions.

Table 1, in which those factors were taken into account, shows the rates of smoking cessation. The factors found to be most influential were cigarette consumption level, age, sex, socieconomic group and the desire to quit. The odds ratios for exposure only to media relative to controls were 1.2 for the percent of smokers who gave up cigarettes and 1.1 for the percentage of non-smokers who took up cigarettes. The comparison between media plus network and the controls gave odds ratios of 1.7 for smokers who quit and 0.58 for non-smokers who started. None was significant; however, the odds ratio of 1.2 for people exposed to media only means that 25% were more likely to quit smoking than in the control region, and the odds ratio of 1.7 for the key test region, West Yorkshire, means that the odds of smokers quitting were 70% higher than in the control region. This ratio is similar to those achieved with intensive clinical interventions.

Two factors, age and previous smoking, predicted that non-smokers would start smoking. When these were taken into account, there was no evidence of an effect of media only, but people exposed to both the media and the local network were about half as likely to take up smoking or to relapse.

Conclusions

The changes in smoking prevalence, which appear to be due to changes in rates of cessation and uptake, indicate that an intensive media campaign supported by an active local tobacco control network can be effective. The dose–response effect observed in the preliminary analysis of prevalence suggests that there is a threshold of television

Table 1. Effects of the interventions on smoking status after 18 months

Intervention	Smokers giving up cigarettes (%)	Non-smokers taking up cigarettes (%)
Control	8.6 (27/314)	3.1 (37/1187)
Media only	9.7 (71/735)	3.3 (62/1903)
Media + network	12 (26/212)	2.0 (11/547)

advertising below which changes in smoking behaviour are unlikely to be observed. Inclusion of a local network clearly enhanced the impact of the media intervention.

The network in West Yorkshire generated maximum publicity on smoking and health in all the media, through press releases, creating launch opportunities and photocalls and providing the media with spokespeople. It also responded opportunistically to other tobacco issues as they arose in the press, providing comment. The network was supported by local councils, health authorities and public transport authorities and by other tobacco control organizations. The cessation activities included a free help line to back up the national Quitline, a pack of materials to help smokers quit, a programme for general practitioners to encourage their involvement in smoking cessation, resources for health visitors and midwives to encourage them to raise the issue with smokers who have children and small grants to encourage community-based anti-smoking activity. The network also created an award named after a Yorkshire entertainer who died of lung cancer attributed to environmental tobacco smoke, and gave it to restaurants and pubs that met certain smoke-free criteria. It then published 'The Yorkshire Guide to Smoke Free Eating and Drinking', which were widely distributed in the region and to tourist information centres.

Which media to use to promote your message about smoking

K. Aston

Health Education Authority, London, United Kingdom

The importance of integrated campaigning

The influence of the media on people's attitudes to health is well documented, both for the general public and in reaching opinion-formers who determine the structural changes that are required to influence changes in health behaviour. Media interventions are considered to be particularly effective when supported by community activity. What this means in practice is that the national media are most effective at providing a 'noise', which generally has an awareness-raising function. By providing the key themes and messages, it also provides the backdrop against which communities can target their own constituents most effectively. For example, a local smoking education campaign targeting children will make primary prevention a priority. Similarly, someone working with elderly smokers would probably want to focus on the benefits of stopping smoking at any age. It is therefore important when developing national media stories and activities to consider whether they can be adapted to local use. This can be achieved in a number of ways, for instance by providing a regional breakdown of data or simply by supporting a national story with local case studies.

Some thought must also be given to whether targeted communications, such as those for pregnant women smokers, are as effective without a backdrop of mass media. There is an increasing view that unless there is a critical mass of investment in national media more targeted communications will not be particularly effective. This happens for two reasons. First, individuals are most likely to respond to communications that reflect their attitudes and beliefs rather than to those that treat them as a population target group. Secondly, the population cannot be easily segmented in a simplistic way; for example, pregnant women could also fall into a number of other population categories, such as the economically disadvantaged. It is therefore important to target from a number of different angles.

Which media to use when targeting the public

The Health Education Authority's smoking education campaign involves a mix of advertising, press and public relations activity, which is delivered through national,

local and specialist print and broadcast media. Its communications address the basic medical and physiological facts and issues associated with smoking in order to remind smokers and professionals of the toll that smoking has on both individuals and society as a whole. The campaign communications strategy is made up of the following elements, which provide the messages that are used to target smokers throughout the year:
* Providing a rationale for smokers to quit: "Quitting smoking is the single most effective action you can take to improve your health." "You won't have to worry about being the only smoker when you're out socializing." "Think of the money you'll save."
* Providing motivation for smokers to quit: "You can do it." "Take one day at a time." and providing identification for smokers, including personal testimonies of quitters and those who haven't quit but wish they had.
* Supporting smokers in their efforts to quit with tips on dealing with difficult situations while reinforcing immediate and on-going benefits and promoting support for smokers, including the Quitline.
* The non-smoker vision: aspirational and conceptual, i.e. the 'non-smoker' within; tapping into the emotions , "You'll be around to see your grandchildren"and assuring recent ex-quitters that they have made the right decision.

Accordingly, there are a number of elements within the simple 'giving up smoking' message, and consideration is required as to which media or communications device is most effective in delivering each message. For example, television is the most effective medium for providing emotional engagement and feeling. Similarly, tips for smokers who want to stay non-smokers are probably best communicated through a magazine or leaflet in which the readers have access to the information whenever they need it. Motivation for smokers to quit can be provided through a case study in a magazine of through an interview with an ex-smoker on the radio. This approach takes into account not only the messages for smokers but also how different media are received. We know, for example, that consumers have a far more intimate relationship with radio than television. Similarly, we know that women respond to media that target them as a population group, whereas men tend to favour media that reflect their interests, such as computers and sports. By using this method, communications have more impact and value is achieved for money by using the most effective media or communications delivery system available.

Getting your message across

Regardless of the medium—television, radio or print—the principles of newsworthiness include some of the following key criteria: human interest, new information, conflict or a story occurring in a local community. When considering which messages are to be sent to whom, it is essential also to think about the context in which the media will have the most impact. If the message is 'high risk' and the consequences of it not being reported properly are considerable, it may be appropriate to pay for the message to be communicated through the media. This could include advertising, planned product placement and endorsement schemes. This is obviously expensive, but the degree of control obtained may mean that the money is well spent.

Managing public perception and risk

Health risks are big news, and people often use the media as their primary source of information on health issues, such as food scares, pollution, and cancer. A recent study by the Health Education Authority into public perception of air pollution (including environmental tobacco smoke) showed that most people do not understand that chemical and biological pollution harm health. Far fewer understand how this happens, for instance the link between asthma and air pollution is widely misunderstood. Much of the media coverage of air pollution and asthma has been alarmist and dramatic. What consumers are asking for are simple tips on air pollution, its impact on their lives and what they can do. A worrying consequence of an alarmist approach in the media is that people are beginning to switch off or feel confused by the information. This has obvious consequences for work in smoking education. With regard to asthma, health professionals are left with the dilemma of having to reassure those people who are not at risk while alerting those who are. It is therefore important to consider other sources of information to back up media activity, which in this case could include general practitioners or specialist voluntary agencies.

Using the media to influence opinion formers

The role of the media in influencing opinion-formers who determine health policy is well documented. Media advocacy is being used increasingly as a method of achieving maximum media publicity to add to the changing climate of opinion on public health issues. The publicity achieved raises the profile and status of the issues both locally and nationally. Media advocacy can also broaden health alliances. For example, *The Smoking Epidemic* used smoking mortality statistics to gain unpaid publicity. The Prime Minister asked for a personal briefing after reading an article in a newspaper, and the issues were taken up during *Question Time* (an important current affairs television programme in the United Kingdom) and featured in popular comedy programmes. Unpaid publicity reaches audiences that run into millions and is therefore a crucial health promotion tool.

Using the media in strategic planning

Analysis of the media can also be used in strategic planning, as it is possible to track not only one's own media coverage but also that of other agencies involved in the smoking debate, both pro and anti. For example, it would be possible to counter a 'considerate smoker' media campaign supported by the tobacco industry with coverage describing the overwhelming support for controls on smoking in public places. Similarly, during a campaign in the United Kingdom in which images were used to promote Embassy cigarettes in a way that was considered to be appealing to children and young adults, the media were used to publicize research commissioned by the Health Education Authority which confirmed the appeal of both the image and character to children. A consequent complaint to the Advertising Authorities Commission resulted in withdrawal of the advertisement.

Conclusion

Use of the media by health professionals raises a central contradiction: on the one hand, unpaid publicity is of crucial value in communicating health messages and generating debate; on the other hand, news by its very nature can be sensational and we are at risk of confusing, or, worse, alienating those whom we wish to reach. Our ability to achieve the best results from the media is not dependent on chance but on strategic planning, using various media in different ways and taking a long-term view.

A most potent weapon: Three case studies of media advocacy by the medical profession in the fight for tobacco control

K. Woollard

Australian Medical Association, Australia

The Australian Medical Association is a professional organization representing more than 25 000 Australian doctors. One part of our work involves the promotion of public health, and a significant part of that is devoted to eliminating the incidence of death and sickness caused by the consumption of cigarettes. Governments are best placed to bring about changes that decrease the consumption of cigarettes, as it is the government that has its hands on the levers of power. It alone can make the radical and necessary changes that can dramatically reduce the carnage caused by smoking. But governments are naturally cautious. They need a great deal of persuasion to do anything that either costs money or upsets powerful interest groups, such as tobacco companies.

So, how do we put pressure on governments to adopt positive changes that reduce cigarette consumption? The most potent weapon at our disposal is the media. In my experience, the first thing health ministers do every morning is pick up their press clippings and read the issues of the day. They worry about what is in the media because journalists will ring them up and ask difficult questions. And when they are asked those questions, they go to their bureaucrats and demand answers. A politician once told me that one strong headline in a newspaper is far more effective than a very detailed 500-page submission that took months of painstaking work to produce. Rightly or wrongly, it's the squeaky wheel that gets the oil. So, what can we do to generate media interest in our cause?

A few observations about the media

Journalists portray issues in black and white. In the case of smoking, the public health lobby is almost always portrayed as 'good' and the tobacco companies as the personification of evil. But not always. We must try and avoid the label of public health authoritarians who seek to control the lifestyles of others.

The media never tire of news on smoking. Media organizations conduct many surveys to find out what their readers, viewers and listeners want, and health nearly always tops the list. Smoking is a significant story, because so many readers are smokers and are engaged in an activity which, in many cases, will kill them. A survey of a major Australian newspaper showed that smoking ranked alongside cancer as the leading health topic covered by that paper, ahead of issues such as AIDS, environmental health, road trauma and diet.

The media love statistics. They have a permanent thirst for facts and figures and especially new or local statistics. Facts and figures must be made available in small packages. Journalists must not be drowned in unnecessary detail.

The media love colour and conflict. Anything that is clever, colourful or involves conflict is much more likely to be taken up than something mundane, drab and dull.

Be prepared. When approaching the media, it is important to be know exactly what message you want to sell. It is useful to anticipate the questions journalists are likely to ask and to have the answers ready. One can think of a headline that the media could use, making sure it is sufficiently colourful, newsworthy and succinct for the journalist.

I shall describe three short case studies that show how potent a weapon the media can be, how easy and inexpensive it is to gain positive media exposure and how important it is to be creative and to spend time planning for success.

Warnings on cigarette packs

My first case study involves the use of simple objects to help secure the introduction of tough new warnings on Australian cigarette packs. In 1993, the Australian Medical Association and other public health groups were lobbying for tougher warnings on cigarette packs, as the old warnings were barely visible. To win the new warnings, we had to get the agreement not only of our national government but also of all eight state and territorial governments. At first, each government indicated support, but then the Victorian State Government said it wished to back out of the agreement, which would have been a public health disaster. The Australian Medical Association worked out a tactic that would bring the issue to national attention: It contrasted the very clear labelling on a pack of household rat poison with the low-key warnings on cigarette packs. The rat poison packet clearly states that the contents kill rats and mice, but the warning on the cigarette pack was barely visible. The story made front-page news across the country and was featured on national television news and current affairs programmes. Shortly afterwards, the Federal Government used its powers to enforce the new warnings on cigarette packs. The Federal Health Minister became a convert to the cause of tobacco control. The total cost of the exercise was about AUS$ 4 for the rat poison and AUS$ 5 for the cigarette pack.

National tobacco scoreboard

Our second case study involves a simple scoreboard. The Australian Medical Association has joined with the Australian Council on Smoking and Health to launch an annual scoreboard, which rates the performance of all state and territorial governments on a range of tobacco control measures. The results are released on World No Tobacco Day. The scoreboard has achieved some spectacular media cover. We present prizes to the health minister who has achieved the best score for tobacco control and give an encouragement award to the minister who has tried hardest. The minister with the worst score wins the infamous Australian Medical Association Dirty Ashtray Award. Health ministers try very hard to avoid winning the dirty ashtray, and those who win the top awards display them prominently in their ministerial offices. This is another cheap and easy exercise to undertake and has helped to put real pressure on our health minsters to do the right thing.

The inside story

The third case study demonstrates how the media can be used to turn a cheap, simple poster and brochure campaign into a campaign of national significance. In this case, our audience is not so much government but the general public. The Australian Medical Association and two Australian medical colleges launched a low-budget campaign aimed at curbing smoking among young people and particularly among young women. We used material developed by the American Cancer Society but not previously seen in Australia. The poster features the face of a young woman covered in tar and gunk. The slogan says: "If what happened on your inside happened on your outside, would you still smoke?" The campaign was designed to de-glamourize the image of smoking among young women. Focus group sessions held with young women showed that the image had real credibility and impact. The American Cancer Society very generously provided the artwork free of charge.

We had a small Federal Government grant of about AUS$ 5000 to reproduce posters and brochures in Australia, and the Royal Australian Colleges of Surgeons and Physicians each contributed a further $2500. But this campaign would inevitably be a low-profile exercise unless we could generate real community interest. As we did not have the budget to advertise, we had to rely on the media to spread our message. A high-profile launch with a newsworthy event was the answer, and we decided to set up a macabre fashion show, featuring four women smokers, a student, a businesswoman, a social smoker and a pregnant smoker. Each of the models, who were volunteer Australian Medical Association staff members, was made up to resemble the woman on the poster; the fifth and final model was a non-smoker who, of course, had an unblemished face. This simple but colourful and unusual event was a big hit with the media and was mentioned on the evening news on all five national television networks. It also received extensive newspaper coverage. In addition, one of Australia's leading cartoonists chose to illustrated the story.

The Medical Association was inundated with calls from schools, health agencies and government departments which wanted to use the material. We still get daily calls for the poster and brochure. The material has been used in New Zealand, other parts of the Pacific and Sweden. This was a good example of a low-cost, high-impact campaign which worked because of a simple idea that attracted the media. The campaign was also effective for lobbying, reminding the government that the medical profession was not only criticizing the government health policy but was also participating actively in health promotion programmes.

We used similar tactics in 1996 to launch a special poster which promotes a public health message to Australia's indigenous people, a group that has not had access to public health messages in the same way as the rest of the community, and their smoking rates are double the national average. The poster features three top Australian football players all of whom are Aboriginal, and the poster was launched just before the grand final series, which involved all three players. The poster has been distributed throughout Aboriginal communities, schools, hospitals and prisons. Again, the media played a key role in promoting what has been a low-cost but very popular campaign. Significantly, the campaign has also helped put pressure on the Federal Government to develop a national smoking strategy for our indigenous population. That must be a priority for the Australian Government.

Conclusion

These case studies show how the media can be used as a potent, cost-effective public health tool. Good preparation, clear thinking and imagination are essential to successful use of the media. I conclude by quoting that great medical educator, Sir William Osler, who in 1905 cautioned doctors not to 'dally with the Delilah of the press'. In my experience, his advice was completely wrong. Perhaps he should have said, 'Do dally with the Delilah of the press, but for goodness' sake, go well prepared.'

Using television and other mass media to counter the threat of tobacco to women and children

M. Palmer[1], S. Palmer[1], W. Zatoński[2] & D. Zaridze[3]

[1]The Center for Communications, Health and the Environment, Washington DC, United States; [2]Centre of Oncology, Warsaw, Poland, and [3]National Institute of Carcinogenesis, Moscow, Russian Federation

While tobacco consumption is falling in most western countries, it is rising in the developing world and particularly among women and children. The decline in western tobacco use is no accident: it is the result of massive information and public education, which in turn has led to action by governments and individuals. The participants in the workshop on 'Using television and other mass media to counter tobacco's threat to women and children' shared approaches and lessons, especially those used in central Europe, and stimulated discussion on building partnerships for a global effort to counter the growth of tobacco use through mass media and information, especially among women and children in developing countries and the newly independent states of the former Soviet Union.

Ambassador Mark Palmer led the workshop with a brief introduction to the global problem of tobacco use, emphasizing the potential for mass media to counteract the onslaught of advertising by the tobacco industry. He presented the archives of programmes of the Center for Communications, Health and the Environment and experience with production and airing of anti-tobacco programmes on nationwide television in 17 central European countries. He proposed a coalition of global media giants and a sustained television campaign.

Dr Witold Zatoński of the Centre of Oncology in Warsaw and Dr David Zaridze of the National Institute of Carcinogenesis in the Russian Federation shared their contrasting experiences—both successes and failures—and sought recommendations for halting the onslaught of tobacco promotion in their countries, especially to women. Dr Zatoński demonstrated the challenge and the success of using the mass media in Poland to combat tobacco advertising, whereas David Zaridze made it clear that, despite his Institute's extensive efforts, obtaining the cooperation and the interest of the Russian media still remains a challenge.

Sushma Palmer of the Center for Communications, Health and the Environment used the results of an ongoing programme on heart disease in the Czech Republic to demonstrate the experience of her Center and to stimulate discussion on successful use of the mass media for health education and awareness. She showed a series of anti-smoking public service announcements and screened a portion of a five-part television series, *A Family Year*, which focuses on the use of tobacco and alcohol among adolescents in the newly independent States.

Ambassador Palmer led an extensive discussion on a proposal for a global media campaign and use of regional demonstration programmes for building indigenous capacity, heightening public awareness and catalysing anti-tobacco legislation, especially targeted at three key audiences: the local tobacco control community, influential groups including media professionals, employers and policy-makers and tens of millions of women and children. The workshop culminated in support from anti-tobacco leaders from around the globe who attended the workshop for the following letter to President Clinton and selected members of the United States Congress, urging them to embrace media campaigns and other means of supporting the international tobacco-or-health struggle.

28 September 1997

The Honorable William Clinton
President of the United States
The White House,
Washington DC

Dear Mr President
    The United States has a unique opportunity to benefit from its extraordinary domestic revolution by leading a worldwide revolution against smoking. The United States also has a unique responsibility: American tobacco companies and American marketing genius are major causes of the sharp increases in smoking among women and children throughout the world. In fact, as smoking and the market in the United States have leveled off, American tobacco companies are primarily targeting women and children in Russia, China, India, and other emerging nations of Africa, Asia, Latin America, and Central and Eastern Europe.
    As the advertising campaigns of the tobacco companies themselves have demonstrated, the most powerful way to affect individual behavior is television, radio and the print media. This is the basis for the provision in the agreement with the American tobacco industry "to spend $ 500 million annually for multi-media campaigns designed to discourage and deglamorize the use of tobacco products" in the United States. We propose that the United States take the lead in forging an alliance of global media companies (most of which are American) and national media organizations and antismoking activists throughout the world in a massive, persistent campaign to keep children from starting to smoke and to help others kick the habit.
    The campaign will kick off with an hour-long splashy television program with globally known entertainment, political and spiritual figures and hard hitting investigative reporting on the industry and the effects of smoking. The mix of star quality, great popular music and revelation of new information will appeal to a younger as well as an older audience and be usable both on satellite and terrestrial networks throughout the world. More generally, we will work with the multinational and national media companies to train their people in antismoking programming and to tie this programming into on-the-ground campaigns by governments, communities, professional associations and other NGOs and activists in schools, workplaces, legislatures, clinics and so forth. Just as American cigarettes can be exported, so can America's leading expertise in tobacco control—using our Madison Avenue skills to combat rather than promote this deadly addiction. The tools which will be used to achieve these ends in addition to training and coproduction must include direct grants to non-governmental entities.
    If $500 million annually is needed to conduct such a media program in the United States (and if the tobacco industry itself spends much more on marketing), then clearly at least one-tenth that amount as America's contribution to this global campaign is required. We will leverage these

funds many times. One of the best features of this program is that we will negotiate free air time and space—whereas the tobacco industry has to pay for its space. Furthermore, media companies would be expected to contribute to coproduction costs.

This program would not be dependent on whether there is a settlement with the tobacco industry. It also could be funded from a portion of the proceeds from a cigarette tax increase.

The signers of the proposal are leading antismoking activists from India, Russia, Hungary, Poland, Ukraine and China. The American signer is the Center for Communications, Health and the Environment (CECHE)—which has been working with global media companies and anti-smoking activists to train and coproduce effective antismoking media programming. We would like to work with you to make this global campaign a reality and to save tens of millions of lives around the globe.

Respectfully yours,

GLOBALink

R.J. Israel

GLOBALink Information Services, International Union against Cancer, Geneva, Switzerland

History of the international tobacco control network
The international tobacco control network was launched in Perth at the 'Trade for Life' conference. At that time, tobacco control advocates were isolated and often alone in the face of of a powerful, rich, well-organized opponent. After several technological upgrades and the rapid growth, spread and use of Internet, GLOBALink was made available to all advocates.

Information services provided by GLOBALink
The network consists of a variety of news bulletins, documents and technical functions that make it a powerful tool for the exchange and delivery of messages among members. GLOBALink offers a selection of regional and thematic news bulletins. It also relays bulletins from organizations that would not publish outside their country or region and thus allows worldwide coverage. We collect documents from many sources and archive them in what will become the memory of the tobacco control movement. These documents consist of texts, images, sound, video clips, etc. GLOBALink offers a series of discussion groups, enabling network members to discuss important events, share information and receive international support. GLOBALink played a key role in the European advertising ban initiative. We offer several full-text databases and a chat service which lets members discuss in real time. For more information: http://www.globalink.org/glob/

Free home pages
As part of its communication strategy, GLOBALink offers a free home page hosting service to all its members. This way it ensures better visibility of tobacco control organizations on the World Wide Web.

Event coverage on the Internet–World Wide Web
GLOBALink has demonstrated its ability to improve communications in the organization and operation of various tobacco-control events. The most important to date is certainly the World Conference on Tobacco or Health held in Beijing in August

1997. GLOBALink was the official website of the conference and published daily information on the Internet, including photographs and press releases. GLOBALink, with the support of commercial sponsors, offered all conference delegates access to the Internet with electronic mail, World Wide Web and other online services. GLOBALink promotes every tobacco-control event in the online calendar: http://www.globalink.org/calendar/

A document describing how GLOBALink can help the organizers of tobacco-control conferences, *Organising World Conferences on Tobacco or Health: An Electronic Manual*, has been written by Dr Judith Mackay, Director, Asian Consultancy on Tobacco Control, and can be obtained on GLOBALink or by e-mail: mackay@globalink.org

Future plans

GLOBALink is THE network for tobacco control experts and will continue to provide its members with valuable and timely information. GLOBALink is continuously seeking partnerships with other tobacco control organizations in order better to serve the actors for a tobacco-free world. For more information, you may visit the GLOBALink website: http://www.globalink.org/glob or send an electronic mail to Ruben Israel, Head, UICC GLOBALink Information Services: israel@globalink.org

Consumer pressure as a counter-measure to tobacco promotion

K. Mulvey, L. Wykle-Rosenberg & W. Fassett

INFACT, Boston, Massachusetts, United States

INFACT, a United States organization that fosters corporate accountability, launched a campaign in 1993 to stop the tobacco industry from addicting new young customers around the world and to stop manipulating public policy to enhance their profits. INFACT's boycott of the tobacco industry, started in 1994, is a growing liability for Philip Morris' Kraft and RJR Nabisco's food brands, as the boycott has fostered pressure from shareholders to free these businesses from their tobacco interests. Both companies have experienced stable or declining tobacco markers in the United States, increased public opposition to the advertising and promotion of tobacco, massive litigation and regulatory pressure, which have spurred them to expand into international markets.

Philip Morris, maker of Marlboro, the world's leading brand of cigarettes, is the largest and most profitable tobacco corporation in the world, with an annual revenue in 1996 of US\$ 54.6 thousand million. It is also the largest food corporation in the United States and owns well-known brands such as Kraft, Jell-O and Maxwell House. Revenues from sales of its food products in the United States have, however, decreased by 22% since INFACT launched its consumer boycott campaign. More than half of its revenues now come from international sales, which accounted for 66% of its tobacco revenue in 1996 and an increasing proportion of that from foods. France and Germany are two of Philip Morris' largest markets for coffee. Other large markets for foods are central and eastern Europe, Hong Kong, the Philippines, Taiwan and Argentina, Brazil and Mexico.

In 1993, most of RJR Nabisco's revenue came from tobacco, but by 1996 most came from its food businesses. As both of these sources of revenue declined in the United States, RJR Nabisco also became more dependent on international revenue, its largest market (56%) being Latin America, followed by Canada, China, Indonesia and Spain.

This increased dependency of the tobacco giants on international revenue from foods is an important tool for consumers in those markets to use against their marketing and promotion of tobacco. The effectiveness of consumer pressure to challenge the expansion of the tobacco industry is enhanced further when combined with existing strategies such as government regulations, litigation, public health education and divestment campaigns. Our first campaign, a boycott against Nestlé from 1977 to 1984, resulted in significant reforms in the aggressive marketing of infant formula in poor countries. INFACT also contributed to the development of the World Health Organization's International Code of Marketing for Breast-milk Substitutes in 1981. Nestlé agreed to abide by the Code after intense pressure changed the cost–benefit ratio for the corporation of abusing public health. In our next campaign, we succeeded in pushing General Electric out of its involvement in nuclear weapons.

The tobacco industry offers similar opportunities for consumer pressure. We first called upon Philip Morris, RJR Nabisco and British–American Tobacco to stop abusing public health. In the absence of a satisfactory answer, we launched a boycott and issued a challenge to the tobacco industry, outlining the changes that must be made before we would stop the campaign pressure:

- stop tobacco marketing and promotion that appeals to children and young people;
- stop spreading tobacco addiction internationally;
- stop influencing and interfering with public policy on issues of tobacco and health;
- stop deceiving people about the dangers of tobacco and
- pay the high costs of health care associated with the tobacco epidemic.

Boycotts are effective when they involve millions of people acting together, when they are part of a strategic campaign and when they affect a corporation's revenues. The efficacy of a boycott is measured not only in lost sales, but also in the effect on the corporation's public image—one of its most valuable assets. Kraft and Nabisco give Philip Morris and RJR Nabisco a legitimacy and influence that they would not otherwise have. We identified the food brands that would maximize the financial impact of our campaign and make it easy for millions of people to participate. We therefore chose brands for their value and visibility, including Kraft, Nabisco, Post and Maxwell House.

Participation in a boycott is simple: Don't buy the corporation's products, and let the corporation know why. RJR Nabisco and Philip Morris must hear from people around the world that their abusive tobacco marketing practices will cost them sales of seemingly unrelated products. Transnational corporations depend on us to succeed. By using that power in an organized effort with others around the world, we can bring about change to prevent the needless deaths of millions of people each year.

Note: Since 1997, when this paper was presented, RJR Nabisco has sold its international tobacco business to Japan Tobacco and split its food and United States tobacco business into separate companies. INFACT's consumer boycott, combined with shareholder pressure, helped shift the business and public climate around RJR Nabisco, which forced the move. With the completion of these transactions, INFACT removed Nabisco as a target of the tobacco industry boycott on 16 June 1999. Philip Morris's Kraft is now the focus of the boycott.

Advocating for a total ban on tobacco advertising in Hong Kong

S.H. Lee

Hong Kong Council on Smoking and Health, Department of Community and Family Medicine, Chinese University of Hong Kong, Hong Kong SAR, China

The Hong Kong Council on Smoking and Health (COSH) was established in 1987 on the recommendation of WHO. It is a statutory body, funded by the Government. The mission of COSH is a smoke-free community in Hong Kong by promoting a smoke-free lifestyle. The Council aims to promote, publicize, educate, plan and coordinate all activities related to smoking and health and advise on the relevant legislation issues.

Members of the Council include Government officials and professionals from many areas, including health care, public relations and legal offices.

The control measures taken by the Council have followed a step-by-step approach, taking into account changing world trends and local views. In 1988, COSH submitted to the Hong Kong Government 24 recommendations, which included six recommendations for banning smoking in public areas such as cinemas, theatres, concert halls and public transport; three recommendations for controlling the sale of tobacco products, including increasing the size of health warnings on cigarette packs and health warnings for all tobacco products; nine recommendations for banning tobacco advertising on television, radio, cinema, printed media, public transport, all outdoor displays and indirect advertising; and five other recommendations concerning tar and nicotine group designations and an increase in the tobacco tax.

Between 1988 and 1994, the laws passed included banning tobacco advertising on television, radio and cinema, banning smoking on public transport, a 100% increase in the tobacco tax and prohibiting the sale of tobacco products to people under age 18.

In April 1994, the WHO Regional Office for the Western Pacific promulgated a five-year action plan which called for a 'Tobacco advertising-free Region by the year 2000'. In support of this plan, proposals were submitted to the Hong Kong Legislative Council to introduce further anti-smoking legislation.

COSH has adopted a 'multi-dimensional approach' combining political lobbying, scientific research and media publicity in urging the Government to ban all tobacco advertisements.

- A special ad-hoc working group was set up in COSH to work out the strategies for lobbying with legislative councillors and professional bodies. These included meetings with individual legislative councillors, attendance at the Legislative Council sessions to present our views and mobilizing support from medical associations, sporting organizations, public transport and major utility companies and banking organizations.
- COSH, in conjunction with academic institutions, undertook research to determine the status of smoking and health in Hong Kong. A survey of smoking and health among young people in 1994 showed that the smoking rate was increasing and that 60% of male students and 40% of female students had tried smoking before the age of 16; 20% of boys were current smokers, which was higher than the adult smoking rate of 15%. The same survey also indicated that tobacco advertisements had a strong influence on the attitude of young people towards smoking. A public opinion survey indicated that most Hong Kong citizens supported a ban on tobacco advertisement. The results of the surveys were made known to the public through press conferences.
- As the electronic and printed media can play a very important role in anti-tobacco work, various activities for the media were organized. These included media interviews, press conference, editors' briefings, press releases, printed advertisements and feature articles. Through these activities, the need to ban tobacco advertisements was fully explained to the media, and any misconceptions about the effect of banning tobacco advertisements, such as reductions in revenue and unemployment, were dispelled.

In June 1997, the Legislative Council of Hong Kong passed the Smoking (Public Health) (Amendment) Bill, 1997. The areas of amendment included: more no-smoking areas; greater control on sales of tobacco products; greater control on tobacco advertising; restaurants with more than 200 seats are required to designate not less than one-third of the area as a no-smoking area; smoking will not be permitted in supermarkets, banks, department stores and shopping malls; the sale of cigarettes in packs of less than 20 will be prohibited; tobacco display advertisements were to be banned after two years of the passage of legislation; tobacco advertisements in printed medial were to be prohibited after 31 December 1997; the placing of tobacco advertisements on the Internet was prohibited; and the use of tobacco brand names in sponsoring sport and cultural activities was banned.

It took COSH some 10 years to achieve compliance with 85% of the 24 recommendations made in 1988 for bringing tobacco under effective control. The road to success is long and arduous, but step by step we have come closer to our goal of making Hong Kong a smoke-free and tobacco advertising-free city. There is, however, no room for complacency. We must continue to monitor enforcement of tthe laws and the effectiveness of the measures. We must close any loopholes in the legislation if they are found. We will continue to press Government to set up a health promotion fund to replace tobacco company sponsorship. We will also double our efforts to ban indirect tobacco advertisements. Our battle for a total tobacco advertising ban in Hong Kong will not be won until there is a continuous reduction in the smoking rate of young people in our community. Fortunately, we have an understanding, enlightened, support-ive Government. We shall continue our fight in all directions until the battle is won.

Evidence-based lobbying for stronger legislation: Inputs versus outcomes

H. Glasgow[1], B. Swinburn[2] & M. Laugesen[3]

[1]*Cancer Society of New Zealand, Wellington, [2]National Heart Foundation, Auckland, and [3]Health New Zealand, Auckland, New Zealand*

Abstract
    The Smoke-free Coalition of over 20 national health agencies lobbied Government from mid-1995 to mid-1996, starting six months behind tobacco lobbyists. A weak Smoke-free Environments Amendment Bill was introduced to Parliament in late 1995. The challenge was to get it strengthened.
    The inputs were an experienced tobacco specialist, an advocate and researcher, experienced executive guidance and NZ$ 55 000 annual funding (NZ$ 1 equals US$ 0.7). The outputs were research and publication of a lobbying book of fact sheets; encouraging health groups to make written submissions; assisting groups making oral submissions; lobbying Parliamentarians; and suggesting legislative wording to the Parliamentary Committee.
    The outcome was the bill reported back to Parliament in August 1996, which was strengthened, and the bill passed in July 1997, which put the onus of checking the age of tobacco purchasers on retailers; banned packs of fewer than 20 cigarettes; banned tobacco advertising inside shops from December 1998, achieving a total ban on all advertising; added new clauses to enable effective regulation of nicotine, tar and packaging; and banned incentives to retailers either to advertise or to place tobacco products favourably for sale inside their shop.
    The conclusion is that evidence-based lobbying is essential and cost-effective.

Introduction
    The *Smoke-free Environments Act 1990* banned almost all tobacco advertising and smoking in offices. By July 1995, virtually all tobacco advertising and sponsorship had disappeared, except for product advertising in shops. Tobacco consumption per adult fell from 1957 cigarettes in 1990 to 1520 in 1994. The prevalence of smoking dropped from 27% in 1990 to 26% in 1991 but remained at 27% between 1992 and 1994.
    In October 1994, in the face of little Government action against tobacco, the National Heart Foundation called together a coalition of over 20 health agencies to urge Government to renew efforts for tobacco control. This coincided with the Minister of Health's plan for an amendment bill, limited to restricting access of young people to tobacco. The Smoke-free Coalition was formed to research and publicize tobacco issues from September 1995. An executive group, based in three cities, included representatives

of the National Heart Foundation, the Cancer Society, ASH, the Asthma and Respiratory Foundation, Te Hotu Manawa Maori and the Smoke-free Workers Network. The executive teleconferenced regularly to plan strategies and coordinate research, advocacy and publicity. The total funding (contributed mainly by the National Heart Foundation and the Cancer Society) was approximately NZ$ 55 000 (US$ 37 000) per year.

Phase 1: Research and publicity

The many issues in the bill were researched and published in a lobbying booklet of 24 fact sheets, *The (Not Very) Smokefree Book*, which was widely distributed to health workers throughout New Zealand. Steady efforts were made to generate publicity on the issues covered in the bill.

The research methods included studying the texts of legislation in other countries, a medical student's survey of retailers, surveys of public opinion, analysis of manufacturers' tests on cigarette smoke by brand, reference to the scientific literature, a survey of tobacco advertising in shops, legal advice and requests under the Official Information Act for tobacco industry correspondence.

The publicity methods included publication and wide distribution of a book on lobbying in which the left-hand pages displayed excerpts from the bill and the right-hand pages provided the relevant fact sheets, with references listed at the foot of each page; media releases with fact sheets attached; parliamentary questions; tobacco advertisements photocopied for display by opposition parliamentarians during question time; and the results of a public opinion poll (NZ$ 5000).

Phase 2: Submissions on the bill

Written submissions on the bill were encouraged from November to December 1995 at meetings of public health groups in three main cities: 90% of the 130 written submissions supported the Coalition's views. We encouraged groups to make oral submissions between March and April 1996. Individuals and health agencies were encouraged to speak of their own interests and expertise and to obtain publicity. In 1996, a new group of public health service units sent staff to testify on the workings of the 1990 Act.

Visits to Parliamentarians were made March and April 1996. Some 15 legislators were approached in their electorates, and 20 approached by Coalition staff at Parliament, out of a total of 99 legislators. Further submissions were made in June and July 1996. After considering the submissions, the Parliamentary Select Committee prepared to make its recommendations. The Smoke-free Coalition suggested precise wordings for proposed legislative changes.

Outcomes

As in 1990, the evidence of young people was highly valued by Parliamentary Committee members. The issues in the 1995 bill were matters of detail, less divisive than in 1990, and grabbed fewer headlines. The 1995 bill required detailed evidence-based arguments on sales, advertising, harmful constituents and smoking restrictions. Submissions that were not knowledgeable were ineffective. The Select Committee members were knowledgeable because of tobacco legislative hearings from 1990 onwards. They accepted that 'smoking is bad for health', wanted to know how young people's smoking could be discouraged and cooperated across party lines on this issue. As a result of the research, advocacy and publicity, the Bill passed was considerably stronger than that originally introduced (see Table 1). Government has now provided funding for the Coalition and a director has been employed.

Conclusions

Evidence-based advocacy and lobbying is cost-effective: a small amount of funding produced significant changes, but it required subject and research expertise and media skills. We also found that the advocacy group should be located close to Parliament. Partial success is still success; gains should be collected, despite lack of progress in

Table 1. Lobbying for stronger legislation: Inputs versus outcomes

Bill introduced	Inputs	Bill reported back
Retailers required to prove only that they believed on reasonable grounds that the person was aged ≥ 18	Fact sheet[a] quoted stronger wording from the United Kingdom law	Retailers required to take reasonable precautions and exercise due diligence to determine the age of person buying cigarettes
No fewer than 10 cigarettes per pack	Surveys of retailers, adolescents; cost comparisons; fact sheets[b,c]	No fewer than 20 cigarettes per pack
Voluntary code permits advertising in shops	Fact sheets[d] [g]; new advertisements displayed by opposition Members of Parliament	Tobacco advertising in shops to cease from December 1998
No ban on incentives for retailers place and promote tobacco products	Manufacturers' incentive schemes for retailers tabled with the Parliamentary Committee	Ban on incentive schemes for retailers
No tar or nicotine regulation	Increased tar yields publicized; fact sheets[h,i]	Penalties for manufacturers inserted; regulation-making powers strengthened
No provision for smoke-free work areas for non-office workers	Fact sheets[j-l]	No progress: outside scope of Bill; Health Minister has announced provision in next amendment bill
Vending machines can be placed in hotels	Fact sheet[m]; a 15-year-old testified that she had bought cigarettes from vending machines	Vending machines limited to supervised areas of hotels: only slight gain

a   Ending tobaco sales to under 18s: effective law needed. Fact sheet. Smokefree Coalition 1996
b   Outlaw 'kiddie'packs of less than 20 cigarettes. Smokefree Coalition 1995
c   Outlaw 'kiddie'packs of less than 20 cigarettes: 1996 update. Smokefree Coalition 1996
d   Rescind the proposed advertsiing code and end tobacco advertising to children. Fact sheet. Smokefree Coalition 1995
e   Tobacco advertising codes: discredited, ineffectual, defective, oudated. Regulation needed to end the heavy shop promotion of tobacco. Fact sheet. Smokefree Coalition 1996
f   Tobacco advertising and promotions as powerful as peer pressure in increasing adolescent susceptibility to smoking: new evidence. Fact sheet. Smokefree Coalition 1996
g   Evidence: Cigarette advertising closely linked to adolescent smoking. Fact sheet. Smokefree Coalition 1996
h   Lower the high tar in New Zealand cigarettes. Fact sheet. Smokefree Coalition 1995
i   Regulate to lower the ceilings on the high tar and nicotine levels in New Zealand cigarettes: new evidence. Fact sheet. Smokefree Coalition 1996
j   Smokefree working conditions as of right by law for all. Fact sheet. Smokefree Coalition 1995
k   A one-word change to the Act, by extending smokefree work areas to all workers, can avert over 100 smokers' deaths a year. Fact sheet. Smokefree Coalition 1996
l   Smokefree workplaces for all New Zealand workers; and for gaming, drinking, outdoor events and children in cars. Fact sheet. Smokefree Coalition 1996
m   A complete ban on cigarette vending machines is required to protect young people from cigarette addiction. Fact sheet. Smokefree Coalition 1996

some areas. But there is no room for complacency: victory gains only an illusion of peace for a few years. Lobbying must be ongoing, to educate new parliamentarians and to counter tobacco lobbying.

Postscript

Owing to a change of government in late 1996, the Bill first drafted in October 1994 was not passed until July 1997. Tobacco consumption per adult rose by an average of 1% per year in 1994–96, and the prevalence fell to 26%. The Smoke-free Coalition is now a charitable trust, with its own part-time director (Roger Booth). Although there were imperfections in the final Bill, the Smoke-free Coalition decided to support its quick passage in 1997. In 1997, the Coalition also asked for increased prevention campaigns, for an increase in the tobacco tax and for work to begin on the next smoke-free environments amendment bill, to incorporate outstanding issues.

Reducing passive smoking in public places

R. Burton[1] & S. Woodward[2]

[1]Anti-cancer Council of Victoria, Carlton South, and [2]Protocol Management Group, Melbourne, Victoria, Australia

Introduction

The health consequences of passive smoking have been recognized for a long time. Harlap and Davies (1974) reported in *The Lancet* 25 years ago that children of mothers who smoked were more likely to be admitted to hospital with respiratory-tract infections. A body of evidence has followed that makes the case that passive smoking causes a number of diseases, including lung cancer in adults, attacks of asthma in adults and children, other respiratory diseases, coronary heart disease and irritation of the eyes, nose and throat. It is not the purpose of this paper to review the health effects of passive smoking, as several excellent reviews have been published, including those of the International Agency for Research on Cancer (1985), the United States Surgeon General (Department of Health and Human Services, 1986), the United States National Research Council (Committee on Passive Smoking, 1986), the United Kingdom's Independent Scientific Committee on Smoking and Health (1988) and Australia's National Health and Medical Research Council (1987) and the more recent reports of the United States Environmental Protection Agency (1992) and the Californian Environmental Protection Agency, and there are more.

The knowledge that passive smoking can harm others causes us to give consideration to the 'neighbour principle' described by the British judge, Lord Atkin, in the case of Donoghue versus Stevenson (1932), as follows:

'You must take reasonable care to avoid acts or omissions which you can reasonably foresee would be likely to injure your neighbour. Who, then, in law is my neighbour? The answer seems to be—persons who are so closely and directly affected by my act that I ought reasonably have them in contemplation as being so affected when I am directing my mind to the acts and omissions which are being called into question.'

The principle was adopted by most of the English-speaking world, and other jurisdictions have similar legal rules. Even if this is a legal principle in some countries, the moral principle applies in all countries that you should not do things or allow things to happen that can harm others.

So, now that we know that passive smoking is dangerous, how can we lessen or, preferably, eliminate exposure, so that the incidence of the diseases it causes are reduced? Strategies can take two forms: a voluntary approach and a legislative approach. Much can be done to change the situation without laws. For example, few laws specifically on smoking in public places and workplaces exist in either Britain or the United States, yet there is a substantial difference in restrictions on smoking. Americans have been far more active in using existing laws and customs to pressure people to eliminate smoking at work and elsewhere. There has been less activity in the United Kingdom, and smoking in public is commoner there.

Voluntary restrictions

Several elements are important in persuading proprietors to make their premises smoke free, the most important probably being public opinion. Public opinion must first be measured by a poll and measured periodically thereafter. The results should be broken down by smokers and non-smokers and also given as a total. It may be important to examine the results for males and females separately, if one or the other group is more heavily exposed to smoke; the results of the poll should be publicized in newspapers and magazines and elsewhere, to bring the information to the attention of the community. Each successive poll should be publicized in the ways that have been found to be successful. At the same time, health agencies should be publicizing the dangers of passive smoking to health, by a special publicity campaign or by a health professional commenting on the results of a recent study published in a scientific journal.

As soon as the public statements start to have an effect, the tobacco industry will make statements that passive smoking is not a problem. This is known as the 'scream test': when the tobacco industry begins complaining and complaining loudly, you can be sure you are having an effect; the silence or relative silence of the tobacco industry is a sure sign of an inactive or ineffective anti-tobacco programme.

Legislative approach

New legislation may not be needed; often, existing laws can be re-interpreted in the light of new medical evidence that passive smoking is dangerous. In Australia, for example, there are five sets of laws which have no specific mention of tobacco smoking but which can be interpreted with passive smoking in mind to bring about a positive result. Some of these are related to occupational health and safety and conditions of employment.

In countries where litigation is important, individuals who are injured by passive smoking can sue, and this has been a successful way of reducing the prevalence of smoking in Australia. In countries where class actions are easy to initiate, they can be a successful approach to achieving government measures to protect non-smokers from the harmful effects of passive smoking, as the current 'American tobacco settlement' illustrates.

In conclusion, smoking in public places can be changed by applying these strategies in any country. It will take time, but change will occur.

References

Committee on Passive Smoking (1986) *Environmental Tobacco Smoke—Measuring Exposures and Assessing Health Effects*, Washington DC: National Academy Press
Department of Health and Human Services (1986) *The Health Consequences of Involuntary Smoking. A Report of the Surgeon General* (DHSS Publication No. (CDC)87-8398), Rockville, Maryland: Office on Smoking and Health
Donoghue v Stevenson (1932) AC 562
Environmental Protection Agency (1992) *Respiratory Health Effects of Passive Smoking: Lung Cancer and Other Disorders* (EPA/600/6-90/006F), Washington DC
Harlap, S. & Davies, A.M. (1974) Infant admissions to hospital and maternal smoking. *Lancet*, **i**, 529–532
Independent Scientific Committee on Smoking and Health (1988) *Fourth Report*, London: Her Majesty's Stationery Office
International Agency for Research on Cancer (1985) *IARC Monographs on the Carcinogenic Risk of Chemicals to Humans*, Vol. 38, *Tobacco Smoking*, Lyon
National Health and Medical Research Council (1987) *Effects of Passive Smoking on Health. Report of the NH & MRC Working Party*, Canberra: Australian Government Publishing Service

The Swedish war against the tobacco industry: A Non Smoking Generation

G. Steinwall

A Non Smoking Generation, Stockholm, Sweden

The new campaign of the organization 'A Non Smoking Generation' was conducted during one week in May 1997. On 1090 pillars throughout Sweden, the organization went to war against the world's largest brand: Marlboro. The campaign showed the frightening face of smoking: the real Marlboro men—young, innocent children who have been seduced by the message that the tobacco industry is spreading with its increasingly aggressive marketing. This campaign is a follow-up to campaigns in 1994, 1995 and 1996.

One goal of he campaign was to call attention to the way in which the tobacco industry recruits smokers; another was to continue to fight the tobacco industry and a third was to exert pressure on politicians to pass the bill that is before Parliament regarding prohibition of indirect tobacco advertising. A Non Smoking Generation would have had to pay about US$ 250 000 if it had had to pay the full price for renting the pillars and the advertisment and printing, but it has been able to carry out its campaigns with the support of advertising agencies, printers and newspapers.

The results were huge media attention and continuing focus on the subject in the media ever since. Campaigns of this aggressive type are therefore necessary to wake up politicians, convince them to become more involved in this important matter and to make laws that forbid the tobacco industry to continue their aggressive indirect advertising to recruit children and young people as smokers.

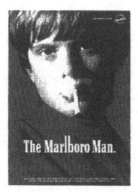

The Marlboro Man.

Lobbying for tobacco control:
Attitudes and experiences of Canadian legislators

J.E. Cohen, M.J. Ashley, R.G. Ferrence, D.A. Northrup, J.S. Pollard
& D.L. Alexander

Ontario Tobacco Research Unit, University of Toronto, and the Institute for Social
Research, York University, Toronto, Canada

Background: Tobacco control policies are ultimately shaped by legislators, and lobbying activities can influence the development of public policies. We describe Canadian legislators' attitudes and experiences regarding lobbying on tobacco issues.

Methods: All 1044 Canadian Federal, provincial and territorial legislators were invited to participate in a 25-min, structured telephone interview. Ten of the 12 provinces and territories had response rates of at least 60%.

Results: Legislators had the most contact with non-profit health groups and the least contact with tobacco companies. Significant numbers of legislators said they had too little contact with medical associations (42%) and non-profit health groups (31%) about tobacco-related issues. Overall, 10–12 times more legislators said they could be persuaded on tobacco issues by lobbyists from non-profit health (41%) and medical associations (49%) than by tobacco industry lobbyists (4%).

Discussion: Significant proportions of Canadian legislators would be receptive to increased lobbying by representatives of non-profit health and medical associations about tobacco-related issues.

THE ROLE OF HEALTH PROFESSIONALS

Practising health professionals

The role of doctors in tobacco prevention

G. Boëthius

Doctors Against Tobacco, Stockholm, Sweden

Just as a battery of measures is used in a comprehensive tobacco control policy to diminish the use of tobacco, medical doctors should play several roles in their fight against tobacco. Just as no single part of a control policy replaces another, none of the roles of the doctor can be singled out as more important than another. In both cases, it is a question of consistent and comprehensive action.

The role model

Regardless of their position, doctors are important role models, for younger colleagues, for other health workers, for patients and for the public in general. People take it for granted that the doctors' training has made them well aware of the hazards of smoking and expect them to act accordingly. If they don't, they provide a perfect 'excuse' for other people. Young doctors usually do not realize their importance as role models, but that kind of modesty does not pay.

Doctors who smoke are obviously not good role models. The smoking habits of doctors vary among countries. In some, the prevalence of smoking among doctors is said even to exceed that of the general population. In my country, there has been a favourable development over the past few decades, the prevalence of daily smoking having decreased from 46% in 1969 to 6% in 1996, although about the same proportion, 6%, reported in 1996 that they used snuff as a source of nicotine. In that same survey, smoking was found to be less frequent among younger than older doctors. Another important finding was that those who gave 'wishing to be a role model' as the reason for not smoking had increased from 10 to 71%.

The clinician

Clinical doctors have many competing tasks to perform. On a busy day on a ward or in an out-patient department, it may be easy to forget to ask patients about tobacco use, unless it is considered to be a very firm routine in the doctor's mind. Today, knowing that smoking affects virtually all organs of the body, doctors should ask all patients about their smoking habits, regardless of their symptoms. By such constant questioning, people's perception of the importance of smoking will increase. If the doctor does not ask, they may think, 'Why worry?' Asking about smoking takes little time. What takes time is advising and assisting patients to change their habits. This can often be left to nurses, who are generally much better in this capacity, after some training.

Increasing demands and decreasing resources mean that priorities must be set, constituting a real challenge for doctors, forcing them to balance costs, benefits, quality of life and integrity. The clinician's role is to explain differences between medical and ethical aspects to patients and their families: 'My decision not to operate on your narrowed vessel is a medical decision and not a moral one. Only if you succeed in quitting smoking will an operation be effective.' Rational argumentation combined with truly professional help in quitting are essential for the credibility of a clinician.

The teacher

Most doctors, whether in university or other clinics, have teaching responsibilities in their daily routine. Teaching in cardiology and pulmonology, for instance, often makes medical students aware of the many negative effects of smoking. An important task for teachers is to summarize the extent of the problem and to explain the content of a comprehensive tobacco control programme, thereby demonstrating the role of doctors in its implementation. For this purpose, teachers and students can make use of the increasing number of tobacco databases that are now accessible all over the world. Perhaps most importantly, the medical school curriculum should also stimulate discussion on how to relate knowledge about the tobacco epidemic to changing attitudes and making doctors devoted health workers after leaving school (Richmond, 1996) .

The leader

Doctors are often leaders of groups or teams which may include persons in other professions. They expect doctors to be knowledgeable about the tobacco issue and to initiate and lead tobacco prevention activities, for instance, a smoke-free hospital project. Often, however, this does not happen. Instead, a nurse or a hospital administrator may take the initiative, sometimes to find that the doctors—shamed by their negligence—do not provide support. This must not happen!

The opinion maker and health lobbyist

Facts and opinions must also reach the community, to influence decision-makers at various levels to agree on a policy or to facilitate implementation of tobacco control measures in general. For example, the creation of Doctors against Tobacco in Sweden in 1992 was prompted mainly because legislators considered that there was no demand for a Tobacco Act. After successful lobbying, with other public health workers, we saw how effective and credible doctors can be. Of course, they must first learn the game: a 40-min lecture will not persuade busy politicians!

To summarize, the tobacco epidemic is a health issue and a political issue. I believe we have the right to demand increased awareness in the medical profession about the extent and character of the problem. We also have the right to demand more active participation in the implementation of tobacco control programmes. I urge all national medical associations to accept increased responsibility and encourage their members to fight against tobacco through instruments such as policy declarations.

The role of health professionals: Caring for the victims

L. Sarna[1] & P. McCarthy[2]

[1]School of Nursing, University of California, Los Angeles, California, United States
[2]ALCASE

Despite the heroic efforts at tobacco control, millions of people will die from tobacco-related diseases within the next decade (Murray & Lopez, 1996). Although almost unknown as a serious public health problem at the beginning of the century, tobacco will become a major cause of preventable death in the world in the next millennium (Peto et al., 1994). One of the most lethal forms of tobacco-related disease is lung cancer. It is the tenth leading cause of death in the world today and in the next 20 years is projected to become the fifth leading cause. Lung cancer is now the first cause of cancer-related death in the world, and its incidence is increasing in developing countries. Currently, 945 000 people die from lung cancer every year, and the number of deaths from lung cancer is projected to double by the year 2020, resulting in 2.4 million deaths, largely because of an 82% increase in the number in developing countries. In comparison with other diseases, lung cancer will move up in the rank order of projected years of life lost from premature death, from No. 22 to No. 12 in the next 25 years, and for disability-adjusted-life years (an indication of premature death and living with disability) will move from No. 33 to No. 15. In developing regions, the impact of lung cancer is escalating, and this disease is already the 48th cause of disability-adjusted-life years (Murray & Lopez, 1996).

Because of past differences in smoking rates between the sexes, lung cancer is currently disproportionately diagnosed in men, the highest global rates being found in Hungary (81.6 per 100 000), the Czech Republic (75.3), the Russian Federation (72.8) and Poland (71.3). Lung cancer continues to be a major cause of death among women in developed countries, although it is often ignored in treatises on women's reproductive issues. The United States currently has the highest rate in the world of death from lung cancer among women (25.6), followed closely by Denmark (24.8), Canada (21.8) and the United Kingdom (21.0) (Parker et al., 1997). China is ranked ninth. In 1990, however, almost 48% of all lung cancer deaths among women occurred in developing regions, and this proportion is projected to increase in the aftermath of increased smoking among women throughout the world (Murray & Lopez, 1996).

In this paper, we focus on the 'victims' of tobacco, particularly patients and families affected by lung cancer, and the important roles of health professionals in providing care, treatment, comfort and solace. The health professional's roles in the interplay of tobacco and lung cancer is discussed as a recurring theme: at diagnosis, during treatment and during rehabilitation or palliation. The word 'victim' is defined in *Webster's New Twentieth Century Dictionary* as 'someone killed, destroyed, injured, or otherwise harmed by or suffering from some act, condition, agency, or circumstance'. Although we are reluctant to label patients with cancer as 'victims', in this case, childhood addiction to tobacco results in overwhelming pain and suffering, 'victimizing' patients, families and society.

At diagnosis

The diagnosis of any cancer can contribute to an existential crisis. 'Why me?' is a frequent question asked of health-care professionals. Unlike cancers such as that of the breast, in which the cause is often unknown, the cause of lung cancer in a patient with a history of smoking may be all too apparent. The role of health professionals includes helping patients and families cope with the diagnosis. In the case of a tobacco-related disease such as lung cancer, issues of guilt and blame about smoking complicate this resolution. In addition, there are limited data about smoking patterns and withdrawal symptoms experienced by patients after a diagnosis of lung cancer (Gritz, 1991).

As not all smokers get lung cancer, many smokers may underestimate their chances of premature death (Schoenbaum, 1997). Both patients who currently smoke and those with a history of smoking commonly grapple with the reality of the relationship between their own smoking and the diagnosis of lung cancer. Patients may experience rage at themselves and others because of their habit and their inability to quit. Despite a long history of smoking, some patients may deny the relationship, citing numerous relatives, colleagues and celebrities who have continued to smoke without developing cancer (Sell et al., 1993; Faller et al., 1995). At the time of diagnosis, the degree of distress with regard to current and former smoking should be assessed. One instrument for routine assessment of quality of life in people with lung cancer (Cella et al., 1995) even includes a question on guilt and smoking.

Blame for smoking from family members and even from health-care professionals is not helpful for patients at this time. It is important to remember that most people become addicted to tobacco when young, before they are aware of or concerned about the devastation caused by lung cancer. People in whom lung cancer is diagnosed have often been exposed to tobacco 30–40 years earlier (Peto et al., 1994; Murray & Lopez, 1996). Many became addicted before the link between tobacco and lung cancer was revealed in scientific reports, over 30 years ago (US Department of Health, Education, and Welfare, 1964). Women who continued to smoke in increasing numbers during the 1970s thought that the data (derived primarily for male smokers) did not apply to them.

The period of risk for lung cancer continues long after cessation. Almost half of all people in whom lung cancer is diagnosed may have stopped smoking, in either the distant or recent past (Richardson et al., 1993; Strauss et al., 1995). These patients may be very resentful and angry about their diagnosis, after they have made efforts to improve their health. For example, one woman with lung cancer said that she had quit five years previously and thought that she would be 'as pure as the driven snow' (Sarna, 1995). Recent evidence suggests that women with a shorter smoking history than men may be at the same risk for lung cancer (Zang & Wynder, 1996).

Benefits can be derived from smoking cessation even at the time of diagnosis. Patients may mourn the habit, which was an important part of their everyday lives, and health professionals should be aware that the absence of this major coping mechanism and the withdrawal that accompanies cessation may make it even more difficult to deal with the diagnosis.

Smoking cessation efforts by family, friends and colleagues and strategies to decrease exposure to environmental tobacco smoke may be part of a health promotion plan after diagnosis (Schilling et al., 1997). The relationship between lung cancer and environmental tobacco smoke can cause anger and conflict in family situations, especially for the almost 30% of women in the United States with lung cancer who have no history of smoking (Zang & Wynder, 1996). A diagnosis of lung cancer for a family member may be pivotal event for others in the family and spur attempts to quit (Sarna, 1995), but the diagnosis is not a panacea. Continued smoking by family members and friends may cause additional distress and concern for the patient.

Many health-care professionals are not adequately prepared to engage in tobacco control and smoking cessation efforts. These interventions may become even more complicated in a hospital setting and when a patient is faced with a life-threatening illness such as lung cancer (Schoenbaum, 1997). The Smoking Cessation Clinical Practice Guidelines, published by the Agency for Health Care Policy Research, provides a research-based approach to the delivery of effective smoking cessation (Fiore et al., 1996). Systematic documentation of smoking status, use of nicotine replacement therapy, emotional support from clinicians and training in skills and strategies for problem solving are all critical elements of successful cessation. The skills training and emotional support recommended by the guidelines are essential components of a smoking cessation programme for patients with potentially life-threatening disease.

During treatment

The roles of health professionals during treatment for lung cancer include strategies to optimize survival and management of side-effects and symptoms. Assessments of quality of life during clinical trials are crucial adjuncts in determining the overall impact and benefit of treatment beyond tumour response and length of survival (Ganz et al., 1991; Sarna, 1993a). One of the reasons for the high rate of mortality from lung cancer is the lack of effective early detection of small, curable lesions. As a result, diagnosis occurs when the cancer is in advanced stages, when treatment is largely palliative; in the Unites States, only 13% of patients survive more than five years (Parker et al., 1997). Cancer is generally a disease of older adults, and tobacco-related co-morbidity from a lifetime of smoking may complicate treatment options, eliminating some that require adequate cardiovascular and pulmonary function. Women generally have a better survival rate, perhaps because of shorter smoking histories (Zang & Wynder, 1996).

Different issues accompany lung cancer treatment in developed and developing countries. In developing countries, less than 50% of patients with pre-terminal cancer are treated, and cancers such as those of the lung may be left untreated in favour of cases with a better prognosis (Murray & Lopez, 1996). Even in developed countries, treatment of advanced lung cancer is controversial because of modest advances in treatment and because therapeutic nihilism might affect clinical care (Brundage & Mackillop, 1996; McVie, 1996)..

Tobacco-related concerns continue during the treatment phase of lung cancer. Patients who continue to smoke after diagnosis should be advised to quit in order to minimize the side-effects of treatment and to decrease the risk of recurrence. Continued smoking during treatment has been linked to increased risks of symptoms, including weight loss (Ganz et al., 1989; Geddes et al., 1990).

Rehabilitation

Long-term survivors of lung cancer are rare, and recurrence is common. Those who do survive may still be faced with the co-morbiditiy from a lifetime of smoking, but data on their quality of life are limited (Schag *et al.*, 1994). Rehabilitation programmes may be necessary for people whose pulmonary status is compromised by surgical resection. Continued cessation is an essential component of any recovery programme for patients who have had lung cancer and a history of smoking.

Palliation

Despite attempts at earlier diagnosis and more effective treatment, most people with lung cancer will die of their disease. The distress experienced by people with incurable lung cancer can be severe, and a wide range of symptoms and physical effects can be experienced, including weight loss, fatigue, functional decline, pain, cough, respiratory distress and impaired cognitive functioning (Hyde *et al.*, 1973; Hurny *et al.*, 1993; Sarna, 1993b; Cull *et al.*, 1994; Mercadante *et al.*, 1994; Sarna *et al.*, 1994; Hopwood & Stephens, 1995; Meyers *et al.*, 1995). Skilled and compassionate nurses and physicians caring for these patients can make a profound impact on symptom management and quality of life (McCorkle *et al.*, 1989).

In both developed and developing countries, a large burden of lung cancer deaths and the accompanying burden of care on the family and society have important implications for health-care policy. The loss of an increasing number of women from lung cancer will have a significant impact on the day-to-day structure of family lives (Sarna, 1993a). Like research funding for other cancers, that for lung cancer is directed primarily at the prevention, cause and treatment of this lethal disease, but for the majority of patients research is needed to maximize function, minimize distress due to symptoms and enhance the quality of life when there is no cure (WHO, 1990; Sarna & McCorkle, 1996). The research priorities for care must be valued to the same degree as those for cure. In 1990, WHO suggested a paradigm for palliative care and allocation of resources which may be applied to the care of lung cancer patients, for whom the need for resources for care increases as the prognosis worsens.

The issue of smoking cessation is more complicated when palliation is the goal. The data on the cost–benefit relationship in terms of symptoms or disease progression are limited (Sarna, 1995; Schoenbaum, 1997). In the face of the numerous losses experienced by patients with a life-threatening illness such as lung cancer, the loss of a familiar habit such as smoking can be significant.

Advocacy

Although a diagnosis of lung cancer can be a rallying cry for people who want to prevent this dreaded disease, unlike the cases of breast cancer and AIDS, there are few public forums for people affected by tobacco-related disease. Health-care professionals can assist interested patients and family members in moving from the role of 'victim' to 'advocate' for people with lung cancer. Despite the prevalence of mortality from this disease, no ribbons are worn or quilts made as a testimony. Blame may be focused on the patients rather than on the cause of their fatal illness, tobacco. ALCASE, an international coalition focused on the treatment and support of people living with lung cancer, may provide additional support. This unique programme offers education, support and an avenue for political advocacy for lung cancer patients which may affect health policy in the next century.

In conclusion, we have focused on the multiple challenges in caring for 'victims' of tobacco. Despite many encouraging scientific advances, the lung cancer epidemic demands compassionate palliative care for the majority of the people of the world,. Health professionals, especially nurses, can play a pivotal role in providing this care. It is to be hoped that the next century will bring more effective methods for early diagnosis and for treatment, but for now prevention is the key to cure.

References

Brundage, M.D. & Mackillop, W.J. (1996) Locally advanced non-small cell lung cancer: Do we know the questions? Survey of randomized trials from 1966–1993. *J. Clin. Epidemiol.*, **49**, 183–192

Cella, D.F., Bonomi, A.E., Lloyd, S.R., Tulsky, D.S., Kaplan, E. & Bonomi, P. (1995) Reliability and validity of the functional assessment of cancer therapy—lung (FACT-L) quality of life instrument. *Lung Cancer*, **12**, 199–220

Cull, A., Gregor, A., Hopwood, P., Macbeth, F. et al. (1994) Neurological and cognitive impairment in long-term survivors of small cell lung cancer. *Eur. J. Cancer*, 30A, 1067–1074

Faller, H., Schilling & Lang, H. 9!((%0 Causal attribution and adaptation among lung cancer patients. *J. Psychsom. Res.*, **39**, 619–627

Fiore, M.C., Bailey, W.C., Cohen, S.J. et al. (1996) *Smoking Cessation* (Clinical Practice Guideline No. 18, Publication No. 96–0692. 60), Rockville, Maryland, US Department of Health and Human Services, Agency for Health Care Policy and Research

Ganz, P.A., Figlin, R.A., Haskell, C.M., La Soto, N. & Siau, J. (1989) Supportive care versus supportive care and combination chemotherapy in metastatic non-small cell lung cancer. Does chemotherapy make a difference? *Cancer*, **63**, 1271–1278

Ganz, P.A., Lee, J.J. & Siau, J. (1991) Quality of life assessment: An independent prognostic variable for survival in lung cancer. *Cancer*, **67**, 3131–3135

Gritz, E.R. (1991) Smoking and smoking cessation in cancer patients. *Br. J. Addict.*, **86**, 549–554

Geddes, D.M., Dones, L., Hill, E., Law, K., Harper, P.G., Spiro, S.G., Tobias, J.S. & Souhami, R.L. (1990) Quality of life during chemotherapy for small cell lung cancer: Assessment and use of a daily diary card in a randomized trial. *Eur. J. Cancer*, **26**, 484–492

Hopwood, P. & Stephens, R.J. (1995) Symptoms at presentation for treatment in patients with lung cancer: Implications for the evaluation of palliative treatment. *Br. J. Cancer*, **71**, 633–636

Hurny, C., Bernhard, J., Joss, R., Schatzmann, E., Cavalli, F., Brunner, K., Alberto, P., Senn, H.J. & Metzger, U. (1993) 'Fatigue and malaise' as a quality-of-life indicator in small-cell lung cancer patients. *Support Care Cancer*, **1**, 316–320

Hyde, L., Wolf, J., McCracken, S. & Yesner, R. (1973) Natural course of inoperable lung cancer. *Chest*, **64**, 309–312

McCorkle, R., Benoliel, J.Q., Donaldson, G., Georgiadou, F., Moinpour, C. & Goodell, B. (1989) A randomized clinical trial of home nursing care for lung cancer patients. *Cancer*, **64**, 199–206

McVie, J.G. (1996) Non-small lung cancer: Meta-analysis of efficacy of chemotherapy. *Semin. Oncol.*, 23 (Suppl. 7), 12–16

Mercadante, S., Armata, M. & Salvaggio, L. (1994) Pain characteristics of advanced lung cancer patients referred to a palliative care service. *Pain*, **59**, 141–145

Meyers, C.A., Byrne, K.S. & Komaki, R. (1995) Cognitive deficits in patients with small cell lung cancer before and after chemotherapy. *Lung Cancer*, **12**, 231–235

Murray, C.J.L. & Lopez, A.D. (1996) The Global Burden of Disease, Vol. 1, Boston, Harvard University Press, pp. 117–200, 247–294, 325–396, 417

Parker, S.L., Tong, T., Bolden, S. & Wingo, P.A. (1997) Cancer statistics. *CA Cancer J. Clin.*, **47**, 5–27

Peto, R., Lopez, A.D., Boreham, J. et al. (1994) *Mortality in Relation to Smoking in Developed Countries, 1950–2000: Indirect Estimates from National Vital Statistics*, New York, Oxford University Press

Richardson, G.E., Tucker, M.A., Venzon, D.J., Linnoila, I., Phelps, R., Phares, J.C., Edison, M. & Ihde, D.C. (1993) Smoking cessation after successful treatment of small-cell lung cancer is associated with fewer smoking-related second primary cancers. *Ann. Intern. Med.*, **119**, 383–390

Sarna, L. (1993a) Women with lung cancer: Impact on quality of life. *Qual. Life Res.*, **2**, 13–22

Sarna, L. (1993b) Correlates of symptom distress in women with lung cancer. *Cancer Pract.*, **1**, 21–28

Sarna, L. (1995) Smoking behaviors of women after diagnosis with lung cancer. *Image*, **27**, 35–41

Sarna, L. & McCorkle, R. (1996) Burden of care and lung cancer. *Cancer Pract.*, **4**, 245–251

Sarna, L., Lindsey, A.M., Dean, H., Brecht, M.L. & McCorkle, R. (1994) Weight change and lung cancer: Relationships with symptom distress, functional status, and smoking. *Res. Nurs. Health*, **17**, 371–379

Schag, C.A.C., Ganz, P.A., Wing, D.S., Sim, M.S. & Lee, J.J. (1994) Quality of life in adult survivors of lung, colon and prostate cancer. *Qual. Life Res.*, **3**, 127–141

Schilling, A., Conaway, M.R., Wingate, P.J., Atkins, J.N., Berkowitz, I.M., Clamon, G.H., DiFino, S.M. & Vinciguerra, V. (1997) Recruiting cancer patients to participate in motivating their relatives to quit smoking. *Cancer*, **79**, 152–160

Schoenbaum, M. (1997) Do smokers understand the mortality effects of smoking? Evidence from the health and retirement survey. *Am. J. Public Health*, **87**, 755–759

Sell, L., Devlin, B., Bourke, S.J., Munro, N.C. et al. (1993) Communicating the diagnosis of lung cancer. *Respir. Med.*, **87**, 61–63

Strauss, G., DeCamp, M., Dibiccaro, E., Richards, W., Harpole, D., Healey, E. & Sugarbaker, D. (1995) Lung cancer diagnosis is being made with increasing frequency in former cigarette smokers. *Proc. Am. Soc. Clin. Oncol.*, **14**, 1106

US Department of Health, Education, and Welfare (1964) *Smoking and Health. Report of the Advisory Committee to the Surgeon General of the Public Health Service* (PHS pub.No. 1103), Washington DC: US Government Printing Office

WHO (1990) *Report of a WHO Expert Committee: Cancer Pain Relief and Palliative Care* (Technical Report Series 804), Geneva

Zang, E.A. & Wynder, E.L. (1996) Differences in lung cancer risk between men and women: Examination of the evidence. *J. Natl Cancer Inst.*, **88**, 183–192

Teaching about tobacco in medical schools

R. Richmond

School of Community Medicine, University of New South Wales, Sydney, Australia

The Tobacco Prevention Section of the International Union Against Tuberculosis and Lung Disease (IUATLD) consists of a Committee of representatives from many countries around the world. The aims of the Section are to stimulate the interest of medical students in tobacco control and influence teachers in medical schools to teach smoking and cessation techniques and to conduct a series of studies in medical schools. Two series of surveys have been conducted by the Tobacco Prevention Section. The first consisted of studies conducted in medical schools worldwide on the smoking behaviour, knowledge of and attitudes to tobacco smoking of medical students (Tessier et al., 1989, 1992a,b, 1993; Crofton et al., 1994)). The second is a worldwide survey on the education of medical students about tobacco (Richmond et al., 1997, 1998).

The objectives of this paper are to report on the smoking rates of medical students; their knowledge about smoking as a major cause of disease; whether they believe that they can counsel patients about smoking; the extent of teaching about tobacco, tobacco-related diseases and smoking cessation techniques to students in medical schools around the world and the barriers to and problems of getting teaching about tobacco onto the medical curriculum.

First series: International studies of medical students

The Tobacco Prevention Section of the IUATLD initiated international studies of first- and final-year medical students on their smoking rates, their knowledge about smoking as a major cause of disease and their attitudes to counselling patients about smoking. Surveys were conducted among more than 9000 students in 51 medical schools in 42 countries. The questionnaire used was developed by the IUATLD, WHO, the American Cancer Society and the International Union against Cancer.

The prevalence of smoking among medical students ranges from 0 to 48% for men and 0 to 22% for women. In Asia and Africa, the rates of smoking were lower among female than among male students. The lowest rates of smoking were in Australia, some European countries and the United States. The prevalence among medical students is lower than in the general population of their age and sex and among doctors in their countries. The rates are affected by the smoking behaviour and attitudes of their teachers and reflect the history of the tobacco epidemic and the national response to tobacco control. For example, in Australia, the United Kingdom and the United States, use of tobacco is long-standing, but much has been done in tobacco control, whereas in African and Asian countries tobacco use is more recent and counter-action is in its infancy.

The surveys of medical students' attitudes showed that most of those in their final year would advise their patients to quit smoking if they had a smoking-related disease, and most would advise quitting if the patient raised the subject of smoking. Few would advise all patients who smoked to quit, particularly if they had no smoking-related disease. Medical students who smoked were less serious than non-smoking students about advising patients who smoked to quit. Overall, the students did not appreciate the important responsibility that doctors have in disease prevention.

When students in their final year were asked whether they believed that they had sufficient knowledge about smoking cessation techniques, a positive response was given by 45% of students in medical schools in Africa and the Middle East, 29% of those in Asia, 27% in Europe, 16% in the countries of the former Soviet Union, 10% in Australia, 8% in the United States and 6% in Japan. The percentage of students who knew that coronary artery disease is a major result of smoking ranged from 11 to 43%. Of students in their final year, 62–100% in most countries knew that smoking causes lung cancer.

The exceptions were those in Japan and the Community of Independent States, where only 53 and 51%, respectively, had this knowledge. Chronic bronchitis was known to be caused by smoking by 57–84% of students, except in Japan, where only 35% were aware of the relationship. Pulmonary emphysema was known to be caused by smoking by 12–75% of students in most countries; the percentage was 67–75% in Australia, Chile and the United States. Peripheral vascular disease was known to be caused by smoking by only 4–45% o students, except in Australia where a higher percentage was found. Oral cancer was recognized as associated with tobacco use by 22–45% of the students, but only 3–7% knew that smokingwas related to neonatal death.

Although the results of these studies are almost 10 years old, they show that medical students have little knowledge of smoking as a major cause of diseases, even coronary artery disease, lung cancer and peripheral vascular disease. These results should pose a major challenge to medical educators around the world.

Second series: Worldwide survey on the education of medical students about tobacco

The objectives were to determine the extent of teaching about tobacco, tobacco-related diseases and smoking cessation techniques to students in medical schools around the world and to ascertain the barriers and problems of getting teaching about tobacco onto the medical curriculum. On the basis of the WHO Directory of Medical Schools, three mailings were made to 1353 medical schools in 1995. The questionnaires were translated into French, Japanese, Mandarin and Russian. Responses were received from 493 medical schools (36% response rate). Europe and the countries of the former Soviet Union had the highest response rate (45%), and the Middle East had the lowest (28%); the other geographic regions had similar response rates: Africa, 36%; Asia, 32%; Australia/Pacific, 36%; North America, 35%; and South America, 32% (Richmond et al., 1998).

Most medical schools give teaching about tobacco and related diseases at some level. Only 12% indicated that the topic was not covered at all in the curriculum, this percentage including almost one-fourth of the medical schools in Africa and Asia. Only 11% of the respondents indicated that they had a specific teaching module for tobacco issues. The commonest method of teaching about tobacco (58%) was non-systematic, the topic being mentioned during the teaching of other subjects. The other method of teaching about tobacco (40%) was by systematically integrating it with related modules, covering areas such as the health effects, health education and smoking cessation.

In courses on tobacco, 98% taught about major diseases related to tobacco use; 71% included pharmacological issues and the harmful components of tobacco smoke; 685 included the effects of passive smoking; 64% the psychology and physical addiction related to tobacco (70% in developed and 53% in developing countries); 39% taught smoking cessation techniques, including those delivered by doctors and 30% covered smoking by adolescents.

Among the medical schools that included tobacco in their curricula, 22% reported having had moderate to severe problems in introducing the topic. The commonest problems were difficulty in motivating students and lack of enthusiasm among staff. The latter problem was not helped by having smokers on the staff. Other problems were administrative, which included lack of cooperation and coordination between departments; lack of knowledge about training and teaching about tobacco-related diseases and cessation techniques; lack of government legislation restricting smoking in public places; and tobacco being the country's main cash crop.

Conclusions

Teachers in medical schools should counteract social pressures to smoke exerted by friends, the family and the mass media. They should present non-smoking models and actively educate medical students about tobacco-related diseases and smoking cessation techniques. Almost all (97%) of the medical schools expressed interest in obtaining a copy of the book, *Educating Medical Students about Tobacco: Planning and Implementation* (Richmond, 1997), which is a further initiative of the Tobacco Prevention section.

References

Crofton, J.W., Freour, P.P. & Tessier, J.F. (1994) Medical education on tobacco: Implications of a worldwide survey. *Med. Educ.*, **28**, 187–196

Richmond R., ed. (1997) *Educating Medical Students about Tobacco: Planning and Implementation.* Paris: International Union Against Tuberculosis and Lung Disease

Richmond, R., Larcos, D. & Debono, D. (1997) A worldwide survey of teaching about tobacco in medical schools. In: Richmond, R., ed., *Educating Medical Students about Tobacco: Planning and Implementation.* Paris: International Union Against Tuberculosis and Lung Disease, pp. 281–298

Richmond, R.L., Debono, D.S., Larcos, D. & Kehoe, L. (1998) Worldwide survey of education on tobacco in medical schools. *Tobacco Control* (in press)

Tessier, J.F., Freour, P.P., Crofton, J. & Kombou, L. (1989) Smoking habits and attitudes of medical students towards smoking and anti-smoking campaigns in fourteen European countries. *Eur. J. Epidemiol.*, **5**, 311–321

Tessier, J.F., Freour, P.P., Nejjari, C., Belougne, D. & Crofton, J. (1992a) Smoking behaviour and attitudes of medical students towards smoking and anti-smoking campaigns: A survey in ten African and Middle Eastern countries. *Tobacco Control*, **1**, 95–101

Tessier, J.F., Freour, P.P., Belougne, D. & Crofton, J. (1992b) Smoking habits and attitudes of medical students towards smoking and anti-smoking campaigns in nine Asian countries. *Int. J .Epidemiol.*, **21**, 298–304

Tessier, J.F., Freour, P.P., Nejjari, C., Belougne, D. & Crofton, J.W. (1993) Smoking behaviour and attitudes of medical students towards smoking and anti-smoking campaigns, in Australia, Japan, USA and the former USSR (Russia and Estonia). *Tobacco Control*, **2**, 24–29

Putting an end to tobacco use in hospitals:
A tribute to Dr Takeshi Hirayama

L.L. Fairbanks

Arizonans Concerned about Smoking, Tempe, Arizona, United States

" Smoke-free health care campuses must be the starting point of whole anti-smoking activities. I wish you would propose to the WHO, and to each country, that 100% of health care campuses in the world become smoke-free." (correspondence of September 1992 from Takeshi Hirayama). "A smoke-free medical centre protects both employees and patients from exposure to environmental tobacco smoke by lowering risks for lung cancer, breast cancer and ischaemic heart disease, and by protecting babies and children from getting pulmonary disease." (Takeshi Hirayama, Ninth World Conference on Tobacco or Health, 1994).

The large-scale prospective population studies conducted by Dr Hirayama in Japan between 1965 and 1982 were of worldwide significance. They showed a clear-cut dose–response relationship between the number of cigarettes smoked and the risk of lung cancer among active smokers. Even more noteworthy was the epidemiological evidence about the hazards of 'passive smoking' (Hirayama, 1981, 1983). Tobacco smoking could no longer be considered merely as an addictive personal habit for individuals. By applying Boyle's Law (which describes how gas diffuses immediately to fill an enclosed space), smoke in the air was shown to be a community public health problem, harming those who share an enclosed air space with a smoker. The large-scale prospective study conducted in six prefectures in Japan between 1965 and 1982 included 265 118 adults (122 261 males and 142 857 females) (Hirayama & Hoel, 1985; Hirayama, 1987).

Dr Hirayama reported that the most noteworthy findings of the study were the significant risks of cancers of the lung, nasal sinus, breast and brain and leukaemia and ischaemic heart disease among non-smoking wives of smoking husbands (Table 1).

Table 1. Relative risks for selected causes of death among non-smoking wives due to their husbands' smoking habits; cohort study in Japan, 1966–81

Cause of death	Husbands' cigarette consumption			Mantel-extension chi	One-tailed p
	Non-smoker	1–19 daily	≥ 20 daily		
Cancer					
Lung	1.00	1.11	1.21	3.143	0.000
Nasal	1.00	1.44	1.90	2.990	0.001
Sinus	1.00	2.28	3.29	2.064	0.019
Brain	1.00	4.01	4.78	2.069	0.019
Breast	1.00	1.12	1.73	1.795	0.036
Leukaemia	1.00	1.79	2.04	2.009	0.022
Ischaemic heart disease	1.00	1.14	1.31	2.164	0.015
Subarachnoid haemorrhage	1.00	1.52	1.69	1.846	0.032
Cerebral haemorrhage	1.00	1.31	1.25	2.680	0.036
Suicide	1.00	1.34	1.46	2.030	0.021
All causes	1.00	1.15	1.19	5.449	0.000

In the United States in the early 1980s, as we moved forwards from the embarrassment of unhealthy tobacco smoke-filled hospitals to totally smoke-free hospitals, reports on the hazards of passive smoking from several other countries were helpful to us. None, however was as helpful and well-publicized as the epidemiological evidence reported by Dr Hirayama. Dr Hirayama and Dr Martin Kawano of Japan were both very supportive of our early efforts, under the Surgeon-General Dr C. Everett Koop, to eliminate smoking in all public places by the year 2000 (Koop, 1985) and not only create smoke-free hospitals (Welty et al., 1987) but avoid captive, involuntary smoking anywhere in any public location with shared airspace (see Department of Health and Human Services, 1986).

We defeat our credibility as health-care professionals if we allow staff, patients and visitors to commit slow suicide anywhere in hospitals grounds, on health-care campuses and near entrances. This is a realistic standard and can be achieved with good education and good planning and by providing smoking cessation support to smokers, as shown by the leadership of the Mayo Clinic and its affiliated hospitals in Rochester, Minnesota, Jacksonville, Florida, amd Scottsdale, Arizona, and of other health-related organizations. Smoke-free campuses, both indoors and outdoors, are a realistic, attainable and effective goal in health promotion and help in addiction control and treatment (Offord et al., 1992; Hurt, 1997). As smoking is a major contributor to air pollution in shared airspace, it cannot be allowed in a safe workplace (Stillman et al., 1990; Environmental Protection Agency, 1992).

Smoking in public is not a right (Banzhaf, 1985). Several international groups have recognized that smoke-free hospitals must be role models if we are to be credible in helping other segments of society to control tobacco use. One such resource organization is the International Network towards Smoke-free Hospitals in the United Kingdom.

At an international symposium in Kita-Kyushu, Japan, after the Sixth World Conference in Tokyo in 1987, the following 10 goals were endorsed (Kawano, 1997):
1. Leaders of all kinds should set a good example to young people by not smoking.
2. Education on smoking should be started at an early age and continued to protect children from the habit of smoking.
3. All advertising and promotion of cigarettes should be banned.
4. All vending machines for cigarettes should be banned.
5. Smoking should be eliminated in schools, hospitals, government buildings and all other public places.
6. Non-smoking policies should be established in the workplace.
7. Smoking should be banned from all forms of transportation.
8. Non-smokers, children in particular, must be protected from cigarette smoke.
9. Clear, definite warnings should be printed on the packages of tobacco.
10. Taxes on tobacco products should be raised periodically.

Progress towards achieving these goals will vary by country, depending on cultural circumstances. There could be no more fitting tribute to Dr Hirayama and his work than for us to endorse these goals and work vigorously until they are achieved. A prospective study in the United States confirms the finding of Hirayama that passive smoking contributes not only to cancer and respiratory disease but also to heart disease (Kawachi *et al.*, 1997).

A leader in pointing out the causal relationship between passive smoking and heart disease and the efforts of the tobacco industry to hide this connection is Dr Stanton Glantz of the University of California at San Francisco (Glantz & Parmley, 1995). At the Sixth World Conference in Tokyo, Dr Glantz led the audience in a standing ovation to thank and pay tribute to the pioneering work of Dr Takeshi Hirayama.

References

Banzhaf, J.F., III (1985) Public smoking is not a right. *ASH Smoking Health Rev.*, 11
Department of Health and Human Services (1986) *The Health Consequences of Involuntary Smoking; A Report of the Surgeon General*, Atlanta, Centers for Disease Control
Environmental Protection Agency (1992) *Respiratory Health Effects of Passive Smoking: Lung Cancer and Other Disorders*, Washington DC, Indoor Air Division, Office of Atmospheric and Indoor Air Pollution and Indoor Air Programs, Office of Air and Radiation
Glantz, S.A. & Parmley, W.W. (1995) Passive smoking and heart disease. *J. Am. Med. Assoc.*, 273, 1047–1053
Hirayama, T. (1981) Non-smoking wives of heavy smokers have a higher risk of lung cancer: A study from Japan. *Br. Med. J.*, 282, 183–185
Hirayama, T. (1983) Passive smoking and lung cancer, consistency of association. *Lancet*, ii, 1425–1426
Hirayama, T. (1987) *Gann Monogr.*, 33, 127–135
Hirayama, T. (1988) Health effects of active and passive smoking. In: Aoki, M. *et al.*, eds, *Smoking and Health, 1987*, Amstrdam, Elsevier, pp. 75–86
Hirayama, T. (1995) Epidemiology of tobacco in Asia. In: Slama, K., ed., *Tobacco and Health, 1995*, New York, Plenum Press, pp. 247–250
Hirayama, T. & Hoel, D.G., eds (1985) *Statistical Methods in Cancer Epidemiology*, Hiroshima, Radiation Effects Research Fopundation, pp. 73–91
Hurt, R.D. (1997) Toward smoke-free medical facilities (editorial). *Chest*, 1027–1028
Kawachi, I. et al. (1997) A prospective study of passive smoking and coronary heart disease. *Circulation*, 95, 2374–2379
Kawano, M. (1997) *The Cloud and the Light* (English edition translated from 1993 Japanese edition), Notre Dame, Indiana, Cross Cultural Publication, p. 218
Koop, C.E. (1985) A Smoke Free Society by the Year 2000. *New York J. Med.*, 290–292
Offord, K.P., Hurt, R.D., Berge, K.G., Frusti, D.K. & Schmidt, L. (1992) Effects of the implementation of a smoke-free policy in a medical center. *Chest*, 102, 1531–1536
Stillman, F.A., Becker, D.M., Swank, R.T., Hantula, D., Moses, H. & Glantz, S. (1990) Ending smoking at the Johns Hopkins medical institutions: An evaluation of smoking prevalence and indoor air pollution. *J. Am. Med. Assoc.*, 264, 1565–1569
Welty, T.K., Tanaka, E.S., Leonard, B., Rhoades, E.R., Hulburt, W.B. & Fairbanks, L. (1987) Indian health service facilities become smoke-free. *J. Am. Med. Assoc.*, 258, 185

Changes in tobacco habits and attitudes to tobacco prevention among Swedish dental personnel, 1991–96

E. Uhrbom

Dentistry against Tobacco, Department of Preventive Dentistry, Public Dental Health Service, Falun, Sweden

Why 'Dentistry against Tobacco'? The oral cavity is the principal target for both smoke and snuff. If a person smokes 20 cigarettes a day for 20 years, for a total of about 150 000 cigarettes, and each cigarette represents 15 puffs through the mouth down into the lungs and then out again, the oral cavity will be exposed more than 4 million times during the 20-year period. If a person places snuff under his or her upper lip for 6 h per day, which is not unusual in Sweden, especially among young men, the oral cavity will be exposed for a total of five years during a 20-year period.

As dentists are experts in examining the mouth and related structures, we are well placed to recognize early signs of abnormal changes. Even if those changes do not always cause oral cancer, we have a good opportunity to show the lesions to patients in a mirror and ask them what they think might be happening to the unprotected tissues of the lungs.

Another reason for Dentistry against Tobacco is the contact we have with the population. People see dental practitioners routinely more frequently then they see other health professionals. In Sweden, we regularly see about 85% of the adult population and nearly all of the population under the age of 20. Furthermore, dental personnel have long experience with prevention, changing patients' behaviour to a healthier pattern. Finally, we are regarded as health authorities by our patients.

The Swedish association 'Dentistry against Tobacco' was founded in May 1992 and consists of dentists, dental hygienists and dental assistants. We have more than 300 individual members, all of the public health organizations in Sweden's 24 counties and the largest organization for private practitioners. Thus, we are in regular contact with about 10 000 Swedish dental personnel. These organizations distribute a periodical to their members four times a year which gives information from our association. In Sweden, there are also associations of doctors, nurses, teachers and pharmacists against tobacco, and we have established a common organization, 'Health Professionals against Tobacco', comprising about 1500 members, which has become a powerful influence on Swedish politicians.

In order to obtain more information about smoking habits and attitudes towards tobacco prevention among Swedish dental personnel, we conducted two surveys, in 191 and 1996, by postal questionnaire. For each study, 1000 dentists, 1000 dental hygienists and 1000 dental assistants were chosen randomly to receive the questionnaire, which elicited information on occupation, age, sex, tobacco habits and attitudes to tobacco prevention. The response rates in the two surveys were 90 and 85%.

In 1991, the prevalence of smoking was 13% among dentists and 17% among both dental hygienists and dental assistants. In 1996, the prevalence had decreased significantly, from 13 to 8% among dentists, from 17 to 10% among dental hygienists and from 17 to 13% among dental assistants. This decrease is crucial, as our patients regard us as health models; it is difficult to give advice to patients when you smell of tobacco and have yellow fingers. No difference in the prevalence of snuffing was seen: about 8% were daily snuffers, almost all among male dentists.

Regular questioning about tobacco habits was reported by about 30% of the dentists in 1991 and 50% in 1996; the corresponding figures for dental hygienists were 68 and 82%.

In 1996, we asked some questions about problems encountered in counselling tobacco users. The most frequent problem was lack of training in tobacco prevention. Few said that tobacco prevention was not a matter for dentistry, and a minority was concerned about 'worrying their patients'. When asked for ideas to improve tobacco prevention in daily practice, most wanted folders for themselves and pamphlets for thie patients. The dental hygienists also asked for seminars on tobacco prevention.

In conclusion, we found a positive trend in tobacco habits among Swedish dental personnel and an increasing interest in giving advice about tobacco in daily practice. The survey in 1996 also shows a demand for further improvement. These surveys show that dental personnel are a valuable supplement to other health professionals in reducing tobacco use.

World Dentistry against Tobacco

O. Akerberg

Center for Public Health, Mariestad, Sweden

The association World Dentistry against Tobacco was first discussed at the Eighth World Conference on Tobacco or Health in 1992. At that time we were six dentists; now we reach more than 500 000 dentists around the world.

Dentists are well placed to conduct tobacco control, as in most countries dentists see most children and adolescents about once a year; they have long experience in prevention, for example in preventing dental caries; and the consequences of tobacco use on dental and oral health are easy to recognize, especially with use of smokeless tobacco, where the effects on the oral mucosa can be devastating.

The involvement of dental services in tobacco prevention and counselling differs markedly from country to country, ranging from nothing to highly skilled work. In the United States, the dental profession has been working strategically against tobacco use for many years. A manual on tobacco prevention for use by dentists was published in the United States in 1989 and was accompanied by the formation of a national dental tobacco-free steering committee. Japan has had a Medical–Dental Association for Tobacco Control for many years, and in Finland dentists now belong to Doctors against Tobacco.

We found after discussions that there were many advantages to forming an international network for the dental profession's work against tobacco as a section within the Féderation Dentaire International, which was formed in Paris in 1900. This Federation groups 112 national dental associations, 24 dental and other health organizations and about 30 000 individual members. The eight sections of the Federation are organized for individual members with common interests. A section representing World Dentistry against Tobacco was formed in 1995, at the annual World Dental Congress, and an agenda for action was adopted. One of the goals was "... to make it possible for every dentist in the world to, as a professional, work with tobacco prevention and counselling and thus diminish the number of tobacco-related deaths in the world."

The section also wished to form the basis for work against tobacco by the dental profession throughout the world, and a position statement was adopted at the World Dental Conference in 1996. This document involves all of the Federation's associations and individual members, comprising more than 500 000 dentists. Furthermore, although the Federation is a dentists' group, the position statement recognizes and gives responsibility for work against tobacco use to 'all oral health professionals'. In many countries, dental hygienists are at the forefront in counselling and cessation services. The position statement on tobacco covers daily practice, education, protection of children and prevention of initiation and stipulates that all the congresses, educational programmes, business meetings and head office of the Federation must be smoke-free. World Dentistry against Tobacco also organizes scientific programmes for exchange of knowledge and experience at every World Dental Congress.

Dental patients can be helped to achieve a tobacco-free life in many ways. Demonstrating the oral consequences of tobacco use, such as stained teeth, periodontitis and halitosis, are as effective as the fear of cancer in motivating people to eliminate the habit. merely being asked about their tobacco habits and being made aware of the consequences of smoking may make many dental patients think about quitting. Of course, we should set a good example for our patients. In 1949, over half of all doctors and dentists were smokers; in the United States, the number of dentist smokers has fallen steadily, so that by 1994 the prevalence was only 7%. In Sweden, the percentage of dentists who smoke regularly decreased from 13% in 1991 to 8% in 1996.

The dental profession is making a growing contribution to slowing the tobacco pandemic. Their contribution is important in many developing countries where various forms of smokeless tobacco are used, creating serious medical problems. Working with tobacco prevention and cessation services improves the quality of the work of oral health professionals and provides an opportunity to reach new patients seeking advice on stopping smoking. As health professionals, we should participate in the public debate that shapes community tobacco policies and improves education on tobacco use. In working against the tobacco pandemic, oral health professionals will improve the overall health of their patients.

Habits and opinions about smoking among health professionals in Denmark

T. Clement

The Danish Council on Smoking and Health, Copenhagen, Denmark

The percentage of daily smokers in Denmark decreased in the period 1989–96 among doctors from 24 to 19%, among nurses from 29 to 22% and among midwives from 30 to 22%, in comparison with 44 and 33% of the general population.

The Danish Council on Smoking and Health (established in 1988) has appointed health professionals as key persons in campaigns on smoking issues. It was therefore necessary to study the smoking habits and knowledge on smoking in this target group. The study was carried out in 1989 and repeated in 1996.

The questionnaire contained about 25 questions and was mailed to 1000 health professionals in each group.

The Danish Council on Smoking and Health calls on other countries to carry out similar studies in order to organize a multinational study. The questionnaire is available in English and can be ordered from the Council.

New approach to improving the effectiveness of anti-smoking interventions in primary health care

W.K. Drygas & W. Sapiński

Department of Social and Preventive Medicine, Medical University, Lodz, Poland

Non-communicable diseases such as coronary heart disease, hypertension, neoplasms, diabetes and liver diseases are closely related to lifestyle and pose a major threat to the European population, in which 70–80% of all deaths are attributed to diseases that could be treated or even prevented. Unfortunately, few doctors in many countries are really involved in effective disease prevention and health promotion.

The situation is especially bad in many countries of central and eastern Europe. In contrast to most countries of the European Union, the rates of premature death and 'man-made' diseases are increasing steadily, leading to a dramatic health gap between western and eastern European countries. The average life expectancy of men is about 58 years in Estonia and 57 years in the Russian Federation, while in 1970s and 1980s, these values were 66–67 years. Life expectancy in Poland is 67.5 years for men and 75.5 years for women. In sharp contrast, the life expectancy in countries of the European Union is 73–75 years for men and 80–82 years for women. Risk factors like heavy smoking, bad nutrition, heavy alcohol consumption, overweight and obesity and lack of adequate physical activity are recorded frequently in population surveys in central and eastern Europe. Thus, it is not surprising that the rates of coronary heart disease, hypertension, stroke, lung cancer and liver cirrhosis in this region are extremely high.

Physicians working in primary health care can have a strong influence on the health behaviour of a population. These doctors, who see patients from three to six times a year, are in a privileged position to monitor and positively affect many of the risk factors responsible for the high rates of morbidity and premature death. Unfortunately, most primary health-care physicians are mainly involved in routine curative work and have little motivation or time to address their patients' smoking and alcohol habits or control their blood pressure or lipid concentration. Thus, simple disorders such as sore throats, colds, stomach aches and sprains, which are usually not life-threatening, are well diagnosed and treated, while serious diseases such as lipid disorders, hypertension, early phases of coronary heart disease and diabetes, and their risk factors, including smoking, are not identified or managed.

In Poland, as in the United Kingdom, most primary health care physicians see 30 or more patients per day, for a short time (in the United Kingdom, the average visit lasts 7–8 min). Although many doctors are overwhelmed with routine activities, they could devote some time to disease prevention and health promotion. The necessary prerequisite is that these additional activities do not take too much time and the financial incentive is attractive and adequate to cover the extra work.

Aim of the project
The aim of our project is to strengthen the preventive and health promotion activities of primary health-care doctors. The steps involved are preparing a system of financial incentives; preparing the organizational framework, including investigation methods, financial resources, administration and data management; estimating the direct and indirect costs for implementation; implementation of the project in selected region(s) in a pilot study; a cost–benefit analysis and implementation of the project in other regions if the health benefits and economic evaluation justify such a decision.

Because of the complexity of the project and its time limits, we present only the preliminary assumptions and proposed methods.

Methods
Many different methods are used to motivate professionals to intensify or change their methods of work. Experiences in other countries and cultures indicate that the best method of motivating doctors to enhance their activities is a target-orientated financial incentive. The system of incentives should take into account not only the quantity of preventive work but also its quality and effectiveness. The population covered by the project and the methods of surveying health behaviour should be well defined, in line with international standards and guidelines. The doctors and other health professionals involved, such as nurses and technical assistants, should receive clear instructions and the necessary training. Data sampling, analysis and the methods of administration and management should be well prepared. The educational materials for patients should be carefully selected.

Although many preventive activities are important, efforts should be concentrated on well-defined risk factors. The choice should be made on the basis of: relevance, whether diagnosis is possible, reliable and simple, whether intervention is possible and cost-effective and whether the effects are measurable and can be achieved in a relatively short time. The risk factors chosen should be universal, i.e. responsible for many diseases, including coronary heart disease, common neoplasms and other man-made diseases responsible for high morbidity rates and premature death. We suggest that the scope of the intervention be limited to the following factors:
- smoking (the most important single risk factor),
- hypertension,
- cholesterol, high- and low-density lipproteins and triglycerides,
- obesity and excess weight,
- physical inactivity,
- alcohol consumption and
- poor nutrition.

For women, simple breast tumour screening might be included. Many published studies indicate that these options are the best buys in public health today.

The next important question is the number, age and sex of the population selected. From the point of view of health economics, it seems reasonable to restrict the study to middle-aged men, who are the most threatened by these risk factors of premature death; however, if the financial resources are adequate and for both ethical reasons and pragmatic considerations (women influence the nutritional and other habits and leisure time of the family), both men and women aged 25–55 will be included in the project.

The proposed system of incentives is shown in Table 1. Theoretically, the maximum score a doctor may achieve for effective intervention (as opposed to treatment) in patients with all of the risk factors being analysed is $5 + 5 + 2 + 18 = 30$ points. As most patients have only one to three risk factors, the total number of points per patient will be 12–18. The bonus would be US$ 0.2 per point in middle- to low-income countries. If the bonus system is accepted in countries in this category, such as the Czech Republic, Estonia, Hungary, Poland and Slovakia, the bonus for effective prevention could be US$ 1200–2500 per year, or 25–60% of the regular salary of primary health-care doctors. The bonuses could represent up to 20–25% of the regular salary of nurses and assistants.

Cost analysis

Both direct and indirect costs will be included in the cost analysis of the project. Apart from the financial incentives for the doctors and other medical professionals involved, the direct costs necessary to implement should cover: training of the staff involved, educational resources for the patients (leaflets, booklets), mailing, printing of check-up cards and surveys, data sampling and analysis, hardware and software, administration, management and laboratory costs for cholesterol determinations.

Preliminary analysis of the direct costs for the 15 000 patients enrolled in the project indicate that US$ 90 000–100 000 will be necessary to implement it in Poland, assuming a direct cost per patient per year of US$ 6.0–6.6. About 50% of all direct costs are for the financial incentives for the health professionals. It is diffciult to calculate the indirect costs, such as for medication and additional medical services for the patients in the programme.

Time scale

If the preliminary results are positive, the study should be continued for at least three to five years to allow analysis of the long-term health changes in risk factors and morbidity and mortality rates and an economic evaluation of the project. The proposed system of incentives for preventive activities may represent a stable bonus system for general practitioners. Because the salaries of physicians in Poland and in some other central and eastern European countries are very low, the system of incentives might be included in the reform of the payment system in primary health care in these countries.

Table 1. Principles of proposed incentive system for primary health care physicians

Intervention	Bonus (no. of points)
Bonuses for activities	
First examination (analysis of risk factors and advice)	5
Last examination (analysis of risk factors)	5
Any other visits	1–2 per visit
Bonuses for effectiveness (on the grounds of comparsion of risk factors at first and last visits)	
Quitting smoking	1–5
Reduction in blood pressure	1–3
Reduction in cholesterol	1–3
Reduction in body weight and body mass index	1–3
Reduction in alcohol consumption	max. 2
Increase in physical activity	max. 1
Improvement in nutrition	max. 1

Doctors' opinions about education for smoking control in Nairobi, 1996

B. Fiévez, W. Lore, H. de Vries & H. Adriaanse

Faculty of Health Sciences, University of Maastricht, Maastricht, Netherlands

As doctors are seen as role models by their patients, it is important that they give their patients education on smoking control. We examined the extent to which 82 doctors in Nairobi, Kenya, were advising those of their patients who smoked to quit and their opinions about this activity. This information was obtained by distributing a questionnaire based on a model designed by H. de Vries, which assumes that behaviour is influenced by intention, barriers and skills and indirectly by attitude, social influences and self-efficacy through intention.

In order to determine differences or correlations between the respondents, demographic variables were collected: 33% were Protestant, 64% lived in the city, 58% were specialists and 67% were black. Statistical analysis was performed with the t test, with a significance level of 5%. Of the 82 respondents, 73% were male, of whom nine were smokers; none of the 22 female doctors smoked.

Almost all the doctors (95%) advised their patients to stop smoking, and 53% provided information on smoking cessation, but 40% thought that their efforst would have no results and 50% said that their patients would probably not respond to smoking control education. The majority (71%) considered that they had sufficient knowledge to counsel patients on quitting smoking.

The only significant difference between doctors who never provided smoking control education and those who did was social support. Those who did educate their patients had the support of partners, colleagues, friends and associations. A supportive environment could be created by increasing the role of the Government, for instance by advertising on television and radio, and of medical boards and universities and by organizing a conference on smoking control education.

Developing the contribution of health professionals to smoking cessation

M. Raw[1], A. McNeill[2], L. Owen[2] & K. Aston[2]

[1] Kings College School of Medicine and Dentistry, University of London, and
[2] Health Education Authority, London, United Kingdom

In spite of good published evidence that health professionals can help smokers to stop by routinely giving advice and support, they still have not integrated smoking cessation advice into their clinical routines. There are many reasons for this, structural and motivational, including lack of time, skills and confidence and a failure of the health system to make smoking cessation a priority, despite the huge costs of smoking. The Health Education Authority is developing an integrated programme to increase the involvement of health professionals in giving smoking cessation advice and support. The programme includes providing clinical guidance, evidence of the cost–effectiveness of smoking cessation for smokers, assessing training and education needs and opportunities and developing a strategic, integrated approach to cessation at the community level.

The problem

Health professionals in the United Kingdom can get support from training (for example, *Helping People Change*[Mason *et al.*, 1993]) and leaflets (especially from the Health Education Authority, a Government agency), but this support is fragmented. It is not based on a strategic overview or on consensus and is not integrated in routine professional practice. For example, whether practice nurses receive training in cessation counselling depends on the attitudes and budgets of their employers and funding for locum replacements, on whether there is a suitable course near them and if they hear about it.

Various data sources (Health Education Authority, 1996; Bolling & Owen, 1997; Owen & McNeill, 1997) suggest that the situation may be getting worse, that general practitioners are even less likely to offer advice and support to smokers who wish to stop than they were several years ago. There is also evidence that the same is true of midwives, and that many advise women to cut down rather than stop, thus decreasing attempts to stop by pregnant women. Another survey showed that health professionals oversestimate the extent to which they routinely give advice to smokers.

There are several key reasons why smoking cessation is still not part of routine care in the British health-care system. Most health professionals are still not obliged to do so; others consider that they do not have the confidence or skills and cannot take time for training; others do not see it as part of clinical medicine; and many health professionals simply plead lack of time. Furthermore, the message given by the regulatory authorities undermines the seriousness of smoking as a problem; for example, a proven treatment, vicotine replacement therapy, is not reimbursed.

There is thus a clear need to improve the quality and quantity of advice and support given to smokers through the health-care system. Not only better training and resources but also changed attitudes, new structures and more logical strategic planning are needed.

Solutions

The Health Education Authority in England is developing a number of interrelated projects to address these problems. They are supporting two large projects to improve the quality and quantity of smoking cessation advice and support given by health professionals to smokers in the course of their routine work, and to influence health-care purchasers to buy smoking cessation interventions. Further plans are to look at the implications of these projects for training—basic, postgraduate and professional—and for integrated cessation services at community level.

Smoking cessation guidelines for the use of health professionals are being developed on the basis of the best evidence available for good practice and drawing on the work of the United States Department of Health's Agency for Health Care Policy and Research (Fiore *et al.*, 1996). Formal endorsement of these guidelines will be sought from the professions, and we hope that they will play an active role in adapting and promoting them to their own professionals.

Guidelines for action have been available for two decades or more; Russell *et al.* in 1979 showed the potential of simple advice given by general practitioners for achieveing wothwhile rates of smoking cessation. Yet, our surveys indicaqte that such advice has not been integrated into routine clinical practice. One of the aims of our second project was to address structural factors.

Many providers of health care are now bound by contracts with purchasrs. Although this system will be changed in England to promote more cooperation between commissioners and providers, the need to balance budgets will not change; we must still get the best value for money to achieve gains in population health. The second project will provide health authorities with data on the cost–effectiveness of various smoking cessation interventions, so that they will be incorporated into service provision contracts. The evidence will permit local health authorities to choose from a range of interventions and show them that smoking cessation is extremely cost–effective in producing health gain in comparison with other health interventions.

The two projects combine 'bottom-up' and 'top-down approaches: more and better guidance for health professionals on how to intervene and influencing the content of purchasing contracts with evidence of what works and is cost–effective. We shall do this by reviewing current practice, both through the literature and by consulting professionals, reviewing purchase contracts and the processes that determine their content, looking at the resources currently available, including training, and then working with the professions to develop and disseminate new cessation guidelines.

The Health Education Authority will be working with as many relevant professions as possible, including the Royal College of Physicians, the National Pharmaceutical Association, the Community Practitioners and Health Visitors Association, the Faculty of dental Practitioners, the Royal College of General Practitioners, the British Medical Association, the Royal College of Midwives, the Royal College of Obstetrics and Gynaecology and the Royal College of Nurses.

Resources will also have to be made available to back up health professionals, including training, to be determined with the professions. We must examine the organization of cessation services in the community. The need for staff to receive support and motivation to intervene more implies the development of a strategic, integrated plan to deliver smoking cessation support throughout local communities, involving all relevant parts of the health system and support from smoking policies in work and public places.

References

Bolling, K. & Owen, K. (1997) *Smoking and Pregnancy. A Survey of Knowledge, Attitudes and Behaviour,* London: Health Education Authority

Fiore, M., Bailey, W.C., Cohen, S.J., *et al.* (1996) *Smoking Cessation* (Clinical Practice Guideline No. 18; AHCPR Publication No. 96-0692), Washington DC: US Department of Health and Human Services

Health Education Authority (1996) *National Adult Smoking Campaign. Health Professionals,* London

Mason, P., Hunt, P., Raw, M. & Sills, M. (1993) *Helping People Change. A Training Course for Primary Health Care Professionals,* London: Health Education Authority

Owen, L. & McNeill, A. (1997) Trends in smoking and pregnancy: 1992–1997. Is there a role for health professionals in reducing smoking in pregnancy? (submitted for publication)

Russell, M., Wilson, C.., Taylor, C. & Baker, C. (1979) Effect of general practitioners' advice against smoking. *Br. Med. J.,* ii, 231–235

Role of paediatricians and obstetricians in preventing and combating tobacco smoking

J. Szymborski[1], W. Zatonski[2] & B. Chazan[2]

[1] National Research Institute for the Mother and Child and [2] Department of Epidemiology, Cancer Centre and Institute of Oncology, Warsaw, Poland

Prenatal and postnatal health care at counselling centres and hospitals in Poland involves tobacco control efforts during a number of visits. At the first visit of an expectant mother, background information is obtained, and the woman is given information about the consequences of cigarette smoking and assistance is she has stopped smoking. Women at high risk are given assistance and are monitored. At subsequent visits, assistance and advice is given to women who have stopped smoking. Those who have not are advised of the importance of involving their partners and close friends in helping them to quit. They are given information and shown the embryo's movements on ultrasound monitors. During the visit at the third trimester or in hospital, their anti-smoking attitude is consolidated and they are given assistance in coping with stress and provided with information about the harmful effects of tobacco smoke.

The role of paediatricians in preventing and combatting tobacco smoking involves a number of activities. They should be aware of the risk associated with tobacco smoking in each age group, ask questions about exposure to cigarette smoke and smoking, advise parents on how to stop smoking and advise children how to avoid starting and plan follow-up visits, if necessary.

Anti-tobacco activities for children aged 0–4 involve anticipating exposure of babies and young children to tobacco smoke by asking about smoking at home, in kindergarten and in preschool; advising parents on how to stop smoking by telling them about the effects of tobacco smoke on children's health and assisting them to quit by providing educational materials and advice. The activities of paediatricians for children aged 5–12 should anticipate the first experimentation with smoking by carrying out preventive activities with the children and their parents; they should ask about smoking by the child, brothers and sisters and parents and about anti-tobacco programmes at school. They should advise children not to start smoking, help them to say 'No' to smokers and help both children and parents to stop smoking. Frequent visits should be planned for children who have tried smoking cigarettes.

Anti-tobacco activities for children aged 13–19 include anticipating that many youngsters in this age group will have tried smoking. A good paediatrician–patient contact is necessary, so that information about the harmful effects of smoking can be given. Questions should be asked about the patient's smoking habits, opinions on a healthy lifestyle and school anti-tobacco programmes. They should give advice to non-smoking patients, raise awareness of the influence of the media and advertising, and emphasize the right to say 'No'. Smokers should be given assistance in quitting and anti-tobacco programmes. The paediatrician might visit the patient's school and environment.

An approach by community physicians to quitting smoking

D.Y. Yan[1] & L.Q. Cheng[2]

[1]*Chinese Academy of Preventive Medicine and* [2]*Dong Cheng Epidemic Station, Beijing, China*

Abstract

In order to promote quitting activities in communities, we developed a kind of voluntary contract between smokers and physicians in a community in Beijing. Doctors responsible for primary health care gave regular health education programmes and monitored smokers who had entered into a contract to quit. Data were obtained during 1992–94 for 340 smokers with an average consumption of 13 cigarettes per day; 53% of the smokers were retired. After personal education sessions, 65 smokers succeeded in stopping (19%) and 187 reduced their consumption (55%). The results suggest that this method is successful, especially among older persons.

Introduction

All hospitals in large cities in China have a community health department, in which the physicians are responsible for disease prevention and public health services. Each physician is in charge of the health care of 2500–4000 residents. We conducted a pilot study to determine whether community doctors could participate in smoking control through voluntary contracts with smokers.

Methods

The target population was selected by oral communications from doctors and community leaders. The physicians interviewed smokers to determine their attitudes and behaviour and selected those who wished to cooperate with doctors and would accept supervision and consultation. The doctors then informed the smokers about the hazards of their habit, the importance of quitting and the meaning of the contract. They gave each smoker a contract signed by both the smoker and the doctor, and also educational material. They then trained them in methods for quitting, such as making a resolution, selecting a date for quitting, drinking a cup of tea or eating instead of smoking and taking exercise. The doctors made home visits every three months and provided advice and encouragement; they kept a record of these visits.

Results

Of the 340 people who signed a contract, 292 did so in 1992, 43 in 1993 and five in 1994; a total of 23 smokers withdrew from the study, 10 in 1993 and 13 in 1994. The age distribution is shown in Table 1. Most of the participants were elderly. Women comprised 28% of the population. Table 2 shows that most of the particpants were retired, cadres and housewives. The participants had smoked for 1–74 years, for an average of 33 years. The number of cigarettes smoked per day varied from 1 to 50, with an average of 13.

Table 2. Distribution of occupations of participants in a quit campaign, 1992–94

Occupation	Male	Female	Total
Student	1		1
Worker	59	3	62
Cadre	73	2	75
Retired	102	38	140
Housewife		43	43
Other	9	10	19

After the intervention, to of the participants (60 men and 17 women) stopped smoking, but six men and one woman (11%) relapsed subsequently, so that the rate of quitting was 19%. A reduction in the number of cigarettes smoked was achieved by 187 persons (55%; 141 men and 46 women). The extent of reduction was associated with the number of follow-up visits that had been paid by the doctor.

Conclusion

The method of establishing a contract between smokers and community physicians appears to be effective in helping them to quit and is acceptable to the population. Other surveys in the same district showed a quitting rate of only 3–8%, whereas we achieved a rate of 19%. The reasons for our success may include the fact that older people suffer from a number of disorders and accept the opinion of doctors; community physicians have a good relationship with the residents, and they can visit the families and provide practical advice.

Integrating tobacco education and provider advice into clinical practice in community-orientated primary care settings

D.I. Bahrs

Tobacco Free project, San Francisco Department of Health, San Francisco, California, United States

Introduction

Designing a method for physicians and other health-care providers to integrate tobacco education into their existing clinical practice is a challenge to those trying to change health care. The active, busy clinical environment, where productivity may be antithetical with the quality of patient care, can be a formidable barrier. Providers' attitudes to smoking, their academic training and focus and cultural and family environments add to the complexity of the problem. Furthermore, the desire to address smoking and other addictions in a routine practice wanes when a patient presents an acute problem which can be remedied with fast-acting medications, whereas long-term behavioural actions are required for cessation. Providers must be cognizant of the role of nicotine in exacerbating many health problems. They must also believe that people can change their behaviour. As physicians, they must be able to address their patients' questions and concerns confidently in order to empower the patient to quit smoking. The goal of the project described here was to assist nine clinics to create an environment conducive to education, health promotion and smoking cessation.

Methods

Over a two-year period, a six-phase approach was developed to integrate smoking cessation services into primary care. The first phase consisted of introducing the project and observing and assessing current practices and the staff's level of interest and needs. In the second phase, we conducted a review of medical charts to determine the clinicians' involvement in education, assessment and assistance to patients. The third phase was an environmental assessment and development of cues; the fourth consisted of consultation and environmental change; the fifth phase involved staff training and development, and the sixth was a final programme evaluation.

The staff of the project met with the administrative team at each of the nine health-care clinics to obtain input for the objectives of the programme and revise them to meet realistic outcomes. Clinic staff were also involved in the second phase, and their ideas were incorporated. A contact person was identified at each site. The review of charts was conducted in cooperation with other departmental actions for changing programmes. On the basis of the initial observational environmental review, promotional and educational materials were bought to raise awareness of smoking as a health-care problem. Racks of brochures were installed, and educational materials were placed in waiting rooms and examination rooms. The front page of the medical records was altered to prompt the clinicians to assess their patients for smoking, exposure to environmental tobacco smoke and ex-smoker and non-smoker status. The staff of the project were available for consultation about signs, policy issues and problems with implementation. At each location, training for clinicians was available, which involved both didactic and experential components, with role-playing and modelling activities. A final two-part evaluation was conducted at each site, which consisted of interviewing patients when they left the clinic and matching their medical charts with the result of the interview in order to assess the clinicians' reports.

Results

We compared 168 interviews and 160 charts for the patients. In seven of the nine clinics, 51% of the charts did not match the patients' reports, but there was greater consistency between patient reports and medical notations in centres where clinicians had received training earlier in the cycle than in those who had received training later in the year. One clinic in which predominantly HIV-positive patients are treated showed the least consistency between the clinicians' and the patients' reports, even though it was one of the facilities that had received earlier training.

Discussion

Clinicians are willing to change their interventions and interactions when they are involved in all stages of planning of a project and when the programme responds to their needs. The approach must be slow and deliberate; pushing forwards with no regard for the history of the establishment and issues of external organization can only hinder the development of new working patterns. The clinicians learnt to discuss the short- and long-term effects of smoking in their own way and gained confidence that they were capable of delivering a concise but sensitive message even when their time with a patient was limited. With their new interest in education, prevention and health promotion, they may become receptive to other behavioural approaches to health care that could improve the health status of public health patients.

Cigarette smoking and anti smoking counselling among Chinese physicians

H.Z. Li[1], D. Fish[1] & X. Zhou[2]

*[1]Faculty of Health and Human Sciences, University of Northern British Columbia, Prince George, British Columbia, Canada
[2]Hubei Medical University, Wuhan, Hubei Province, China*

We surveyed 493 Chinese physicians about their cigarette smoking patterns and frequency and methods of anti-smoking counselling in Wuhan, the capital city of Hubei Province, in early 1996. We found that 61% of the male and 12% of the female physicians were current cigarette smokers—an increase of 20% for men and 150% for women in comparison with findings among physicians in the same city nine years previously. About one-third of the smokers reported a daily consumption of 20 cigarettes or more, and 45% consumed fewer than five cigarettes daily. Two-thirds of the physicians had counselled their patients about smoking in the past year, and 57% of them had done so 'often' or 'always'.

Four variables were predictive of the frequency of counselling on anti-smoking by the physicians: whether they perceived it to be their responsibility to advise patients about cigarette smoking, whether they thought they should set an example for their patients by not smoking, whether they perceived themselves as the most influential people in helping people to quit smoking and whether they perceived their previous counselling services as successful.

The findings of this study provided valuable information on the smoking patterns of Chinese physicians and their anti-smoking counselling practices. The dramatic increase in the prevalence of smoking among Chinese physicians within the past nine years, especially among women, is alarming. As more physicians become cigarette smokers, fewer will care about counselling their patients not to smoke. This critical change indicates new themes for future anti-smoking strategies in China.

Categorical, clear and helpful approach of health professionals to smoking cessation in the Czech Republic

E. Králíková[1] & J.T. Kozák[2]

[1]Charles University and [2]Hospital Kutná Hora, Prague, Czech Republic

Doctors, nurses and pharmacists should ask all patients about their smoking habits, clearly recommend that they stop and treat them. The prevalence of smoking among health professionals in the Czech Republic is shown in Table 1.

It can be seen that only 15% of medical students in their fifth year are smokers. All of the medical faculties are involved in control of smoking, with 2–6 h of seminars in the basic curriculum (Crofton, 1996) and epidemiological studies on the prevalence of health professionals to smoking, smoking among pregnant women, smoking among

Table 1. Prevalence of smoking among health professionals and the general population in the Czech Republic

Population	Prevalence (%)			
	Occasional smokers	Regular smokers	Ex-smokers smokers	Non-smokers
Women				
General population	5	22	11	62
Doctors	5	21	13	61
Nurses	6	35	14	45
Men				
General population	3	29	22	46
Doctors	5	26	16	53
Total				
General population	4	25	17	54
Doctors	5	24	15	56
Fifth-year medical students	6	3	3	82

Population sample (n = 1118) from Opinion Poll Institute, 1997
Doctors and nurses (n = 920) from First Faculty of Medicine, Charles University, 1997
Medical students (n = 209) from First Faculty of Medicine, 1996–97

schoolchildren and other topics, including smoking and anaesthetics. An intervention is performed in the first and fifth years of study, and a textbook is provided, entitled *Smoking Cessation Methods in Doctors' Everyday Practice.*

The Table also shows that 29% of doctors are smokers. A number of steps have been taken to reduce the prevalence. A two-day course is run to train health professionals in smoking cessation methods for their patients. There are now about 60 smoking cessation clinics in the country, and the Czech Medical Association is preparing its own guidelines for smoking cessation. The basic guidelines are published in a magazine for all 40 000 doctors in the country. In 1993, the Czech Committee of the European Medical Association Smoking or Health had 200 members. Furthermore, excerpts from articles on tobacco in the foreign literature are published in the leading Czech medical journal, which has been published continuously for the last 20 years.

It may be seen that 41% of nurses are smokers. An organization of 'Nurses against Tobacco' is being created, and a two-day course in smoking cessation methods is held at the Postgraduate Education Institute for Health Professionals. Publications on smoking appear regularly in the magazine *Nurse.*

The WHO programme on smoking cessation in pharmacies is presented to pharmacists by the Chamber of Pharmacists and there about 10 pharmacies are now involved. Courses on the use of nicotine replacement therapy are run in pharmacies and in the postgraduate institute, and a chapter on the topic is published in *The Pharmacists' Manual,* which reaches every pharmacy in the country.

Reference
Crofton, J. (1996) Guidelines for teaching medical students about the health effect of tobacco: A checklist. In: Richmond, R., ed., *Educating Medical Students about Tobacco: Planning and Implementation,* Paris: Tobacco Prevention Section, International Union Against Tuberculosis and Lung Disease, p. 371

Quantitative research among doctors in Nairobi, Kenya, about their smoking behaviour and their opinions on smoking control education

H. de Vries, B. Lore, B. Fiévez & H. Adriaanse

kenyan Medical Association, Nairobi, Kenya, and Department of Health Education, University of Limburg, Maastricht, Netherlands

Introduction

Doctors in Kenya are important role models for quitting smoking. In order to improve smoking control in Kenya, it is therefore important to find out what doctors believe about smoking control policies and what their smoking habits are. The main objectives of this study were to determine the extent to which doctors in Nairobi are encouraging their patients to quit, their opinions about these practices and the prevalence of smoking among the doctors. In order to do this, we designed a questionnaire on the basis of a model which posits that behaviour is influenced by intention, attitude, social influences, self-efficacy, barriers and skills. The model is based on the theory that behaviour is a function of a person's intention, which in turn is determined by attitude and social norms (De Vries et al., 1995).

'Attitude' is what a person thinks of a behaviour as a result of the perceived advantages and disadvantages of that behaviour. 'Social influences' are those that a person experiences from others, what they think, do and expect. 'Self-efficacy' refers to the expectations people have of their own ability to behave in a certain way. 'Intention' is that which a person has to behave in a certain way, such as quitting smoking. 'Barriers' are the perceived obstacles to behaving in a certain way. 'Skills' qre the abilities people need to behave in that way. 'Behaviour' is the sum of the observable acts of individuals.

Method

We selected 82 respondents randomly from among about 350 in Nairobi. Of these, 33% worked in private clinics, 27% in hospitals and 26% in both. The survey was carried out between 11 February and 17 May 1996, with formal consent from the Office of the President and under the supervision of the Chairman of the Kenyan Medical Association, who was at that time Dr Lore. A qualitative study was performed first, in which the doctors were asked to define their experience and opinions of smoking cessation education and their own smoking behaviour. Subsequently, they were given a questionnaire to fill in within three weeks, either at work or at home. To enhance their validity, the questionnaires were anonymous. Smokers took 20–30 min to fill in the questionnqires and non-smokers 15–20 min, as fewer questions were relevant to non-smokers. The results were analysed in The Netherlands.

The content of the questionnaire was based on qualitative research performed in Nairobi in 1996 and on that of other, quantitative questionnaires. The content, comprising 29 questions, was divided into blocks that addressed attitude, social influences and self-efficacy, for both quitting smoking and providing education of smoking control. Many were incompletely filled in.

Results

In 1992, there were 3554 doctors in Kenya, of whom 15% were female. In the absence of data, it had previously been assumed that the prevalence of smoking among doctors in Nairobi was 10% and that very few female doctors smoked. Of the 82 questionnaires that were returned, 60 were from male and 22 from female doctors. Of the total, 73 were non-smokers; none of the women smoked. The doctors ranged in age from 20 to 74; 71% lived in the city; 33% were Protestants, 20% Catholics and 14% Anglicans. Of the 82 doctors, 67% were black, 18% Asian and 9.8% white.

With regard to social influences, we found that 64% of the partners of the doctors who smoked did not smoke; 54% answered however that a minority of their family, friends, staff and colleagues were smokers. With respect to self-efficacy, 86% thought that it   would be difficult not to smoke when they were drinking alcoholic beverages, 57% foresaw difficulty while they were drinking tea or coffee, 62% cited after dinner, 62% cited at a party and 78% thought that it would be easy when other people supported them in not smoking. When asked about stressful situations, 38% thought that it would be difficult not to smoke and 38% thought that it would be easy.

General questions about smoking control education showed that 71% considered their current knowledge to be sufficient to counsel patients about quitting smoking, 96% agreed that they should not smoke at work, 47% agreed that smoking control education is effective in helping people to quit smoking and 46% thought that doctors are the right people to give smoking control education to patients. The patients to whom the doctors always gave training in smoking control were those with symptoms of smoking-related diseases (90%) and those who asked about smoking (65%); 30% sometimes gave advice to patients who had no symptoms and who did not ask. For smoking control, 76% never gave out leaflets on smoking or smoking cessation, 53% never provided information on smoking cessation courses, 51% never promoted cessation aids such as nicotine chewing-gum, 49% never made an appointment to help a patient to quit, and 61% never called a patient back after a quit attempt. Nevertheless, 95% sometimes often or always advised patients to stop smoking, 91% told patients about the advantages of quitting, 58% told them how to obtain support from others and 54% discussed how to handle barriers.

We found that 40% of the doctors thought they would probably see no results and 50% thought that the patients would probably not respond to the smoking control education. With regard to social influences, 39% said that they did not know whether colleagues were giving such education to their patients, and 36% said that they received no support from colleagues in this activity. With respect to their self-efficacy, 80% said that they found it difficult to provide education on smoking in the absence of support, 64% found it difficult in the absence of funds for audiovisual aids, 59% found it difficult when they saw no result, 65% found it difficult when the patient was too sick, 70% found it difficult when the patient was too old, 60% found it difficult when campaigns against alcohol and tobacco were being run, 64% found it difficult with patients who have a low level of education and 76% found it difficult when patients were influenced by their friends to smoke.

Discussion

We found that 89% of our sample did not smoke, which confirms the estimate of a 10% smoking prevalence in this profession in Nairobi. We also found that only a minority of the partners, friends, staff and colleagues of the doctors smoked. The nine doctors who smoked considered that they would be given support by others if they tried to give up smoking, but most thought that it would be difficult not to smoke after dinner or when drinking tea, coffee or alcoholic beverages.

The only smoking control activity practised by most of the doctors was to advise their patients to quit smoking; about half told them how to obtain support from others and how to handle barriers to quitting. Doctors who never provided information on smoking cessation courses said that they thought patients might avoid further contact if they were given smoking control education; this group also said that few of their colleagues supported them in this activity. Those who considered that smoking control education is ineffective in helping people to quit smoking also found that this activity took up too much time. This group also considered that they received little support from their colleagues.

The main finding of this study is therefore that doctors who perceive that they are receiving support from their colleagues are more likely to give smoking control education and provide information about smoking cessation courses. This finding is in agreement with that of Bandura (1986), who reported that social influences play an important role in the development of behaviour.

References
Bandura, A. (1986) *Social Foundations of Thought and Actiob: A Social Cognitive Theory*, New York: Prentice-Hall
De Vries, H., Backbier, E., Kok, G. & Dijkstra, M. (1995) The impact of social influences in the context of attitude, self efficacy, intention, and previous behavior as predictors of smoking onset. *J. Appl. Soc. Psychol.*, **25**, 237–257

Smoking cessation in general practice

R. Borge, D. Skylstad & E. Aaserud

Kokstad Occupational Health Services, Bergen and Nordaas General Practice, Bergen, Norway

About 70% of all smokers see a physician every year (Ockene, 1987). The consultation is therefore a unique opportunity for soctors to motivate and help smokers to quit. Even simple questions like "Do you smoke?" and "Would you like to quit?" have an effect on smoking behaviour when they come from a doctor (Russel *et al.*, 1979). Many doctors would like to do more but consider that they lack suitable training.

To give doctors a tool to use during consultations, we designed a smoking cessation programme, which we have called 'Flipover'. The programme involves four consultations: the first two constitute the motivation phase with a gradual reduction in nicotine intake, and the third and fourth represent the maintenance phase in which patients are taught how to handle abstinence and craving, keep up their motivation and avoid gaining weight.

About 1500 Flipovers have been distributed in Norway by the pharmaceutical company Novartis on request. About 600 of the recipients are doctors, and the others are mainly nurses and pharmacists. This indicates widespread interest in smoking cessation among health professionals.

The Flipover does not cover all of the physical and psychological problems that may be associated with smoking cessation. It is meant to give health professionals a more structured approach to helping smokers to quit. It is hoped that the Flipover will eventually result in increased interest and competence in responding to patients who smoke and who wish or need to quit.

Acknowledgement
We thank Novartis for financing and distributing the Flipover.

References
Ockene, J.K. (1987) Smoking intervention: The expanding role of the physician. *Am. J. Public Health*, **7**, 782–783
Russel, M.A., Wislon, G., Taylor, G. & Baker, C.D. (1979) Effect of general practitioners' advice against smoking. *Br. Med. J.*, ii, 231–235

Behaviour and attitude of Turkish physicians to smoking

N. Bilir, A. Naci Yyldyz, B. Güçiz Doðan &S. Emri

Department of Public Health, Hacettepe University, Ankara, Turkey

Rationale

The prevalence of smoking is high in Turkey, even among physicians, and the percentage of smokers is increasing, in contrast to developed countries. Smoking among health personnel is especially dangerous in view of their role as a model for the community. Furthermore, physicians are key persons in smoking control programmes. In a study conducted in Elazyg Province in Turkey in 1988, the prevalence of smoking among physicians and dentists was 55% in men and 40% in women, and 57% of them smoked in front of their patients.

Method

Ankara Province was chosen as the site for a descriptive study. Of 2021 general practitioners and 1775 specialists registered with the Ankara Chamber of the Turkish Medical Association, 130 general practitioners or residents and 120 specialists were chosen by simple random sampling; the final study population consisted of 132 general practitioners and 105 specialists. Data were collected from a self-administered questionnaire developed by examining sample questionnaires recommended by various international institutions and finalized after pre-testing on 20 officials working in Hacettepe University hospitals. The physicians were visited at their workplaces, and forms were either collected immediately or at a subsequent visit.

Results

The mean age of the physicians was 36.3 ± 9.1 years, and the male:female ratio was 1.1; most were married (77%), with a mean of 1.2 ± 0.8 children. The prevalence of smoking was 44%, with rates of 51.2% for men and 34% for women. The percentage of female physicians who had never smoked was 54%, while only one male physician out of four was a non-smoker; 25% of the men and 12% of the women had quit smoking.

Among male physicians, the highest prevalence of smoking (56%) was in the 30–44-year age group. After 45 years of age, the prevalence was nearly same in female and male physicians (42 and 43%, respectively). Most (74–100%) of the physicians did not approve of smoking in public and/or enclosed places, but nearly 80% of physicians who smoked approved of smoking in restaurants and offices under certain conditions. The physicians who smoked disapproved of smoking in airplanes (71%). Almost all of them said that a physician should not smoke when examining a patient, and also considered that teachers should not smoke in front of students, and sportsmen should never smoke. Nevertheless, 68% of the physicians who smoked stated that they smoked while working, 84% had smoked at home, 49% in front of children, 68% while working, 66% while having a drink, 72% from boredom and 75% at a restaurant. About one-fourth of the physicians stated that they did not regret smoking, while 77% had regrets and 69% said they would be non-smokers if they were born again.

One-half of male and one-third of female physicians in Turkey are thus regular smokers, the frequency increasing by age. Most of them had begun smoking at a relatively advanced age when compared with the average for the general population. Twenty-two percent smoked fewer than five cigarettes per day, but about 40% smoked about one pack per day.

Helping health professionals to help smokers

F. Bass

British Columbia Doctors' Stop Smoking Programme, Vancouver, British Columbia, Canada

Tobacco addiction results from five determinants: biochemical, behavioural, psychological, social and economic. Strategic action against each of these factors is needed to reduce the prevalence of tobacco use. Knowledge of the epidemiology of tobacco addiction is basic to controlling it; thus, surveys of the population are required to identify the prevalence and trends of smoking and smoking cessation. The 'epidemiological triad' of agent, host and environment applies to tobacco addiction. The agent, tobacco, provides benefits to the addict; the host is identified by the smoker's demographic characteristics, level of addiction and readiness to stop smoking; the environment includes physical access to tobacco and tobacco smoke, the social environment of family, friends and co-workers, and the economic environment.

Considerable clinical research has identified the components of effective assistance to smokers, which can be summarized as ask, advise, assist and follow up. The clinician should *ask* each patient (as early as nine years of age) about whether and how much they smoke and their readiness to stop. Next, the clinician should label the medical records with 'Smoker', 'Smoker ready to stop', 'Recent ex-smoker', 'Long-term ex-smoker' or 'Never smoked'.

The clinician should *advise* each smoker with a strong, personalized message to quit and provide up-to-date information on the dangers of smoking. Smokers should be advised to tell their children not to start smoking. Part of advising patients is motivating them, since most smokers are not ready to stop. Motivation includes asking them "How do you feel about stopping smoking?" or "Tell me about stopping smoking." and then listening to the answer. Afterwards, printed information can be offered on the dangers of smoking and how to stop.

The clinician should *assist* smokers who are ready to stop by helping them to set a quit date, recommending use of nicotine chewing-gum or patches or other proven treatment and warning them that after they have stopped smoking it will be important to avoid even one puff on a cigarette and to be careful when drinking alcohol and near other smokers. Assistance in stopping should take the form of stepped care, level one being self-management of smoking (the way in which most smokers stop smoking), level two being help from a health professional and level three being help from an expert in nicotine addiction. For the clinician to ask, advise and assist smokers consistently, a team approach involving multiple health professionals is best. Office staff can ask about smoking, keep medical records and follow-up and give support to smokers.

Clinicians should *follow up* smokers at scheduled visits, using labels to identify smoking status on each medical record and evaluate the programme periodically. Clinicians should also advise all their patients about environmental tobacco smoke: tell smokers to avoid smoking near non-smokers and around children and encourage non-smokers to ask for clean indoor air.

Health professionals can be motivated to deliver effective clinical intervention by being told that it is one of the most effective ways of saving lives and that clinical help is particularly effective (8–20% of smokers per year stop smoking with help from health professionals and only 2–4% without such help). Health professionals can also be offered training in the clinical management of nicotine addiction, printed materials on clinical procedures, educational materials for patients and follow-up support. To help women avoid the dangers of smoking, tobacco intervention should be part of family planning and all routine medical care. This should involve prenatal and postnatal care and the care of children with ear infections, bronchitis or asthma.

Creating awareness about the effects of smoking through community-based health-care providers in Nigeria

O.A. Abosede[1], E. Bandele[2], G. Essien[3] & N. Olupona[4]

[1]*Institute of Child Health and Primary Care, College of Medicine, University of Lagos;* [2]*Department of Medicine, College of Medicine, University of Lagos;* [3]*Child Association of Nigeria;* [4]*Baptist Medical Services, Ogbomoso, Oyo State, Nigeria*

Abstract

Aggressive cigarette advertising prompted this successful attempt at creating awareness of the dangers of tobacco use through community-based health-care givers. The medium chosen—mostly women and community development committees—is very relevant at the grassroots level of the traditional Nigerian infrastructure and primary health care.

At refresher courses on health, 297 village health workers, traditional birth attendants and community-based distributors of family spacing devices did not associate direct or passive smoking with many of its hazards. Assuming that their lack of knowledge reflected the level of awareness in their communities, an health education programme was critical. A survey one year after the intervention showed enhanced knowledge in the participating communities when compared with nearby controls.

Introduction

Advertising of tobacco products and especially cigarettes in Nigeria is very aggressive. Billboards are placed in strategic places, television networks show advertisements at prime time, movies and popular musical entertainment is sponsored by tobacco companies, there are advertisments on police kiosks and bus shelters, and large umbrellas are distributed bearing familiar colours and messages.

Our project targeted women, for several reasons. The 1991 national census showed a high proportion of women in Nigeria, and even though the prevalence of smoking among women is generally lower than that among men (bandele & Abosede, 1997), many women live with a husband or son who smokes or are exposed to tobacco smoke at work. They are usually ignorant of the dangers of environmental tobacco smoke to family members and especially pregnant women and infants (Davis, 1989; Kawachi et al., 1989). Adolescednt girls are beginning to smoke more than boys in some countries (Wells, 1989), and female smokers have high rates of morbidity and mortality from cervical cancer, spontaneous abortions, abruptio placentae, antepartum haemorrhage and premature delivery (Colditz et al., 1988; Andriassen et al., 1989; Asmussen, 1989; Pandey et al., 1989).

Group counselling and radio are more appropriate in Nigeria than written information, as the literacy rate is still lower in the female population (39%) than the male (51%), especially in the rural population (70%). The purpose of this project was to create awareness and disseminate information about the dangers of tobacco use. The target audience was the whole community, but women of child-bearing age in particular.

Methods

The states selected for the pilot project are representative of the rural southern and northern parts of the country; Oyo and Osun were still one state at the time the project was conducted. The study population comprised 297 community-based health-care providers, made up of 25 distributors of family spacing devices and 168 village health workers and traditional birth attendants from Oyo/Osun and 104 from Jigawa State. These women mobilized their community development committees and primary health care staff for the health education programmes.

After showing a 20-min film on breast-feeding and infant nutrition in the local language, the women explained the dangers of tobacco use to 3546 people in the communities, from community leaders to schoolchildren. The impact of the programme was assessed one year later in a community survey, by interviewing 200 selected participants and 200 unexposed people from another community nearby about the health problems associated with smoking and exposure to environmental tobacco smoke, the effects of tobacco on breast milk production and birth weight and attempts to quit or helping someone to quit tobacco use.

Results and discussion

The participants showed enhanced knowledge about the dangers of both direct and indirect exposure to tobacco smoke (Table 1), and 78% of them had advised other members of their communities against tobacco use within the past year. Only one person had quit smoking.

The project was successful in enhancing knowledge about the dangers of tobacco use, including less well-known effects such as cancer of the cervix and lung, heart disease, low birth weight, reduced breast-milk volume and sudden death. Neither participants nor controls related cot deaths to tobacco use, as in rural Nigeria most people attribute such deaths to evil spirits.

In order to broaden the coverage of this project, we hope to involve women's organizations and various philanthropic organizations in anti-tobacco activities.

Table 1. Knowledge about the dangers of tobacco use among 200 participants in a tobacco control intervention and among 200 controls

Harmful effect	Participants		Controls	
	No.	%	No.	%
Chest infection	169	84	116	58
Poverty	100	50	15	7.5
Use of hemp or hard drugs	76	38	6	3.0
Mental problems	179	90	31	16
Sudden death	199	100	99	50
Lung cancer	129	64	11	5.5
Heart disease	108	54	28	14
Cot death	1	0.5	0	0
Itchy, bloodshot eyes	145	72	139	70
Loss of appetite	152	76	136	68
Loss of weight	174	87	164	82
Irresponsibility	94	47	69	34
Addiction	84	42	75	38
Violence and crime	36	18	9	4.5
Cancer of the cervix	92	46	24	12
Effect on birth weight				
No effect	10	5.0	13	6.5
Small baby	146	74	43	22
Large baby	5	2.5	0	0
Effect on breast-milk volume from environmental tobacco smoke				
No effect	26	13	74	37
Greater than normal	31	16	2	1.0
Less than normal	122	61	74	37

References

Andriassen, H., Cox, H., Knottnerus, J.A., Essed, G.G.M. & Delgado, L.R. (1989) One ounce per cigarette: Smoking in Dutch pregnant women and birthweight. In: Durston, B. & Jamrozik, K., eds, *The Global War. Proceedings of the 7th World Conference on Tobacco and Health, Perth, Australia*, p. 436

Asmussen, I. (1989) Why do smokers deliver preterm? Because foetal membrances rupture more easily in smokers. In: Durston, B. & Jamrozik, K., eds, *The Global War. Proceedings of the 7th World Conference on Tobacco and Health, Perth, Australia*, pp. 101–108

Bandele, E. & Abosede, O.A. (1997) Prevalence of smoking in a low socio-economic area of Lagos State, Nigeria (in press)

Colditz, G.A., Bonita, R. & Stampter, M.J. (1988) Cigarette smoking and risk of stroke in middle-aged women. *New Engl. J. Med.*, **318**, 937–941

Davis, R.M. (1989) Women and smoking in the United States: How lung cancer became an 'equal opportunity' disease. Washington DC: US Office on Smoking and Health

Kawachi, I., Pearce, N.C. & Jackson, R.T. (1989) Deaths from lung cancer and ischaemic heart disease due to passive smoking in New Zealand. *N.Z. Med. J.*, **102**, 337–340

Pandey, M.R., Sharma, T.R. & Neupane, R.P. (1989) Parental smoking and acute respiratory infection in Nepal. In: Durston, B. & Jamrozik, K., eds, *The Global War. Proceedings of the 7th World Conference on Tobacco and Health, Perth, Australia*, pp. 511–513

Wells, A.J. (1989) Passive smoking and adult mortality. In: Durston, B. & Jamrozik, K., eds, *The Global War. Proceedings of the 7th World Conference on Tobacco and Health, Perth, Australia*, pp. 516–519

General practitioners' role in preventive medicine: Scenario analysis with smoking as a case study

C. Doran[1], B. Pekarsky[2], M. Gordon[3] & R. Sanson-Fisher[1]

[1] New South Wales Cancer Council Cancer Education Research Program, Newcastle; [2] Flinders Medical Centre, Adelaide, and [3] Economics Department, University of Newcastle, Australia

The purpose of this study was to develop a model that can be used in conjunction with scenario analysis to evaluate the strategies that are available to assist general practitioners in reducing smoking among their patients. The scenario analysis involves a four-step procedure for identifying opportunities for detection, intervention and efficacy and assigning probabilities to outcomes, so that a range of prevention strategies can be examined both in isolation and in combination.

This study specifically addresses general practice in Australia, and the model is based on information on smokers who visited their general practitioner within a six-month period and on empirical evidence for the rates of detection, intervention and efficacy.

The outcome measurements, which are evaluated in terms of marginal effectiveness, include the number of smokers among the doctors' patients, the number of smokers who were offered an intervention, the number of smokers who quit as a result of the intervention and the additional years of life saved as a result of the intervention.

The results show that the most significant factor in reducing smoking rates among patients is improving the efficacy of interventions. The results also suggest that, although improving the rate of detection of patients' smoking status by general practitioners has a potentially greater effect on quit rates than increasing the level of intervention; increasing both detection and intervention levels had a greater effect than either strategy alone.

General practitioners have an important role to play in preventive medicine. Their knowledge, skill and attitude towards smoking are significant, and they can be the prime motivators in persuading their patients to stop smoking. Detection, intervention and efficacious strategies are all key elements in achieving this result.

A full report of this study has been published in *Addiction* 1998; 93(7):1013–1022.

Prevalence of smoking among pneumologists in Romania

F. Mihaltan

M. Nasta Institute of Pneumophtisiology, Bucharest, Romania

The alarming incidence of smoking among physicians and patients in Romania incited us to conduct this study. We distributed questionnaires on smoking to 250 pneumologists, who were a representative sample of the specialists in the country; 232 (94%) returned the forms. The group consisted of 167 women and 65 men, 70% of whom were 31–50 years old.

The prevalence of smoking was 60% among men and 40% among women. Of the smokers, 40% had begun smoking to emulate their school friends. Most of the smokers were aged 31–50. Forty percent of the pneumologists expressed concern about smoking among university students and among their patients, and 53% expressed concern about the lack of methods for stopping smoking. Only 7.1% of pneumologists stopped smoking when they became ill, only 7.3% asked for assistance in stopping smoking, and very few (4.4%) asked for an anti-smoking consultation.

These findings indicate the irresponsibility of Romanian pneumologists who smoke, as their attitude makes it difficult for them to advise patients who smoke. The situation in the Romanian medical corps is thus dramatic. As women predominate among pneumologists of Romania, the prevalence of smokers is greater than the average for the total female population of the country. Removing this dependence should begin with the medical corps.

Smoking among professors at medical schools in Spain

I. Nerin

Department of Medicine and Psychiatry, Faculty of Medicine, Zaragoza, Spain

The objective of this study was to determine the prevalence of smoking among professors at medical schools and their attitudes towards smoking. A study on smoking was therefore carried out among teachers at the school of medicine in Zaragoza, Spain. A questionnaire was distributed to 363 persons, comprising 262 men (73%) and 99 women (27%), and 229 were returned, 155 from men (68%) and 74 from women (32%). The mean age of the study population was 44.9, with a standard deviation of 6.8.

The results showed that 35% smoked daily, 10% smoked less than one cigarette per day, and 55% did not smoke. No difference was observed by sex. Only 78% of the teachers considered that smoking is dangerous for health; 81% believed that most patients affected by lung cancer are (or were) smokers and 75% considered that passive smoking represented a risk for health. Smoking was seen as a risk factor for lung disease by 96% of this population, for coronary ischaemia by 90%, for urinary bladder cancer by 50% and for osteoporosis and early menopause by 11%. Smoking was considered to be addictive by 45%, and 83% thought that more information about smoking should be included in degree studies at university level.

The prevalence of smoking among professors at medical schools is similar to that in the general population. This study shows the necessity of increasing information about the relationship between smoking and health and emphasizing on the role of health professionals in this area.

This study was supported by the University of Zaragoza research programme.

General practitioners and smoking prevention

C.M. Doran[1], B. Pekarsky[2], M. Gordon[3] & R.W. Sanson-Fisher[1]

[1]New South Wales Cancer Council Cancer Education Research Program;
[2]Department of General Practice, Flinders Medical Centre; and [3]Department of
Economics, University of Newcastle, Australia

The purpose of the study described here was to develop a model for analysing the various strategies that are available to assist general practitioners to reduce smoking among their patients. The scenario analysis involves four steps. The first is to identify the opportunities for detection, intervention and efficacy and to express them as a decision process. The second step is to assign probabilities to each node in the decision process. During the third step, the outcomes for current (base case) levels of decision, intervention and efficacy are estimated, and a number of scenarios in which these rates are increased are drawn up. The final step is a 'break-even' analysis of the outcomes of the scenarios. The results are expressed in a table which emphasizes incremental differences between strategies for detection, intervention and efficacy.

The literature tends to suggest that techniques which involve more resources are generally more effective than those which use fewer resources in bringing about abstinence from smoking. The results of this analysis suggest, however, that improvements in the rate of detection by general practitioners of their patients' smoking status can have a potentially greater effect on quit rates than increasing the level of intervention.

Health education on tobacco or health:
The role of professional nurses in Hong Kong

S. Chan[1,2], C. Betson[2] & T.H. Lam[2]

[1]Department of Nursing Studies and [2]Department of Community Medicine, The
University of Hong Kong, Hong Kong

Nurses are in a key position to carry out health education. There are more nurses in the Department of Health of the Hong Kong Government than any other kind of health care professionals, and they have the most contact with clients. It is generally accepted that health education can influence individual choices and raise awareness of many health issues, such as the use of tobacco; however, there is little data about nurses' health education in Hong Kong.

The aim of this study was to explore the knowledge, attitudes and practice of nurses in health education and how these relate to their present tasks in general out-patient clinics in Hong Kong. This study has provided valuable information for our understanding of their preparation, roles, perceptions, competence, frequency of practice and educational needs and the helping and hindering forces in conducting health education.

Methods

The study was a cross-sectional survey in which a self-administered questionnaire was used. The subjects are all 296 registered nurses working in the general out-patient clinics of the Department of Health in Hong Kong. Questionnaires were posted to all of the nurses with a covering letter explaining the aims of the study. A letter explaining the distribution procedure was circulated the nursing officer in charge of each clinic to solicit support, after the questionnaires had been sent out to ensure that they understand the procedure and that they had received the questionnaires. Serial numbers were assigned to the questionnaires so that non-responders could be identified. The initial response rate was 50%, but after a written reminder and numerous telephone calls, the response rate was increased to 80%.

Results

The majority of the nurses were female (99.5%) and were aged 26–40. Over two-thirds of them (71.2%) were married. More than half (54%) of the nurses had completed secondary education; 32% had attended school up to form 6 and 14% up to form 7. Only about 10% had a degree in nursing; the rest had either a certificate or a diploma. Only about 20% had taken the course in public health nursing, but 22% were currently taking various post-registration courses. Of the 296, 81% were registered nurses, and 14% were nursing officers. Nearly two-thirds of the registered nurses had been qualified for 5–15 years. About 64% had worked in the Department of Health for up to five years and 21% for 6–10 years. Almost all (90%) had worked in their current general out-patient clinic for less than five years.

Most of the nurses seemed to have a good grasp of the concepts of health education, and their attitudes were positive. Their self-perceived knowledge and ability were satisfactory, but nearly two-thirds (29%) did not think they were the most appropriate health professional to conduct health education. Only 47% thought they were able to develop new methods and materials for health education, and 66% doubted their ability to evaluate the outcome of their efforts.

The frequency of performance of health education activities varied. The focus was on providing information, such as giving pamphlets, showing videos, counselling patients and giving advice about medical treatment. These activities were most frequently performed by nurses, but primary health education activities such as health promotion, disease prevention, advising a healthy lifestyle, smoking cessation and prevention of exposure to environmental tobacco smoke received less attention and were less frequently practised by nurses.

Over two-thirds of the respondents expressed some interest in acquiring more knowledge and skills in health education, and 87% indicatied interest in learning how to do research. Over half of the respondents expressed a desire for continuing education in areas such as new trends in health education, interpersonal skills, development of health education programmes and preparation of health education materials. Almost all (96%) indicated they would attend seminars or workshops if offered.

The nurses said that the most important forms of help in conducting health education were knowledge of health education, support from patients, skills in conducting health education, resources and a reasonable workload. The factors that most hindered nurses in the performance of health education were lack of resources, lack of time, a heavy workload, lack of knowledge and lack of support from patients.

Discussion

Although the nurses' concepts and perceptions of health education were generally positive and most thought they were able to conduct health education, 29% thought they were not the most appropriate health professionals to do so. In meeting the challenge of increasing emphasis on primary health care in Hong Kong, which should be characterized by health promotion and disease prevention, the role of nurses should be redefined and reorientated (Working Party on Primary Health Care, 1990). Furthermore, the practice of primary health education activities aimed at health promotion and illness prevention, maintaining a healthy lifestyle and smoking cessation should be emphasized.

Most nurses thought they were able to conduct health education, but only 47% thought they were able to develop new methods and materials for this purpose. A large percentage (87%) indicated that they would like to learn how to carry out research, but

66% thatdoubted whether they could evaluate the outcome of their efforts. Research is vital for gathering evidence to improve nursing practice, education and health policy (Burns & Grove, 1997). More importantly, research on health promotion and illness prevention is crucial in improving people's quality of life. Currently, little local research exists to document the effectiveness of health promotion and illness prevention interventions. This implies a need to educate and refine the new knowledge and skills of nurses in their expanded roles in health education and research.

The nurses recognized the importance of health education and were keen to obtain more knowledge and skills in this area. The fact that nearly all of them indicated their willingness to attend workshops or seminars if offered reflects the need for continuing professional education in preparation for the changing role of nurses. A study by Twinn and Lee (1997) demonstrated a similar need among nurses working in acute care settings in Hong Kong.

The three most important hindering factors identified in the performance of health education activities were lack of resources, lack of time and a heavy workload, consistent with the findings of Macleod Clark et al. (1992) and Twinn and Lee (1997). Macleod Clark et al. (1992) argued that such hindrances are related to nurses' understanding of health education. While health education is perceived as an isolated activity added on to care rather than integrated into it, it is unlikely that health education will be integrated into nursing activities. If nurses can be taught to integrate health education into other nursing activities, the importance of these hindering factors may be diminished.

Conclusion

This study has provided some important basic information for the development of professional nursing practice in health education. Although the nurses' concepts and attitudes to health education were quite positive and there are ample opportunities for practising it in general out-patient clinics, the nature and extent to which they are appropriately practised is doubtful. Nurses should make the best use of any available opportunities to engage in such activities, as they are an essential part of nursing practice. Furthermore, the emphasis of health education needs to be reorientated to highlight health promotion and illness prevention. This study has also provided important findings for the future planning and development of professional and continuing education for nurses. If nurses can be educated to understand the philosophy upon which health education is based, they will have an enormous potential for fulfilling a vital role in health promotion and health education.

Acknowledgements

We would like to thank the Health Services Research Committee for funding this project. We are grateful to The Department of Health and Ms. Betty Wu, Principal Nursing Officer, who assisted us in this project. Thanks must also go to the nurses who assisted and participated in this research, without whom the study would not have been possible. Lastly, I would like to thank Dr Y. He and Ms S.F. Chung who provided assistance in data analysis.

References

Burns, N. & Grove, S.K. (1997) *The Practice of Nursing Research. Conduct, Critique and Utilization*, 3rd Ed., Philadelphia: W.B. Saunders

Macleod Clark, J., Wilson Barnett, J., Latter, S. & Maben, J. (1992) *Health Education and Health Promotion in Nursing: A Study of Practice in Acute Areas*, London: Department of Health

Twinn, S.F. & Lee, D.T.F. (1997) The practice of health education in acute care settings in Hong Kong: An exploratory study of the contribution of registered nurses. *J. Adv. Nurs.*, 25, 178–185

Working Party on Primary Health Care (1990) *Health for All. The Way Ahead. Report of the Working Party on Primary Health Care*, Hong Kong: Government Printer

Smoking habits of Finnish public health nurses

A.-E. Liimatainen-Lamberg

Finnish Union of Public Health Nurses, Helsinki, Finland

Public health nurses have an essential role in basic health care and health education. In public health terms, reducing the prevalence of smoking by inviduals is one of the most important goals of health education. Accordingly, public health nurses should use their model influence to change their clients' attitudes.

The purpose of this study was to investigate the smoking habits of public health nurses. Data were collected on 1430 public health nurses who worked in maternity health care, child health clinics, school health care, occupational health care and nursing care in homes and in hospitals. The study was carried out at the University of Kuopio with a WHO questionnaire adapted to the Finnish culture.

The results indicated that 93% of the public health nurses were non-smokers; only 2.6% smoked daily and 4.1% occasionally, the younger nurses (under 35 years of age) smoking slighly more than the older ones. The number of smokers was very low in comparison with, for instance, the frequency among teachers in health care institutions (24%).

The most important reasons for not smoking included caring about health and avoidance of unpleasant symptoms, being a good role model and consideration for others. Public health nurses estimated that they had adequate knowledge for giving health education about smoking, but considered that health-care personnel needed special training in helping clients and patients to quit smoking. The non-smoking public health nurses were more definitive on this point than those who smoked. According to these nurses, prevention of smoking should be a part of the basic education of health-care personnel.

Swedish Nurses against Tobacco: How to build an organization

Y. Höijer[1] & I. Nordström Torpenberg[2]

[1]Department of Cancer Prevention, Karolinska Hospital, Stockholm, and
[2]Tobacco Prevention Centre, Novum, Huddinge, Sweden

As nurses, we take care of an increasing number of patients with tobacco-related diseases. We can no longer silently accept the growing number of tobacco victims. Although continuous information to the Swedish people about the damage caused by tobacco has led to a decrease in the number of users, women and nursing staff are still heavy smokers. There are about 95 000 trained nurses and midwives in Sweden.

Various branch associations against tobacco have been established independently. We decided to establish 'Nurses against Tobacco' in May 1992, with the purpose of building a strong, active network. In our profession, we work with people from the first phase of life to the last, and can therefore act in preventing tobacco use.

Our board includes registered nurses with a wide network of contacts, both among colleagues and in society. Competences in child health, school health and occupational health are represented, as well as competences in smoking cessation, education and national campaign activities. The trade unions of nurses and midwives support the association.

Marketing and building the network

Efforts were initially concentrated on marketing the association to all nurses in Sweden. The magazine of the nurses union, *Vårdfacket*, was contacted and ran a story on the recently formed association. Applications for membership flowed in. Together with other anti-tobacco associations, we then demonstrated and advertised and finally brought about the enactment of a Swedish Tobacco Control Act, in July 1993. Newspapers and television showed interest in the organization, and Nurses against Tobacco produced articles, served on a panel of experts for one of our major evening papers and participated in a television production on tobacco throughout one entire evening. The lobbying and demonstrations continue with undiminished strength.

There are now five branch associations against tobacco in health and nursing care in Sweden: Nurses against Tobacco, Doctors against Tobacco, Dentistry against Tobacco, Teachers against Tobacco and Pharmacists against Tobacco. The five organizations share a secretariat, where the work is coordinated. The National Institute of Public Health and The Swedish Cancer Society are our main partners and financial supporters. The association participates in health care congress, where we draw attention to the tobacco issue and the effects of tobacco in various ways and remind our colleagues that we nurse an increasing number of tobacco victims. We also offer smoking cessation support to colleagues.

A network of contacts has been established within the branch associations throughout Sweden, who receive information on the latest findings in tobacco-related issues. These persons act locally to provide education and various activities. All members receive an information letter at least four times a year. A subscription to the magazine *Tobaccofront* is included in the membership fee.

What Swedish nurses and midwives do in tobacco prevention

Nurses and midwives have vast knowledge of and opportunities for working in tobacco prevention. Midwives meet expectant mothers throughout pregnancy and can give them support and encouragement to give up smoking, without apportioning blame. They can influence teenagers to have a smoke-free life through work at medical centres for young people. Nurses at child health clinics can influence parents to give their children a smoke-free environment and continue the work by supporting parents in staying smoke-free. Conversation methods that focus on the parents' knowledge and motivation have begun to be used in these situations.

School nurses have an important role to play in encouraging pupils not to begin to use tobacco and in supporting pupils who have begun smoking or snuffing. They have conversations about health with all pupils, and many schools also have smoke cessation support. Public health nurses are closest to the local inhabitants; health centres are often in the middle of town. Public health nurses can provide individual advice and support and run smoking or snuffing cessation groups. Occupational health nurses have a key role in health consciousness at places of work. They often participate in group discussions on policy issues at places of work.

Practical nurses, for instance, in wards for heart and lung diseases, can run disease-orientated support groups. There are many opportunities for instigating discussions about stopping smoking in those groups. Ward sisters give individual advice to patients who should give up tobacco or take the opportunity of providing additional support when patients change environment. They have access to nicotine substitutes to ease cessation. One of the duties of the health planning officer in tobacco prevention is to support the local network.

Members of Nurses against Tobacco thus work actively to reach their colleagues to create a smoke-free society. There is still much left to do, but showing a good example and taking all opportunities to work preventively are essential for reaching the goal.

Swedish Nurses against Tobacco
see it as their duty to ....
• increase knowledge about tobacco among their colleagues
• motivate nurses to refrain from tobacco use and
act as role models for their patients
• promote tobacco-free pregnancies and start of life for children
and tobacco-free environments for adolescents
• encourage nurses worldwide to start organizations against tobacco
• continue to work with the international network of Nurses against Tobacco
to keep in touch and share experiences

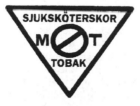

Nurses against Tobacco in Sweden
Office: Gamla Brogatan 13, Stockholm
Mail: Box 298, S-101 25 Stockholm, Sweden
Tel +46-8-677 10 90; fax +46-8-677 10 93

Smoking behaviour among midwives in some hospitals in Japan

F. Fukushima[1], K. Miyasato[2], Y. Osaki[3] & M. Minowa[3]

[1] Department of Public Health Nursing, National Institute of Public Health,
[2] Department of Nursing, University of Kitazato, and [3] Department of Epidemiology,
National Institute of Public Health, Tokyo, Japan

Stop-smoking policies among persons engaged in medical care in Japan are still deficient in comparison with those in western countries. The prevalence of smoking among women in their twenties and thirties is rising, and an increase in the proportion of smokers among adolescents is predicted. This will lead to an increase among women of reproductive age, resulting in a serious problem of smoking mothers, which will also harm the health of their foetusus and infants. Persons engaged in medical care who have contact with mothers throughout pregnancy and delivery thus play an important role in helping mothers to stop smoking and prevent them from starting to smoke.

The smoking status of health professionals affects their advice and actions with regard to patients. Research is needed for planning stop-smoking campaigns in hospitals, by determining the smoking status of nursing staff in obstetrics and gynaecology wards, investigating their attitudes to and awareness of the hazards of smoking and clarifying the problems of their smoking behaviour.

Methods
We approached the nursing staff of the obstetrics wards in one hospitals in Tokyo and six in Shizuoka Prefecture. An anonymous, self-administered questionnaire was distributed to each midwife and registered nurse; after they had completed the forms at the hospital, they placed them in previously provided small blank envelopes, sealed

them, placed them in larger envelopes on which their names were written and gave them to the head nurse of the ward. The head nurse checked only the large envelopes, to ensure that all the nurses and midwives had handed in the questionnaires, and then posted the small envelopes to the National Institute of Public Health without opening them. The survey was conducted in March and April 1997.

The percentage of forms collected was 99% (175/177); since none was incomplete, all were used in the analysis. Smoking status was classified as: daily smoker, occasional smoker, ex-smoker (persons who had smoked continuously for over six months but no longer smoked), 'ever smoker' (persons who had tried smoking but had not smoked continuously for over six months and did not smoke currently) and 'never smoker' (persons who had never tried smoking).

Results and discussion

The rate of smoking among midwives was low (Table 1) and a strong relationship was seen between smoking status and the attitude towards smoking. Surprisingly, no relationship was seen between knowledge about the hazards of smoking and giving advice to pregnant women on quitting smoking. A relationship was found between opinions about regulating smoking in hospitals and smoking status. Thus, many of those who thought there should be a complete ban on smoking did not smoke (21% of midwives and 11% of registered nurses) and many of those who thought an area should be designated for smokers (79% of midwives and 87% of nurses) were themselves smokers. In an analysis of knowledge about illnesses caused by smoking, a high percentage of correct answers was obtained with respect to lung cancer and cancer of the larynx and a low percentage with respect to pancreatic cancer, cervical cancer and urinary bladder cancer. No relationship was found between smoking status and knowledge of other diseases associated with smoking, i.e. cancer of the oesophagus, chronic bronchitis, emphysema and stroke, and the smoking rates were high among those who correctly identified gastric ulcer and myocardial infarct. Incorrect answers were given about the relationship with low-weight babies, mainly by women who smoked. Knowledge about passive smoking was not related to smoking status, but those who were uninterested in passive smoking were likely to smoke .

There was a strong relationship between the attitude towards smoking and smoking status. There was a high smoking rate among those who answered 'Do not know' to the attitude 'Pregnant women should not smoke for the well-being of their foetus and baby.' Agreement with the attitude 'People should not smoke for social reasons' was higher among people who smoked. Of the three questions about smoking by women, the relationship with smoking was strongest with the attitude 'Smoking should be allowed without discrimination between males and females'. The smoking rate was high among nurses who disagreed with the attitude 'Health professionals should not smoke'. The smoking rate tended to be high among those who agreed that 'Smoking should be allowed for people involved in medical care outside working hours' and 'Smoking

Table 1. Smoking status of 102 midwives and 60 registered nurses in Japan

Profession	Smoking status	Prevalence (%)
Midwife	Daily	5.9
	Occasional	< 2
	Ex-smoker	< 2
	'Ever smoker'	38.2
	'Never smoker'	52
Registered nurse	Daily	28.3
	Occasional	6.0
	Ex-smoker	< 2
	'Ever smoker'	16.7
	'Never smoker'	46.7

should be allowed as in other occupations'. The relationship between attitudes towards smoking and smoking status might be due to smokers tending to justify their habit.

Smoking status was weakly correlated with opinions about giving advice to pregnant women to stop smoking. Thus, the smoking rate was lower among those who gave advice frequently. The rate was high among those who had received no education about smoking. Satisfaction at being a nurse had little relation to smoking status.

To sum up, we found a low rate of smoking among midwives, and even smokers agreed that smoking should be restricted in hospitals. As smoking status affected opinions about giving advice to pregnant women to stop smoking, it is important that steps be taken to reduce smoking among nursing staff in obststrics and gynaecology wards.

Comparison of results with those of national surveys

We compared our results with those of surveys on the smoking behaviour of nursing staff in national hospitals. The smoking rate in our survey was slightly higher among nurses aged 40–50. In a comparison of the smoking rates of nursing staff in obstetrics and gynaecology wards, although the number of samples of our survey was insufficient for detailed analysis, the smoking rate in our study tended to be higher among nurses aged 40–50. The major differences between our survey and the national surveys were the extremely low proportion in our survey of those who replied 'to regain health' as the reason for stopping smoking; a slightly higher proportion of those who gave a correct answer about low-weight babies; and the lack of relationship satisfaction at being a nurse and smoking status. Most of the other results of the surveys were similar. Accordingly, although the sampling for our survey was not random, the results were broadly consistent with those of national research.

Nurses and tobacco control: Need for a strategic plan

L. Sarna

School of Nursing, University of California, Los Angeles, California, United States

The purpose of this communication is to highlight the efforts of nurses in tobacco-related education, practice, research and policy in the United States and to initiate discussion on the need for a global, strategic plan for the activity of nurses in tobacco control. In collaboration with the American Nurses' Association's Nursing Coalition for Tobacco Control, a nursing centre for tobacco intervention has been established, with a web site, for dissemination of information. Educational programmes directed at student nurses, school nurses and other special groups have been offered, and new educational materials are being developed. The tobacco control policies of the American Nurses' Association, the Oncology Nursing Society, the nursing sub-committee of the International Union Against Cancer and the International Society for Nurses in Cancer Care will be used as models. Strategies and research are being used to enhance use of the smoking cessation guidelines of the AHCPR. Barriers to national and international collaboration exist, but potential solutions are being developed for strategic planning.

Prevalence of smoking among staff in chemists' shops in Romania

F. Mihaltan

M. Nasta Institute of Pneumophtisiology, Bucharest, Romania

The pupose of the study reported here was to determine the prevalence of and the attitude towards smoking of pharmacists and assistant pharmacists in Romanian chemists' shops. On the basis of a questionnaire distributed in two districts of the country, a representative sample of 169 individuals (54 chemists and 115 attendants and sisters) was selected, most of whom were women (94%).

Active smokers represented 22% of the sample, ex-smokers, 11% and passive smokers, 8.9%. On average, the staff of chemists' shops had smoked 4.5 cigarettes per day for 6.8 years. The prevalence of smoking in their families was 68%. Only half of the pharmacists and assistant pharmacists had received information about smoking at university or at school, but 88% considered it to be harmful. Although 78% regarded smoking as an addiction, only 14% knew methods for stopping smoking, and only 32% had tried to stop smoking. The staff showed little interest in obtaining more knowledge about smoking (32%), although 57% considered that conferences on the topic were useful.

The prevalence of smoking among chemists' shop staff generally exceeded the average for the female population of Romania. As they lack knowledge about the dependence induced by smoking, training courses should be organized, both at university and afterwards. They should also be informed about techniques for stopping smoking, if the relevant products are available in chemists' shops in Romania.

Health-care students

Evaluation of smoking prevention and cessation support programme for student nurses and their patients

K. Okada[1], C. Kawata[2], M. Nakamura[3] & A. Oshima[4]

[1]Chiba University, [2]University of Tokyo, [3]Osaka Cancer Prevention and Detection Center and [4]Osaka Medical Center for Cancer and Cardiovascular Diseases, Japan

Purpose

Education about smoking must be directed towards health professionals and especially nurses, because of their numbers and their roles. Women in their 20s and 30s in Japan appear to be smoking in greater numbers than previously (Ministry of Health and Welfare, 1987, 1993), and the prevalence of smoking among female nurses and student nurses is even higher (Okada & Kawata, 1995). We tried to involve student nurses in a smoking prevention programme with the view that elimination of smoking in nursing schools would not only be beneficial to student nurses but would also encourage them to help their patients to quit smoking.

We have already published results on the effectiveness of this programme among student nurses during the first year (Okada et al., 1996). Here, we evaluate the programme for longer-term smoking prevention and cessation among both the student nurses and their patients.

Methods

The study was conducted between 1994 and 1997 among 220 first-year female student nurses. A self-administered, multiple-choice questionnaire was given to all the nurses at the beginning of their first year and at the end of their third year. The programme consisted of an 80-min lesson for the students at the beginning of the first year, then advice for smokers; two lessons during the second year and cessation support while studying in a hospital. One group of 41 nurses followed the entire programme and 71 received only the lesson and advice during the first year; the other 108 served as the comparison group. We also provided cessation support to 52 patients or smokers who had been in contact with the student nurses.

Results and discussion

There was no difference in the percentage of smokers in the three groups of student nurses at the end of three years, indicating that it is difficult to change behaviour with only three lessons and cessation advice and support. The percentages who were occasional smokers, smoking 1–29 cigarettes per week, at the time of the first questionnaire and were non-smokers at the end of the programme was, however, 47% among those who had participated in the programme and 32% in the comparison group (Okada et al., 1996).

When the student nurses were asked, "Do you think nurses should provide cessation support to smokers?", 44% of those who had followed the entire programme and only 12% of the comparison group agreed strongly (Table 1). Analysis of the cigarette consumption of patients or smokers who had received cessation support from the student nurses showed that 54.2% smoked fewer cigarettes after receiving support, indicating that the programme was effective.

References

Okada, K. & Kawata, C. (1995) Correlation between smoking behavior and school life satisfaction among students of nursing in Japan. In: *Tobacco and Health*, New York: Plenum Press, pp. 717–720

Okada, K., Kawata, C., Nakamura, M. & Oshima, A .(1996) The short-term effectiveness of a smoking prevention program for student nurse. In: *Health Promotion and Education. Bringing Health to Life*, Tokyo: Hoken-Dojin sha., pp. 234–235

Ministry of Health and Welfare (1987) *Smoking and Health*, First Edition, Tokyo

Ministry of Health and Welfare (1993) *Smoking and Health*, Second Editio, Tokyo

Table 1. Reactions to the question, "Do you think nurses should provide cessation support to smokers?" among student nurses according to participation in the programme

Participation	Agreement (%)			
	Strong	Agreement	Some	Disagreement
Full	18	19	3	1
1st year	15	33	16	6
None	13	49	31	15

Cigarette smoking among Polish medical students

R. Palusiński, A. Bilan, J. Mosiewicz, W. Myslíński & J. Hanzlik

Department of Internal Medicine, University School of Medicine, Lublin, Poland

Introduction

Despite widespread knowledge about the risks of tobacco smoking, nearly half of the adults in Poland continue to smoke (Zatonski, 1995). Moreover, at the beginning of 1990s, the cigarette consumption among adults was the highest in the world (World Health Organization, 1997). Health-care professionals can play an important role in supporting smoking cessation, as physicians are uniquely placed to aid people who smoke. They are also important role models of appropriate health behaviour, so that smoking by physicians undermines the message to patients about the adverse health effects of smoking (Dawley et al., 1981) and makes tobacco control more difficult. Most physicians are not trained to treat patients who are addicted to nicotine (Wechsler et al., 1983). One reason is that only 8% of medical faculties in Europe and none in Poland have specific teaching modules on tobacco (Crofton et al., 1996).

The aim of this study was to assess the prevalence of tobacco smoking among medical students of our university during their first, third and fifth years of training.

Methods

A questionnaire designed to elicit information on the prevalence and intensity of smoking was filled in anonymously by 565 students (85% of the total), comprising 310 women and 255 men. There were 211 students in the first year, 156 in the third and 198 in the fifth year. The criteria for smoking status were those described in the guidelines of the World Health Organization (1980). The degree of addiction level was estimated from the Fagerström nicotine dependence chart.

Results

The overall prevalence of smoking increased between the first and the fifth year, from 14% to 29%, and the percentage of non-smokers decreased progressively, from 84% among the first-year students to 65% among those in the fifth year. In spite of the increasing number of ex-smokers, the percentages of daily smokers and occasional smokers increased. The results for smoking prevalence are presented in Table 1.

There was a higher percentage of female than male non-smokers. Among male fifth-year students, only 52% were non-smokers. The male rates for daily smoking were 9.8% in the first year and 22% in the fifth year, and a pronounced increase was observed among female students (from 2.2 to 10%). The sex differences are presented in Table 2.

The fifth-year students were also more strongly addicted than those in other years, with Fageström scores of 1.2 ± 1.8 for first-year students, 0.6 ± 1.2 for third-year students and 2.4 ± 2.5 for fifth-year students.

Table 1. Prevalence of smoking among Polish medical students

Year	Non-smokers		Ex- smokers		Daily smokers		Occasional smokers	
	No.	%	No.	%	No.	%	No.	%
I	192	84	4	1.8	12	5.3	20	8.8
III	120	77	8	5.1	8	5.1	20	13
V	128	65	13	6.6	31	16	26	13
I, III, V	440	76	25	4.3	51	8.8	66	11

Table 2. Prevalence of smoking among female and male medical students in Poland

Year	Sex	Non-smokers		Ex-smokers		Daily smokers		Occasional smokers	
		No.	%	No.	%	No.	%	No.	%
I	Female	121	89	1	0.74	3	2.2	11	8.1
	Male	71	77	3	3.3	9	9.8	9	9.8
III	Female	69	81	3	3.5	5	5.9	8	9.4
	Male	51	72	5	7.0	3	4.2	12	17
V	Female	80	76	4	3.8	11	10	10	9.5
	Male	48	52	9	9.7	20	22	16	17
I, III, V	Female	270	83	8	2.5	19	5.8	29	8.9
	Male	170	66	17	6.7	32	12	37	14

Discussion and conclusion

We studied only students at our home university; however, the relatively high response rate and the fact that the study population is a cross-section of Polish society lead us to believe that our results are reliable. The percentage of medical students who smoked was the same as that in our study in 1992 (Bilan et al., 1996), i.e. 20%. The incidence of daily cigarette smoking among medical students and the substantial increase in the number of daily and occasional smokers between the first and the fifth year are consistent with other reports (Tessier et al., 1989, 1992). This unfavourable trend may be due to the lack of specific teaching on tobacco (Crofton et al., 1996), and neither basic nor clinical classes provide sufficient information about nicotine addiction. We found a great number of occasional smokers, especially among male students, and this group is a potential target for an anti-smoking campaign. Although the total number of daily smokers is higher among male than female students, the prevalence appeared to increase more rapidly in the female population. The most striking finding is that the fifth-year students smoke more heavily than those at the beginning of medical training.

The prevalence of cigarette smoking among Polish medical students is still high, especially among men, and more fifth-year students smoke and smoke more heavily than those in lower years. An anti-smoking campaign should be targeted mainly at first-year students.

References

Bilan, A., Palusinski, R., Mosiewicz, J., Ostrowski, S., Mysliński, W., Rymarz, E. & Hanzlik, J. (1996) Tobacco smoking among Polish students of medicine. In: *Abstract Book. Smoke Free Europe Conference on Tobacco or Health 1996*, p. 195

Crofton, J.W., Tessier, J.F., Freour, P. & Piha, T. (1996) European medical schools and tobacco. *Med. Educ.*, **30**, 424

Dawley, H.H., Carrol, S.F. & Morrison, J.E. (1981) The discouragement of smoking in a hospital setting: The importance of modeled behavior. *Int. J. Addict.*, **16**, 905

Tessier, J.F., Freour, P., Crofton, J. & Kombou, L. (1989) Smoking habits and attitudes of medical students towards smoking and antismoking campaigns in fourteen European countries. *Eur. J. Epidemiol.*, **5**, 311

Tessier, J.F., Freour, P., Belougne, D. & Crofton, J. (1992) Smoking habits and attitudes of medical students towards smoking and antismoking campaigns in nine Asian countries. *Int. J. Epidemiol.*, **21**, 298

Wechsler, H., Levine, S., Idelson, R.K., Rohman, M. & Taylor, J.O. (1983) The physician's role in health promotion. *New Engl. J. Med.*, **308**, 97

World Health Organization (1980) *Guidelines for Smoking Control*, Geneva

World Health Organization (1997) *Tobacco or Health: A Global Status Report*, Geneva

Zatonski, W. (1995) The health of the Polish population. *Public Health Rev.*, **23**, 139

Social environment and tobacco smoking among Polish medical students

A. Bilan, R. Palusiński, A. Witczak, S. Ostrowski, E. Rymarz, J. Zdanowska & J. Hanzlik

1st Department of Internal Medicine, University School of Medicine, Lublin, Poland

Abstract
The aim of this study was to assess the social and environmental factors associated with smoking among Polish medical students and their level of knowledge about the effects of tobacco on health. The study group consisted of 326 women and 256 men, and there were 117 smokers (20%). Of the smokers, 84% reported that at least one of their parents smoked; among the non-smokers, this percentage was 68% ($p = 0.008$). The main reasons for smoking reported by smokers were pleasure, soothing effect, social pressure and activity for the hands. Knowledge of the hazards of tobacco smoking in our group of students did not differ between smokers and non-smokers. Many students realized that smoking increases mortality from cardiovascular and respiratory diseases, but there remained a great number of lacunae about the other consequences of smoking.

Introduction
Scientists, medical staff and health promotors have made more and more people aware of the hazards of tobacco smoking. As physicians are important role models of appropriate health behaviour, they should not smoke. Unfortunately, many investigators have reported substantial increases in the number of smokers between the first and the final year of medical studies (Tessier *et al.*, 1989, 1992). The aim of the study was to assess the social and environmental factors associated with tobacco smoking among Polish medical students.

Methods
A questionnaire designed to evaluate the prevalence and intensity of smoking and habits and the social environment was filled in anonymously by 582 students (85% of the total). The study group consisted of 326 women and 256 men, with 117 smokers (20%); 25 ex-smokers were excluded from the analysis. The study criteria of smoking status were those of WHO (1980). The statistical analysis was performed with the χ^2 test.

Results
At least one parent was reported to be a smoker by 84% of the students who smoked and 68% of the non-smokers ($p = 0.008$). The largest differences between the groups were in relation to the percentage of fathers (40 vs. 32%) and both parents (32 vs. 23%) who smoked.
The responses to the questionnaire eliciting knowledge about tobacco-related diseases are presented in Table 1. Nearly all of the students (99%) knew about the harmful effects of environmental tobacco smoke. Belief that there is a 'safe cigarette' was expressed by 5.8% of the smokers and only 1.3% of the non-smokers ($p = 0.019$). As many as 67% of the smokers thought that doctors should be allowed to smoke as compared with 33% of the non-smokers ($p = 0.0000$).
The main reasons for smoking reported by the smokers were for pleasure (40.1%), for a soothing effect (35%), social pressure (6.1%) and activity for the hands (6.1)%. Tobacco advertising was cited by 14% of the students as the influence to start smoking.
We also found that the smokers were more frequently overweight (15%) than the non-smokers (8.6%), but the difference was not statistically significant.

Table 1. Knowledge of Polish medical students about the
hazards of cigarette smoking

Disease	Smokers (%)	Non-smokers (%)
Lung cancer	95	98
Chronic bronchitis	93	90
Myocardial infarction	89	87
Neonatal death	87	93
Infertility	42	40
Premature menopause	32	38

Discussion

Our findings indicate that smoking among medical students depends heavily on the smoking habits in their families, especially that of their fathers, which is consistent with other findings (Vlajinac *et al.*, 19898; Prokhorov & Aleksandrov, 1992). Flynn (1961) and Morrison and Medovy (1961) noted in the early 1960s that smoking was almost twice as frequent among children whose two parents smoked than when neither smoked. Health education campaigns should thus be started as early as possible and directed not only to smokers but also to their families.

Knowledge about the hazards of tobacco smoking in our group of students did not differ between smokers and non-smokers, although it was incomplete. In the study of Tessier *et al.* (1992) in nine Asian countries, over 80% of non- or ex-smokers but only 60% of smokers thought that smoking is harmful to health. European medical students also had many defects in their knowledge about tobacco and its effects (Tessier *et al.*, 1989; Crofton *et al.*, 1994). In our study, nearly all of the students knew about the harmful effects of passive smoking, but a significantly larger percentage of smokers thought that there was such a thing as a 'safe cigarette'. The students who smoked were more likely to accept doctors' smoking, yet, doctors who are addicted to nicotine cannot reliably persuade their patients to give up smoking (Chapman, 1995).

The main reasons given for smoking were pleasure, a soothing effect, social pressure and manual activity, and these should form the target for anti-smoking campaigns.

References

Chapman, S. (1995) Doctors who smoke. *Br. Med. J.*, 311, 142–143
Crofton, J.W., Freour, P.P. & Tessier, J.F. (1994) Medical education on tobacco: Implications of a worldwide survey. *Med. Educ.*, 28, 187–196
Flynn, M.P. (1961) *J. Irish Med. Assoc.*, 48, 87 Prokhorov, A.V. & Aleksandrov, A.A. (1992) Tobacco smoking in Moscow school students. *Br. J. Addict.*, 87, 1469
Morrison, J.B. & Medovy, H. (1961) *Can. Med. Assoc. J.*, 84, 1006
Tessier, J.F., Freour, P., Crofton, J. & Kombou, L. (1989) Smoking habits and attitudes of medical students towards smoking and antismoking campaigns in fourteen European countries. *Eur. J. Epidemiol.*, 5, 311
Tessier, J.F., Freour, P., Belougne, D. & Crofton, J. (1992) Smoking habits and attitudes of medical students towards smoking and antismoking campaigns in nine Asian countries. *Int. J. Epidemiol.*, 21, 298
Vlajinac, H., Adanja, B. & Jarebinski, M. (1989) Cigarette smoking among medical students in Belgrade related to parental smoking habits. *Soc. Sci. Med.*, 29, 891–894
WHO (1980) *Guidelines for Smoking Control*, Geneva

Smoking habits and knowledge of its harmful effects among medical students in the Slovak Republic

E. Kavcová, E. Rozborilová, R. Vysehradsky, J. Kollár, J. Zucha & M. Bronis

Department of Tuberculosis and Respiratory Diseases, Jessenius Medical Faculty of the Comenian University and Faculty Hospital, Martin, Institute of Experimental and Clinical Medicine of the P.J. Safarik University, Kosice, Institute of Medical Education, Bratislava, Slovak Republic

Introduction

Medical doctors should be the leaders in tobacco prevention activities. As role models for their patients and as helpers, leaders and activists, they are needed in campaigns to reduce smoking. We were interested in the smoking behaviour and attitudes towards smoking of Slovak medical students, who represent the next generation of medical doctors. The aims of the study were:

- to investigate the smoking habits of medical students and define the factors that influence smoking
- to determine the role of doctors in preventing smoking,
- to determine the general knowledge of medical students about tobacco-related diseases and
- to determine their attitudes to legislative measures.

Materials and methods

A modified, anonymous version of the questionnaire of WHO and the International Union against Tuberculosis and Lung Disease was given to 350 first- and fifth-year students at the medical faculties in Martin and Kosice (Tessier *et al.*, 1989) at lectures and seminars during two months in 1995. The response rate was 95.1% (333 respondents). Of these, 72 men and 107 women were in the first year of their studies and 63 men and 91 women were in the fifth year. Differences between groups were analysed by the chi-squared test.

Results

There were 19% current smokers, 74% non-smokers and 7.3% ex-smokers in this group of medical students. Of the smokers, 8% were regular smokers and 11% occasional smokers. The prevalence of smoking was significantly higher in the fifth (26%) than in the first year of study (12%; $p < 0.001$), and 43% of the respondents had started to smoke while at university. Male students smoked more (22%) than females (16%), but the difference is not significant. Most of the students said that their main motivation for smoking was that their friends smoked (60%) and because they wanted to belong to a group (21%). Peer pressure and peer bonding thus played important roles in our respondents' decision to smoke.

Only 2.7% of the students thought that they would probably or certainly smoke daily within five years. Health issues were the main reasons for wishing to quit. The reasons for wishing to start smoking among non-smokers were 'None' for 71% of students, 'Don't know' for 7% and stress, society, problems, nervousness, psychological problems, trauma and other reasons were each cited by about 6% of the students.

More than 99% of the students strongly or mildly agreed with the statement that smoking is harmful for health, with no difference between first- and fifth-year students, but the students' knowledge about smoking-related diseases differed. Almost 100% of all students indicated that smoking causes lung cancer, but few were aware that it causes other diseases, such as bladder cancer, pulmonary emphysema, leukoplakia, soft-tissue lesions and neonatal death. The most erroneous and absent responses were given by first-year students, but small proportions existed among those in their fifth year.

Between 80 and 94% of all students agreed that it is doctors' responsibility to convince people to stop smoking and that they should set a good example by not smoking, but less than half of the fifth-year students (49%) have sufficient knowledge to counsel patients who wish to stop smoking.

Nearly all the students (99%) agreed with smoking restrictions in closed public places, 97% agreed that sales of tobacco to children should be prohibited, 94% agreed that there should be health warnings on cigarette packs, 93% agreed with restrictions on smoking in hospitals except in special rooms, 83% agreed with a complete ban on tobacco advertising, but only 65% of students agreed with a sharp price increase for tobacco products. Most of the students agreed (78%) that health professionals should receive special training on how to help patients who wish to stop smoking.

Conclusions

The results of this study should not only provide information about the prevalence of smoking among medical students in the Slovak Republic and their knowledge and attitudes towards tobacco, but should also serve as a basis for changes and challenges to medical education and postgraduate education for doctors (Waalkens *et al.*, 1992). We recommend the following:

- to improve teaching about smoking and health,
- to provide students with the results of successful smoking prevention policies in developed countries,
- to stress the importance of legislative measures,
- to train students and doctors in smoking cessation programmes and
- to emphasize the positive example that medical doctors should set for patients and the public.

It is everyone's responsibility to support students in deciding to be non-smokers and to create a non-smoking environment so that being a non-smoker becomes the norm.

References

Tessier, J.F., Freour, P., Crofton, J. & Kombou, L. (1989) Smoking habits and attitudes of medical students towards smoking and antismoking campaigns in fourteen European countries. *Eur. J. Epidemiol..*, **5**, 311–321

Waalkens, H.J., Schotanus, J.C., Adriaanse, H. & Knol, K. (1992) Smoking habits in medical students and physicians in Groningen, The Netherlands. *Eur. Respir. J.*, **5**, 49–52

Tobacco habits among medical students in Spain: An 11-year study

A. Montes-Martínez[1] & J.J. Gestal-Otero[1,2]

[1]Department of Preventive Medicine, University of Santiago de Compostela, and [2]Unit of Preventive Medicine, Complexo Hospitalario de Santiago, Spain

Medical students in the last year of their studies can nearly be regarded as health professionals. Thus, it is interesting to determine the attitudes that they will soon implement. Follow-up of such a well -defined population is very accurate because the students are enrolled in an administrative structure and are easy to trace. This population is thus optimal for predicting the future tobacco habits of young health workers.

The starting age and the evolution of tobacco habits was studied among students registered in the course for preventive medicine in the final year of medical studies at the University of Santiago de Compostela between 1985 and 1996, in a cross-sectional study carried out during each academic year. The questionnaire was formulated on the basis of the recommendations of the World Health Organization for this type of study.

The prevalence of tobacco use decreased significantly between 1985 and 1996: 56% (95% confidence interval [CI], 54–62) of students were habitual smokers in 1985 and only 20% (95% CI, 14–25) in 1996, although the proportion of occasional smokers remained more or less constant during this period. The decrease in prevalence was due to a doubling in the number of occasional smokers in 1996 compared with 1985 and a tripling of the number of those who had never smoked (Figure 1).

The decrease in smoking prevalence was greater among men than women: the prevalence of habitual smokers dropped from 61% (95% CI, 55–66) to 17% (10–27) among men and from 54% (49–61) to 22% (14–29) among women. The age at starting habitual smoking increased from 17 years in 1985 to 18 in 1996, but this evolution differed for men and women, women starting to smoke later in life, although the differences are not statistically significant. The percentage of usual smokers (both current and ex-smokers) who started smoking during their medical studies increased from 5.5% (95% CI, 3.8–7.8) in 1985 to 10% (6.3–15) in 1996.

A large, significant reduction in the consumption of tobacco was thus seen between 1985 and 1996, and the age at starting appears to be delayed. More than half of the current or ex-smokers acquired their habit while students in the Faculty of Medicine.

Figure 1. Prevalence of smoking among final-year medical students in Spain, 1985–96

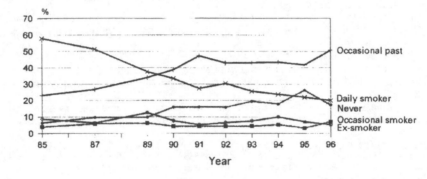

Smoking among medical students in Spain

I. Nerin, I. Sánchez Agudo, D. Guillén, C. Toyas, R. Vicente & A. Más

Faculty of Medicine, University of Zaragoza, Spain

Objectives: To determine the prevalence and attitudes of fourth-year medical students towards tobacco and to sensitize future health professionals to the importance of being a non-smoker.

Methods: A survey was carried out among 332 fourth-year medical students, 124 male (37%) and 208 female (63%). Each received a questionnaire in class, and 158 (48%) were returned, 54 from men (34%) and 104 from women (66%).

Results: Of the total, 65% had ever smoked, 20% smoked daily, 13% smoked < 1 cigarette per day, and 67% were non-smokers. There was no difference by sex. Of the smokers, 32% started to smoke during their medical studies. Smoking was considered to be dangerous for health by 92% of the students, 93% thought that most patients with lung cancer had been smokers and 90% considered that passive smoking was a risk for health. With regard to smoking as a risk factor, 99% of this population related smoking to lung disease, 95% to coronary ischaemia and 55% to urinary bladder cancer. Smoking was considered to be addictive behaviour by 42%; 68% thought that professors should avoid smoking, and 62% considered that health professionals have an exemplary role

Conclusions: The prevalence of smoking in this group is lower than in the general population (34%) or among the staff at the same school (35%; $p = 0.001$). The students had extensive knowledge about the effects of tobacco on health, but they must be convinced of the exemplary role that doctors play in improving health.

This study was supported by the University of Zaragoza research programme.

Prevalence and attitudes of medical students in Spain towards smoking

I. Nerin, L. Sánchez Agudo, A. Más, D. Guillén, C. Toyas & R. Vicente

Faculty of Medicine, University of Zaragoza, Spain

Objectives: To determine the prevalence and attitudes in a group of medical students between the fourth and sixth years of their studies.

Methods: A study was carried out among fourth-year medical students and was repeated during the sixth year. There were 332 students in the fourth year, 37% male and 63% female, 158 of whom returned the questionnaire (34% of men and 66% of women; mean age, 22 years). In the sixth year, there were 339 students (37% male and 63% female) and 175 questionnaires were returned (30% males and 70% females; mean age, 23). The groups differed slightly, as some students had not continued to the sixth year.

Results: Daily smoking was reported by 20% of students in the fourth year and 30% in the sixth year; 13% in the fourth year and 12% in the sixth year smoked less than one cigarette per day, and 67% in the fourth year and 58% in the sixth year were non-smokers.

Conclusions: A statistically significant increase ($p < 0.05$) was found in the prevalence of smoking between the fourth and the sixth year of medical studies. Schools of medicine should be the centres for imparting knowledge about smoking and for emphasizing the exemplary roles that health professionals should play in this regard. Intervention should be carried out during the first years of study, when the age of the students makes them more receptive to infromation that will change their attitudes.

This study was supported by the University of Zaragoza research programme.

Smoking among medical students and student nurses in the Russian Federation: Educational problems

K.P. Hanson, A.S. Barchuck & M.A. Zabezhinski

N.N. Petrov Research Institute of Oncology, St Petersburg, Russian Federation

The study reported here was part of a special programme on tobacco control developed at the N.N. Petrov Research Institute of Oncology in collaboration with the City Centre of Medical Prevention. We reported the general principles and directions of the activities in an earlier publication (Hanson *et al.*, 1995).

The most urgent problem was to obtain a ban on tobacco advertising. A law was finally passed by Parliament (State Duma) in which tobacco advertising is banned in all mass media. We also tried to involve journalists in anti-tobacco activities, with the result that information about the hazards of tobacco smoking and smoking cessation methods were published regularly.

The important problem now is health education. In a survey of doctors at our Institute (Hanson *et al.*, 1996), we found that although they were all aware of the carcinogenic risk of smoking, the prevalence was high, reaching 50% of men. Nevertheless, the majority advised their patients to stop smoking.

We have now studied the prevalence of smoking among medical students. Anonymous questionnaires were distributed to medical students (mean age, 23 years) and student nurses (mean age, 18 years) which included items concerning their smoking pattern, the health hazards of smoking and tobacco control. No significant differences were found between the two groups. The prevalence of smoking was 56% among male medical students, 35% among female medical students, 60% among male student nurses and 27% among female student nurses. This prevalence was higher than that among doctors in our previous study.

All of the students smoked filter cigarettes, at a rate of 10 cigarettes per day among men and seven per day among women; these rates were lower than among doctors. The mean age at starting to smoke was 16 years for men and 18 for women. Of the smokers, 67% wanted to stop, and most had already tried to do so, but success in quitting was seen only among women, and all had stopped without outside help. Of the women who quit smoking, 13% had not smoked for more than six months. Of the smokers who had not succedded in quitting, 22% intended to reduce their consumption of cigarettes, and 11% intended to quit. The main reasons for wishing to stop were to avoid respiratory disorders and for cosmetic reasons (among women). Of the whole population, 68% intended to recommend stopping smoking to their parents.

Knowledge about the health consequences of smoking was limited mainly to cancer in both groups. They had little knowledge about the risk to embryos, the hazard associated with exposure to enviromental tobacco smoke or therapy for nicotine dependence. There was no relationship between level of knowledge and smoking status.

The students considered that the most effective measures for tobacco control included information on the hazards of tobacco, the benefits of stopping smoking and methods of smoking cessation.

After the results of this survey had been analysed, seminars on the problems of health promotion were organized for professors at the medical institute and the medical college, and posters on tobacco hazards and tobacco control were prepared with the students. We conclude that if all health professionals are to be involved in health education and tobacco control, special courses on these topics should be included in the curricula of medical students and student nurses.

References

Hanson, K.P., Barchuk, A.S. & Zabezhinski, M.A. (1995) Tobacco control in St Petersburg. Problems and perspectives. In: Slama, K., ed., *Tobacco and Health*, New York: Plenum Press, pp. 879–880
Hanson, K.P., Zabezhinski, M.A., Barchuk, A.S. & Berstein, L.M. (1996) Tobacco use among doctors, attitude and prevention. In: *Abstracts of the 'Smoke Free Europe' Conference on Tobacco or Health, Helsinki, Finland, 2–4 October 1996*, p. 119

Prevalence of smoking among medical students at Makerere University, Kampala, Uganda

E.K. Kanyesigye[1], R. Basiraha[2], A. Ampaire[2], G. Wabwire[2], J.B. Waniaye[2], S. Muchuro[2] & E. Nkangi[3]

[1]*Health Services and* [3]*Nutrition Department, Ministry of Health, Masaka, and* [2]*Makerere University, Kampala, Uganda*

Introduction

In developing countries, life expectancy is about 20 years lower than that in industrialized countries because of the high prevalence of infectious and parasitic diseases, and this has masked the effects of cigarette smoking on health. Furthermore, the prevalence of cigarette smoking has been low, especially among rural peasants. Smoking has therefore not been regarded as a serious public health problem in developing countries such as Uganda. Now, however, tobacco companies are fleeing the shrinking market in industrialized countries and have moved into developing countries, with intensified marketing tactics and cheap, high-nicotine and high-tar products. Governments derive considerable revenue from the excise duties levied on cigarette sales, and tobacco farmers often get better prices for tobacco than for other cash crops such as coffee, cotton and tea.

When the head of a household smokes, a sizeable proportion of the household budget is spent on cigarettes, which exerts unfair competition on budget allocations for food, clothing, health care and children's school fees. Tobacco farmers use up wood from natural forests to process (flue-cure) raw tobacco, posing a threat to the local and global environment in a situation in which there is inadequate land for reforestation and wood is also needed for domestic purposes such as cooking.

With intensified programmes for the control of infectious diseases, life expectancy is increasing: for example, in Uganda, from 45 years in 1978 to 51 years in 1988. Many smokers will therefore live to take part in the tobacco epidemic, with rates of cancer, cardiovascular disease and other smoking-related health problems which may approach those of industrialized nations.

Adolescents, a particularly vulnerable group, are usually the target of the tobacco industry's marketing strategies, and the prevalence of smoking in this group in Uganda may rise in view of the relaxed anti-smoking measures that characterize post-independence public schools (in contrast to the pre-independence missionary education). Health education is now an optional subject in these schools, and many adolescents begin smoking without being made aware of the implications for their health.

Few recent studies are available on the prevalence of smoking in Uganda. Mbaziira (1984) found in a random survey that the prevalence of smoking in Kampala was 10% among men and 3% among women. Males were reported to start smoking at the age of 15, with a maximum prevalence at the age of 30. Masironi and Rothwell (1985) reported that the national prevalence was 33%. Kanyesigye (1990) reported an overall smoking prevalence among secondary-school pupils in Uganda of 15%, with 19% among boys and 2.3% among girls. In a survey of students at Makerere University in 1969, Arya and Bennett (1970) found that 33% of men and 7% of women smoked. The purpose of our study was to determine the prevalence of cigarette smoking among medical students at Makerere University and their attitudes and beliefs about tobacco consumption.

Methods

A survey was conducted at the Makerere University campus by a group of five medical students, one from each year of the medical curriculum. Every other name was selected from class lists, so that 250 of the 500 students were chosen and given a self-administered standard WHO questionnaire adjusted to suit the students. The answers were entered into a d-Basc III programme in a personal computer and analysed with Epi Info software.

Results

Of the 250 students surveyed, 146 (58%) were from up-country, 83 (33%) were from Kampala and 21 (8.4%) were from a district capital. The sex distribution was 168 (67%) male and 82 (33%) female. The age distribution was 92% between the ages of 19 and 25; of the 20 who were over 25, 15 were aged 26–30, four in their early 30s, one aged 40 and one aged 52.

Smoking at least once in their lives was reported by 97 (39%) of the respondents. Of these, 50 said that they smoked at least once a week and had done so for three months or more; 28 said that they had smoked daily during the past three months, 7 had done so at least once a week and the remainder less than once a week. Of 40 respondents who smoked every week, 22 (55%) smoked one cigarette per week, five smoked 4–10 cigarettes per week and 13 smoked 20–40 cigarettes per week. Only three smoked hand-rolled cigarettes, and one smoked hand-rolled cigars. All of the 43 respondents who smoked cigarettes said that they smoked filter-tipped cigarettes; of these, 37 bought cigarettes one by one and only six bought them by the pack.

Of the 50 students who replied that they smoked at least once a week and had done so for three months or more, 41 had tried to stop smoking; 11 of these had tried once, 10 twice and the remainder three times or more.

Fathers were reported to smoke by 14% of the participants, mothers by 4.4%, older brothers by 30%, older sisters by 2.0% and best friends by 20%.

The results of the test of knowledge about the hazards of smoking and the opinions of the students about tobacco use are shown in Table 1.

Discussion

A significant association was found between the age of the students and their smoking status ($p = 0.002$) but no difference with regard to socioeconomic status. Whereas the smoking status of the father was significantly associated with that of the student ($p = 0.00003$), that of the mother or older brother or sister was not strongly related; the smoking status of the best friend did show a correlation. The purchase of cigarettes one by one rather than by packs encourages young people to smoke, as they would otherwise be unable to afford the product.

We have gained important information about the prevalence of smoking among medical students in Uganda. More detailed analyses of the results will be published elsewhere.

Acknowledgements

We are grateful to the WHO country office in Uganda for sponsoring this study, to all the medical students who responded and to our fellow investigators for preparing the survey and the interviews.

References

Arya, O.P. & Bennett, F.J. (1970) Smoking amongst university students in Uganda: An analysis of prevalence and attitudes. *East Afr. Med, J.*, 47
Kanyesigye, E.K. (1990) *The Tobacco Industry, and Smoking among Ugandan Teenage Students*, MPH Thesis, Department of Community Medicine, University of Adelaide
Masironi, R. & Rothwell, K. (1988) World trends and effects of tobacco smoking. *World Hlth Stat. Q.*, 41
Mbaziira, M. (1984) Country report, Uganda. In: *Conference on Smoking and Health Issues in Selected English Speaking Countries, Lusaka, Zambia, 26–28 June 1984* (WHO/SMO/84.5)

Table 1. Knowledge and opinions of medical students in Uganda about tobacco use

Statement	Answer (%)		
Knowledge	True	False	Don't know
If you smoke, you are more likely to cough.	86	8.5	15
Smoking is bad for you only if you smoke a lot every day.	32	63	13
Smokers usually die younger than non-smokers.	51	26	24
Breathing smoky air harms babies and young children.	98	0	2.0
A pregnant woman can harm her baby if she smokes.	97	0	2.8
Some cigarettes are not dangerous.	7.3	68	24
Smoking is bad for you if you smoke for a long time.	88	10	2
Opinion	Agree	Disagree	Don't know
Smoking makes you feel good.	38	28	34
You have to smoke if you are with friends who smoke.	12	90	4.0
If you smoke, you worry about being told about it.	43	65	35
Parents shouldn't allow their children to smoke.	86	12	2.0
Teachers should be allowed to smoke at school.	8.8	90	1.2
Cigarettes should be made more expensive to stop young people from smoking.	56	37	5.6
Smoking should not be permitted in public places.	89	10	0.8
Smoking makes you appear grown up.	13	80	6.8

Smoking behaviour of first-year student nurses in Canada

A. Draffin Jones

University of Manitoba, Winnipeg, Canada

We examined the smoking behaviour of students in the first-year programme in the four schools of nursing of Winnipeg. Of the 240 students registered in the programme, 119 volunteered to participate. Information was obtained from their responses to a 35-item questionnaire, presented during a regular class. The students were assured of anonymity.

The data collected indicated that 21% of the respondents reported smoking cigarettes. The majority of the smokers were single females aged 19–33. Of particular concern is the fact that 10 of the 119 students (40% of the current smokers) reported having started to smoke or having increased the number of cigarettes smoked after entry to the school of nursing. Stress was cited by all smokers as a factor for starting.

Although 52% of the smokers stated that they would like to quit within the coming 12 months, none of the schools offered a cessation programme specifically targeted to student nurses or young women. An opportunity exists for schools of nursing to address this issue.

RELIGION AND TOBACCO

Islamic beliefs and practices in tobacco control

E. Dagli

Marmara University, Istanbul, Turkey

Islam began in the Middle East nine centuries before the tobacco plant was introduced into Europe. Tobacco use was therefore not part of the religious rules during the establishment of the religion in the seventh century. Information on tobacco appeared in Islamic literature only after 1606. The Islamic world therefore met tobacco about 1000 years after the birth of this religion. Understanding and acceptance of tobacco use was developed by religious leaders only after the seventeenth century, within the general rules for evaluating attitudes in Islam.

Islam evaluates the acceptability of behaviour at three levels: allowed, unwarranted and forbidden as a sin. Although religious leaders have argued about the acceptability of tobacco use for centuries and have been unable to reach a consensus, the present tendency is to label it as unwarranted. The arguments of religious leaders for categorization of tobacco use into each of the three levels are discussed below.

'Tobacco is allowed'

El Echuri and Abdulgan en-Nablusi both declared that tobacco use should be allowed, and Nablusi (1640–1731) wrote a book about the benefits of smoking. The evidence that these and subsequent leaders have used in coming to the conclusion that tobacco is allowed is as follows:

- In principle, everything is allowed unless otherwise stated in the Koran (*Sure Baqara*). God forbids anything evil. As tobacco was not forbidden in the Koran, the assumption is that it is allowed.
- God created everything for the benefit of the human race. God could not have created a substance that harms people. Humans should not have the right to ban objects and substances that God created.
- Substances that cause loss of consciousness or intoxicate should not be consumed, and their use is considered to be a sin and is forbidden. Tobacco does not cause loss of consciousness.
- If a person uses tobacco and is harmed by it, that is the concern of that individual. It should not be forbidden for other people.
- The evidence that tobacco is harmful is conflicting; in the absence of adequate evidence, smoking should not be declared a sin.

Many of these arguments date from before the 1950s and have not been revised in the light of information on health effects obtained since then. At present, no Islamic religious leader supports the premise that tobacco is harmless and therefore allowed.

'Tobacco use is unwarranted'

Most authorities now consider that tobacco use is unwarranted. The arguments include the following:

- Tobacco has an irritating smell, and the public should not be irritated.
- Islam assumes that a behaviour is unwarranted if there is still debate about whether it is forbidden or allowed. Smoking is still considered a debatable issue.

'Tobacco use is forbidden as a sin'

There have been proponents of the view that tobacco use is a sin for centuries, but there has never been consensus on this view. The arguments for forbidding it as a sin are:

- Torturing people is a sin. As smokers irritate and disturb non-smokers, they are sinful.

- In Islamic literature and the Koran, punishment is frequently referred to as eating fire. Smoking involves smoke and fire.
- Waste is sinful. Buying cigarettes is a waste of money.
- All harmful things are forbidden in Islam. The body is given use of the soul only transiently. Humans do not have the right to harm their bodies. The Koran *Sure Nisa* says "Do not kill yourself." The Sure Baqara says "Do not put yourself in dangerous situations." Smoking is harmful to health.
- Although smoking does not intoxicate, it sedates and relâxes people like other drugs.
- One caliph in the past declared that tobacco use was forbidden, and that ruling should be accepted.
- Smoking stops people from praying, fasting and doing their job properly.

Although many tobacco control advocates would agree with these arguments, the religious authorities cannot yet arrive at a consensus.

Our survey

In order to judge the effect of religious observance on tobacco consumption objectively, we carried out a face-to-face interview survey in Istanbul in 1996 among 538 women from various social and economic backgrounds. The overall prevalence of smoking was 48%, the lowest being found among those who had completed only primary-school education ($p < 0.05$). The rates were similar for women who had been married in a religious ceremony and those who had had only an official ceremony; women who were for and those who were against women's rights activities; women who believed in family planning and those who did not; and women who performed their religious duties regularly and those who did not. Thus, regardless of whether they have modern or conservative religious attitudes, women tend to have similar attitudes to smoking.

There is a need for collaboration with Islamic religious authorities to re-evaluate the perception of tobacco use in the light of recent medical information. It would also be important for Islamic communities to have a better understanding of the effects of tobacco use.

Buddhist belief in tobacco control

Phramaha Chanya Khongchinda

Wat Umong, Chiangmai, Thailand

Introduction

Tobacco is one of the greatest killers in the world, and I am appalled at the death, ill-health, sorrow, lamentation, despair and suffering that tobacco brings to humanity. It is estimated that corrently tobacco kills 3 million people a year—that is one death every 10 seconds. The tobacco war is more powerful, harmful, destructive and violent than all of the wars of this century. Conventional wars are limited in time and space, and other conditions can control war. This is not true for the undeclared tobacco war, which is worldwide and difficult to control. furthermore, it is not just a tragedy of the past, but our future is threatened by smoking as it becomnes popular with the young.

The health, economic, environmental and social problems caused by addiction to smoking are not only of personal concern; smoking is a global problem linked through cause and effect with the way society functions. In Buddhism, this is called the interdependent origination process. Capitalism, materialism, consumerism, socialization, medernization, industrialization, taxation, attitude, education, tradition, culture, scientific and technological progress, the development of communication, advertising and political policy are all part of the promotion of tobacco production and use. We must exchange experiences and knowledge and share responsibility across all sectors of society if we are to find appropriate ways to save the human race from the tobacco epidemic.

The role of religion

All religions and beliefs have strategies to pull people back from the lure of intoxicants and can play a role in alerting people to the evil of tobacco. Buddhism is a world religion that influences the thought, tradition, culture, behaviour and lives of many millions of people. Many schools and temples in which Buddhist training and meditation take place insist that their members not smoke or use other intoxicants or addictive drugs. Many Buddhists practice and teach outdoors, consciously promoting an environment with clean air and free of smoke and persuading smokers that smoking pollutes and will affect both their spiritual and physical well-being.

The 'Four Noble Truths' constitute the central message of Buddhism (Horner, 1987). The truths relate to suffering, the cause of suffering, the possibility of extinguishing suffering and the noble eightfold path to the extinction of suffering. Suffering is a universal problem and is the obstacle that everyone struggles to overcome; non-suffering is the goal to which everyone attains. The natural law of causation, the interdependent origin, is that human life, body and mind are all interlinked, and it is these links that cause suffering and allow its extinction. Defilements—ignorance, craving and attachment—are the main sources of greed, hatred and delusion, which are the causes of suffering. The steps in the noble eightfold path that must be taken to end suffering are a right view, right aspiration, right speech, right action, right livelihood, right effort, right mindfulness and right insight.

The human mission is to investigate, study, review, note and understand the causes and effects of phenomena. The positive and negative effects of causes must be noted on real experiences in daily life. Studying cause and effect in daily life will result in sufficient wisdom to find solutions to life's problems. Physical, verbal and mental behaviour, right or wrong, determine whether there is peace or crisis. Action, speech and thought are the crucial gates to a good or a bad destiny. It is these elemnts in our lives that must be addressed by appropriate training and control. Morality, insight and wisdom are appropriate ways within which there is no room for defilement.

'Mindfulness' involves contemplation of the body, feelings and mind and all perpetually changing natural phenomena as they really are. This is the starting point of self-training for development and the origin of all of the wholesome truths that allow human beings to find the right path, get rid of all evil deeds, attain purification, overcome sorrow and grief, decrease suffering and misery and realize everlasting peace.

Human beings and their behaviour are the place for the study and practice of Buddhism. Study, awareness, development, training, control to prevent selfishness, realization, confidence, liberation and refuge by the self are the main concepts of Buddhist training. Use of the word 'self' does not mean that Buddhism prones self-centredness. In the Buddhist sense, 'self' means that solutions to all the problems of life, health, society, country and the world should begin at the level of the individual, which can then be extended. This involves awakening people by ensuring good information to improve their knowledge and experience and allow them to make behavioural decisions that are safe for themselves and others.

Buddhism is not just concerned with internal, individual issues but also with external factors, such as social, economic, political, environmental, physical and spiritual health, the environment and human rights. Individual glory is a benefit to society. Harmony, mutual understanding, compassion and unity among all who take the right path are important forces for accumulating all individual potential to make a strong, stable society.

Application of Buddhism to tobacco control

Tobacco control in Buddhism means applying Buddhist principles and finding a way to emancipate people from the slavery of tobacco. Although tobacco addiction is not stated in Buddhist texts as positive or negative, tobacco addiction and related behaviour can be analysed by the principles of the four noble truths and interdependent origination. The principle of interdependent origination is searching for and solving real problems in detail, earnestly and step by step in accordance with the condition of causation. In evaluation, the middle way must be used to complete the process, because it presents the right way to observe all things in balance. When one understands the origin and the end, the attractions, dangers and the way to salvation, one is more readily concerned with things as they really are (Muler, 1977). In this way, other kinds of problems in human behaviour can be understood because all are based on causes, effects and balance.

Tobacco addiction starts with human behaviour and is then extended. In order to overcome tobacco addiction, human thought and behaviour must be studied. All human behaviour derives from thought. Whether the thought is right or wrong depends on its basis: if the basis is a defilement, such as ignorance, sensation, craving and attachment, then the thought is wrong and is the cause of all wrong verbal and physical behaviour, which lead to suffering. If the basis is associated with truth, involving mindfulness, insight and wisdom, the thought is right and results in the extinction of suffering.

Tobacco control can be done at both the individual and the social level. No one can use the law or the threat of punishment to compel people to stop smoking. Most smokers stop because of their own solemn intention or because they are inspired by some outside condition. Firstly, they realize that smoking cigarettes causes danger and suffering for themselves. Then, they think that must free themselves of it. Thirdly, they consider that their spiritual and physical condition is prepared. Fourthly, they make the decision by themselves, with no pressure. Fifthly, they try to find the appropriate and effective way to stop. Sixthly, they do the best they can.

Examination of the processes of thought and human behaviour according to Buddhism shows that the defilements that maintain smoking are ignorance, delusion, sensation, craving and attachment. The process of smoking can be seen as follows: certain conditions result in the idea (associated with ignorance and delusion) that smoking is attractive (sensation), and the desire to smoke (craving) arises. When this process is repeated, smoking becomes an attachment. As long as nothing breaks into the process, the vicious circle is maintained. The power of truth—mindfulness, awareness, right understanding, insight and wisdom—can destroy the vicious circle.

The method for destroying the vicious circle is as follows: certain conditions make an individual think about smoking. Mindfulness and awareness must be used to awaken and remind individuals that smoking is dangerous. The, right understanding and insight (calm reflection and thinking about things systematically) must be used to look at all the dangers of smoking. When this type of thinking is mastered, developed and practised in daily life, until the person becomes very pure, strong and stable, the vicious circle will be broken. There is no more thinking about smoking. The right process is preserved and practised until it becomes a skill, and the individual maintains perfect freedom from smoking.

In order to preserve this free spirit, people must live with self-care by carrying our the following activities:
• self-discipline: People must decide to abstain from all that endangers life and observe this rule strictly.
• self-protection: People should avoid other persons and places that stimulate a desire to smoke.
• self-awakening: People should be minful, careful and aware of all of the phenomena of daily life and learn to separate what is beneficial and what is detrimental.
• self-support: Information and knowledge about tobacco should be collected and studied to learn about the negative effects on human life, society and the world.
• self-respect: People should be proud of their ability to save themselves and others from the risk for untimely death and ill-health.
• self-examination: People should examine themselves regularly to continue with their good actions. When more people become winners, fewer people will be addicted to tobacco.

Shared social responsibility

Society. The social environment plays an important role in tobacco addiction. In Buddhism, the process of thought, learning and behaviour arises from the contact between the inner and outer sense organs. Right understanding causes right thought. Right thought causes right conduct and right behaviour. Right undertsanding also leads to knowledge, wisdom and freedom of mind. The two conditions necessary for having right understanding are utterance to another and wise attention (Horner, 1987). Providing a good social environment to allow people to gain good knowledge and create good thought is a form of utterance to others. When the social environment becomes complex, it is difficult for people whose minds are not strong, stable and pure enough to separate what is beneficial and what is evil. When the bad stream is stronger than the good one, it has a greater influence in shaping bad thoughts and behaviour. Tobacco addiction is influenced by the social environment, In order to reduce the number of people who smoke, everyone must join together to create a good social environment and strong minds to shape the new generation of non-smokers. All individuals and social entities must participate in the best way they can.

Family. Parents must be good role models and therefore non-smokers. They should watch their children closely: if they start smoking, the parents should gently advise them and give them good information so that they are aware of the positive and negative aspects. They can then evaluate the information and shape their behaviour appropriately to be free of tobacco addiction.

Educational institutions. Parents send their children to school to study, to acquire knowledge and to emulate the behaviour of their teachers. As the teachers' behaviour has a strong influence on the behaviour of children, the teachers' ethical code should guide them to be non-smokers. Lessons on smoking and non-smoking should be part of the curriculum at every level. All education should be conducted in non-smoking areas.

Mass media. In this time of globalization and progress in science and technology, people from different parts of the world can share experiences. The mass media become an important source of knowledge and have a strong influence on the thoughts of people, thus shaping their character and behaviour. The media should stop advertising all tobacco products and, instead, should be used to communicate information that shows people how to avoid smoking and life a healthy life.

Religious institutions. All religions have a common emphasis on 'salvation' as a goal for life. This concept should be extended to include emancipation from all evils, including tobacco addiction. Religious institutions have always played a leading role in instruction and imparting the concepts of virtue, morality, ethical codes for good conduct and spiritual encouragement. All religious activities should be free of tobacco, all holy and religious places no-smoking zones, and all spiritual leaders be free of tobacco, as models for the people. Religious organizations should support no-smoking campaigns and take the lead in forming groups to combat smoking.

Youth groups. Youth groups can play key roles in determining the orientation of a society. They are often influential in political change. They should be allowed to participate as leading activists, especially in tobacco control.

Farmers and tobacco companies. Knowing the dangers of tobacco addiction, these groups should support the process of reduction of tobacco use. They should think of the danger of their product to their fellow man rather than thinking of self-benefit, and they should change their business to one that contributes to the health and well-being of people.

Government. All governments have a direct duty to promote health and well-being and to protect against ill-health. As smoking results in ill-health, governments must use their powers to reduce tobacco use. A united policy is required to educate people to reduce tobacco use and release themselves from smoking.

Conclusion

Tobacco addiction is perpetual crisis for human beings. We must cooperate, join our hands and hearts, exchange ideas, knowledge and experience and make friends with all arms of the fight against tobacco. Innovations from science and technology must be used. In Buddhism, tobacco addiction derives from defilement caused by ignorance, craving and attachment. Mindfulness, awareness, insight and wisdom must be practised and developed to remove the defilement. We must be confident that right knowledge and wisdom would be a bright light to lead the human race to freedom and safety from the greatest killer in the world.

References
Horner, I.B., translator (1987) *The Collection of the Middle Length Sayings*, Vol. 1, London, Pali Text Society
Muler, M., translator (1977) *Sacred Books of the Buddhists*. London, Pali Text Society

Survey of the knowledge, attitudes and practices of Cambodian Buddhist monks with regard to tobacco

M. Smith[1], T. Umenai[1] & C. Radford[2]

[1]*Tokyo University, Tokyo, Japan;* [2]*Adra Cambodia, Phnom Penh, Cambodia*

Introduction

As Cambodia a predominantly Buddhist country, Buddhist monks have great influence and elicit great respect in Cambodia. Their knowledge, attitudes and practices towards tobacco therefore have a tremendous bearing on the population at large.

Thailand, with a similar Buddhist tradition, has had much success in enlisting its monks in tobacco control efforts. According to Pra Thepwethee, a well-known monk who is a leader in the anti-smoking campaign in Thailand, monks are the best persons to help boost the campaign because Thai people are used to consulting a monk when they have problems. The monks are respected and have close contact with the people. Dr Uthai Dulyakasem, a lecturer at Silpakorn University in Thailand, agrees that monks may make better teachers than educators or legislators in the sense that they understand the peoples' way of life best of all. According to Buddha, monks should teach 'good things' to people. Thus, teaching and warning people about the harm that can result from cigarette smoking is a duty of every monk. Monks can therefore be a great help to the anti-smoking campaign. A detailed survey conducted by the Thai Ministry of Public Health revealed that the encouragement of a monk was a more important reason for quitting smoking than was encouragement by physicians and other health-care personnel or even family members.

Because of its similar Buddhist tradition, the same type of cooperation could be achieved in neighbouring Cambodia.

Methods

With this long-term objective in mind, a 30-cluster survey was designed, as a first step, to measure the prevalence, knowledge, attitudes and practices of Buddhist monks with regard to tobacco in the capital city of Phnom Penh, Cambodia. All of the temples in the city were listed and, according to the number of monks residing at them, 30 were randomly selected for conducting interviews with seven to 11 monks in each, for a total of 318 interviews.

In designing the survey questionnaire, care was taken to include, for comparative purposes, the WHO standardized core questions for tobacco control. During pre-testing, however, hesitancy was detected among interviewers and interviewees about the straightforward WHO questions, because of the underlying stigma of smoking in relation to Buddhist principles. For this reason, control questions were included to obtain a more accurate measure of actual tobacco consumption.

Results and discussion

According to the survey results and responses to the WHO standardized questions, 62% of monks interviewed had ever smoked, and 45% had smoked at least 100 cigarettes in their lifetime. They hesitated, however, when asked if they were current smokers or ex-smoker; only 19% responded that they were current smokers, and 38% said that they were ex-smokers. Of the monks who had ever smoked, 56% did or had done so daily and 35% did or had done so occasionally.

The figure for current smoking raises some serious questions. The prevalence of smoking among the general male population in Phnom Penh is almost 65%, and the prevalence of smoking among monks in Thailand is 56%.

When asked in another part of the survey, "Do you want to quit smoking?", 44% of all interviewees gave some type of response; 37% said "Yes", 3% said "No" and 4% replied "Not sure". The rest replied "Not applicable". When asked, "Why do you want to quit?", 44% of all respondents gave some reason. Of these, 60% cited health. This figure is significant, showing that health education alone does not bring about behavioural change. Among other reasons given, 29% of the respondents said that smoking was a waste of money, 5% said it was a waste of time, and 6% gave other reasons.

When asked what they did with tobacco received as gifts, 44% of all the monks interviewed said that they smoked the cigarettes themselves, and 50% said they gave the cigarettes away. This result indicates that the true prevalence of current smoking among Cambodian Buddhist monks is closer to 44%. It is significant that 33% of the monks interviewed were receiving 10 or more packs of cigarettes per month.

The average age of the monks interviewed was 28, which is relatively young; 53% of the smokers had smoked for five years or less and 19% for six to 10 years. The influences that made them start smoking was stated to be a friend by 27% of respondents, and 18% cited group pressure from friends or other monks. These two influences alone—individual friends and group pressure—were responsible for almost half of all the factors cited; 21% of the monks said that they had started because they received free cigarettes, 12% mentioned work and stress, 8% cited their father's influence, 3% said advertising and 12% gave other reasons.

When asked what the teachings of Buddha said about smoking, 91% of respondents said said that nothing was mentioned about smoking, but when they were asked if there should be a Buddhist law against smoking by monks, 71% said "Yes". When asked if the Government should require warning messages on all tobacco advertising, 94% agreed, and an equal number agreed that the Government should ban all tobacco advertising.

Only 34% thought that people should not offer cigarettes to monks, while 38% thought they should; about one-third were not sure. As the average income in Phnom Penh is less than the equivalent of US$ 100 per month, cigarettes given as are probably sold or bartered for extra income, although it would not be appropriate according to Buddhist principles to admit this.

Direct assistance for smoking cessation is urgently needed, as 84% of the smokers wanted to quit. If a programme were offered in the vicinity to help people stop smoking, 96% of smokers said they would attend; 86% of all respondents said they would be willing to teach people about the effects of smoking.

Conclusions

The pattern of responses to the questionnaire indicates that even though the teachings of Buddha say nothing directly about smoking, there is a stigma tied to smoking that inhibits many monks from admitting their smoking habits. The large majority of monks considered that smoking is not an appropriate practice and that there should be a Buddhist law prohibiting them from smoking.

The survey revealed that although health awareness is high, most monks have little understanding about the specific detrimental effects of smoking or the effects of environmental tobacco smoke. In addition to health awareness, other methods such as tax-pricing policies and cessation programmes are needed to bring about the desired behavioural changes.

The small scale of this research does not allow generalization of the conclusions to monks throughout the country, but it does provide useful insights into trends in tobacco use among monks in Cambodia and highlights a number of issues for further research. Most importantly, this study reveals the potential that exists for successful cooperation with monks in tobacco control in Cambodia.

Religious influences on tobacco investments: The Judaeo–Christian perspective

M.H. Crosby

Corporate Responsibility Program, Beatitudes Program, St Benedict Friary, Milwaukee, Wisconsin, United States

The main scriptural mandate in the Hebrew scriptures against smoking, which kills and injures, arises from the Fifth Commandment, "You shall not kill." (Exodus 20: 13). Because of the wording, this can be interpreted as a prohibition of those activities that take one's own life or those of others. Smoking is a form of slow suicide at the most; at the least, it compromises the health of the body. Taking the lives of others would cover the manufacture of a product which, if used as intended or after intentional exposure, kills or diminishes health. Adults who smoke in front of children would be affected by this commandment as well.

Other passages from the Hebrew scriptures that are related to the ways in which large tobacco companies advertise are those from the prophets condemning people who exploit little ones or the powerless. For instance, through the Prophet Isaiah, the Lord scorned Israel for 'your crimes that separate you from God ... your hands are stained with blood, your fingers with guilt; your lips speak falsehood, and your tongue utters deceit. No one brings suit justly, no one pleads truthfully" (Isaiah 59: 2–4).

While the Christian scriptures build on the hebrew scriptures' admonitions not to kill or exploit, Jesus urged his followers to follow those admonitions. In addition, He warned against what today would be called addictive patterns of behaviour: 'being given over' to such things as would be taken into the body or put into the body (see Matthew 6: 24–34). He also warned against exploiting the little ones (Matthew 18: 1–11). The Apostle Paul reminded the early Christians that their bodies were temples of the spirit of God and should therefore not be defiled (2 Corinthians 6:19; see 4: 16–17).

Traditionally, following St Paul's admonition, many Protestant churches have refrained from involvement with or investing in what have become known as 'the sin stocks': tobacco, alcohol and gambling. The Catholics have not considered smoking itself as sinful. The catholic Church has operated from the position that considers that all things are good unless offocially stated otherwise in the scriptures: "What God has purified you are not to call unclean." (Acts 11: 9). The official Catholic approach is to consider smoking within the virtue of temperance or moderation. The only mention of tobacco in the most recent *Catechism of the Catholic Church* is in the statement "The virtue of temperance disposes us to avoid every kind of excess: the abuse of food, alcohol, tobacco or medicine."

In an effort to determine how Jewish and Christian (Protestant and Catholic) institutions addressed the issue of tobacco, I designed a questionnaire eliciting information and views in several areas: the morality of smoking, whether prohibition or divestment was used to keep tobacco concerns out of their investment portfolio, whether tobacco stocks were used to challenge tobacco companies, whether the institutions accepted money from or feted tobacco company executives or interests, smoke-free policies in their buildings and whether the respondent considered that religious leaders were silent on tobacco-related issues. The questionnaire was sent to all major Protestant denominations in the United States, a representative sample of Catholic (Arch)dioceses, religious orders of women and of men and a representative sample of Catholic, Jewish and Protestant health-care systems. Since none of the Jewish health-care systems responded, the data refer only to Christian respondents. Participants were given a paper describing the findings.

More groups with a stronger position against tobacco tended to respond, and 47% of the Protestant groups and 36% of the Catholic groups responded. Among the Protestants, the most actively anti-smoking group, the Seventh Day Adventists, responded best (71%). Less than a third of the institutions had denominational positions, probably because a high percentage of Catholic institutions were included. Only 14% of these had any kind of statement, and none of these came clearly from 'official' Catholic groups like dioceses. In contrast, 67% of the Protestant groups said that their denomination had a moral position regarding tobacco. Half of the the Adventist groups considered that their moral statement was effective, in comparison with an overall percentage of 13%, indicating that religious leaders in general consider that their moral statements have little effect.

Restrictions on including tobacco stocks were reported by 70% of the Protestant groups and 40% of the Catholic groups. Of the catholics, restrictions were reported by 20% of the dioceses, 55% of women's congregations, 14% of men's congregations and 50% of the health-care entities. Every Protestant denomination sampled (seven of the 15) said they had some kind of restriction. None of the groups acknowledged receiving money from tobacco interests, and none said that they had feted tobacco company executives.

Because of the restrictions on tobacco stocks, no data were available for many of the Protestant groups about whether they had used their stocks to take action against tobacco interests; however, the Episcopal Church in America (which has restrictions) reported that it had challenged other health-related entities in which it held stock to become 'tobacco-free'. One catholic group, Maryknoll, reported that, as a result of publicity about its efforts to persuade RJR Nabisco Holdings to 'spin-off' its non-tobacco businesses, it had received many complaints about the morality of holding such stock in the first place. As a result, a decision was taken to divest itself of all tobacco stock.

While the Protestant groups varied in their responses about whether religious leaders had been silent on the issue of tobacco, 80% of the religious orders of women and all of the other Catholic groups answered affirmatively. The reasons ranged from surmising that many of the leaders were or had been smokers, the acceptance of smoking in society and the "difficulty of separating the morality of tobacco use from moral judgements about tobacco users." Very few groups raised moral judgements of corporations involved in the promotion of tobacco use; most limited their moral concerns to individuals, including themselves.

Smoking control and religion

H. Gimbel

China Project, Redlands, California, United States

Tobacco companies deliberately lie. They tell young people that smoking has social advantages that outweigh the health hazards. Tobacco companies try to persuade young people to do something wrong for their health, wrong for their future, wrong for their families and wrong for the good of their country. The tobacco companies try to get young people to believe in and behave on the basis of lies. As smoking control workers, we are trying to get young people to believe in and act on the truth. Can there be a starker contrast between wrong and right?

Recent surveys have shown that religion can play a useful role in smoking control. Many of the world's major religions urge non-smoking, and it has been shown in several countries that people of all ages who hold strong religious beliefs are less likely to take up smoking and are more likeley to quit if they smoke. Thus, among students in Saudi Arabia, religion was given as the main reason for not taking up smoking (Taha *et al.*, 1991). In a study of schoolchildren in The Netherlands, it was concluded that religion was a powerful influence on young people's attitude against tobacco (Mullen & Francis, 1995). A survey of secondary-school pupils in Ireland showed that children more closely bonded to religion were less involved in smoking (Grube *et al.*, 1989). Among Turkish undergraduate students, religious belief was an important characteristic that distinguished smokers from non-smokers (Torabi 1989–90). In the United States, African–American men who went to church regularly had lower use of tobacco (Brown & Gary, 1994).

Smoking control workers in various countries have made attempts to appeal to moral sensibilities. When monks in Thailand conducted anti-smoking activities, the success rate was 50% greater than in a control group (Anon., 1993). The 'five-day plan to stop smoking', the 'breathe-free plan' and the 'twelve step plan' all appeal to the moral principle of preserving health and life and offer practical suggestions for using spiritual resources to overcome tobacco addiction (Orleans & Slade, 1993).

Almost all small children believe that smoking is bad. Why do the same children, when they become adolescents, believe that smoking is good? Beliefs and values are learnt from parents and other adults who are important to children. The strength of children's bonding to those adults determines how fully they will accept and adhere to those beliefs and values. If children's bonds with their families and adult social groups are weakened or are weak to begin with, they are more likely to seek bonding support from other role models, and their childhood beliefs and values may be gradually exchanged for new ones (DeFronzo & Pawlak, 1993).

During the unstable transition time of adolescence, the idols of tobacco advertising frequently become the new objects of worship for young people. The appeal to independence often successfully lures young people into self-destructuve smoking behaviour. They adopt the cigarette as the symbol of their grown-up status and their bond with their friends who smoke. They accept the false belief that smoking is a normal and necessary part of their young lives (Eiser, 1985).

The belief that smoking is wrong tends to deter young people from smoking. Internalization of the belief is the key, when they adopt the values and beliefs of their parents and other adults as their own. Strong, prolonged bonding between parents or other important adults and children increases the probability that beliefs and values 'taught' by one generation will be 'caught' by the next.

Another vital element is conscience—the inner voice to which a person answers "Yes" or "No". Over the past 30 years, psychologists have developed techniques to study conscience and moral development. Raymon B. Cattell, probably the contemporary pyschologist most often cited in the United States on the subject, describes conscience as an influence inside the mind rather than as social pressure from outside. He says that conscience is an innate sense of what is right and what is wrong (Cattell, 1994). He presented data on the moral structure of societies in 52 countries, which showed that there is a sense in all societies of what is morally right. They all have similar prohibitions against lying, stealing, sexual misconduct and killing, including self-destructive behaviour. Other psychologists also say that conscience is not social pressure but is the spiritual, supernatural principle in humans, of divine origin. A conscience that is not irreparably damaged urges the individual to non-destructive behaviour.

As smoking control workers, we attempt to help young people not to begin smoking and to help those who smoke to quit. We cannot motivate people to change their beliefs, values and behaviour. Motivation comes from within the individual. We can, however, assist people to recognize and respond to their inner core of moral principles. Once people choose not to smoke, we can assist them to maintain that behaviour. This could appropriately include internal and external spiritual resources. As smoking control workers, we have the privilege and the responsibility to appeal to the conscience of those we try to influence against taking up smoking. It is also appropriate, I think, to help smokers respond to their basic, innate principles as a protection against self-destructive bahaviour. The tobacco companies use immoral and evil strategies to persuade young people to begin smoking. We could well use moral persuasion to counteract the lies of the tobacco companies.

Health workers tend to separate the spirit and mind from the body. We feel most comfortable working with factors that affect only the body and prefer to leave matters of conscience to religious leaders. But people are not divided up in that way: body, mind and spirit are one and inseparable.

Tobacco companies are wrong. Smoking control workers are right. Smoking is harmful and wrong. Not smoking is healthy and right. Let us strike iron with iron, fire with fire and make better use of moral influences and spiritual resources. We would do well to recognize the power of a good conscience. In the struggle against the evil of tobacco, we should encourage young people and adults to respond positively to their source of inner strength. Religion used judiciously and sensitively has a useful role in smoking control.

References

Anon. (1993) Influence of religious leaders on smoking cessation in a rural population—Thailand. *Morbid. Mortal Wkly Rep.*, **42**, 367–369

Brown, D.R. & Gary, L.E. (1994) Religious involvement and health status among African–American males. *J. Natl Med. Assoc.*, **86**, 825–831

Cattell, R.B. (1994) *How Good Is Your Country? What You Should Know*, Washington DC: Institute for the Study of Man

DeFronzo, J. & Pawlak, R. (1993) Effects of social bonds and childhood experiences on alcohol abuse and smoking. *J. Soc. Psychol.*, **133**, 635–642

Eiser, J.R. (1985) Smoking: The social leaqrning of aan addiction. *J. Soc. Clin. Psychol.*, **3**, 446–457

Grube, J.W., Morgan, M. & Kearnye, A. (1989) Use of self-generated identification codes to match questionnaires in panel studies of adolescent substance abuse. *Addict, behav.*, **14**, 159–171

Mullen, K. & Francis, L.J. (1995) Religiosity and attitudes toward drug use among Dutch school children. *J. Alcohol Drug Educ.*, **41**, 16–25

Orleans, C.T. & Slade, J., eds (1993) *Nicotine Addiction: Principles and management*, New York: Oxford University Press

Taha, A., *et al.* (1991) Smoking habits of King Saud University students in Riyadh. *Ann. Saudi Med.*, **11**, 141–143

The tobacco plantation system in the extreme south of Brazil

L. Prado

The Anglican Church of Brazil, Pelotas, Rio Grande do Sul, Brazil

Tobacco is cultivated everywhere in Brazil, but the largest producer if the State of Rio Grande do Sul. It is situated between 27° 04' 49" south and 57° 38' 34" west—no longer in the tropical belt but with freezing temperatures in winter. The population is 9 730 000, of whom 76% live in the cities. Our State income is US$ 40 thousand million, representing 8.1% of the Brazilian gross national product. We hold third place in exports from Brazil, and tobacco is the main product. In 1994, 251 out of a total of 427 municipalities produced tobacco, involving 60 150 producers, who cultivated an area of 135 700 ha, harvesting 230 000 tonnes of tobacco with an average commercial value of US$ 1.20 per kilogram. This represents about 11% of the total tobacco harvest of Brazil.

Tobacco is tending to replace 'survival' crops such as beans, potatoes, corn, vegetables, fruit and honey and, most importantly, dairy products. In 1994, 157 000 ha of beans were planted and 140 000 tonnes were harvested, with an average commercial value for the producer of US$ 0.35 per kilogram. The food industry is also suffering from this gradual changeover; the remaining few companies are in serious difficulties.

The country is suffering from the oppression of the so-called globalization of the economy. The Government is obliged to obey the proposals of the International Monetary Fund and the World Bank for 'alleviation of poverty' and 'austerity plans'. The tobacco industry thus has convincing arguments for recruiting new producers. Cash is the first one, but one of the main ones is that the tobacco produced is sold directly to the industry, with no intermediates. This results in a large difference in price. With other, traditional crops, the 'middle man' increases the price by 10 times or more.

The tobacco companies draw up contracts with the producers, commiting themselves to give technical assistance. All the seeds, fertlizers, pesticides and installations such as heaters and sheds are built with financing from banks. The farmers are committed to deliver their entire production to the companies, but they take three to five years to pay back the bank loans, and during that time they are committed to the companies. Many producers manage to pay off their debts, but many others do not and they lose their lands. On the pretext of introducing new technology, the companies try to replace the traditonal production methods with more expensive ones, resulting in even greater indebtedness. These rising debts can result in breaking-up of farming families, gambling and prostitution.

The growing numbers of tobacco plantations are resulting in a monoculture, which increases the number of pests, soil erosion and the accumulation of pesticides in the soil, water and air. Although this agroindustrial complex uses mainly family labour, the Government collects 70% of the capital that is generated as taxes, 25% is kept by the industry, and the remaining 5% is divided between the merchants and the farmers. This may appear to be profitable for the Government, but the damage that tobacco causes, in the form of tobacco-related diseases, the risks of the producers and the destruction of the environment, is greater than any monetary profit.

A national forum has been held to discuss use of child labour on tobacco farms. Furthermore, the tobacco farmers and their families, from children to the elderly, are exposed to huge amounts of pesticides, starting with the preparation of the seeds. Hardly any use protective equipment. As wood is needed for the heaters that are used to dry tobacco, the native forests are being destroyed. Each harvest results in the consumption of 2 275 000 m^3 of wood, equivalent to cutting down 6000 ha of forest. This means that 30% of the native trees, over 1800 ha, are cut down each year. The result is erosion, silting up of rivers, contamination of water and disease among animal life.

In regions with widespread tobacco production, there is a high rate of suicide, especially among men ages 40–60. New studies indicate that this may be due neurological dysfunction due to cholinergic toxicity in the central nervous system, which is known to be caused by organophosphate pesticides.

The Christian churches and our Anglican Diocese of Pelotas have been conducting an open battle against the tobacco plantation system and its consequences. The tobacco issue is a theological matter: not for reasons of morality but for life or death. Our motto is 'Milk or tobacco'. As a rural diocese (only two large urban areas and three universities), we are committed to deprived people living in the countryside. Some three dozen small congregations, priests and myself, the Bishop, have formed a number of community groups to provide encouragement, technical advice and some modest agricultural projects, such as new cows, new seeds and plants, tools, education for young people and support to women and childre. Our alternative to the tobacco companies is to link all these activities and groups to a regional cooperative producing milk and cheese. The cooperative works only with small farmers. It provides many different needs, such as medical assistance, supermarket items, clothes and refrigerators, without the need for cash: milk is the accepted currency! A medical appointment costs about 50 L of milk, the average daily production. A new cow or a milk cooler can be bought and paid for over many months, with the family's production of milk.

About 15 community groups look to the Church as a reference for planning for the future. Spreading awareness about the hazards of tobacco is a hard fight, but the diocesan education programmes gives priority to young farmers and their children. Churches are not equipped to compete with the powerful companies' funding system, agronomists and their tools (cars, television and the cash approach), but we are not giving up. Several non-governmental organizations and the Brazilian Medical Association are helping us in our struggle. One important thing that is lacking is a closer national network to link all of the isolated efforts at resistance to the tobacco companies. Step by step, we hope to be able to change the wrong thinking of our farmers, politicians and consumers.

DISCUSSANTS' REMARKS

The tobacco holocausts

T.H. Lam

Department of Community Medicine
The University of Hong Kong
Pokfulam, Hong Kong SAR, China

The theme of this conference is 'Tobacco: The Growing Epidemic'. After hearing the presentations on this theme and trying to be a bit provocative, I would argue that the term, although scientifically correct, is not politically stimulating. Since we are talking about over 3 million deaths each year at present and 10 million a year by the years 2025–30, we need a better phrase to describe these huge numbers of death, a phrase that would attract more attention, arouse stronger emotions and, one hopes, result in more effective control. I therefore respectfully suggest that we call the massive scale of killing of the human race by tobacco 'the expanding global holocausts' or, in brief, 'the tobacco holocausts'.

We must emphasize that these figures for global mortality are conservative estimates based on evidence mainly from the United Kingdom and the United States and the untested assumption that smoking is less dangerous in developing than developed countries. We have heard that China has a very high prevalence of smoking, but early results from the Chinese prospective study show lower relative risks than those in the United Kingdom and the United States. Such findings for developing countries might be falsely interpreted as supportive of this untested assumption. That assumption and findings could be potentially dangerous, because the tobacco industry could exploit them fully in pushing tobacco into developing countries. We must make sure that the people and governments are not led to believe that the risks due to smoking are low and therefore acceptable. We must repeatedly point out that the results reflect only the early stage of the tobacco holocaust. I therefore suggest that we should also use another assumption in future estimates, which, until proven otherwise and despite some variations in the pattern of specific causes of death, is that smoking in developing countries is as dangerous as it is in developed countries.

We must remember that the two important sub-themes of this conference are women and developing countries. At the last World Conference in Paris, it was stated that 'Women who smoke like men die like men'. I agree with that statement, even though results from the west tend to find lower relative risks due to smoking in women. To modify the statement, I suggest we also say 'People in developing countries who smoke like people in developed countries, die like those in developed countries'. To apply this general statement to specific countries like China, we can then say 'Chinese who smoke like Americans die like Americans' or 'Hungarians who smoke like the British die like the British'.

If the early results of epidemiological studies in developing countries do not appear to support this assumption, it is probably because the time has not yet come. We therefore need epidemiological studies to monitor this holocaust.

At the Paris Conference, Professor Judith Mackay and I used the term 'the new opium war' to describe the situation in Asia. It is now obvious that this new war is not confined to particular countries or regions. My last question is whether we can win this world war and, if so, how and when? We have the global enemies—tobacco and the multinational tobacco companies. Do we have a world ally, an ally in the real sense, a united force fighting this Third World War? I don't think we do at the moment. Do we need one? I sincerely think so Let us start building up this world ally against the tobacco holocausts today!

Note: *Holocaust*: complete destruction, especially of a large number of persons; a great slaughter or massacre. *The Oxford English Dictionary* (Oxford Clarendon Press, 1933, Volume V, p. 344)

Tobacco use in the developing world

J.P. Koplan

The Prudential Center for Health Care Research, Atlanta, Georgia, United States

The presentations on tobacco use in the developing world by Dr Jha, Professor Weng and Professor Muna provide very thoughtful and informative perspectives on this major international public health challenge. Dr Jha of the World Bank described economic studies of tobacco use and their impact on society, but most of these studies take a broad societal perspective. The better to influence the decision-makers in the tobacco policy debate and the better to understand and design effective interventions, we need also to analyse the economics of tobacco use by the individual players, the affected population, comprising smokers and non-smokers, tobacco farmers, insurance programmes, industry, government and the health-care system. I would also like to thank Dr Jha and the agency he represents, the World Bank, for sponsoring a major health loan to China, 'Health VII', which supports health promotion and anti-tobacco activities, in particular, in eight Chinese cities. Professor Weng provided us with a history of tobacco control efforts in China, illustrating the increasing commitment of the Ministry of Public Health to this issue. He also illustrated the very important role of voluntary organizations in furthering tobacco control. Using Cameroon as an example, Professor Muna has shown an early stage of tobacco intrusion into a developing country and the opportunities to fight this hazard at this early stage rather than wait until a more entrenched tobacco industry and addicted populace make control efforts more difficult. He has noted the considerable differences between African nations in the nature and future trajectory of tobacco use, in part influenced by whether a nation is a tobacco producer or not.

One aspect that I'd like to emphasize is that tobacco use is not genetically programmed in any particular population. Mankind has not needed tobacco for its evolutionary development or for better adaptation to the environment. Its growth and harvesting are not native to most parts of the world. Rather, smoking is an acquired behaviour and one that is not even immediately pleasurable. Thus, while it is alien to most nations of the world, all of our populations are at risk of its allure and addictive potential.

This conference is specifically focused on tobacco. But permit me to take a broader perspective, one that builds on our interests in all of the components of health promotion and disease prevention. In global history, many societies have drifted from essentially healthy behaviour, of diets low in fat, high in fibre and appropriate in total caloric intake, of work and transport needs that make us physically active daily, and an absence of tobacco use (except for ceremonial or celebratory purposes) to new, acquired unhealthy behaviour that includes diets high in fats and excess calories, a more sedentary lifestyle and common tobacco use.

In public health, various 'transitions' have been described, particularly the epidemiological and demographic transitions, but I would ask you to consider a third transition, 'the behavioural transition'. The 'pre'-behavioural transition state involves accepting the elements of modern or western life, which has essentially evolved during the twentieth century in many of the richest countries of the world. This lifestyle can be characterized by unhealthy diets, inadequate physical activity and tobacco use. Many of these western nations are now trying to achieve a 'post-behavioural' transition state, trying to improve diet, increase physical activity and decrease tobacco use.

A challenge for developing countries is to maintain traditional healthy behaviour, including resisting further inroads by the tobacco industry, preventing new smokers and encouraging current smokers to quit. It should not be necessary for developing nations to repeat western patterns of behaviour with their disastrous health outcomes.

China has shown itself an excellent example of compressing the epidemiological transition and addressing the demographic transition strategically. Since liberation in 1949, overall mortality has decreased and longevity increased, the burden of infectious diseases and malnutrition have decreased, and progress has been made in controlling the size of the population. With regard to the behavioural transition, however, we have seen a rapid increase in smoking prevalence and per capita cigarette consumption in China. What took over 50 years to achieve in smoking rates and quantity in the United States has occurred with accelerated speed in China. This is a problem and a great danger.

Let's look at the health of the world's nations in 2025. There will be pre-behavioural transition nations and post-transition nations. Post-transition nations will have robust health education programmes—not pamphlets and posters, but real comprehensive health promotion. They will have extremely restrictive governmental tobacco policies, including high taxation, environmental smoking restrictions and rigorous enforcement of such regulations. They will actively support, through policies and environmental structures, increased physical activity and healthy diets. Pre-behavioural transition nations will be found grappling with deteriorating health status, marked by unabated epidemics of lung cancer and heart disease. They will struggle with deeply entrenched tobacco interests that manipulate their governments and strongly influence public opinion and the social norm towards unhealthy behaviour and outcomes. These countries will be able to look back on the Ninth, Tenth and Eleventh World Conferences and recognize that they had the opportunity to build significant barriers to this evil invasion of the 1990s and early twenty-first century. But having failed to do so, they will find it very difficult to expel these foreign invaders and occupiers and their domestic allies from their midst. They will be doomed to repeat the painful and costly experience of the post-transition nations.

My hope and expectation is that all those attending this conference will take a leading role in ensuring that their countries fall in the post-transition category before 2025.

Passive smoking:
The industry sows doubt behind epidemiology's plough

A.J. Hedley

Department of Community Medicine, The University of Hong Kong, Hong Kong SAR, China

This session can perhaps claim to be the most novel of the conference. It provided an opportunity, by invitation, for the tobacco industry to present its own sponsored views on an issue of tobacco control. We came to this session with a well-established background of disputatious reports on environmental tobacco smoke in the scientific literature, industry-sponsored publications and the lay press. From the public health perspective, the issue is to weigh the burden of evidence and take whatever precautionary action is indicated by suppressing the hazard and thus reducing the predictable avoidable morbidity and mortality. The banning of smoking in public places, restaurants and various forms of transport is now well established as a necessary response to the accumulating evidence of health risks. From the tobacco industry's perspective, however, any community action that is taken to avoid health risks resulting from exposure to environmental tobacco smoke represents a serious threat to their frenetic efforts to maintain the social acceptability of smoking.

The public health views have been very clearly and emphatically stated in seminal reports from the United Kingdom, the United States and several hundred painstaking epidemiological studies published around the globe. Much of this work was reiterated, summarized and added to by S. Glantz, J. Samet and D. Zaridze at this symposium. We heard from Stanton Glantz a spirited defence of the work of Glantz and Parmley, published in *Circulation* (Glantz & Parmley, 1991) and *The Journal of the American Medical* Association (Glantz & Parmley, 1995) on the effects of environmental tobacco smoke on the circulatory system and heart disease; an update on Jonathan Samet's paper at the Fifth World Conference on foetal and childhood exposure (Overpeck & Moss, 1991; Rush *et al.*, 1992; Samet *et al.*, 1994) and a review of studies on exposure to environmental tobacco smoke and lung cancer with a new Russian study by David Zaridze (Zaridze *et al.*, 1998). In my view, it is important to emphasize that these and other workers have taken a rigorous approach to the study of the effects of environmental tobacco smoke on health and can be said to represent the best scientifically based advocacy available from the fields of epidemiology, public health and clinical sciences.

My own bias should also be externalized before I move to the next part of my critique. My views concur with those expressed by Law and Hackshaw (1996), namely, 'The overall hazard is sufficient to justify measures to prohibit or restrict smoking in public places and workplaces, and health education to discourage people from smoking in their homes.'

Peter Lee, who is a declared consultant to the tobacco industry, invariably produces reports which perhaps unsurprisingly are very favourable to the industry's cause. Peter Lee was the main authority referred to by the industry-sponsored European Working Group which published in 1995 their report *Environmental Tobacco Smoke and Lung Cancer: An Evaluation of the Risk*. The report centres on interpretation of the reported risks of lung cancer in declared non-smoking spouses of smokers. Davey Smith and Phillips (1996) commented in detail on the omissions and distortions of the report, pointing out that Lee's misclassification model does not take account of the 'underestimation of the association between exposure to environmental tobacco smoke and lung cancer risk which will be generated by the use of spousal smoking as an indicator of exposure'. The European Working Group's meta-analysis indicated a relative risk estimate of 1.16 (95% confidence interval, 1.08–1.25) which was down-sized to 1.08 (1.00–1.16) by applying Lee's method. In the approach recommended by Davey Smith and Phillips to take account of the misclassification of exposure arising from the inhalation of environmental tobacco smoke when using a proxy measure of exposure, namely marriage to a smoker, the association would be 'considerably larger than the estimate from the meta-analysis' published by the industry's European Working Group. Lee's response (Lee, 1997) was that, as there is no significant association between spouses' smoking and lung cancer after misclassification is taken into account, there is no need to ask by how much any such association is an underestimate of the relationship with total exposure. Many would not agree.

One problem is that people who present perspectives favourable to the industry focus on selected outcomes, such as lung cancer, where they busily exploit issues of uncertainty without considering the whole spectrum of evidence on the adverse health effects of environmental tobacco smoke and weighing the accumulating burden of this evidence. Lee complained that not only did Davey Smith and Phillips wrongly criticize his work but also 'insinuated that he distorted evidence for money' because he is (according to Davey Smith and Phillips) 'an enthusiastic recipient of tobacco industry financial support....' Peter Lee then argues that because he is 'widely consulted on many issues and attempts always to provide an unbiased assessment' he must be regarded as an *bone fide* independent scientist. Most workers in the public health sciences would question whether any individual or organization that receives very substantial support from the tobacco industry should be given the privilege of being regarded as independent and intellectually honest sources of informed opinion. Many journals (including the *British Medical Journal*, which afforded Lee the right of reply to Davey Smith and Phillips) require their authors to declare conflicts of interest. I suggested (Hedley, 1997) that Lee did not fully comply with this requirement and invited him to tell us what proportion of the gross income of P.N. Lee Statistics and Computing Ltd over the past five years came from the tobacco industry. I still extend this invitation to him and reiterate that unless we know what he stands to lose we will always be obliged to question how and why certain inferences are drawn in his work. It is clearly a major problem for him, because it seems certain that the industry would not buy his product unless it clearly supported their global strategy to promote the uptake and maintenance of tobacco smoking and its social acceptability.

Lee's commitment to the view that environmental tobacco smoke is not a health hazard is clearly signalled in his monograph *Environmental Tobacco Smoke and Mortality* (Lee, 1992). In his conclusion to the preface of that book, he states that 'There is no convincing evidence that exposure to environmental tobacco smoke results in an increased risk of death from cancer, heart disease or any other disease in non-smokers.' (I understand that the publication of the book was underwritten by the tobacco industry through its purchase of the majority of the copies.)

I have reason to be sceptical about the evidence that is presented in this book. Lee actually visited my department in Hong Kong to gather some of his information. On page 57, Lee quotes a 'personal communication' from a member of my staff who has published papers which question a direct causal relationship between environmental tobacco smoke and lung cancer in non-smoking Chinese women. The staff member made a gratuitous criticism of a study published by another member of my staff, which purports to show a causal association between environmental tobacco smoke and cancer in non-smoking Chinese women. Although Lee had travelled 6000 miles for this interview, he was apparently unwilling to take one further step to the room next door where he would have heard a different point of view from the author. The result is a deliberately biased view of an important piece of evidence.

Peter Lee's submission to this symposium begins with the assertion that, for lung cancer, his meta-analysis shows a 'modest association with lung cancer' of 1.16 (95% confidence interval, 1.09–1.25). The implication of the term 'modest' in this context is that relatively small excess risks can be ignored simply because they are numerically small. The industry may be able to mount dismissive arguments against them relatively easily. But what is the meaning of 'modest' when it is applied to a significant excess risk which results from a ubiquitous hazard and thus in public health terms may be associated with an important preventable fraction? Lee's position is that methodological weaknesses can be identified which explain the observed excess risks and dose–response relationships. Lee's paper goes on to argue that these problems include: misclassification of 'ever' smokers as 'never' smokers; uncontrolled confounding; publication bias and recall bias. He also adds the caution that there is no experimental evidence and implies that the 'concentrations of chemicals in environmental tobacco smoke' are too low to be harmful.

I suggest that a more objective review of the health effects of environmental tobacco smoke would acknowledge that (i) active cigarette smoking is indisputably the cause of cancer and cardiovascular disease and that *a priori* it is entirely plausible that both the mainstream and sidestream smoke, which form environmental tobacco smoke and contain a wide spectrum of toxic chemicals, have carcinogenic effects, among other adverse health outcomes; and that (ii) there is overwhelming evidence that exposure to environmental tobacco smoke does take place in ordinary social settings such as the home and results in both acute and chronic illness. Unfortunately, children are the most sensitive sentinels in whom we can observe this pattern of morbidity but it is measurable in adults too. Nowhere in the extensive documents (P.N. Lee, A review of the epidemiology of ETS and lung cancer; P.N. Lee, A review of the epidemiology of ETS and heart disease; P.N. Lee, Environmental tobacco smoke (ETS), lung cancer and heart disease: Set of overhead projection plates presented (in part) at 10th World Congress on Tobacco or Health) which Lee submitted to this symposium does he refer to the conclusive evidence that these exposures clearly occur and damage the respiratory system of both children and adults, causing reliably reported symptoms of cough, phlegm and wheeze. Lee could in my opinion have been a little less disingenuous in his description of environmental tobacco smoke as simply diluted mainstream smoke. There is no reference in his paper or overheads to the composition or concentrations of sidestream smoke, which is a critically important characteristic of environmental tobacco smoke.

Lee claims that 'most toxicologists' disagree with the statement that 'there is no safe level of exposure to cancer-causing agents' (Kraus et al., 1992). This assertion is derived from a report on 'intuitive toxicology' (sic), in which Lee states that 47% disagreed and 28% agreed with the statement. It seems in fact that 53% agreed or were unsure or non-responders. What I am unsure about is the independent standing of toxicologists who are quoted by industry advocates; many are themselves long-standing, paid tobacco consultants who have, for example, set up with others indoor air quality associations and journals as a front for industry disinformation activities.

The general tenor of P.N. Lee's paper is disparaging of other work and publications. For example, he states 'although most studies have been presented in published papers, some have been reported only in abstracts, in an abstract plus a review paper, in a thesis or as a letter'. The implication is that these sources and therefore their content are in some way inferior and not to be regarded as credible vehicles of valid scientific information. Oddly enough, elsewhere in his paper Lee is actually concerned about publication bias. I would have thought that the capture of each and every report on this topic would tend to minimize this problem. Lee himself treats us to a feast of unpublished documents, personal papers (including review articles) and industry-sponsored publications as the sole references to support many of his claims. For example, Lee states that 'The excess in the prospective studies [on lung cancer and spouses' smoking] arises from the high RR in the large Hirayama study, a study which has been widely criticized'. The 'wide criticism' (unspecified) is that in two publications by P.N. Lee, one of which was directly funded by the tobacco industry and the other of which is unpublished but available on request from Lee's headquarters.

Lee makes the interesting point that inaccurate diagnosis of lung cancer may be a source of incorrect estimates, including underestimates of any true relationship between exposure to environmental tobacco smoke and lung cancer. Lee states, 'as histological confirmation was not insisted upon in over half of 44 studies ... a proportion of cases ... is likely ... to have been misdiagnosed'. This focus on only one aspect of clinical decision-making and death certification is supported by a single reference—a review by Lee published in a supplement of Acta Pathologica, Microbiologica et Immunologica Scandinavica (Lee, 1994). Good, but may I ask who funded the supplement and why? I confess to being deeply suspicious about the motivation for published articles on uncertainties in health and medical science when they originate from industry-supported sources. How would P.N. Lee reassure me that my concerns are unfounded? Incidentally, most worthwhile journals are now wary of inadvertently publishing industry-funded supplements. This includes The International Journal of Epidemiology, which once unwittingly produced a supplement (Anon., 1990) with funds from the Centre for Indoor Air Research. It will not happen again.

P.N. Lee is an able biostatistician. Why then does he couch his descriptions of statistical test results in such vague, ambiguous and misleading terms? For example, we are asked to accept that in studies that were rated as 'inferior' by Lee, using his own in-house criteria, the environmental tobacco smoke-related (husband smoking) relative risk for lung cancer 'was almost (my emphasis) significantly higher than that in superior studies'. Playing with statistical inference, rather than considering overall plausibility and burden of evidence, is the main plank of the industry's campaign to sow doubt about causal relationships in tobacco-related disease.

Lee discusses the possible influence of misclassification of smokers in some detail. He suggests that misclassified 'ever' smokers, particularly ex-smokers, are a major problem for studies of exposure to environmental tobacco smoke. This focus on misclassification of adult smoking histories is apparently contrary to Lee's belief that his own work in the conduct of major retrospective and cross-sectional population-based surveys of smoking is entirely reliable (e.g. Lee, undated).

Misclassification of current smoking by Asian women is, according to Lee, a critical issue in the interpretation of studies on environmental tobacco smoke in Asia. So what evidence is offered? One estimate (from a paper by Lee) based on measurement of cotinine studies is 21% among married Japanese women (Lee, 1995). Another (referred to in Lee's presentation) claims that 62% of Cambodian, Laotian and Vietnamese women under-declare their smoking (Wewers et al., 1995). I thought this was a fascinating revelation until I read in his paper that these were emigrants living in Ohio (United States)! When I asked P.N. Lee about the provenance of this remarkable report and who the authors were (Wewer et al.), he told me that he did not know. To be fair, Lee's interpretation of this form of misclassification is more cautious. While a 2.5% rate reduces the RR in the United States from 1.12 to 1.01 and that in Europe from 1.19 to 1.12, it 'has little effect' in Asia. A 'more plausible 10% rate' is chosen by Lee, which is then shown to reduce the RR from 1.20 to 1.12, 'making it only marginally significant'. I conclude that, after the best effort Lee could make to down-size the risk in Asia (and still appear to stay within the bounds of reasonableness in his methods), the point estimates for relative risk remain significant with conventional levels of confidence. Other biases are invoked as explanations for dose–response relationships, both referenced to papers by Lee (Lee, 1987), one of which is unpublished. In particular, we are invited to accept as plausible 'that lung cancer cases may overstate spousal cigarette consumption or duration of smoking, relative to controls, in an attempt to rationalize their disease state, so causing a spurious dose–response relationship'. No evidence is offered for this interesting supposition, but apparently Lee states, 'Recently it has been clearly shown that it would only take a modest recall bias to explain the significant association between lung cancer and pack years of exposure from the husband reported in the large study by Fontham et al. (1994)'. The reference to this so-called clear demonstration is an unpublished paper by M. LeVois and P. Switzer (LeVois, M. & Switzer, P. [cited by Lee as 'submitted for publication'] Exposure misclassification effects on trend statistics for case–control exposure–response data: A sensitivity analysis). Sounds interesting, but how and why does Lee know about this paper, what is the basis of this enquiry and what is the source of funding for the work? In other words, are there any possible conflicts of interest here, such as those which the rest of us are obliged to declare when we argue our case in peer-reviewed publications? How many of the publications listed in P.N. Lee's reference list were funded in some way by the tobacco industry? As Lee states, 'Adjustment for bias due to misclassification is a very complex issue, involving various uncertainties. However, the analyses presented certainly suggest that misclassification bias is important, thus weakening the inference of causality'. Granted, this is possibly true, but, as Lee clearly demonstrates, the inference of causality remains entirely justifiable as a precautionary public health measure.

Lee's paper concludes with reference to a report by Dr F.J.C. Roe, who dismisses the argument of Glantz and Parmley (1991) about the effects of environmental tobacco smoke on exposure to carbon monoxide and free radicals, platelet function, endothelial cells and blood lipids. All of the studies in laboratory animals are also uniformly dismissed. I was surprised to find Lee and Roe's review so selective. For example, on what grounds did they choose to ignore the report by Celermajer et al. (1996) in the New England Journal of Medicine which demonstrates dose-related impairment of endothelium-dependent arterial dilatation after exposure to environmental tobacco smoke of young healthy adults who were free from other risk factors for atherosclerosis? Dr F.J.C. Roe was formerly a medical scientist at the United Kingdom Medical Research Council, now retired. I feel obliged to ask why he is now described as a 'colleague' by P.N. Lee. Is this because he is now working as a consultant to the tobacco industry and supporting activities coordinated by P.N. Lee Statistics and Computing Ltd? This is his prerogative if it is true, but we should have been told.

The observations of P.N. Lee and F.J.C. Roe might be interesting to workers in this field if their conclusions were not so patently influenced by other, non-scientific considerations. Why do they think it is reasonable from their current positions so confidently and cavalierly to demolish the work of others, who are actively engaged in the field in institutions that ensure that their intellectual honesty is constantly under scrutiny? Do Lee and Roe seek to imply that all evidence-based health and medicine is flawed, or just the areas of vested interest to the tobacco industry? When Lee and Roe are able to pass peer review by *The Journal of the American Medical Association* or *The New England Journal of Medicine* and other front-line, rigorously peer-reviewed journals, as Glantz, Parmley and others have done, then we might accept that they have established a platform for debate. But so long as their musings remain on the shelf in the leafy glades of Cedar Avenue, Sutton in Surrey (or appear in a miscellany of other sources), we should exercise caution and discretion.

Finally I should, on P.N. Lee's behalf, acknowledge that he was extremely unhappy about the style and content of my contribution to this symposium and considered that he was unfairly treated. In particular, he complained that my stance 'was silly, and did not address the science'; that 'before this session he had never heard of me' (strange, considering that he surreptitiously visited my department) and that I had done no work in the field of the health effects of environmental tobacco smoke. Perhaps then I should conclude this piece by inviting conference delegates to draw their own conclusions about both the validity and strength of P.N. Lee's arguments. All his documents are available from his office, and he can hardly complain about the publicity I have given to his work in this paper. I apologize for my low profile and promise to raise this in the forthcoming battles over the tobacco industry's disinformation campaigns in Asia. I should like to remind P.N. Lee that in my department we are at the cutting edge in defining the impact of environmental tobacco smoke and active smoking on the health of young children, their parents and others in the community in Hong Kong and China (He *et al.*, 1994; Lam *et al.*, 1994, 1995; Peters *et al.*, 1996; Lam *et al.*, 1998; Peters *et al.*, 1998). We shall continue to support the development of public policy in the Special Administrative Region of Hong Kong, China, to prevent exposure to environmental tobacco smoke in all public areas, eating places and the home and to reduce the avoidable morbidity and mortality which results from this hazard.

Acknowledgement

I have quoted extensively from the paper of Davey Smith and Phillips and recommend it as a very useful source on the nefarious activities of the tobacco industry in the promotion of their special brand of disinformation on passive smoking.

References

Anon. (1990) Assessing low risk agents for lung cancer: Methodological aspects. *Int. J. Epidemiol.*, **19** (Suppl. 1)

Celermajer, D.S., Adams, M.R. & Clarkson, P. (1996) Passive smoking and impaired endothelium-dependent arterial dilatation in healthy young adults. *New Engl. J. Med.*, **334**, 150–154

Davey Smith, G. & Phillips, A.N. (1996) Passive smoking and health: Should we believe Phillip Morris's 'experts'? *Br. Med. J.*, **313**, 929–933

European Working Group (1996) *Environmental Tobacco Smoke and Lung Cancer: An Evaluation of the Risk*, Trondheim: European Working Group

Fontham, E., Correa, P., Wu-Williams, A., Reynolds, P., Greenberg, R.S., Buffler, P.A., Chen, V.W., Boyd, P., Alterman, T., Austin, D.F., Liff, J. & Greenberg, S.D. (1994) Environmental tobacco smoke and lung cancer in non-smoking women. A multicenter study. *J. Am. Med. Assoc.*, **271**, 1752–1759

Glantz, S.A. & Parmley, W.W. (1991) Passive smoking and heart disease: Epidemiology, physiology and biochemistry. *Circulation*, **8**, 1–12

Glantz, S.A. & Parmley, W.W. (1995) Passive smoking and heart disease. Mechanisms and risk. *J. Am. Med. Assoc.*, **273**, 1047–1053

He, Y., Lam, T.H., Li, L.S., Li, L.S., Du, R.Y., Jia, G.L., Huang, J.Y. & Zheng, J.S. (1994) Passive smoking at work as a risk factor for coronary heart disease in Chinese women who have never smoked. *Br. Med. J.*, **308**, 380–384

Hedley, A.J. (1997) The tobacco industry and scientific publications. *Br. Med. J.*, **314**, 1350

Kraus, N., *et al.* (1992) Intuitive toxicology: Expert and lay judgements of chemical risks. *Risk Anal.*, **12**, 215–232

Lam, T.H., Chung, S.F., Wong, C.M., Hedley, A.J. & Betson, C.L. (1994) *Youth Smoking, Health and Tobacco Promotion* (Hong Kong Council on Smoking and Health (COSH) Report No. 1), Hong Kong: Hong Kong Council on Smoking and Health

Lam, T.H., Chung, S.F., Wong, C.M., Hedley, A.J. & Betson, C.L. (1995) *Youth Smoking: Knowledge, Attitudes, Smoking in Schools and Families, and Symptoms Due to Passive Smoking* (Hong Kong Council on Smoking and Health (COSH) Report No. 2), Hong Kong: Hong Kong Council on Smoking and Health

Lam, T.H., Chung, S.F., Betson, C.L., Wong, C.M. & Hedley, A.J. (1998) Respiratory symptoms due to active and passive smoking in junior secondary school students in Hong Kong. *Int. J. Epidemiol.*, **27**, 41–48

Law, M.R. & Hackshaw, A.K. (1996) Environmental tobacco smoke. *Br. Med. Bull.*, **52**, 22–34

Lee, P.N. (1987) Passive smoking and lung cancer association: A result of bias? *Hum. Toxicol.*, **6**, 517–524

Lee, P.N. (1994) Comparison of autopsy, clinical and death certificate diagnosis with particular reference to lung cancer: A review of the published data. *APMIS*, **102** (Suppl. 45), 42

Lee, P.N. (1995) Marriage to a smoker may not be a valid marker of exposure in studies relating environmental tobacco smoke to risk of lung cancer in Japanese non-smoking women. *Int. Arch. Occup. Environ. Health*, **67**, 287–294.

Lee, P.N. (1997) Many claims about passive smoking are inadequately justified. *Br. Med. J.*, **314**, 371

Lee, P.N., ed. (undated) *Statistics of Smoking in the United Kingdom* (Research Paper 1), 7th Ed., London: Tobacco Research Council

Overpeck, M.D. & Moss, A.J. (1991) *Children's Exposure to Environmental Cigarette Smoke Before and After Birth*, Hyattsville, Maryland: US Department of Health and Human Services

Peters, J., Hedley, A.J., Wong, C.M., Lam, T.H., Ong, S.G., Liu, J. & Spiegelhalter, D.J. (1996) Effects of an ambient air pollution intervention and environmental tobacco smoke on children's respiratory health in Hong Kong. *Int. J. Epidemiol.*, **25**, 821–828

Peters, J., McCabe, C.J., Hedley, A.J., Lam, T.H. & Wong, C.M. (1998) The economic burden of environmental tobacco smoke on Hong Kong families: Scale and impact. *J. Epidemiol. Commun. Health*, **52**, 53–58

Rush, D., Poswillo, D. & Alberman, E., eds (1992) *Effects of Smoking on the Fetus, Neonate and Child. Exposure to Passive Cigarette Smoking and Child Development: An Updated Critical Review*, New York: Oxford University Press

Samet, J.M., Lewitt, E.M. & Warner, K.E. (1994) Involuntary smoking and children's health. *Crit. Health Issues Child. Youth*, **4**, 94–114

Wewers, M., *et al.* (1995) Misclassification of smoking status among Southeast Asian adult immigrants. *Am. J. Respir. Care Med.*, **152**, 1917–1921

Zaridze, D., Maximovitch, D., Zemlyanaya, G., Aitakov, Z.N. & Boffetta, P. (1998) Exposure to environmental tobacco smoke and risk of lung cancer in non-smoking women from Moscow, Russia. *Int. J. Cancer*, **75**, 335–338

The strategic role of smoking cessation

L.M. Ramström

Institute for Tobacco Studies, Stockholm, Sweden

Behavioural and pharmacological approaches to cessation have now become well established means for health professionals to deliver support to large numbers of smokers. In order to make the best possible use of this knowledge, we should further analyse the role of smoking cessation in the framework of tobacco control as an issue of public health.

Tobacco control : A brief goal analysis

The generally agreed overall goal for tobacco control is reduction of smoking-related morbidity and mortality. This may be achieved to some extent by various product modification procedures, but a major target will always be a lower prevalence of tobacco use. On the way towards this target, two intermediate objectives are: preventing the onset of tobacco use and promoting cessation of tobacco use. It is important to notice that these two objectives are complementary and not mutually exclusive. Both deal with prevention at some level, since cessation of smoking serves as prevention of disease. For example, smoking cessation by a still-healthy smoker is primary prevention of lung cancer, by removing the major cause of this disease. For a patient with a myocardial infarct, smoking cessation serves as secondary prevention by reducing the risk of a second infarct. Prevention of onset also serves as prevention of disease, but only in the future. During the next 30 years, virtually all smoking-related deaths will occur among people who already smoke. Obviously, deaths among current smokers cannot be reduced by preventing other people from starting to smoke. Consequently, up to the year 2025, smoking cessation will be the only effective means of reducing the number of smoking-related deaths.

We have also learnt that successful cessation requires both motivation to stop and ability to overcome the dependence. Strengthening motivation is primarily a matter of health education. Reducing the dependence-related obstacles is usually a matter of suitable treatments.

The global need for smoking cessation

Large-scale success in smoking cessation is indeed an urgent matter in all parts of the world. It is true that cigarette consumption is no longer rising in the industrialized world, as it is in less developed countries, but smoking-related mortality as a percentage of total mortality is still also rising in developed countries (Figure 1). The curves in Figure 1 represent an average for all developed countries, but there are wide variations between countries in this category, as may be seen in Figure 2.

In most of the countries shown in Figure 2, there is a continuing rise in smoking-related mortality, Sweden is the only country in which the smoking-related proportion of all male deaths is no longer increasing but has actually started to decrease. The reason seems to be that an unusually high proportion of male Swedish smokers have quit, including not only light smokers but also, which is unusual, many heavy smokers as well. The example of Sweden demonstrates that large-scale smoking cessation can yield measurable reductions in smoking-related mortality.

There is no country in which the smoking-related proportion of female deaths is decreasing. The reason is that smoking, as well as smoking cessation, became common so much later among women than among men in all countries that no female population has yet reached the stage of a decrease in smoking-related mortality.

In a global perspective, most countries are still at an early stage of dissemination of smoking habits, which means that the natural development will be a dramatic worsening of the health injuries caused by smoking. It has been calculated that, if current smoking patterns persist, the numbers of deaths due to smoking will be:

- in the whole world: 3 million/year in the 1990s
                           10 million/year around 2025
- in China: 0.5 million/year in the 1990s
                           2 million/year around 2025

These are figures for individual years. For the whole period 1996–2025, they will add up to about 200 million of today's smokers in the whole world and 35 million of today's smokers in China.

If current smoking patterns are changed by large-scale cessation, some 30–70% of current smokers, i.e. some 100 million people, will be spared from dying prematurely. Thus, there are good reasons to make implementation of large-scale cessation programmes the top priority in tobacco control, at least for the next few decades.

Figure 1. Smoking-related deaths as a percentage of deaths from all causes in all developed countries

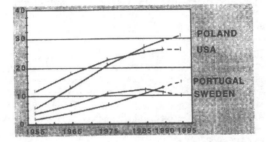

Figures for 1995 are a projection

Figure 2. Smoking-related deaths as a percentage of deaths from all causes among males in four developed countries

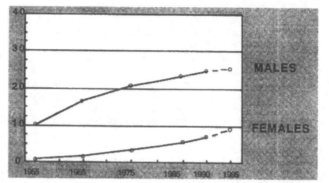

Figures for 1995 are a projection

Practical approaches to smoking cessation

A. Hillhouse

No-Smoking Day (UK), Edinburgh, Scotland

Cessation is often the most neglected part of an overall tobacco control strategy. Helping people to quit smoking is often seen as expensive, not cost effective and, quite frankly, boring. Other tobacco control activities, such as fiscal measures and eliminating tobacco promotion, are seen as more effective in reducing smoking prevalence. I have been an activist and advocate for tobacco control for over 20 years, and I used to share this view in some respects; my views have changed, however, as a result of practical experience in tobacco control and cessation, and I am convinced that an effective strategy to help smokers quit is an important part of any effective tobacco control strategy. I was struck by Richard Peto's powerful reminder of the vital necessity to help more people to quit if we are to prevent millions of premature deaths in the next two or three decades among people who have already started smoking. Nigel Gray made a similar important point when he stressed the need to make serious attempts to help those addicted to tobacco.

The aim of a cessation strategy must be to improve cessation rates generally as well as to help individual smokers. To ensure that cessation rates improve, however, the programmes must be effective and above all practical, and we must recognize that what is effective and practical is different in different countries and cultures. Since I am not a scientist, I do not presume to comment in depth on the papers on smoking cessation but will rather try to draw out one or two general points and make some suggestions about the essential elements of a successful cessation programme.

Professor Yan Di-ying described the very practical and cost-effective use of an existing infrastructure, that of primary care, to deliver not just cessation advice but also health education within a community. This approach will be of interest to many, and not only to those in developing countries. I was impressed by his results, particularly those among older people, who are often neglected in cessation programmes in developed countries, in spite of the fact that we know how much quality of life as well as longevity can be improved by quitting smoking.

Dr Pechachek's paper strongly supports my own view that for large-scale cessation programmes to be effective they must be delivered as an integral part of an overall tobacco-control strategy and within a supportive social and political environment. His conclusions are sobering and it is important that we learn from them.

Professor Kunze's paper demonstrated graphically the opportunities and the dilemmas created by advances in our scientific understanding of the processes of addiction and of quitting smoking. We should base our programmes on the best available science if they are to be effective, and although for many people, particularly in developing countries, the sophisticated approaches described by Professor Kunze may not be practical at the moment, developing science will eventually benefit us all.

Dr Glynn focused on cessation for young people, a group which is receiving increasing attention, at least in developing countries. He suggests what I have come to believe from practical experience: that we do not yet know how to devise practical, effective, cost-effective programmes for young people. But I know that, at least in my country, there is a strong demand for help from young people, and that we need to learn how to respond.

I would like to draw on the papers we have heard to make a few general points. First of all, why should we spend time and resources on helping people to stop smoking? Why have a strategy on cessation? As I indicated before, there are arguments for thinking that cessation is not as important as other parts of national tobacco control strategies. This is an attractive argument, particularly in countries where resources are limited and smoking rates are still low. The papers we have heard illustrate some of the issues involved, but they also demonstrate some of the reasons why cessation programmes are important. Here are five reasons for making cessation an integral part of a comprehensive tobacco control strategy.

1. Richard Peto reminded us, and I will repeat, that 'political' tobacco control, public education and prevention programmes alone will not enable us to achieve our public health goals in the first quarter of the next millennium, and that large numbers of existing smokers must be persuaded to quit if millions of deaths in the next 20–30 years are to be avoided.
2. Most developed countries are finding that prevention programmes aimed at young people are simply not effective in the absence of a powerful cessation programme aimed at adults. Young people who choose whether to smoke or not seem to respond to an environment in which adults are seen to be anxious to quit. In developing countries, where smoking rates among children and women are still low, we could find that by increasing quit rates among adult men we are making a significant contribution to prevention among women and children.
3. The third reason is ethical, and perhaps should have come first. Public awareness campaigns inevitably produce a demand for help from smokers, to which, I am sure you agree, we have a duty to respond.
4. In recent years, research has resulted in significant advances in our understanding of addiction, of the processes involved in quitting and of the personal, social and environmental factors that affect individuals' ability to quit. We know a great deal more than we did a few years ago about effectiveness in cessation and what is likely to work with different target groups. So, if we plan carefully and apply what we already know in a practical way, we should be confident of increasingly satisfactory results. I should stress of course, that, as Dr Pechachek suggested, cessation programmes will be more effective if implemented alongside other tobacco control measures.
5. Finally, an important point that is not often discussed by tobacco-control advocates is that successful strategies in the end depend on public support, and that the more ex-smokers and people wanting to stop there are in any society, the more support there is for effective tobacco control measures. I do not think that the tobacco industry in the United States would discuss a settlement or in the United Kingdom would face a complete ban on tobacco promotion without the support of the millions of people who have quit smoking and the millions more who would do so if they could.

I do not apologize for going over familiar arguments. What I want to do is to encourage all of us who are engaged at any level in the rewarding but unglamorous task of helping people to quit smoking to remind our colleagues who are engaged in the political, fiscal or legal aspects of tobacco control why cessation programmes matter and why a tobacco-control strategy without an effective and practical cessation component will be less successful than it could be.

To conclude, I should like to make a few comments on what makes a comprehensive cessation strategy practical and effective. A strategy to help the maximum number of smokers to quit will include:

• public information and activities designed to inform and motivate smokers, delivered within the context of an integrated tobacco control strategy;
• appropriate and accessible support to help motivated smokers through the immediate attempt to quit and the longer-term process of becoming a non-smoker;
• special programmes targeted at key groups and those who find it hardest to quit.

The form the strategy will take will of course vary with local or national circumstances and resources, but the methods used will be based on the best available science.

I have one final suggestion on how to ensure that a cessation strategy is effective, which is to start with the consumer or potential consumer of cessation help and advice, rather than with the individual method to be used. We must not only use the best methods available for the target group we are addressing, but we must ensure that they think the methods are appropriate and that we have found the best routes through which to deliver them. I believe that one reason why cessation has become the 'poor relation' in tobacco control is that practitioners and planners have tended to concentrate more on cessation methods than on delivery mechanisms. Looking at the problem in another way, in marketing jargon, we tend to start with the producers of cessation services rather than with the consumers. The best possible methods will not deliver results if the consumer is unaware of what is available, doesn't think it is appropriate or can't reach the help that is available because of lack of social support. In other words, we need to consider both the efficacy and the reach of programmes. To increase reach we must study our market very closely and consider the needs of different groups. We must also be creative in finding routes through which to deliver services, whether through primary care, community networks, religious agencies, schools, the voluntary sector, telephone help lines or whatever routes are practical and affordable in our own circumstances. I think that if we can do this, then, with the knowledge we already have, quit rates in both developed and developing countries will increase and our work will be seen to make an essential contribution to the worldwide campaign against the tobacco epidemic.

Tobacco control programmes

K. Bjartveit

International Union Against Tuberculosis and Lung Disease, Paris, France

Presentations were made on global, legislative and community approaches, which represent the fundamental aspects of tobacco control. Bung-On Ritthiphakdee underlined that smoking rates in Thailand have decreased although an increase was expected. This is in agreement with experience in Norway: per capita consumption peaked in 1975, and we should have experienced an increase after that, for the same reasons as in Thailand. Thus, if tobacco consumption had continued to rise at the same rate as before 1970, it would have been about 50% higher than it actually is today. Our peak occurred at a level of consumption that is only half that experienced in Canada, the United Kingdom and the United States. What happened was that we introduced our advertising ban in the same year, 1975, and, contrary to what has been reported at this conference, smoking rates among adolescents fell after that ban was enforced and sales levelled off at the time Parliament decided to introduce legislation. This was emphasized by the Norwegian Minister of Health in a letter to Dr Judith Mackay: "... there is no doubt that the Norwegian advertising ban has had a clear and substantial influence on total consumption in general, and smoking rates among schoolchildren in particular. In my view, the reduction brought about by the advertising ban will have a positive and marked impact on the future incidence of smoking-related diseases and consequent mortality."

I agree completely with Garfield Mahood that we should not be satisfied with our results. We should recognize our failures and hunt unceasingly for new and radical approaches to tobacco control. We should, however, guard against the attitude that nothing has been achieved, as such a view is dangerous and may be contagious. It could put us in a corner, where the tobacco industry wants us to be: frustrated, paralysed campaigners who have lost faith and their fighting spirit. We started off as a relatively small group 30 years ago at the First World Conference, in New York, United States. In my view, an amazing amount has been achieved in many parts of the world in the intervening years. One striking example is the clearly decreasing trend in mortality from lung cancer among men in the United Kingdom, shown by Richard Peto; good news was also brought from Canada, New Zealand and Poland, and now Thailand.

My first message is therefore 'Keep the faith.' Far greater challenges lie ahead, and much more emphasis will have to be placed on a global approach. Tobacco control, however, includes steps other than the traditional public health measures. Some years ago, I presented a paper on tobacco control in a low-income tobacco-producing country. The immediate response of the audience was that an efficient tobacco control programme would eliminate the income of poor people who had no other alternative. We should not be fooled by this argument, however, and it should not be allowed to obstruct an aggressive tobacco control programme. Tobacco as a source of income will not disappear overnight; it will happen gradually, and during that time governments should actively set up a programme to help poor people find other sources of income. Today, the opposite is often true: tobacco growing is subsidized. A global programme must find radical solutions to the many economic problems involved.

In 1993, at a conference in Oslo, Mike Daube presented his dream: the 2010 report of the United Nations Tobacco Control Authority, which would be established in the 1990s by a resolution of the United Nations General Assembly. It would be given full support and comprehensive powers by all governments and a substantial budget. The 2010 report summarizes the activities of the Authority, which introduced measures step by step in all countries, resulting in a dramatic fall in cigarette smoking. In 1999, a special international fund would be established to support crop diversification for tobacco growers and to reimburse developing countries for losses from declining tobacco sales. In 2009, the ageing but still active British epidemiologist, Sir Richard Peto, concludes that "on the basis of current trends, the smoking epidemic will cease to be an important cause of premature death by the middle of this century". The publication reaches its climax by reporting a joint statement from the chairpersons of the major multinational tobacco companies, who throw in the towel, declaring that the time has come to put conscience before finance.

Today, Mike Daube's dream has actually started to come true, although the timetable and details differ slightly. The World Health Organization has begun preparing an international framework convention for tobacco control, presented at this conference. Our task is to urge our governments to take up this vital matter at the highest level in the United Nations system, in particular to secure adequate funding for this global task. We are in a state of emergency. It is therefore necessary to cut through all of the bureaucracy, at both national and international levels, so that action can be taken immediately. We should provoke our top politicians to be the first to take an initiative. My second message is therefore 'Global tobacco control is a United Nations concern.'

During the conference, we were constantly confronted with data on present and future mortality due to tobacco. Mortality today tells us about risks in the past. Risk today tells us about mortality in the future. The past is the past, and nothing can be done about it; but the future is in our hands. The pessimistic predictions do not need to happen. We can influence today's risk and alter the future. The fundamental question is, 'In whose hands?' In the hands of the tobacco industry swearing that they would tell the truth, the whole truth and nothing but the truth? Do we want to have those hands on the steering wheel of tobacco control? Do we even want to shake those hands, in an agreement or a settlement, to reach our goal? Let me remind you of a statement made by a World Health Organization Expert Committee in 1978 in which Nigel Gray and I participated: "The tobacco industry has invariably sought to reduce the impact of virtually all smoking control measures and, in general, does not willingly agree to any legislation or voluntary codes likely to have an adverse effect on tobacco sales. It would be surprising commercial practice if it did." That's the main reason for my scepticism about the settlement with the tobacco industry. These people will hardly agree to an arrangement that in the long run will have catastrophic consequences on their sales, and that is exactly what we want.

There is only one thing I fear more than the settlement: that the settlement will divide our forces. Then, our enemy will really have succeeded, with us in a corner not only as frustrated campaigners but also as divided campaigners. United we are strong.

The future is therefore in the hands of the United Nations General Assembly. Their hands should be raised in a vote which commits all nations of the world to a radical global programme that could stem the wave of the growing epidemic.

Health promotion in tobacco control

E. Protacio-Marcelino

Department of Psychology, University of the Philippines, Manila, Philippines

Most efforts in tobacco control begin with a 'medical' model, or a concept of health as merely the 'absence of disease'. Thus, initial efforts have focused on various types of smoking cessation programmes. Recent years have seen, however, the growth of a new public health movement that has a holistic, integrated approach to health that goes beyond healthy lifestyles and emphasizes a state of physical, mental and social well-being. Health is seen as a resource for everyday life and not just a goal. Good health is seen as a major resource for social, economic and personal development. Health is considered to be a basic human right, and good health to be an important aspect of quality of life. Thus, health is created and lived by people in their everyday lives. It is created by caring for oneself and others, by being able to take decisions and have control over one's life and by ensuring that society creates conditions that allow the attainment of health by all its members.

Health promotion is the process of enabling people to increase their control over their health and to improve it. It is a practical approach to achieving greater equity in health—reducing differences in health status and ensuring equal opportunity and resources to enable people to achieve their full health potential. Research and case studies around the world provide convincing evidence that health promotion works. Thus, health promotion strategies are being applied in all aspects of tobacco control.

For example, research suggests that the economic benefits of health promotion at the work site are likely to exceed the costs, making it a wise financial investment. Such programmes generally involve periodic or continuous provision of materials and activities for education and behavioural change, designed to maintain or improve the fitness, health and well-being of workers, changes in organizational practices and policies conducive to health promotion.

Dr James Terborg has used the techniques of cost–effectiveness and cost–benefit analysis to evaluate health promotion programmes and interventions in economic terms. These are especially useful in making policy decisions that involve the allocation of scarce financial resources. Economic benefits resulting from health promotion strategies at the work place have been clearly demonstrated with regard to absenteeism, occupational injuries, health-care costs and productivity. Thus, health promotion activities at the work site are good business and good national policy.

In another light, the American Cancer Society suggests that we go beyond traditional health promotion at an accelerated pace in order to stem the tide of tobacco-related illness. They propose a paradigm shift in the prevalence of tobacco use in order to achieve more dramatic reductions in other countries. Thus shift is towards changing the social norm of the acceptance of tobacco. To do this, they suggest that we focus on three areas of concern: access of young people to tobacco, environmental tobacco smoke and the 'high-tech' marketing and influence-wielding of the tobacco industry. Experience in the United States has shown that such strategies work well in tandem with tax increases and litigation to recover present and future tobacco-related costs.

Africa, according to Dr Yussuf Saloojee, may still be in the unique position of being able to avoid the worst ravages of the unfolding tobacco epidemic. The urgent need is to develop human and institutional capacity for tobacco control. Health promotion efforts thus become the necessary first step in taking advantage of this situation.

Health promotion in tobacco control means:
* building healthy public policy, such as banning tobacco advertising, increasing taxes on tobacco, strengthening community action by enhancing self-help and social support systems and encouraging public participation in directing health agencies;
* reorientating health services from an emphasis on curative and clinical services to promotion of a more holistic, integrated, culturally-sensitive approach, with a focus on training and research;
* developing personal skills for making healthy choices on the basis of information on the health hazards and other issues in tobacco control and
* creating supportive environments.

In the final analysis, health cannot be separated from other goals. The link between people and their environment requires a bio-psycho-socio-ecological approach to health. We must take care of ourselves, our communities and our natural environment.

Effective use of the mass media for tobacco control

J. Watt

Victorian Smoking and Health Programme, Melbourne, Victoria, Australia

In this symposium, the co-chairs were Ms Katie Aston (Health Education Authority, United Kingdom) and Professor Jingheng Huang (Shanghai Medical University, China). The speakers were Professor Rob Donovan (University of Western Australia), Dr Lesley Owen (Health Education Authority, United Kingdom), Dr Kishore Chaudhry (Indian Council of Medical Research) and Ms Judith Watt (Victorian Smoking and Health Programme, Australia). The discussants were Mr James Fox (Department of Health and Family Services, Australia) and Dr Ron Borland (Centre for Behavioural Research in Cancer, Anti-Cancer Council of Victoria, Australia).

Whether developed or developing, all countries engaged in tobacco control activities aim to communicate the health consequences of smoking to the widest possible audience. To do so effectively means using the mass media (television, radio, press, outdoor posters etc.) as well as traditional health education programmes in schools and health services. Health agencies in many countries have long experience in communicating anti-smoking messages through the mass media, whether by buying advertising time, using public or community service slots or creating publicity that is reported for free. The extent to which these efforts are effective has been the subject of intense scrutiny by researchers and evaluators around the world.

Professor Rob Donovan opened the symposium with an overview of mass media and tobacco control. The 1940s and 1950s saw large-scale use of the mass media for public 'information' campaigns. Since then, the advent of sophisticated electronic media and better understanding of communication processes has led to the development of campaigns that not only provide health information but also attempt to persuade individuals to adopt recommended healthy behaviours. Much recent research has been directed to understanding and detailing the circumstances in which the media and media messages are effective and the circumstances in which various aspects of health can be influenced.

The effectiveness of the media in tobacco control, via both publicity and paid advertising, is now well established for well-designed and implemented campaigns. A number of researchers in health promotion and communications have attempted to identify the conditions under which the media are most effective in promoting health. Distilling these analyses, Professor Donovan offered practical recommendations for designing a successful campaign and offered a practical model for using the media in tobacco control and for evaluating a communications strategy. He concluded by observing that the effective application of the techniques and principles of marketing to health promotion requires an understanding of both consumer decision-making and health issues. In practical terms, this requires close cooperation between marketing experts, public health professionals and, for mass media campaign components, behavioural scientists with expertise in communication theory and attitude and behavioural change. Realization of this need has been a long time coming.

Dr Lesley Owen discussed the Health Education Authority's family smoking campaign, which was begun in 1992. The aim was to test the impact on smoking prevalence of a mass media campaign supported by local activities and to try to establish the optimal (cost-effective) amount of television advertising required to bring about a change in smoking behaviour. The campaign had three major components: television advertising, a national telephone help-line which offered advice and support to smokers who wanted to quit and a local tobacco control alliance to generate as much unpaid publicity and public relations as possible on smoking and health and to support local health professionals. The comprehensive programme of research and evaluation included surveys of the general population, pre- and post-testing of the television advertisements, evaluation of the local activity network, evaluation of the telephone help-line and monitoring of unpaid media coverage. Changes in smoking behaviour were measured in a large-scale panel survey. The first survey was carried out before the campaign began, and the two follow-up surveys were carried out after each television campaign (about six and 18 months after the first survey).

There was good evidence that the campaign had an effect. In fact, the research showed a clear dose–response effect, whereby the region with the greatest input showed the greatest change and regions with little or no input showed virtually no change. Thus, West Yorkshire, which received a double weight of advertising and was supported by a local network, showed the greatest change in smoking prevalence. Over the two-year period, the prevalence in this region fell by 3.5%; 8.6% had quit in the control region, 9.7% in the region with media only and 12% in the region with media and a local network. The dose–response effect observed in the preliminary analysis of prevalence suggests that there is a minimum amount of television advertising below which positive changes in smoking behaviour are unlikely to be observed. The inclusion of a local activity network clearly enhanced the impact of the heavy mass media intervention.

Dr Kishore Chaudhry of the Indian Council of Medical Research described the project Radio DATE, a collaborative effort of the Council and All India Radio run in

1990. The acronym DATE stands for Drugs, Alcohol and Tobacco Education. In 1990, television covered about 15% of the population, while radio covered about 97%. The intervention was in the form of 30 weekly episodes of 20 min each. The episodes were broadcast from 84 stations of All India Radio (out of 104 existing at that time) at prime time, simultaneously in 16 languages, and were repeated on all the stations during the week, generally in the evening. The programme was heard by up to 32% of the potential listeners, and immediately after the programme 4–6% of tobacco users quit their habit. The programme was extensively reviewed in other media and became the subject of a television programme.

Judith Watt from the Victorian Smoking and Health Programme in Australia concluded the session with observations on the importance of research to the development of media campaigns and on the importance of using mass media to reach disadvantaged groups of the population, citing the new Australian campaign on smoking as an example.

Tobacco economics

D.J. Collins

School of Economic and Financial Studies, Macquarie University, Sydney, New South Wales, Australia

Introduction

In recent years, the emphasis of policy discussion on tobacco has moved increasingly into the area of economics. Epidemiological evidence on the health impact of tobacco is now largely unchallenged, even by the tobacco industry. For example, the Chairman of Philip Morris has been reported as saying that thousands of Americans might have died of diseases caused at least in part by smoking. The Chairman of RJR Nabisco is reported as saying that he believed smoking played a part in causing cancer. Note that the tobacco industry is now using phrases such as 'caused by' rather than 'associated with'.

There remains substantial epidemiological disagreement over the impact of passive smoking, and the tobacco industry has yet to agree that nicotine has addictive properties; in the main, however, the epidemiological arguments are over, and both sides are increasingly resorting to arguments based upon economic analysis and data.

Professor Jin's paper

Many countries have produced estimates of the costs of smoking to the health care system and to society as a whole. Some of the countries for which estimates have been produced are Australia, Canada, Japan, New Zealand, South Africa and the United States. Professor Jin Shuigao's paper 'Estimation of direct smoking-related costs in China' has produced some frightening estimates of the direct health care costs of smoking in China. They are frightening not so much because of their absolute level—indeed, to western eyes they appear comparatively low, perhaps because of low *per capita* income, health costs and health expenditure in China—but because Professor Jin estimates that they will rise fast in the next few years. Western experience would suggest that they may rise even faster than Professor Jin predicts. Furthermore, these estimates do not take account of other important costs of tobacco related mortality and morbidity, for example, tangible production losses and the intangible costs of loss of life.

This type of cost information is largely unavailable for developing countries. In 1996, the Canadian Centre of Substance Abuse produced *International Guidelines for Estimating the Costs of Substance Abuse* (Single et al., 1996) with the intention of encouraging the use of a standard cost estimation method. The hope was to encourage internationally comparable estimates. Unfortunately, these guidelines have not been as widely disseminated as was hoped, and their objective has remained largely unrealized.

Professor Warner's paper

The tobacco industry's response to tobacco cost estimates of this type has been threefold:

- to query the technical basis of the calculations and to produce alternative estimates, almost without exception suggesting lower costs and higher benefits of tobacco consumption. An internationally accepted method for estimating the cost of tobacco use would reduce the strength of these attacks.
- to query the interpretation of the results. Professor Warner drew attention to some of the problems of interpreting social cost estimates, including the issue of whether gross or net health-care costs (after taking account of the 'benefits' to health expenditure of the premature deaths of smokers) should be calculated. For a variety of reasons, social cost estimates are not easy to interpret, and misinterpretation is common by both the tobacco industry and tobacco control advocates. Economists have an important role in clarifying the meaning of cost estimates. Helen Lapsley and I, in our work on the social costs of drug abuse in Australia (Collins & Lapsley, 1996), estimated that the net health-care costs attributable to tobacco in a particular year (adjusting for the health-care savings resulting from premature deaths of smokers) are still high, even after deducting these 'benefits'. In terms of health-care costs, smokers live and die very expensively.
- to produce evidence for the asserted economic benefits of the tobacco industry, which include: increased national income; increased tax revenue; higher employment; consumer surplus benefits and improved balance of payments (in appropriate circumstances). Professor Warner evaluated these claimed benefits and showed them to be based largely on inadequate or incomplete economic analysis. Industry studies usually assume, explicitly or implicitly, that the resources used in tobacco and cigarette production have no alternative uses, and so, in the absence of the tobacco industry, would remain unemployed; and that the money saved as a result of reduced smoking would not be spent elsewhere (and so create employment or income elsewhere). Indeed, in the industry studies I have seen, the money saved seems to disappear into a black hole, since any effects of higher savings on interest rates are ignored. Both these assumptions are highly implausible.

Another claim frequently made by the tobacco industry but not mentioned by Professor Warner is that cigarette tax revenues create productive resources for the community. They do not. They simply reallocate existing resources. As Professor Warner says, it is most important that the inadequacies or omissions of the industry's economic arguments be exposed. These inadequacies are well known to economists but not to the wider community (for further consideration of these issues, see Collins & Lapsley, 1997).

Professor Townsend's paper

Economic analysis is a powerful instrument for developing appropriate policies to counter the smoking epidemic. Professor Townsend's paper presented evidence on the effectiveness of tobacco taxes in reducing consumption in certain countries and target community groups (for example, the young). It is especially important to use this type of information to identify effective policies for reducing smoking among young people, since almost all smokers take up the habit during adolescence or earlier. It is also important, however, to dissuade current smokers from continuing their habit since, as Professor Peto showed so clearly, there are great health benefits to be achieved by giving up smoking. Professor Townsend's paper demonstrates that considerable information on the elasticity of tobacco demand and income exists for developed countries, but that there is still a great scarcity of such information for developing nations.

We do know that tobacco tax policies are, in all countries, relatively cheap to implement and need not impose high costs for compliance. Indeed, these taxes, while being effective in reducing tobacco consumption, can be very lucrative for governments. The evidence that the price elasticity of demand for tobacco is almost universally low means that there is a free lunch for governments which impose tobacco taxes. It is possible simultaneously to reduce tobacco consumption and increase tobacco tax revenue. Governments are frequently accused of paying lip service to the need for reduced tobacco consumption while in reality their actual objective is to increase tax revenue. But what do motives matter if the two targets can be achieved simultaneously?

Dr Stamps' paper

Where does this leave countries, such as Zimbabwe, which are genuinely dependent on tobacco production? Dr Stamp's paper, 'Tobacco or health: The grower's perspective', illustrates the problems of countries that have difficulty in finding replacement export cash crops that can offer the same levels and stability of prices as tobacco.

It is not acceptable for tobacco-consuming countries to adopt the moral stance that countries such as Zimbabwe should reduce their tobacco production, unless the necessary practical and financial assistance to do so is provided at the same time. There do not seem to be any grounds for optimism in this regard. It is significant that the proposed United States tobacco settlement agreement, as it stands at the time of writing, does not propose any restriction on exports by the US tobacco industry. Zimbabwe can be confident that not only will it receive little international assistance to reduce the reliance of its balance of payments on tobacco exports, but also that any attempt to do so will be actively exploited by other tobacco-exporting countries. Perhaps the only advice that we can reasonably offer to tobacco-producing countries such as Zimbabwe is that it will be unequivocally in their interests to reduce the *domestic* prevalence of smoking. This will undoubtedly yield benefits for health-care and public expenditure and could even result in a favourable balance of payments.

Conclusion

Economics has a significant contribution to make to tobacco policy. Economic analysis and policies represent important weapons in the anti-tobacco armoury. Unfortunately, too few economists have enlisted in this conflict.

References
Collins, D.J. & Lapsley, H.M. (1996) *The Social Costs of Drug Abuse in Australia in 1988 and 1992* (National Drug Strategy Monograph Series No. 30), Canberra: Australian Government Publishing Service
Collins, D.J. & Lapsley, H.M. (1997)*The Economic Impact of Tobacco Smoking in Pacific Islands*, Pacific Tobacco and Health Project
Single, E., Collins, D., Easton, B., Harwood, H., Lapsley, H. & Maynard, A. (1996) *International Guidelines for Estimating the Costs of Substance Abuse*, Ottawa: Canadian Centre on Substance Abuse

Litigation for tobacco control

P. Boucher

Comité National contre le Tabagisme, Versailles, France

As a discussant in this very lively symposium about litigation for tobacco control, I was captivated. The obvious lessons we can draw are that the tobacco industry is very devious indeed and ready to do almost anything—legal or not—to improve its sales. There is no limit (for the moment) to what they can spend, while health advocates very often operate on limited funding, if any. Still, we heard about many victories, and many more are yet to come. This is good news, but we should know what the costs can be if we do not win.

Stephen Woodward described graphically how he has been harassed by tobacco industry law suits and lawyers. Stephen is courageous and resilient, but not everybody is as strong. From my own experience with lawsuits against the tobacco industry and its allies in France, where I supervised more than 200 such cases in six years, I suggest that one must first find the best lawyers to have a chance of winning.

Listening to Dick Daynard, Cliff Douglas, Matt Myers and John Banzhaf, we had the opportunity to hear good lawyers, and we must look for the equivalent in our own countries. Of course, the legislation, regulations and rules of procedure vary from one country to another. What is won in one may be impossible to obtain elsewhere. Still, there are many opportunities for international cooperation, and we can rely on Globalink to share key information and ask for help. Recently we have been able to provide our foreign friends with information about the marketing plans of various cigarette companies, which we obtained through an aggressive investigative judge. Since the multinationals operate in similar ways all over the world, it can be very interesting to learn about their activities in other countries.

A major problem of tobacco control legislation is its enforcement. When drafting new legislation, one must be very precise about enforcement procedures and sanctions. I am very pleased that the French anti-tobacco groups have obtained legal standing in cases involving tobacco control. As a result, we have been able to win sizeable punitive damages. Unfortunately, in many countries, non-profit organizations do not have legal standing.

As we heard, there are many reasons for litigation: former smokers can sue, as can non-smokers, but we must be ready to be very patient. Many of the few big victories we can enjoy now were prepared over many years, with many defeats or very small victories. But we now know that finally we have no choice. As John Banzhaf would say, we must "Sue the bastards", again and again.

Settlements with the tobacco industry

R. Weissman

Essential Action, Washington DC, United States

The growing tobacco epidemic which is the subject of this conference is spread by identifiable agents: the multinational tobacco companies. Two of the three leading global tobacco companies, Philip Morris and R.J. Reynolds , are based in the United States. Two-thirds of their sales and about half of their profits come from overseas sales, but the United States deal with the tobacco companies to settle existing and future lawsuits says nothing about the global operations of Philip Morris and RJR. It does nothing to restrict their overseas activities. The deal is completely compatible with the companies' global strategy and ambitions: to maintain constant or slowly declining sales at home while expanding massively abroad. The deal would sacrifice many of the most powerful tools available to discipline the tobacco multinationals—most importantly, litigation in United States courts—without doing anything to curtail the tobacco epidemic in the companies' target regions: the Third World, eastern Europe and the former Soviet Union.

To compound the problem, the deal may actually intensify the global epidemic in a series of ways.

1. The deal will enable and perhaps encourage the tobacco companies to intensify their predatory behaviour abroad. It requires the tobacco companies to pay US$ 368 thousand million over 25 years, and in exchange it grants the industry a comprehensive peace in the United States, an end to the lawsuits and myriad hassles it now faces. Whether or not international sales end up subsidizing the company's payment obligations under

the deal, there is little doubt that peace at home will enable the companies to intensify their invasion of oveseas markets. The lawsuits and growing public controversies about the behaviour of the tobacco companies are a drain on the time and energy of company executives and on the resources of the companies; with that diversion eliminated, if the deal is approved, we may expect to see them adopt a laser-like focus on overseas expansion.

There is no question that corporate expansion of United States tobacco companies means not only an enlarged market share for the companies, but also higher smoking rates. From the Republic of Korea to the Russian Federation, smoking rates increased rapidly after the United States companies entered the market.

2. The deal will absolutely or effectively preclude lawsuits by non-United States victims in United States courts. It states that it settles 'all' medical cost reimbursement and aggregated suits by governmental entities against the tobacco companies. On the face of it, this provision would block other governments from bringing suit in United States courts on the same theories as those used in state cases. Similarly, the deal's limitations on private suits, which preclude victims from joining together in class actions or other means to sue the industry collectively, appear to apply to lawsuits filed in United States courts by non-United States citizens. But while United States victims and the United States public are presumably receiving benefits in exchange for this grant of effective immunity, overseas victims and non-United States populations are receiving nothing.

The deal will interfere with the efforts of foreign governments and foreign victims to collect judgements in United States courts. Even if foreign governments or victims choose to sue in their home courts, the deal will still restrict their rights. If the foreign government or victims win judgement in their home country and then seek to collect their money from the parent company in the United States, they are likely to run up against the restrictions on liability in the deal.

3. The deal appears to preclude the United States Food and Drug Administration from equally regulating products made for domestic consumption and for export. The deal defines the scope of the Administration as 'all products sold in United States commerce', specifying that it covers imports but not mentioning exports. Leading United States regulatory law authorities believe that this provision would preclude the Food and Drug Administration from regulating cigarettes manufactured in the United States for export. That would enshrine into law a double standard. Cigarettes manufactured in United States factories for domestic consumption would be subject to warning requirements included in the deal or tougher warning, labelling, ingredient disclosure or ingredient regulations potentially later required by the Food and Drug Administration. Cigarettes made in the same factories, but for export, would not be subject to these rules.

4. A bankruptcy loophole in the deal could give the tobacco companies a means of ravaging the Third World, eastern Europe and the former Soviet Union. The deal specifies that, in the event of bankruptcy, the United States companies must continue to meet their payment obligations under the deal, but it stipulates that those obligations do not apply to subsidiaries selling overseas. This means that the companies' overseas earnings would go directly into the shareholders' pockets, without being diverted to the settlement payment. It is easy to imagine disturbing scenarios in which the companies might exploit this provision, especially if United States consumption rates decline significantly in the coming years.

5. The deal would effectively end the disclosure in the United States of damning internal company documents. The proposed terms of the deal would enable the tobacco industry to continue to conceal its most important documents for years and perhaps permanently. Those tobacco control advocates outside of the United States who find industry disclosures in the United States helpful would be out of luck if the deal is enacted.

6. The deal will end the United States political momentum against the industry and the media focus on tobacco, much of which stimulates similar political and media interest in other countries.

Conclusion

The so-called 'global settlement' is really a United States settlement, but it has global implications. The proponents of the deal have not given sufficient attention to international tobacco control issues; they have not appropriately consulted with their international allies. They need to hear a clear message from international tobacco control advocates: Don't accept a deal that hurts the rest of the world.

CLOSING REMARKS

Lessons from the conference: The next 25 years

J. Mackay

Asian Consultancy on Tobacco Control, Hong Kong SAR, China

Introduction

We have been privileged to hear outstanding presentations at this conference by colleagues from around the world on a wide range of issues in the tobacco epidemic. Rather than list these one by one, in this closing keynote address I shall describe some major points that emerged and use these to predict the status of the tobacco epidemic in the year 2025.

Deaths: Three times as many people will die from tobacco-related causes in 2025

The number of tobacco-attributable deaths will continue to rise from today's 3 million to 10 million a year by 2025 (Peto *et al.*, this volume). China will be the leading country for these deaths. Passive smoking will persist in harming a significant number of non-smokers. The good news is that tobacco-attributable deaths will continue to fall among males in developed countries with small populations.

Developing countries will suffer the most

By 2025, the transfer of the tobacco epidemic from rich to poor countries will be well advanced, with only 15% of the world's smokers living in the rich countries. Health-care facilities will be hopelessly inadequate to cope with this epidemic.

Smoking prevalence: Bad news for women—better news for men

In developing countries, the prevalence of smoking among women will rise from 8% to 20% by 2025. By then, women will be dying from tobacco in substantial and ever-increasing numbers. The good news is that the prevalence of smoking among men will fall to 25% in developed countries (possibly even as low as 15% in some) and from 60% to 45% in developing countries by 2025.

The total numbers of smokers will go up

There are 1.1 thousand million smokers in the world today. This number will increase to over 1.64 thousand million by 2025, because (i) the world's population will rise from the current 6 thousand million to 8.5 thousand million, (ii) people will live longer (United Nations, 1991) and (iii) more women will be smoking.

Women: Gloomy prospects

The huge increases in the number of women smokers will have enormous consequences on health, income, the foetus and the family. Women's organizations and women's magazines have singularly failed both to understand that smoking is a feminist issue and to take an appropriate role. The 10th World Conference made an unprecedented effort to involve women at all levels—on committees, as chairs, speakers, discussants and funded delegates. Every invited speaker was asked to include a perspective on tobacco and women in their presentation. Perhaps when women are involved at core decision-making level (e.g. at future conferences, on the WHO Expert Panel), the issues of women and tobacco will be properly addressed.

Economics: Tobacco use will have severe economic effects

Already, the economic costs of tobacco are at least US$ 200 thousand million greater than the economic gain, with one-third of this loss being incurred by developing countries

(The Bellagio statement on tobacco and sustainable development at the Rockefeller Foundation's Bellagio Study and Conference Centre, Italy, 26–30 June 1995). This toll can only get worse. Yet, the World Bank states that tobacco control efforts could contribute to economic development in low- and middle-income countries. Before 2025, governments will finally understand that tobacco control is good for the economy and that no tobacco farmers, retailers or tobacco workers will be out of a job because of tobacco control measures.

Treatment and care

This conference hardly touched on the possibilities of spectacular advances in diagnosis, investigation and treatment of tobacco-attributable diseases, for example in genetics, surgery, nanotechnology, telemedicine, targeted pharmaceuticals and radiotherapy. In 2025, individuals who are genetically prone to tobacco-attributable diseases could be identified at birth. Secondary cancers, currently untreatable, could be treated. Most of this technology will be expensive, but some, such as automated sputum cytology, will be cheaper. Medical advances will have almost no impact on global mortality statistics but will help individual smokers, especially in the rich countries.

Tobacco control action
Globally

By 2025, the WHO international framework convention on tobacco control should have been adopted, ratified and implemented. WHO may have a major department on tobacco or health at Headquarters, appropriately staffed and financed, with a staff member in each regional office. All other United Nations agencies may recognize their role. There will be the need for:

- global policies and legislation on supra-national tobacco advertising *via* satellite and internet, tar and nicotine yields, additives, tax and smuggling;
- greater regional coordination, for example in the European Community and the Association of South East Asian Nations;
- restriction on trade pressures from one government to another; and
- electronic networking, such as Globalink.

Nationally

Many conference presentations showed that tobacco control is clearly a low priority for most governments, illustrated by negligible funding. Few people are working on tobacco control: for example, there are fewer than 10 full-time people in the Asia–Pacific region, covering more than half the world's smokers.

In future, a major distinction will evolve between nations that have and have not made the 'transition' to committed and vigorous preventive health measures and practices (J. Koplan, this volume). By 2025, 'post-transition' nations will have robust health education programmes and extremely restrictive tobacco policies, with active promotion of and increased support for physical activity and a low-fat, high-fibre, high-fruit and mainly vegetarian diet. 'Pre-transition' nations will be grappling with deteriorating health status, an unabated epidemic of lung cancer, heart disease, obesity and industrial and road accidents. They will struggle with deeply entrenched tobacco interests that manipulate their governments, the media and public opinion. They will have made an extremely costly mistake by missing the opportunity to build significant barriers to tobacco in the late twentieth and early twenty-first century, and will then find it very difficult to expel the powerful foreign tobacco companies and their domestic allies from their midst. They will be doomed to repeat the painful and costly experience of the 'post- transition' nations, which laboured for 30–50 years to achieve significant gains over tobacco pedlars.

The following will be attained in nations that take serious tobacco control action now:
- establishment of a national office to coordinate tobacco control efforts;

- licensing of nicotine as an addictive drug, with its manufacture, promotion and sale under regulatory control by agencies such as the Food and Drug Administration in the United States;
- smoke-free areas in workplaces, indoor public areas and public transport;
- bans on all promotion: sports and arts bodies will look back with amazement at the time in history when their predecessors accepted money from the tobacco industry;
- cigarette packs will be plain black and white and bear only the brand name, tar and nicotine levels and health warnings;
- tar levels will be below 15 mg all over the world and 10 mg in 'post-transition' countries;
- health education will be carried out by all nations, in some more effectively than in others: the failure of schools programmes in the twentieth century will force health educators to turn to social marketers for professional help;
- prices will be higher in real terms in comparison with today's. 'Duty-free' tobacco will have long disappeared. Smuggling (currently 30% of all traded cigarettes) will continue to undermine the price policy. As the smuggling trade expands, tobacco will have become a predominantly illegal product in many markets. The tobacco industry may have been hit by several spectacular legal cases proving their involvement in smuggling of their own cigarettes.
- core funding for tobacco control and health promotion will come from governments and tobacco taxes, although it will become fashionable in future for big business to contribute, in the same way it is beginning to contribute to environmental issues today;
- partners in fighting the tobacco epidemic will include a wide range of youth leaders, environmentalists, religious leaders, consumer pressure groups, sports bodies and many others. By 2025, the backlash will be more intense, with smoking firmly entrenched among rebellious youth.

Cessation

If efforts are concentrated only on preventing children from smoking, there will be no reduction in the up to 200 million smoking-related deaths expected to occur before 2025 among people who already smoke. Papers presented at this conference showed that few countries, especially developing countries, are sufficiently energetic about assisting cessation. By 2025, medical schools will have systematically incorporated tobacco issues into their curricula, and health professionals will be competent and effective in advising patients about quitting smoking.

The tobacco industry

Many papers illustrated how the commercial transnational companies are expanding their empires, denying the evidence on health effects, advertising and promoting their products in every corner of the earth, obstructing government action, overpowering national monopolies and selling more and more cigarettes. Their grip on the big markets in developing countries will become stronger as they move their growing and manufacturing processes out of the United States, where by 2025 there may be no tobacco grown.

The 20th World Conference on Tobacco or Health may see discussions of the domination of the world tobacco market by the largest exporter (China) and by Japan and the reversal of fortunes of the American and British tobacco companies. How will the tobacco companies behave in 2025? Who would have imagined 30 years ago that they would engage in settlement talks with governments today? An ex-tobacco industry executive has made the interesting prediction that tobacco production could be reduced by the global demand for food, brought about by the increasing population and a century of ecological abuse and mismanagement of the planet's food and water supply. He pointed out that, as many of the tobacco companies are involved in the transnational food business, their corporate and personal pockets, previously lined with tobacco gold, will now likewise be lined with gold from wheat, corn and rice.

The litigation flurry will have run its course. Much of the developed world will have moved to a managed tobacco industry, with liability automatically paid for tobacco-attributable health-care costs to individual smokers who have been harmed by tobacco. The United States settlement agreement with the tobacco industry produced unique interest at this meeting: the Resolutions Committee received more submissions on this topic than on any other, and the specific recommendations differed quite considerably. There was, however, broad consensus on the principles that should apply to all countries, and these are reflected in the resolutions, which apply not only to the United States but also to Indonesia, Japan, the United Kingdom and other large exporting countries. Delegates with specific ideas will be able to draw on these principles for their own campaigns, for example, the current United States settlement.

Conclusion

It was clearly shown at this conference that the global tobacco epidemic is worse today than it was 30 years ago. The extraordinary effort needed to prevent the epidemic from becoming even worse in another 30 years is not being made. Several countries have already shown that smoking rates can be reduced. These successes can be reproduced in any responsible nation only by determined, immediate and sustained governmental and community action. This requires encouragement and guidance by the delegates to this conference and our colleagues from around the world. We know it can be done....

Reference
United Nations (1991) *World Population Prospects 1990* (Population Studies No. 120), New York, Department of International Economic and Social Affairs

AUTHOR INDEX

A

Aaserud, E., 897
Abdus Sattar, S.M., 450
Abe, M., 716
Abedian, I., 699
Abosede, O.A., 900
Abrams, D.B., 770
Adriaanse, H., 205, 212, 887, 895
Adrianza, M., 47, 501
Aghi, M.B., 231, 233, 301
Ah-Song, R., 252, 604
Ainetdin, T., 743
Aizik-Kelem, A., 750
Akerberg, O., 883
Alexander, D.L., 633, 634, 865
Alexandrov, A.A., 266
Alexandrova, V.Yu., 266
Alexeev, O.L., 518
Alexeeva, N.V., 518
Allen, M., 464
Amos, A., 260, 336, 542, 544
Ampaire, A., 924
Andress, W.C., 728
Andrews, J.A., 761
Annett, N., 699
Appleby, P., 111
Asgari, S., 278
Ashley, M.J., 172, 246, 453, 633, 634, 865
Assunta, M., 635
Aston, K., 685, 849, 887
Athanasiou, K., 295
Azinge, R.C., 325

B

Bagheri, M., 158
Bahrs, D.I., 891
Baigi, A., 255
Bakker, M.J., 758
Bal, D.G., 497, 796
Baldwin Radford, K., 451
Bales, S., 33
Bandele, E., 900
Banzhaf, J., 817
Barchuk, A.S., 923
Barnes, M., 573
Barreiro-Carracedo, A., 100
Barros-Dios, J., 100
Barton, J., 111
Basiraha, R., 924
Bass, F., 898
Batra, A., 213, 229
Bechmann Jensen, T., 309

Becker, K., 5
Becoña, E., 735
Behera, D., 137
Bell, R., 260
Benhaïm-Luzon, V., 252
Beral, V., 104
Bergmark-Bröske, Y., 844
Berstein, L.M., 123
Betson, C.L., 163, 338, 751, 904
Bevc Stankovic, M., 619
Biczysko, W., 129
Bilan, A., 916, 918
Bilir, N., 57, 234, 897
Bittoun, R., 205
Bjartveit, K., 959
Blackburn, M., 443
de Blij, B., 842
Blitner, M., 750
Boëthius, G., 844, 871
Bolling, K., 258, 847
Bondy, S., 172
Bonet Gorbea, M., 45
Boreham, J., 10
Borge, R., 897
Borland, R., 627, 645
Borski, H.R., 781
Borthwick, C., 443
Boschiero, M., 521
Boshtam, M., 138, 139, 140, 278
Bostock, C., 336
Bostock, Y., 336
Boucher, P., 966
Bourdès, V., 604
Bourgeois, F., 561
Boulter, J., 805
Bozwoda, W., 104
Bronis, M., 920
Buchkremer, G., 213, 229
Buckler, J., 493
Buda, B., 159
Buist, S., 78
Bull, S.B., 172, 453
Buller, D., 353
Burns, L., 676
Burton, R., 863
Burton, S.L., 713

C

Callard, C., 610
Calvo, J., 170, 263, 739
Calvo, J.R., 170, 263, 347, 739
Calvo-Rosales, J., 347

Carr, A., 768
Carrara, H.R.O., 104
Carreras-Castellet, J.M., 762, 764
Carroll, A.M., 357
Catalan-Vazquez, M., 191
Cederhom-Williams, S., 111
Chaloupka, F.J., 387, 697
Chan, S., 904
Chapman, S., 447
Charoenca, N., 811
Chassin, L., 353
Chaudhry, K., 459
Chazan, B., 235, 889
Chen, C., 103
Chen, M., 435
Chen, T., 579
Chen, Z., 84
Chen, Z. M., 10
Cheng, L.Q., 890
Chiu, N.Y., 274
Chng, C.Y., 480
Choi, E., 783
Chou, H.-H., 282
Chun, W., 137
Chung, S.F., 167, 306, 338, 751
Chung, T.W.H., 751
Clarke, R., 111
Clement, T., 884
Co, N.V., 102
Cohen, J.E., 172, 453, 633, 634, 865
Cohen, S.B., 667
Collins, D.J., 964
Collins, R., 84, 111
Collishaw, N.E., 410
Connolly, G.N., 379
Consuegra Manzanares, M.J., 708, 734
Cook, J., 497, 796
Cotter, T., 805
Courant, P.N., 48
Crosby, M.H., 938
Crossan, E., 542
Crowe, J.W., 268
Csémy, L., 197
Cunningham, R., 392, 608, 689
Cunningham-Burley, S., 260

D
Dagli, E., 931
Dai, P.X., 33
Dartau, L., 478
Dashzeveg, G., 277
Daynard, R.A., 821

Demjén, T., 159
Deng, J., 90
Deva, D., 137
De Wet, T., 308
Denisova, D., 270
Didilescu, C., 691, 692
Dizdarevic, S., 619
Dmitriev, D.A., 62
Dobrowolska, A., 589
Dobson, A., 241, 243
Dols, M., 205
Donovan, R.J., 845
Doran, C.M., 594, 902, 904
Douglas, C.E., 209
Draffin Jones, A., 927
Drojachih, V., 51
Drygas, W.K., 745, 884
Du, R.Y., 153
Dubois, G., 617
Duckmark, A., 540
Dugdill, L., 303
Dung, T.K., 102
Dydamony, M., 807
Dzhumasultanova, S.V., 123
Dziankowska-Stachowiak, E., 745

E
Eadie, D.R., 351, 686
Eckert, B., 229
Edler, L., 291
Eensoo, D., 190, 285
Efroymson, D., 624
El Fehri, V., 289, 592
El-Shahat, H.M., 746
Elovainio, L., 458
Emri, S., 897
Erben, R., 553
Eriksson, L., 743
Erilsen, M., 682
Essien, G., 900
Esterhuysen, P., 799, 803
Eyre, H., 796

F
Fagerstrom, K.O., 218
Fairbanks, L.L., 666, 879
Fan, L., 5
Farger, G., 213
Farren, C., 515, 833
Fassett, W., 857
Fawzy, M.H., 746
Feachem, R.G.A., 425

Fedichkina, T., 51
Feigelman, W., 278
Feng, L.N., 130
Ferrence, R.G., 172, 246, 453, 633, 634, 865
Fiévez, B., 887, 895
Fish, D., 893
Fleitmann, S., 456
Florek, E., 128, 129
Flores-Sanchez, S., 718
Flórez, S., 263
Forbes, E.R., 585
Forouzeah, M., 278
Fourie, J.M., 528
Fox, B., 826
Fraser, T., 569
Frazier, E.A., 78
Fridegotto, M., 521
Frizzell, S.K., 357
Fukushima, F., 909

G
Gajalakshmi, C.K., 40
Galbally, R., 441, 443
Galley, L., 159
Gamajunova, V.B., 123
Gan, C.-Y., 236
Gan-Noy, S., 750
Gao, X.J., 163
Gao, Y.-T., 90
García, A., 733
García, M.P., 739
García Baena, E.I.D., 708
Garfami, I., 213
Gaunt-Richardson, P., 542
Gelband, H., 43
Geller, A., 573
Gendre, I., 252, 604
Gestal-Otero, J.J., 921
Gillies, P., 759
Gimbel, H., 939
Giovino, G., 373, 682
Girgis, A., 594
Gitchell, J., 713, 715
Glantz, S.A., 826
Glasgow, H., 72, 860
Glover, M., 468
Glynn, T., 789
Godfrey, A.A., 390
Goldstein, S., 799, 803
Gonzàlez, J., 733
Gonzàlez Quintana, J., 708, 734
Gordon, J.S., 761

Gordon, M., 902
Goto, K., 369
Graham, P., 686
Grande, D., 570
Grant, C., 812
Gray, N., 401
Grossman, M., 697
Güçiz Doğan, B., 57, 234, 897
Guillén, D., 246, 922, 923
Guldbrandsson, K., 743
Guo, M.-R., 90
Gupta, P.C., 20

H
Habil, H., 39
Haglund, M., 18, 539, 540
Hale, M., 104
Hamann, S., 439, 811
Han, J.-J., 90
Hanafiah, L.A., 565
Hänggi, D., 289
Hanson, K.P., 923
Hanzlik, J., 916, 918
Hassan, F., 43
Hastings, G.B., 351, 686
Hayley, R., 768
Haywant, A.D., 78
He, J.M., 319
He, X.-Z., 10
He, Y., 94, 111, 130, 153
Hedley, A.J., 67, 150, 313, 338, 949
Hehl, I., 213
Helgason, A.R., 175, 176
Heloma, A., 159
Henningfield, J.E., 218
Hernandez-Garduno, E., 191
Herrera, N., 47, 501
Hessult, B., 175
Heuer-Jung, V., 229
Hilder, C., 840
Hill, D., 309, 627, 805
Hillhouse, A., 957
Hjalmarson, A., 716
Ho, A., 462
Ho, L., 488
Ho, S.Y., 67, 319
Hoang, T.T., 33
Hoffman, M.N., 528
Höijer, Y., 907
Holm, C., 529
Hong Tiy, Mrs, 633
Honzátková, K., 483

Hooper, P., 531, 593, 663
Houghtling, R.A., 125
van den Hout, M., 205
Hrubá, D., 217
Hsieh, L.-Y., 274
Hu, B.-Y., 90
Hu, T., 698
Hu, Y., 564
Hu, Z.G., 150
Huang, J., 111, 113
Huang, J.-H., 523
Huang, J.Y., 153
Huang, S.-J., 281
Huang, S.-Y., 282
Hudtloff, A.P., 175
Hung, D.K., 102
Hurt, R.D. , 666
Husten, C., 373, 374

I

Iñigo-Barrera, F.J., 762
Islam, N., 271
Israel, R.J., 856
Ivanova, E.I., 266
Izumi, T., 135

J

Jackiewicz, T., 673
Jacobsen, S., 473
Jakovljevic, D., 505
Jamrozik, K., 447
Japhet, G., 799, 803
Jarvis, M.J., 705
Jayne, K. , 111
Jenkins, C.N.H., 33
Jha, P., 425
Jia, G.L., 113, 153
Jiang, B., 130
Jiang, C.Q., 319
Jiang, Y., 369
Jiménez, C., 170, 263, 739
Jimenez-Santolaya, M.P., 762
Jin, S., 369
Joao Maia, A., 37
Jones, K., 655
Jones, T.E., 711
Joossens, L., 381, 685
Jøsendal, O., 592
Juczyński, Z., 589
Juul Anderson, E., 470, 473

K

Kachlík, P., 217
Kähkönen, E., 159
Kaiserman, M.J., 678
Kalyoncu, F., 57
Kamantina, T.V., 62
Kanyesigye, E.K., 924
Karasikova, T.B., 62
Kavcová, E., 920
Kawata, C., 915
Kellar, K.J., 125
Kemper, K.E., 713
Kemppainen, U., 299
Khan, S.M., 104
Khanduja, K.L., 137
Khongchinda, P.C., 932
Khurelbaatar, N., 277
King, J., 678
Kinh, H.V., 33
Kinoshita, T., 756
Kobayashi, Y.M., 371
Kolandai, M.A., 272
Kolesnik, O.S., 123
Kollár, J., 920
Kolser, T., 175
Komar-Szymborski, M., 235
Konno, K., 716
Koplan, J.P., 948
Koplan, K., 288
Koranteng, S., 348
Kovalenko, T.A., 518
Kowalczyk, T., 235, 589
Kowalska, A., 745
Kozák, J.T., 893
Králíková, E., 893
Krasovsky, K., 623
Krebs, H., 289, 592
Krjukova, O.G., 123
Kronenfeld, J., 353
Krstic, N., 699
Kunze, M., 771, 773
Kyle, K., 838

L

Laikier, R., 104
Laixuthai, A., 387
Lam, C., 37
Lam, T.H., 67, 94, 150, 153, 163, 167, 313,
        319, 338, 751, 904, 947
Lancaster, T., 714
Laugesen, M., 72, 681, 860

Lee, H., 353
Lee, J., 278
Lee, P.N., 145
Lee, S.H., 858
Legetic, B., 505
Legl, T., 214, 216
Lehofer, M., 214, 216
Leong, C.H., 606
Levashov, S.U., 62
Levin, A.M., 62
Levitt, N.S., 528
Levshin, V., 51
Lewandowska, M., 589
Lhkaijav, D., 275
Li, H.Z., 893
Li, L., 111, 113
Li, L.S., 153
Li, S.Y., 163
Li, W.-X., 84
Liao, W.K., 580
Liaw, K., 72
Librett, J.J., 781
Lichtenstein, E., 761
Liebmann, P.M., 215, 216
Lightwood, J., 826
Liimatainen-Lamberg, A.-E., 563, 631, 907
Lin, C.-L., 488
Lindblad, B.-M., 844
Lins, N., 497, 796
Lipponen, S., 458
Liu, J.L.Y., 710
Liu, W.W., 319
Lo, T.-P., 282
Loh, C., 181
López, A., 170, 263, 739
López, B., 47
López, M., 170, 263, 347, 739
López-Cabanas, A., 347
Lore, W., 887, 895
Luha, J., 55
Lund, A., 772
Lund, A.B., 769
Lund, K.E., 175, 176
Lyon, V., 111

M
Ma, A.-P., 282
Ma, H., 564
Mackay, J., 973
MacKinnon, D., 353
MacKintosh, A.M., 351, 686
Mahood, G., 599

Majewski, J., 115
Mak, K.H., 67
Maldonado-Arostegui, B., 764
Malyutina, S.K., 518
Marica, C., 691, 692
Marin, T., 733
Marín Tuyà, D., 708, 734
Markham, P., 840
Marrero, M., 170, 263, 347
Marshall, J., 111
Marszalek, A., 128, 129
Martin, J., 172
Martinez-Rossier, L., 191, 718
Más, A., 922, 923
Masui, S., 812
Masuyer, E., 81
McCabe, P., 731
McCarthy, P., 872
McIntyre, D., 658
McNeill, A., 227, 847, 887
McPhee, S.J., 33
McVey, D., 847
Mehl, G.L., 60
Melin, T., 255
Méndez, D., 48
van der Merwe, R., 699
Meyer, E.L., 125
Michaeli, M., 750
Michieletto, F., 521
Midorikawa, E., 716
Milhaltan, F., 903, 912
Miller, C., 625
Minowa, M., 284, 909
Mishra, G., 241, 243
Miyasato, K., 909
Mo, S., 274
Mobasher, A.A.M.T., 746
Mochizuki-Kobayashi, Y., 27, 331
Moczurad, K., 115
Mohammad, Y., 236
Mohammadifar, N., 138, 158
Molokov, A.L., 518
Montes, A., 735
Montes-Martinez, A., 100, 921
Montes-Vizuet, R., 718
Moore, M., 542
Morand, M., 172
Morra, M., 497, 796
Moser, M., 214, 216
Mosiewicz, J., 916
Mostafa, S., 807
Mostafavi, S., 138, 139, 171

Mowery, P., 682
Moyer, C.A., 582
Muchuro, S., 924
Mullins, R., 172, 759
Mulvéy, K., 857
Muna, W., 439
Murad, J.E., 211
Myllylvoma, J., 682
Myśliński, W., 916

N

Naci Yildiz (Yyldyz), A., 57, 234, 897
Naderi, G.R., 278
Nagai, A., 716
Nagai, S., 135
Naik, U.D., 360
Naing, N.N., 343
Nakahara, T., 371
Nakamura, M., 756, 812, 915
Nakano, N., 335
Nasreen, S., 104
Navarro, M.C., 170, 263, 347, 739
Nerin, I., 246, 903, 922, 923
Newton, R., 104
Ngoc, D.H., 33
Nhung, N.V., 102
Niaura, R.S. , 770
Niezurawski, J., 235
Nishida, H., 137
Niu, S.-R., 10
Nkangi, E., 924
Nordström Torpenberg, I., 907
Northrup, D.A., 633, 634, 865
Nour, E.I.D., 746
Nová, E., 217
Novelli, W.D., 558
Novotny, T.E., 425
Nurkkala, H., 757

O

Ogbulu, H.C.O., 325
Ogińska-Bulik, N., 589
O'Hara, B., 676
Ohida, T., 284
Okada, K., 915
Olupona, N., 900
Omeruwa, V.I., 325
O'Neil, C., 676
Orengo, J.C., 170, 263, 347
Osaki, Y., 284, 909
Oshima, A., 915
Ostrowski, S., 918

Otto, C., 59
Ouynbileg, Sh., 275
Owen, L., 227, 258, 491, 847, 887
Owen, P., 325
Owens, C., 494

P

Paavola, M., 568
Palmer, M., 854
Palmer, S., 854
Palusiński, R., 308, 916, 918
Pan, H.-C., 10
Pan, S.C., 163
Pandey, M.R., 348
Pantelejev, V., 299
Parish, S., 111
Parkin, D.M., 81
Parkin, S., 184
Pärna, K., 190, 285
Parrott, S., 278
Patel, M., 104 Pattison, P., 309
Pavis, S., 260
Pechacek, T., 373, 374, 682
Pederson, L.L., 172, 453
Pekarsky, B., 902
Pentillä, U.-R., 757
Perez Neria, J., 192
Pernhaupt, G., 214, 216
Peters, J., 150, 313
Peto, R., 10, 40, 43, 84, 111
Phat, H.L., 102
Phillips, Dr, 633
Phuong, D.T., 624
Pierce, J.P., 341
Pilati, G., 521, 653
Pilz, L.R., 291
Pisani, P., 81
Planojevic, M., 505
Pnomareva, S.U., 62
Poland, B., 172
Poland, P.D., 453
Pollard, J.S., 633, 634, 865
Poncet, M., 252
Pope, M., 246
Porcellato, L., 303
Posluszna, J., 308
Pötschke-Langer, M., 291
Prado, L., 941
Protacio-Marcelino, E., 961
Pun, S., 451
Purcell, K., 676
Puška, P., 299, 458, 568

Q

Quesnelle, G.M., 713
Quezada-Zambrano, R., 191
Qi, G., 5

R

Radford, C., 451, 936
Rafie, M., 140
Ramos, A., 170, 263, 739
Ramström, L.M., 955
Ratte, S., 555
Rautama, P., 297
Raw, M., 887
Razlan, M., 343
Reagan, G., 528
Reddy, P., 488
van Reek, J., 212
Rehar, V., 485
Reid, Y., 759
Reijula, K., 159
Reimers, A., 743
Reynolds, C., 625
Richmond, R., 874
Richter, I., 308
Rios-Dalenz, J., 450
Ritthiphakdee, B.-O., 525, 732
Roberts, L., 520, 625, 759
Robinson, R.G., 508
Roche, G., 45
Rodrigo, E.K., 60
Roemer, R., 407
Rogayah, J., 343
Rojas, O., 170, 263, 739
Romand, R., 740
Romo, M., 757
Rossouw, K., 528
Rothberg, M., 159
Rozborilová, E., 920
Ruan, Z.-X., 98
Ruff, P., 104
Ruiz, M.J., 246
Russell, M.A.H., 715
Rymarz, E., 918

S

Saava, A., 190, 285
Sadegi, K., 138
Sadek, R., 807
Saffer, H., 692
Sakagami, K., 137
Saloojee, Y., 488, 794
Samet, J., 5

Sánchez-Agudo, L., 246, 762, 764, 922, 923
Sanderson, F., 303
Sanner, T., 75, 470, 473
Sano, A., 137
Sanson-Fisher, R.W., 594, 902
Sapiński, W., 884
Sarna, L., 872, 911
Sarrafzadegan, N., 138, 139, 140, 158,
   171, 278
Sasco, A.J., 14, 252, 604
Sätterberg, C., 576
Sawyer, D.E., 325
Schauenstein, K., 214
Schoepff, H., 10
Shiffman, S., 218, 715
Schioldborg, P., 456, 669
Schoberberger, R., 771
Schofield, M., 241, 243
Schofield, P., 309
Schupp, P.E., 229
Seffrin, J., 495, 497
Segura, J.M., 170, 263, 347, 739
Seimon, T., 60
Selin, H., 535, 774
Severson, H.H., 761
Shanta, V., 40
Sharma, R., 137
Sharp, D., 682
Shi, Q., 111, 113
Shi, Q.L., 153
Shiffman, S., 218, 715
Shongwe, T., 799, 803
Shrivastava, B.M., 325
Silagy, C., 714
Silva, K.T., 60
Sitas, F., 104
Skrondal, A., 176
Skylstad, D., 897
Slade, J., 199
Slama, K., 723
Sleight, P., 111
Slepchenko, N., 51
Smith, M., 936
Sodnompil, T.S., 275
Solano, S., 170, 263, 739
Song, Y.Y., 163
Sovinová, H., 197
Spedding, M., 451
Spiik, M., 743
Springett, J., 303
Stamps, T.J., 376
Stanikas, T., 636

Stapleton, J.A., 715, 847
Stead, M., 686
Steinwall, G., 577, 844, 864
Stenmarck, S., 470, 473
Stergar, E., 264, 619
Stewart, S., 33
Steyn, K., 308, 488, 528
Stjerna, M.-L., 743
Strecher, V., 715
Suarez Lugo, N., 45, 454, 590, 616
Sukhbat, G., 277
Sullivan, D., 673, 783
Sun, C., 111
Supakorn, B., 808
Supawongse, C., 664
Sutherland, G., 715
Sutherland-Brown, C., 582
Suwanrasami, S., 732
Svinhufvud, J., 159
Swanson, M.G., 440
Swart, D., 488
Sweanor, D.T., 199, 641
Swinburn, B., 860
Szymborski, J., 235, 589, 889

T
Tafazoli, F., 171
Tafazzoly, F., 171
Takubo, T., 716
Takahashi, Y., 770
Takeuchi, M., 135
Takkouche, B., 100
Talmud, J., 813
Talu, I., 560, 844
Tamang, E., 521, 653
Tan, D., 793
Tanaka, H., 167
Tang, J.-L., 710
Tapia-Conyer, R., 58
Taylor, A.L., 422
Taylor, C.E., 5
Taylor, M.C., 202
Teng, W.-K., 90
Teran-Ortiz, L., 718
Terborg, J.R., 797
Teusner, D., 655
Thanhawla, R., 41
Thanseia, R., 41
Thomas, S., 783
Thompson, C., 783
Thompson, J.M., 125
Thuy, T.T., 503

Tillgren, P., 743
Tkachenko, G.B., 62
Todd, R., 497, 796
Tomori, M., 264
Tong, S.H., 306
Torabi, M.R., 268
Torres, M., 170, 263, 347, 739
Tossavainen, K., 299
Tostain, J., 326
Toyas, C., 246, 922, 923
Trangbek, K., 594
Tsai, S.P., 69, 98
Tsang, G.Y., 581
Tsang, L.C.V., 767
Tsang, S.L., 306
Tsang, Y.H., 306
Tsyrlina, E.V., 123
Turnbull, D., 655
Tvaermose, P., 767

U
Uhrbom, E., 881
Umenai, T., 936
Unnikrishnan, K.P., 459
Urano, S., 137
Urban, S., 55
Usdin, S., 799, 803
Uyanwatte, R., 60

V
Vaidya, J.S., 360
Vaidya, S.G., 360
Vakacegu, A., 633
Van-Santos, A.E., 325
Varona Perez, P., 45
Vartianinen, E., 299, 568
Vázquez, F.L., 735
Vateesatokit, P., 621
Vergeer, F., 212
Vertio, H., 458
Vicente, R., 246, 922, 923
Vierthaler, B., 530
Villalba-Caloca, J., 191, 718
Villamizar, T., 47, 501
Volkova, E.G., 62
Voller, W.M., 78
de Vries, H., 758, 887, 895
Vysehradsky, R., 920

W
Wabwire, G., 924
Wakefield, M., 520, 625, 655, 759

Wang, G.-H., 10
Wang, J.-L., 10
Wang, Z.-X., 90
Waniaye, J.B., 924
Warner, K.E., 48, 199, 365
Wasowicz, M., 129
Wat, Z.M., 306
Watanabe, B., 666
Watanabe, S., 27, 369
Watt, J., 805, 962
Weissman, R., 967
Wen, C.-P., 69, 98
Weng, X., 436
Whidden, M., 155, 819
White, P., 685
Willems, B., 205
Willemsen, M.C., 321
Wilson, S.R., 78
Winder, A., 573
Wiseman, L., 574
Witczak, A., 918
Wong, C.H., 306
Wong, C.M., 150, 313, 338
Wong, C.Y., 306
Wong, H., 306
Wong, H.S., 30
Wong, K.C., 306
Wong, M.K., 306
Wong, S.H., 306
Wong, S.T., 306
Wong, W.Y., 306
Woodward, A., 447
Woodward, S., 863
Woollard, K., 851
Wu, R., 278
Wykle-Rosenberg, L., 857

X

Xia, H.-F., 523
Xiang, Y.-B., 90
Xiao, Y., 125
Xiong, F.-J., 523
Xu, D., 113
Xu, Z., 84
Xuan, Q.S., 163

Y

Yach, D., 308
Yamaguchi, N., 27, 369
Yan, D.-Y., 890
Yang, G., 5
Yang, G.H., 10
Yang, M.-H., 282
Yao, H., 113
Yao, T., 523
Yavuz, K., 587
Yen, D.D., 69, 98, 282
Yoshino, K., 716
Youngman, L., 111
Yu-Chan, M.M.H., 566
Yuen Loke, A., 163

Z

Zabezhiński, M.A., 923
Zai, S., 104
Zain, Z. M., 635
Zaki, L.A., 746
Zapotoczky, H.G., 216
Zaridze, D., 143, 854
Zarief, L., 807
Zatoński, W., 235, 589, 854, 889
Zdanowska, J., 918
Zeeman, G., 323, 741
Zhang, B.-Y., 564
Zhang, P., 373, 374
Zhang, W.S., 319
Zhang, Y., 5
Zhang, Y.-S., 90
Zheng, J.S., 153
Zhou, L., 523
Zhou, X., 893
Zhu, C.Q., 319
Zolty, B., 429
Zubritsky, A.N., 103, 476
Zucha, J., 920
Zulkifli, A., 343

SUBJECT INDEX

A

Addiction to tobacco (see also Nicotine)
   modification of by context stimuli, 205–9
Advertising of tobacco products (see also
   individual regions and countries)
   and women, 18, 335–8
   and young people, 338–50, 353–7
   bans (see Legislation)
   international control of, 418–9
Advocacy for tobacco control, 833–65
Africa (see also individual countries)
   tobacco use in, 794–5
   tobacco control in, 439, 508–10, 512, 795
Age
   at starting to smoke
      in Bangladesh, 271
      in China, 5–7, 13, 436
      in Cuba, 455, 590–1
      in Greece, 296
      in Mongolia, 275
      in the Russian Federation, 268–9
      in Slovenia, 265
      in Spain, 263
      in Taiwan, 274
      in Turkey, 56–7
      in Venezuela, 46–7
      in Viet Nam, 33–4
   prevalence of smoking according to, 6,
      28–32, 54, 320
Albania, cigarette smuggling in, 385
Alcohol, association of with tobacco use,
   103, 217, 218–22, 235
   among young people, 253–5, 262, 265,
      278, 292
Alternative uses of tobacco, 183, 188–9
Andorra, cigarette smuggling in, 385
Argentina, cigarette smuggling in, 382, 420
Asia, tobacco control in, 439–40
Attitudes
   to smoking
      in China, 8–9, 164–5
      in Cuba, 46
      in France, 813
      in Hong Kong, 305–8, 338–41
      in Macao, 38
      in Mongolia, 277
      in the Russian Federation, 52–3, 61–2
      in Turkey, 57, 898
      of young people, 281–310, 353–7
   to exposure to environmental tobacco
      smoke, 172, 176–7
   to tobacco control, 8–9, 453, 625–33,
      633–4, 897–8
Australia
   attitudes to exposure to environmental
      tobacco smoke in, 172
   attitudes to smoking in, 309
   control of tobacco use in, 413–4, 440–7,
      574–6, 594–5, 655–8, 673–8
   health education in, 805–6
   health sponsorship of sport in, 357–9

Australia (contd)
   programmes for smoking cessation in,
      520–1, 711–3, 783–9
   reproductive effects of smoking in, 241–
      6
   role of general practitioners in tobacco
      control, 902, 904
Austria
   cigarette smuggling in, 384 –5
   programmes for smoking cessation in,
      771–2, 773–4

B

Bangladesh
   anti-smoking education in, 450
   prevalence of smoking among
      adolescents in, 271–2
Belgium
   cigarette smuggling in, 384–5
   control of tobacco use in, 561–3
Benefits of smoking, perceived, 39, 232,
   234, 302, 325, 355–6
Bidi, use of, 20, 40–1, 60, 137, 231–4, 325,
   459–60
Bolivia, control of tobacco use in, 450
Brazil
   control of tobacco use in, 412
   cultivation of tobacco in, 211–2, 941–3
Bulgaria, cigarette smuggling in, 382

C

Cambodia
   knowledge, attitudes and practices of
      Buddhist monks in, 936–8
   prevalence of tobacco use in, 452
   tobacco advertising in, 452
   tobacco control in, 451–2
Canada
   control of tobacco use in, 413, 415–6,
      453, 535–8, 582–5, 641–5, 678–80
   exposure to environmental tobacco
      smoke in, 172
   health education in, 812–3
   mortality attributable to use of tobacco
      by women in, 246
   prevalence of smoking among student
      nurses in, 927
   programmes for smoking cessation in,
      774–7, 898–9
Cancers, and tobacco use, 81–107
   all sites, 70–1
   hepatocellular carcinoma, 103
   of the lung
      among women, 14–5, 31–2, 70
      and cigarette consumption, 31–2, 295–
         6
      attributable to environmental tobacco
         smoke, 143–50
      attributable to tobacco smoking, 81–3,
         94–100, 102–3
   of the oral cavity, 15, 20–1, 41, 104, 232

Cancers, and tobacco use (contd)
    of the upper aerodigestive tract, 15, 103–4
    of urinary sites, 15
Cardiovascular disease, and tobacco use,
    111–7
    among women, 16, 71, 153–5
    attributable to environmental tobacco
        smoke, 145–50, 153–5, 158
    effects of smoking on lipid profile, blood
        pressure and glucose, 137–40
    in China, 86–94, 111–5, 153–5
    in Egypt, 42–5
    in India, 41
    in Poland, 115–7
    in Taiwan, 71
    in the United Kingdom, 111
    programmes for smoking cessation in
        patients with, 757
Cartoons in tobacco control, 587–8
Cessation, 705–89, 975
    attitudes to, 46, 52–3
    behavioural methods, 723–77
    during pregnancy, 227–30, 247
    pharmacological methods, 705–19
    practical approaches to, 957–9
    programmes for (see also individual
        regions and countries), 302–3, 481,
        507, 522, 768–9
        at the worksite, 321–3
    strategic role of, 955–7
Change, 'trans-theoretical' model of
    behavioural, 429–30, 725
Children (see Young people)
China
    cigarette consumption in, 6, 11, 13, 84–5
    cigarette smuggling in, 382
    control of tobacco use in, 412, 435–8,
        523–5, 564–5, 580–2, 698, 890–1, 893
    exposure of non-smoking pregnant
        women to environmental tobacco
        smoke in, 163–6
    mortality from tobacco-related disease in,
        5, 10–3, 67–9, 84–94, 111–5
    prevalence of smoking in, 5–10, 11, 85–6,
        181, 319–20, 438, 893
    production of tobacco in, 438
    smoking and occupational exposure in,
        319–21
Consumer pressure in tobacco control, 857–8
Control of tobacco use (see also individual
    regions and countries), 435–595, 959–61
    attitudes to, 8–9, 625–33, 633–4
    directed towards women, 19, 466, 489,
        535–49
    directed towards young people, 435, 450,
        452, 466, 472–3, 489, 507, 523, 530,
        553–95, 673–82
    funding for, 441, 444, 446, 457, 466,
        472, 475, 480, 482–3, 528, 594–5
    international, 401–30, 974
    role of governments in, 425–8, 974–5
    use of computers in, 478–9

Costa Rica, control of tobacco use in, 412
Côte d'Ivoire, control of tobacco use in, 412
Cotinine, determination of, 716–9
Cuba
    control of tobacco use in, 412, 454–5,
        590–1
    prevalence of smoking in, 45–6, 455, 590
    tobacco consumption in, 45–6, 455
Cultural factors and tobacco use, 39, 42, 59–
    60, 231–2, 451
Cyprus, control of tobacco use in, 412
Czech Republic
    cigarette consumption in, 197–8
    nicotine dependence in, 197–9
    prevalence of smoking in, 197–9, 893–4
    risk behaviour in, 217
    role of health professionals in tobacco
        control in, 893–4

D
Denmark
    attitudes of young people to smoking in,
        309–10
    cigarette smuggling in, 384–5
    control of tobacco use in, 594
    prevalence of smoking among health
        professionals in, 884
    programmes for smoking cessation in,
        767, 769
Duty-free sales of tobacco products, 393,
    420

E
Economic burden of tobacco use, 365–76,
    426, 964–6, 973–4
    in China, 369, 438
    in Hong Kong, 181
    in Japan, 334, 369–73
    in New Zealand, 464
    in Norway, 76–7
    in the Russian Federation, 62
    in Slovakia, 484
    in the United States of America, 76–7
    in Viet Nam, 36
Economic measures to control tobacco use,
    685–700
Education, level of
    and attitudes to smoking, 8, 171, 227–9
    and knowledge about hazards of smoking, 8
    and prevalence of tobacco use, 5–6, 34,
        37, 41, 52–3, 55, 198–9, 265, 320, 463
Egypt
    health education in, 807–8
    prevalence of smoking in, 42–5
    programmes for smoking cessation in,
        746–9
Environment, effects of tobacco cultivation,
    production and use on, 181–93
Environmental tobacco smoke, exposure to,
    143–77, 949–55
    and cancer, 15, 143–50, 879–10, 949–55
    and cardiovascular disease, 145–50, 949–55

Environmental tobacco smoke, exposure to (contd)
  and lung function, 313–5
  attitudes to, 172–4
  control of, 411
    in Australia, 863–4
    in Finland, 415
    in Norway, 415
    in Singapore, 415
    in the United States of America, 380
  effect in guinea-pig eustachian tube, 130–2
  effects on fibrinogen and lipids, 158
  in China, 5, 70–1, 313–5, 320
  in Japan, 27, 371–3
  in Turkey, 56
  in the workplace, 320
  interference with research on in Australia, 447–50
  legislation against, 449, 450, 461, 463, 465–7, 481, 484–5, 488
  lesser known and minor effects of, 155–8
  measurement of, 159
  social costs of, 371–3
Estonia
  attitiudes to the environment associated with smoking status in, 190–1
  prevalence of smoking among adolescents in, 285–7
Ethnic group and prevalence of smoking, 5–6, 46, 74, 236, 254, 270, 468–70
Europe
  attitudes to tobacco-related disease in, 456
  cigarette smuggling in, 383–6
  control of tobacco use in, 456–9, 555–7
  prevalence of smoking in, 295
  tobacco promotion directed at women in, 336–8

F
Family
  attitudes of to smoking, 306–8
  effect on smoking status of smoking by 37, 40, 52–3, 60–1, 212–3, 271, 275, 277, 283, 290–1, 300, 339–40, 472, 591
  in control of tobacco use, 579–82
  structure and smoking, 286, 356
Fiji, legislation to control smoking in, 633
Finland
  cigarette smuggling in, 384–5
  control of tobacco use in, 413, 415–6, 563–4, 568–9
  influences on smoking behaviour in, 297
  prevalence of smoking in, 298, 907
  programmes for smoking cessation in, 757
Foreign brands of cigarettes, preference for
  in Hong Kong, 182–3
  in Viet Nam, 35–6
France
  control of tobacco use in, 413–4
  cigarette smuggling in, 384–5
  prevalence of smoking among adolescents in, 253–5

France (contd)
  programmes for smoking cessation in, 740–1
Friends, effect on smoking status of smoking by, 37, 52–3, 271, 281, 283, 286, 290, 300, 339–41, 452

G
Germany
  attitudes to smoking in, 291–4
  cigarette smuggling in, 384–5
  prevalence of smoking in, 229–30, 292
Ghana, tobacco promotion in, 348
Greece
  cigarette consumption in, 295
  cigarette smuggling in, 384–5
  mortality from lung cancer in, 295–6

H
Health-care students
  prevalence of smoking among, 916–27
  role of in tobacco control, 915–6
Health education, 793–813, 904–6
  for women, 19
  for young people, 39, 414, 465, 553, 563–4,
Health professionals
  attitudes of to legislation, 9
  attitudes of to tobacco control, 887, 895–7
  prevalence of tobacco use among, 6, 52, 235, 506, 882, 884, 893–4, 895–7, 897–8, 903, 907, 909–11, 912
  programmes for smoking cessation in, 762–6
  role of in smoking cessation, 887–9, 890–1, 897, 898–9, 902, 904
  role of in tobacco control, 871–6, 882–4, 884–6, 889–93, 900–2, 904–6, 907–9, 911
  teaching about tobacco in medical schools, 877–9
Health promotion
  cost–benefit of, 797–9
  foundations for, 350, 357–9, 411, 414, 441–7, 810
  in tobacco control, 793, 961–2
Heroin (see Opiate dependence)
Hong Kong
  attitudes to smoking in, 306–8, 338–41
  cigarette smuggling in, 390–2, 438
  control of tobacco use in, 566–7
  exposure of children to environmental tobacco smoke in, 167–9, 313–5
  health education in, 904–6
  incidence of lung cancer in, 94–8
  prevalence of smoking in, 307, 313–4
  programmes for smoking cessation in, 728–31, 751–6, 767–8
  tobacco advertising in, 182, 338–41, 858–60
Hungary, awareness of exposure to environmental tobacco smoke in, 159

I

Iceland, control of tobacco use in, 413
Immunity, effect of tobacco smoke on, 135–6
Income and prevalence of smoking, 35, 39, 46, 60–1, 351–3, 468–70, 542–4, 686–9
India
    advertising of tobacco products in, 21, 360–1
    cessation programmes in, 302–3
    control of tobacco use in, 412, 459–62
    tobacco use in, 20–1, 40–2, 301–3, 325, 460
        by women, 231–4
Indonesia, control of tobacco use in, 565
International Framework Convention for Tobacco Control, 381, 405, 407–25
Internet sources for tobacco control, 840–1, 856–7
Iran
    exposure of children to environmental tobacco smoke in, 171
    prevalence of tobacco use among adolescents in, 278
Ireland, cigarette smuggling in, 384–5
Israel, programmes for smoking cessation in, 750–1
Italy
    cigarette smuggling in, 382, 384–5
    control of tobacco use in, 521–3
    prevalence of smoking in, 521

J

Japan
    cigarette consumption in, 27, 29–32
    control of tobacco use in, 413, 548
    health education in, 812
    mortality from tobacco-related diseases in, 27
    prevalence of tobacco use in, 27–33, 909–11
    programmes for smoking cessation in, 756–7, 770–1, 915–6
    tobacco promotion directed at women in, 331–6

K

Kenya
    prevalence of smoking in, 895–7
    role of health professionals in tobacco control, 887, 895–7
Knowledge about hazards
    of environmental tobacco smoke, 176–7
    of smokeless tobacco, 812–3
    of smoking
        in Canada, 453, 634
        in China, 8–9, 164–5
        in Cuba, 46
        in Macao, 38
        in Mongolia, 275
        in Nigeria, 901
        in the Russian Federation, 52–3, 924
        in Slovakia, 920–1

Korea, Republic of, control of tobacco use in, 413
Kuwait, control of tobacco use in, 412–3

L

Latin America, control of tobacco use in, 508–9
Legislation against smoking, 408, 415–6, 420, 436, 438, 599–638
    attitudes towards, 8–9, 453, 625–33, 633–4
    in Australia, 414, 625–31, 673–4, 677, 864
    in Canada, 413, 599–603, 610–6, 678–80, 837
    in China, 435–7
    in Cuba, 455, 616–7
    in the European Union, 604–6
    in Fiji, 633
    in Finland, 408
    in France, 414, 617–8
    in Hong Kong, 182–3, 606–8
    in India, 459
    in Macao, 463
    in Malaysia, 39, 635–6
    in New Zealand, 414, 465–7, 469
    in Norway, 408
    in Slovakia, 484–5
    in Slovenia, 619–20
    in Taiwan, 490
    in Thailand, 414–5, 621–3
    in Ukraine, 623–4
    in the United States of America, 692–3
    in Viet Nam, 624–5
Lithuania
    control of tobacco use in, 412, 636–8
    prevalence of smoking in, 18
Litigation against the tobacco industry, 379–8, 817–29, 966–7
Lobbying for tobacco control, 833–65
    in Canada, 836–40, 865
    in the Netherlands, 842–4
    in New Zealand, 74, 860–2
    in Sweden, 844–5
    in the United Kingdom, 833–6
Lung function, and exposure to environmental toacco smoke, 313–5
Luxembourg, cigarette smuggling in, 384–5

M

Macao
    control of tobacco use in, 462–4
    prevalence of smoking in, 463
    tobacco consumption in, 37, 463
Malaysia
    cigarette advertising in, 343
    control of tobacco use in, 39, 635–6
    prevalence of tobacco use in, 39–40, 236, 272–4
Media, use of for tobacco control, 845–56, 864–5, 962–4
Mexico
    carbon dioxide in expired air in, 192–4

Mexico (contd)
  epidemiological transition in, 59–60
Mongolia
  control of tobacco use in, 412
  prevalence of tobacco use among
      adolescents in, 275–7
Mortality and morbidity from tobacco-related
    diseases (see individual regions and
    countries and individual causes), 67–117,
    947, 973

N
Nepal
  control of tobacco use in, 412
  prevalence of smoking in, 349
  tobacco promotion in, 348–50
Netherlands
  cigarette smuggling in, 384–5
  programmes for smoking cessation in,
      321–4, 741–2, 758–9
New Zealand
  control of tobacco use in, 74, 413–6, 464–
      70, 569–70
  mortality due to cigarette smoking in, 72–4
  prevalence of tobacco use in, 73–4, 464
  specific problems of Maori in, 72–4, 464–
      70
Nicotine
  action of in rats, 125–8
  addiction to, 39, 380, 403
    in psychiatric patients, 213–4
  content of tobacco products, 41, 209–12,
      403–4, 455, 681–2
  delivery systems, future of, 199–205
  dependence score, 52, 197–9, 218, 708
  regulation of, 403–4, 641–50
  replacement therapy, 705–19
Nigeria, tobacco control in, 900–2
Nordic countries, exposure of children to
    environmental tobacco smoke in, 175
Norway
  control of tobacco use in, 413, 415, 470–6,
      592
  mortality due to cigarette smoking in, 75–7
  prevalence of smoking in, 426, 471
  programmes for smoking cessation in,
      772–3, 897

O
Occupation
  and knowledge about hazards of smoking, 8
  and prevalence of smoking, 5–6, 319–21
Opiate dependence
  association of smoking with, 40, 214–5,
      218–22
  potentiating effect of on smoking rates,
      216–7

P
Packaging of tobacco products
  for taxation, 393
  generic, 401–2

Pakistan, use of snuff and oral cancer in,
    104
Palau
  control of tobacco use in, 59
  prevalence of tobacco use in, 59
Passive smoking (see Environmental
    tobacco smoke)
Pipe smoking, 7, 143
  water, 6–7, 33, 42, 102, 137, 236–7
Poland
  attitudes to smoking in, 235, 308–9, 426
  control of tobacco use in, 412, 589–90,
      884–6, 889–90
  prevalence of smoking in, 916–9
  programmes for smoking cessation in,
      745–6
  smoking and coronary changes in, 115–7
Portugal
  cigarette smuggling in, 384–5
  control of tobacco use in, 413
Pregnancy
  exposure to environmental tobacco
      smoke during, 163–6
  programmes for smoking cessation
      during, 227–30, 247, 758–61
  smoking during
    animal models of effects on offspring,
        128–30
    health effects on offspring, 17, 156–7,
        167, 227
    in China, 9
    in England, 227–9
    in Germany, 229–30
    in Spain, 246–7
Prevalence of tobacco use (see also
    individual regions and countries), 27–62,
    973
Price of tobacco products (see also Income),
    414, 418–20, 427, 455, 471, 481, 558
  to control tobacco use, 658–63, 681–2,
      686–91, 697–8, 834
Production of tobacco, 41, 373–6, 376, 428,
    438, 462, 503–6, 941–3
Profit control, 689–91
Promotion of tobacco products, 331–61
Public places, smoking in
  in Australia, 172–4, 863–4
  in China, 181, 438
  in France, 414
  in India, 460
  in Taiwan, 71

R
Radon, additive effect with smoking on
    lung cancer, 100–2
Reasons for smoking
  in Cambodia, 452
  in China, 7
  in Finland, 298, 300
  in Hong Kong, 341
  in India, 42, 300–2, 325
  in Malaysia, 273

Reasons for smoking (contd)
  in the Russian Federation, 300
  in Sweden, 256–7
  in Switzerland, 290
  in Taiwan, 281
Regulatory measures against tobacco use,
  641–50
Religion
  and tobacco control, 527, 931–43
  and tobacco use, 6, 39–42, 272–3
Reproductive health and tobacco use, 17
  effect of cigarette smoke on oestrogens in
    rats, 123–5
  rate of miscarriage, 241–3
  risk for early menopause, 243–6
Respiratory disease
  and tobacco use among women, 16, 236–7
  and free radical production, 137
  attributable to environmental tobacco
    smoke, 150–3, 236
  in China, 86–94
  in the United States, 78
Risk behaviour, association with smoking,
  217, 266, 292, 354, 441
Romania
  control of tobacco use in, 691–2
  prevalence of tobacco use in, 691, 903,
    912
  production of tobacco in, 692
Russian Federation
  control of tobacco use in, 476–9, 518–9
  exposure to environmental tobacco
    smoke in, 144
  laryngeal cancer in, 103–4
  prevalence of smoking in, 52–4, 62–3,
    923–4
  prevalence of smoking among
    adolescents in, 266–71
  smoking behaviour among young people
    in, 300

S
Sales of tobacco
  government-controlled, 27, 415
  to minors, 32, 58, 401, 481, 484, 488,
    558, 673–82, 834–5
School
  control programmes in, 42, 267, 275,
    435, 450, 460, 465–6, 507, 522–3, 526,
    553–5, 560–1, 563–70, 574–9, 580–1,
    582–5, 589–92, 594
  smoking in, 32, 56–7, 284–5, 631–3
Scotland
  control of tobacco use in, 542–4
  prevalence of smoking among
    adolescents in, 260–3
  smoke-free bars in, 658–63
Sex (see also Women)
  and prevalence of smoking, 5–6, 54, 102,
    234–5, 254, 300, 463

Singapore
  control of tobacco use in, 413, 480–3
  prevalence of tobacco use in, 481–2
Slovakia
  cigarette consumption in, 55, 484
  control of tobacco use in, 483–5
  mortality attributable to smoking in, 483–4
  prevalence of smoking in, 55–6, 483,
    920–1
  tobacco production in, 484
Slovenia
  control of tobacco use in, 412, 485–8
  prevalence of smoking in, 264–6, 486
Smokebusters, 526, 561
Smoke-free
  bars, 658–63
  cities, 653–5, 663–4
  Europe, 458–9, 484
  facilities, 666–9
  hospitals, 450, 522, 879–81
  nation, 71, 487
  public places, 402, 450, 455, 461, 481,
    490
  restaurants, 173–4, 402, 465, 655–8, 664–6
  schools and universities, 402, 435, 455,
    465, 523–5, 569–70, 669
  sport, 531
  transport, 414, 450, 455, 475–6, 490
  workplaces, 326–7, 402, 465
Smokeless tobacco
  programmes for cessation of use of, 761–2
  use of, 20–1, 37, 40–2, 60, 104, 231–4,
    236, 257, 350, 477
Smuggling of tobacco products, 379–95,
  415, 420, 462, 504
  control of, 392–5, 418–9, 428
  investigation and prosecution of, 390 –2
Socioeconomic status
  and attitudes to smoking, 54, 171, 227–
    30, 286, 301–2
  and exposure to environmental tobacco
    smoke, 314–5
South Africa
  attitudes of children to smoking in, 308
  control of tobacco use in, 412, 488, 528–
    9, 699
  health promotion in, 799–804
  prevalence of smoking in, 439
  smoking-related cancer in, 104–7
Spain
  cigarette smuggling in, 384–5
  exposure of children to environmental
    tobacco smoke in, 170–1
  prevalence of smoking in, 170–1, 263–4,
    903, 921–3
  programmes for smoking cessation in,
    708–9, 734–40, 762–6
  targeting of young people in, 347–8
  telephone counseling for cessation in,
    733–4

Sponsorship
  of arts for health, 442–7, 465
  of sports and arts by tobacco companies,
    36, 272, 347–50, 360–1, 481, 498–9,
    592–3, 636
  of sports for health, 357–9, 414, 440, 442–
    7, 465, 531
Sri Lanka, tobacco use in, 60–61
Sweden
  cigarette smuggling in, 384–5
  control of tobacco use in, 257–8, 413–4,
    529–30, 540–2, 548, 560–1, 576–9,
    864–5, 881–4, 907–9
  prevalence of tobacco use in, 18, 255–8,
    881–2
  programmes for smoking cessation in,
    716, 743–5
Switzerland
  cigarette smuggling in, 385
  control of tobacco use in, 592–3
  smoking among adolescents in, 289–91,
    592
Syria, female pattern of smoking in, 236–7

T
Taiwan
  cigarette consumption in, 70
  control of tobacco use in, 71, 488–90
  hepatocellular carcinoma in, 103
  lung cancer in, 98–100
  mortality from tobacco smoking in, 69–72
  prevalence of smoking in, 70
  prevalence of smoking among adolescents
    in, 274–5
Tar
  content of tobacco products, 41, 403, 455
  regulation of, 647
  yield and myocardial infarct, 111
Tax on tobacco products, use of
  to control smuggling, 392–3
  to control tobacco use, 401–3, 411, 414,
    420, 427–8, 440–7, 465–6, 481, 504,
    685–6, 689–91, 697–700
  to promote health, 350, 357–9, 411, 441–2
Telephone counseling for cessation, 481, 527,
  731–4
Thailand
  control of tobacco use in, 413–5, 525–8
  health promotion in, 808–12
  smuggling in, 415
  telephone counseling for cessation in,
    732–3
Tobacco loyalty programme, 351–3
Turkey
  cigarette consumption in, 57–8
  control of tobacco use in, 412
  mortality from tobacco-related disease in,
    56
  prevalence of smoking in, 57–8, 234–5,
    897–8

U
Uganda, prevalence of smoking among
  medical students in, 924–6
United Kingdom
  attitudes of young people to smoking in,
    303–5
  cigarette smuggling in, 384–5
  control of tobacco use in, 491–5, 515–8,
    531, 548, 593–4, 685–6, 887–9
  effects of targeted advertising in, 341–3
  prevalence of smoking in, 258–60
  programmes for smoking cessation in,
    759–61
  telephone counseling for cessation in,
    731–2
United States of America
  cigarette consumption in, 387
  cigarette promotion in, 353–7
  cigarette smuggling in, 420
  control of tobacco use in, 379–81, 412,
    495–501, 508–12, 530, 548, 558–60,
    570–4, 579–80, 585–7, 891–3, 911
  health promotion in, 796–7, 891–3
  impact of tobacco farm policy on
    cigarette consumption in, 373–6
  mortality from tobacco-related disease,
    12, 19, 75–6, 78
  prevalence of smoking in, 12, 49–52,
    278
  programmes for smoking cessation in,
    713–6, 770, 781–3, 789
  settlement with tobacco companies in,
    181, 183, 386, 405, 407, 821–9, 967–9

V
Venezuela
  control of tobacco use in, 501–3
  prevalence of tobacco use in, 47–8
Viet Nam
  advertising of tobacco products in, 36
  cigarette smuggling in, 504
  control of tobacco use in, 503–5
  mortality from tobacco-related diseases
    in, 36, 102–3
  prevalence of tobacco use in, 33–6, 102,
    504
  production of tobacco in, 503–4

W
Warning labels, 411, 414
  in Australia, 627–31
  in Bolivia, 450
  in Canada, 536–7
  in India, 460–1
  in New Zealand, 465
  in the Russuan Federation, 477
  in Singapore, 481
  in Taiwan, 71
  in the United States of America, 692–3

Women, 227–47
  as targets of tobacco promotion, 18,
    331–4, 445, 485, 537–8
  cessation programmes directed towards,
    743–4, 783–9
  control programmes directed towards,
    19, 175
  health effects of tobacco use in, 14–20
  International Network of Women Against
    Tobacco, 19, 539, 548
  mortality from tobacco-related diseases
    in, 18, 88
  prevalence of tobacco use among (see
    also individual regions and countries),
    331–2, 973
  risk behaviour among, 217
World No-Tobacco Day
  in Cambodia, 452
  in China, 437
  in Ghana, 348
  in India, 42
  in Macao, 463
  in Singapore, 480
  in Venezuela, 501–3

World trade in tobacco products, 379–95,
  418–9

Y
Young people, 253–315
  as targets of tobacco promotion, 338–50,
    353–7, 360–1, 485
  attitudes of to the environment in relation
    to smoking status, 190–1
  effects of exposure to environmental
    tobacco smoke in, 163–77
  prevalence of tobacco use among (see
    also individual regions and countries),
    253–78
  programmes for smoking cessation in,
    750–1, 781–9
  risk behaviour among, 217
Youth access (see Sales of tobacco to
  minors)
Yugoslavia
  cigarette smuggling in, 385
  control of tobacco use in, 505–7
  prevalence of tobacco use in, 506
  tobacco production in, 505–6